Stefan Dhein
Friedrich Wilhelm Mohr
Mario Delmar

Practical Methods in Cardiovascular Research

Stefan Dhein (Editor)
Friedrich Wilhelm Mohr (Editor)
Mario Delmar (Editor)

Practical Methods in Cardiovascular Research

With 33 Tables and 290 Figures

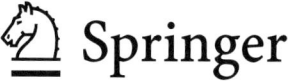

Prof. Dr. Stefan Dhein
Klinik für Herzchirurgie
Universität Leipzig
Herzzentrum
Strümpellstraße 39
04289 Leipzig
Germany

Prof. Dr. Friedrich Wilhelm Mohr
Klinik für Herzchirurgie
Universität Leipzig
Herzzentrum
Strümpellstraße 39
04289 Leipzig
Germany

Mario Delmar, MD PhD
Department of Pharmacology
SUNY Upstate Medical University
766 Irving Avenue
Syracuse NY 13210
USA

Library of Congress Control Number: 2004105045

ISBN 3-540-40763-4   Springer Berlin Heidelberg New York

This work is subject to copyright. All rights are reserved, whether the whole or part of the material is concerned, specifically the rights of translation, reprinting, reuse of illustrations, recitation, broadcasting, reproduction on microfilm or in any other way, in storage in data banks. Duplications of this publication or parts thereof is permitted only under the provision of the German Copyright Law of September 9, 1965, in its current version, and permission for use must always be obtained from Springer-Verlag. Violations are liable for prosecution under the German Copyright Law.

Springer is a part of Springer Science+Business Media
springeronline.com
© Springer-Verlag Berlin Heidelberg 2005
Printed in Germany

The use of general descriptive names, registered names, trademarks, etc. in this publication does not imply, even in the absence of a specific statement, that such names are exempt from the relevant protective laws and regulations and therefore free for general use.

Product liability: The publisher cannot guarantee the accuracy of any information about dosage and application thereof contained in this book. In every individual case the user must check such information by consulting the relevant literature.

Editor: Dr. Thomas Mager, Heidelberg
Development Editor: Natasja Sheriff, Heidelberg
Production: Frank Krabbes, Heidelberg
Cover Design: deblik, Berlin
Page makeup: Hilger VerlagsService, Heidelberg
Printing: Krips BV, Meppel, Niederlande

Printed on acid-free paper   SPIN: 10891623   14/3109 – 5 4 3 2 1 0

Preface

Cardiovascular disease is among the most common causes of death in Western industrialized countries. Although a number of diagnostic and therapeutic possibilities exist today, many problems remain unsolved. This implies the urgent need for future cardiovascular research. The present book gives an overview of a number of available techniques most often used in cardiovascular sciences, especially for investigators coming from other fields of research.

The book is divided into three sections. In the first part, the focus is on techniques used for in vivo experimentation. This field has regained great interest, given the availability of knock-out models which now await in-vivo testing. The book describes the most commonly used procedures for anesthesia and analgesia in laboratory animals as well as „classical" isolated organ techniques, including electrophysiological methods now – again – in common use.

In the second part of the book, we move from the organ and tissue level to the cellular domain. Topics covered include electrophysiology, histology and cell culture techniques as well as biochemical methods such as HPLC, protein biochemistry and binding assays. This part closes with a brief chapter on how to register and analyze concentration response curves giving briefly the mathematics and basic analysis techniques. In the final part, the focus narrows further into molecular procedures such as surface plasmon resonance, nuclear magnetic resonance, RNA methods and DNA arrays. Finally, a chapter is devoted to the molecular aspects of transgenic mice technology as well as an overview of procedures and regulations applicable to housing and transfer of transgenic animals.

The novelty of this book is in the description of practical protocols and troubleshooting procedures. It is our intention to provide a basic guide for investigators interested in applying these techniques in their own laboratories. The book also aims to close the gap between the integrative in-vivo and organ-based methods and the reductionist cellular and molecular approaches. We wish all researchers every success with their experiments and that this book may help them start their way toward new frontiers.

Stefan Dhein
Mario Delmar
Friedrich Wilhelm Mohr

Table of Contents

In-Vivo Techniques

1   Models of Cardiovascular Diseases

1.1   Anaesthesia (Inhalative or i.v. Narcosis) of Laboratory Animals 5
      Katja Schneider
1.2   Extracorporeal Circulation 26
      Cris W. Ullmann
1.3   Open-chest Models of Acute Myocardial Ischemia and Reperfusion 37
      Kai Zacharowski, Thomas Hohlfeld and Ulrich K.M. Decking
1.4   Models of Chronic Ischemia and Infarction 58
      Nicolas Doll, Heike Aupperle, Fabian Stahl and Thomas Walther
1.5   Models on Left Ventricular Hypertrophy (LVH) 72
      Thomas Walther and Volkmar Falk
1.6   Experimental Models of Heart Failure 83
      Volkmar Falk, Jens Garbade and Thomas Walther
1.7   In-Vivo Models of Arrhythmias: a Canine Model of Sudden Cardiac Death 111
      George E. Billman
1.8   In-Vivo Models of Atrial Fibrillation 129
      Ulrich Schotten, Yuri Blaauw and Maurits Allessie

In-Vitro Techniques

2   Isolated Organs

2.1   The Langendorff Heart 155
      Stefan Dhein
2.2   The Working Heart 173
      Marc W. Merx and Jürgen Schrader
2.3   Isolated Papillary Muscles 190
      Stefan Dhein
2.4   Isolated Vessels 198
      Rudolf Schubert

3 Electrophysiological Techniques

- 3.1 Optical Techniques for the Recording of Action Potentials 215
  Helmut A. Tritthart
- 3.2 Recording Action Potentials Using Voltage-Sensitive Dyes 233
  Vladimir G. Fast
- 3.3 Epicardial Mapping in Isolated Hearts – Use in Safety Pharmacology, Analysis of Torsade de Pointes Arrhythmia and Ischemia-Reperfusion-Related Arrhythmia 256
  Stefan Dhein
- 3.4 Voltage-Clamp and Patch-Clamp Techniques 272
  Hans Reiner Polder, Martin Weskamp, Klaus Linz, Rainer Meyer
- 3.5 L-Type Calcium Channel Recording 324
  Uta C. Hoppe, Mathias C. Brandt, Guido Michels and Michael Lindner
- 3.6 Recording Cardiac Potassium Currents with the Whole-Cell Voltage Clamp Technique 355
  Erich Wettwer and Ursula Ravens
- 3.7 Recording the Pacemaker Current If 381
  Uta C. Hoppe, Fikret Er and Mathias C. Brandt
- 3.8 Recording Gap Junction Currents 397
  Ardawan J. Rastan and Stefan Dhein
- 3.9 Recording Monophasic Action Potentials 417
  Paulus Kirchhof, Larissa Fabritz and Michael R. Franz
- 3.10 Heart on a Chip – Extracellular Multielectrode Recordings from Cardiac Myocytes in Vitro 432
  Ulrich Egert and Thomas Meyer

4 Histological Techniques

- 4.1 Immunohistochemistry for Structural and Functional Analysis in Cardiovascular Research 457
  Wilhelm Bloch, Yüksel Korkmaz and Dirk Steinritz
- 4.2 Classical Histological Staining Procedures in Cardiovascular Research 485
  Wilhelm Bloch and Yüksel Korkmaz
- 4.3 Practical Use of in situ Hybridisation and RT in situ PCR in Cardiovascular Research 500
  Yüksel Korkmaz, Dirk Steinritz and Wilhelm Bloch
- 4.4 Practical Use of Transmission Electron Microscopy for Analysis of Structures and Molecules in Cardiovascular Research 525
  Wilhelm Bloch, Christian Hoffmann, Eveline Janssen and Yüksel Korkmaz
- 4.5 DAF Technique for Real-Time NO Imaging in the Human Myocardium 546
  Dirk Steinritz and Wilhelm Bloch

5 Cell Culture Techniques

5.1 Isolation and Culture of Adult Ventricular Cardiomyocytes 557
Klaus-Dieter Schlüter and Hans Michael Piper

5.2 Culture of Neonatal Cardiomyocytes 568
Aida Salameh and Stefan Dhein

5.3 Culture of Embryoid Bodies 577
Cornelia Gissel, Dirk Nierhoff, Bernd Fleischmann, Jürgen Hescheler
and Agapios Sachinidis

5.4 Culturing and Differentiation of Embryonic and Adult Stem Cells
for Heart Research and Transplantation Therapy 592
Marcel AG van der Heyden and Henk Rozemuller

5.5 Preparation of Endothelial Cells from Micro- and Macrovascular Origin 610
Saskia C. Peters, Anna Reis and Thomas Noll

5.6 In Vitro Cultivation of Vascular Smooth Muscle Cells 630
Daniel G. Sedding and Ruediger C. Braun-Dullaeus

5.7 Engineering Heart Tissue for In Vitro and In Vivo Studies 640
Wolfram-Hubertus Zimmermann, Ivan Melnychenko, Michael Didié,
Ali El-Armouche and Thomas Eschenhagen

6 Biochemical and Analytical Techniques

6.1 High-Performance Liquid Chromatography (HPLC) 661
Veronika R. Meyer

6.2 Protein Biochemistry 686
Aida Salameh, Stefan Lehr, Jürgen Weiss and Peter Rösen

6.3 Receptor and Binding Studies 723
Peter Hein, Martin C. Michel, Kirsten Leineweber, Thomas Wieland,
Nina Wettschureck and Stefan Offermanns

6.4 Recording and Analysing Concentration-Response Curves 784
Stefan Dhein

6.5 Measurement of NO and Endothelial Function in Cardiovascular Research ... 799
Renate Roesen, Anke Rosenkranz, Dirk Taubert and Reinhard Berkels

6.6 Biomechanical Stimulation of Vascular Cells In Vitro 813
Henning Morawietz and Andreas Schubert

6.7 Measurement of Function and Regulation of Adrenergic Receptors 829
Marc Brede, Melanie Philipp and Lutz Hein

6.8 Measurement of Function and Regulation
of Muscarinic Acetylcholine Receptors 848
Björn Kaiser and Chris J. van Koppen

6.9 Cytometry in Cardiovascular Research 863
Attila Tárnok

Molecular Biology in Cardiovascular Research

7 Molecular Biology Techniques

7.1 Real-Time PCR Analysis of Cardiac Samples 891
Dalton A. Foster and Steven M. Taffet

7.2 Use of cDNA Arrays to Explore Gene Expression
in Genetically Manipulated Mice and Cell Lines 907
Dumitru A. Iacobas, Sandra Iacobas and David C. Spray

7.3 Using Antibody Arrays to Detect Protein-Protein Interactions 916
Heather S. Duffy, Ionela Iacobas, David C. Spray and Anthony W. Ashton

7.4 Surface Plasmon Resonance as a Method to Study the Kinetics
and Amplitude of Protein-Protein Binding 936
Brian D. Lang, Mario Delmar and Wanda Coombs

7.5 How to Solve a Protein Structure by Nuclear Magnetic Resonance –
The Connexin43 Carboxyl Terminal Domain 948
Paul L. Sorgen

7.6 Managing a Transgenic Mouse Colony: A Guide for the Novice 959
Robert H. Quinn and Karen L. Vikstrom

Appendix

Colour Plates 979
Index 997

List of Abbreviations

AP	action potential		COMT	catechol-O-methyltransferase
1D	one-dimensional		COS cells	kidney cells from the monkey Cercopithecus aethiops
2D	two-dimensional			
3D	three-Dimensional		CPB	cardiopulmonary bypass
5-HT	serotonin		CS	cell signaling
α_1AR	α_1-Adrenoceptor		CSD	cell cycle-shape-differentiation
AADC	aromatic L-amino acid decarboxylase		CV	superior caval vein
ABC	avidin-biotin peroxidase complex		Cx43	connexin43
AC	adenylyl cyclase		CY	cytoskeletal
Ach	acetylcholine			
ACT	activated clotting time		DA	diacetate
AEC	3-amino-9-ethylcarbazole		DAB	diaminobenzidine tetrahydrochloride
AF	atrial fibrillation			
AMI	acute myocardial infarction		DAFs	diaminofluoresceins
Ao	Aorta		DAF-T	triazole-fluoresceins
APHIS	Agriculture Animal and Plant Health Inspection Service		Daun	daunorubicin
			DβH	dopamine β-hydroxylase
Ara-C	cytosine-β-D-arabinofuranoside		dd	double-distilled
ARI	activation-recovery-interval		DDSA	dodecenyl succinic anhydride
AT-1	angiotensin type 1 receptor		DEPC	diethylpyrocarbonate
AT-2	angiotensin type 2 receptor		DMEM	Dulbecco's modified Eagle medium
			DMEM-F12	Dulbecco's Modified Medium
B0	the static magnetic field		DMP	tri(dimethylaminomethyl)phenol
β3-AR	β3-adrenoceptors		DMSO	dimethylsulfoxide
BCIP	5-bromo-4-chloro-3-indolylphosphate		Dox	doxorubicin
			dP/dt_{max}	maximum rate of left ventricular pressure development
BCL	basic cycle length			
BDM	2,3-butanedione-monoxime		dP/dt_{min}	maximum relaxation velocity
BM	bone marrow		dP/dt_{min}	minimum rate of pressure development
BrdU	5-bromo-2-desoxyuridine			
BSA	bovine serum albumin		DSEVC	discontinuous single electrode voltage clamp amplifier
BSA	biotin-streptavidin			
BSS	balanced salt saline		DSS	Dahl salt sensitive rat
BTP	breakthrough-points		DTT	dithiothreitol
C	capacitance		EBNA-LP	Epstein-Barr virus nuclear antigen-leader protein
CABG	coronary artery bypass grafting			
CARB	carbachol		EBs	embryoid bodies
CARD	catalyzed reporter deposition		EC	embryonal carcinoma
CCD	charge-coupled device		EC	endothelial cells
CDC	Centers for Disease Control		ECG	electrocardiogram
CF	coronary flow		ECL HRP	enhanced chemiluminescence horseradish peroxidase
CHO	Chinese hamster ovary cells			
CK	creatine kinase		EDC	1-Ethyl 3-3-dimethylaminopropyl carbodiimide
CK/CKMB	cCreatine kinase/cardiospecific CK			
CK-MB	cardiospecific CK		EDP	end-diastolic pressure
CN	cellulose nitrate		EDTA	ethylenediaminetetraacetate
CNBD	cyclic nucleotide-binding domain		EGF	epidermal growth factor
CNS	crystallography & NMR systems		EGFP	enhanced green fluorescent protein
CO	cardiac output		EnMet	Energy and Metabolism

eNOS	endothelial nitric oxide synthase	IUPAC	The International Union of Pure and Applied Chemistry
EPC	endothelial progenitor cells		
Epi	epirubicin	IV	intravenous
ERP	effective refractory period		
ES	embryonic stem	JAE	junction-adhesion-extracellular matrix
ESI	electrospray-ionisation		
ESTs	expressed sequence tags		
ET-1	endothelin-1	Kv-channels	voltage-gated potassium channels
ET$_A$R	endothelin-1 receptor subtype A		
EtOH	ethanol	LA	left atrium
		LAD	left anterior descending coronary artery
FACS	fluorescence activated cell sorter		
FCS	foetal calf serum	LCX	left circumflex artery
FISH	fluorescence in situ hybridisation	LDH	lactate dehydrogenase
FITC-	fluorescein-isothiocyanate-	LIF	leukemia inhibitory factor
FOC	force of contraction	LV	left ventricle
FP	field potentials	LVDP	left ventricular developed pressure
		LVEF	left ventricular ejection fraction
Gab	Grb-associated binder	LVP	left ventricular pressure
GAP	GTPase-activating protein		
GFP	green fluorescent protein	MACS	magnetic activated cell sorting
GPCR	G protein coupled receptor	MALDI	matrix-assisted-laser-desorption-ionisation
HBSS	Hank's balanced salt solution	MAO	monoamine oxidase
HCN channels	hyperpolarisation-activated cyclic nucleotide-gated cation channels	MAP	mean arterial pressure
		MAP	mitogen activated protein
HE	hematoxylin-eosin	MAP	monophasic action potentials
HEK	human embryonic kidney cells	MAPC	multipotent adult progenitor cell
HEPA-filter	high efficiency particulate air filter	Mb	myoglobin
HEPES-Na	2-[4-(2-Hydroxyethyl)-1-piperazinyl]-ethanesulphonic acid sodium salt	MBF	myocardial blood flow
		MEA	microelectrode arrays
HR	Heart rate	MEF	mouse embryonic fibroblast
HRP	horseradish peroxidase	MEM	non-essential amino acids
HSC	haematopoietic stem cells	MHC	myosin heavy chain
HSQC	$^1H^{15}N$-heteronuclear single quantum coherence	MI	myocardial infarction
		MLP	muscle LIM-domain protein
HW	heart weight	MNC	mononucleated cells
		MOI	multiplicity of infection
IACUC	Institutional Animal Care and Use Committees	MRI	magnetic resonance imaging
		MS	mass spectrometry
IC	intracoronary	MS/MS	tandem mass spectrometry
ICM	inner cell mass	MSC	mesenchymal stem cells
IMAC	immobilized metal ion affinity chromatography		
		NA	noradrenalin
IMDM	Iscove's modified Dulbecco's medium	NAT	nordadrenaline transporter
		NBT	nitro blue tetrazolium chloride
IP	intraperitoneal	NCS	newborn calf serum
IPPV	intermittent positive pressure ventilation	NHS	N-hydroxysuccinimide
		NMR	nuclear magnetic resonance
ITO	indium-tin oxide	NO	nitric oxide

NOE	nuclear overhauser effect	RCX	circumflex artery
NOS	NO-synthases	REV	relative estimated (transcription) variability
Ntg	non-transgenic		
		RGS	regulators of G protein signalling
OG	organelle genetics	ROS	reactive oxygen species
		RP	reverse-phase
PAP	peroxidase anti-peroxidase	rpm	revolutions per minute
PAR1	thrombin activated protease receptor type 1	RT	room temperature
		RT	reverse transcription
PBS	phosphate buffered saline	$RT_{1/2}$	relaxation halftime
PCNA	proliferating nuclear antigen	RU	response units
PCR	polymerase chain reaction		
PD	proportional distance	S/N	signal-to-noise ratio
PDA	photodiode arrays	SAN	sino-atrial node
PDEA	(2-(2-pyridinylthio)ethanamine hydrochloride)	SC	subcutaneous
		SCX	strong cation exchange
PDGF	platelet derived growth factor	SECV	single electrode voltage clamp
PE	phycoerythrin	sGC	soluble guanyl cyclase
PE	phenylephrine	SHR	spontaneously hypertensive rats
PEEP	positive end expiratory pressure	SMC	smooth muscle cell
PEG	polyethylene glycol	SM-MHC	smooth muscle myosin heavy chain
PEI	polyethylenimine	SNR	signal-to-noise ratio
PenStrep	penicillin/streptomycin solution	SO	Symmetrical Optimum
PET	positron emission	SP	side population
PFA	para-formaldehyde	SP	systolic pressure
P-I	proportional integral	SPF	specific-pathogen-free
PIPES	piperazine-N'-N'-bis[2-ethane-sulfonic acid	SPR	surface plasmon resonance
		SSC	standard saline citrate
PKA	cAMP-dependent protein kinase	synthase	L-NNA
PL	intrapleural		
PLC-β	β-isoforms of phospholipase C	T	tesla
PLD	phospholipase D	T1	transport into the cell
		T2	transport within the cell
PMMA	polymethylmethacrylate	TAT	total activation time
PNMT	phenylethanolamine-N-methyl-transferase	TB	Tris buffer
		TBS	Tris-buffered saline
PPM	parts per million	TBST	150 mM NaCl, 25 mM Tris-HCl, 0.05% Tween20, pH 7.5
PQ	atrioventricular conduction time		
PSD	post source decay	TD	trypsin-diluted
PTCA	percutaneous transluminal coronary angioplasty	TdP	torsade de pointes
		TE	expiratory ventilation time
PTK	protein tyrosine kinase	TEA	tetraethylammonium aspartate
PTP	protein tyrosine phosphatase	TEVC	two-electrode voltage clamp
PVDF	polyvinylidendifluoride	Tg	transgenic
		TH	tyrosine hydroxylase
QTc	frequency corrected QT time	TI	inspiratory ventilation time
		TMR	transmyocardial laser revascularisation
R	resistance		
RA	right atrium	TPP	time to peak pressure
RCA	right coronary artery	TR	transcriptional

Tris	trishydroxymethylaminomethane	VMAT	vesicular monoamine transporter
TSA	tyramide signal amplification	V_{rev}	reversal potential
TSP	3-(Trimethylsilyl)- Propionic acid-D4	VT	transverse ventricular propagation velocity
tTA	tetracycline-controlled transactivation		
TTX	tetrodotoxin	VWF	von Willebrand factor
USDA	United States Department of Agriculture	WPW	Wolff-Parkinson-White syndrome
		WT	wildtype
VDCC	voltage dependent calcium channel	YAC	yeast artificial chromosome
V_L	longitudinal ventricular propagation velocity		

List of Contributors

Allessie, Maurits A.
University Maastricht
Department of Physiology
PO Box 616
6200 MD Maastricht
The Netherlands

Ashton, Anthony W.
Albert Einstein College
of Medicine
Department of Neuroscience
Bronx, New York 10461
USA

Aupperle, Heike
Universität Leipzig
Herzzentrum
Klinik für Herzchirurgie
Strümpellstraße 39
04289 Leipzig
Germany

Berkels, Reinhard
Universität zu Köln
Institut für Pharmakologie
Gleueler Straße 24
50931 Köln
Germany

Billman, George E.
The Ohio State University
Department of Physiology
and Cell Biology
304 Hamilton Hall
1645 Neil Ave.
Columbus OH 43210-1218
USA

Blaauw, Yuri
University Maastricht
Department of Physiology
PO Box 616
6200 MD Maastricht
The Netherlands

Bloch, Wilhelm
Deutsche Sporthochschule Köln
Institut für Kreislaufforschung
und Sportmedizin
Carl-Diem-Weg 6
50933 Köln
Germany

Brandt, Mathias C.
Universität zu Köln
Klinik für Innere Medizin III
Joseph-Stelzmann Straße 9
50924 Köln
Germany

Braun-Dullaeus, Ruediger C.
Technische Universität Dresden
Klinik für Innere Medizin
Fetscherstraße 76
01307 Dresden
Germany

Brede, Marc
Bayerische Julius-Maximilians-
Universität Würzburg
Institut für Pharmakologie
und Toxikologie
Versbacher Straße 9
97078 Würzburg
Germany

Coombs, Wanda
SUNY Upstate Medical University
Department of Pharmacology
766 Irving Ave.
Syracuse NY 13210
USA

Decking, Ulrich
Heinrich-Heine-Universität
Universitätsklinikum
Institut für Herz- und Kreislauf-
physiologie
Universitätsstraße 1
40225 Düsseldorf
Germany

Delmar, Mario
SUNY Upstate Medical University
Department of Pharmacology
766 Irving Ave.
Syracuse NY 13210
USA

Dhein, Stefan
Universität Leipzig
Herzzentrum
Klinik für Herzchirurgie
Strümpellstraße 39
04289 Leipzig
Germany

Didié, Michael
Universitätsklinikum Hamburg-
Eppendorf
Zentrum für Experimentelle
Medizin
Institut für Experimentelle
und Klinische Pharmakologie
Martinistraße 52
20246 Hamburg
Germany

Doll, Nicolas
Universität Leipzig
Herzzentrum
Klinik für Herzchirurgie
Strümpellstraße 39
04289 Leipzig
Germany

Duffy, Heather S.
Albert Einstein College
of Medicine
Department of Neuroscience
Bronx, New York 10461
USA

Egert, Ulrich
Universität Freiburg
Neurobiologie und Biophysik
Institut für Biologie III
Schänzlestraße 1
79104 Freiburg
Germany

El-Armouche, Ali
Universitätsklinikum Hamburg-
Eppendorf
Zentrum für Experimentelle
Medizin
Institut für Experimentelle
und Klinische Pharmakologie
Martinistraße 52
20246 Hamburg
Germany

Er, Fikret
Universität zu Köln
Klinik für Innere Medizin III
Joseph-Stelzmann-Straße 9
50924 Köln
Germany

Eschenhagen, Thomas
Universitätsklinikum Hamburg-
Eppendorf
Zentrum für Experimentelle
Medizin
Institut für Experimentelle
und Klinische Pharmakologie
Martinistraße 52
20246 Hamburg
Germany

Fabritz, Larissa
Universitätsklinikum Münster
Medizinische Klinik
und Poliklinik C
Kardiologie und Angiologie
und Institut für Arteriosklerose-
forschung
Albert-Schweitzer-Straße 33
48149 Münster
Germany

Falk, Volkmar
Universität Leipzig
Herzzentrum
Klinik für Herzchirurgie
Strümpellstraße 39
04289 Leipzig
Germany

Fast, Vladimir G.
University of Alabama
at Birmingham
1670 University Blvd., VH B126
Birmingham, AL 35294
USA

Fleischmann, Bernd
Rheinische-Friedrich-Wilhelms-
Universität Bonn
Institut für Physiologie I
Argelander Straße 2a
53115 Bonn
Germany

Franz, Michael
Georgetown University
and Veterans Administrations
Medical Centers
Departments of Cardiology
and Pharmacology
50 Irving Street, NW
Washington DC 20422
USA

Foster, Dalton A.
SUNY Upstate Medical University
Department of Microbiology
and Immunology
750 E. Adams St
Syracuse, NY 13210
USA

Garbade, Jens
Universität Leipzig
Herzzentrum
Klinik für Herzchirurgie
Strümpellstraße 39
04289 Leipzig
Germany

Gissel, Cornelia
Universität zu Köln
Institut für Neurophysiologie
Robert-Koch-Straße 39
50931 Köln
Germany

Hein, Lutz
Bayerische Julius-Maximilians-
Universität Würzburg
Institut für Pharmakologie
und Toxikologie
Versbacher Straße 9
97078 Würzburg
Germany

Hein, Peter
Bayerische Julius-Maximilians-
Universität Würzburg
Institut für Pharmakologie
und Toxikologie
Versbacher Straße 9
97078 Würzburg
Germany

Hescheler, Jürgen
Universität zu Köln
Institut für Neurophysiologie
Robert-Koch-Straße 39
50931 Köln
Germany

van der Heyden, Marcel A.G.
University Medical Center
Department of Medical
Physiology
Universiteitsweg 100
3584 CG Utrecht
The Netherlands

Hoffmann, Christian
Universität zu Köln
Zentrum Anatomie
Institut I für Anatomie
Joseph-Stelzmann-Straße 9
50931 Köln
Germany

Hohlfeld, Thomas
Universität Düsseldorf
Institut für Pharmakologie
Moorenstraße 5
40225 Düsseldorf
Germany

List of Contributors

Hoppe, Uta C.
Universität zu Köln
Klinik für Innere Medizin III
Joseph-Stelzmann Str. 9
50924 Köln
Germany

Iacobas, Dumitru A.
Albert Einstein College
of Medicine
Department of Neuroscience
Bronx, New York 10461
USA

Iacobas, Ionela
Albert Einstein College
of Medicine
Department of Neuroscience
Bronx, New York 10461
USA

Iacobas, Sandra
Albert Einstein College
of Medicine
Department of Neuroscience
Bronx, New York 10461
USA

Janssen, Eveline
Universität zu Köln
Zentrum Anatomie
Institut I für Anatomie
Joseph-Stelzmann-Straße 9
50931 Köln
Germany

Kaiser, Björn
Universitätsklinikum Essen
Institut für Pharmakologie
Hufelandstraße 55
45122 Essen
Germany

Kirchhof, Paulus
Universitätsklinikum Münster
Medizinische Klinik
und Poliklinik C
Albert-Schweitzer-Straße 33
48129 Münster
Germany

van Koppen, Chris J.
Universitätsklinikum Essen
Institut für Pharmakologie
Hufelandstraße 55
45122 Essen
Germany

Korkmaz, Yüksel
Universität zu Köln
Zentrum Anatomie
Institut I für Anatomie
Joseph Stelzmann Straße 9
50931 Köln
Germany

Lang, Brian D.
Biacore Inc.,
Piscataway, New Jersey
USA

Lehr, Stefan
Heinrich-Heine-Universität
Düsseldorf
Institut für Klinische Biochemie
und Pathobiochemie
Diabetes Forschungszentrum
Leibniz-Zentrum für Diabetes-Forschung
Auf'm Hennekamp 65
40225 Düsseldorf
Germany

Leineweber, Kirsten
Universitätsklinikum Essen
Institut für Pathophysiologie
Hufelandstraße 55
45147 Essen
Germany

Lindner, Michael
Universität zu Köln
Klinik für Innere Medizin III
Joseph-Stelzmann-Straße 9
50924 Köln
Germany

Linz, Klaus
Grünenthal GmbH
Safety Pharmacology
Zieglerstraße 6
52078 Aachen
Germany

Melnychenko, Ivan
Universitätsklinikum Hamburg-Eppendorf
Zentrum für Experimentelle
Medizin
Institut für Experimentelle
und Klinische Pharmakologie
Martinistraße 52
20246 Hamburg
Germany

Merx, Marc W.
Universitätsklinikum Aachen
Medizinische Klinik 1
Kardiologie und Pneumologie
Pauwelstraße 30
52074 Aachen
Germany

Meyer, Rainer
Rheinische-Friedrich-Wilhelms-Universität Bonn
Institut für Physiologie II
Wilhelmstraße 31
53111 Bonn
Germany

Meyer, Thomas
Multi Channel Systems
MCS GmbH
Aspenhaustraße 21
72770 Reutlingen
Germany

Meyer, Veronika R.
EMPA St. Gallen
Eidgenössische
Materialprüfungs- und
Forschungsanstalt
Metrologie in der Chemie
Lerchenfeldstrasse 5
9014 St. Gallen
Switzerland

List of Contributors

Michels, Guido
Universität zu Köln
Klinik für Innere Medizin III
Joseph-Stelzmann-Straße 9
50924 Köln
Germany

Michel, Martin C.
University of Amsterdam
Academic Medical Center
Dept. Pharmacology
& Pharmacotherapy
Meibergdreef 15
1105 AZ Amsterdam
The Netherlands

Morawietz, Henning
Technische Universität Dresden
Medizinische Klinik
und Poliklinik III
Bereich Gefäßendothel/
Mikrozirkulation
Fetscherstraße 74
01307 Dresden
Germany

Nierhoff, Dirk
Universität zu Köln
Institut für Neurophysiologie
Robert-Koch-Straße 39
50931 Köln
Germany

Noll, Thomas
Justus-Liebig-Universität Giessen
Physiologisches Institut
Aulweg 129
35392 Giessen
Germany

Offermanns, Stefan
Universität Heidelberg
Pharmakologisches Institut
Im Neuenheimer Feld 366
69120 Heidelberg
Germany

Peters, Saskia C.
Justus-Liebig-Universität Giessen
Physiologisches Institut
Aulweg 129
35392 Giessen
Germany

Philipp, Melanie
Universität Zürich
Institut für Zoologie
Winterthurerstrasse 190
8057 Zürich
Switzerland

Piper, Hans Michael
Justus-Liebig-Universität Giessen
Physiologisches Institut
Aulweg 129
35392 Giessen
Germany

Polder, Hans Reiner
npi electronic GmbH
Hauptstraße 96
71732 Tamm
Germany

Quinn, Robert H.
SUNY Upstate Medical University
Department of Laboratory
Animal Resources
750 East Adams Street
Syracuse, NY 13210
USA

Rastan, Ardawan J.
Universität Leipzig
Klinik für Herzchirurgie
Herzzentrum
Strümpellstraße 39
04289 Leipzig
Germany

Ravens, Ursula
Technische Universität Dresden
Institut für Pharmakologie
und Toxikologie
Fetscherstraße 74
01307 Dresden
Germany

Reis, Anna
Justus-Liebig-Universität Giessen
Physiologisches Institut
Aulweg 129
35392 Giessen
Germany

Rösen, Peter
Heinrich-Heine-Universität
Düsseldorf
Institut für Klinische Biochemie
und Pathobiochemie
Leibniz-Zentrum für Diabetes-
Forschung
Auf'm Hennekamp 65
40225 Düsseldorf
Germany

Rösen, Renate
Universität zu Köln
Institut für Pharmakologie
Gleueler Straße 24
50931 Köln
Germany

Rosenkranz, Anke
Universität zu Köln
Institut für Pharmakologie
Gleueler Straße 24
50931 Köln
Germany

Rozemuller, Henk
Jordan Laboratory
University Medical Center
Department of Heamatology
Universiteitsweg 100
3584 CG Utrecht
The Netherlands

Sachinidis, Agapios
Universität zu Köln
Institut für Neurophysiologie
Robert-Koch-Straße 39
50931 Köln
Germany

List of Contributors

Salameh, Aida
Universität Leipzig
Klinik I für Innere Medizin
Johannisallee 32
04103 Leipzig
Germany

Schlüter, Klaus-Dieter
Justus-Liebig-Universität
Giessen
Physiologisches Institut
Aulweg 129
35392 Giessen
Germany

Schneider, Katja
Universität Leipzig
Herzzentrum
Klinik für Herzchirurgie
Strümpellstraße 39
04289 Leipzig

Schotten, Ulrich
University Maastricht
Department of Physiology
PO Box 616
6200 MD Maastricht
The Netherlands

Schrader, Jürgen
Heinrich-Heine-Universität
Düsseldorf
Institut für Physiologie
Postfach 10 10 07
40001 Düsseldorf
Germany

Schubert, Andreas
Universität Leipzig
Herzzentrum
Russenstraße 19
04289 Leipzig
Germany

Schubert, Rudolf
Universität Rostock
Institut für Physiologie
Postfach 10 08 88
18055 Rostock
Germany

Sedding, Daniel G.
Justus-Liebig-Universität Giessen
Medizinische Klinik I
Innere Medizin/Kardiologie
Klinikstraße 36
35392 Giessen
Germany

Sorgen, Paul. L.
University of Nebraska
Medical Center
Department of Biochemistry
and Molecular Biology
Omaha, NE 68198
USA

Spray, David C.
Albert Einstein College
of Medicine
Department of Neuroscience
Bronx, New York 10461
USA

Stahl, Fabian
Universität Leipzig
Herzzentrum
Klinik für Herzchirurgie
Strümpellstraße 39
Germany
04289 Leipzig

Steinritz, Dirk
Universität zu Köln
Zentrum Anatomie
Institut I für Anatomie
Joseph-Stelzmann-Straße 9
50931 Köln
Germany

Taffet, Steven M.
SUNY Upstate Medical University
Department of Microbiology
and Immunology
750 E. Adams St
Syracuse, NY 13210
USA

Tárnok, Attila
Universität Leipzig
Herzzentrum
Klinik für Kinderkardiologie
Strümpellstraße 39
04289 Leipzig
Germany

Taubert, Dirk
Universität zu Köln
Institut für Pharmakologie
Gleueler Straße 24
50931 Köln
Germany

Tritthart, Helmut A.
Karl-Franzens-Universität Graz
Institut für Medizinische Physik
und Biophysik
Harrachgasse 21
8010 Graz
Austria

Ullmann, Cris W.
Universität Leipzig
Herzzentrum
Klinik für Herzchirurgie
Strümpellstraße 39
04289 Leipzig
Germany

Vikstrom, Karen L.
SUNY Upstate Medical University
Department of Laboratory
Animal Resources
750 East Adams Street
Syracuse, NY 13210
USA

Walther, Thomas
Universität Leipzig
Herzzentrum
Klinik für Herzchirurgie
Strümpellstraße 39
04289 Leipzig
Germany

Weiß, Jürgen
Heinrich-Heine-Universität
Düsseldorf
Institut für Klinische Biochemie
und Pathobiochemie
Leibniz-Zentrum für Diabetes-
Forschung
Auf'm Hennekamp 65
40225 Düsseldorf
Germany

Weskamp, Martin
npi electronic GmbH,
Hauptstraße 96,
71732 Tamm
Germany

Wettschureck, Nina
Universität Heidelberg
Pharmakologisches Institut
Im Neuenheimer Feld 366
69120 Heidelberg
Germany

Wettwer, Erich
Technische Universität Dresden
Institut für Pharmakologie
und Toxikologie
Fetscherstraße 74
01307 Dresden
Germany

Wieland, Thomas
Universität Heidelberg
Fakultät für Klinische Medizin
Mannheim
Institut für Pharmakologie
und Toxikologie
Maybachstraße 14–16
68169 Mannheim
Germany

Zacharowski, Kai
Heinrich-Heine-Universität
Düsseldorf
Universitätsklinikum
Klinik für Anästhesiologie
und Intensivmedizin
Moorenstraße 5
40225 Düsseldorf
Germany

Zimmermann, Wolfram-Hubertus
Universitätsklinikum Hamburg-Eppendorf
Zentrum für Experimentelle
Medizin
Institut für Experimentelle
und Klinische Pharmakologie
Martinistraße 52
20246 Hamburg
Germany

In-Vivo Techniques

1 Models of Cardiovascular Disease — 3

1 Models of Cardiovascular Disease

1.1 **Anaesthesia (Inhalative or i.v. Narcosis) of Laboratory Animals** — 5
Katja Schneider

1.2 **Extracorporeal Circulation** — 26
Cris W. Ullmann

1.3 **Open-chest Models of Acute Myocardial Ischemia and Reperfusion** — 37
Kai Zacharowski, Thomas Hohlfeld and Ulrich K.M. Decking

1.4 **Models of Chronic Ischemia and Infarction** — 58
Nicolas Doll, Heike Aupperle, Fabian Stahl and Thomas Walther

1.5 **Models on Left Ventricular Hypertrophy (LVH)** — 72
Thomas Walther and Volkmar Falk

1.6 **Experimental Models of Heart Failure** — 83
Volkmar Falk, Jens Garbade and Thomas Walther

1.7 **In-Vivo Models of Arrhythmias: a Canine Model of Sudden Cardiac Death** — 111
George E. Billman

1.8 **In-Vivo Models of Atrial Fibrillation** — 129
Ulrich Schotten, Yuri Blaauw and Maurits Allessie

Anaesthesia (Inhalative or i.v. Narcosis) of Laboratory Animals

Katja Schneider

Introduction

Sufficient anaesthesia is a prerequisite for any intervention using laboratory animals for scientific purposes. In most countries there are strict regulations and laws for the use and handling of laboratory animals. Thus, in several countries, e.g. in Germany, it is necessary that general anaesthesia is performed by a veterinarian. This has to be checked with the local authority.

In the following chapters, protocols for general anaesthesia will be described for those animals which are most often used for scientific purposes in cardiovascular research. The reader will see that these protocols in many aspects are similar to those used for human beings. Thus, for further and more detailed reading, textbooks of anaesthesia for humans can be recommended. The protocols given in this chapter are protocols as they are used many times in our laboratory at Leipzig. These are examples of how general anaesthesia can be achieved in a certain species; however, other protocols may also be suitable.

The protocols as they are given here are designed and tested for use in cardiovascular scientific research and therefore are different from those used in common veterinarian practice. The problem encountered in cardiovascular research is that it is necessary to maintain all hemodynamic parameters in a stable range and to prevent variations in the depth of anaesthesia. This is in most cases best achieved with an inhalation anaesthesia with controlled ventilation. Another aspect is that in some cases it is desired that the animal survives the operation to allow a postoperative chronic phase of the experiment. Therefore, it is necessary to use a protocol which allows good control of anaesthesia and hemodynamics for the duration of the – in many cases long – operation and allows good and quick recovery.

Each protocol of anaesthesia comprises the five phases of treatment: premedication, induction of anaesthesia, maintenance of anaesthesia, termination of anaesthesia, and postoperative treatment. This will be given for each animal species. On the other hand, we have to distinguish between short termed operations and operations of longer duration. For short anaesthesia normally intravenous anaesthesia is used. This can be recommended for operations of 15 min maximum duration, e.g. for punctures or sample excision. In specific protocols it is possible to prolong intravenous anaesthesia but this cannot generally be recommended. If the operative treatment needs more time, i.e. more than 30 min, generally inhalation anaesthesia protocols should be used.

In many cases premedication is recommended in order to prevent bradycardia, which often is associated with general anaesthesia, and to prevent bronchial hypersecretion or bronchospasms. Mostly, atropine is the drug of choice for premedication. Alternatively, scopolamine can be used. In certain circumstances it might be necessary to induce sedation of the animal prior to transport to the operation room. For this purpose, ketamine and xylazine may be used, because it will induce deep sedation with spontaneous respiration and allow intubation. For pigs, normally the neuroleptic drug azaperone (e.g. Stresnil®) is used for premedication to induce sleep for transportation. For intubation the pig has to be treated with thiopental.

In principle there are several forms of intravenous anaesthesia. First of all, the so-called neuroleptanaesthesia may be used under certain circumstances, e.g. for short operations. The principle is to combine an opioid analgesic drug such as fentanyl with a high potency neuroleptic drug such as droperidol. Since under this narcosis uncontrolled movements of the animal may occur this is not suitable for most experimental purposes except sample excisions.

The most commonly used intravenous anaesthetic drug is the barbiturate derivative thiopental or pentobarbital. Barbiturates are good narcotics but lack analgesic properties, so they must be combined with some analgesic treatment, e.g. fentanyl.

Another drug which is often used in veterinarian medicine for intravenous anaesthesia is the benzodiazepine midazolam (e.g. Dormicum®) and medetomidine (e.g. Dormitor®) which induce sleepiness and sedation. For intravenous general anaesthesia these drugs have to be combined with an opioid such as fentanyl.

For intravenous analgesia, especially in ruminants xylazine (e.g. Rompun®) is recommended as an opioid-like analgesic drug which normally is combined with the narcotic drug ketaminee. Although xylazinee was first developed for use in ruminants this can also be used in other species.

Regarding forms of inhalation anaesthesia, in former times the most commonly used form of anaesthesia was the use of diethylether. Pharmacologically this is the classical general anaesthetic drug since this substance combines the three properties a good anaesthetic drug should possess, i.e. diethylether has good narcotic, analgesic and relaxant properties. However, today this is no longer preferred for several reasons (see below). The advantage of diethylether is the simplicity of use (by a Schimmelbusch's mask or by putting the animal [rat, mouse] in a closed cage with paper soaked with diethylether). Another advantage especially for cardiovascular research is that diethylether – in contrast to fluorinated hydrocarbons- does not induce sensitization of the heart against catecholamines. However, although its pharmacological properties are suitable and the use is simple, this drug is highly explosive and therefore cannot be used in an operation room when a cautery is used. Another disadvantage is a possible long excitation state. Today diethylether in some labs is still used for rats, guinea pigs or mice to induce general anaesthesia for the removal of an organ, e.g. preparation of an isolated heart according to Langendorff. It cannot be generally recommended for prolonged operations. If it is used it is necessary to test the depth of anaesthesia in short intervals and if necessary to repeat application of diethylether.

N_2O is often used as an analgesic drug in humans. However, in veterinarian medicine about 80% N_2O would be needed for suitable analgesia, so that the remaining 20% O_2 may not be sufficient. N_2O can be used as an analgesic in combination with halogenated or fluorinated hydrocarbons such as halothane or isoflurane.

For inhalation anaesthesia the most suitable drugs are fluorinated hydrocarbons which are applied by a vaporizer. Typical drugs used in veterinarian practice are halothane and isoflurane. Due to the physical and pharmacological properties of these drugs anaesthesia, using these drugs can be easily controlled and narcosis can be terminated without prolonged sedation or sleep.

Finally a possible combination of intravenous and inhalation anaesthesia should be briefly discussed. Although in principle a combination of barbiturate and N_2O would be useful to circumvent the lack of analgesic properties of the barbiturate component, such a treatment is unusual in veterinarian medicine.

If extracorporeal circulation is used during the experiment inhalation anaesthesia cannot be used during this period and one has to switch for the duration of extracorporeal circulation to intravenous anaesthesia e.g. with fentanyl and midazolam or thiopental.

For a more detailed description of the pharmacological properties of the drugs used in the protocols described here, we recommend the classical textbooks of pharmacology or anaesthesiology for further reading.

Description of Methods and Practical Approach

Anaesthesia of Pigs

Pigs are often used in cardiovascular research, especially in models of acute and chronic ischemia or infarction. Depending on the goal of the experiments pigs of different size are used ranging from piglets of 5–8 kg to adult pigs of 80 kg. However, it should be noted that with increasing weight pigs are more critical in narcosis. Common problems are cardiac arrhythmia, and spontaneous cardiac arrest especially during transport and initial manipulation/positioning in the operation room due to their susceptibility to stress. From our experience this seems to be related to weight and obesity. Therefore, we recommend the use of smaller pigs. One possibility to circumvent this problem at least in part is the use of the so-called mini-pigs or micro-pigs both of which are not so susceptible to stress and often are used for chronic experiments.

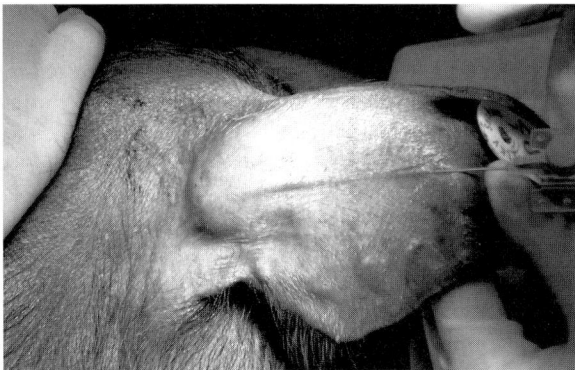

Figure 1
Demonstration of a punction of the porcine V. auricularis

As mentioned, a general peculiarity of pigs is that these animals are very susceptible to stress and therefore have to be pretreated with some sedative drug prior to any other intervention. Normally azaperone is the preferred drug of choice.

For intramuscular injections the muscle layer between ear and processus mastoideus can be used. The pig has not many superficial veins and therefore the intravenous injection is performed into V. auricularis (Fig. 1). Instead, the V. cephalica, V. saphena and V. jugularis can be used.

Intravenous Anaesthesia (pigs)

For premedication atropine is injected intramuscularly. Thereafter, azaperone is applied in the muscle layer between ear and processus mastoideus. If this premedication is not sufficient azaperone can be used in combination with ketaminee, especially if the animal was exposed preoperativley to any form of stress. Ten minutes after this application the animal should be transportable. It should be noted that – if a transport is necessary – the duration should not be longer than 30 min. Otherwise a second application of azaperone would be necessary because pigs are sensitive to transport stress even during premedication.

After premedication an application of metomidate into the auricular vein is suggested by the literature, which should result in a mild (not deep) narcosis for about 30 min, sufficient to last the duration of the surgery. If the duration of surgery is longer, metomidate can be applied a second time. A disadvantage of metomidate is that the recovery from narcosis is prolonged.

In most cases additional application of ketamine is needed. An alternative to metomidate is the use of barbiturates like pentobarbital and thiopental. Pento-barbital should be dosed precisely because of the danger of overdosing (Blonait et al. 1988). Typical side effects are respiratory depression, decreased blood pressure, vasodilation, spleen swelling and a decrease of digestive functions (Blonait et al. 1988).

In contrast, thiopental which exhibits a faster pharmacokinetic with faster onset of effect, can be controlled better and does not lead to decreased blood pressure but – as all barbituric acid derivatives – depresses respiration (Blonait et al. 1988). Thus, the effect of a second application must be carefully controlled by the veterinarian because of an enhanced effect due to accumulation of the barbiturates in adipose tissue and its redistribution. As a consequence, all barbiturates should be given in several small doses.

- Option 1
    - 0.02 mg/kg atropin sulfate (i.m)
    - 2 mg/kg azaperone (i.m.)
    - 5–10 mg/kg ketamine (i.m.)
    - 2–4 mg/kg metomidate (i.v)
- Option 2
    - 0.02 mg/kg atropin sulfate (i.m)
    - 2 mg/kg azaperone (i.m.)
    - 10–25 mg/kg pentobarbital (i.v) or
    - 4–6 mg/kg thiopental (i.v)

Inhalation Anaesthesia (Pigs)

If there is a possibility for inhalative anaesthesia this form should be preferred (Swindle 1998). For premedication azaperone (e.g. for transport) and thiopental (for intubation) should be applied. After depression of the swallowing reflex the pig is intubated in ventral position (pig laying on the belly) which simplifies the procedure of intubating. This position is advantageous since the relatively large tongue drops down (to the mandible) due to gravity allowing intubation using a spatula (specially designed for pigs). In dorsal position this procedure is hard to perform since one has to move away the heavy tongue. Owing to the anatomical situation, animals above 50 kg should be intubated in sight control. In the case that the epiglottis is fixed behind the velum palatinum it must be moved away using the spatula (Fig. 2).

Magill tubes (size 7–10) can be used but it should be checked whether tubes are long enough. In case of animals with a weight of 5 kg (with a small rima glottidis) or above 100 kg (with an elongated skull) tracheotomy can be performed (as an alternative). However, in that case local anaesthesia is needed. After intubating, the tubes are connected with the lung ventilator and ventilated with isofluran and oxygen. For infusion isotonic NaCl, G5 or Ringer solution is suggested (500 ml/h).

Inhalation Anaesthesia:
- premedication:
    - 0.02 mg/kg atropin sulfate (i.m)
    - 2 mg/kg azaperon (i.m.)
- for intubation:
    - 4 mg/kg thiopental (i.v.)
- inhalation:
    - 3–5 vol% isofluran (begin)
    - 0.8–1.5 vol% (later)

The following parameters should be controlled and set to the suggested values for a pig (30–50 kg):
- intermittent positive pressure ventilation (IPPV)
- % O_2: 40–60
- respiratory minute volume: 2.5–6 L/min
- respiratory volume: kg×10 ml
- respiratory rate: 12–17 min^{-1}
- inspiratory ventilation time (TI) : expiratory ventilation time (TE): 1:2
- positive end expiratory pressure (PEEP): 3 mbar
- P_{max}: 25 mbar

If the animal is connected with the cardiopulmonary bypass for extracorporeal circulation the inhalative narcosis must be stopped and instead anaesthesia is continued with injection of fentanyl and midazolam. To stop narcosis isofluran is progressively decreased and oxygen increased. Moreover, the animal should be brought back into a ventral position. With the beginning of independent breathing the extubation can be performed.

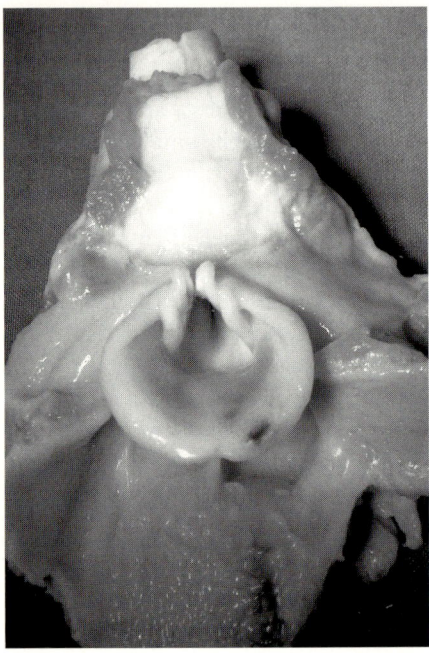

Figure 2
Demonstration of the pharyngeal area of a pig

Postoperative Treatment

After surgery the pig should be kept in a box without other animals. Possible analgesics are metamizol (20–50 mg/kg) or fentanyl (0.05 mg/kg) or a plaster with fentanyl. The plaster is a useful method because the applied concentration does not change and injections are not necessary. A broad spectrum antibiotic (such as amoxicilline) should be given for one week.

Troubleshooting

The possibility for thermoregulation is not well developed in the pig as it does not have many sweat glands. Thus, it is necessary to control temperature carefully during anaesthesia and after the operation until mobilization of the animal. A genetic condition in certain breeds of domestic swine is malignant hyperthermia (e.g. Pietrain, Landrace and Yorkshire). The condition is induced by stress or by many anaesthetic and paralytic agents and some veterinarians give prophylactic intramuscular 5 mg/kg dantrolene (Swindle 1998).

A typical problem of anaesthesia in pigs is the intubation, which should be performed in the ventral position as described. Possible mistakes may be a small tubus (air leaking) or a big tubus which leads to injuries. Furthermore, intubation of only one lung is possible which results in assymetric breathing. An intubation of the oesophagus will result in inflation of the abdomen, and can be detected by a lack of rib motion and a missing CO_2 increase in the expiratory gas.

Another problem in narcosis of pigs is a predisposition for ventricular fibrillation, which is treatable with conventional methods (electrical defibrillation, or lidocaine, or flecainide). A closure of LAD proximal to the last third in most cases will lead to ventricular arrhythmia. If only a manipulation at the LAD is intended without inducing infarction, it is advisable to construct a bypass between the mammary artery and the distal LAD. Moreover reoperations are risky and problematic because the pigs may have developed adhesions in the pericard, epicard and the lungs. In order to prevent such adhesions it is possible to use goretex foil (Table 1).

Table 1
Clinical parameters and blood parameters of pigs

Parameter	Unit
Clinical parameter	
Body temperature	38.0–39.5 °C
Heart rate	60–80
Respiratory rate	14–36
Blood pressure	100/70
Blood volume	61–69 ml/kg
Cardiac output	3–4 l/min
Blood parameter	
Erythrocyte	5.8–8.1 T/l
Haematocrit	33–45%
Haemoglobin	6.7–9.2 mmol/l
Leucocyte	10.5–21.3 G/l
Calcium	2.5–3.3 mmol/l
Chloride	100–110 mmol/l
Sodium	130–170 mmol/l
Potassium	4.5–6.5 mmol/l
Magnesium	0.9–1.7 mmol/l
Glucose	4.0–6.4 mmol/l
Urea	2.9–8.1 mmol/l
Creatinine	0–2.5 mg/l
Bilirubin	0.1–4.1 µmol/l
Protein	55.4–85.4 g/l
Alkaline phosphatase	140–250 U/l
GOT	8–22 U/l
Creatinine kinase	0–1500 U/l

Anaesthesia of Sheep

Sheep are widely used in acute and chronic animal experiments. For intramuscular injections M. glutaeus superficialis as well as M. semimembranosus or M. semitendinosus can be used. Per depot, a maximum of 20 ml should be injected.

Intravenous injections are performed with the same vessels as in the pig: V. jugularis, V. auricularis, V. cephalica and V. saphena. For mean arterial pressure (MAP) monitoring A. auricularis as well as A. femoralis can be used.

Intravenous Anaesthesia (Sheep)

Acepromazine is appropriate because of its sedative effect. The induction of narcosis is faster than with other narcotics and, moreover, the awakening is faster. Thus, due to the faster pharmacodynamics many investigators prefer acepromazine in sheep or cows. However, the risk of regurgitation in sheep is increased by acepromazine. Moreover, hypovolemic sheep might develop hypotension.

Due to its strong sedative effect, xylazine is the most suitable sedative for injection in cows and sheep. Depending on the dose the drug can induce mild sedation or deep narcosis (in combination with ketaminee). Xylazine leads to musclular relaxation and moderate analgesia. As side effects depression of respiration and circulation. Moreover, inflation of the belly (paunch or rumen) may occur as well as paralysis of the rumen. In addition, hyperglycemia may be observed. In the last third of gravidity abortion may be induced by the drug.

Another possibility for general anaesthesia is a short intravenous narcosis using trapanal, a single injection resulting in general anaesthesia of about 20 min duration. Because of a possible apnoea during narcosis with trapanal, the experimentor should always keep a tracheal tubus in readiness.
- Option 1
  - 0.2 mg/kg xylazine (i.m.)
  - 10 mg/kg ketamine (i.m.)
- Option 2
  - 10–20 mg/kg thiopental (i.v.)

Inhalation Anaesthesia (Sheep)

For the transport and intubation of the animals ketamine and xylazine is applied. Swallowing reflex must be suppressed and tubes with the size 7.5–9.5 are used for intubation. As described above (for pigs) sheep should be intubated in ventral position.

Mouth wedges are important for transport since the tubus becomes leaky after seconds due to the sheep's chewing. After intubation the sheep is ventilated with isofluran, oxygen (40–60%) and air. Sheep should have an empty stomach for the last 24 h prior to surgery. Nevertheless, these animals will have some food in the gastrointestinal tract even after 24 h fasting. Thus, there is possible danger of aspiration pneumonia due to regurgitation. Therefore, each sheep should receive a gastric tube during narcosis.

Moreover, sheep as typical ruminants might develop tympania. This problem can be solved with a trokar inserted into the paunch. For infusion isotonic NaCl, G5 or Ringer solution is suggested (500 ml/h).

Inhalation anaesthesia:
- premedication:
    - 0.02 mg/kg atropine sulfate
    - 0.22 mg/kg xylazine
    - 11 mg/kg ketamine
- inhalation:
    - 3–5 vol% isofluran (initially)
    - 0.8–1.5 vol% isofluran (for maintenance)
- parameters (sheep 60–80 kg):
    - intermittent positive pressure ventilation (IPPV) % O_2: 40–60
    - respiratory minute volume: 6–12 L/min
    - respiratory volume: kg×10 ml
    - respiratory rate: 12–17 min^{-1}
    - inspiratory ventilation time (TI): expiratory ventilation time (TE): 1:2
    - positive end expiratory pressure (PEEP): 3 mbar
    - P_{max}: 25 mbar

To end narcosis, the dosage of isofluran is progressively decreased and oxygen increased. Moreover, the animal should be brought back into ventral position. With the beginning of independent breathing the extubation can be performed.

Postoperative Treatment

Extubation can be performed when reflexes have returned to normal and spontaneous chewing starts. Since sheep are gregarious animals they should not be alone even after surgery. For postoperative analgesia in sheep metamizol (20–50 mg/kg) or fentanyl (0.05 mg) can be applied. A broad spectrum antibiotic (e.g. amoxicilline) should be administered for one week.

Troubleshooting

During the surgical manipulations sheep should be preferably placed in a lateral position (rather than in a dorsal or ventral position), since in lateral position venous backflow to the heart is better. However, since cardiac surgery is best performed in dorsal position, in some cases the sheep have to be placed in dorsal position. In these cases, the whole animal has to be placed in an oblique position with the abdomen or caudal part of the animal in a lower position than the heart and the head higher. Otherwise, it is very problematic to ventilate the sheep correctly since the gastrointestinal tract may press on the diaphragm thereby impeding easy ventilation. Also, the sheep should not be kept in one position for long periods, because dependent lung lobes become oedematous and poorly perfused (Lumley et al. 1990). However, in that position venous backflow has to monitored carefully.

Table 2
Clinical parameters and blood parameters of sheep (50 kg)

Parameter	Unit
Clinical parameter	
Body temperature	38.0–39.5
Heart rate	60–80
Respiratory rate	16–30
Blood pressure	103/85
Blood volume	55–80 ml/kg
Cardiac output	3.9 l
Blood parameter	
Erythrocyte	7.3–11.3 T/l
Haematocrit	30–40%
Haemoglobin	6.4–11.0 mmol/l
Leucocyte	4.2–9.0 mmol/l
Calcium	2.4–3.0 mmol/l
Chloride	105–115 mmol/l
Sodium	130–154 mmol/l
Potassium	3.8–5.8 mmol/l
Magnesium	0.9–1.3 mmol/l
Glucose	2.5–5.2 mmol/l
Urea	2.5–7.0 mmol/l
Creatinine	36–120 mmol/l
Bilirubin	0.7–4.8 µmol/l
Protein	51–73 g/l
Alkaline phosphatase	50–250 U/l
GOT	25–80 U/l

For chronic trials a lateral thoracotomy is preferred because sheep often lie in ventral position which could lead to problems in wound healing (in case of sternotomy). In sheep, no peripheral muscle relaxants should be administered since the effect on the breathing muscular system is more effective than in other animals (Table 2).

Anaesthesia of Dogs

Intravenous injections are performed into V. cephalica antebrachii and V. saphena lateralis, for intramuscular injections the femoral muscles (M. semimembranosus and M. biceps femoris) and for subcutaneous injections the lateral thorax is applied.

Intravenous Anaesthesia (Dogs)

For short surgical operations (e.g. wound treatment, punctions) barbiturates can be used (5–10 mg/kg). The dose can be given again a second time, but it should not exceed more than one third of the initial dose.

As side effects of barbiturates breathing depression, arrhythmia and a decrease in the cardiac output have been observed. For analgesia xylazine and medetomidine can be used.

Propofol is another drug for short general anaesthesia in dogs. It is effective after 30 s and lasts for 4–8 min. Propofol has no analgesic effect (and therefore should be combined with an analgetic drug), and causes a dose-dependent breathing depression. Without premedication 4–7 mg/kg should be given, with premedication 2–4 mg/kg. The narcosis with propofol can be prolonged as often as necessary using a dose of 2–4 mg/kg.

For short and painful encroachments a combination of ketamine and xylazine should be used. The sedative hypnotic effect of xylazinee is enhanced by the premedication with diazepam. Ketamine is prefered for anaesthesia regarding operations at the surface of the body, while xylazine produces a good visceral analgesia. For maintenance of narcosis ketamine and xylazine are given every 10–20 min.

Typical doses as used in our lab are:
- 0.5–1 mg/kg diazepam (premedication)
- 0.03–0.05 mg/kg atropine sulfate (premedication)
- 3 mg/kg ketamine
- 0.3 mg/kg xylazine

For longer surgical interventions a combination of acepromazine, levomethadon, ketamine and xylazine can be used.
- Option 1
  - premedication:
    0.2–0.75 mg/kg levomethadon (i.v.)
    0.05–0.1 mg/kg acepromazine (i.v)
  - maintenance:
    3 mg/kg ketaminee
    0.03–0.08 mg/kg xylazine
- Option 2
  - 40 µg/kg medetomidin (i.v.)
  - 2–3 mg/kg ketamine (i.v.)
  - 0.2–0.4 mg/kg diazepam if needed

Inhalation Anaesthesia in Dogs)

- premedication:
  - 0.03 mg/kg atropin sulfate
  - 3 mg/kg ketamine
  - 0.3 mg/kg xylazine
- inhalation:
  - 2.5 vol% isofluran (initially)
  - 0.8–2 vol% isofluran (maintenance)
- parameters (dogs 20–30 kg):
  - intermittent positive pressure ventilation (IPPV)
  - % O_2: 40–60
  - respiratory minute volume: 3–6 L/min
  - respiratory volume: kg×10 ml
  - respiratory rate: 12–17 min^{-1}
  - inspiratory ventilation time (TI): expiratory ventilation time (TE): 1:2
  - positive end expiratory pressure (PEEP): 3 mbar
  - P_{max}: 25 mbar

Postoperative Treatment

Extubation can be performed when reflexes have returned to normal and spontaneous chewing starts. After surgery the pig should be kept in a box without other animals. Possible analgesics are, e.g., metamizol (20–50 mg/kg) or buprenorphine (0,01–0,02 mg/kg every 8–12 h) (Lumley et al. 1990).

Troubleshooting

Dogs are often used in cardiovascular research, because they have no typical problems of anaesthesia.

Anaesthesia of Rabbits

Blood withdrawal is possible out of V. jugularis, V. auricularis (Fig. 3) and V. saphena lateralis or just from the claw. To advance the sight of the vessel that is treated it is possible to shave the hair or to amass the vessel with an alcohol swab. General anaesthesia in rabbits is not easy to perform since surgical tolerance and asphyxia occur at nearly the same dose of the anaesthetic in this species. Fasting prior to surgery is not advisable since hypoglycemia and changes in the acid-base status may appear (Schall 2001).

Rabbits are very sensitive during the induction of narcosis and cardiac arrest or deep hypotension may develop. Prior to surgery the animal should be examined carefully to exclude lung injuries which may lead to ventilation problems during surgery.

Barbiturates are the only anaesthetic which are not recommended because of the development of deep hypotension and the small therapeutic width (see Fig. 3).

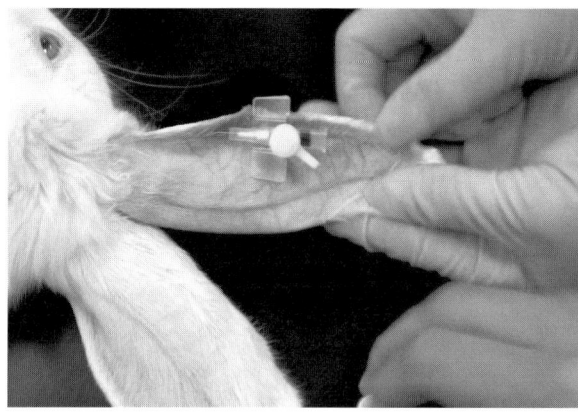

Figure 3
Punction of the V. auricularis of the rabbit

Intravenous anaesthesia (rabbits)

Intramuscularly administered neuroleptanalgetics do not cause surgical tolerance in rabbits, thus these drugs should be given i.v.

We have good experince with a combination of ketaminee and xylazine. The combination of ketamine and xylazine can be administered i.v. as well as i.m. For the i.m. administration a ratio of 1:5 should be given.

For injection narcosis there are two possibilities: one possibility which can be antagonised, the other which cannot. The i.m. administration of ketamine and xylazine is not antagonisable. Effect begins after 5–10 min and lasts for 20–60 min. For prolongation of narcosis a fifth of the initial dose can be given.

The other possibility (which also cannot be antagonised) is a combination of ketamine and meditomidine. After intramuscular administration of ketamine and meditomidine surgical tolerance is achieved after 2–5 min and lasts for 20 to 60 min. Intravenous prolongation of narcosis can be performed with diluted ketamine only.

Alternatively, a protocol resulting in narcosis which can be antagonised, consists of a combination of medetomidine, midazolam and fentanyl. Surgical tolerance is achieved after 5–10 min and lasts for about 2 h. For antagonising atipamezol, flumazenil and naloxon may be administrated i.m.

Xylazine and medetomidine exhibit a sedative and muscle relaxing effect but are cardio-depressant and suppress breathing.

- Option 1
  - narcosis (which can be antagonised):
    0.2 mg/kg medetomidine
    1.0 mg/kg midazolam
    0.02 mg/kg fentanyl
  - antagonists:
    1.0 mg/kg atipemazol
    0.1 mg/kg flumazenil
    0.03 mg/kg naloxon

- Option 2
    - narcosis (which cannot be antagonised):
        0.1 mg/kg atropine
        50 mg/kg ketamine
        4 mg/kg xylazine
- Option 3
    - narcosis (which cannot be antagonised):
        30 mg/kg ketaminee
        0.3 mg/kg meditomidine

Inhalation Anaesthesia (Rabbits)

For premedication atropine is administered i.m., thereafter a combination of ketaminee and medetomidine is administered. In case of preoperative excitation of the rabbit a premedication with medetomidine should be considered (and for narcosis the medetomidine dose has to be reduced).

After 10–20 min an intravenous canula has to be inserted (e.g. in the auricular vein) and connected with the perfusor to administer ketamine and medetomidine. Intubation is performed using a tubus (size 3–3.5) in ventral position or reclination of the head. Therafter, the rabbit is ventilated. Spontaneous ventilation is stopped by hyperventilation or by pancuronium. For infusion therapy NaCl (50 ml/h) may be used.

We have good experience with the following regimen:
- premedication:
    - 0.05 mg/kg atropine
    - 0.186 mg/kg medetomidine
    - 26.25 mg/kg ketaminee
- inhalation:
    - 2–3 vol% isofluran (initially for general anaesthesia)
    - 0.8–1 vol% isofluran (maintenance)
- parameters (rabbit 3 kg):
    - intermittent positive pressure ventilation (IPPV) % O_2: 40
    - respiratory minute volume: 0.4–1.0 L/min
    - respiratory volume: 30–50 ml
    - respiratory rate: 15–20 min^{-1}
    - inspiratory ventilation time (TI) : expiratory ventilation time (TE): 1:2
    - positive end expiratory pressure (PEEP): 0–5 mbar
    - P_{max}: 25 mbar

Postoperative Treatment

During and even after surgery the rabbit should be warmed, e.g. with an electric pad, since thermoregulation is discontinued in small animals during narcosis and due to the small body size these animals may cool very fast. Thus, shaving and washing should be reduced to a minimum in these animals.

Postoperative analgesia with metamizol (30 mg/kg i.v.) or fentanyl (0.002 mg/kg) can be started already during waking in order to reduce postoperative pain and to improve the overall condition, it may help the animal to begin feeding (Schall 2001).

Troubleshooting

Postoperatively, the animal should be ventilated since there is a predisposition for hypoxia. A typical problem in anaesthesia of rabbits is the development of deep hypotension. This can be circumvented by avoidance of barbiturates. Sometimes the animals do not start feeding after undergoing surgery. In these cases very often

Table 4
Clinical parameters and blood parameters of rabbits

Parameter	Unit
Clinical parameter	
Body temperature	37.5–39.5
Heart rate	120–250
Respiratory rate	32–60
Blood pressure	110/80
Blood volume	40–70 ml/kg
Cardiac output	140 ml/kg/min
Blood parameter	
Erythrocyte	4.0–7.0 T/l
Haematocrit	36–48%
Haemoglobin	100–155 g/l
Leucocyte	9–11 G/l
Calcium	1.4–3.1 mmol/l
Chloride	92–112 mmol/l
Sodium	138–155 mmol/l
Potassium	3.7–6.8 mmol/l
Magnesium	2.0–5.4 mmol/l
Glucose	4.1–8.7 mmol/l
Urea	2.8–3.9 mmol/l
Creatinine	70.7–159 µmol/l
Bilirubin	4.3–12.6 µmol/l
Protein	54–75 g/l

the animals experience postoperative pain, which should be treated using metamizol (see above). If the rabbit does not eat after surgery (which sometimes occurs) a parenteral nutrition is advised (Table 4).

Anaesthesia of Rats

The localization of choice for i.m. injection is the M. semitendinosus and M. semimembranosus. The maximum volume to be injected should not exceed 0.25 ml (Wijnbergen 2001). For blood withdrawal V. saphena is used (or the retroorbital vein plexus). If retroorbital punction (Fig. 4) is used it is necessary to apply pressure after the manipulation in order to avoid bleeding in the retroorbital situs. Moreover, dexpanthenol salve should be applied to the eye in order to avoid desiccation. I.m. injection should be preferred compared to i.v. since the stress for the rat is less. Attention should be paid to the fact that the effect after i.m. administration appears slower. However, in animals below 50 g (i.e. in newborn rats) the dosage is difficult. Moreover, very often toxic effects of the anaesthetics may appear and, thus, it is better to choose anaesthetics which can be antagonised.

Intravenous Anaesthesia (Rats)

Narcosis which cannot be antagonised is achieved using i.m. administration of ketamine and xylazine. This will result in general anaesthesia lasting for 30–60 min. For prolongation a fifth of the initial dose is given. As side effects depression of circulation and ventilation may be observed. For stimulation of the ventilation doxapram and for stimulation of the heart ephedrine can be used.

Alternatively, narcosis, which can be antagonised, is achieved by a combination of medetomidine, midazolam and fentanyl. Surgical tolerance is achieved after 5–10 min and the effect lasts for about 1 h. For antagonisation atipamezol, flumazenil and naloxon can be used. Antagonists are applied s.c. in contrast to the i.m. administration of the drugs for narcosis.

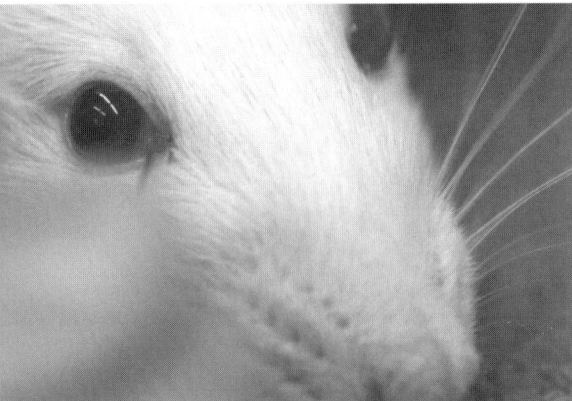

Figure 4
Retroorbital punction of the vein plexus of the rat eye

We have good experience with the following regimens:
- Option 1
  - narcosis which can be antagonised (drugs can be administered either intraperitoneal or i.m.):
  0.15 mg/kg medetomidine
  2 mg/kg midazolam
  0.005 mg/kg fentanyl
  antagonists (s.c.):
  0.75 mg/kg atipamezol
  0.2 mg/kg flumazenil
  0.12 mg/kg naloxon
- Option 2
  - narcosis which cannot be antagonised:
  0.1 mg/kg atropine (i.p. or i.m.)
  100 mg/kg ketamine (i.p. or i.m.)
  1.5 mg/kg xylazine (i.p. or i.m.)

Inhalation Anaesthesia (Rats)

For suppression of bronchial secretion, salivation and vagal influences on circulation the parasympatholytic atropine should be administered for premedication. Possibilities for inhalative narcosis in rats are either closed chambers (e.g. for administration of diethylether), a mask, or intubation with ventilation. Induction and recovery from anaesthesia are both slow because ether is highly solubile in water and blood. For induction a concentration of 10–20% and for maintenance 4–5% are needed (Lumley et al. 1990).

Since intubation may be difficult, in acute experiments many investigators recommend the use of tracheotomy. Instead, a Schimmelbusch mask may be used although this has the disadvantage that the narcotic may be dissolved in the room air as well. The closed chamber could be a glass barrel where the gas is filled in (this is normally used with diethylether or CO_2). After reaching the state of surgical tolerance the animal can be operated. Disadvantages are a high price and a difficult dosage of the anaesthetics.

Plastic tubes may serve as a mask which is supplied with a swab soaked with the narcotic (e.g. diethylether). The open drop evaporator (modified Schimmelbusch mask) serves for maintaining the state of narcosis.

In our lab we have good experience with the following protocol:
- % O_2: 40
- respiratory minute volume: 0.15–0.3 L/min
- respiratory volume: 10 ml
- respiratory rate: 15–25 min^{-1}
- inspiratory ventilation time (TI) : expiratory ventilation time (TE): 1:2
- positive end expiratory pressure (PEEP): 0–5 mbar
- P_{max}: 25 mbar
- premedication:

- 0.1 mg/kg atropine (i.p. or i.m.)
- 80–100 mg/kg ketamine (i.p. or i.m.)
- 1.5 mg/kg xylazine (i.p. or i.m.)
- inhalation:
    - 3 vol% isofluran (initially)
    - 0.8–1.5 vol% isofluran (maintenance)

Alternatively, a mixture of NO_2 and halothane may be used:
- parameters:
    - % O_2: 50
    - % NO_2: 49
    - % halothan 0,5–1
    - respiratory volume: 10–20 ml
    - respiratory rate: 15–25 min^{-1}
    - inspiratory ventilation time (TI) : expiratory ventilation time (TE): 1:2
    - positive end expiratory pressure (PEEP): 0–5 mbar
    - P_{max}: 25 mbar

Postoperative Treatment

During and even after surgery the rat should be warmed, e.g. with an electric pad since thermoregulation is discontinued in small animals during narcosis. Therefore shaving and washing should be reduced to a minimum in these animals. Postoperative analgetics can be given with drinking water in these animals. We recommend buprenorphin 0,1–1 mg/kg s.c. every 8–12 h (Lumley et al. 1990).

Troubleshooting

Animals should not have been fed prior to surgery. It should be controlled whether there are remnants of food in the mouth (Wijnbergen 2001). During examination the lungs must be investigated very carefully since older rats often suffer from diseases of their lungs (Table 5).

Anaesthesia of Mice

For blood withdrawal V. saphena or retroorbital punction can be used. For intramuscular injections the femoral muscles can be used.

Intravenous Anaesthesia (Mice)

Narcosis which cannot be anagonised is achieved using i.m. administration of ketamine and xylazine. This will result in general anaesthesia lasting for 60 min. For prolongation a fifth of the initial dose is given. Alternatively, narcosis, which can be antagonised, is achieved by a combination of medetomidine, midazolam and fentanyl. Surgical tolerance is achieved after 10–20 min and the effect lasts for about

Table 5
Clinical parameters and blood parameters of rats

Parameter	Unit
Clinical parameter	
Body temperature	37.0–38.9
Heart rate	250–500
Respiratory rate	63–179
Blood pressure	145/105
Blood volume	50–70 ml/kg
Cardiac output	70–120 ml/min
Blood parameter	
Erythrocyte	6.0–10.0 T/l
Haematocrit	36–48%
Haemoglobin	110–180 g/l
Leucocyte	6–17 G/l
Chloride	100–110 mmol/l
Sodium	143–156 mmol/l
Potassium	5.0–6.3 mmol/l
Magnesium	1.6–4.4 mmol/l
Glucose	2.8–7.5 mmol/l
Urea	0.8–3.5 mmol/l
Creatinine	17.5–70.8 µmol/l
Protein	56–76 g/l

1 hour. For antagonisation atipamezol, flumazenil and naloxon can be used. Antagonists are applied s.c. in contrast to the i.m. administration of the drugs for narcosis.
- Option 1
  - narcosis (which can be antagonised):
    0.5 mg/kg medetomidine
    5 mg/kg midazolam
    0.005 mg/kg fentanyl
  - antagonists (s.c.):
    2.5 mg/kg atipamezol
    0.5 mg/kg flumazenil
    1.2 mg/kg naloxon

- Option 2
  - narcosis (which cannot be antagonised, i.m. or i.p):
    0.1 mg/kg atropine sulfate
    100 mg/kg ketamine
    5 mg/kg xylazine

Inhalation Anaesthesia

Possibilities for inhalative narcosis in mice are either closed chambers (e.g. for administration of diethylether or CO_2) and a mask. It is difficult to intubate a mouse and therefore an inhalation anaesthesia with isofluran is not used.

Table 6
Clinical parameters and blood parameters of mice

Parameter	Unit
Clinical parameter	
Body temperature	36.5–38.0
Heart rate	325–780
Respiratory rate	94–163
Blood pressure	147/106
Blood volume	70–80 ml/kg
Cardiac output	60–100 ml/kg/min
Blood parameter	
Erythrocyte	7.0–11.0 T/l
Haematocrit	35–50%
Haemoglobin	120–150 g/l
Leucocyte	4–14 G/l
Chloride	105–110 mmol/l
Sodium	128–145 mmol/l
Potassium	4.8–5.8 mmol/l
Magnesium	1.0–3.9 mmol/l
Glucose	5.9–10.6 mmol/l
Creatinine	44.2 µmol/l
Bilirubin	3.1–9.2 µmol/l
Protein	50–86 g/l

Postoperative Treatment

During and even after surgery the mice should be warmed, e.g. with an electric pad, since thermoregulation is discontinued in small animals during narcosis (Visser 2001). Therefore shaving and washing should be reduced to a minimum in those animals. Postoperative analgesics such as fentanyl or metamizol can be given with drinking water in these animals. Postoperative analgesia with buprenorphin (2,5 mg/kg s.c. or i.p.) can also be used (Table 6).

Troubleshooting

There are similar problems in mice as in rats. Therefore, the reader is referred to the respective section of this chapter in which rates are discussed.

References

Blonait-H, Bickhardt-K: Lehrbuch der Schweinekrankheiten. Kap. Therapeutische Technik, Berlin and Hamburg, Paul Parey Verlag, 1988, pp 42–49

Lumbley-JSP, Green-CJ, Lear-P, Angell-James-JE: Essentials of Experimental Surgery. Chapter: Anaesthesia. London, Boston, Singapore, Sydney, Toronto, Wellington, Butterworth & Co, 1990, pp 46–79

Schall-H, Kaninchen in: Gabrisch-K, Zwart-P, Krankheiten der Heimtiere, Hannover, Schlütersche, 2001, pp 1–45

Swindle-MM: Surgery, Anaesthesia, & Experimental Techniques in Swine. Chapter: Anaesthesia and Analgesia, Iowa, Iowa State Press, 1998, pp 33–64

Visser-CJM, Mäuse in: Gabrisch-K, Zwart-P, Krankheiten der Heimtiere, Hannover, Schlütersche, 2001, pp 101–124

Wijnbergen-A, Ratten in: Gabrisch-K, Zwart-P, Krankheiten der Heimtiere, Hannover, Schlütersche, 2001, pp 125–149

Extracorporeal Circulation

Cris W. Ullmann

Introduction

Many methods of artificial oxygenation of blood have been investigated over the last century starting from the direct injection of oxygen into the bloodstream and proceeding to the use of chemicals to generate oxygen, to the film oxygenators which were used in the heyday of cardiac surgery and finally to the modern bubble and membrane oxygenators in use today.

Cross-circulation for total body perfusion utilized what became known as the "azygos principle". Lillehei reported the use of cross-circulation technique to repair intracardiac defects in 32 patients in 1955.

The development of modern extracorporeal circulation began in 1953 when Gibbon performed the first open heart operation using a 45 min period of extracorporeal perfusion at the Massachusetts General Hospital. He realized that the key to extracorporeal circulation was the oxygenator and developed a disc-oxygenating device with a 4 m^2 exchange surface. Since then the technology of extracorporeal circulation has developed rapidly.

In 1955 Lillehei used the first bubble oxygenator. A year later Rygg developed a disposable bubble oxygenator, from which time developments in extracorporeal circulation have aimed at achieving completely disposable products.

Description of Methods and Practical Approach

Components of Extracorporeal Circuit

The extracorporeal system consists of interconnected devices for the oxygenation and circulation of blood, temporarily replacing the functions of the heart and the lungs. The main components of the circuit are a pump (artificial heart), an oxygenator (artificial lungs), a cardiotomy reservoir, a heat exchanger, cannulae, filters and inter-connecting tubing (Fig. 1).

The venous blood arrives at the venous reservoir by gravity drainage. The venous reservoir has a storage capacity of between 3.5 and 4.5 l enabling the operation to meet the flow variation requirements. The reservoir must be of a highly transparent

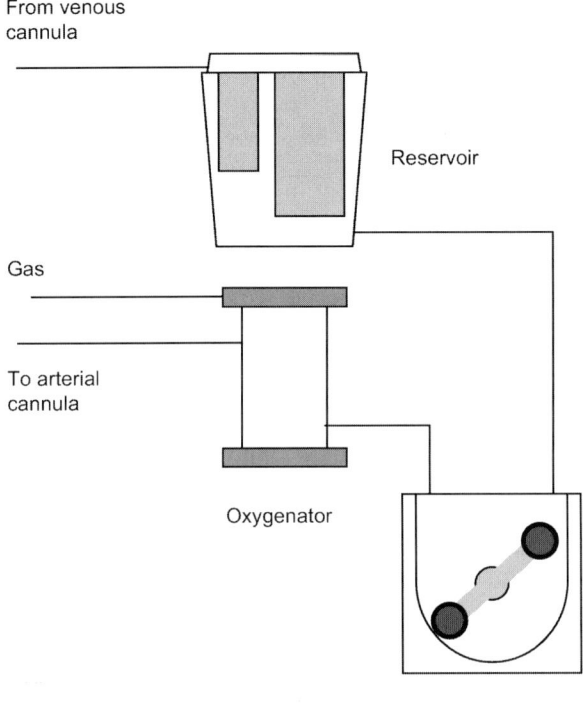

Figure 1
Schematic of extracorporeal circuit

material permitting early detection of level variations. The defoaming section serves to remove bubbles from the blood *via* the surface, which is coated with an antifoam compound. This can either be made of silicone or sponge coated with surfactants to perform an anti-bubble action. A 120 μm filter removes particles of higher calibre. The geometric configuration is also important to allow laminar progress of the blood flow.

In the membrane oxygenators, the oxygenating gas is separated from the blood by a permeable membrane. There is no direct contact between blood and gas. The membrane is normally made from either silicone rubber or polypropylene. The transmembrane pressure causes gas to diffuse from the higher pressure area into the lower pressure one.

The rate of transfer depends on both the pressure gradient across the membrane and the permeability of the membrane.

The membrane oxygenator is superior to the bubble oxygenator having reduced trauma to the elementary constituents of blood, no direct blood gas contact, independent control of pO_2 and pCO_2, low priming volumes and high efficiency of gas and temperature exchange.

A heat exchanger is generally integrated into all membrane oxygenators in the form of metallic tubes or additional plastic fibres.

Pumps

While the oxygenator performs the task of the lungs during cardiopulmonary bypass, the pump takes over the role of the heart. Its sole function is to provide an adequate flow of oxygenated blood to the patient's arterial circulation. The main technical requirements of the pump are as follows:
1. Wide flow range (up to 7 l/min)
2. Low haemolytic effect
3. Minimum turbulence and blood stagnation
4. Simplicity and safety of use
5. Capacity for pulsatile flow
6. Cost effectiveness

There are two principle types of pumps available for use.

Roller Pumps

At present the roller pump is the most common type of pump used in extracorporeal circuits. The pump comprises a semicircular stator and a rotor with twin rollers at 180° to each other. The blood tubing is compressed between the stator and the rotor. The flow is unidirectional as one of the rollers keeps compressing the tube at all times. A partially occlusive pump setting is preferable (Fig. 2).

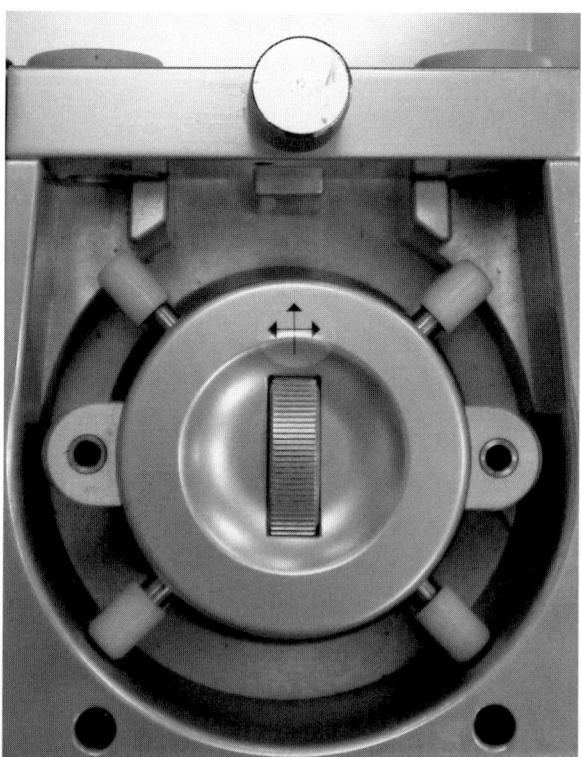

Figure 1.2-2
Rollerpump

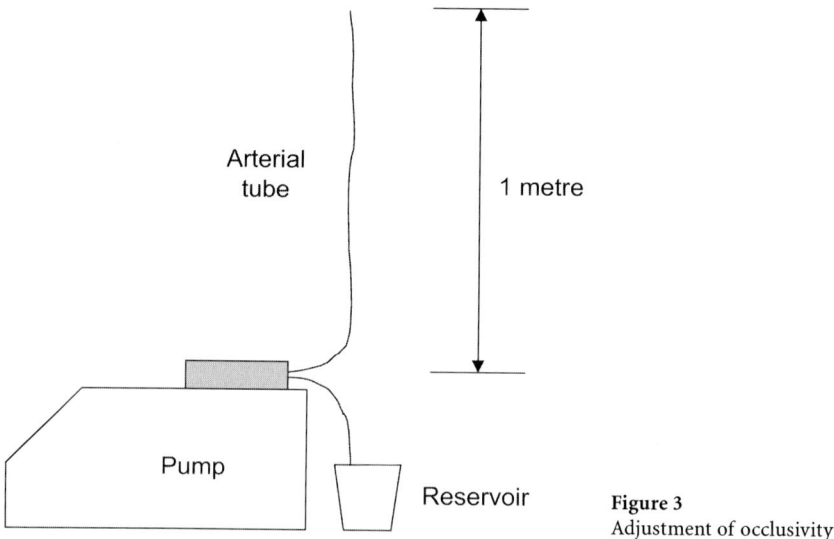

Figure 3
Adjustment of occlusivity

Pump occlusivity is calibrated to allow a 1 cm/min drop along a 1 m high saline column (Fig. 3).

Pump function must be monitored carefully at all times. A line restriction upstream (e. g. caused by kinked tubes) would create an excessive vacuum leading to degassing of the blood. Conversely a line restriction downstream would lead to excessive pressure build-up and a rupture of the line itself. Safety features include adequate pressure monitors (pre- and post oxygenator) and an ultrasonic bubble sensor placed in the arterial line.

Centrifugal Pumps

With the centrifugal pump, blood is driven through a rotating impeller creating a centrifugal force which imparts kinetic energy to the blood. The driving motor and the spinning impeller are coupled by a magnetic linkage, which makes hermetic sealing of the pump head possible (Fig. 4).

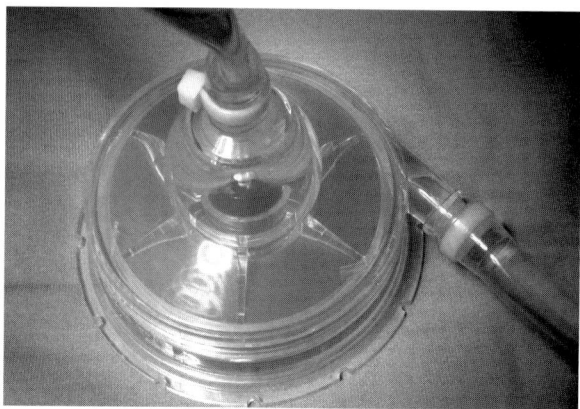

Figure 4
Centrifugal pump

Centrifugal pumps are not occlusive and are therefore load-sensitive, i. e. if the resistance to flow increases the blood flow decreases. During operation, centrifugal pumps require strict flow measurements. Electromagnetic or ultrasonic flow probes are normally used. This measurement enables pump speed adjustments to achieve constant flow. Centrifugal pumps cause minimal haemolysis compared with roller pumps and have a further advantage. If air enters the system, the pump is no longer able to transmit kinetic energy to the blood. The fluid motion will stop immediately. The incidence of massive air embolism is minimised.

Venous Reservoir

Venous reservoirs have two principal functions. These are to accumulate blood from the patient's venous system and to remove air and micro-emboli from the venous blood.

The setup of the extracorporeal pump system may be either open or closed. An open setup requires a hardshell reservoir, a closed setup a softshell reservoir.

Open System with Rigid Hardshell Reservoir

Rigid hardshell reservoirs are used as an open system. Both the venous and the aspirated blood are filtered and defoamed in a single reservoir. The reservoir capacity may range between 1 l and 4.5 l.

In the event of a sudden emptying of the reservoir there is no intrinsic safety mechanism against massive gaseous emboli.

Closed System with Softshell Reservoir

A closed system incorporates a collapsible softshell reservoir (bag), entered by venous blood and an additional cardiotomy reservoir receiving the blood from the cardiotomy suckers and vents. This serves as a storage area and also filters out the large number of solid and gaseous microemboli. The defoamer is comprised of layers of open-cell polyurethane foam or polyester screens. The screens incorporate a filter of between 20 μm and 40 μm.

The "bag" consists of soft PVC with a 100–200 μm filtering screen and a defoaming polyurethane layer. Bag capacity may range between 200 ml and 3000 ml.

The advantage of soft reservoirs is that they can be used as a closed system. As the reservoir empties the venous bag collapses preventing gaseous emboli.

Cannulas and Cannulation Techniques

Mechanical factors affecting bypass flow rates include the size and position of venous and arterial cannulae. The flow obtained in total bypass is a function of the blood volume and the diameter of the tubing used for the venous line and the diameter of the venous cannula. Assuming that 100 cm H_2O of siphon suction is applied to the venous cannula, the maximal possible flow increases with the fourth power of the tubing size and cannula diameter (Hagen-Poiseuille's law).

$$Q = \frac{\Delta p \times r^4}{l \times \eta} \times \frac{\pi}{8}$$

Under conditions of inadequate venous return, whether due to low blood volume or low arterial perfusion with sequestration, the flow through the venous line is regulated by the collapsing of the vena cavae around the venous cannula. Under conditions of adequate venous return, the bypass flow is limited by the size and length of the venous drainage lines.

Two Stage Cannulation

Venous cannulation with a two-stage cannula usually enables an adequate venous drainage. This technique is preferred in bypass and aortic valve surgery. This cannula incorporates two inlets for the drainage of both the vena cavae.

Bicaval Cannulation

Most of cardiac surgery can be performed using bicaval cannulation. This technique is essential if the right heart is opened.

Arterial Cannulation

Theoretically, the size of the arterial cannula is not a major consideration during non-pulsatile flow. If 5 l/min is pumped then 5 l/min will flow through the arterial cannula. However, the flow rate will be maintained only at the expense of higher pressures and greater turbulence in the perfusion system. These factors may lead to haemolysis and increase the risk of tubing separation or rupture. Arterial cannulae which are capable of providing adequate flow with a pressure gradient across the cannula of <100 mmHg and arterial line pressures of <250 mmHg have been recommended.

Intraoperative Myocardial Protection

Under aerobic conditions, oxidation of a variety of substrates, predominantly free fatty acids, but also glucose, pyruvate, acetate, ketone bodies and amino acids, occurs in the mitochondria with the generation by oxidative phosphorylation of the high energy phosphates ATP and creatine phosphate. Their subsequent degradation to ADP, AMP and creatine is associated with energy release in the form of heat and muscle activity, both isometric and isotonic. In this process 1 mole of glucose is consumed in the production of 36 moles of ATP. The rate of metabolism in the contracting heart depends on a number of factors including heart rate, wall tension and the action of catecholamines.

There is 75% oxygen extraction from the coronary blood, higher than in any other organ, and an increased demand for oxygen must be met by increasing coronary flow rather than by increasing extraction. When pO_2 is reduced to <5 mmHg, oxidative phosphorylation ceases and ATP production falls. Glycogenolysis and anaerobic glycolysis take over, with the formation of glycolytic intermediaries. Anaerobic glycolysis only yields 2 moles ATP per mole glucose in comparison with aerobic glycolysis.

Hypothermic Cardiopulmonary Bypass

Electromechanical work accounts for approximately 80–85% of the oxygen demand of the myocardium, with the remaining 20–25% representing basal metabolism. Cardiopulmonary bypass reduces myocardial oxygen consumption by approximately 50–70% in the beating, non-tachycardiac, adequately perfused, non-hypertrophied, empty heart at 37 °C. As the heart is cooled there is a progressive slowing of metabolism and oxygen uptake is further reduced by almost 40% at 28 °C and 50% at 22 °C. Thus, hypothermic cardiopulmonary bypass can reduce myocardial oxygen consumption to approximately 25% of that of the working heart at 37 °C.

Systemic hypothermia can be combined with induction of ventricular fibrillation for additional reduction of myocardial oxygen consumption.

Cardioplegic Techniques

Cold chemical cardioplegia has become almost universally adopted by surgeons as the standard intra-operative protective measure. The objectives of cardioplegia are to achieve mechanical and electrical arrest of the heart as quickly as possible, to cool it to the optimal temperature, to provide substrates to meet the reduced metabolic demands, buffer adverse changes in pH and to prevent intracellular and interstitial oedema developing.

Cardioplegia may be induced in a number of ways, most commonly by raising the concentration of potassium in the solution, but also by removing calcium, lowering sodium, raising magnesium and adding procaine. Controversy still exists over the composition of the solutions and over the details of their administration. These include whether the solutions should be blood or crystalloid based, their electrolyte composition and pH, the addition of agents designed to maintain the concentration of high energy phosphates, reduce cell and interstitial oedema, increase coronary flow and avoid accumulation of toxic metabolites and free radicals and the temperature, frequency, volume and method of administration.

Minimized Perfusion Systems

A significant trend towards minimizing trauma related to cardiac surgery is aimed at modifications or elimination of cardiopulmonary bypass (CPB) altogether. Minimizing neurocognitive outcomes are of keen interest due to the high human cost associated with stroke and neurocognitive deficits. Recently efforts to completely eliminate CPB have resulted in potential risks in cardiovascular procedures that may offset any real or perceived benefits. Specifically, neurological benefits of off-pump bypass have not yet been clearly demonstrated relative to the risk of a more technically challenging operation. Therefore, new technology designed to provide incremental improvements in the gold standard of CPB are rapidly developing, offering features such as reduced priming volume and elimination of cardiotomy reservoirs.

Examples

Open Extracorporeal Perfusion System

The main feature of an open perfusion system is the hardshell reservoir (Fig. 5). Both the venous and sucked blood are filtered and defoamed in a single reservoir. The reservoir capacity may range between 1 l and 4.5 l depending on the animal's blood volume (ref. chapter "Anaesthesia" for blood volume and cardiac index).

The blood can be pumped by either a roller pump or a centrifugal pump. The use of a centrifugal pump offers more safety features and less blood damage. This pump drives the blood through a membrane oxygenator. The maximum flow rate of the oxygenator depends on the animal's weight and size. In humans the target flow should be approximately the body surface area multiplied by the factor 2.4 l/(min × m^2). Due to differences of opinion, constants for animals are very varied (ref. chapter "Anaesthesiology"). The recommended maximum blood flow through the oxygenator should be at least 150% of the target flow.

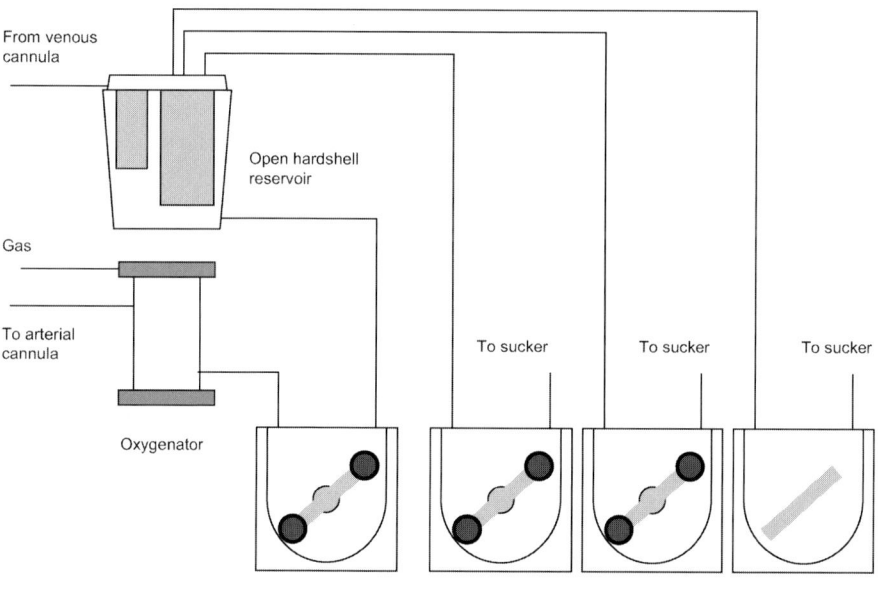

Figure 5
Schematic of open perfusion system

The use of an arterial filter can be considered. It offers further safety against gaseous emboli but requires an additional priming volume (and hemodilution) of nearly 100 cc.

Closed Extracorporeal Perfusion System

A closed system incorporates a collapsible softshell reservoir (bag), entered by venous blood and an additional cardiotomy reservoir receiving the blood from the cardiotomy suckers and vents. This serves as a storage area and also filters out the large number of solid and gaseous microemboli. Softshell reservoir capacity may range between 200 ml and 3000 ml. The pump, oxygenator and arterial filter are similar to the open system.

The advantages of closed systems are that, if the reservoir empties the venous bag collapses thereby preventing gaseous emboli (Fig. 6).

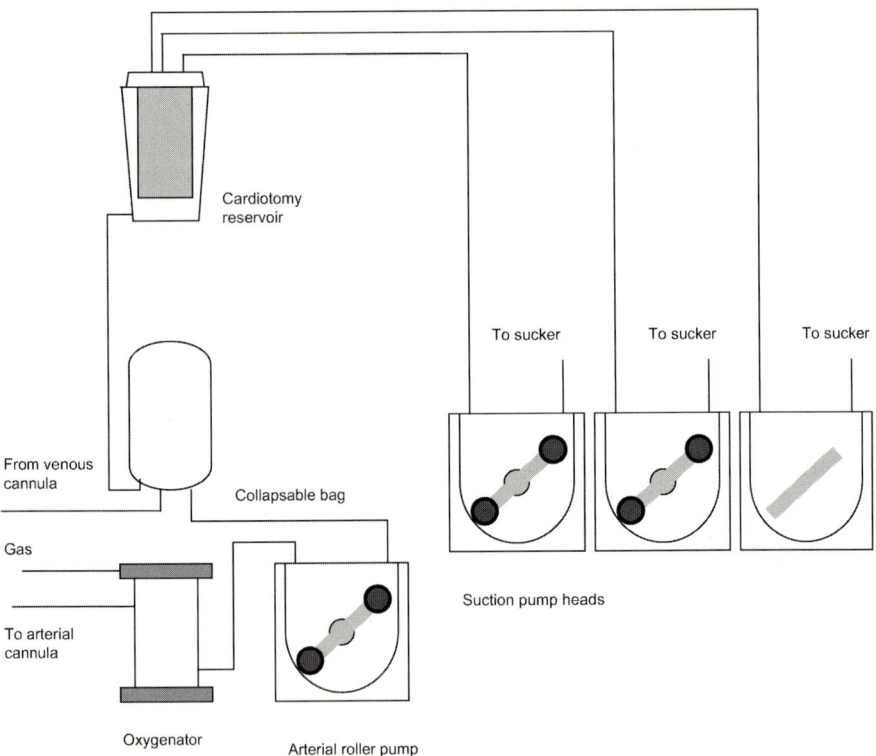

Figure 6
Schematic of closed perfusion system

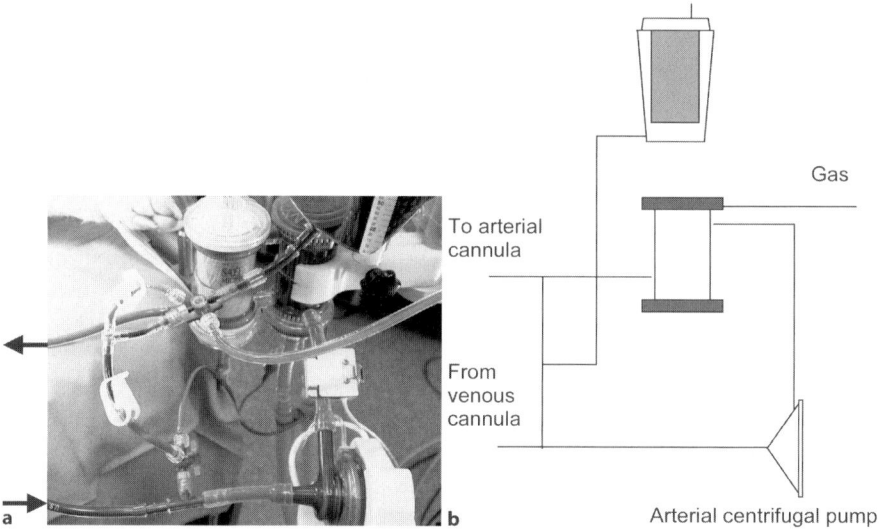

Figure 7
Schematic of minimized perfusion system

Minimized System for Perfusion of Small Animals

As mentioned in the chapter "Anaesthesia" the blood volume of some animals is very small. Special care has to be taken on haemodilution. Because of this the system does not contain a venous reservoir. The blood is drained actively by the centrifugal pump directly from the venous cannula. The collapsible blood-transfer bag serves as volume storage. The active venous drainage allows the use of smaller tubes and the system does not need a siphon drain with a height difference. The tubes can be very short (Fig. 7).

The priming volume of the whole system is approximately 80 cc. The recommended maximum blood flow is 800 cc/min.

Troubleshooting

In all cases of trouble during extracorporeal circulation troubleshooting decisions have to be made very quickly depending on the current situation. Therefore it is practical to have a step-by-step protocol for the setting up and operation of the entire circuit.

Setup:
1. Connect up all the disposables of the extracorporeal circuit! Fix high-pressure connections by tie straps.

Check:
- oxygen inlet of the oxygenator connected to the gas mixer
- Heat exchanger connected to heater/cooler
- Pump direction of arterial and vent pumps
- Occlusion of all pumps
- Kinking of any tubes
2. Prime the reservoir, de-air oxygenator and filter
   - Check: watch the entire arterial tubing for bubbles and micro air
3. Warm the priming solution to 35 °C, wait for the cannulation, recirculate the priming solution
   - Check: hematocrit of the animal, replace priming solution partly by blood if necessary
4. When the surgeons are ready for cannulation, stop the arterial pump and clamp both arterial and venous lines.
   - Check: Occlusion of arterial pump
   - Anti-coagulation, e. g. measure the activated clotting time (ACT)
5. When cannulation is achieved, declamp the arterial line and start pumping at a low flow rate. Declamp the venous line partially and induce cardiopulmonary bypass. Watch the reservoir level. Keep the blood of the animal constant. Increase arterial flow slowly until 100% flow.
   - Check: venous drainage
   - Arterial line pressure

Monitor ACT, arterial line pressure and venous drainage very carefully all the time. If necessary replace venous or arterial cannulae, add volume and adjust flow to the hemodynamic situation. If possible, monitor blood gas values and venous saturation.

References

Kay PH (1992) (ed) Techniques in extracorporeal circulation. 3rd rev. edn. Arnold, London
Tschaut RJ (1999) (ed) Extrakorporale Zirkulation in Theorie und Praxis. Pabst Science Publishers, Lengerich
Lauterbach G (2002) Handbuch der Kardiotechnik. Urban & Fischer, München
Brandt L (1996) Handbuch der Kardioanästhesie: Grundlagen, Theorie und Praxis für die Weiterbildung. Wissenschaftliche Verlagsgesellschaft, Stuttgart

Open-chest Models of Acute Myocardial Ischemia and Reperfusion

Kai Zacharowski, Thomas Hohlfeld and Ulrich K.M. Decking

Introduction

In acute myocardial ischemia and reperfusion, open chest models allow a) the investigation of cardiac physiology, b) the elucidation of biochemical, functional and morphological changes and c) the evaluation of therapeutic interventions. In chronic studies, open-chest surgery is carried out for instrumentation of animals and as a final step at the end of the study to perform invasive measurements and obtain myocardial tissue. The present overview aims to discuss surgical procedures and steps of open-chest preparations. A selection of techniques to measure parameters of cardiovascular function in open-chest preparations is also discussed.

Description of Methods and Practical Approach

Experimental Set-Up and Procedures

To study ischemia and reperfusion in open-chest models, the laboratory needs to be appropriately equipped for surgery, including an adjustable operating table and cold-light lamps for adequate lighting of the operating area. A complete set of preferably sterile surgical instruments; threads, needles, swabs etc. must be prepared and set out before the start of the experiment. To minimize blood loss during surgery, bleeding can be stopped by careful cauterization or ligature around the relevant vessel. Once the chest is opened, thorax retractors are fitted to keep it open during the experiment.

For open-chest surgery in experimental animals, anesthesia, ventilation, thoracotomy and intrathoracic surgical manipulation are steps of primary importance. These will be discussed in the following.

Anesthesia and Mechanical Ventilation

For ethical and experimental reasons, open-chest models can only be performed under deep anesthesia. A wide range of anesthetics has been used with success in open-chest models. However, anesthetics can cause unwanted side effects, such as hemodynamic depression, and can compromise the outcome of the experiment. Therefore, the phar-

Table 1
Selection of drugs commonly used in open-chest studies and their potential to interfere with experimental models of ischemia and reperfusion

Indication	Drug	Mechanism of action	Practical importance
sedation	azaperone and other neuroleptics	inhibition of α-adrenergic effects of endo- and exogenous catecholamines	hypotension, loss of baroreceptor reflex
anesthesia	barbiturates	depression of vasomotor control and myocardial contractility	hypotension, loss of baroreceptor reflex
	opioids (morphine and congeners)	histamine liberation, preconditioning of myocardium against ischemia via activation of myocardial δ-opioid receptors	hypotension, decrease of ischemic myocardial injury
	halothane	decreased control of body temperature, cardiodepression preconditioning against ischemia	malignant hyperthermia in some breeds of pigs alteration of myocardial function reduction of experimental infarct size
	isoflurane	arterial dilation, preconditioning (like halothane), vasodilation	systemic hypotension and impairment of coronary autoregulation, reduction of experimental infarct size, hypotension
	sevoflurane	preconditioning (like halothane) minor vasodilatation minor cardiodepression	reduction of experimental infarct size
	propofol	protection against ischemia	reduction of experimental infarct size
muscle relaxation	pancuronium	ganglionic and peripheral anticholinergic action	hypotension, tachycardia
	succinylcholine	slight sympathetic stimulation	increase of heart rate
anti-coagulation	heparins	platelet activation or inhibition anti-inflammatory effects	surgical bleeding, alteration of thrombogenesis and microcirculation, reduction of ischemic injury

macological properties of an anesthetic and the species in which it will be used should be carefully considered. Examples are summarized in Table 1 and information about specific anesthetics is given as described below.

Surgical opening of the thorax immediately causes the lungs to collapse; this can be prevented by mechanical ventilation following intubation of the trachea. The ventilator should be set to apply a positive end-expiratory pressure of 1–6 mmHg, to prevent airway collapse and atelectasis. Single-sided opening of the pleura may lead to respiratory problems by asymmetric ventilation.

The most useful indicator for the appropriate control of tidal volume and respiratory rate is the end-expiratory CO_2. Arterial pH, pO_2 and pCO_2 can additionally be determined at regular intervals. Depending on the duration of the experiment, pre-wetting and -warming of the inhalation gasses are useful to prevent airway dehydration. Special precautions should also be taken to prevent hypothermia, which may ensue due to loss of endogenous temperature control and excessive heat loss via ventilation and dissipation from the open chest.

Surgical Preparation

Open-chest models require invasive surgery and therefore some experience in basic surgical techniques is essential. Common steps in open-chest preparations are thoracotomy (usually left-side or midsternal), incision of the pericardium and the applica-

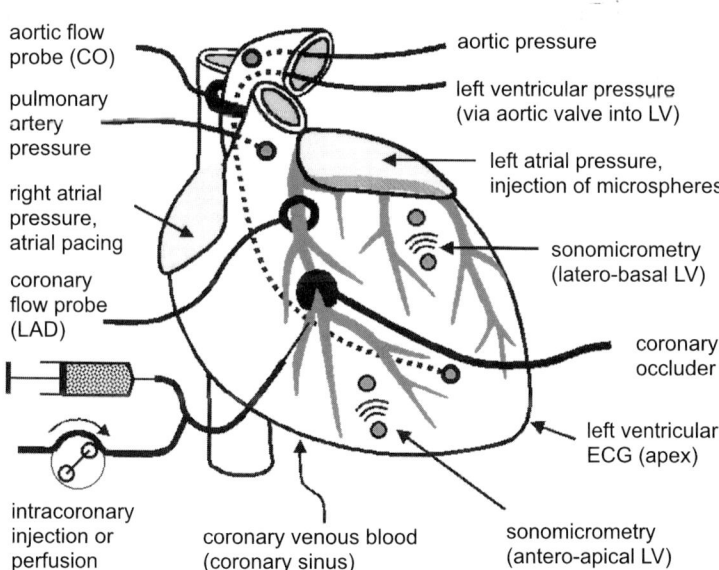

Figure 1
Schematic example of an open chest preparation for induction of myocardial ischemia and reperfusion in a larger animal, such as a dog or a pig. Generally, many physiological parameters are assessed in parallel. More detailed information about the depicted experimental techniques and measurements is given in the text. Abbreviations: *CO* cardiac output, *ECG* electrocardiogram, *LAD* left anterior descending coronary artery, *LV* left ventricle

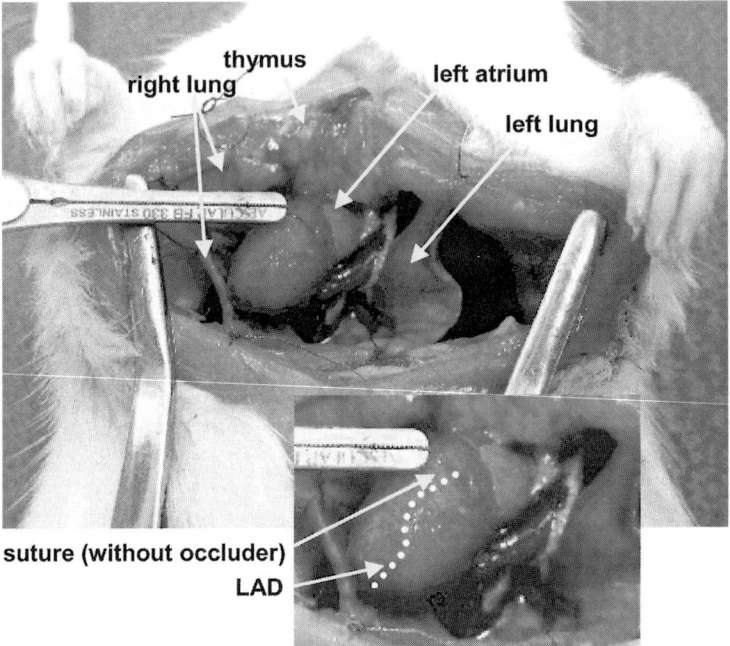

Figure 2
Open chest preparation of a rat, achieved by mid-sternal thoracotomy (Zacharowski et al. 1999). The chest is kept open by the branches of a retractor. The LAD is represented by a dotted line (inset). A hairline suture around the proximal LAD allows experimental coronary occlusion, resulting in myocardial ischemia and infarction

tions of various catheters for blood collection and drug administration. In addition, probes are applied or inserted for data acquisition. Additional surgery is required to perform experimental interventions such as the positioning of coronary occluders or the connection of extracorporal perfusion systems (Fig. 1).

Many steps of the surgical procedure must be adapted to the species and the particular aims of the experiment. For example, median thoracotomy may be preferable when access to the anterior wall of the ventricles is intended (e. g., occlusion of the left anterior descending coronary artery, LAD), while left lateral thoracotomy may be preferred for access to the left lateral and posterior left ventricular wall, including the circumflex coronary artery.

After the completion of surgery, a stabilization period is required before experimental interventions or data acquisition are initiated. Figure 1 summarizes a selection of well-established experimental techniques commonly used in open-chest preparations of larger animal species, such as dogs and pigs. A typical small animal preparation is shown in Fig. 2.

Experimental Manipulation of Coronary Perfusion

A significant number of experiments involving open-chest preparations aim to measure and manipulate coronary blood flow. Obviously, these experiments are of considerable value for the investigation of the pathophysiology of myocardial ischemia and help to develop new or improved therapeutic strategies.

Controlled Perfusion

In larger animal species (dog, pig), the main branches of the common left coronary artery can be cannulated and supplied by a coronary bypass, withdrawing blood at a predefined rate from another arterial vessel (e. g. carotid or femoral artery). This allows the perfusion of a segment of the left ventricle at a defined flow rate or perfusion pressure (see Fig. 1). This technique has greatly contributed to an improved understanding of coronary autoregulation. Moreover, the tight control of the flow rate enables the intracoronary infusion of drugs or substrates at well-defined arterial concentrations. This may be important for drugs with a small therapeutic range. The approach can also be employed to selectively modify vascular tone or myocardial contractility in the area supplied by a bypass or to provide a metabolic substrate at a given concentration to this region (Decking 2001).

Subtotal Ischemia

When studying the effects of flow reduction on myocardial contractility and metabolism, the bypass technique described above enables reduction in coronary flow in a step-wise manner in order to investigate functional and metabolic adaptation processes, such as perfusion-contraction-matching (Ross 1991) and myocardial hibernation (Heusch 1998). In these studies, flow was classically reduced by 50% of baseline, and the effects on contractile function and myocardial energetics were analyzed. Using a similar approach, the sensitivity of cytosolic adenosine to an imbalance in the oxygen-supply to -demand ratio was demonstrated (Deussen 1998). Open-chest models with reduced coronary flow and controlled reperfusion have also been extensively used to define and study the phenomena of stunning and preconditioning, including pharmacotherapeutic strategies to improve myocardial function and biochemical outcome after subtotal ischemia.

Intracoronary Thrombosis

Open-chest preparations are useful to simulate myocardial ischemia in conjunction with its pathophysiological "trigger", coronary thrombosis. Several experimental techniques are available to induce coronary arterial thrombi. One of the more popular models, originally introduced by Folts (1991), combines an acute injury of the coronary artery (transient clamping at a defined force) with a critical stenosis of the injured segment (plastic cylinder around the injured region). Stenosis and vessel wall injury will cause a mural thrombus to develop within minutes to hours, depending on the extent of arterial injury. This results in a gradual decline in coronary flow. Blood flow often suddenly recovers due to the mobilization of the thrombus into the distal circulation, causing recurrent ("cyclic") coronary flow variations. Intravenous administration of adrenaline can be used to exacerbate thrombosis.

Other strategies aim to injure the endothelium by intracoronary injections of concentrated saline, alcohol or hot solutions with consequent formation of an intracoronary thrombus. Arterial thrombosis can also be induced by the administration of an electrical current (about 150 µA) to the endothelial surface of an artery (Romson et al. 1980). This is done by inserting an electrode (anode) into the artery. The electrical current results in local platelet adhesion and thrombus development. The electrical cathode may be applied to the adventitia of the vessel.

Open-chest models of coronary thrombosis have contributed to the development and investigation of anticoagulants, inhibitors of platelet function and thrombolytics, of which many have become indispensable agents for antithrombotic treatment in clinical medicine.

Coronary Occlusion

The surgical occlusion of a coronary artery (see Figs. 1 and 2) with consequent myocardial infarction has been performed in many species during the past 50 years, including dogs, pigs, cats and rabbits. Since the use of small rodents is less expensive and keeps drug consumption low, models of coronary occlusion have also been developed for smaller species, including rats and mice. Genetically manipulated mice offer new possibilities of characterizing the pathomechanisms of ischemia-reperfusion injury.

It must be realized, however, that the experimental occlusion of a coronary artery does not ideally simulate the natural course of myocardial infarction, which often involves subtotal thrombotic occlusion and intermittent phases of spontaneous thrombus dislocation or thrombolysis. Nevertheless, this technique can provide valuable insight into the functional, morphological, biochemical and molecular events that lead to the development of ischemic myocardial injury.

Many techniques have been used to occlude a coronary artery. A simple suture around the vessel can only be recommended for continuous ischemia without reperfusion.

If reperfusion is intended, a surgical "snare" should be applied, consisting of a thread sling placed around the artery with both ends pulled through a piece of soft silicon tubing. The snare is tightened for induction of ischemia. Care must be taken not to injure the artery by pulling the occluded segment into the tubing. Soft arterial clamps and hydraulic occluders are also available and may be less traumatic.

Assessment of Myocardial Integrity and Function

Open-chest preparations with access to the intrathoracic cavity allow for an almost unlimited evaluation of alterations in myocardial tissue integrity and function. Blood and tissue samples can be analyzed for biochemical and morphological parameters.

Plasma Markers of Myocardial Injury

Acute models of myocardial ischemia and reperfusion often require the quantitative determination of infarct size. This may prove to be difficult, because some myocytes are clearly viable or necrotic, while others are still in the process of recovery or transition from viable to necrotic or apoptotic cell death. Therefore, terminal infarct size should ideally be determined after stabilization for several days of survival. However, many studies have obtained a reasonable differentiation of necrotic from viable tissue after much shorter periods, but it must be kept in mind that long-term processes such as ischemia-induced inflammation, thrombosis and apoptosis may not be adequately reflected in these studies. It depends on the experimental aims whether or not short- or long-term effects on myocardial viability are of primary interest.

Cytosolic or myofibril-bound markers released into plasma from the ischemic-reperfused myocardium are commonly used to estimate infarct size. These include lactate dehydrogenase (LDH), creatine kinase (CK), myoglobin, cardiospecific CK (CK-MB) and cardiac troponins. Commercial enzymatic assays are available for routine measurements. During reperfusion after severe ischemia, the concentration (or activity) of these markers rapidly rises in peripheral blood. Depending on collateral coronary blood flow during ischemia, this rise may already become evident during ischemia.

Morphological Infarct Size

A widely accepted technique for measuring infarct size is histochemistry. Many studies have determined the loss of myocardial dehydrogenase activity by tetrazolium dyes in order to detect severe and probably irreversible myocardial injury. In the presence of intact dehydrogenase enzyme systems (viable myocardium), tetrazolium salts form blue or red formazan pigments, whilst areas of necrosis lack dehydrogenase activity and therefore fail to stain. Since the dehydrogenase activity slowly disappears when myocardial tissue becomes necrotic, relevant results can only be expected after several hours of reperfusion (Fishbein et al. 1981). Tetrazolium staining is inexpensive and requires the reperfused ischemic tissue to be incubated in aqueous solutions of triphenyl or nitroblue tetrazolium. *Ex vivo* perfusion with tetrazolium salts is also possible. Vital (stained) and necrotic tissues (unstained) are easily distinguished (Fig. 3).

In order to quantitate infarct volume, the heart must be cut into slices, which are analyzed by computer-assisted planimetry to provide a representative measure over the entire heart.

As important additional information, many studies have also determined the amount of tissue, which is subjected to ischemia and reperfusion and within which necrosis is expected. This "area at risk" is identified *ex vivo* by re-occlusion of the coronary artery and subsequent perfusion with Evans Blue or other dyes, which results in staining of the perfused myocardium and leaves the formerly ischemic area unstained (see Fig. 3).

Infarct size can be expressed as a fraction/percentage of the entire heart, of the left ventricle or of the area at risk.

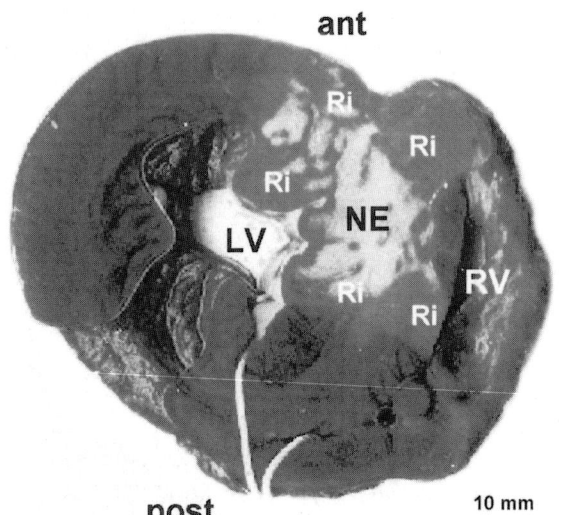

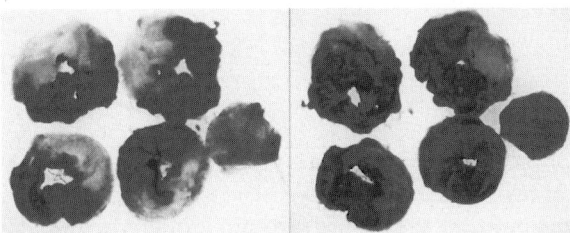

Figure 3
Top: transversal slice of a pig heart after 1 h of LAD occlusion, followed by 3 h of reperfusion. At the end of reperfusion, the coronary artery has been re-occluded and saline with Evans Blue dye perfused into the coronary ostia. Non-ischemic myocardium is stained dark blue within the posterior (post) and lateral wall of the left ventricle (LV). The anterior (ant) septum and a small part of the anterior left ventricular wall, located distal to the occluded coronary artery (area at risk, Ri), remained unstained. The risk area amounted to about 30% of the left ventricle. Additional staining of vital myocardium with triphenyl tetrazolium delineated the necrotic tissue (Ne), which was approximately 50% of the area at risk in this experiment. *Bottom:* determination of the area at risk and infarct size in a rat heart by a modified technique (Zacharowski et al. 1999b). Rats were subjected to 25 min of LAD occlusion and 2 h of reperfusion. After re-occlusion of the LAD, Evans blue dye was injected, staining perfused tissue blue (non-perfused area stains red; *left panel*). Subsequent incubation of the heart slices with nitro-blue tetrazolium stained vital tissue (normally perfused plus area at risk) dark-blue. Necrotic myocardium is not stained (*right panel*). *For coloured version see appendix*

There are additional techniques to measure irreversible myocardial injury. For example, myocardial cell integrity has been determined by perfusion with horseradish peroxidase, followed by *in vitro* detection of intracellular peroxidase after transition of the enzyme through the injured plasma membrane into the intracellular space. This procedure appears to identify infarcted myocardium after rather short periods of reperfusion (Farb et al. 1993).

As compared with histochemical staining, light and electron microscopy do not usually quantify myocardial infarct size. Nevertheless, histology provides invaluable morphological information about ischemia-induced myocardial injury.

Myocardial Contractile Function

As in closed-chest models, global measures of myocardial contractile function can be assessed by catheter-based manometers. Open-chest preparations allow direct insertion of miniature pressure tip catheters into the atria and ventricles for the sensitive detection of pressures and dP/dt. Myocardial contractile function can nowadays be assessed by imaging techniques such as ultrasound and magnetic resonance. These techniques usually achieve better signal-to-noise ratios and thus a higher spatial resolution in the open-chest animal.

The measurement of regional ventricular dynamics is usually performed by sonomicrometry, which has developed as a common standard to measure ventricular segment length, wall thickness or vessel diameters. The devices commercially available allow a high resolution of time (milliseconds) and dimensions (micrometers). Traditionally, a pair of piezoelectric crystals (emitter and receiver) is applied to the tissue of interest (often the ventricular wall) and the transit times of repetitive ultrasound pulses (1 MHz or higher) are recorded. These are automatically converted into distances, assuming a constant speed of ultrasound propagation (1540 m/s) in biological tissue.

Single crystal systems, which measure pulse reflection from interfaces between different tissues (e. g., blood/myocardium), are also available. Two- and three-dimensional arrangements of ultrasound crystals are used to estimate ventricular volumes. Sonomicrometry can provide very valuable information about regional myocardial function in open-chest preparations (see below).

Electrophysiological Measurements

The conventional ECG (chest wall) is often difficult to interpret in open-chest preparations due to the altered electrical environment of the heart. Therefore, ECG recordings are frequently derived from uni- or bi-polar electrodes attached to the epicardium.

Open-chest preparations also provide an opportunity to simultaneously record many ECG signals from the epicardial surface with high geometrical resolution, in order to map the propagation of action potentials across the surface of the heart under normal and pathological conditions. The origin and spreading of arrhythmias can also be investigated, giving valuable information about the effects of antiarrhythmic drugs. A large number of channels (> 1000) on an epicardial surface of about 50 cm^2 can be achieved in larger species (pigs or dogs), with a resolution of about 2 mm^2.

In addition to ECG recordings, it is possible to derive cardiac monophasic action potentials (MAP) from almost any ventricular location (Franz 1999). The MAP signal is thought to represent a local injury potential, which is created between the normal tissue beneath a reference electrode and the locally injured (depolarized) area beneath another electrode. The depolarization can be generated by exerting a gentle mechanical pressure on the tissue under one of the electrodes. Different designs apply KCl solutions locally. More recently, catheter-based MAP electrodes have become available for closed-chest experiments and human use. A general problem is that a relative rather than the absolute action potential voltage is recorded. There is also a limitation in time, because stable signals are obtained only over minutes to hours. Nevertheless, MAP measurements can provide information about depolarization, refractory period and after-depolarizations. They are well suited for the *in vivo* evaluation of antiarrhythmic drugs.

Techniques to Measure Coronary Blood Flow and Perfusion

Coronary blood flow is of great importance for numerous types of studies and mandatory to calculate myocardial consumption of substrates or oxygen and the release of metabolites. The open-chest preparation provides excellent means in this context, because arterial and coronary venous blood from the coronary sinus or an epicardial coronary vein are easily accessible for the transcardiac measurement of metabolites and elaborate techniques are available to determine coronary perfusion with high precision. In the open-chest animal, coronary flow and myocardial perfusion are conventionally studied using 1) flow probes or 2) microspheres.

Flow Probes

Until 20 years ago, electromagnetic flow probes were the state-of-the-art for determinations of vascular volume flow (ml/min). The current standard equipment is ultrasound transit time flow probes. These probes cover vessel diameters from about 0.5 to 16 mm. Perivascular flow probes measure local volume flow with high temporal resolution and precision. Since a perivascular probe has to surround the interrogated vessel, the relevant arterial vessel has to be carefully dissected, which can injure smaller side branches and impair local sympathetic control. Due to size constraints, flow probes in mice and rats have only been employed in the assessment of cardiac output (ascending aorta) or carotid or femoral artery flow. In larger animals (e. g. dogs and pigs), coronary flow can also be assessed at the level of the left anterior descending or left circumflex artery. Many of the flow probes available are not only suitable for measurement in open-chest models, but can be chronically implanted for monitoring of cardiac output or coronary artery flow.

Microspheres

Without quantitative knowledge of the region supplied by a given vessel, the vascular volume flow, e. g. of a coronary artery, is not a direct measure of local myocardial perfusion, which is generally given in ml/min/g. In the open-chest animal this is most frequently assessed using microspheres of 10 to 15 µm in diameter. In the context of ischemia and reperfusion, microsphere flow measurements are almost mandatory to define the extent of residual collateral flow during coronary artery occlusion or stenosis in the area at risk and also to determine local flow in the border zone.

Microspheres (e. g. 0.2 million/kg) are usually injected during a period of 5–30 s into the left atrium. Following natural mixing in the atrium and ventricle they are homogeneously distributed in the cardiac output and are distributed to all arterially supplied organs in proportion to their respective share of cardiac output. Since the microspheres are clearly greater than the internal diameter of any capillary (5–7 µm), they are almost completely extracted during the first pass of organ perfusion, most probably in pre-capillary arterioles and capillaries. The number of microspheres per organ is therefore a relative measure of arterial blood supply. To obtain an absolute measure of flow, a virtual reference organ is frequently employed by withdrawing blood from a central artery (e. g., aorta) at a given volume flow (e. g., 10 ml/min) for

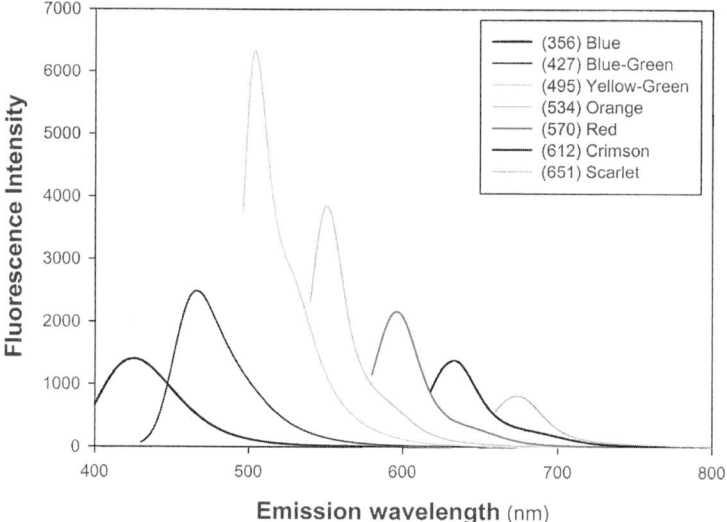

Figure 4
Fluorescence emission spectra of 7 differently labeled fluorescent microspheres (Molecular Probes), dissolved in 2-ethoxyethylacetate. Excitation wavelengths in nm are given in brackets. *For coloured version see appendix*

2 to 3 min into a syringe during and after microsphere application. Thus, if 10,000 microspheres are deposited in the reference organ (10 ml/min), 1000 microspheres in a given organ would represent a blood supply of 1 ml/min.

The technique required to measure microsphere deposition depends on their labeling. Commercially available radioactive microspheres are labeled with ^{46}Sc, ^{85}Sr, ^{113}Sn, ^{153}Gd (all γ-radiation), display a uniform activity per microsphere (e. g. 1 Bq/sphere) and can be detected in tissue or tissue samples using a γ-counter without additional preparation.

The measurement of fluorescent (Fig. 4) and colored (absorbing) spheres, which are available from different manufacturers, requires tissue degradation in KOH (4 mol/l, 50 °C, 4 h, > 5 ml KOH/g tissue) and the separation of the microspheres from the tissue digest by 8 μm polyethylene filters. Thereafter, filters and fluorescent microspheres are quantitatively transferred into cups and the microspheres are dissolved by 2-ethoxyethylacetate, enabling the detection of fluorescent emission intensities at defined excitation wavelengths. Similar protocols apply for colored microspheres.

The choice of microspheres depends on the available detection equipment and the number of measurements required. Radioactive microspheres require little manipulation but are more expensive, expose the laboratory to radiation and require the disposal of radioactive waste. For colored microspheres, only 3 different colors can be reliably quantified in one sample, which limits the number of time points that can be measured in one experiment.

Since in the microsphere technique local blood perfusion is inferred from the deposition of discrete particles, there are two caveats of practical importance:

1. The stochastic nature of the particle distribution pattern in tissue requires a given number of counted spheres for a desired precision of measurement. It has been calculated that about 400 spheres are required to estimate local deposition density with 5% precision (Buckberg et al. 1971). This already limits on theoretical grounds the spatial resolution of flow measurements attainable using microspheres.
2. In the arterial vascular tree, the deposition of microspheres may not be identical to plasma or erythrocyte flow. Indeed, Bassingthwaighte et al. compared microsphere deposition with the uptake of methylimipramine, which is almost completely extracted during its first capillary passage, and observed a small bias of microspheres towards areas of higher flow. Most probably, the bias will increase at higher spatial resolution, where flow at small arterial bifurcations may control the direction of deposition of an individual microsphere. In general, however, microsphere deposition correlates well with local plasma flow (reviewed by Prinzen and Bassingthwaighte 2000).

Microsphere studies revealed that the distribution of myocardial blood flow is not entirely homogenous. There is a transmural gradient, with higher subendocardial and lower subepicardial values, the ratio being about 1.2–1.4/1. Moreover, microsphere measurements at high spatial resolution revealed in several species a substantial spatial variability within each myocardial layer. For example, at a resolution of 0.3 g, about 6% of samples receive less than 50% and another 6% more than 150% of the average flow, which cannot be explained by the transmural gradient. This spatial heterogeneity is temporally stable for weeks (Decking et al. 2002) and correlates with indices of substrate uptake, energy turnover and local protein expression (reviewed by Deussen 1998 and Decking 2002). Hence, when applying microspheres for flow determinations, the microsphere density in small myocardial samples may not be a valid measure of the average myocardial blood flow, e. g. in the LV free wall or a distinct myocardial region. However, providing the number of counted spheres exceeds 400 and the tissue size is greater than 1 g per sample, the flow value determined may be representative of a larger area of myocardium under similar experimental conditions.

Methods to determine myocardial perfusion are not limited to microsphere deposition. Uptake of radioactive molecular markers would be an alternative, but most (e.g. K^+ or Rb^+) suffer from incomplete first pass extraction or rapid wash-in and wash-out kinetics (e.g. ^3H_2O). Local perfusion measures using positron emission (PET), magnetic resonance imaging (MRI) or echocardiography are also available.

Examples

Experimental Preparation

Anesthesia and Mechanical Ventilation

Many anesthetics with different pharmacological properties have been used in open-chest studies. Examples are barbiturates, propofol, opioids and the volatile anesthetics halothane, isoflurane and sevoflurane. Chloralose, while obsolete in clinical medicine, has occasionally been preferred for cardiovascular studies because the vasomotor tone is less affected than by many other anesthetics. The anesthetic is of great importance for the desired experiments and can be a source of severe problems. As in clinical anesthesia, experimental protocols often use a combination of different anesthetics, allowing for an acceptable narcotic and anesthetic effect with a minimum of circulatory depression.

Numerous anesthetics have been used with good success in open-chest experiments. For acute studies with open-chest rats, for example, the authors routinely use barbiturates, such as thiopentone sodium (120 mg/kg, i.p.) or pentobarbitone (60 mg/kg i.p.), followed by supplementary small doses, as required. Artificial ventilation is mandatory during anesthesia. Thiopentone has a longer anesthetic effect than pentobarbital but tends to reduce blood pressure. For chronic experiments with intended survival, midazolame (5 mg/kg, i.p.) with the neuroleptanalgesic combination of fentanyl (0.1 mg/kg, i.m.) plus fluanisone (3 mg/kg, i.m.) is a better alternative, because spontaneous respiration recovers more rapidly at the end of the experiment.

For open-chest studies with larger animals, such as swine, the authors start anesthesia by an i.m. injection of azaperone (4 mg/kg), followed by i.m. ketamine (10 mg/kg). Atropine (0.02 mg/kg) may be helpful to prevent excessive tracheobronchial mucus production. After tracheal intubation and start of artificial ventilation, pancuronium bromide (0.1 mg/kg) is given i.v. for skeletal muscle relaxation. Thereafter, fentanyl (0.01–0.02 mg/kg) is injected i.v. to provide sufficient analgesia, later re-administration being required for longer surgical procedures. Anesthesia is maintained by isoflurane (1–1.5%). Food should be withheld for 12 h before anesthesia with free access to water.

In chronic experiments, the administration of prolonged acting opioids (e.g. piritramide) may be required to prevent pain during the recovery from surgery. Additional information about anesthesia is also given below.

Surgical Preparation

The surgical procedure, as described above, must remember that the intrathoracic anatomy may differ between species. For example, the left coronary artery is predominant in rats without a true equivalent of a circumflex artery. Most of the blood of the left coronary artery is carried by the left descending branch, which runs in an almost straight line from its origin towards the apex of the heart and supplies the left ventricular wall by almost horizontal, lateral branches. Species differences in coronary anatomy also include the degree of collateral blood supply during ischemia, which is high in dogs and much lower in pigs (Hearse 2000).

Manipulation of Coronary Perfusion

The duration of ischemia required to achieve a certain degree of injury is determined by many experimental variables. Examples are species differences in collateral supply, anesthetics, hemodynamic parameters and body temperature. Pilot experiments are usually needed for adjustment of the experimental conditions to achieve the desired degree of experimental ischemic injury. Fig. 5 shows an example of a series of experi-

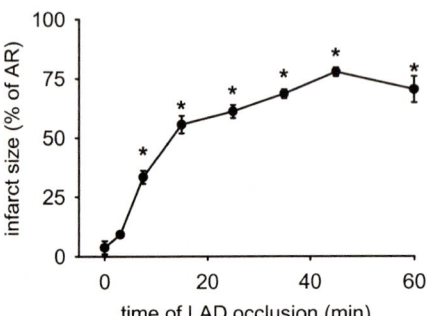

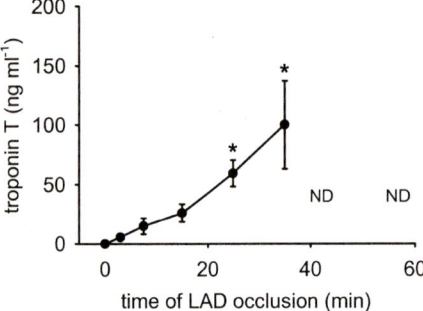

Figure 5
Effects of varying lengths of regional myocardial ischemia (LAD occlusion for 0–60 min) followed by 2 h of reperfusion in anesthetized rats. Each group n = 5–11. *Top:* Infarct size expressed as percentage of the area at risk (AR), which amounted to approximately 50% of the left ventricle in these experiments. *Bottom:* cardiac troponin T release expressed as plasma concentrations. *, p < 0.05 vs. control experiments without ischemia. *ND* not done

ments that have been performed to characterize the time-dependent increase of infarction. There is a steep interrelation between the duration of ischemia and injury, as measured by the release of cardiac troponin T into the plasma or morphological infarct size.

Moreover, the experiments show that parameters of ischemic injury respond clearly with different temporal kinetics (see below for further discussion). Therefore, assessment of more than one parameter of ischemic myocardial injury is generally re-commended, if this is an important endpoint in a particular study.

Many studies have suggested that the re-introduction of oxygen or the occurrence of inflammation during reperfusion may aggravate ischemic myocardial injury ("reperfusion injury"). The amount of reperfusion-induced injury also depends on the particular experimental conditions and is probably most prominent within the first minutes of reperfusion. An aggravation of myocardial injury during the first minutes of reperfusion is, however, difficult to detect because the methodology to identify infarcted myocardium (e. g., tetrazolium staining) requires a minimum duration of reperfusion (hours).

Nevertheless, the viability of ischemic myocardium before re-perfusion is of little practical interest, because reperfusion is a *conditio sine qua non* for tissue survival. Longer times of reperfusion may be less critical. In a systematic evaluation in open-chest rats, an increase of the reperfusion period from 2 to 8 h did not result to a major increase in infarct size (K. Z., unpublished).

Assessment of Myocardial Integrity and Function

Measurement of Myocardial Infarct Size

Regional ischemia induces myocardial infarction, the extent of which correlates to the duration of ischemia. For example, coronary artery occlusion in the rat causes necrosis after several minutes of ischemia, with a continuous increase until approximately 45 min. At this time, about 75% of the area at risk has become necrotic. Longer periods of ischemia often do not lead to a further increase in infarct size, because marginal regions of the area at risk may be supplied by diffusional oxygen or collateral blood flow from the surrounding normally perfused tissue, the lumen or the epicardial surface. Figure 5 shows representative examples from open-chest rats.

There is also a positive correlation between plasma markers of ischemic injury and soluble markers of ischemia, such as cardiac troponin T (see Fig. 5). Nevertheless, the time courses of troponin T in plasma and morphological infarct size are not identical. Obviously, the kinetics of troponin release following impairment of myocardial cell membrane permeability on the one hand, and the release and degradation of myocardial dehydrogenases (used for tetrazolium staining) on the other hand are only loosely related to one another.

Similar considerations may apply to reperfusion. In open-chest rats, for example, morphological infarct size remains almost unchanged between 2 and 8 h of reperfusion, while there is a remarkable (more than 50%) decline in the plasma concentration of cardiac troponin T within the same time (K.Z., unpublished). The clearance or redistribution of troponin is apparently high enough to cause a decrease in plasma troponin within only a few hours.

Sonomicrometry

Measurements of regional contractile function with sonomicrometric crystals usually require larger animal species, mostly pigs or dogs. Within the ventricular wall, distances between two crystals may be measured circumferentially in a short-axis plane, longitudinally (base to apex) or in a diagonal orientation. Which one gives the best results depends on the local fiber orientation. In addition, endo- and epicardial placement of crystals enables the measurement of wall thickness, which is preferred by many investigators because it is independent of the local fiber direction. Epicardial single-crystal devices, which determine wall thickness from the endocardial echo signal, are particularly convenient.

Sonomicrometric measurements are very useful in evaluating regional myocardial contractile function during ischemia and reperfusion, whereas global parameters, such as intraventricular pressures or cardiac output, may not adequately reflect myocardial function within an ischemic area. This is demonstrated in Fig. 6, where LAD occlusion in an open-chest pig causes only moderate changes of left ventricular pressure and aortic flow. In contrast, the sonomicrometric registration of left ventricular wall thickness within the ischemic area shows a dramatic decline in the systolic increase in wall thickness (contraction), which is already completely lost 2 min after coronary occlusion. At this time, the ischemic ventricular wall is passively stretched

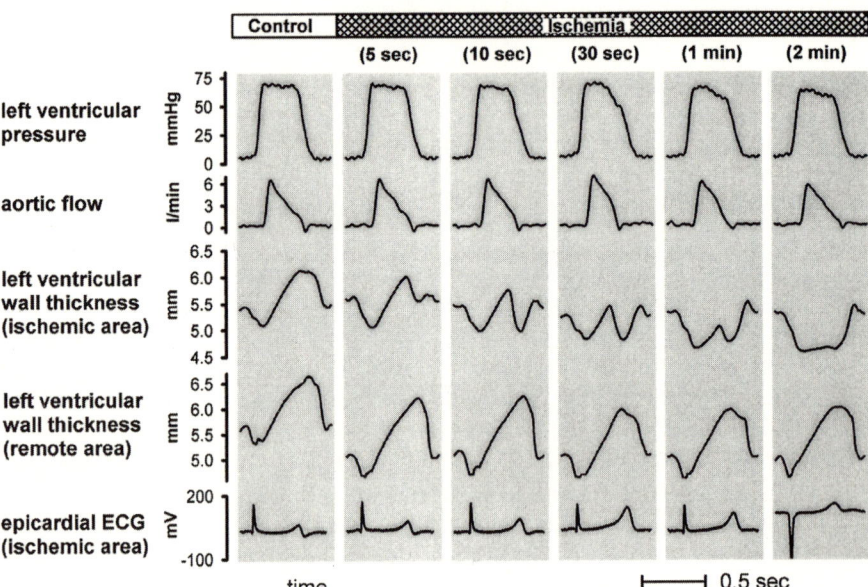

Figure 6
Registrations of left ventricular pressure, aortic flow, wall thickness (sonomicrometry) and epicardial ECG in an anesthetized open-chest pig immediately before (control) and different times after experimental occlusion of the LAD. Myocardial ischemia, which comprised about 20% of the left ventricle in this experiment, resulted in only minor changes of global ventricular function (left ventricular pressure, aortic flow), while regional function measured by sonomicrometry (wall thickness) reveals the deterioration of left ventricular systolic contraction with progressive thinning during systole. Regional contractile function in an area remote from ischemia was preserved, except for a decrease in end-diastolic wall thickness (increasing end-diastolic volume). The epicardial ECG shows the characteristic signs of acute myocardial ischemia (increase of T, loss of R wave)

by the intraventricular pressure, as shown by a systolic decrease in wall thickness (bulging). There is also a decrease in the end-diastolic wall thickness of the non-ischemic ventricular wall, which results from an increase in the end-diastolic left ventricular volume due to a moderate degree of ventricular failure.

Microspheres

Microsphere measurements are, as outlined above, generally stochastic and a sufficient amount of microspheres needs to be trapped within a given volume of myocardial tissue. As long as the number of spheres in the sample of interest exceeds 400, the precision of the measurement in the sample of interest will be > 95%, which conventionally requires (at 200.000 microspheres/kg) a sample size of 0.5–1 g wet weight. Nevertheless, due to the physiological phenomenon of spatial perfusion heterogeneity, the perfusion of an individual 1 g sample may still not be representative of average myocardial blood flow. Transmural analysis of > 10% of the total LV tissue will

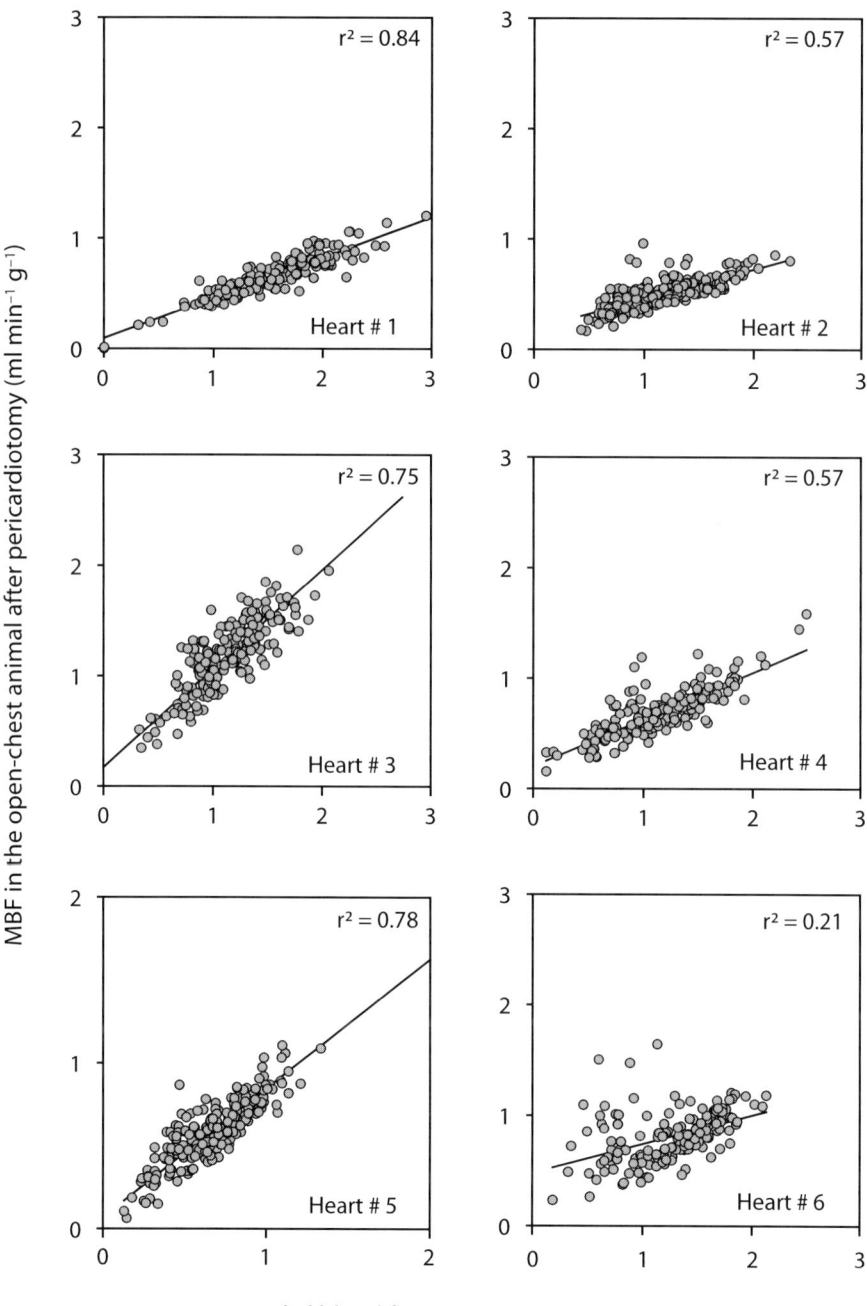

Figure 7
Myocardial blood flow (MBF) following midazolam-piritramide anesthesia, open-chest surgery and pericardiotomy as compared to blood flow under resting conditions (awake) in chronically instrumented beagle dogs. Each data point represents the local perfusion of an individual left ventricular tissue sample (300 mg) determined in the anesthetized and conscious animal, respectively

be necessary to obtain a valid measurement of LV perfusion even under physiological conditions. Special attention is required when perfusion is to be measured in models of local ischemia and reperfusion, where the extent of spatial heterogeneity is substantially increased.

Figure 7 shows examples of LV free wall flow measurements by microspheres. Microspheres were given first in conscious, chronically instrumented beagle dogs, and thereafter in the anesthetized animal following open-chest surgery and pericardiotomy. Following myocardial excision, the local perfusion of individual 300 mg myocardial samples was determined. The perfusion of each individual sample under anesthesia is related to the basal perfusion in the conscious animal. Two important features become apparent. First, local myocardial blood flow already varies substantially in the conscious animal despite the absence of any coronary stenosis, reflecting spatial heterogeneity of flow. Secondly, in most hearts, areas receiving little flow under basal conditions displayed low flow during anesthesia, and high flow areas remained on average high flow areas during anesthesia. However, on average anesthesia resulted in a decrease in local perfusion since the slope of a linear regression was < 1 in each of the experiments. The lower average blood flow most probably reflects the lower energy demand due to a reduced global workload.

While in most hearts flow under anesthesia correlated closely to that under basal conditions, in some hearts flow under anesthesia was almost independent of basal perfusion (see heart #6 in Fig. 7), reflecting a redistribution of perfusion. These factors have to be taken into account in the interpretation of myocardial blood flow in open-chest models.

Troubleshooting

Anesthesia and Mechanical Ventilation

Anesthesia in general and the pharmacological properties of anesthetics specifically exert a profound influence on cardiovascular control. One problem frequently encountered is the potential depression of blood pressure and myocardial contractility. Anesthetics may directly reduce myocardial contractility and alter the autonomic tone with profound effects on myocardial oxygen consumption in normal and underperfused tissue. Hence, the anesthetic agents must be carefully selected according to potential interference with the experiment (see Table 1).

The dosing strategy should also consider the pharmacokinetic properties of anesthetics. Depending on the drug, administration by continuous infusion is better than a bolus injection, particularly if constant hemodynamic conditions are required. Nevertheless, the pharmacological properties of some compounds are complex. For example, with pentobarbitone the dosing regimen is critical, because redistribution within the body during early anesthesia may favor underdosing, while longer administration (hours) may lead to accumulation and overdosage. If anesthetics are not given with a loading dose, a duration of at least 4 times the compound's terminal half-life will be required to achieve a pharmacokinetic steady state.

Volatile anesthetics are frequently used in open-chest preparations. However, there is some indirect evidence that halogenated compounds (e. g., halothane, isoflurane), even when administered for a short period (minutes), may alter myocardial tolerance to ischemia, potentially by acting via myocardial K^+_{ATP} channels (Kwok 2002). Intravenous agents such as pentobarbital, ketamine-xylacine and propofol do not appear to have this property. Nevertheless, ketamine may interfere with ischemic preconditioning (Walsh et al. 1994).

Mechanical ventilation can change hemodynamic parameters, in particular by increasing the intrathoracic pressure, which decreases venous blood return into the thorax and reduces ventricular preload and cardiac output. This may be of particular significance if insufficient amounts of fluid are administered and can be prevented by infusing sufficient amounts of fluid.

Experimental Preparation

Open-chest preparations require major surgical experience. A typical complication during thoracotomy is the injury of a large cranial vein near the cranial thorax aperture with severe venous bleeding and lethal air embolism. In some species (e. g., pigs) the anterior ventricular wall is very close behind the sternum, resulting in risk of injury to the heart during sternotomy. Moreover, the dissection of coronary arteries may injure unrecognized diagonal or marginal branches, particularly when the anatomy is complex. In larger species (dogs, pigs), it is helpful to keep heart rate low (< 100 beats per min) by appropriate anesthesia.

Surgical blood loss increases the tendency of open chest preparations to develop hypovolemia and, therefore, must be minimized. Minor unrecognized bleeding may cause significant blood loss into the thoracic cavity. Whenever possible, blunt dissection should be preferred to sharp incision and anticoagulants should not be administered until surgical manipulations are completed.

Surgery generally causes an inflammatory response. This may be of particular importance for manipulations at the epicardial surface of the heart, such as are required to apply epicardial electrodes, flow probes, vascular cannulas or sonomicrometric crystals (see Fig. 1). Within only a few hours, an accumulation of neutrophil granulocytes can be observed within the subepicardial layers of the ventricles. It may therefore be difficult to distinguish between an inflammatory response caused by an experimental intervention (e. g., ischemia and reperfusion) and one caused by an artifact of surgery.

Tilting of the heart, as sometimes required to expose structures which are difficult to access (lateral segments of coronary arteries, posterolateral biopsies, coronary sinus) may cause deterioration in myocardial function and circulatory stress, which can profoundly alter coronary blood flow and cause an unwanted preconditioning of the heart against ischemia.

An open pericardium can also change ventricular geometry, for example diastolic over-distension of the ventricles at higher end-diastolic pressures. An intact or reclosed pericardium is, hence, recommended if increased ventricular filling pressures are expected.

The open chest represents a large wound, making it vulnerable to the development of hypothermia. Mechanical ventilation and infusion of cold solutions contributes to this condition. The continuous monitoring of body temperature and, if necessary, external heating (infrared lamp, heating pads) are required. Hypothermia can critically influence the experimental outcome. For example, a fall in temperature by only 1°C reduces infarct size by 10% (Chien et al. 1994).

Manipulation of Coronary Perfusion

Extensive manipulation of a coronary artery, often required in open-chest studies for cannulation or placement of occluders, can induce vasospasm with myocardial ischemia, arrhythmias and infarction. It can be helpful to administer a short-acting local vasorelaxant such as glycerol trinitrate topically to prevent or terminate arterial spasm. Vascular compression must be avoided to prevent injury to the vascular wall with subsequent spasm or intravascular thrombosis.

Assessment of Myocardial Integrity and Function

Markers of Myocardial Injury

Plasma markers of ischemic injury (e.g., troponins) may correlate with morphological infarct size, such as tetrazolium staining (O'Brien et al. 1997), but disparities between cardiac troponins and infarct size have also been reported (Kawakami et al. 1999). These may be explained by delayed washout of the markers from injured myocardium during ischemia, as demonstrated in Fig. 5. In addition, the plasma levels of soluble infarct markers are also influenced by the excretion and distribution kinetics, both of which are poorly defined in experimental animals. The estimation of ischemic injury from plasma markers can also be limited by insufficient myocardial perfusion during reperfusion ("no reflow phenomenon"), potentially preventing marker washout from infarcted tissue. The relation between plasma markers and myocardial injury is also complex in clinical myocardial infarction (Omura et al. 1995).

Microspheres

All types of microspheres may form aggregates during storage, which can prevent stochastic distribution in the microcirculation. This is particularly important for radioactive microspheres due to their higher specific density. Microsphere aggregation can be prevented by careful sonication (5–10 min) immediately before application. Commercial microsphere preparations may contain low concentrations of detergents to prevent aggregation. Moreover, homogenous distribution within the syringe should always be ensured by rapid shaking or vortexing the syringe before use, because microspheres tend to sediment rapidly. Microspheres may cause hemodynamic changes due to microvascular blockade, limiting the number of spheres that can be injected. In dogs, for example, repeated measurements with left atrial injection of

15 µm spheres, totaling up to 48×10^6, are unlikely to cause significant changes in systemic hemodynamics or regional myocardial flow. Larger numbers of spheres may impair circulation, which results, for example, in a depression of myocardial function.

Long-term studies with an intended survival for days, weeks or months must also take into account the possible release of label from the microspheres. While fluorescent microspheres appear to be physically stable and to continue to reside at the location of their first deposition (Van Oosterhout 1998), radioactive microspheres may clearly leak. Their use cannot be recommended for chronic studies.

References

Buckberg GD, Luck JC, Payne DB, Hoffman JIE, Archie JP, Fixler DE (1971) Some sources of error in measuring regional blood flow with radioactive microspheres. J Appl Physiol 31: 598–604

Chien GL, Wolff RA, Davis RF, van Winkle DM (1994) "Normothermic range" temperature affects myocardial infarct size. Cardiovasc Res 28: 1014–1017

Decking, UKM, Skwirba S, Zimmermann MF, Preckel B, Thamer V, Deussen A, Schrader J (2001) Spatial heterogeneity of energy turnover in the heart. Pflügers Arch 441: 663–673

Decking UKM (2002) Spatial heterogeneity in the heart: recent insights and open questions. News Physiol Sci 17: 246–250

Deussen A (1998) Blood flow heterogeneity in the heart. Bas Res Cardiol 93: 430–438

Farb A, Kolodgie FD, Jones RM, Jenkins M, Virmani R (1993) Early detection and measurement of experimental myocardial infarcts with horseradish peroxidase. J Mol Cell Cardiol 25: 343–353

Fishbein, MC, Meerbaum S, Rit J, Lando U, Kanmatsuse K, Mercier JC, Corday E, Ganz W (1981) Early phase acute myocardial infarct size quantification: validation of the triphenyl tetrazolium chloride tissue enzyme staining technique. Am Heart J 101: 593–600

Folts J (1991) An in vivo model of experimental arterial stenosis, intimal damage, and periodic thrombosis. Circulation 83 [Suppl IV]: 3–14

Franz MR (1999) Current status of monophasic action potential recording: theories, measurements and interpretations. Cardiovasc Res 41: 25–40

Hearse DJ (2000) Species variation in the coronary collateral circulation during regional myocardial ischaemia: a critical determinant of the rate of evolution and extent of myocardial infarction. Cardiovasc Res 45: 213–219

Heusch G (1998) Hibernating myocardium. Physiol Rev 78: 1055–1058

Kawakami T, Lowberg C, Valen G, Vaage J (1999) Mechanical conversion of post-ischaemic ventricular fibrillation: effects on function and myocyte injury in isolated rat hearts. Scand J Clin Lab Invest 59: 9–16

Kwok WM, Martinelli AT, Fujimoto K, Suzuki A, Stadnicka A, Bosnjak ZJ (2002) Differential modulation of the cardiac adenosine triphosphate-sensitive potassium channel by isoflurane and halothane. Anesthesiology 97: 50–56

O'Brien PJ, Dameron GW, Beck ML, Kang YJ, Erickson BK, Di Battista TH, Miller KE, Jackson KN, Mittelstadt S (1997) Cardiac troponin T is a sensitive, specific biomarker of cardiac injury in laboratory animals. Lab Anim Sci: 47: 486–495

Omura T, Teragaki M, Takagi M, Tani T, Nishida Y, Yamagishi H, Yanagi S, Nishikimi T, Yoshiyama M, Toda I (1995) Myocardial infarct size by serum troponin T and myosin light chain 1 concentration. Jpn Circ J: 59: 154–159

Prinzen FW, Bassingthwhaighte JB (2000) Blood flow distributions by microsphere deposition methods. Cardiovasc Res 45: 13–21

Romson JL, Haack, DW, Lucchesi B (1980) Electrical induction of coronary artery thrombosis in the ambulatory canine: a model for in vivo evaluation of anti-thrombotic agents. Thromb Res 17: 841–853

Ross J (1991) Myocardial perfusion-contraction matching. Implications for coronary heart disease and hibernation. Circulation 83: 1076–1083

Van Oosterhout MFM, Prinzen FW, Sakurada S, Glenny RW, and Hales JRS (1998) Fluorescent microspheres are superior to radioactive microspheres in chronic blood flow measurements. Am J Physiol 275: H110–H115

Walsh RS, Tsuchida A, Daly JJ, Thornton JD, Cohen MV, Downey JM (1994) Ketamine-xylazine anaesthesia permits a K_{ATP} channel antagonist to attenuate preconditioning in rabbit myocardium. Cardiovasc Res 28: 1337–1341

Zacharowski K, Olbrich A, Piper J, Hafner G, Kondo K, Thiemermann C (1999a) Selective activation of the prostanoid EP_3 receptor reduces myocardial infarct size in rodents. Arterioscler Thromb Vasc Biol 19: 2141–2147

Zacharowski K, Olbrich A, Otto M, Hafner G, Thiemermann C (1999b) Effects of the prostanoid EP_3-receptor agonists M&B 28767 and GR 63799X on infarct size caused by regional myocardial ischaemia in the anaesthetized rat. Br J Pharmacol 126: 849–58

Models of Chronic Ischemia and Infarction

Nicolas Doll, Heike Aupperle, Fabian Stahl and Thomas Walther

Introduction

Progressive atherosclerotic coronary obstruction results in ischemic heart disease and myocardial infarction. The degree of cardiac damage is mainly determined by the degree of collateral circulation that developed either before the occlusion or within a short period thereafter. Ischemia and potentially the size of myocardial infarction may thus be reduced by coronary collateral circulation, leading to an ultimately improved long-term outcome (Charney and Cohen 1993). The majority of patients with coronary artery disease are treated by coronary artery bypass grafting (CABG) or percutaneous transluminal coronary angioplasty (PTCA). A growing number of patients have survived multiple bypass operations and/or multiple angioplasty procedures and are not amenable to any repeat intervention due to severely diseased or totally occluded vessels.

The quality of life in these patients is impaired by persistent angina pectoris, progressive ischemic heart failure and the absence of a reasonable prospect of improvement of their symptoms. For these patients, new alternative therapeutic strategies are required. Such new therapeutic strategies need to be tested by chronic experiments before clinical application. For such experiments, effective animal models resembling severe myocardial ischemia with chronic ischemic myocardium are required.

Chronic myocardial ischemia has already been studied in species such as pigs, dogs, rabbits and rats (Operschall et al. 2000; Schaper et al. 1976; Scheel et al. 1977; White et al. 1992). These models allow for detailed investigations of collateral circulation and angiogenesis. To date the ameroid constrictor is the instrument of choice for inducing myocardial ischemia in species like pigs or dogs. It has been used for various types of chronic animal *in vivo* studies, for example mechanisms and quantification of collateral blood flow, investigation of the effects of angiogenic growth factors, determination of coronary reactivity and analysis of concomitant myocardial infarction (Harada et al. 1996; Lazarous et al. 1996; Lopez et al. 1998; Maxwell et al. 1987).

Description of Methods and Practical Approach

The chronic ischemic swine model is suitable to examine new alternative therapeutic strategies for the treatment of coronary artery disease, because myocardial morphology, coronary anatomy and especially collateral development in pigs are very similar to the situations in humans (White et al. 1986). Several examples of the use of pigs for different studies on myocardial ischemia are described below.

Studies on Physical Exercise (Training)

Experimental studies demonstrated that one important factor in the induction of ischemia was the presence of myocyte hypoxia. In clinical studies, patients with an occluded coronary artery and chronic myocardial ischemia often have extensive collateral development into the ischemic myocardium. Animal studies have shown that the number and function of these collaterals can be increased significantly by regular physical exercise, resulting in increased myocardial perfusion and also in improved myocardial function in the dependent regions. Histologically an increase in vascular density could be demonstrated (Bloor et al. 1984; Roth et al. 1990, 1997; White et al. 1998a,b).

In patients with chronically occluded coronary arteries, increased collateral perfusion after training has not yet been demonstrated. These studies evaluated collateral perfusion only under resting conditions using angiographic visualization. Studies investigating collateral perfusion under exercise conditions are not yet available.

Studies on Myocardial Laser Revascularisation

Transmyocardial laser revascularisation (TMR), is used to create transmural channels from the epicardial surface to the ventricular chamber. Histological studies have provided evidence for neoangiogenesis in the vicinity of such laser channels, resulting in increased formation of new blood vessels in the laser treated areas, so that increased perfusion *via* these new vessels is thought to represent a possible pathophysiological mechanism which accounts for the clinical improvement of patients after TMR (Diegeler et al. 1998; Lazarous et al. 1996). The intention of providing additional perfusion channels to the ischemic myocardium had to be reconsidered soon after this form of treatment was introduced into clinical practice, because nearly all channels were found to be occluded by coagulated and thrombotic material soon after their creation.

Studies on Angiogenetic Factors

Neoangiogenesis is the development of new vessels from blood islands that occurs physiologically during embryonic development or during wound healing. It is a complex process that is still not fully understood, but it is thought to occur in a sequence including:

1. endothelial cell and pericyte activation,
2. basement membrane disruption and degradation of the extracellular matrix by cell-derived proteases,
3. endothelial cell migration, sprouting and proliferation,
4. organization of endothelial cells into tubelike structures and re-establishment of cell-cell interactions with the existing vessels, and
5. endothelial cell conversion back into a quiescent vascular phenotype.

Neoangiogenesis is an integral component of a wide variety of biological activities such as wound healing and pathological processes such as proliferative retinopathy or development of neoplasms. Neoangiogenesis is controlled by intracellular and extracellular signaling pathways. The mediators that induce angiogenesis are referred to as angiogenes.

In the last few years, several angiogenetic factors have been detected by basic biochemical and molecular biological studies (VEGF family, FGF family, angiopoetin, angiostatin, angiogenin, TGF-α and -β, TNF-α, scatter factor, HIV_1-alpha) and their biological functions and molecular physiologic mechanisms have been analyzed. These factors seem to play a role in the cascade of events leading to angiogenesis. Studies could demonstrate that these growth factors were upregulated in ischemic conditions and neovascularisation was suppressed by antagonists of these mediators (Hrada et al. 1996; Lopez et al. 1998).

Several of these angiogenetic substances are already available for experimental therapeutic studies of angiogenesis in acute or chronic ischemia. For the first time, these substances offer the possibility of influencing new vessel formation, i.e. angiogenesis, in various experimental and also clinical settings.

Experimental studies in various animal models demonstrated a significant angiogenetic effect of these substances (Hrada et al. 1996; Lopez et al. 1998). In initial clinical studies on a small number of patients with peripheral arterial disease as well as coronary artery disease, increased vascularization and improvement of clinical symptoms was reported.

However, large, well-documented and controlled studies on the angiogenetic effect of these substances are not yet available.

Several basic questions concerning the therapeutic application of angiogenetic factors in patients with chronic ischemia still remain to be answered:
- Is a one-time single-shot application of one angiogenetic factor enough to result in therapeutic angiogenesis or will a sequential administration of the factor at various time points prove to be more efficient?
- Is the application of only one angiogenetic factor enough or will the administration of a combination of angiogenetic factors yield better results?
- Are there possible side effects (development of malignomas or increased growth of occult cancers)?

Furthermore, several questions remain about the optimal way of applying these angiogenetic factors. Several studies have used direct administration of the angiogenetic factor as a protein into the myocardium; in other experimental studies, gene transfer has been used to induce expression of the angiogenetic factor into the muscle.

Studies on Autologous Endothelial Progenitor Cells/Stem Cell Therapy

Catheter-based, intramyocardial transplantation of autologous endothelial progenitor cells, which are able to enhance neovascularization in myocardial ischemia, can be sufficiently investigated using a chronic ischemic swine model. It has been shown already, that this kind of therapy is effective in an animal model (Kawamoto et al. 2003).

Further studies with stem cell therapy in a chronic ischemic animal model may show effectiveness and one day it could be possible to transfer this concept to humans. Ongoing studies will have to demonstrate the safety and efficacy of these new therapeutic strategies for treating patients with coronary artery disease, who are not suitable for standard options like coronary artery bypass grafting or percutaneously coronary angioplasty.

The Ameroid Constrictor

Chronic ischemia will be produced in the myocardial territory supplied by the left circumflex artery by use of an ameroid constrictor (Fig. 1). By this slowly progressive ischemia sufficient collateral growth will be allowed to prevent myocardial necrosis (Shen et al. 1996) (Fig. 2).

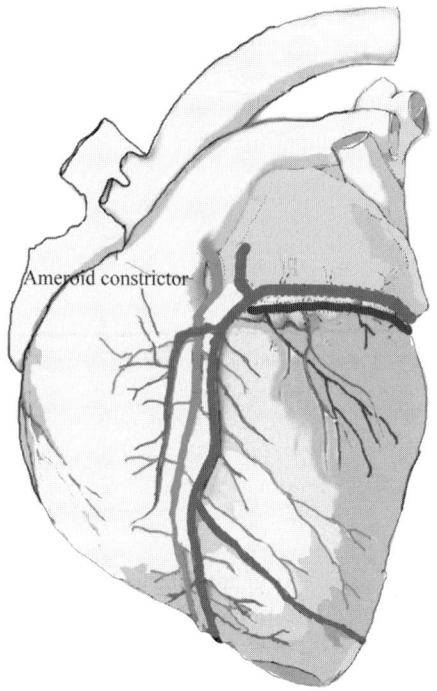

Figure 1
Schematic illustration of the position of the ameroid constrictor close to the origin of the circumflex artery (RCX). The chronic ischemic area is shown by yellow-brown color. *For coloured version see appendix*

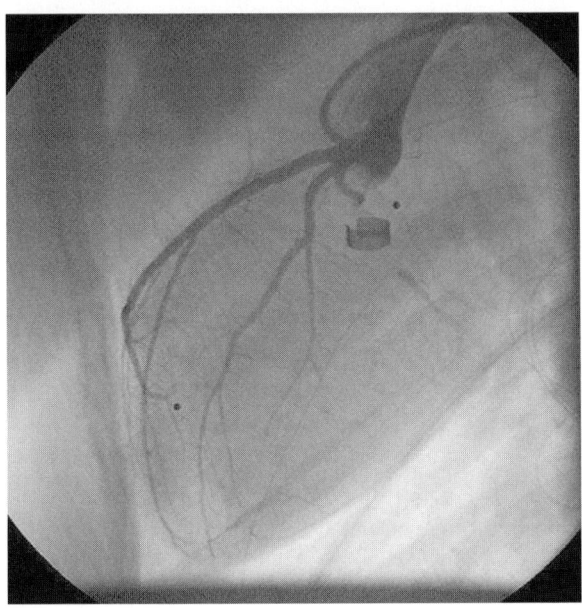

Figure 2
Injection of contrast medium into the left coronary artery. The ameroid constrictor had occluded the circumflex artery. The distal parts of the circumflex artery are refilled *via* small antegrade collaterals

The ameroid material is hygroscopic and slowly swells, leading gradually to complete closure of the artery after a period of 2–3 weeks post-placement (Fig. 3), with minimal infarction (< 1% of the left ventricle) (O'Konski et al. 1987) because of the development of collateral blood vessels. Myocardial function and blood flow are normal at rest in the region previously perfused by the occluded artery (the ischemic region), but blood flow is insufficient to prevent ischemia when myocardial oxygen demand increases. Collateral vessel development is completed within 21 days of ameroid placement and remains unchanged for at least 4 months (White et al. 1992).

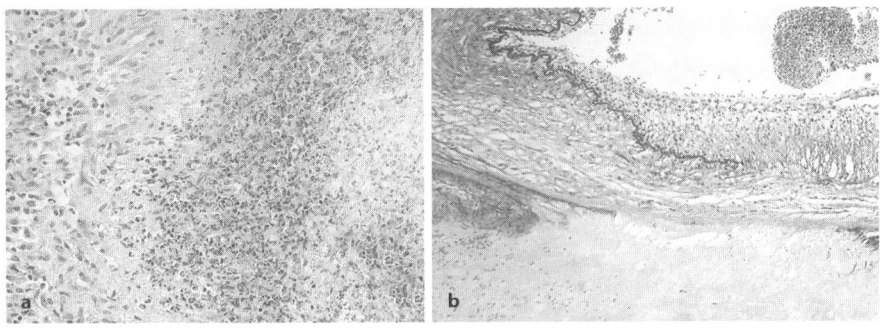

Figure 3a,b
Histology of the constrictor: **a** 3 weeks after implantation of the ameroid constrictor the coronary artery is necrotic with purulent inflammation and granulation tissue is spreading from the periphery (H.-E. stain). **b** 3 weeks after implantation of the ameroid constrictor the distal part of the coronary artery shows segmental inflammatory and degenerative lesions: transmural vacuolization and destruction, severe intimal hyperplasia and mild purulent inflammation (Picro Sirius Red stain). *For coloured version see appendix*

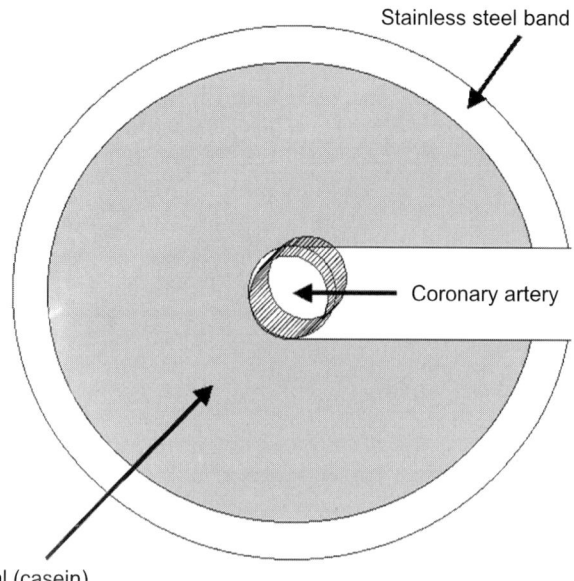

Figure 4
The ameroid constrictor consists of a stainless steel band that has to be placed around the ameroid material. The coronary artery should be placed at the end of the ameroid groove

Placement of the Ameroid Constrictor on the Left Circumflex Artery (LCX)

The constrictors are not sterile when shipped and sterilization with ethylene oxide is recommended. Two different sizes of the constrictors are available: 9×4 mm (mostly used) and 10×5 mm. The ameroid constrictor consists of a stainless steel band that has to be placed around the ameroid material (Fig. 4). A special pie-shaped ameroid configuration was designed by Professor Dan Mc Kirnan (San Diego, California) (Figs. 5 and 6). The classic ameroid constrictor does not lead to complete obstruction of the vessel in some animals. With the new pie shaped constrictor (Ameroid constrictor; Clifford L.Gwin; Research Instruments; P.O. Box 1959, Corvalis OR 97339), complete occlusion of the coronary artery can be safely achieved.

Technical details of the operative procedure:
- premedication, beginning of anesthesia
- left lateral thoracotomy
- preparation of the circumflex artery (RCX)
- placement of the ameroid constrictor
- placement of left atrial pacemaker leads, leads will be tunneled subcutaneously to the right thorax
- implantation of telemetric unit for ECG monitoring
- closure of the thorax

As a premedication, one day prior to the operation a cutaneous fentanyl adhesive plaster can be placed at a cleaned and shaved spot on the back of the animal.

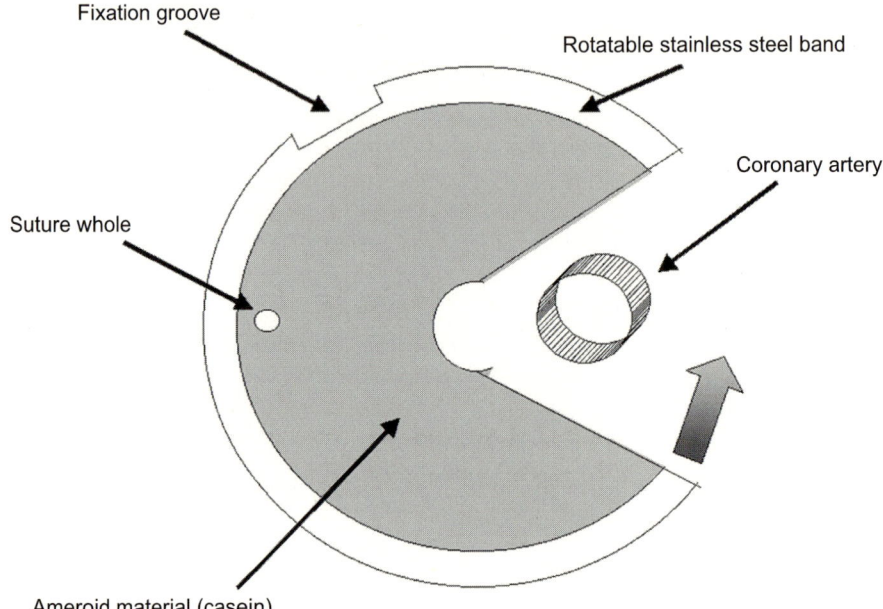

Figure 5
A special pie shaped ameroid constrictor configuration designed by Professor Dan Mc Kirnan (San Diego, California)

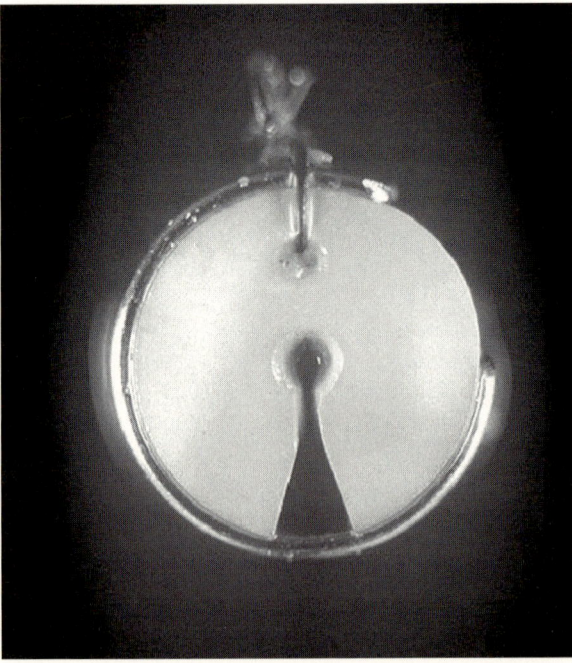

Figure 6
An explanted ameroid constrictor 5 days after implantation. A non-absorbable suture is placed to fix the ring to avoid a dislocation of the coronary artery

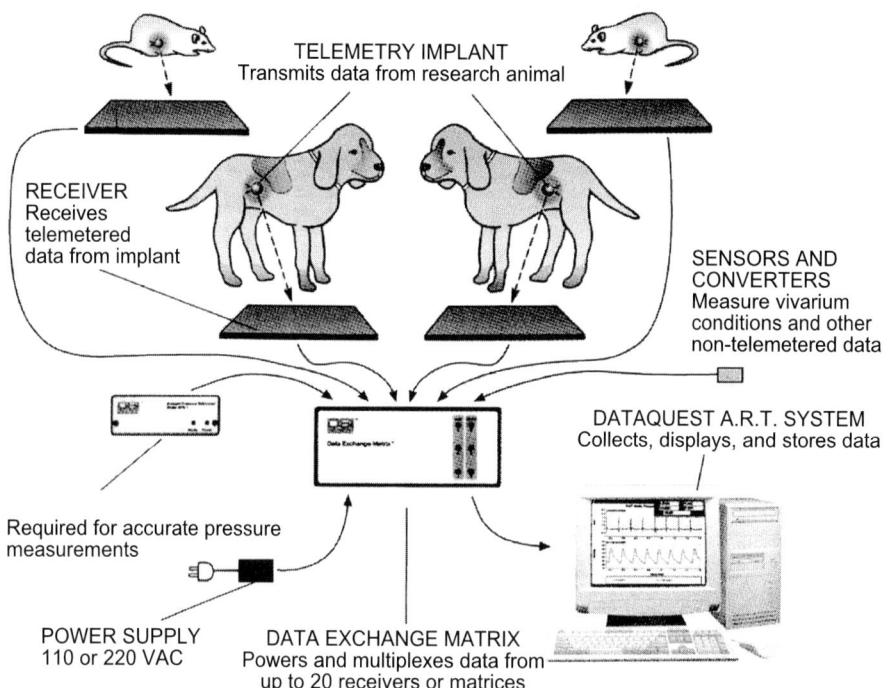

Figure 7
Schematic illustration of the telemetry unit

During such experiments in our own laboratory an anterolateral left-sided thoracotomy in the 4th intercostal space was performed using sterile techniques under general anesthesia.

Underneath the left atrial appendage, the bifurcation of the main stem into the left anterior descending (LAD) and the circumflex artery (RCX), and the corresponding vein were dissected. An ameroid constrictor was placed on the proximal part of the left circumflex artery before the takeoff of the first marginal branch. The size of the constrictor was matched to the weight of the pig. In a 30 kg animal, a 9×4 mm constrictor was usually used. The ring of the constrictor was secured with a 5×0 Prolene suture.

Two pacing leads were sutured on the left atrial appendage and were tested with a stimulation of 200 beats/min. The leads were tunneled through the intercostal spaces into a subcutaneous pocket for later use during follow-up examinations.

The telemetric unit of the ECG (Fig. 7) was implanted into the left chest cavity. The antennas of the unit were also tunneled through the intercostal spaces into a subcutaneous pocket. The vector in between the two antennas should be positioned from the base to the apex of the heart, to reveal best telemetric results.

A temporary left sided chest tube was inserted. Adaptation of the ribs and closure of the subcutaneous tissue followed. The skin was sutured with a non-absorbable intracutaneous suture. All animals were treated intraoperatively with antibiotics.

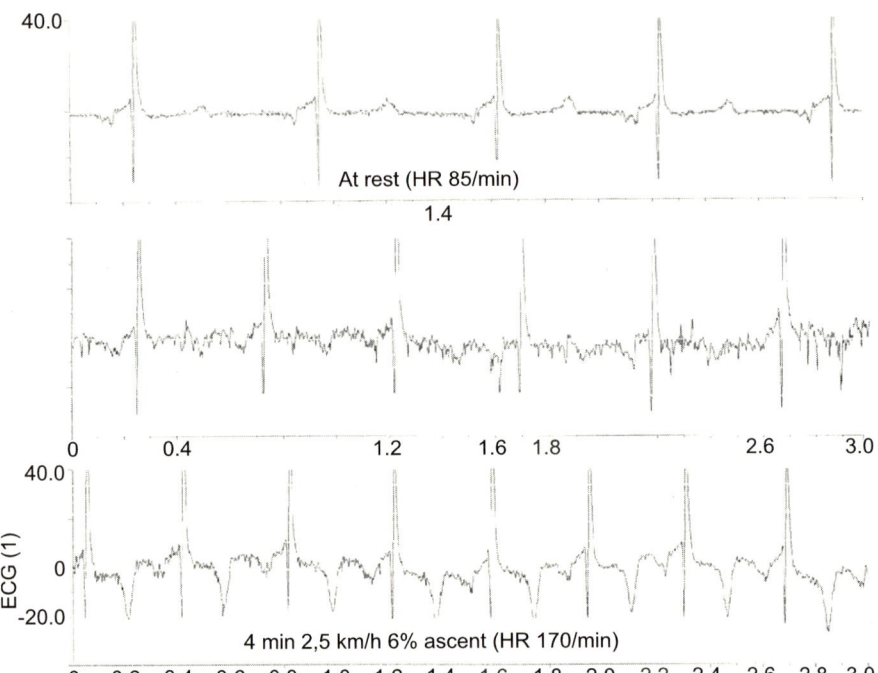

Figure 8
Telemetric ECG at rest and at effort with significant ST-level changes due to chronic ischemia

Soon after the animal was awake and breathing spontaneously the chest tube was removed under suction. Normal blood gas parameters should be achieved at this point.

During our chronic training study, animals were exercised on the special treadmill ergometer for 25 min daily during the first week with an increase of 5 min every week until 50 min per day was reached. The training intensity was targeted to achieve a heart rate of 70–80% of the maximum heart rate; for the mini-pigs we assumed 160–200 beats/min as the targeted heart rate for endurance training. The heart rate was measured via implanted electrodes and telemetric transfer of ECG once a week for adjustment of the training level by increasing the speed and/or elevation of the treadmill.

Exercise tests were performed before and at various periods within the trial. For the exercise test, pigs started with a 3% elevation with the speed necessary for reaching the daily training heart rate. Increase of the load was reached by increasing the elevation by 1% every 2 min. ECG-waves were saved digitally and were analyzed with a special software program to measure ST-changes (Fig. 8).

In addition the aortic and left ventricular pressures at rest and exercise can be recorded; these data are measured and telemetrically transmitted via pressure leads for continuous registration.

Examples

Quantification of Myocardial Perfusion

Myocardial perfusion can be assessed by colored microspheres at rest and under exercise. Myocardial perfusion before intervention can be compared to perfusion after intervention (myocardial laser revascularisation, angiogenetic factors, physical exercise).

The exercise test is performed under telemetric supervision using the implanted ECG electrodes and pressure leads on the aorta and left ventricle.

Neoangiogenesis and Collateral Development

Neoangiogenesis and collateral development can be analyzed by coronary angiography and histological analysis. Visible collaterals on coronary angiography are quantitated using the Rentrop score. For further analysis of the results of experiments inducing chronic ischemia, histomorphometrical evaluation of routine hematoxylin-eosin stained slides can be performed. This is especially helpful in quantifying the extension of fibrotic areas (Fig. 9) and the number and diameter of blood vessels/capillaries in the ischemic region and for comparison to non-ischemic regions of the heart. Blood vessels are identified by marked immunohistological methods using antibodies against smooth muscle cells (smooth muscle actin) (Hughes et al. 1998; Fig. 9) and endothelial cells (v. Willebrandt factor, CD31) (Krabatsch et al. 1996; Horvath et al. 1999). New vessels, but also other mesenchymal cells that may have developed during the study period, can be identified immunohistochemically by Ki-67 antigen or Proliferating Nuclear Antigen (PCNA) (Yu et al. 1992).

Another method for identifying *de novo* cells is the detection of bromodeoxyuridine (BrDU). Daily subcutaneous injection of BrDU leads to an incorporation of BrDU into the nuclei of new cells instead of thymidine. At the end of the study BrDU can be detected by immunohistochemical methods (Green et al. 1998; Hardonk and Harms 1990).

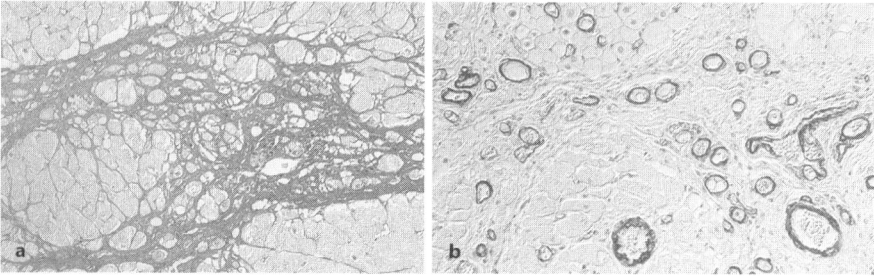

Figure 9a,b
Histology of the myocardium distal to the constrictor position: **a** 3 months after implantation of the ameroid constrictor the myocardium shows a patchy fibrosis. (Picro Sirius Red stain). **b** 3 months after implantation of the ameroid constrictor an intensive vascularization appears in areas of myocardial degeneration and fibrosis. The vascular smooth muscle cells express smooth muscle actin. (Immunohistochemistry, smooth muscle actin)

Furthermore the composition of newly developed extracellular matrix (collagen, fibronectin, laminin) can be investigated by immunohistochemical techniques (Weihrauch et al. 1994). Evaluations possible in a chronic ischemic swine model are:

Myocardial perfusion

- Coronary angiogram
- Application of microspheres
- Treadmill ergometry with continuous ECG registration

Myocardial function

- Echocardiography at rest
- Echocardiography in stress by rapid atrial stimulation (200/min)
- Left ventricular angiogram

Hemodynamics

- Cardiac output measurement by PICO-catheter
- Cardiac output measurement by Swan Ganz (pulmonary artery) catheter (PCWP, CVP, CO, PVR, SVR, PA and RV pressures)
- Pressure-volume measurements by "conductance catheter"

Laboratory

- Creatine kinase (CK/CKMB) postoperatively and post > 6 h
- Lactatedehydrogenase (LDH) post 3 weeks
- Tropinin

Histopathology

- Histopathological examination of the myocardium
- Quantitation of the fibrotic areas in the myocardium
- Histomorphometrical analysis of vascular density/neoangiogenesis
- Immunohistochemical detection of vessels (smooth muscle actin, v. Willebrandt factor)
- Immunohistochemical investigation of proliferation markers (Ki-67 antigen, PCNA, BrDU)
- Electron microscopy of the ischemic areas/neoangiogenesis

Other investigations

- Integrin receptor $\alpha v\beta 3$
- Tyrosine kinase receptor Flk-1/KDR and Flt-1
- Tie-1, Tie-2, TNF-α-receptor
- Molecular genetic detection of growth factors

Troubleshooting

Wound Infections

Wound infections in animals occur in the first postoperative week. It is very important to close the skin very exactly, so that primary wound healing is enabled. To avoid a second manipulation we recommend the use of absorbable sutures, which adapt to the skin, with an intracutaneous suture technique.

The use of bandages is not recommended, because the animals are able to get rid of these uncomfortable wrappings. Depending on the localization of the wound, a wound closing spray can sometimes protect the incision against flies and dirt in the pen.

Avoid Stress!

Underfeeding of animals can cause acute stress-induced myopathy. If the hungry animals realize persons are working in the vicinity and making some noise, they get so excited that this fact could be responsible for ventricular arrhythmias, myocardial infarctions and sudden cardiac death.

Furthermore it is known that pigs in general are very sensitive to stress of any kind and may suddenly die of a generalized myopathy. Some groups used normal pigs and had to learn, that underfeeding, to avoid unmanageable bodyweights in the animals (which can reach 100 kg), can cause myopathy and myocardial necrosis. The most critical period is the first two weeks after insertion of the ameroid constrictor. During this time the myocardium is very vulnerable, due to the progressive chronic ischemia. We learned to spend more money for the much smaller and more robust mini-pigs, which reach a maximum weight of 35–40 kg.

Development of Collaterals

The development of collaterals depends on the coronary morphology. If a right dominant coronary artery supplies most of the posterior wall, a constrictor to the small circumflex artery is not able to induce a region of chronic myocardial ischemia. On the other hand, it is dangerous to occlude a dominant left coronary artery with a large circumflex vessel with an ameroid constrictor. The pig will not die immediately, but the constrictor could provoke left heart failure, because the area of chronic ischemia may become too big.

To be sure to have a sufficient model of chronic ischemia, one has to perform previous coronary angiography.

The development of collaterals to the ischemic region also depends on the coronary artery flow distribution. With a right dominant system, the collaterals will spread retrogradely from the right side up to the circumflex artery; in case of a small right coronary artery, the collaterals will grow anterogradely from the left artery.

Damage to Arteries and Veins during Implantation

If a side branch of the circumflex artery is incidentally damaged during dissection of the circumflex artery, many authors record, that ligature of small vessels will be tolerated by the animal without any myocardial deficiencies. If the main circumflex artery is damaged or torn, there are no reports of any ongoing successful experiments. Most of the pigs died at once or on the same day after transferring them into their pen. Damaged veins can usually be ligated without any problems.

Immunohistochemical Methods

The investigators should be aware that the detection of proliferation markers is limited by the half-life of the antigens (about 30–60 min) and an immediate fixation of the specimens is necessary to prevent false negative results.

Electronmicroscopical Methods

The preparation of specimens for electron microscopy needs very fast fixation of the tissue to prevent autolytic alterations in the cells. After about 10 min post-mortem the first signs of autolysis (swollen mitochondria and reticulum as well as myelin figures) can be detected and can no longer be distinguished from intra-vital degenerative lesions.

References

Bloor CM, White FC, Sanders TM (1984) Effects of exercise on collateral development in myocardial ischemia in pigs. J Appl Physiol 56: 656–665

Charney R, Cohen M (1993) The role of coronary collateral circulation in limiting myocardial ischemia and infarct size. Am Heart J 126: 937–943

Diegeler A, Schneider J, Laier B, Mohr FW, Kluge R (1998) Transmyocardial laser revascularisation using the Helium – YAG laser for treatment of end stage coronary artery disease. Eur J Cardiothorac Surg 13: 3927

Green JA, Edwards RE, Manson M (1998) Immunohistochemical detection of bromodeoxyuridine-labeled nuclei for *in vivo* cell kinetic studies. Methods Mol Biol 80: 251–254

Harada K, Friedmann M, Lopez JJ, Wang SY, Li J, Prasad J, Pearlman PV, Edelmann JD, Sellke ER, Simons M (1996) Vascular endothelial growth factor administration in chronic myocardial ischemia. Am J Physiol Herat Circ Physiol 270: H1791–H1802

Hardonk MJ, Harms G (1990) The use of 5'-bromodoxyuridine in the study of cell proliferation. Acta histochemica [Suppl XXXIX]: 99–100

Horvath KA, Chiu E, Maun DC, Lomasney JW, Greene R, Pearce WH, Fullerton DA (1999) Up-regulation of vascular endothelial growth factor mRNA and angiogenesis after transmyocardial laser revascularization. Ann Thorac Surg 68: 825–829

Hughes GC, Lowe JE, Kypson AP, Louis JDST, Pippen AM, Peters KG, Coleman RE, DeGrado TR, Donovan CL, Annex BH, Landolfo KP (1998) Neovascularization after transmyocardial laser revascularizatiom in a model of chronic ischemia. Ann Thorac Surg 66: 2029–203

Kawamoto A, Tkebuchava T, Yamaguchi J et al. (2003) Intramyocardial transplantation of auto-logous endothelial progenitor cells for therapeutic neovascularization of myocardial ischemia. Circulation 107: 461–468

Krabatsch T, Schäper F, Leder C, Tülsner J, Thalmann U, Hetzer R (1996) Histological findings after transmyocardial laser revascularization. J Card Surg 11: 326–331

Lazarous DF, Shou M, Scheinowitz M, Hodge E, Thirumurti V, Kitsiou AN, Stiber JA, Lobo AD, Hunsberger S, Guetta E, Epstein SE, Unger EF (1996) Comparative effects of basic fibroblast growth factor and vascular endothelial growth factor on coronary collateral development and the arterial response to injury. Circulation 94: 1074–1082

Lopez JJ, Laham RJ, Stamler A, Bunting S, Kaplan A, Carrozza JP, Sellke FW, Simons M (1998) VEGF administration in chronic myocardial ischemia in pigs. Cardiovasc Res 40: 272–281

Maxwell M, Hearse D, Yellon D (1987) Species variation in the coronary collateral circulation during regional myocardial ischemia: A critical determinant of the rate of evolution and extent of myocardial infarction. Cardiovasc Res 21: 737–746

O'Konski MS, White FC, Longhurst J, Roth D, Bloor CM (1987) Ameroid constriction of the proximal left circumflex coronary artery in swine. A model of limited coronary collateral circulation. Am J Cardiovasc Pathol 1: 69–77

Operschall C, Falivene L, Clozel J-P, Roux S (2000) A new model of chronic cardiac ischemia in rabbits. J Appl Physiol 88: 1438–1445

Roth DM, White FC, Nichols ML, Dobbs SL, Longhurst JC, Bloor CM (1990) Effect of long-term exercise on regional myocardial function and coronary collateral development after gradual coronary artery occlusion in pigs. Circulation 82: 1778–1789

Roth DM, Maruoka Y, Rogers J, White FC, Longhurst JC, Bloor CM (1997) Development of coronary collateral circulation in left circumflex ameroid-occluded swine myocardium. Am J Physiol 253: 1279–1288

Schaper W, Flameng W, Winkler B, Wusten B, Turschmann W, Neugebauer G, Carl M, Pasyk S (1976) Quantification of collateral resistance in acute and chronic experimental coronary occlusion in the dog. Circ Res 39: 1377

Scheel KW, Rodriques RJ, Ingram LA (1977) Directional coronary collateral growth with chronic circumflex occlusion in the dog. Circ Res 40: 384–390

Shen YT, Kudej RK, Bishop SP, Vatner SF (1996) Inotropic reserve and histological appearance of hibernating myocardium in conscious pigs with ameroid-induced coronary stenosis. Basic Res Cardiol 91: 479–485

Weihrauch D, Zimmermann R, Arras M, Schaper J (1994) Expression of extracelllar matrix proteins and the role of fibroblast and macrophages in repair processes in ischemic porcine myocardium. Cell Mol Biol Res 40: 105–116

White FC, Bloor CM, McKirnan MD, Carroll SM (1998a) Exercise training in swine promotes growth of arteriolar bed and capillary angiogenesis in heart. J Appl Physiol 85: 1160–1168

White FC, Carroll SM, Magnet A, Bloor CM (1992) Coronary collateral development in swine after coronary artery occlusion. Circ Res 71: 1490–1500

White FC, Roth DM, Bloor CM (1998b) Coronary collateral reserve during exercise induced ischemia in swine. Basic Res Cardiol 84: 42–54

White FC, Roth DM, Bloor CM (1986) The pig as a model for myocardial ischemia and exercise. Lab Anim Sci 36: 351–356

Yu CC-W, Woods AL, Levison DA (1992) The assessment of cellular proliferation by immunohistochemistry: a review of currently available methods and their applications. Histochemical J 24: 121–131

Models on Left Ventricular Hypertrophy (LVH)

Thomas Walther and Volkmar Falk

Introduction

Left ventricular hypertrophy (LVH) is defined as an increase in left ventricular mass. Myocyte growth as well as changes in interstitial tissue (extracellular matrix) contributes to the development of LVH. Concentric LVH is characterized by a similar increase of all diameters, namely the anterior, posterior, lateral, septal and apical parts of the left ventricle. The increase in myocardial mass is caused by an enlargement of the myocytes. In mammals (rat, rabbit, dog, whale, humans) non hypertrophied myocytes constantly measure 10–12 μm in diameter whereas in LVH they are >15 μm (Poche et al. 1996).

Pressure overload leads to concentric LVH which can be clinically diagnosed in parallel to arterial hypertension, valvular aortic stenosis and coarctation of the aorta. Development of LVH involves pathological changes. Initially LVH coincides with preserved left ventricular function but ultimately may lead to ventricular failure. As proven by a large scale population study, the Framingham study, LVH coincides with an increased incidence of cardiac morbid events, namely sudden cardiac death, cardiac failure, myocardial infarction and stroke. Thus LVH is an independent cardiac risk factor and a major determinant for patient outcome as it is associated with increased morbidity and mortality (Levy et al. 1990; Yacoub 2001).

The process of myocardial remodeling has many causes, including changes in pressure load conditions and an interplay of different growth effectors and inhibitors.

Reverse remodeling with normalization of left ventricular mass can be anticipated after corrective therapy, for example, aortic valve replacement in patients having severe aortic stenosis. Reverse remodeling has been clinically documented by serial echocardiographic follow-up studies (Krayenbuehl et al. 1989; Walther et al. 1999). However, the underlying cellular and molecular changes in the myocardium are not yet completely understood. We performed experimental studies to prove reverse remodeling of myocardial gene expression after corrective surgical therapy resembling myocardial restoration after aortic valve replacement (Walther et al. 2001, 2002).

The high incidence of patients having LVH (approximately 25% of the population suffer from arterial hypertension in western civilizations and aortic stenosis is the most frequent heart valve disease) and its potentially severe consequences documented by the Framingham study, underline the importance of further research in this field. For thorough analysis, sufficient experimental models mimicking LVH are required to further study potential therapeutic approaches.

Methods and practical approach

Experimental models for studying LVH can be divided into studies on small (mouse, rat, rabbit, cat) and large (pig, sheep, dog, monkey) animals. The use of any of these animals has individual advantages and disadvantages. Small animals are cheaper and easier to handle. Usually a larger number of interventions can be performed without too many restrictions. However, some measurements and interventions, comparable to common medical practice on humans, are not possible on small animals. Repeated surgical interventions are difficult; technically all interventions require sufficient expertise.

In contrast, the use of large animals is restricted by practical problems such as having sufficient capabilities for animal care, stalls, a large operative theatre etc. These animals are more expensive and require special peri-operative handling. The advantage is, the close similarity to human heart size and function, leading to meaningful results when extrapolating to future patient therapies.

There are several different models to establish LVH, all aiming at an increase in ventricular workload. Ultimately an increase in ventricular workload can lead to ventricular failure, thus there are several aspects where LVH and heart failure models are overlapping. LVH can be induced by creating pressure or volume overload. Common models for pressure overload include banding of the aorta or the pulmonary artery, or creation of aortic valve or pulmonary valve stenosis (Burrington 1978; Copeland et al. 1974; Rodger et al. 1971; Walther et al. 2000). Volume overload can be achieved by any arterio-venous shunt of the femoral, jugular and/or abdominal vessels or by creating valvular insufficiency. Some difficulties, shortcomings and limitations exist for all these models.

When inducing LVH, the ventricle must compensate for the increased workload. This will lead to hypertrophy and/or dilatation and can lead to, but must not ultimately lead to heart failure. Several individual factors are decisive, mostly the amount of pressure or volume overload implemented within a distinct period of time. When aiming at chronic experiments, a gradual increase in workload would be best to achieve a gra-dual adaptation and compensation of the ventricle without failure.

The optimal strategy to achieve a gradual increase in ventricular workload is to take advantage of animal growth. As such, pressure or volume overload should be induced when the animals weigh about one third to one half of their final body weight. With gradual further growth, any fixed banding, for example, will lead to a functionally smaller and smaller lumen.

Growth may lead to perforations but these adverse events are relatively rare and usually 80 to 90% of the animals will be available for further studies (Walther et al. 2000, 2001). Thus only moderate stricture is applied initially, with subsequently increasing pressure load over time.

Development of LVH will not always be possible within a distinct period of time. To achieve relatively fast changes, a combination of pressure and volume overload can be applied. However, this may ultimately lead to earlier ventricular failure.

The usual time frame for significant LVH to develop is difficult to predict. We applied routine monthly echocardiographic control examinations. After applying supracoronary banding in 6 to 8 month old sheep (body weight about half of the full grown weight) we were able to induce a highly significant increase in left ventricular mass after 8.3 ±1 month. This led to compensated LVH without a significant increase in episodes of heart failure (Walther et al. 2000, 2001). Overall, the time frame may be variable and serial echocardiographic examinations are required.

Anesthesia should be performed according to the special needs of the species chosen. General anesthesia is usually recommended with mechanical ventilation while performing the thoracotomy. Induction can be easily accomplished using intramuscular Ketamine, together with a dose of benzodiazepines. For intubation specially prolonged blades of the laryngoscope are helpful. Inhalative agents such as Isoflurane are convenient for sustained anaesthesia, some morphine analgesic (e. g. Fentanyl) and eventually a small dose of muscle relaxant will be required. All these should be discontinued with chest closure at the latest. Low dosages of all anesthetics are recommended in order to achieve an early extubation and then reintegration of the animal with others of their species. Any adequately sized tube (between 8 and 16 mm in large animals, otherwise smaller) will serve as a nasogastric tube. This is essential if sternotomy is performed in order to prevent aspiration. Temporary chest tube insertion (approximately 1 to 3 hours) with persistent suction will be required to avoid pneumothorax and atelectasis before extubation. Use of a redon drain connected to a premade vacuum bottle is helpful whenever continuous suction is not available or in case the animals are already mobilized. Extubation should be performed as soon as the animals are sufficiently breathing, awake and almost chewing their tube out.

Hemodynamic measurements should be performed as required. These may include central venous access and pressure as well as an arterial line for continuous pressure monitoring and blood gas analyses. These lines can be partially introduced using common percutaneous techniques. However, in some instances surgical incision after cutdown of the vessel is required. Whenever banding is performed, direct pressure measurement before the banding (done eventually with a temporary needle introduced intraoperatively) and after the banding for direct measurements of the pressure gradient, is highly recommended.

Echocardiography should be applied whenever available. Immediate evaluation of the amount of pressure or volume overload induced, as well as an assessment of ventricular function, can be performed. Acute deterioration of ventricular function diagnosed by echocardiographic measurements early after banding should lead to immediate reversal. Otherwise early heart failure may result. Transthoracic echocardiographic measurements can be performed with an unsterile probe out of, or with a sterilely draped probe within the surgical field. Transesophageal echocardiography allows an excellent visualization of the ascending aorta in most animals (Walther et al. 2000). However, assessment of ventricular function is difficult because of reduced visualization due to the shape of the thorax of different species. Another option is to use a sub-xiphoid transdiaphragmal approach with a small intraperitoneal incision for advancing the sterilely draped echocardiographic probe. Almost optimal visualization can be achieved with the transabdominal approach.

Surgical access for inducing LVH should be chosen according to personal experience, species related factors, as well as the type of procedure planned. Aortic or pulmonary artery banding should be performed via a lateral minithoracotomy whenever possible. A left sided anterolateral thoracotomy in the fourth or the fifth intercostal space will provide optimal exposure of the main pulmonary artery and of the ascending aorta that lies more posteriorly. The descending thoracic aorta can be easily reached via a left posterolateral thoracotomy. In both instances the lung can be temporarily retracted with a swab. Performing additional partial rib resection will provide optimal visualization for further transthoracic echocardiographic studies. A sternotomy in comparison to a lateral thoracotomy would provide a wide and thus optimal access. However, there are several advantages of avoiding a sternotomy: Wound healing will be much improved with a lateral thoracotomy. Most of the animals usually lie directly upon their sternum. Due to constant pressure, wound healing problems would have to be anticipated. To avoid this a far lateral incision (about 5 to 7 cm paramedian in sheep for example) and a large skin and muscle flap is highly recommended whenever a sternotomy cannot be avoided. Furthermore whenever a study with repeated operations is planned, it is helpful to preserve the sternotomy approach for the reoperation. This can then usually be performed later without severe adhesions.

Banding should be performed using slightly pliable material that can eventually be easily detached from the vessel. Easy detachment is very helpful if repeat interventions with debanding are planned. We were able to successfully detach a 5 mm wide polyester band (Mersilene®, Ethicon, Norderstedt, Germany) from the aorta in sheep (Walther et al. 2001). From our clinical experience, especially for the treatment of congenital heart defects, any silicone material, for example silicone elastomer is advantageous.

During the operation the pleural space (especially the right one in a left anterolateral thoracotomy) should not be opened if possible. This will prevent pleural adhesions and reduce the risk of pneumothorax. The pericardium is opened longitudinally just over the target vessels. Two to four pericardial stay sutures will improve surgical exposure. Later pericardial closure should be performed whenever tolerated, to prevent severe adhesions.

Positioning of the band should be performed after careful blunt dissection between the aorta and the main pulmonary artery. A stay suture around the main pulmonary artery can be helpful to improve exposure of the ascending aorta. The band should then be positioned by using a blunt instrument and gentle traction only.

Tying the band can be performed down to preset circumference markers to achieve a standardized reduction of the cross-sectional area of the ascending aorta. These were calculated to reduce the cross-sectional area of the ascending aorta by 25% in our growing sheep model (Walther et al. 2000). The clinical effect of the band is then controlled by measuring the direct pressure gradients. Titan clips are helpful for initial adjustment before measuring the pressure gradient and then finally tying the band. A schematic view of supracoronary banding in sheep via a left anterolateral minithoracotomy is given in Figure 1.

Creation of valvular incompetence can be accomplished in different ways (Gross 1994; Morais et al. 1957; Spratt et al. 1983). With catheter interventions, perforations could be established, however, these are quite unpredictable in severity. Thus they are not very helpful to establish a controlled and reliable amount model of LVH. The surgical approach is feasible in a more or less blind fashion via the atrial appendages or with extra-corporal circulation (ECC) with or without cardiac arrest. ECC could be established via the femoral vessels in larger animals or by direct thoracic cannulation

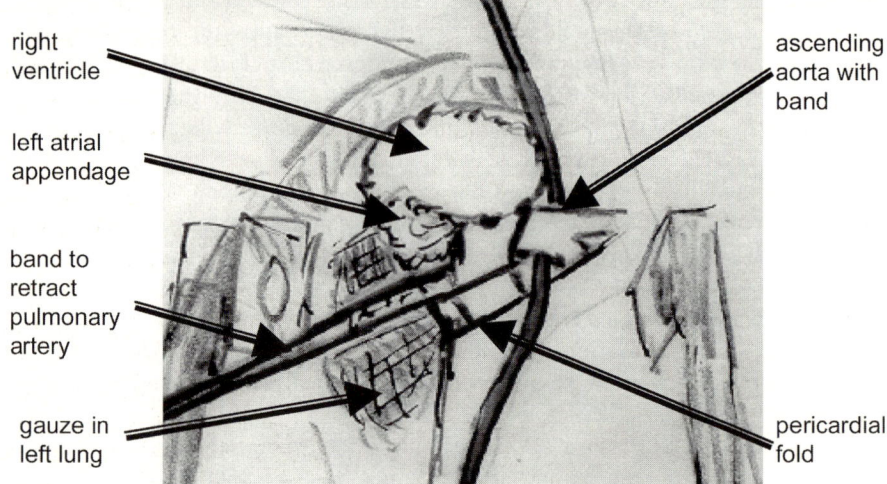

Figure 1
Schematic drawing of supracoronary aortic banding in sheep via a left anterolateral minithoracotomy. The edges of the rib retractor can be seen at both inferior and lateral aspects of the image

when using sternotomy or lateral thoracotomy. All approaches have special advantages and disadvantages, the most invasive strategy applying ECC will lead to the most reproducible results and vice versa.

Access for surgical induction of valvular incompetence should be similar as described for banding of the aorta. The left atrial appendage can be easily reached via a left lateral thoracotomy, the right one from the right side. Thus mitral and tricuspid valves can be targeted. When attempting to induce aortic valve incompetence a sternotomy, approach should be considered.

Shunt models to establish volume overload are relatively straight forward to apply (Gross 1994; Flaim et al. 1979). The femoral or the jugular vein can be directly anastomosed end to side to the corresponding artery. Measurement of shunt flow can be accomplished with a flow probe intraoperatively. Eventually two shunts are required. Postoperative control of shunt flow can be easily performed with palpation and/or echocardiographic examinations. As mentioned before, the generation of shunts may lead to progressive heart failure.

Examples

In the following paragraph different examples of models to achieve LVH will be given. Basically the different techniques available to generate an increased ventricular workload can be combined in whatever species is to be studied. Technical details for inducing LVH as well as shortcomings and pitfalls of the different models have also been mentioned previously. Initially different methods to induce pressure overload hypertrophy and models to achieve volume overload will be mentioned:

- Ventricular pressure overload can be induced using banding of the aorta or the pulmonary artery. These techniques have been applied to different species successfully (Bishop et al. 1976; Burrington et al. 1978; Cooper et al. 1984; Mirsky et al. 1980; Olivetti et al. 1989; Walther et al. 2000; Walther et al. 2001; Welham et al. 1978). Materials for banding include nylon, polyester, silicone or even a dacron tube.
- Acute pressure overload can be induced by applying a side biting clamp to the ascending aorta. Acute effects can then be studied on the open chest (Pirzada et al. 1976). Theoretically the aorta can be plicated leading to prolonged overload, eventually resulting in a chronic condition.
- An inflatable cuff or a hydraulic occluder can be applied around the aorta or the main pulmonary artery (Crozatier et al. 1984).
- In the aortic position it is important to decide upon supracoronary banding leading to atypical coronary blood flow or infracoronary (supravalvular) banding. Supracoronary banding is easier to achieve and carries a low risk of myocardial ischemia, however it does not completely represent the clinical situation of aortic stenosis. Infracoronary banding is technically much more difficult to induce. In most animals the left main stem descends deep down close to the aortic valve. The right coronary artery may still be perfused under high pressure thus changing the relation of myocardial blood supply (Iyengar et al. 1973; Rodger et al. 1971).
- An ameroid clip has been used around the aorta, leading to increased obstruction due to gradual swelling. However, the amount of constriction is difficult to control with this model, leading to a great variability in the experimental result (Schwartz 1973).
- Banding of the aorta or pulmonary artery, done in young animals to take advantage of further growth, has also been described by several studies (Ishihara et al. 1992; O'Kane et al. 1973; Rodger et al. 1971). This is our method of choice as well and we would strongly recommend planning any experiments in such a manner (Walther et al. 2000, 2001).
- Shunts usually lead to high output cardiac failure, possibly associated with left ventricular hypertrophy. Timing of the optimal period for further studies as well as the amount of cardiac output shunted is critical. Different shunt positions are feasible. However, creation of a modified Blalock-Taussig shunt for example, would be technically more demanding than a peripheral one. Thus this cannot be recommended. Aorto-caval shunts have been used in rats to redirect about 50% of the total cardiac output (Flaim 1979). Two months were allowed for recovery before the animals were further used.
- More peripheral shunts are a standard model for the initial induction of LVH, as such unilateral or bilateral femoral artery vein shunts can be applied to induce left ventricular overload (Conway et al. 1975). This results in myocardial hypertrophy and later on, heart failure. In our own laboratory we used unilateral jugular vein to carotid artery shunts. To increase the volume overload and achieve faster ventricular dilatation and deterioration towards heart failure, we applied bilateral jugular vein to common carotid artery shunts in sheep. These measure approximately 4 to 6 mm in diameter, flow measurements showed about 1 l/min shunt

volume. The time frame to deterioration is variable, serial echocardiographic examinations are helpful and a period of 3 to 8 months has to be anticipated. Models on heart failure will be discussed in detail in another chapter.

- Models on valve failure comprise another option to increase left ventricular workload by volume overload and thus induce LVH. Quite comparable to shunts the exact amount of volume overload is difficult to measure and control. Thus all these models may result in different degrees of hypertrophy and/or failure of the ventricle. As mentioned earlier, there is a fluent transition from compensated hypertrophy to ventricular failure.

  On the mitral or tricuspid valves distinct chordae can be cut in order to obtain significant regurgitation (Morais et al. 1957). The exact amount of chordae to be cut is difficult to assess. Other models imply perforations of the valve with blades or punches that are available in selected sizes. The instruments can be guided with a finger through the atrium. As pointed out earlier induction of valvular insufficiency can be performed in a more controlled setting when using ECC. However, this is a much more complex procedure.

- Simulation of mitral valve incompetence can be performed by implanting a shunt between the left ventricle and the left atrium (Spratt 1983). Negative side effects are a high left atrial pressure with pulmonary congestion and eventually pulmonary edema. This may lead to early and/or sudden heart failure in several cases.

- Aortic valve incompetence can be induced by similar puncture techniques or under direct vision requiring a much greater effort (ECC etc.) as described previously (Ito et al. 1974). A standard punch of 4 or 5 mm instead of a wire or blade would be more precise to create reliable and repeatable results. However, this will be difficult if not impossible to perform without ECC.

- Aortic valve stenosis can be achieved by direct clipping or suturing of the cusps (Copeland et al. 1974). Tearing of the thin cusp tissue can lead to additional valve incompetence. The amount of valvular lesion is always difficult to control with these models.

Whenever planning for one of these models individual factors have to be taken into account. All animals are individuals and studies in different laboratories show at least some slight discrepancies.

Quantification of the effects created should be performed whenever possible using direct pressure measurements, flow measurements or routine echocardiographic controls. Combinations of different models are feasible to achieve an accelerated effect. However, earlier heart failure may be the result.

Regarding the choice of animals, individual and species related factors as well as local availabilities have to be taken into account. Dogs for example are more difficult to control than pigs or sheep after an intervention. Among all large animals sheep are relatively easy to handle and are quite tolerant in terms of wound healing, nutrition, preoperative fasting, housing and postoperative care. Furthermore, in sheep there is a low risk of cardiac arrhythmia during open heart operations. When planning such experiments, ethical issues must be considered, especially when considering dogs or even monkeys the primary choice.

We performed serial experiments in sheep inducing LVH initially in growing animals 6 to 8 months of age, performing surgical therapy after a mean interval of 8 months and examining reverse remodeling of the left ventricle after another 9 months. In the following paragraph we will give our protocol as a step by step example:

All surgical interventions were performed under general anesthesia with central venous access and endotracheal intubation as described earlier. The animals were positioned in theatre according to the access chosen. For the initial left lateral thoracotomy they were positioned on the right side. The thoracotomy was performed in the fourth intercostal space. Step by step control of any bleeding is important, this can be easily performed using electro-cautery. Usually, the left pleural space was opened, then the pericardium was dissected bluntly. The pericardium was incised for about 5 cm just above the main pulmonary artery, then the edges were fixed with stay sutures. Then the main pulmonary artery was dissected further and entrapped with a blunt retraction tape. Left ventricular biopsies were taken through the left atrial appendage and secured with a purse-string using conventional biopsy forceps. Afterwards the aorta was mobilized. We then measured the diameter to calculate the length of the band required for a reduction of 25% of crossectional area. Banding of the ascending aorta was then performed using a 5 mm wide Polyester-Band (Mersilene®, Ethicon, Norderstedt, Germany). Left ventricular and common carotid artery pressures were measured online for further control. An instantaneous gradient between 20 and 30 mmHg was achieved.

After control of bleeding the pericardium was closed, a chest drain inserted (see above), the ribs attached and the wound closed. After banding the animals were extubated early and were brought back to their flock of sheep within one hour. Daily wound control was performed. The chest drains were kept for approximately one day.

On our model, repeated surgical interventions were performed via a median sternotomy. We performed a right paramedian incision (about 5 cm) and performed a skin and muscle flap to the left side. Then a median sternotomy was performed. With this incision we did not observe any wound infections later on. The left femoral artery was dissected in case ECC support was required during debanding. The pericardium was opened and retracted using stay sutures. There were moderate to severe adhesions around the ascending aorta. After careful dissection we were able to detach the band from the aortic wall without destroying its integrity. The band was resected at a length of at least two thirds of the circumference of the aorta. In case of severe adhesions an end to end anastomosis of the aorta under right atrial to femoral artery ECC, moderate hypothermia of 32 °C and cardioplegic cardiac arrest (blood cardioplegia) was performed. Left ventricular biopsies were obtained via the left apex after securing it with a purse-string.

After control of the bleeding the pericardium was closed, the sternum was fixed using steel wires, and then the incision was closed carefully.

After this operation we aimed at early extubation again. All animals received sufficient pain medication. They were supervised for one night close to the theatre and then returned to their flock of sheep the next morning. Chest drains were usually removed by then.

We performed the third and final intervention via a repeated median sternotomy approach. This time there were dense adhesions requiring careful dissection. All repeat measurements were performed similarly to the first two interventions. Biopsies were obtained after retrieving the whole heart. The animals were then sacrificed.

This gives only one example on how to surgically induce LVH and on how to perform repeated interventions. Any modifications can be performed according to individual requirements.

Troubleshooting

All models on LVH described imply surgical techniques to manipulate normal hemodynamic function. These can be complicated by different factors, initially related to surgical intervention, to the species chosen or to the increased hemodynamic workload created. Some of the possible complications have already been mentioned.

Most of these pitfalls are common complications that can happen during any surgical intervention. These include all kinds of infections and wound healing problems, hemodynamic instabilities, respiratory problems or post-intervention organ dysfunction. Listing all of them is beyond the scope of this review.

Species related factors should be considered when planning any project. Surgical access has to be planned carefully as most laboratory animals directly lie upon their sternum. Thus a sternotomy approach should be avoided whenever planning on chronic experiments. The possible alternative of using a large skin and muscle flap has been described above.

Some model related factors have already been described previously. We think that banding is the best and most convenient method to achieve controlled isolated LVH. Progression to heart failure usually occurs later. Thus banding can be much better controlled than any shunt or valvular incompetence model, the latter usually leading to progressive heart failure.

Generation of increased ventricular workload may be complicated by problems such as inconsistent degrees of LVH or aortic rupture and eventually development of heart failure (Crozatier et al. 1984; Gross 1994; Mercadier et al. 1981; O'Kane et al. 1973). These problems, especially aortic rupture, are difficult to avoid completely. The use of a relatively wide band of at least 4 to 5 mm is advantageous. Additional wrapping of the aorta with a dacron tube has not shown any additional benefit. Thus it has to be accepted that when using a banding model during the development of significant LVH there may be a loss of up to 20% of the animals (Gross 1994). This has to be included in the initial calculation.

Acute cardiac failure during banding can be diagnosed by hemodynamic monitoring, control echocardiography and direct visualization. Careful adaptation of the band in order to prevent failure should be performed. In the case of acute degeneration a fixed band can be easily cut and the heart will recover almost immediately. Acute failure after generating a valvular defect would be difficult to treat and would require surgical intervention. Standard medication such as volume therapy, eventually ACE Inhibitors and temporary inotropic support can be applied. The anesthetist should always be prepared when inducing acute hemodynamic changes. When using shunt models decompensation should occur less frequently. Temporary closure of the shunt with a snare or a clamp will be the immediate and best therapy.

Pulmonary failure after the initial operation may occur as a consequence of the operative intervention (pneumothorax, infection) or as a consequence of the hemodynamic changes (pulmonary congestion, pulmonary edema). Chest drainage, antibiotic therapy and medication such as ACE inhibitors or temporary inotropic support can be applied.

Measurement of the direct effects generated can sometimes be difficult due to variable hemodynamic conditions and the fact that the animals usually are under general anaesthesia during the surgical interventions. It has to be considered that the hemodynamic effects induced may be aggravated later on as soon as the animals are awake and under physical exercise or stress conditions.

Whenever possible, invasive hemodynamic measurements should be performed for quantification of the effect induced. In addition, echocardiographic baseline data are very helpful for ambulatory follow-up measurements during chronic experiments.

The optimal amount of increased ventricular workload to be induced is difficult to predict. With all methods available and presented some degree of LVH can be achieved but the final amount is mostly beyond practical control.

References

Bishop SP, Melsen LR (1976) Myocardial necrosis, fibrosis and DNA synthesis in experimental cardiac hypertrophy induced by sudden pressure overload. Circ Res 39: 238–45

Burrington JD (1978) Response to experimental coarctation of aorta and pulmonic stenosis in fetal lamb. J Thorac Cardiovasc Surg 75: 819–826

Conway G, Heazlitt RA, Montag J, Mattingly SF (1975) The ATPase activity of cardiac myosin from failing and hypertrophied hearts. J Mol Cell Cardiol 7: 817–822

Cooper G, Marino TA (1984) Complete reversibility of cat right ventricular chronic progressive pressure overload. Circ Res 54: 323–331

Copeland JG, Marm BJ, Luka NL, Ferrans VJ, Michaelis LL (1974) Experimental production of aortic valvular stenosis: short-term and long-term studies in dogs. J Thorac Cardiovasc Surg 67: 361–379

Crozatier B, Caillet D, Bical O (1984) Left ventricular adaption to sustained pressure overload in the conscious dog: Circ Res 54: 21–29

Flaim SF, Minteer WJ, Nellis SH, Clark DP (1979) Chronic arteriovenous shunt: evaluation of a model for heart failure in rat. Am J Physiol 236: H698–H704

Gross DR (1994) Iatrogenic models for studying heart disease. In Gross DR: Animal models in cardiovascular research, 2nd edn. Kluwer, Dordrecht Boston London

Ishihara K, Zile MR, Tomita M, Tanaka R, Kanazawa S, Carabello BA (1992) Left ventricular hypertrophy in a canine model of reversible pressure overload. Cardiovasc Res 26: 580–585

Ito J, Suko J, Chidsey CA (1974) Intracellular calcium and myocardial contractility. V. Calcium uptake of sarcoplasmatic reticulum fractions in hypertrophied and failing rabbit hearts. J Mol Cell Cardiol 6: 237–243

Iyengar SR, Charrette EJ, Iyengar CK, Lynn RB (1973) An experimental model with left ventricular hypertrophy caused by subcoronary aortic stenosis in dogs. J Thorac Cardiovasc Surg 66: 823–827

Krayenbuehl HP, Hess OM, Monrad ES, Schneider J, Mall G, Turina M (1989) Left ventricular myocardial structure in aortic valve disease before, intermediate, and late after aortic valve replacement. Circulation 79: 744–755

Levy D, Garrison RJ, Savage DD, Kannel WB, Castelli WP (1990) Prognostic Implications of echocardiographically determined left ventricular mass in the Framingham heart study. N Engl J Med 322: 1561–1566

Mercadier JJ, Lompre AM, Wisnewski C, Samuel JL, Bercovivi J, Swynghedauw B, Schwartz K (1981) Myosin isoenzyme changes in several models of rat cardiac hypertrophy. Circ Res 49: 525–532

Mirsky I, Laks MM (1980) Time course of changes in the mechanical properties of the canine right and left ventricles during hypertrophy caused by pressure overload. Circ Res 46: 530–542

Morais DJ, Richart TS, Fritz AJ, Acree PW, Davila JC, Glover RP (1957) The production of chronic experimental mitral insufficiency. Ann Surg 145: 500–508

O'Kane HO, Geha AS, Kleiger RE, Abe T, Salaymeh MT, Malik AB (1973) Stable left ventricular hypertrophy in the dog. J Thorac Cardiovasc Surg 65: 264–271

Olivetti G, Lagrasta C, Ricci R, Sonnenblick EH, Capasso JM, Anversa P (1989) Long-term pressure-induced cardiac hypertrophy: capillary and mast cell proliferation. Am J Physiol 257: H1766–1772

Pirzada FA, Ekong EA, Vokonas PS, Apstein CS, Hood WB Jr (1976) Experimental myocardial infarction. XIII. Sequential changes in left ventricular pressure-length relationships in the acute phase. Circulation 53: 970–975

Poche R, Hauptmann S, Poche-de-Vos F (1996) Strukturelle Veränderungen des druck- und volumenüberlasteten Herzens. In Roskamm H, Reindell H (eds) Herzkrankheiten, Springer, Berlin Heidelberg New York, pp 131–139

Rodger WA, Bishop SP, Hamlin RL (1971) Experimental production of supravalvular aortic stenosis in the dog. J Appl Physiol 30: 917–920

Schwartz A (1973) Biochemical studies concerning etiology of hypertrophy, heart failure and cardiomyopathy. Rec Adv Stud Cardiac Struct Metab 2: 501–502

Spratt JA, Olsen CO, Tyson GS Jr, Glower DD Jr, Davis JW, Rankin JS (1983) Experimental mitral regurgitation. Physiological effects of correction on left ventricular dynamics. J Thorac Cardiovasc Surg 86: 479–489

Walther T, Falk V, Langebartels G, Krüger M, Bernhardt U, Diegeler A, Gummert J, Autschbach R, Mohr FW (1999) Prospectively randomized evaluation of stentless versus conventional biological aortic valves: Impact on early regression of left ventricular hypertrophy. Circulation 100 [Suppl II]: II6–II10

Walther T, Schubert A, Falk V, Binner C, Kanev A, Bleiziffer S, Walther C, Doll N, Autschbach R, Mohr FW (2001) Regression of left ventricular hypertrophy after surgical therapy for aortic stenosis is associated with changes in extracellular matrix gene expression. Circulation 104 [Suppl 1]: I-54-I-58

Walther T, Schubert A, Falk V, Binner C, Walther C, Doll N, Fabricius A, Dhein S, Gummert J, Mohr FW (2002) Left ventricular reverse remodeling after surgical therapy for aortic stenosis: correlation to Renin-Angiotensin system gene expression. Circulation 106 [Suppl 1]: I23–26

Walther T, Falk V, Binner C, Löscher N, Schubert A, Rauch T, von Oppel U, Autschbach R, Mohr FW (2000) Experimental aortic stenosis and corresponding left ventricular hypertrophy in sheep. J Invest Surg 13: 327–331

Welham KC, Silove ED, Wyse RK (1978) Experimental right ventricular hypertrophy and failure in swine. Cardiovasc Res 12: 61–65

Yacoub MH (2001) A novel strategy to maximize the efficacy of left ventricular assist devices as a bridge to recovery. Eur Heart J 22: 534–540

Experimental Models of Heart Failure

Volkmar Falk, Jens Garbade and Thomas Walther

Introduction

Congestive heart failure is one of the leading causes of cardiovascular morbidity and mortality. In the United States alone 550,000 new cases are diagnosed each year. Heart failure causes approximately 40,000 deaths a year and is a contributing factor in another 225,000 deaths in the US, where the death rate attributed to heart failure rose by 148% from 1979 to 2000. Hospital discharges for CHF in the US rose from 377,000 in 1979 to 990,000 in 2000, an increase of 165% causing a substantial economic burden.

Congestive heart failure is a clinical syndrome caused by left ventricular dysfunction, remodelling and activation of neurohormonal systems. CHF is caused by a variety of underlying diseases that alter left ventricular function, geometry and structure. Substantial pharmacological as well as surgical research is performed to treat and to alter the cause of CHF, generating the need for small and large animal models of heart failure (Hongo et al. 1997, Roos and Ikeda 2002, Yarbrough and Spinale 2003).

A number of animal models that mimic heart failure exist and will be discussed in this chapter. Besides some naturally occurring models, heart failure can be induced by acute or chronic coronary artery occlusion, coronary artery embolization, pressure overload (induced hypertrophy by aortic banding), volume overload (arterio-venous shunts), valvular disruption or tachycardia-induced ventricular dilatation. Other models include the induction of heart failure by applying toxic agents or viral infection. Recently, genetically manipulated animals that develop heart failure have become available.

Following an injury (myocardial infarct, viral infection) myocardial function declines. Initially, a number of adaptive mechanisms are activated to maintain adequate cardiac output and tissue perfusion. Among these are the Frank-Starling mechanism to maintain cardiac output by an increase in preload, compensatory myocardial hypertrophy of unaffected myocardium, activation of the sympathetic system and activation of the renin-angiotensin-aldosterone system to maintain arterial pressure and organ perfusion. Prolonged activation of the neurohormonal systems eventually results in an increase in afterload and enhances structural and functional changes that further reduce cardiac function. This process is termed ventricular remodelling. Chronic sympathetic stimulation leads to desensitization and a decrease in myocardial beta-adrenoreceptor density. As cardiac performance declines, redistribution of blood to vital organs will cause underperfusion of skeletal muscle and kidneys, causing metabolic acidosis and renal failure. Endothelial dysfunction in heart failure contributes to the impaired vasodilator capacity. Functional abnormalities in contractile protein function, excitation-contraction coupling, and myocardial energetics occur with heart failure. As the heart progressively dilates, lysis of myofibrils, distortion of the sarcoplasmic reticulum, myocyte necrosis and alterations in extracellular matrix proteins causing cardiac fibrosis can be observed. In overt heart failure, cardiac output is no longer sufficient to meet the metabolic demands, resulting in end organ damage.

The interaction among the contributing factors for heart failure and ventricular remodelling – cardiac damage, hemodynamic overload and secondary compensating effects – is complex. While pharmacological therapy mainly targets the neurohormonal axis, surgical research focuses on reducing wall stress and myocardial stretch and unloading of the failing ventricle by the use of mechanical assist systems or other means to restore a more favourable left ventricular geometry.

Description of Methods and Practical Approach

Spontaneous Development of Heart Failure Models

In a number of animals heart failure occurs naturally with ageing. Except for some small animal strains like the spontaneously hypertensive rat or the Syrian hamster, the incidence of heart failure in large animal models such as the dog is too unpredictable to make these models useful for laboratory use.

Spontaneously Hypertensive Rats

Spontaneously hypertensive rats (SHR) are widely used as naturally occurring models of heart failure. Introduced in 1963 the rat presents a model of genetic systemic hypertension that leads to heart failure with ageing. Vascular lesions attributed to hypertension in SHR develop early around 6 to 7 weeks. The severity and distribution of affected arteries is greater in SHR males than in females. By week 28, blood pressure is usually increased above 240 mm Hg and the rat has reached advanced stages of hypertension. Following a stable period of compensated hypertrophy with preserved contractility, SHR progress to heart failure with senescence. Between 18 and 24 months of age, clinical signs of heart failure such as weight loss, lethargy, poor grooming and respiratory distress can be detected. In end-stage heart failure severe contractile dysfunction is present in SHR. In many ways, and unlike most other animal models, altered active and passive mechanical properties of myocardial tissue that can be found in the ageing human heart are similar in the SHR model. Gross pathological changes include an increase in LV wet weight and an increase in the ratio of lung wet weight/dry weight indicating pulmonary oedema as well as left atrial thrombi and myocardial fibrosis. The arterioles in spontaneous hypertensive rats show a thickening of the media as an adaptive structural response to an increased pressure load. Arteriolar changes in the myocardium include medial hypertrophy and medial fibrin-oid degeneration. The measurement of intracellular calcium and isometric force in left ventricular trabeculae from spontaneously hypertensive rats indicate that in this animal model of heart failure contractile function is compromised by increased collagen and its three-dimensional organization, rather than by reduced availability of intracellular calcium (Bing et al. 2002; Ward et al. 2003).

Dahl Salt Sensitive Rat

As opposed to the SHR, the Dahl salt sensitive rat (DSS) develops heart failure at an earlier age. When fed with a high salt diet (8% NaCl) after weaning at age 5–8 weeks, concentric hypertrophy develops at age 11 weeks followed by congestive heart failure at age 16 to 20 weeks. The animals show global LV dilatation and hypokinesis, elevated wall stress and neurohormonal activation and usually die within one week after the development of pulmonary congestion (Morii et al. 1998). Recently an increase in a troponin T isoform (TnT3) and a decrease in TnT phosphorylation were found in failing Dahl salt-sensitive rat hearts. Native thin filaments from failing hearts demonstrated a reduction in calcium sensitivity compared with controls, which could be prevented by endothelin receptor blocker treatment (Noguchi et al. 2003).

Syrian Cardiomyopathic Hamster

The Syrian cardiomyopathic hamster suffers from an autosomal recessive deficiency of a 50 kDa dystrophin-associated glycoprotein. The resulting disruption of the dystrophin/dystroglycan complex alters the linkage of the subsarcolemmal cytoskeleton and the extracellular matrix. At an age of 20 to 25 weeks the hamsters develop heart failure (compensated state) that decompensates at the age of 35 weeks.

Dog Models

Like humans, dogs develop heart failure with ageing. The most prevalent type of acquired heart disease in dogs is valvular heart disease. While mitral valve disease is the most common cause of heart failure in smaller breeds, a number of larger breeds (Doberman pinschers, great Danes, labrador retrievers, and boxers) develop cardiomyopathies.

Gene Targeted Models of Heart Failure

With the advancement of molecular biology, animals can be genetically manipulated to study the impact of overexpression or deletion of specific genes involved in the pathophysiology of heart failure. It is possible to breed animals with specific gene defects that cause different types of heart failure. Transgenic mice with overexpression or deficiencies of specific myocardial receptors help to generate a better understanding of the molecular biology of heart failure The following are only a few examples from a fast growing field that holds the promise of developing gene-targeted treatment strategies.

MLP Deficient Mice

Muscle LIM protein is expressed and located at the Z-line and is involved in cytoarchitecture organization. Targeted deletion of the muscle LIM-domain (MLP) protein gene by homologous recombination causes dilated cardiomyopathy. Subsequently, MLP (–/–) mice show a disruption in cardiomyocyte cytoarchitecture.

EBNA-LP Transgenic Mice

Transgenic mice carrying the Epstein-Barr virus nuclear antigen-leader protein (EBNA-LP) develop symptoms of heart failure at 4 months to one year. The mice show LV dilatation, left atrial thrombosis and pulmonary oedema.

Transgenic Mice Overexpressing the PRKAG2 cDNA

Mutations in the $\gamma 2$ subunit (PRKAG2) of AMP-activated protein kinase produce an unusual human cardiomyopathy characterized by ventricular hypertrophy and electrophysiological abnormalities, Wolff-Parkinson-White syndrome (WPW) and progressive degenerative conduction system disease. Pathological examinations of affected human hearts reveal vacuoles containing amylopectin, a glycogen-related substance.

Transgenic mice overexpressing the PRKAG2 cDNA show elevated AMP-activated protein kinase activity, and an accumulation of large amounts of cardiac glycogen. The mice develop dramatic left ventricular hypertrophy, and exhibited ventricular preexcitation and sinus node dysfunction. Electrophysiological testing demonstrated alternative atrioventricular conduction pathways consistent with WPW. Cardiac histopathology revealed that the annulus fibrosis, which normally insulates the ventricles from inappropriate excitation by the atria, was disrupted by glycogen-filled myocytes. These anomalous microscopic atrioventricular connections, rather than morphologically distinct bypass tracts, appeared to provide the anatomic substrate for ventricular preexcitation (Arad et al., 2003).

AT2 Receptor-Null (–/–) Mice

Both angiotensin type 1 (AT-1) and type 2 (AT-2) receptors are present in the heart and play an important role in the remodelling process. AT-2 receptor-deficient mice do not express the myocardial angiotensin II receptor that plays a prominent role in the progression of heart failure following acute myocardial infarction. In wild-type mice subjected to acute myocardial infarction by coronary artery ligation, AT-2 re-ceptor immunoreactivity is upregulated in the infarct and border areas. Compared to the wild type, in AT-2 receptor-null (–/–) mice, the 7-day survival rate after acute myocardial infarction (AMI) is significantly lower. 24 h after coronary occlusion, ventricular mRNA levels for brain natriuretic peptide, lung weights and pulmonary congestion were found to be significantly higher in AT2–/– than in wild-type mice. Cardiac function was significantly decreased in AT2–/– mice two days after AMI (Adachi et al. 2003).

Beta (1)-Adrenergic Receptor Overexpression

Transgenic mice with specific overexpression of the beta (1)-adrenergic receptor develop left ventricular hypertrophy followed by heart failure. Using this model it was shown that the beta-adrenergic receptor system not only plays a central role in modulating heart rate and left-ventricular contractility, but is also involved in the development of heart failure. As compared to 4-month-old wild-type mice with identical cardiac performance as well as contractile reserve, the ratio of phosphocreatine to ATP and total creatine content were significantly reduced in transgenic mice with overexpression of beta-1 adrenergic receptor.

In addition, there was a significant decrease in creatine transporter content and mitochondrial and total creatine kinase activity as well as citrate synthase activity, indicating impaired oxidative energy generation in the transgenic mice and demonstrating that changes in myocardial energetics play a central role in the deterioration of cardiac function after chronic beta-adrenergic stimulation (Spindler et al. 2003).

eNOS Overexpression

Congestive heart failure results in decreased vascular nitric oxide production. In transgenic mice overexpressing the human eNOS gene that had infarct-induced (LAD occlusion) congestive heart failure, a reduced extent of contractile dysfunction as compared to controls was found. Survival was increased by 43% in the eNOS overexpressing transgenic mice. By using echocardiography and ultraminiature ventricular pressure catheters, fractional shortening and cardiac output were also found to be significantly greater in the eNOS group.

From this model it was concluded that targeted overexpression of the eNOS gene within the vascular endothelium in mice attenuates both cardiac and pulmonary dysfunction and dramatically improves survival during severe congestive heart failure. (Jones et al. 2003).

Transgenic Mice Overexpressing the Dominant-Negative Form of p21^{ras} (H-rasN17)

It has been demonstrated that mice with ventricular-specific overexpression of constitutively active p21^{ras}, a small GTP binding protein that acts as a key regulator of cell growth in eukaryotic cells, develop marked concentric hypertrophy. Transgenic mice overexpressing the dominant-negative form of p21^{ras} (H-rasN17) show severe progressive cardiac dilation with decreased contractility, leading to death at about ten weeks of age.

Histopathological analysis did not reveal any signs of myocyte disarray, necrosis or interstitial fibrosis. On echocardiography, the left ventricular diastolic diameter was increased (5.5±0.4 vs. 3.4±0.1 mm, $p < 0.001$) and fractional shortening was decreased (25±3 vs. 65±6, $p < 0.001$). Low frequency of TUNEL positive cells were detected, most of which were non-myocytes.

Ischemia-Induced Heart Failure Models

Ischemic heart disease is the leading causes of heart failure and has been well studied in a number of animal experiments. Myocardial infarction induces changes in the ventricular architecture, a process called ventricular remodelling. The infarcted heart progressively dilates and signs of overt heart failure develop. Activation of neurohormonal systems, although initially adaptive, accelerates the deterioration in ventricular function that eventually results in heart failure. To produce myocardial infarction in most animal models, acute ligation of the left anterior descending coronary artery is performed. This will produce an acute anterior myocardial infarct that is followed by a remodelling process. Unlike slowly progressing chronic coronary artery disease in humans, an acute infarct in an otherwise healthy animal will produce a distinct area of infarction with a sharp but irregular transition to unaffected myocardium. A border zone of intermediately injured myocardium or hibernating myocardium around the acutely infarcted area does not exist. In order to mimic a more chronic course of cardiac ischemia avoiding an acute infarct, repetitive left-sided coronary artery microembolization can be performed. Another method frequently applied is the gradual creation of a subtotal stenosis by the use of ameroid constrictors.

The coronary circulation varies among species. The porcine coronary circulation is more similar to the human than the canine, with a dominant right and left anterior descending artery with little collateral circulation. In general, the surgical technique for coronary occlusion is straightforward. The procedure requires general anaesthesia and endotracheal intubation. A sternotomy is avoided whenever possible to minimize the risk of wound infection. Usually, the chest is entered through a left lateral thoracotomy. The pericardium is opened and the LAD identified. Encircling the target coronary with a suture that is securely tied performs occlusion. Care must be taken to minimize the risk of lethal arrhythmia following acute infarction. For this reason the distal third of LAD is to be preferred for coronary occlusion. In addition precautions may include the preventive administration of antiarrhythmic agents such as amiodarone as well as topical application of a local anaesthetic (1% lidocaine) on the surface of the heart.

Acute Myocardial Ischemia/Infarct by Coronary Occlusion

Mouse Model

Anaesthesia is achieved with an intraperitoneal injection of pentobarbital. The mouse is fixed in a supine position and endotracheal intubation is performed. The chest is entered through a thoracotomy in the left fourth intercostal space using a small retractor to enhance exposure. After a limited pericardiotomy, the left anterior descending artery is identified. The artery is ligated proximally using a 7–0 suture that is passed underneath the artery and then tied. The resulting acute ischemia is clearly visible as pallor of the anterior wall of the left ventricle. Left ventricular dilation and impaired cardiac function are clearly visible using echocardiography one week after ligation. Infarct size can be calculated and expressed as a percentage of left ventricular surface area. Animals with less than 30% of infarct size after one week should be excluded from the studies, as they generally do not show typical left ventricular remodelling. In order to evaluate the gene expression profiles that are associated with ventricular remodelling and heart failure after myocardial infarction, some genes may serve as positive control marker genes. Activated foetal-type genes, such as ANP and β-MHC genes are usually found in the more acute stages after myocardial infarction, while collagen types I and III and cytokine gene expression are increased in the more chronic stages of remodelling.

Rat Model

As in mice, the left anterior descending coronary artery can be ligated in rats. Extensive infarction is produced. LV geometry and function can be analyzed by echocardiography and pressure/volume loop analysis with an intracardiac pressure-conductance catheter. Five weeks after ligation, dilatation of the left ventricle is found, with an increase in systolic and diastolic diameter. Thinning of the left ventricular anterior wall is present. The left atrium is enlarged and the E/A wave relation is increased. Signs of increased end-diastolic pressure and secondary pulmonary hypertension can be found.

Canine Model

Historically, the acute infarct model in dogs has been widely used. One- or two-stage ligation of the LAD produces an anterior myocardial infarct followed by left ventricular dysfunction. However, the coronary circulation in canines is different from that in other species in that there is a natural collateral circulation between the LAD and the circumflex artery by two to four collateral branches. While this makes the canine model ideal for revascularization trials on the beating heart, such as endoscopic coronary artery bypass grafting (Falk et al. 2000), the unpredictable extent of myocardial necrosis following acute coronary occlusion makes it an unreliable model for studying the course of LV dysfunction following MI.

Porcine Model

The anatomy and distribution of coronary arteries in pigs are very similar to those of humans. Unlike dogs, pigs lack a significant collateral coronary circulation. Since acute occlusion of the proximal LAD leads to an excessive anterior MI that is usually followed by immediate ventricular fibrillation and loss of the animal, ligation of the circumflex artery is preferred. For chronic studies Spinale et al. (1997) have developed a protocol that has decreased the attrition rate to 15%. Initially, a snare is placed around the circumflex artery via a lateral thoracotomy. After successful instrumentation, the pigs are allowed to recover. After recovery, the snares are tightened to produce myocardial infarction under sedation. Coronary occlusion in the closed chest animal with intact circulatory and neurohormonal function rather than intraoperative occlusion at the exposed heart is considered essential (Yarbrough and Spinale 2003).

Sheep Model

As in other large animals, the sheep are operated on *via* a left thoracotomy. In a recent study, the acute and chronic (3 months) hemodynamic changes following acute ligation of the LAD and the first diagonal branch have been characterized using left ventricular pressure–volume loops. Three months post-operatively deterioration of both systolic and diastolic left ventricular function is present. The left ventricular end-diastolic pressure increased from 3±1 to 7±1 mmHg along with a substantial increase in end-diastolic volume from 78±8 to 121±6 ml and a significant decrease in cardiac output from 2±0.2 to 1.5±0.2 l/min. The left ventricular end-systolic pressure–volume relationship deteriorated from 2.7±0.37 to 0.7±0.16 mmHg/ml along with a significant reduction in the pre-load recruitable stroke work. The ejection fraction decreased from 34±2% to 16±4%. The mean systemic blood pressure, however, was maintained due to a substantial increase in the systemic vascular resistance. This model is well characterized and therefore potentially useful for study of the pathogenesis of remodelling, the surgical management of heart failure and the development of novel treatment strategies (Hasnat et al. 2003).

Using sonomicrometry arrays the dimensions in distinct regions corresponding to the remote, transition, and infarcted regions can be measured. Eight weeks after ligation of the LAD in sheep, segment length increased from baseline in the remote (24.9±5.4%), transition (18.0±2.9%), and infarcted (53.8±11.0%) regions. The changes in regional geometry are accompanied by region- and type-specific changes in metalloproteinases and tissue inhibitors of metalloproteinases levels. A region-specific portfolio of MMPs is induced after MI and is accompanied by a decline in TIMP levels, indicative of a loss of MMP inhibitory control (Wilson et al. 2003).

In sheep, the circumflex coronary artery has three marginal branches and terminates in the posterior descending coronary artery. Occlusion of the obtuse marginals causes variable degrees of myocardial injury. Ligation of the first and second marginal branches infarcts 23%±3.0% of left ventricular mass, does not infarct either papillary muscle, significantly increases left ventricular cavity size by 48% at the high papillary muscle level by 8 weeks, and does not cause mitral regurgitation. Occlusion of the second and third marginal branches infarcts 21.4%±4.0% of the left ventricular mass, including the posterior papillary muscle, leads to significant left ventricular dilatation of up to 75%, and causes severe mitral regurgitation by eight weeks. Ligation of the second and third marginal branches and the posterior descending coronary artery infarcts 35% to 40% of the left ventricular mass, increases left ventricular cavity size by 39% within 1 h, and causes massive mitral regurgitation. Thus, only large posterior wall infarctions that include the posterior papillary muscle and lead to ventricular dilatation produce immediate, severe mitral regurgitation (Llaneras et al. 1997).

Models of Chronic Myocardial Ischemia

As opposed to acute occlusion of a coronary vessel, delayed occlusion by ameroid constrictors or hydraulic occluders allows for the development of collaterals that may serve resting metabolic demands but fail to provide enough blood flow during increasing levels of exercise (White et al. 1986). While techniques of delayed occlusion may provide a consistent, stable level of myocardial stunning with normal resting coronary blood flow and some degree of left ventricular dysfunction, they do not reproduce the congestive heart failure phenotype (including activation of the neurohormonal axis) as effectively as acute coronary occlusion.

Ameroid Constrictor

Chronic gradual, complete coronary occlusion can be produced by implantation of an ameroid constrictor. The constrictor consists of an inner ring of hygroscopic casein that swells as it slowly absorbs body fluid. A stainless steel sheath that forces the casein to swell inwards surrounds the casein ring, eventually occluding the coronary artery. Time to occlusion of the vessel is dependent on the sizes of the vessel and constrictor and the rigidity of the outer ring. Closure is most rapid during the first 3–14 days after implantation; complete occlusion is usually achieved in 4–5 weeks.

The choice of ameroid constrictor size is based on vessel diameter. Dissection of tissue around the coronary should be kept to a minimum to prevent postoperative movement of the ring, which may cause acute occlusion. After blunt dissection of the coronary, the constrictor ring is slipped over the coronary artery. The inner casein ring should be rotated so that its opening faces in the opposite direction from that of the stainless steel ring. A detailed technique for implantation of ameroid constrictors is provided in the chapter of N. Doll of this book (1.4). Despite its wide use, the technique lacks some predictability with regard to the degree of functional stenosis.

Hydraulic Occluders

A left thoracotomy is performed at the fourth intercostal space. The left anterior descending coronary artery or circumflex artery is isolated, and the hydraulic occluder is placed around the target vessel. The device consists of three parts, a banding ring, extension tube, and a self-sealing inflation button. The banding ring is a U-shaped hydraulic cuff that comes with various internal diameters. Its outer layer consists of 1 mm thick rigid silicone, which keeps it from deforming. The inner surface has a deformable layer of silicone that expands and compresses the lumen of the vessel according to the volume injected into the inflation button. The extension tube connects the banding ring with the inflation button. The inflation button is a circular reservoir made of self-sealing silicone that is implanted subcutaneously. The inflation or deflation of the banding ring can be done percutaneously on the conscious animal. If coronary blood flow is to be measured, a transonic flow probe can be implanted distal to the occluder. The wire should be externalised between the scapulae, where it is out of reach for the animal.

In a study in minipigs where a 90% stenosis was induced in the circumflex artery, positron emission tomography and dobutamine stress echocardiography were performed after chronic occlusion to evaluate myocardial blood flow and viability. As early as three days after subtotal occlusion, positron emission tomography demonstrated a significant reduction in myocardial blood flow in the left circumflex distribution that was accompanied by increased glucose use consistent with hibernating myocardium. Dobutamine stress echocardiography 3 days after occlusion demonstrated severely impaired contractility at rest in the ischemic region. Thirty days after occlusion, positron emission tomography demonstrated persistent low flow with increased glucose use in the left circumflex distribution. Regional wall motion improved with low-dose dobutamine followed by deterioration at higher doses, consistent with hibernating myocardium. The results of dobutamine stress echocardiography were unchanged. A mean of 8%±2% infarction of the area-at-risk localized to the endocardial surface was found, along with a loss of contractile elements and large areas of glycogen accumulation within viable cardiomyocytes as shown by electron microscopy (St Louis et al. 2000). Thus, using hydraulic occluders, chronic low-flow myocardial hibernation can be reproduced.

Repetitive Coronary Artery Microembolization

Repetitive coronary artery microembolization not only avoids the risk of a severe acute myocardial infarct in the unconditioned heart but also resembles the course of chronic ischemia by repeated ischemic insults. As opposed to coronary ligation or placement of chronic occluders, heart failure with varying degrees of left ventricular dysfunction can be produced in a closed chest model. The downside is that numerous catheter interventions are required over a distinct period of time subjecting the animals to a substantial number of procedures that precede the final experiment. Malignant arrhythmias may cause an attrition rate of up to 30%.

A canine model of chronic heart failure can be produced by multiple sequential intracoronary embolizations with microspheres. With 3 to 10 intracoronary embolizations performed one to three weeks apart using polystyrene latex microspheres (70 to 100 µm in diameter) left ventricular function can be significantly altered. Access is through the femoral artery and the catheter is placed in the target coronary under fluoroscopy. Embolizations are discontinued when the target left ventricular ejection fraction (< 35%) is reached. With this protocol, the LV ejection fraction could be reduced in a canine model from 64±2% at baseline to 21±1% 3 months after the last embolization. LV end-diastolic pressure increased from 6±1 to 22±3 mmHg and LV end-diastolic volume increased from 64±3 to 101±6 ml. Cardiac output decreased from 2.9±0.2 to 2.3±0.1 l/min (Sabbah et al. 1991). A significant increase of LV sphericity was present at 2 weeks with only minimal changes occurring thereafter. Despite the tendency for LV shape changes to plateau between 2 and 16 weeks, the left ventricular ejection fraction continued to decline. These changes were accompanied by significant increases of pulmonary artery wedge pressure and systemic vascular resistance. Plasma norepinephrine increased from 332±17 pg/ml at baseline to 791±131 pg/ml at 3 months and plasma levels of atrial natriuretic factor increased from 12.7±10.0 to 28.8±8.6 pmol/l, whereas plasma renin activity remained essentially unchanged. Three months after the last embolization, the density and affinity of myocardial beta adrenoceptors and voltage sensitive calcium channels had decreased. Gross and microscopic post-mortem examination showed patchy myocardial fibrosis and LV hypertrophy. The model was considered stable and reproducible and representative of many of the sequelae of heart failure (Sabbah et al. 1991, 1992, 2000; Gengo et al. 1992). This model has been successfully used in a number of pharmacological studies that aim at preventing the remodelling process in left ventricular failure. It was shown that inhibition of dopamine beta-hydroxylase, which results in a decrease in norepinephrine synthesis, prevented progressive LV dysfunction and remodelling, as evidenced by lack of ongoing increase in end-diastolic volume and end-systolic volume in dogs with heart failure induced by intracoronary microembolization (Sabbah et al. 2000). In a similar study, the effects of bosentan, a mixed endothelin-1 type A and type B receptor antagonist on the remodelling process was studied. After three months of therapy in dogs with moderate heart failure, bosentan prevented the progression of LV dysfunction and attenuated left ventricular chamber remodelling (Mishima et al. 2000). The effects of long-term monotherapy with the beta-blocker, metoprolol controlled release/extended release (100 mg once daily), on the progression of LV dysfunction have also been studied in dogs with heart failure induced by intracoronary microembolizations. After three months of oral monotherapy, the ejection fraction increased whereas end-diastolic volume remained unchanged. Compared to controls, treatment with metoprolol showed reduction in replacement fibrosis, reduction in interstitial fibrosis and reduction in myocyte cross-sectional area, as a measure of myocyte hypertrophy (Morita et al. 2002). Jiang examined cardiomyocyte apoptosis in a chronic heart failure model in sheep subjected to sequential coronary microembolization. Six months after embolization with the animals in a stable compensated hemodynamic state of heart failure, apoptosis (determined by expression of Fas/FasL) of left ventricular myocytes was found to correlate with increased wall stress. Immunohistochemical studies localized FasL and caspase-8 to intercalated discs, suggesting that wall stress may play a role in initiating cardiomyocyte apoptosis (Jiang et al. 2003).

Volume Overload-Induced Heart Failure

In addition to ischemia, a commonly used model to induce heart failure is volume overloading. By creating a shunt between the arterial and venous system, high output cardiac failure can be produced. Usually a shunt is created between the aorta and vena cava, the femoral artery and vein or the carotid artery and internal jugular vein. Unlike ischemia-induced models, the time course for the development of heart failure is less predictable. Initially, volume overload leads to hypertrophy rather than dilation. Only in decompensated hypertrophy does heart failure occur.

Cervical A-V Shunt Procedure

After induction of general anaesthesia and endotracheal intubation, 10,000 IU of heparin i.v. are administered. A left cervical skin incision of about 5 cm is performed ventral to the jugular vein. To enhance visibility, a non-sterile assistant may compress the vein at the thoracic inlet so that the jugular vein may be better visualized. The pulsating carotid artery can be easily palpated. The sternomastoideus and cleidomastoideus muscle are separated to expose the carotid sheath, which is then incised. Care must be taken not to injure the vagus nerve that runs along the common carotid artery. Both the internal jugular vein and the left carotid artery are exposed. Both vessels are mobilized over a length of 5 cm and ligated distally. The jugular vein is clamped proximally and transected. The left carotid artery is clamped and an end-to-side anastomosis of approximately 10 mm in diameter is performed between the free end of the vein and the side of carotid artery using 6–0 polypropylene sutures. After removal of the clamps the patency of the fistula is confirmed by pulsatile filling of the jugular vein. The separated muscle layers are apposed with 2–0 nonabsorbable sutures. As early as 30 min after opening of the shunt, a 40% increase in cardiac output is observed. A gradual increase in left ventricular end-diastolic diameter as well as an increase in left ventricular end-diastolic volume is found, with a peak at 8 weeks. However, neither clinical nor hemodynamic signs of overt heart failure, such as tachycardia or an increase in left ventricular end-diastolic pressure occurred with this relatively small shunt in a goat model (50–80 kg). Thus this model is considered a compensatory overload dilation model rather than a heart failure model (Bolotin et al. 1999).

An advantage of the cervical shunt model is that it is possible to evaluate the patency of the shunt by palpating the neck. The shunt is easily accessible to ultrasound evaluation and may be temporarily occluded by applying manual pressure.

Aorto-Caval Shunt

In contrast to the relatively small cervical shunt, chronic volume overload by a larger shunt produced by an infrarenal aorto-caval fistula in mongrel dogs has been shown to increase left ventricular end-diastolic pressure and produce clinical signs of heart failure (Porter et al. 1983). The disadvantage of this approach as opposed to peripheral shunts is that an aorto-caval shunt requires a laparotomy.

Initially, the aorto-caval shunt model was established in a rodent model (Flaim et al. 1979). A simple technique to create an aorto-caval shunt in the rat is the commonly applied needle technique that was developed by Garcia and Diebold. The inferior vena cava and abdominal aorta are exposed through a laparotomy. The aorta is punctured caudal to the left renal artery with an 18 gauge disposable needle, which is advanced into the aorta, perforating the adjacent wall between aorta and vena cava and penetrating the latter. A vascular clamp is placed across the aorta cephalad to the puncture, after which the needle is withdrawn, and the aortic puncture wound is sealed with a drop of cyanoacrylate glue. The clamp can be removed 30 s later. Patency of the shunt is verified visually by swelling of the vena cava and mixing of arterial and venous blood. The procedure can be accomplished in 10 min and is usually well tolerated (Garcia and Diebold 1990).

Recently, the alterations in general characteristics and morphology of the heart, as well as changes in hemodynamics, myosin heavy chain isoforms, and beta-adrenoceptor responsiveness, have been determined in Sprague-Dawley rats at 1, 2, 4, 8, and 16 weeks after creation of an aorto-caval fistula. Within the first two weeks a rapid increase of cardiac mass in both left and right ventricles was noted. Compensated hypertrophy occurred between two and eight weeks with normal or only mild depression in hemodynamic function. Decompensated hypertrophy or heart failure occurred between eight and sixteen weeks after aorto-caval shunting and was characterized by a decline of cardiac function, and a shift in myosin heavy chain isozyme expression. At sixteen weeks failing hearts showed a significant increase in beta (1)-receptor density, whereas beta (2)-receptor density was unchanged. Basal adenylyl cyclase activity as well as isoproterenol- and forskolin-stimulated adenylyl cyclase activities were increased, indicating up-regulation of beta-adrenoceptor signal transduction as a unique feature of cardiac hypertrophy and failure induced by volume overload (Wang et al. 2003).

In another study, the effects of a large arterio-venous fistula on left and right ventricular hemodynamics and cardiac myocyte size were examined in adult rats at one week and one month after surgery. Average heart weight increased by 35% at 1 week and 86% at 1 month in rats with fistulas. In general, myocyte hypertrophy was due to a proportional increase in length and width while the length/width ratio remained constant. This change was more evident in the large hearts from rats with 1 month fistulas. At both the one week and one month intervals, the hypertrophic response of right ventricular myocytes was slightly greater than that observed in the left ventricle or interventricular septum. Left ventricular systolic pressure and dP/dt_{max} were significantly reduced at one week, but returned to normal after one month of overloading. Left ventricular end-diastolic pressure was increased approximately fivefold and twofold at 1 week and 1 month, respectively. Right ventricular systolic pressure and dP/dt_{max} were increased at both intervals. Thus, severe volume overloading from a large aorto-caval fistula in the rat initially leads to depressed left ventricular function followed by a compensatory hypertrophy and near normal function at one month, right ventricular pressure overload, and changes in myocyte shape that resemble normal physiological growth (Liu et al. 1991a). At five months heart rate, left ventricular systolic pressure, left ventricular dP/dt_{max}, and systolic aortic pressure were not changed in rats with fistulas as compared to controls. However, cardiac output, stroke volume, left ventricular end-diastolic pressure, and all measured parameters in the right ventricle were significantly increased. Mean cell volume and the ratio of heart weight to body weight were both elevated by 92%. Cell volume, cell length, and cross-sectional area increased significantly in each heart region examined. Hypertrophy was more pronounced in cells from the right ventricle and the endomyocardium of the left ventricle. Despite evidence of renal and hepatic congestion, most indices of cardiac function were normal or elevated 5 months after creation of a large volume-overload-induced hypertrophy (Liu et al. 1991b).

Not only the duration but also the size of the shunt will determine the onset and severity of heart failure following creation of an aorto-caval shunt in rats. A small shunt induced by a 1.2 mm (outside diameter) disposable needle will yield only a moderate degree of heart failure as opposed to a large shunt created by a 1.8 mm disposable needle. Both heart failure models are characterized by increased cardiac weight, which is significantly higher in the large-shunt model, and an increase in central venous pressure. According to a study by Langenickel, left ventricular end-diastolic pressure is elevated only in the overt heart failure group caused by a large shunt for a period of 30 days (control: 5.7±0.7; small shunt 30 days: 8.6±0.9; large shunt 3 days: 8.5±1.7; large shunt 30 days: 15.9±2.6 mmHg). Cardiac function was also only decreased significantly in the large shunt model with a decrease of dP/dt_{max} from 4.8±0.2 to 3.8±0.2×10^3 mmHg/s. In contrast to the small-shunt model and after 3 days of large shunt with only a small increase in LVEDP, the large-shunt model after

30 days demonstrated the typical characteristics of overt heart failure, such as decreased cardiac contractility, elevated LVEDP, and an increased lung weight as an indicator of pulmonary congestion (Langenickel et al. 2000).

Valvular Insufficiency (Mitral Regurgitation)

Mitral valve insufficiency leads to chronic volume overload causing compensatory left ventricular hypertrophy followed by dilatation with pulmonary oedema. Various models to induce mitral insufficiency have been developed. To avoid the need for a thoracotomy, Kleaveland has established a catheter-based method of chordae disruption. Under fluoroscopic guidance a flexible grasping forceps (i.e. biopsy instrument) is inserted into the carotid artery through the aortic valve into the left ventricle. A number of mitral chordae are disrupted producing mitral regurgitation. In half of the animals severe mitral regurgitation was obtained. At 3 months, end-diastolic volume increased from 48±9 to 85±19 ml. Left ventricular mass increased from 71±13 to 90±10 g due to significant eccentric cardiac hypertrophy and left ventricular end-diastolic pressure increased from 9±3 to 19±6 mmHg. Cardiac output decreased from 2.3±0.61 to 1.8±0.6 l/min. Along with the doubling of end-diastolic volume, there was a fall in cardiac output and a rise in left ventricular end-diastolic pressure, suggesting cardiac decompensation in this closed-chest model of chronic mitral regurgitation (Kleaveland et al., 1988; Kunzelman et al., 1999). On a cellular level, an increase in myocyte length, changes in myofilament architecture and reduced myofibril content were found in a canine model of mitral regurgitation induced by chordal rupture (Spinale et al., 1993).

In dogs with chronic mitral insufficiency, it was shown that chronic beta blockade improves left ventricular function and was associated with an improvement in the innate contractile function of isolated cardiocytes and an increase in the number of contractile elements (Tsutsui et al., 1994). In a similar study, the use of angiotensin 1 receptor blockers on remodelling after subacute mitral in-sufficiency was studied. Although a decrease in systemic vascular resistance and attenuated local expression of the renin-angiotensin system was found, angiotensin 1 receptor blockade could not improve left ventricular remodelling and function in the early myocardial adaptive phase of mitral insufficiency (Perry et al., 2002).

Hypertrophy Heart Failure Models

Increased ventricular workload caused by pressure or volume overload leads to myocardial hypertrophy and or dilatation. Pressure overload is usually accomplished by aortic banding (left ventricular pressure overload) or pulmonary artery banding (right ventricular pressure overload). Once the compensatory mechanisms fail, the hypertrophied ventricle dilates and signs of heart failure may develop. Despite marked left ventricular hypertrophy, increased stiffness, impaired relaxation, diastolic dysfunction, and connective tissue remodelling, models of induced hypertrophy often lack neurohormonal activation. Thus, unless end-stage hypertrophy finally leads to ventricular dilatation and impairment of systolic function, hypertrophy models are not ideal for studying the phenotype of congestive heart failure. The surgical techniques to induce hypertrophy are described in detail in chapter 1.5 (Models of Left Ventricular Hypertrophy).

Rapid Ventricular Pacing

Rapid ventricular pacing is a commonly used method of inducing heart failure. After implantation of an atrial (synchronous) or ventricular (asynchronous) lead, pacing is begun usually at a rate of >200 beats per minute. This creates a high output heart failure with biventricular dilatation, a deterioration of systolic and diastolic function and activation of the neurohormonal axis. Along with progressive heart failure, plasma catecholamine levels increase. In advanced stages, endothelin and renin levels increase and beta-receptor density decreases, closely resembling the phenotype of congestive heart failure. Numerous pacing protocols for synchronous and asynchronous pacing over variable times exist. The degree of heart failure varies with the duration and frequency of pacing and is partially reversible after cessation of pacing. The ventricular dilatation and a global decrease in ventricular function that is observed with rapid pacing resemble the clinical picture that is found in dilated cardiomyopathy.

Canine Model

Rapid pacing-induced cardiomyopathy is well studied, mostly in the canine model. Pacemakers are implanted with the animals anaesthetized and intubated. Through a left thoracotomy, a shielded stimulating electrode is sutured either on to the left atrium (for synchronized pacing) or the right or left ventricle (for asynchronized pacing), and connected to a modified programmable pacemaker that allows for stimulation at high frequencies.

The pacemaker is placed in a subcutaneous pocket. The pericardium is approximated, and the thoracotomy closed. Cardiac auscultation and an ECG should be frequently performed to ensure appropriate function of the pacemaker and the presence of 1:1 conduction. One recent protocol (Takagaki et al. 2002) suggests rapid induction pacing at a rate of 230 beats/min for 4 weeks followed by maintenance pacing at a reduced rate of 190 beats/min for another four weeks. With this protocol, left ventricular systolic function was significantly reduced at week 4 and remained low but stable at week 8, including the slope of the end-systolic pressure-volume relationship (2.4 ± 1.0 *vs.* 0.7 ± 0.2 *vs.* 0.8 ± 0.3 mmHg/ml [baseline *vs.* week 4 *vs.* week 8, respectively]), ejection fraction ($63\pm5\%$ *vs.* $28\pm7\%$ *vs.* $33\pm5\%$), and cardiac output (3.1 ± 0.7 *vs.* 2.0 ± 0.3 *vs.* 2.2 ± 0.7 L/min), (Takagaki et al. 2002). Significant ventricular remodelling was observed with increased ventricular volumes and circumferential wall stress, which again were stable between weeks 4 and 8. Activation of the neurohormonal axis was measured by serum catecholamine and atrial natriuretic polypeptide levels. Both increased from baseline but stabilized between weeks 4 and 8. The end-diastolic pressure-volume relationship also showed stable diastolic function between weeks 4 and 8. This technique of maintenance pacing after a rapid induction phase provided a consistent model of severe heart failure.

Others have studied the impact of catecholamine stimulation in rapid pacing-induced heart failure in dogs. In rapid pacing-induced cardiomyopathy, contractile responses (LV dP/dt) to catecholamines are desensitized and accompanied by a parallel decrease in heart rate-adjusted myocardial O_2 consumption when alpha- or beta- or both alpha/beta-1 receptors are stimulated. This is due to impaired myocardial O_2 extraction rather than limitations in coronary blood flow responses. There is an associated shift in myocardial metabolism, evidenced by an increased preference for glycolytic substrates with adrenergic stimulation in cardiomyopathy (Nikolaidis et al. 2002).

Heart failure is associated with changes in action potentials, arrhythmias and an increased risk of sudden death. It is therefore important not only to study the hemodynamic or metabolic changes of the failing ventricle but also to examine the alterations in currents underlying cardiac repolarization that are produced by heart failure. In a canine model of heart failure induced by rapid ventricular pacing, it was shown that in cardiomyopathic dogs electrophysiological changes could be found in all layers of the left ventricle. A down regulation of inward rectifier K(+) current, transient outward K(+) current and slow component of the delayed rectifier K(+) current was associated with an increase in action potential duration and was found to favour the occurrence of early after-depolarisations (Li et al. 2002).

Sheep Model

Rapid ventricular pacing for 21 days at 160 to 190 bpm resulted in moderate heart failure in adult sheep. Additional pacing at a rate of 205 to 215 bpm for 28 days or 42 days produced advanced and severe heart failure, respectively. Marked increases in left ventricular area, mitral valve regurgitation, and left ventricular end-diastolic pressure and decreases in left ventricular wall thickness, and ejection fraction were demonstrated. The model allows examination of both structural changes and hemodynamic parameters of heart failure during and after exercise challenge (Byrne et al. 2002).

Porcine Model

After 3 weeks of chronic rapid atrial pacing at a frequency of 240 bpm, pigs demonstrated clinical symptoms consistent with congestive heart failure, including tachypnea, lethargy, and reduced appetite during the last week of rapid pacing. Basal resting heart rate increased and mean arterial pressure dropped when compared to control values. Left ventricular end-diastolic dimension increased by up to 65% and fractional shortening decreased by more than 60%. With chronic rapid pacing, left ventricular peak wall stress and pulmonary capillary wedge pressure increased by more than threefold and cardiac output decreased by more than threefold from control values. As a measure of neurohormonal activation plasma norepinephrine and endothelin plasma levels increased by more than fivefold with chronic pacing. This model was used to determine the combined effect of angiotensin converting enzyme inhibition and angiotensin-II receptor blockade in chronic heart failure. It was shown that the beneficial effects of ACE inhibition were augmented by adding an angiotensin II receptor blocker (Spinale et al. 1997).

Current Induced Heart Failure

A method more of historical interest is the induction of heart failure by application of direct current to the myocardium. Closed-chest coronary thrombosis was induced in miniature pigs by means of direct current. The induction electrode was introduced via the common carotid artery into the coronary artery. A current of 1 mA applied for 60 min caused intimal injury that induced coronary thrombosis (Sedlarek et al. 1976).

Pharmacological Induction of Heart Failure

Beta Blockade

Acute heart failure can be induced by beta-blockade, resulting in a decline of all parameters of left ventricular function by 30% as compared to baseline values (Kazmarek et al. 2003). This model is however not useful to induce chronic heart failure.

Epinephrine Infusion

Heart failure can be induced by catecholamine infusion. Three repetitive applications (at 16-day intervals) of high-dose epinephrine (first infusion, 5 µg/kg/min for 60 min; second and third infusions, 4 µg/kg/min for 60 min) caused cardiomyopathy in rabbits. Mean arterial pressure and blood flow velocity, as well as the acceleration of blood flow velocity (df/dt) in the proximal abdominal aorta were progressively reduced, and right atrial pressure was significantly elevated. Repetitive infusions of high doses of epinephrine induced a cardiomyopathy with progressive hemodynamic deterioration, LV dilatation and hypertrophy, depressed systolic function, and different stages of neurohormonal compensation. This model appears to be suitable to study the progression of chronic heart failure by serial measurements in a small conscious animal preparation (Muders et al. 1999).

Inducing Myocarditis

The most important clinical manifestation of myocarditis is congestive heart failure. Various models of viral or autoimmune myocarditis are available. Inoculation of four-week-old mice with encephalomyocarditis virus led to hemodynamic abnormalities consistent with heart failure after one week. Contractile function decreased from days 4 to 14. On day 7, when hemodynamic abnormalities consistent with heart failure culminated, end-diastolic volume, and the end-diastolic pressure-volume relation were significantly higher, whilst cardiac index, ejection fraction and end-systolic pressure were significantly lower in the infected than in control mice. (Nishio et al. 1999).

For a model of experimental autoimmune myocarditis, Lewis rats were immunized with human cardiac myosin suspended in complete Freund's adjuvant. Baseline hemodynamics were measured using an ultraminiature catheter pressure transducer *via* the right internal carotid artery, 4 weeks after immunization in one group of rats (acute phase) and 3 months after immunization in another group (chronic phase). The heart weight to body weight ratios were significantly higher in both the acute-phase group and the chronic-phase group compared with normal control rats. The baseline left ventricular systolic pressure was significantly lower in the chronic phase group than in the control group. Peak dP/dt and peak -dP/dt were significantly lower in both the acute-phase group and the chronic phase group compared with the control group. *In vivo* measurements of hemodynamic variables indicated the presence of left ventricular dysfunction in rats with experimental autoimmune myocarditis (Koyama et al. 1995). Autoimmune myocarditis in rats can also be induced by injection of porcine cardiac myosin. The resulting inflammatory cardiomyopathy leads to chronic heart failure with elevated left ventricular end-diastolic pressure and central venous pressure and cardiac fibrosis (Tachikawa et al. 2003).

Toxic Cardiomyopathy

Anthracycline Induced Non-Ischemic Cardiomyopathy

Different established anthracycline antibiotic agents have been shown to induce a chronic non-ischemic congestive heart failure in animals. Models using anthracycline have been reported in both small animals and in larger animals.

Table 1 provides a summary of studies wherein the animal model, the anthracycline agent and the route and period of medication are described.

The cellular mechanisms by which such anthracyclines induce heart failure are multifactorial (Bristow et al. 1982) and include local release of vasoactive substances (Rhodon et al. 1993), cytotoxic effects of local free radical generation (Singal et al. 1985; Arnolda et al. 1985), inhibition of nucleic acid and protein synthesis, calcium overload, which was facilitated by inhibition of Na-K-ATPase (Olson et al. 1988), enhancement of slow inward Ca^{2+} current and release of Ca^{2+} from the sarcoplasmic reticulum (Sacco et al. 2003; Boucek et al. 1997), direct interaction with the actin–myosin contractile system in terms of alteration of the actin–myosin cross-bridge interaction (Singal et al. 1986; Asayama et al. 1992) and the anthracycline metabolite hypothesis – secondary alcohol metabolites – (Olson et al. 1990; Arai et al. 2000).

Examples

Example of Small Animal Model

Schwarz and co-workers assessed a reliable model of non-ischemic dilated cardiomyopathy produced by the intravenous administration of 2.5 mg/kg adriamycin in the rat once a week over 10 weeks. Transthoracic echocardiographic analysis revealed an increase in end-diastolic and end-systolic diameters and a decrease in fractional shortening whilst electron microscopy demonstrated cellular degeneration and ultrastructural changes including interstitial oedema and myocyte vacuolation, typical for adriamycin-induced cardiotoxicity (Schwarz et al. 1998).

Table 1
Anthracycline induced cardiomyopathy in small and larger animals

Anthra-cycline	Animal	Dosis	Duration	Route	References
Dox	Rat	2–5.0 mg/kg	2–12 weeks	SC/IV/IP	Ambler 1993 Singal 1995 Schwarz 1998 Sayed 2001 Suzuki 2002
Dox	Mice	2–25 mg/kg	1 day–4 weeks	IP	Scorsin 1998 Pacher 2003
Dox	Rabbit	0.4–3 mg/kg	1–18 weeks	IV/PL	Wanless 1987 Elisson 1988 Jones 1990 Shenesa 1990 Calderone 1991 Dodd 1993 Yoshikawa 1994 Pey 1996 Kelso 1997 Boucek 1997 Kawabata 2000
Dox	Dog	0.7–1.0 mg/kg	4–12 weeks	IC	Magovern 1992 Shah 1997 Toyoda 1998 Monnet 1999 Christiansen 2003
Dox	Piglets	1.5 mg/kg	3 weeks	IV	Cassidy 1998
Dox	Sheep	Not specified	4 weeks	n.s.	Chekanov 1999
Epi	Rat	1.5 mg/kg	3 weeks	IV	Germain 2003
Epi	Rabbit	0.4–2.0 mg/kg	1–8 weeks	PL/IV	Ellison 1988 Kelso 1997
Daun	Rabbit	3.0 mg/kg	10 weeks	IV	Klimtova 2002

Kelso et al. (1997) described a useful model of cardiomyopathy in rabbits given a twice-weekly infusion of epirubicin (2 mg/kg) for a period of 6 weeks followed by a wash-out period of 2 weeks. The functional and morphological alterations appeared to be consistent with the development of cardiomyopathy and like those which have been reported to occur in humans.

Suzuki et al. (2001) induced heart failure successfully by 6 equal intraperitoneal injections of doxorubicin in the rat with a total dosage of 15 mg/kg (each injection containing 2.5 mg/kg) over a period of two weeks.

Pacher and co-workers (2003) reported a significant decline in left ventricular function in a mouse model five days after a single injection of doxorubicin at a dose of 25 mg/kg intraperitoneally.

Example of Larger Animal Model

Evaluation of the effects of new therapies, especially surgical treatments such as dynamic cardiomyoplasty and reduction ventriculoplasty cannot be performed in small animal models. Toyoda and co-workers developed a simple and reproducible large animal model of dilated cardiomyopathy. Beagles weighing 8 to 12 kg underwent repeated intracoronary infusion of doxorubicin (0.7 mg/kg) into the left main coronary artery. The infusions were repeated weekly for 5 weeks. Three months after treatment, significant changes in left ventricular geometry and function as well as in neurohormonal state were noted. The fractional shortening, the left ventricular ejection fraction and the stroke volume were decreased. The left ventricular diastolic diameter, the left ventricular end-diastolic volume and the left ventricular end-diastolic pressure were increased (Toyoda et al. 1998).

Christiansen and colleagues produced a heart failure model in adult foxhounds by weekly intracoronary adriamycin administration (10 mg over a 1 h period on 5 occasions). The intracoronary catheter was introduced into the left main stem *via* the first marginal branch and connected to a percutaneous access port that was used for weekly medication. Adriamycin administration resulted in a severe dilated cardiomyopathy (Christiansen et al. 2003).

Anthracycline-induced cardiotoxicity resulted in a marked decrease in cardiac output as well as an increase in chamber size. End-diastolic pressure increased in both left and right ventricles and was in accord with a model of chronic biventricular heart failure (Yoshikawa et al. 1994). Several small and larger animal studies analyzed sympathoneuronal regulation in anthracycline-induced heart failure. Yoshikawa et al. (1994) showed that the number of myocardial beta-adrenoceptors and the myocardial norepinephrine concentration in both ventricles were decreased and the plasma norepinephrine concentration was increased. Furthermore, they also demonstrated that basal as well as isoproterenol-, sodium fluoride-and forskolin-stimulated adenylate cyclase activities were significantly decreased in this animal model of heart failure. Uno and co-workers showed that the number of cardiac beta-adrenoceptors is reduced in doxorubicin-induced congestive heart failure. This might be due to down-regulation of presynaptic beta-adrenoceptors caused by the elevated plasma noradrenaline due to cardiac failure. Histological changes in both the right and left ventricular myocardial biopsy specimens included myocellular hypertrophy, loss of myofibrillar material, and vacuolization (Uno et al. 1993).

The mortality rate caused by anthracycline administration in small animal models ranged from 12% to 37% (Schwarz et al. 1998; Suzuki et al. 2001). In larger animal studies, particularly in dogs, a mortality rate of 41% is reported (Monnet et al., 1999). Furthermore, anthracycline lethal toxicity appeared to be dose-dependent. In one study the mortality rose from 12% (9 mg/kg) to 33% (15 mg/kg) in epirubicin-treated rats (To et al. 2003).

In summary, the small and larger animal models described represent a non-surgical, adequate, cost-effective and reproducible model for anthracycline-induced non-ischemic dilated cardiomyopathy, resembling morphological and functional changes in human patients treated with anthracycline. This experimental model may be used to study the cellular and metabolic effects of anthracycline cardiotoxicity and the avoidance and the reversal of these morphological and functional alterations by use of different new drug and cellular therapies. Furthermore, this model may be useful to evaluate the efficacy of surgical strategies e.g. cardiomyoplasty, mechanical assist devices, transplantation, and reduction ventriculoplasty.

Furazolidone

Furazolidone is a nitrofuran derivative used both therapeutically and prophylactically as an antimicrobial agent in poultry, pigs, rabbits and fish. If given in a toxic dose, the animals show a failure to grow, ascites and signs of heart failure ultimately leading to death. Gross pathological changes include biventricular cardiac dilatation, thinning of cardiac muscle fibres, multifocal myocytolysis, increased connective tissue, and thinning of the walls of both ventricles. Epicardial fibrosis and endocardial fibroelastosis may also be seen (Reed et al. 1987)

If growing turkey poults are given 700 ppm of furazolidone at 1 week of age for 3 weeks, dilated cardiomyopathy will develop. This model has been used to study differential effects on cAMP and caffeine responsiveness as well as changes in intracellular calcium mobilization kinetics and calcium-myofilament interaction in the failing heart (Kim et al. 2000; Okafor et al. 2003).

Experimental Methods to Study Reverse Remodelling

Recent studies have demonstrated cardiac improvement in patients supported with a ventricular assist device, suggesting that reverse remodelling and myocardial recovery are possible even in cases with severe heart failure. The current literature on myocardial responses to left ventricular support devices supports the concept that mechanical overload is a primary factor in sustaining the pathological phenotype of the failing heart and suggests that the study of reverse remodelling provides a valuable opportunity to discover adaptive signalling pathways capable of mediating myocardial recovery. A number of surgical techniques and devices have subsequently been developed that aim at reverse remodelling. Remodelling, increased myocardial stretch and wall stress result from ventricular dilation. Both active and passive ventricular constraints as well as methods for mechanical unloading of the failing ventricle are currently the subjects of extensive clinical and laboratory research (Teerlink and Ratcliffe 2002).

Recently an interesting model has been developed that can be used to study the effects of cardiac unloading on a failing ventricle. This model partially mimics conditions of ventricular assist devices. By adapting a heterotopic transplantation technique, the pattern of functional recovery in the left ventricle of the failing heart could be examined. After heart failure was induced in adult New Zealand rabbits by coronary artery ligation with subsequent myocardial infarction, the failing hearts were transplanted into the necks of recipient rabbits after 4 weeks or 3 months. Repeated physiological analysis of LV function was performed by a left ventricular latex balloon that was connected to subcutaneous tubing. Contractility (left ventricular dP/dt[max]) and relaxation (left ventricular dP/dt[min]) were significantly lower in transplanted post-infarction hearts as compared to control hearts (*in situ* hearts) immediately after transplantation. Both left ventricular dP/dt(max) and left ventricular dP/dt(min) responses to increased preload and to beta-adrenergic stimulation progressively improved to a significantly higher level after 30 days of left ventricular unloading for the hearts that were transplanted 4 weeks after myocardial infarction. However, this functional improvement was not detected in failing hearts transplanted 3 months after infarction (Tevaearai et al. 2002).

Passive Ventricular Constraint

The theoretical concept in applying passive constraints to the failing myocardium is to provide diastolic ventricular support in order to stop progressive remodelling. These devices work on a passive, mechanical level and aim at reducing periodic myocardial over-stretch and wall stress. It is hoped that a down-regulation of increased local neurohormonal activity, and reduction or elimination of cardiomyocyte maladaptive gene expression can be achieved. Some experimental studies have provided evidence of reverse remodelling with demonstrated reductions in heart size and improvements in cardiac function, as well as changes in cardiac myocytes and gene expression.

A passive ventricular containment device was applied in a failing canine heart model induced by repeated intracoronary microembolizations. The animals were studied before and three to six months after surgical implantation of a thin polyester mesh that surrounded both cardiac ventricles. Long-term use of the device significantly lowered end-diastolic and end-systolic volumes by −19±4% and −22±8%, respectively and shifted the end-systolic pressure-volume relation to the left (Saavedra et al. 2002). These findings are compatible with the event of reverse remodelling. End-diastolic pressure and chamber diastolic stiffness did not significantly change. The systolic response to dobutamine markedly improved after passive ventricular containment. There was no change in the density or affinity of beta-adrenergic receptors. Diastolic compliance was not adversely affected, and preload-recruitable function was preserved with the device, consistent with a lack of constriction. This model demonstrated, that reverse remodelling with reduced systolic wall stress and improved adrenergic signalling can be achieved by passive external support without the risk of diastolic constriction (Saavedra et al. 2002).

In a sheep model of severe heart failure induced by high rate ventricular pacing, a polyester mesh cardiac support device was implanted around both ventricles through a lower partial sternotomy. Rapid ventricular pacing was continued thereafter. Cardiovascular function was assessed using echocardiography and a sub-maximal treadmill exercise protocol at base line, moderate, severe, and advanced stages. Left ventricular ejection fraction (LVEF) decreased from 50% to 25% and $+dp/dt_{max}$

declined. Following implantation of the polyester mesh, exercise capacity improved significantly, despite ongoing rapid pacing, with LVEF and +dp/dt slightly increasing. There were no significant changes in left ventricular long axis area and short axis dimensions at the termination of pacing compared with those at the time of CSD implant. Mitral regurgitation improved slightly after containment in animals with a passive containment device but increased in those without. Heart failure with a custom-made polyester mesh device halted the decline in cardiac function seen in untreated animals in this pacing-induced animal model (Raman et al. 2003).

Cardiomyoplasty

Reduction of ventricular dilatation, rather than direct improvement of pump function, has been suggested to be the main working mechanism of dynamic cardiomyoplasty. This working mechanism was examined in the goat using a chronic cardiac dilatation model induced by the creation of a cervical arterio-venous shunt and submitted to passive and active cardiomyoplasty using the left latissimus dorsi muscle wrapped around the heart. Significant ventricular enlargement, as well as persistent increase in filling pressures, were observed after 8 weeks of shunting. Animals in the control group dilated further beyond 2 months while the dilatation process was stopped by passive cardiomyoplasty. Left ventricular end-diastolic diameter significantly decreased after electrical activation of the wrapped skeletal muscle and increased the slope of the end-systolic pressure-volume relation, indicating an improvement in the LV contractile state (Kaulbach et al. 2002).

Troubleshooting

Congestive heart failure is a chronic disease that often develops over years before overt heart failure occurs. Chronic ischemia as the main cause of heart failure is the result of progressive atherosclerosis and multiple infarcts. This condition is difficult to reproduce under laboratory conditions. As a consequence, most experiments to induce heart failure in animals result from an acute injury, which instantaneously affects ventricular function. Even multiple embolizations or chronic occluders are applied in healthy animals to create a terminal injury pattern within a few weeks. Thus, the phenotype of congestive heart failure that can be achieved under experimental conditions may substantially differ from that typically seen in humans. Follow-up data for most animal experiments rarely extend beyond a few weeks or months and thus do not always properly describe the chronic course of a disease that takes years to develop.

Nevertheless, animal experiments are indispensable for a better understanding of the underlying pathophysiology of heart failure. Given the countless number of existing protocols and approaches for induction of heart failure, selection of the right model is of the utmost importance. Researchers need to be familiar with the species-specific response to injury and differences in the adaptive changes. Whenever a species is selected for modelling heart failure, the specific anatomy has to be taken into account. While pigs have a coronary anatomy and gross cardiac structure similar to humans, they lack collateral coronary circulation, which makes them prone to acute ischemia-induced arrhythmias. It is therefore important to minimize the attrition rate by careful planning and selecting a two-step approach whenever feasible. Variations in anatomy do not only occur across species but also within species (for example two major types of coronary circulation have been described in sheep (Llaneras et al. 1994). Depending on where occlusion is performed, not only acute myocardial infarct but also mitral insufficiency will occur.

Ventricular dilation and hypertrophy are normal compensatory mechanisms following cardiac injury. While acute infarct models provide a circumscribed injury, pressure and volume overload models make it difficult to control the degree of heart failure in an experimental setting as the time course and the final degree of heart failure is less predictable. Rapid pacing creates a phenotype that is typical for dilated cardiomyopathy but not other aetiologies such as that seen in chronic ischemia. Whenever a congestive heart failure phenotype is desired, not only an impairment of left ventricular function but also activation of the neurohormonal axis should be demonstrated.

Although some data on normal values for cardiac function and hemodynamics exist (for a reference see Gross 1994), these can be influenced by age and size of the animal, special breeds and to a large degree by the laboratory conditions and the methods under which they have been obtained. Ideally, measurements are obtained in the instrumented but conscious animal. This is often not possible, therefore care must be taken to acknowledge the cardiovascular effects of commonly applied drugs used for anaesthesia and analgesia. Inhalational anaesthetics, but also antiarrhythmic drugs, have negative inotropic effects and thus may yield unreliable results. There are numerous examples of low cardiac output and altered coronary vascular and myocardial responses following the application of inhalational anaesthetics and other commonly applied drugs. Congestive heart failure induced by toxic agents such as doxorubicin have severe acute and chronic side effects such as bone marrow depression that may not only have an impact on overall survival but may also influence the response to injury. At this time it is not clear whether the described mortality rate caused by anthracycline administration in small and large animal models is a result of the induced heart failure or caused by side effects. In addition the application of anthracycline through the ear vein can lead to inflammation and swelling. In conclusion, we have to take into consideration that this animal model is very time-consuming.

Recently various methods for the surgical treatment of end stage heart failure are being discussed as alternatives to medical treatment and transplantation. Passive ventricular containment devices, ventricular reduction surgery and ventricular assist devices are currently being evaluated. With some of these methods, effective reverse remodelling could be demonstrated.

Whenever reverse remodelling is to be studied, the animal model chosen is again very important. Ventricular pacing is a commonly applied method to induce a phenotype similar to dilated cardiomyopathy seen in humans. Upon cessation of pacing, reverse remodelling occurs spontaneously to some degree, which may interfere with the results of any treatment modality.

Transgenic animals lacking or overexpressing isolated factors that play a role in the cascade of events leading to heart failure, present an ideal opportunity to study the pathophysiology and potential pharmacological targets for treatment of the disease. However, heart failure remains a multifactorial entity caused by chronic myocardial injury. Therefore the isolation of single factors in genetically engineered small animals may not obviate the need for large animal models with a more human form of congestive heart failure.

References

Adachi Y, Saito Y, Kishimoto I, Harada M, Kuwahara K, Takahashi N, Kawakami R, Nakanishi M, Nakagawa Y, Tanimoto K, Saitoh Y, Yasuno S, Usami S, Iwai M, Horiuchi M, Nakao K (2003) Angiotensin II Type 2 receptor deficiency exacerbates heart failure and reduces survival after acute myocardial infarction in mice. Circulation 107: 2406–2408

Arad M, Moskowitz IP, Patel VV, Ahmad F, Perez-Atayde AR, Sawyer DB, Walter M, Li GH, Burgon PG, Maguire CT, Stapleton D, Schmitt JP, Guo XX, Pizard A, Kupershmidt S, Roden DM, Berul CI, Seidman CE, Seidman JG (2003) Transgenic mice overexpressing mutant PRKAG2 define the cause of Wolff-Parkinson-White syndrome in glycogen storage cardiomyopathy. Circulation 107: 2850–2856

Arai M, Yoguchi A, Takizawa T, Yokoyama T, Kanda T, Kurabayashi M, Nagai R (2000) Mechanism of doxorubicin-induced inhibition of sarcoplasmic reticulum Ca^{2+}-ATPase gene transcription. Circ Res 86: 8–14

Arnolda L, McGrath B, Cocks M, Sumithran E, Johnston C (1985) Adriamycin cardiomyopathy in the rabbit: an animal model of low output cardiac failure with activation of vasoconstrictor mechanisms. Cardiovasc Res 19: 378–382

Asayama J, Yamahara Y, Matsumoto T, Miyazaki H, Tatsumi T, Inoue M, Ohta B, Omori I, Inoue D, Nakagawa M (1992) Acute and subacute effects of doxorubicin on postextrasystolic potentiation in guinea pig papillary muscles. Pharmacol Toxicol 71: 371–375

Boucek RJ, Dodd DA, Atkinson JB, Oquist N, Olson RD (1997) Contractile failure in chronic doxorubicin-induced cardiomyopathy. J Mol Cell Cardiol 29: 2631–2640

Bing OH, Conrad CH, Boluyt MO, Robinson KG, Brooks WW (2002) Studies of prevention, treatment and mechanisms of heart failure in the aging spontaneously hypertensive rat. Heart Fail Rev 7: 71–88

Bolotin G, Lorusso R, Kaulbach H, Schreuder J, Uretzky G, Van der Veen FH (1999) Acute and chronic heart dilation model-induced in goats by carotid jugular A-V shunt. Basic Appl Myol 9: 219–222

Bristow MR (1982) Toxic cardiomyopathy due to doxorubicin. Hosp Pract (Off Ed) 17: 101–108, 110–111

Byrne MJ, Raman JS, Alferness CA, Esler MD, Kaye DM, Power JM (2002) An ovine model of tachycardia induced degenerative dilated cardiomyopathy and heart failure with prolonged onset. J Card Fail 8: 108–15

Chekanov VS (1999) A stable model of chronic bilateral ventricular insufficiency (dilated cardiomyopathy) induced by arteriovenous anastomosis and doxorubicin administration in sheep. J Thorac Cardiovasc Surg 117: 198–199

Christiansen S, Stypmann JJ, Jahn UR, Redmann K, Fobker M, Gruber AD, Scheld HH, Hammel D (2003) Partial left ventriculectomy in modified adriamycin-induced cardiomyopathy in the dog. J Heart Lung Transplant 22: 301–308

Falk V, Fann JI, Grünenfelder J, Daunt D, Burdon TA (2000) Total endoscopic computer enhanced beating heart coronary artery bypass grafting. Ann Thorac Surg 70: 2029–2033

Flaim SF, Minteer WF, Nellis SH, Clark DP (1979) Chronic arteriovenous shunt: evaluation of a model for heart failure in rat. Am J Physiol 236: H698–H704

Garcia R, Diebold S (1990) Simple, rapid, and effective method of producing aortocaval shunts in the rat. Cardiovasc Res 24: 430–432

Gengo PJ, Sabbah HN, Steffen RP, Sharpe JK, Kono T, Stein PD, Goldstein S (1992) Myocardial beta adrenoceptor and voltage sensitive calcium channel changes in a canine model of chronic heart failure. J Mol Cell Cardiol 11: 1361–1369

Gross RD (1994) Animal models in cardiovascular research, 2nd edn. Kluwer Academic Publisher, New York

Hasnat AK, van der Velde ET, Hon JKF, Yacoub MH (2003) Reproducible model of post-infarction left ventricular dysfunction: haemodynamic characterization by conductance catheter Eur J Cardiothorac Surg 24: 98–104

Hongo M, Ryoke T, Ross J (1997) Animal models of heart failure: Recent developments and perspectives. Trends Cardiovasc Med 7: 161–167

Jiang L, Huang Y, Hunyor S, dos Remedios CG (2003) Cardiomyocyte apoptosis is associated with increased wall stress in chronic failing left ventricle. Eur Heart J 24: 742–751

Jones SP, Greer JJ, van Haperen R, Duncker DJ, de Crom R, Lefer DJ (2003) Endothelial nitric oxide synthase overexpression attenuates congestive heart failure in mice. Proc Natl Acad Sci 100: 4891–4896

Kaczmarek I, Feindt P, Boeken U, Guerler S, Gams E (2003) Effects of direct mechanical ventricular assistance on regional myocardial function in an animal model of acute heart failure. Artif Organs 27: 261–266

Kaulbach HG, Lorusso R, Bolotin G, Schreuder JJ, van der Veen FH (2002) Effects of chronic cardiomyoplasty on ventricular remodeling in a goat model of chronic cardiac dilatation: part 2. Ann Thorac Surg 74: 514–521

Kelso EJ, Geraghty RF, McDermott BJ, Cameron CH, Nicholls DP, Silke B (1997) Characterisation of a cellular model of cardiomyopathy, in the rabbit, produced by chronic administration of the anthracycline, epirubicin. J Mol Cell Cardiol. 29: 3385–3397

Kim CS, Davidoff AJ, Maki TM, Doye AA, Gwathmey JM (2000) Intracellular calcium and the relationship to contractility in an avian model of heart failure. J Comp Physiol B 170: 295–306

Kleaveland JP, Kussmaul WG, Vinciguerra T, Diters R, Carabello BA (1988) Volume overload hypertrophy in a closed-chest model of mitral regurgitation. Am J Physiol 254: H1034–1041

Koyama S, Kodama M, Izumi T, Shibata A (1995) Experimental rat model representing both acute and chronic heart failure related to autoimmune myocarditis. Cardiovasc Drugs Ther 9: 701–707

Kunzelman KS, Linker DT, Sai S, Miyake-Hull C, Quick D, Thomas R, Rothnie C, Cochran RP (1999) Acute mitral valve regurgitation created in sheep using echocardiographic guidance. Heart Valve Dis 8: 637–643

Langenickel T, Pagel I, Höhnel K, Dietz R, Willenbrock R (2000) Differential regulation of cardiac ANP and BNP mRNA in different stages of experimental heart failure Am J Physiol 278: H1500–H1506

Llaneras MR, Nance ML, Streicher JT, Lima JA, Savino JS, Bogen DK, Deac RF, Ratcliffe MB, Edmunds LH Jr (1994) Large animal model of ischemic mitral regurgitation. Ann Thorac Surg. 57: 432–439

Li GR, Lau CP, Ducharme A, Tardif JC, Nattel S (2002) Transmural action potential and ionic current remodeling in ventricles of failing canine hearts. Am J Physiol 283: H1031–1041

Liu Z, Hilbelink DR, Crockett WB, Gerdes AM (1991a) Regional changes in hemodynamics and cardiac myocyte size in rats with aortocaval fistulas 1. Developing and established hypertrophy. Circ Res 69: 52–58

Liu Z, Hilbelink DR, Gerdes AM (1991b) Regional changes in hemodynamics and cardiac myocyte size in rats with aortocaval fistulas. 2. Long-term effects. Circ Res 69: 59–65

Mishima T, Tanimura M, Suzuki G, Todor A, Sharov VG, Goldstein S, Sabbah HN (2000) Effects of long-term therapy with bosentan on the progression of left ventricular dysfunction and remodeling in dogs with heart failure. J Am Coll Cardiol 35: 222–229

Monnet E, Orton EC (1999) A canine model of heart failure by intracoronary adriamycin injection: hemodynamic and energetic results J Card Fail. 5: 255–264

Morita H, Suzuki G, Mishima T, Chaudhry PA, Anagnostopoulos PV, Tanhehco EJ, Sharov VG, Goldstein S, Sabbah HN (2002) Effects of long-term monotherapy with metoprolol CR/XL on the progression of left ventricular dysfunction and remodeling in dogs with chronic heart failure. Cardiovasc Drugs Ther 16: 443–449

Morri I, Kihara Y, Inoko M, Sasayama S (1998) Myocardial contractile efficiency and oxygen cost of contractility are preserved during transition from compensated hypertrophy to failure in rats with salt sensitive hypertension. Hypertension 31: 949–960

Muders F, Friedrich E, Luchner A, Pfeifer M, Ickenstein G, Hamelbeck B, Riegger GA, Elsner D (1999) Hemodynamic changes and neurohumoral regulation during development of congestive heart failure in a model of epinephrine-induced cardiomyopathy in conscious rabbits. J Card Fail 5: 109–116

Nikolaidis LA, Hentosz T, Doverspike A, Huerbin R, Stolarski C, Shen YT, Shannon RP (2002) Catecholamine stimulation is associated with impaired myocardial O(2) utilization in heart failure. Cardiovasc Res 53: 392–404

Nishio R, Sasayama S, Matsumori A (2002) Left entricular pressure-volume relationship in a murine model of congestive heart failure due to acute viral myocarditis. J Am Coll Cardiol 40: 1506–1514

Noguchi T, Kihara Y, Begin KJ, Gorga JA, Palmiter KA, LeWinter MM, VanBuren P (2003) Altered myocardial thin-filament function in the failing Dahl salt-sensitive rat heart Amelioration by endothelin blockade. Circulation 107: 630–635

Okafor CC, Saunders L, Li X, Ito T, Dixon M, Stepenek A, Hajjar RJ, Wood JR, Doye AA, Gwathmey JK (2003) Myofibrillar responsiveness to cAMP, PKA, and caffeine in an animal model of heart failure. Biochem Biophys Res Commun 300: 592–599

Olson RD, Mushlin PS (1990) Doxorubicin cardiotoxicity: analysis of prevailing hypotheses [see comments]. FASEB J 4: 3076–3086

Olson RD, Mushlin PS, Brenner DE, Fleischer S, Cusack BJ, Chang BK, Boucek RJ Jr (1988) Doxorubicin cardiotoxicity may be caused by its metabolite, doxorubicinol. Proc Natl Acad Sci USA 85: 3585–3589

Pacher P, Liaudet L, Bai P, Mabley JG, Kaminski PM, Virag L, Deb A, Szabo E, Ungvari Z, Wolin MS, Groves JT, Szabo C (2003) Potent metalloporphyrin peroxynitrite decomposition catalyst protects against the development of doxorubicin-induced cardiac dysfunction. Circulation 107: 896–904

Perry GJ, Wei CC, Hankes GH, Dillon SR, Rynders P, Mukherjee R, Spinale FG, Dell'Italia LJ (2002) Angiotensin II receptor blockade does not improve left ventricular function and remodeling in subacute mitral regurgitation in the dog. J Am Coll Cardiol 39: 1374–1379

Porter CB, Walsh RA, Badke FR, O'Rourke RA (1983) Differential effects of diltiazem and nitroprusside on left ventricular function in experimental chronic volume overload. Circulation 68: 685–692

Raman JS, Byrne MJ, Power JM, Alferness CA (2003) Ventricular constraint in severe heart failure halts decline in cardiovascular function associated with experimental dilated cardiomyopathy. Ann Thorac Surg 76: 141–147

Reed WM, VanVleet JF, Wigle WL, Fulton RM (1987) Furazolidone-associated cardiomyopathy in two Indiana flocks of ducklings. Avian Diseases 31: 666–672

Rhodon W (1993) Anthracyclines and the heart. Br Heart J 70: 499–502, Review

Ross J, Ikeda Y (2002) Models of dilated cardiomyopathy in the mouse and hamster. Curr Opin Cardiol 15: 197–201

Saavedra WF, Tunin RS, Paolocci N, Mishima T, Suzuki G, Emala CW, Chaudhry PA, Anagnostopoulos P, Gupta RC, Sabbah HN, Kass DA (2002) Reverse remodeling and enhanced adrenergic reserve from passive external support in experimental dilated heart failure. J Am Coll Cardiol 39: 2069–2076

Sabbah HN, Stein PD, Kono T, Gheorghiade M, Levine TB, Jafri S, Hawkins ET, Goldstein S (1991) A canine model of chronic heart failure produced by multiple sequential coronary microembolizations. Am J Physiol 260: H1379–1384

Sabbah HN, Kono T, Stein PD, Mancini GB, Goldstein S (1992) Left ventricular shape changes during the course of evolving heart failure. Am J Physiol 263: H266–270

Sabbah HN, Stanley WC, Sharov VG, Mishima T, Tanimura M, Benedict CR, Hegde S, Goldstein S (2000) Effects of dopamine beta-hydroxylase inhibition with nepicastat on the progression of left ventricular dysfunction and remodeling in dogs with chronic heart failure. Circulation 102: 1990–1995

Sacco G, Giampietro R, Salvatorelli E, Menna P, Bertani N, Graiani G, Animati F, Goso C, Maggi CA, Manzini S, Minotti G (2003) Chronic cardiotoxicity of anticancer anthracyclines in the rat: role of secondary metabolites and reduced toxicity by a novel anthracycline with impaired metabolite formation and reactivity. Br J Pharmacol 139: 641–651

Schwarz ER, Pollick C, Meehan WP, Kloner RA (1998) Evaluation of cardiac structures and function in small experimental animals: transthoracic, transesophageal, and intraventricular echocardiography to assess contractile function in rat heart. Basic Res Cardiol 93: 477–486

Sedlarik K, Eger H, Wilde J, Vollmar F, Reimann G, Schilling B, Seelig G, Fiehring H (1976) Experimental model of coronary thrombosis in the closed thorax in swine. Z Exp Chir 9: 302–315

Singal PK (1985) Adriamycin does have a potentially depressant effect on left ventricular contractility. Int J Cardiol 7: 447–449

Singal PK, Pierce GN (1986) Adriamycin stimulates low-affinity Ca^{2+} binding and lipid peroxidation but depresses myocardial function. Am J Physiol 250: H419–H425

Spinale FG, de Gasparo M, Whitebread S, Hebbar L, Clair MJ, Melton DM, Krombach RS, Mukherjee R, Iannini JP, O SJ (1997) Modulation of the renin-angiotensin pathway through enzyme inhibition and specific receptor blockade in pacing-induced heart failure: I. Effects on left ventricular performance and neurohormonal systems. Circulation 96: 2385–2396

Spinale FG, Ishihra K, Zile M, DeFryte G, Crawford FA, Carabello BA (1993) Structural basis for changes in left ventricular function and geometry because of chronic mitral regurgitation and after correction of volume overload. J Thorac Cardiovasc Surg 106: 1147–1157

Spindler M, Engelhardt S, Niebler R, Wagner H, Hein L, Lohse MJ, Neubauer S (2003) Alterations in the myocardial creatine kinase system precede the development of contractile dysfunction in beta(1)-αdrenergic receptor transgenic mice. J Mol Cell Cardiol 35: 389–397

St Louis JD, Hughes GC, Kypson AP, DeGrado TR, Donovan CL, Coleman RE, Yin B, Steenbergen C, Landolfo KP, Lowe JE (2000) An experimental model of chronic myocardial hibernation. Ann Thorac Surg 69: 1351–1357

Suzuki K, Murtuza B, Suzuki N, Smolenski RT, Yacoub MH (2001) Intracoronary infusion of skeletal myoblasts improves cardiac function in doxorubicin-induced heart failure. Circulation 104: I213–217

Tachikawa H, Kodama M, Hui J, Yoshida T, Hayashi M, Abe S, Kashimura T, Kato K, Hanawa H, Watanabe K, Nakazawa M, Aizawa Y (2003) Angiotensin II type 1 receptor blocker, valsartan, prevented cardiac fibrosis in rat cardiomyopathy after autoimmune myocarditis. J Cardiovasc Pharmacol 41 [Suppl 1]: S105–110

Takagaki M, McCarthy PM, Tabata T, Dessoffy R, Cardon LA, Connor J, Ochiai Y, Thomas JD, Francis GS, Young JB, Fukamachi K (2002) Induction and maintenance of an experimental model of severe cardiomyopathy with a novel protocol of rapid ventricular pacing. J Thorac Cardiovasc Surg 123: 544–549

Teerlink JR, Ratcliffe MB (2002) Ventricular remodeling surgery for heart failure: small animal models and how to measure an improvement in ventricular function. Ann Thorac Surg 73: 1368–1370

Tevaearai HT, Walton GB, Eckhart AD, Keys JR, Koch WJ (2002) Heterotopic transplantation as a model to study functional recovery of unloaded failing hearts. J Thorac Cardiovasc Surg 124: 1149–1156

To H, Ohdo S, Shin M, Uchimaru H, Yukawa E, Higuchi S, Fujimura A, Kobayashi E (2003) Dosing time dependency of doxorubicin-induced cardiotoxicity and bone marrow toxicity in rats. Pharm Pharmacol 55: 803–810

Toyoda Y, Okada M, Kashem MA (1998) A canine model of dilated cardiomyopathy induced by repetitive intracoronary doxorubicin administration. J Thorac Cardiovasc Surg 115: 1367–1374

Tsutsui H, Spinale FG, Nagatsu M, Schmid PG, Ishihara K, DeFreyte G, Cooper G 4th, Carabello BA (1994) Effects of chronic beta-adrenergic blockade on the left ventricular and cardiocyte abnormalities of chronic canine mitral regurgitation. J Clin Invest 93: 2639–2648

Uno Y, Minatoguchi S, Imai Y, Koshiji M, Kakami M, Yokoyama H, Ito H, Hirakawa S (1993) Modulation of noradrenaline release via activation of presynaptic beta-adrenoceptors in rabbits with adriamycin-induced cardiomyopathy. Jpn Circ J 57: 426–433

Wang X, Ren B, Liu S, Sentex E, Tappia PS, Dhalla NS (2003) Characterization of cardiac hypertrophy and heart failure due to volume overload in the rat. J Appl Physiol 94: 752–763

Ward ML, Pope AJ, Loiselle DS, Cannell MB (2003) Reduced contraction strength with increased intracellular $[Ca^{2+}]$ in left ventricular trabeculae from failing rat hearts. J Physiol 546(Pt 2): 537–550

White FC, Roth DM, Bloor CM (1986) The pig as a model for myocardial ischemia and exercise. Lab Anim Sci 36: 351–356

Wilson EM, Moainie SL, Baskin JM et al. (2003) Region- and type-specific induction of matrix metalloproteinases in post-myocardial infarction Remodeling Circulation 107: 2857–2863

Yarbrough WM, Spinale FG (2003) Large animal models of congestive heart failure: A critical step in translating basic observations into clinical applications. J Nucl Cardiol 10: 77–86

Yoshikawa T, Kokura S, Oyamada H, Iinuma S, Nishimura S, Kaneko T, Naito Y, Kondo M (1994) Abnormalities in sympathoneuronal regulation are localized to failing myocardium in rabbit heart. J Am Coll Cardiol 24: 210–215

In-Vivo Models of Arrhythmias: a Canine Model of Sudden Cardiac Death

George E. Billman

Introduction

Sudden cardiac death resulting from ventricular tachyarrhythmias remains the major cause of death in most industrially developed countries, accounting for between 300,000 and 500,000 deaths each year in the United States (Zipes and Wellens 1998). Yet despite the enormity of this problem, the identification of the mechanisms responsible for these untimely deaths, as well as the development of safe and effective anti-arrhythmic therapies, remains elusive. The use of appropriate animal models of ventricular arrhythmias is critical, not only for discovering the mechanisms that trigger lethal cardiac rhythm disorders, but also for the preclinical evaluation of potential anti-arrhythmic drugs. The model used must mimic, as closely as possible, the underlying pathological conditions most often associated with a high risk of sudden cardiac death. Over the years, a number of different animals have been used to investigate the mechanisms responsible for ventricular fibrillation and to assess anti-arrhythmic medications during the preclinical stage of development. The models used have different strengths and weaknesses and have had varying degrees of success. A detailed analysis and comparison of many of these models has recently been reviewed (Billman 2002; Study Group on Experimental Arrhythmia Research 1995) and, as such, will not be discussed in the present chapter. The present chapter will be limited to a detailed description of methods to prepare a canine model of sudden cardiac death that has proven useful in both the identification of factors contributing to ventricular fibrillation, as well as the evaluation of potential anti-arrhythmic therapies.

Description of Methods and Practical Approach

Animal Selection

Canines provide many advantages over other species. The dog has a large heart with large coronary vessels that greatly facilitates instrumentation and the surgical preparation for the studies (see below). The canine heart shares many features in common with man, including a similar autonomic neural regulation and the presence of coronary collateral blood vessels (although it must be acknowledged that these vessels are more extensive in the dog). Dogs have also been used in cardiovascular investigations since the inception of research in this area. Indeed, much of our knowledge about the physiology of the heart has been derived from studies performed in dogs. As such, there is a large body of existing literature that provides a rich tapestry upon which information obtained from additional studies can be stitched. Needless to say, the success of the studies depends upon the selection of healthy animals. The animals selected for any given study must be free of heartworms, intestinal parasites, and any acute infection. Therefore, purpose-bred animals purchased from commercial dealers should be used. These dealers can provide detailed medical histories and often also provide information about the genetic background of the animals (i.e. the breeding history).

Laboratory or purpose-bred mongrel dogs are preferred over pure-bred animals, as mongrel dogs more closely mimic the non-homogeneous genetic background of the human population. It is also critical that animals selected must be well socialized (accustomed to human contact). It is helpful to request animals that have also been trained to walk on a leash. Many years of experience indicate that there are no obvious gender differences with regards to an animal's susceptibility to ventricular fibrillation, so either sex can be used. However, it is logistically much easier to use only one sex at a time. The purpose bred animals used in the sudden death model described in the following sections are typically 7–12 months old and weigh between 15 and 25 kg, but this is more a matter of personal preference than a strict requirement.

Surgical Preparation

Over the years, the anesthesia procedure has changed as better anesthetic agents have become available. The following is the protocol that is currently used. First, the dogs are given morphine sulfate (15 mg i. m.), a catheter is placed into either the left or the right cephalic vein, and thiopental sodium (20 mg/kg, i.v.) is slowly infused to induce anesthesia. The dogs are then intubated and prepared for surgery. The incision site is prepared by first removing all the hair on left side chest to expose the skin surface. This area is then scrubbed with a providone-iodine 10% solution (Betadine, Purdue Frederick Co., Stanford CT) twice and washed with 70% isopropyl alcohol. Finally, the surgical area is sprayed with the 10% iodine solution (Betadine). A surgical plane of anesthesia is maintained by the inhalation of isoflurane (1–1.5%) mixed with 100% oxygen. The level of the anesthesia is closely monitored throughout the surgery and adjusted as need.

Using strict aseptic techniques, the chest is opened using a left thoracotomy made in either the 4th or the 5th intercostal space. The initial incision in made though the skin and subcutaneous muscle using a #22 blade. The latissimus dorsi muscle is bluntly dissected by separating between parallel muscle fibers (i.e., care is taken not to cut this muscle). The intercostal muscles are cut using blunt tipped Mayo general scissors; once the chest cavity has been opened, rib retractors are inserted and the ribs separated to allow exposure of the heart. Any bleeding that results from cutting the skin or the various muscle layers is terminated by coagulating the affected blood ves-

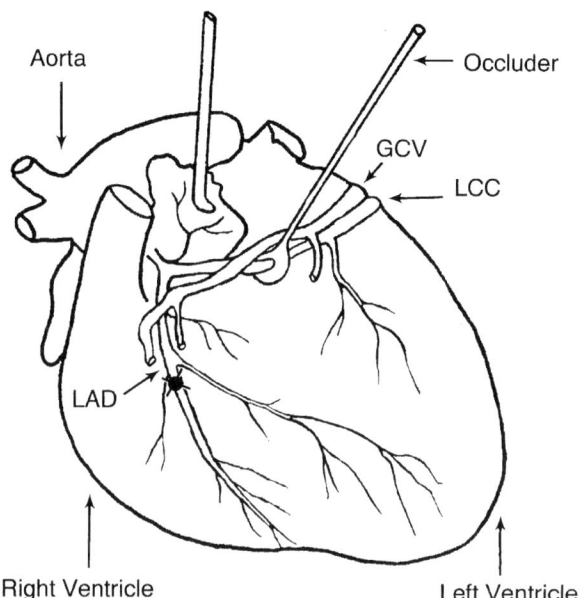

Figure 1
A schematic representation of the instrumentation of the canine heart. A pulsed Doppler flow transducer that would also be placed around the left circumflex coronary artery (LCC) is not shown for the sake of clarity. The *black dot* indicates the point at which the left anterior descending coronary artery (LAD) is ligated. The great cardiac vein (GCV) often must be ligated to facilitate the placement of the flow transducer and occluder

sels using an electrocautery unit. The left lung is wrapped with a cotton gauze sponge that had been moistened with a warm 0.9% saline solution and packed to one side, thereby allowing easy access to the pericardial sac. The pericardial sac is then opened using Metzenbaum curved blunt scissors, being careful to avoid injury to the left phrenic nerve. A pericardial cradle is made to support the heart during the surgery; i.e., the cut edges of the pericardium are temporarily attached to the chest wall with 2–0 silk suture. A suture is also tied around the tip of the left atrial appendage in order to retract this structure, exposing the left circumflex coronary artery. The left circumflex artery is carefully dissected free from the surrounding epicardial fat using slightly curved tonsil forceps. The great cardiac vein often lies on top of the left circumflex artery (Fig. 1). As a consequence, this vessel must frequently be ligated and cut in order to expose the left circumflex vessel.

If this procedure is required, then the great cardiac vein is ligated in two locations and cut between the resulting two ties, preventing any bleeding from this vessel. Approximately 3 cm of the left circumflex artery must be freed from the surrounding tissue in order to place a 20 MHz pulsed Doppler (4 mm diameter, model HDP-20–4.0-S, Crystal Biotech, Hopkinton, MA) flow transducer and a 4 mm diameter hydraulic occluder (vascular occluder model OC4, In Vivo Metric, Inc., Ukiah, CA) around this vessel. The Doppler flow transducer is used to verify that left circumflex coronary blood has been completely interrupted when the hydraulic occluder has been inflated during the exercise plus ischemia test (see below). Insulated silver-coated copper wires or commercially available pacing electrodes are also sutured to the epicardial surface of both the left and right ventricles. These electrodes are used to record a ventricular electrogram or to control heart rate with ventricular pacing.

It is possible at this time to include additional instrumentation of the heart depending upon the needs of a particular experiment. For example, flow transducers could be placed around the ascending aorta to obtain cardiac output, or a solid-state transducer could be placed into the left ventricle (via a stab wound in the apex of the left ventricle and secured with a purse string suture) to record left ventricular pressure and left ventricular dP/dt maximum (an index of ventricular contractility).

Several clinical studies demonstrate that the most important factors associated with an elevated risk for sudden death in patients are alterations in cardiac autonomic regulation (La Rovere et al. 1998), previous myocardial infarction (Davis et al. 1979), and acute ischemia at a site distant from pre-existing ischemic injury (Schuster and Bulkley 1980). Thus, the induction of acute myocardial ischemia in animals with a similar pre-existing ischemic injury would more closely model the clinical situation than ischemia produced in hearts with an entirely normal coronary circulation. For this reason an experimental myocardial infarction is also produced at the time of surgery. A small portion of the left anterior descending coronary artery is dissected free from the surrounding tissue and two ligatures (2–0 silk suture) are placed around this vessel immediately below the first large diagonal branch of this vessel (approximately one third the distance from this vessel's origin from the left main coronary artery, Fig. 1).

A 21 gauge needle with the tip removed and bent to form a right angle is placed next to the vessel and one ligature is tied around the needle and the vessel. The needle is removed thereby creating a restriction or stenosis of the left anterior descending artery. After 20 minutes the second ligature is tied completely obstructing the left anterior descending artery. This two-stage occlusion results in a smaller infarction and better survival than would be elicited by a single stage coronary artery occlusion.

Finally, all the leads to the cardiovascular instrumentation are passed though the 2nd or 3rd intercostal space (i. e., the leads do not exit through the incision site in order to promote healing and reduce the chance of post-operative infection) and are then tunnelled under the skin to exit on the back of the animal's neck. The incision is closed in four successive layers. First, the intercostal muscles are sutured together to seal the chest, followed by the latissimus dorsi muscle, skin muscle, and subcutaneous tissue. All the layers are closed with absorbable suture (e. g., 2–0 chromic gut, 2–0 polyglycolic acid suture, etc.) using a running mattress stitch. Finally the skin is closed using stainless steel skin staples. The incision site is sprayed with an iodine solution and treated with a trypsin spray (Granulex, Bertek Pharmaceuticals, Inc., Morgantown, WV) to prevent infection and promote healing. A 10 French suction catheter is also placed in the chest exiting though the 6th or 7th intercostal space. A 50 ml syringe is used to evacuate any air remaining in the chest. Note that the pericardium is not closed, thereby reducing the chance of cardiac tamponade developing after the surgery.

Post-Operative Care

After completion of the surgery, the anesthesia is turned off and the animals are placed in a quiet recovery area. The endotracheal tube is removed as soon as a swallowing reflex can be elicited in the animal. A transdermal fentanyl patch that delivers 100 µg/h for 72 h (Duragesic, Jansen Pharmaceutical Inc.) is placed on a shaved area on the back of the animal's neck (secured with adhesive tape) 12 h before surgery in order to decrease post-operative discomfort. Morphine sulfate, 1.0 mg/kg subcutaneously, is also given post-operatively as needed. Finally, the long-acting local anesthetic bupivacaine HCl (0.5 ml of 0.25% solution injected at several sites along the incision) is used to block the intercostal nerves in the area of the incision to minimize further discomfort to the animal. All analgesia is adjusted as needed for each animal. The animals are closely monitored during the recovery period and do not return to their home cage until they can support themselves sternally.

The animals are given anti-arrhythmic medication (see troubleshooting section for more details) for the first 24 h after the myocardial infarction. Finally, the animals are given a broad-spectrum antibiotic (e. g., amoxicillin 500 mg BID per os) for seven days post-op. As noted above, the cardiovascular instrument leads exit on the back of the animal's neck. These leads are each wrapped in 4×4 gauze sponge and then the neck is wrapped in medical grade adhesive tape. This neck bandage is changed and the lead exit sites are treated with 70% isopropyl alcohol and iodine spray to prevent the development of infection at least three times per week throughout the study period.

The Exercise Plus Ischemia Test

During a 3–4 week recovery period, dogs are brought to the lab daily to habituate to the laboratory environment. Approximately 2–3 weeks after the surgery the dogs are also trained to run on a motor-driven treadmill. This involves acclimating the animals to the motor noise, placing them in a harness attached to an overhead guide rope, turning the treadmill on and off several times, and finally, gradually increasing the duration and workload of a training session until the animal can complete 15–18 minutes of running. This training period can usually be completed in 2–3 days. Sudden death testing then can be conducted to classify the dogs as being either susceptible or resistant to malignant arrhythmias.

Briefly, the animals run on the treadmill for 15–18 minutes until a criterion heart rate of 210 beats/min has been achieved (~70% of maximum heart rate). The workload is increased every three minutes during this test (initial level, 0% grade 4.8 kph, 0% grade, 6.4 kph, 4% grade, 6.4 kph, 8% grade, 6.4 kph, 12% grade, and finally, 16% grade 6.4 kph). During the last minute of exercise the left circumflex occluder is inflated, the treadmill is then stopped and the occlusion maintained for an additional minute. The occlusion therefore lasts two minutes: one minute during exercise and one minute post exercise. This allows for the differentiation of arrhythmias induced during exercise, post exercise, and post occlusion release. The occlusion is immediately released in those animals that exhibit ventricular tachyarrhythmias (most frequently ventricular flutter that rapidly deteriorates into ventricular fibrillation). Large flexible metal pads (approximately 11 cm diameter) are placed across the animal's chest and are connected to an external defibrillator. A detailed discussion of the defibrillation procedure may be found in the troubleshooting section.

Examples

This model results in two highly stable populations of animals: those resistant and those susceptible to ventricular fibrillation (Billman et al. 1982; Schwartz et al. 1984). Representative recordings obtained from one susceptible and one resistant animal are displayed in Fig. 2. To date, an anterior wall myocardial infarction has been produced in a total of 730 animals. 207 (28.4%) dogs died acutely either during surgery or within the next 4 days following surgery. Thus, 523 dogs survived to be studied; of these dogs, 4 were eliminated (heart worm positive) and 33 experienced instrumentation failure (left circumflex coronary occluder rupture) and could not be classified. The exercise plus ischemia test has been performed on 486 animals. 284 dogs developed ventricular flutter that rapidly deteriorated to ventricular fibrillation (suscep-

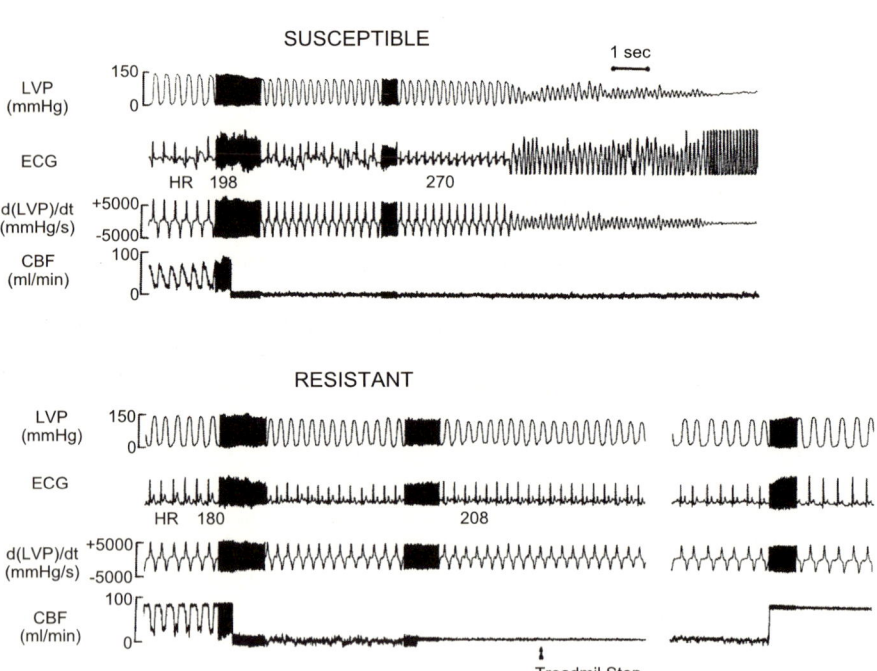

Figure 2
Representative recordings from one susceptible and one resistant animal. The exercise plus ischemia test induced ventricular flutter (that rapidly progresses to ventricular fibrillation) in the susceptible animal. Note the smaller heart rate increase in response to the coronary occlusion in the resistant animal. *LVP* left ventricular pressure, *CBF* coronary blood flow, *HR* heart rate (beats/min)

tible) during this test, while the remaining 207 did not (resistant). Only 15% of the susceptible animals were not successfully resuscitated (see below). The lethal arrhythmias were highly reproducible in the susceptible animals; that is, ventricular fibrillation could be repeatedly induced with *each* presentation of the exercise plus ischemia test. In the initial studies, ventricular fibrillation was induced once a week for up to 8 weeks (n = 8, 8 weeks, the longest period studied). In fact, only 14 of 241 (5.8%) of the susceptible animals failed to develop ventricular fibrillation during either a second or a third exercise plus ischemia test. Conversely, a resistant dog *never* developed ventricular fibrillation during repeated presentations of the exercise plus ischemia test. Therefore, unless other interventions are applied, a susceptible animal remains susceptible to lethal arrhythmias, while the resistant dogs remained resistant to arrhythmia formation throughout the course of a study. It is also important to emphasize another important advantage of this model. Each animal can act as its own control, thereby reducing the number of animals needed to perform the studies. This model was first described over twenty years ago and has proven to be useful for not only the identification of possible mechanisms that can contribute to the development of malignant ventricular arrhythmias, but also for the evaluation of the therapeutic potential of novel anti-arrhythmic drugs. The sections that follow present some representative examples of the results obtained using this model.

Differences in the Autonomic Control of the Heart in Animals Susceptible and Resistant to Ventricular Fibrillation

A number of studies have been completed that indicate that the susceptible animals exhibit alterations in the autonomic control of the heart.

1. The heart rate response to pharmacologically-induced increases in arterial pressure (baroreceptor reflex sensitivity) was significantly reduced in susceptible as compared to resistant animals (Billman et al. 1982; Schwartz et al. 1988). For example, the heart rate reduction induced by a 30 mmHg increase in arterial pressure was -40 ± 12.2 beats/min in resistant animals and -2.9 ± 5 beats/min in susceptible animals. Similar findings have been reported in a number of recent clinical studies (Task Force of the European Society of Cardiology and the North American Society of Pacing and Electrophysiology 1996). To cite just one example, La Rovere et al. (1998) reporting for the ATRAMI (Autonomic Tone and Reflexes After Myocardial Infarction) group found that post-myocardial infarction patients with either low heart rate variability (see below) or a small heart rate response to an increase in blood pressure had a much greater risk of sudden death than those with well preserved cardiac vagal tone. The greatest risk for mortality was observed in patients with a large reduction in both markers of cardiac vagal tone.
2. Time series analysis of the periodic fluctuations in R–R interval (0.24 to 1.04 Hz), a non-invasive marker of cardiac vagal activity (Task Force of the European Society of Cardiology and the North American Society of Pacing and Electrophysiology 1996), was used to evaluate the heart rate response to exercise (Billman and Hoskins 1989; Houle and Billman 1999). The heart rate and heart variability response to submaximal exercise for susceptible and resistant animals are shown in

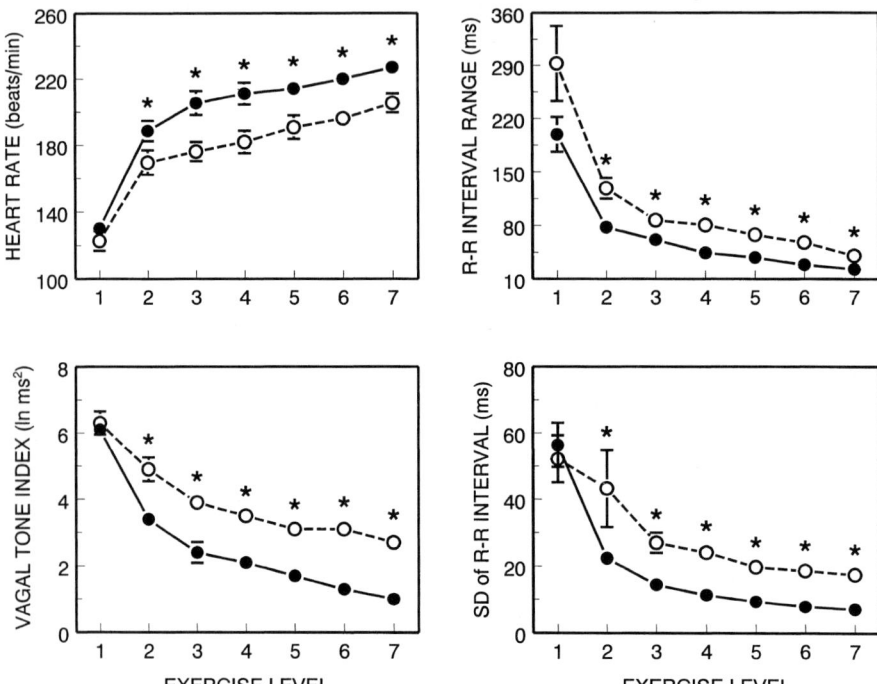

Figure 3
The heart rate and heart variability response to submaximal exercise in susceptible (n = 22, solid line/filled circles) and resistant (n = 14, dashed line/open circles) animals. Note the higher heart rate and greater reductions in all three indices of cardiac parasympathetic activity in response to the exercise for the susceptible animals.
* = p<0.01, exercise levels: level 1 = control 1 minute before the onset of exercise; level 2 = 4.8 kph/0% grade; level 3 = 6.4 kph/0% grade; level 4 = 6.4 kph/4% grade; level 5 = 6.4 kph/8% grade; level 6 = 6.4 kph/12% grade; and level 7 = 6.4 kph/16% grade

Fig. 3. Exercise induced larger increases in heart rate in the susceptible animals as compared to the resistant animals. This greater heart rate increase was accompanied by correspondingly greater reductions in several indices of the cardiac vagal activity in the susceptible animals. Conversely, atropine given during exercise elicited a much greater heart rate increase in the resistant dogs (HR change resistant 54.2±7 versus susceptible 18.7±4.4 beats/ min). β-adrenoceptor blockade attenuated the heart rate increase induced by exercise but exacerbated the reductions in the cardiac vagal tone index. Lower values of cardiac vagal activity were still noted even after β-adrenoceptor blockade in the susceptible dogs.

3. The time series analysis was also performed to evaluate the cardiac response to acute myocardial ischemia at rest (Collins and Billman 1989). The heart rate and heart variability response to a two-minute occlusion of the left circumflex coronary artery for susceptible and resistant animals are shown in Fig. 4. The coronary artery occlusion elicited significantly greater increases in heart rate in the susceptible dogs (control 115.6±5.8, occlusion 176.1±8.7 beats/min) compared to resistant animals (control 114.6±8.9, occlusion 145.7±7.5 beats/min). Correspondingly,

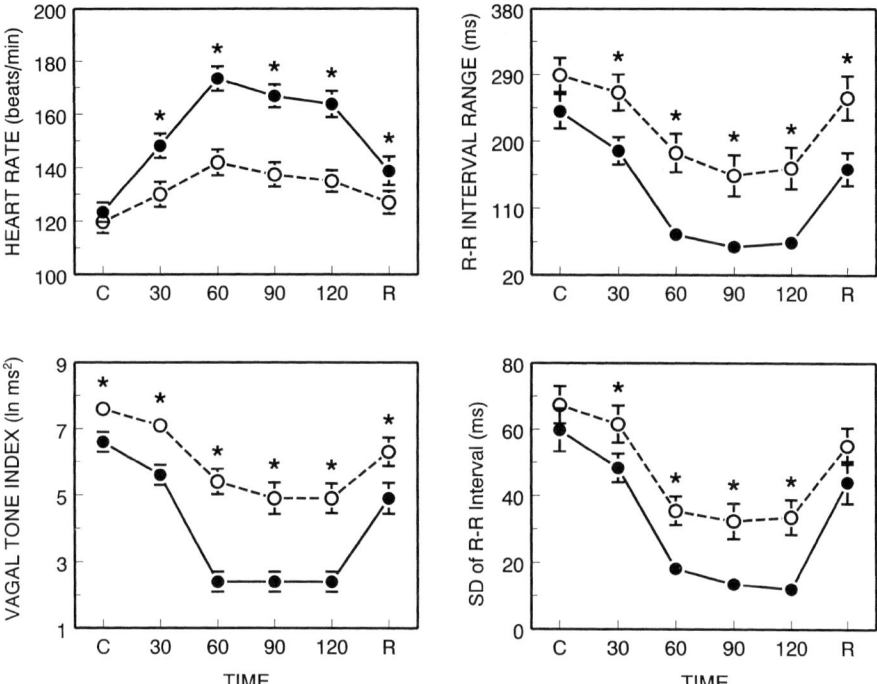

Figure 4
The heart rate and heart variability response to left circumflex coronary artery occlusion at rest in susceptible (n = 40, *solid line/filled circles*) and resistant (n = 23, *dashed line/open circles*) animals. Note the higher heart rate and greater reductions in all three indices of cardiac parasympathetic activity in response to myocardial ischemia in the susceptible animals.
* = $p<0.01$, C = control one minute before the occlusion, R = three minutes after the occlusion release. Time indicated is seconds

the indices of cardiac vagal activity were reduced to a much greater extent in the susceptible animals. β-adrenoceptor blockade reduced but did not eliminate the heart rate differences noted between the groups. In fact, this intervention provoked even greater reductions in the cardiac vagal activity index.

When considered together, these data demonstrate that animals susceptible to malignant arrhythmias exhibit alterations in the autonomic control of the heart: namely, an elevated sympathetic activity accompanied by reductions in parasympathetic activity.

Autonomic Interventions and Susceptibility to Ventricular Fibrillation

The data described above suggest that alterations in the autonomic control of the heart contribute significantly to the development of arrhythmias. If this hypothesis were to be correct, then one would predict that interventions designed either to reduce sympathetic activity or to enhance parasympathetic activity would protect against ventricular fibrillation. Conversely, an increase in sympathetic or a reduction in parasympathetic activity should provoke arrhythmias in resistant animals. Listed below are several studies that largely confirm these predictions:

Parasympathetic Interventions

Cardiac vagal activity was enhanced by the cholinergic agonist carbachol (20 µg/kg, i.v., Billman 1990). This intervention prevented ventricular fibrillation in 11 of 14 susceptible animals. This drug also reduced heart rate. Therefore, studies were repeated with heart rate held constant by means of ventricular pacing. Carbachol prevented ventricular fibrillation in 5 of 6 susceptible animals even with heart rate held constant. These data suggest that heart rate alone cannot account for this drug's protection. In a similar manner, the effects of the cholinergic intracellular second messenger cyclic GMP on susceptibility to ventricular fibrillation were examined using the long acting cyclic GMP analogs, 8-bromo cyclic GMP (n = 9, infused at the rate of 100–150 µg/kg/min, i.v. throughout the exercise test) or dibutyryl cyclic GMP (n = 5, infused at the rate 100–150 µg/kg/min. i.v. throughout the exercise test). Representative recordings from the same susceptible animals before and after 8-bromo cyclic GMP treatment

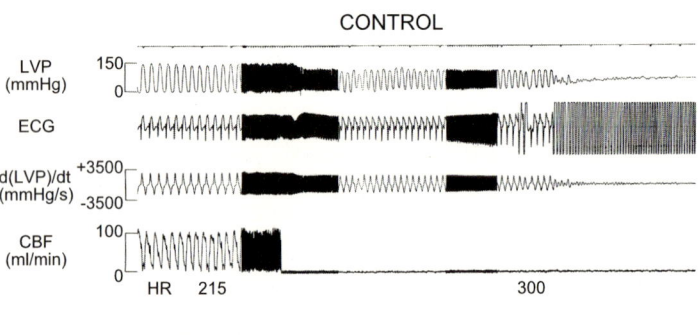

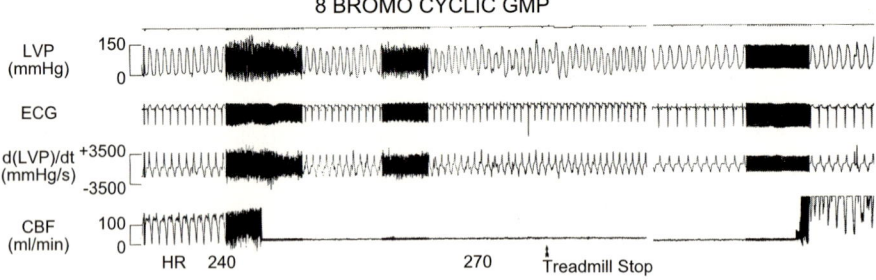

Figure 5
Representative recordings obtained from the same susceptible animal before and after treatment with 8-bromo cyclic GMP (long acting analog of cyclic GMP, parasympathetic intracellular second messenger). Removal of the left stellate ganglion (LSGX). Note absence of ventricular arrhythmias during the 8-bromo cyclic GMP treatment. 8-bromo cyclic GMP prevented ventricular fibrillation in 8 of 9 susceptible animals, dibutyryl cyclic GMP protected 5 of 5 susceptible animals. Thus, cyclic GMP protected 13 of 14 animals tested. *LVP* left ventricular pressure, *CBF* coronary blood flow, *HR* heart rate (beats/min)

are shown in Fig. 5. Increasing cyclic GMP levels reduced the heart rate res-ponse to the coronary artery occlusion and protected 13 of the 14 susceptible animals from malignant arrhythmias (Billman 1990). In contrast, the cholinergic antagonist atropine sulfate (50 µg/kg i.v.) was given three minutes before the coronary occlusion (i.e., while the animals were running) to 21 resistant animals; 3 animals developed ventricular fibrillation while 6 additional dogs showed an increase in arrhythmia formation (unpublished observation). Therefore, a reduction in parasympathetic activity is probably not solely responsible for ventricular fibrillation.

Baseline parasympathetic activity was also increased with low doses (2 µg/kg, i.v.) of atropine sulfate (Halliwill et al. 1998), but the apparent increase in vagal activity was not maintained during myocardial ischemia and, as such, failed to prevent ventricular fibrillation. Thus, baseline or resting increases in vagal activity are insufficient to prevent ventri-cular fibrillation induced by ischemia; only interventions that increase cardiac parasympathetic drive even during ischemia can prevent malignant arrhythmias.

Sympathetic Interventions

Several anti-adrenergic interventions have been shown to protect against ventricular fibrillation. Removal of the left stellate ganglion has proven to be one of the most effective of these interventions (Schwartz et al. 1984). Representative recordings from the same susceptible animal before and after removal of the left stellate ganglion are displayed in Fig. 6. This intervention prevented ventricular fibrillation in all eleven susceptible animals while β-adrenoceptor blockade with propranolol HCl (1 mg/kg, i.v.) only protected 11 of 18 animals tested (unpublished observation). It should be

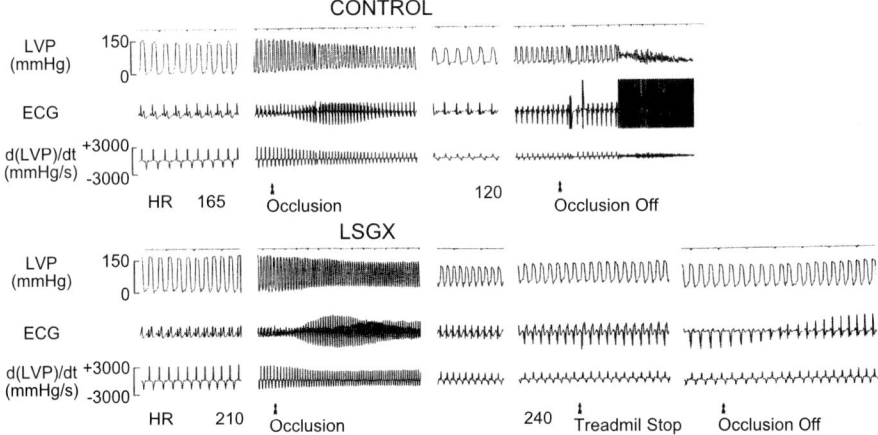

Figure 6
Representative recordings obtained from the same susceptible animal before and after removal of the left stellate ganglion (LSGX). Note that despite the large ischemic ECG changes, the removal of the left stellate ganglion prevented ventricular fibrillation during the second exercise plus ischemia test. LSGX protected 11 of 11 susceptible animals tested. *LVP* left ventricular pressure, *HR* heart rate (beats/min)

noted that 3 of the animals went into acute ventricular pump failure (i.e., ventricular systolic pressure fell to low levels while diastolic pressure increased). Propranolol also decrea-sed heart rate. However, studies have not yet been completed to address the possible contribution of this reduction in heart rate to the protection from ventricular fibrillation. The selective β_2-adrenoceptor antagonist, ICI 118,552 (0.2 mg/kg, i.v.), also prevented ventricular fibrillation 10 of 11 animals tested (Billman et al. 1997). However, the drug also reduced heart rate in 6 animals. Therefore, the ICI 118,551 exercise plus ischemia test was repeated with heart rate held constant by ventricular pacing (n = 3). ICI 118,551 still prevented ventricular fibrillation when heart rate was maintained.

Conversely, the sympathomimic drug, cocaine (1 mg/kg, i.v. given 3 minutes before the coronary occlusion was shown to induce ventricular fibrillation in resistant animals even without the presence of a pre-existing myocardial infarction (Billman and Hoskins 1988).

Effect of Daily Exercise on Susceptibility to Ventricular Fibrillation

It is now well established that aerobic exercise conditioning can alter cardiac autonomic tone, both reducing cardiac sympathetic activity and increasing cardiac parasympathetic activity (Billman 2002) and may, thereby, protect against malignant arrhythmias. In order to test this hypothesis, susceptible animals were assigned to either an exercise (six weeks treadmill running, n = 8) or a sedentary (six week cage rest, n = 8) group (Billman et al. 1984). At the end of the six week period, the animals were re-tested with the exercise plus ischemia test; all 8 exercise treated animals but only 1 of the sedentary animals were protected from ventricular fibrillation. The baroreceptor reflex control of heart rate was evaluated every two weeks during the test period. The heart rate response to an increase in arterial pressure was increased in the exercise treated group but not in the sedentary group; the heart rate response to submaximal exercise was also reduced in the exercise group. Two of the exercised animals were then tested after a six-week cage rest. The heart rate response to an increase in arterial pressure declined toward pre-exercise training levels and the exercise plus ischemia test induced ventricular fibrillation in one animal and non-sustained ventricular tachycardia in the other animal.

These data suggest that daily exercise may alter autonomic tone and thereby protect against ventricular fibrillation induced by myocardial ischemia. However, the mechanisms responsible for the changes in susceptibility remain to be investigated fully. In particular, it must be emphasized that the changes in autonomic cardiac regulation implicated by the baroreceptor reflex changes were not systematically investigated. Thus, the relative contribution of increases in the parasympathetic and/or decreases in sympathetic neural control remains to be determined. One would predict, however, that if exercise-induced increases in vagal tone dominate, then cholinergic antagonists should eliminate this protection. Studies are currently in progress to test this hypothesis.

Effect of Alterations in Calcium Entry and Sarcoplasmic Reticulum Calcium Release in Susceptibility to Ventricular Fibrillation

The studies mentioned above clearly indicate that the autonomic nervous system plays an important role in the genesis of life-threatening arrhythmias. The cellular mediators of this autonomic imbalance probably contribute significantly to ventricular fibrillation. Over the last several years a number of studies have focused on the role that changes in intracellular calcium play in ventricular fibrillation. A brief summary of these studies is as follows:

1. The intracellular calcium chelator BAPTA (delivered as BAPTA-AM, 1.0 mg/kg, i.v.) was shown to prevent ventricular fibrillation induced by either myocardial ischemia (protecting 8 of 12 susceptible animals) or by calcium overload induced by the calcium channel agonist BAY K 8644 (30 µg/kg, i.v., preventing ventricular fibrillation in 5 of 5 resistant animals) (Billman et al. 1991).
2. Calcium channel antagonists (verapamil, 250 µg/kg, i.v.; diltiazem, 1.0 mg/kg, i.v.; mibefradil, 1.0 mg/kg, i.v.; high doses of nifedipine, 100 µg/kg, i.v.; and magnesium, 100 mg/kg, i.v.) prevented ventricular fibrillation in susceptible animals (verapamil 17 of 17, diltiazem, 8 of 8, mibefradil 13 of 17, nifedipine 8 of 9, and magnesium 7 of 9 dogs) while the calcium channel agonist BAY K 8644 (30 µg/kg, i.v.) induced ventricular fibrillation in all nine resistant animals tested (Billman 1989; Billman et al. 1991; Billman and Hamlin 1996). The calcium antagonist studies also demonstrated the important role that acute myocardial ischemia plays in the induction of malignant arrhythmias, which has important implications with regards to the evaluation of potential anti-arrhythmic drugs. Programmed electrical stimulation induced non-sustained ventricular tachycardia in 19 of 25 susceptible animals but failed to induce even single extrasystoles in any resistant animal (n = 23) (Billman and Hamlin 1996). Lidocaine (2 mg/kg i.v., injected three minutes before the occlusion) completely suppressed these electrically-induced arrhythmias, whereas calcium channel antagonists (mibefradil, verapamil and diltizam) not only failed to prevent these arrhythmias, but also increased the duration of the ventricular tachycardia in about half the susceptible animals. In contrast, the same dose of lidocaine failed to prevent arrhythmias induced by the exercise plus ischemia test, while pretreatment with the calcium channel antagonists protected against ventricular fibrillation (Billman and Hamlin 1996). This observation may help explain why so many promising anti-arrhythmic medications have proven to be such dismal failures in the clinical setting. The drugs may have been developed to prevent the wrong arrhythmias; that is, drugs were selected to prevent re-entrant arrhythmias induced by programmed electrical stimulation rather than those potentially life-threatening arrhythmias associated with myocardial ischemia.

It is, therefore, crucial to identify what factor or factors render the *ischemic* myocardium vulnerable to arrhythmia formation in order to develop effective anti-arrhythmic interventions. Once this has been accomplished, it should then be possible to develop therapeutic interventions that correct these ischemically-induced changes in cardiac electrical stability and thereby prevent sudden death. The "ideal" drug would be one that only affects the ischemic tissue with little or no action on the normal cardiac tissue. As a consequence of this selectivity, one would expect that these drugs should also have a low propensity for pro-arrhythmic events.

3. The role of calcium release from the sarcoplasmic reticulum was evaluated using ryanodine (10 µg/kg, i.v.) to deplete sarcoplasmic reticulum calcium. This drug did not prevent ventricular fibrillation induced by ischemia (only 1 of 10 animals was protected), but it significantly decreased left ventricular dP/dt max (Lappi and Billman 1993). In contrast, the same dose of ryanodine prevented ventricular tachycardia (n = 10) induced by ouabain (40 µg/kg i.v., bolus followed by 0.076 µg/kg/min infusion over 1 h, then a second 20 µg/kg bolus) in anesthetized dogs. Thus, alterations in sarcoplasmic reticular calcium release may contribute to arrhythmias resulting from digitalis toxicity but not those arrhythmias induced by myocardial ischemia.

When considered together, these data suggest that alterations in intracellular calcium that result from enhanced calcium entry, rather than from increased calcium release from the sarcoplasmic reticulum, are responsible for ventricular fibrillation induced by myocardial ischemia.

The Role of the ATP-sensitive Potassium Channel in Susceptibility to Ventricular Fibrillation

It is now generally accepted that the activation of the ATP-sensitive potassium channel during myocardial ischemia provokes a potassium efflux and reductions in action potential duration that lead to dispersion of repolarization (Billman 1994). Since heterogeneity of repolarization plays a crucial role in the induction of ventricular fibrillation, drugs that prevent ATP-sensitive potassium channel activation should be particularly effective in the suppression of malignant arrhythmias induced by ischemia. The non-selective ATP-sensitive potassium channel antagonist glibenclamide either at a high (10 mg/kg, i.v.) or at a low dose (1.0 mg/kg i.v.), prevented ventricular fibrillation in 13 of 15 (Billman et al. 1993) and 6 of 7 (Billman et al. 1998) animals, respectively. However, this drug also reduced exercise-induced increases in mean coronary blood flow, depressed left ventricular function, and produced profound hypoglycemia (particularly at the high dose). Recently, drugs selective for the cardiac sarcolemmal cardiac ATP-sensitive potassium channel have been developed (Gogelein 2001). As such, these drugs would attenuate ischemically induced changes in cardiac electrical properties, thereby preventing malignant arrhythmias without the untoward effects of non-selective drugs. HMR 1883 (or its sodium salt HMR 1098) has been shown to block only cardiac sarcolemmal ATP-sensitive potassium channels (Gogelein et al. 1998). This drug attenuated ischemically-induced ST segment changes and prevented ventricular fibrillation in 16 of 20 susceptible animals tested without altering blood glucose levels, mean coronary blood flow, or ventricular function (Billman et al. 1998; unpublished data). Since the ATP-sensitive potassium channel only becomes active as ATP levels fall, HMR 1883 should *only* have effects on ischemic tissue with little or no effect noted on normal tissue. Thus, selective antagonists of the cardiac cell surface ATP-sensitive potassium channel may represent the first truly "ischemia selective" anti-arrhythmic medications, and as such, should be free of the pro-arrhythmic effects that have plagued many of the currently available anti-arrhythmic drugs.

Troubleshooting

The most frequent problems encountered in the model are as follows: early post-myocardial infarction mortality, instrumentation failure, and unsuccessful resuscitation of the animals following the induction of ventricular fibrillation. The selection of the appropriate sample size is also critical for the accurate detection of the effects of the intervention under investigation on the susceptibility to sudden death.

Anti-arrhythmic Therapy

It has proven to be very difficult to control post-operative arrhythmias resulting from the myocardial infarction which remain the primary cause of post-operative death. Over the past several years a variety of different anti-arrhythmic protocols have been used. The following protocol has proven to be the most successful approach. Briefly, procainamide (500 mg i.m.) is injected immediately before the surgery begins. An intravenous drip of normal saline containing 200 μg/ml of lidocaine HCl is started at the rate of 1–2 ml per minute and maintained throughout the surgery period. The dogs also receive bolus injections of lidocaine HCl (60 mg i.v.) during each stage of the two-stage occlusion. It should be noted that additional treatment with anti-arrhythmic medications beyond the first 24 h following the experimental myocardial infarction failed to reduce early mortality. Indeed, these drugs, if anything, increased the early mortality rate. For this reason, anti-arrhythmic medications are now given only during the acute myocardial infarction (peri-operative) period. With the advent of this therapy schedule, at least 70% of the animals routinely survived to be studied.

Defibrillation Procedure

The animal is fitted with large flexible metal pads (Stadz Pads, Zoll Medical Corp., Burlington, MA) placed across its chests. These defibrillation pads are directly connected to a defibrillator (M series, Zoll Medical Corp., Burlington, MA) prior to placement on the treadmill. In order to ensure a good electrical contact, the fur on the left and right side of the chest is removed and the pads are tightly secured next to the skin of the chest on either side of the heart area using adhesive tape and followed by an elastic bandage (ACE bandage). Extra electrode gel is also applied to the defibrillation pads to reduce the electrical resistance between the defibrillation electrodes and the animal. The pad placement is critical; care must be taken to ensure that electrical shock is delivered across the heart. As noted above, the left circumflex occlusion is immediately released in those animals that exhibit ventricular fibrillation. The animal is then disconnected from any recording device and a 300 Joules shock is rapidly delivered to the animal but *only after it loses consciousness* (tested by the absence of an eye blink reflex). As such, the animal does not experience any untoward effects of the electrical defibrillation. If necessary, the animal is placed on its left side and external cardiac massage begun. The external massage facilitates emptying the heart, thereby reducing the heart size and increasing the chance for successful defibrillation. All subsequent shocks are delivered using 360 Joules. Timing is also critical, the faster the shocks can be delivered the greater is the chance for success. Defibrillation often occurs on the first shock and is usually achieved by the third or fourth shock. One week after a successful defibrillation, the exercise plus ischemia test can be repeated. In a typical experimental sequence, the animal first will be classified as being either susceptible or resistant to ventricular fibrillation, one week later the studies will be repeated after pre-treatment with a drug under investigation and then, on a subsequent day, a second control (untreated) exercise plus ischemia test is performed to reconfirm the susceptibility of the animal (i. e., to guarantee that any protection noted resulted from the drug treatment and not as a consequence of a non-specific or a time-dependent healing effect). The number of defibrillation episodes any given animal may experience should also be limited to no more than three. As with any technique, be it learning to ride a bicycle or master a complex piano sonata, practice makes perfect. During the last twenty years, this exercise plus ischemia test has elicited ventricular fibrillation in 284 dogs. The initial resuscitation rate hovered around 70%. However, the current success rate is better than 90%. Overall, only 43 of the 284 animals (15.1%) have not been successfully defibrillated.

Instrumentation Failure

The instrument that is most critical for the success of the experiments is the hydraulic occluder that is placed around the left circumflex coronary artery. It is not possible to classify the animals without a functional coronary occluder. Therefore, care must be taken to ensure that this device remains in a fully operational condition. As noted above, studies could not be completed in several animals due to the failure of this device. The most common problem has been the rupture of the balloon. Many of the failures resulted from an older occluder design; a much lower failure rate is associated with the vascular occluder now in use. Even with the better occluder design, there are a number of steps that further reduce occluder rupture. Firstly, only new occluders should be used. Despite the higher cost, recycled occluders should not be used. Secondly, the occluder should be tested before use by inflating it with air to make sure that there are no leaks. If a leak is detected, or the occluder does not inflate properly, this occluder should be discarded and replaced with a working one. Care should also be taken to make sure that the occluder is not inadvertently "nicked" by a needle during the implantation procedure. Finally, the number of occlusions made with a given occluder should be limited. The balloon tends to weaken with repeated inflation-deflation cycles and, as a result, it may fail if inflated too many times.

A Comment on Sample Size

In addition to the problems described in the proceeding section, sample size is also an important consideration for the accurate interpretation of any experimental results. A power analysis should be performed before any study to determine the optimal number to detect differences between treatment groups. Sample size can also dramatically influence the results obtained for a compound. Trolese-Mongheal and coworkers (Trolese-Mongheal et al. 1985) investigated the effects of sample size on the reproducibility of sudden death using a large series of dogs (n = 648) in which acute myocardial ischemia was produced by ligation of the left anterior descending coronary artery. They then randomly divided these animals into groups of various sizes (n = 10 to n = 100) and found that the pre-treatment rate of sudden death varied widely depending on the sample size. For example, the sudden death rate ranged from 0 to 70% and 5 to 55% if the sample size was 10 or 20 dogs, respectively. In contrast, a much smaller range (14 to 36%) was found in groups that contained 100 animals. Stable values were obtained with a sample size of between 50 and 60 dogs. This wide disparity in the incidence of sudden death may explain the often-conflicting results that have been obtained with the same compound.

In other words, the risk for a false positive result was inversely related to the sample size; that is, the smaller the sample size, the greater the risk was to conclude falsely that a given treatment protected against sudden death. These authors (Trolese-Mongheal et al. 1985), therefore, concluded that a reliable assessment of the anti-arrhythmic potential for a given drug could only be made with at least 50 animals per treatment group.

However, it is not always possible to use large numbers of animals in the pre-clinical evaluation of test compounds, due to both the high costs and the long periods of time that would be necessary to complete studies. Approaches that employ the same animals in both the control and treated groups (i.e., provide an internal control) would reduce the total number of animals required and thereby expedite the evaluation of a compound or set of compounds. Thus, an appropriate model must not only closely mimic the pathology responsible for sudden death in patients but also use a sufficient number of animals so that the anti-arrhythmic properties of a given drug can be accurately assessed.

References

Billman GE (1989) The effect of calcium channel antagonists on susceptibility to sudden cardiac death: protection from ventricular fibrillation. J Pharmacol Exp Therap 248: 1334–1342

Billman GE (1990) The effect of carbachol and cyclic GMP on susceptibility to ventricular fibrillation. FASEB J 4: 1668–1673

Billman GE (1994) The role of the ATP-sensitive K^+ channel in K^+ accumulation and cardiac arrhythmias during myocardial ischemia. Cardiovasc Res 28: 762–769

Billman GE (2002a) Aerobic exercise conditioning: a non-pharmacological antiarrhythmic intervention. J Appl Physiol 92: 446–454

Billman GE (2002b) Animal Models of Lethal Arrhythmias. Drug Dev Res 55: 59–72

Billman GE, Hoskins RS (1988) Cocaine induced ventricular fibrillation: Protection afforded by the calcium channel antagonist verapamil. FASEB J 2: 2990–2995

Billman GE, Hoskins RS (1989) Time-series analysis of heart rate variability during submaximal exercise. Evidence for reduced cardiac vagal tone in animals susceptible to ventricular fibrillation. Circulation 80: 146–157

Billman GE, Hamlin RL (1996) The effects of a novel calcium channel antagonist, mibefradil, on refractory period and arrhythmias induced by programmed electrical stimulation and myocardial ischemia: a comparison with diltiazem and verapamil. J Pharmacol Exp Therap 277: 1517–1526

Billman GE, Schwartz PJ, Stone HL (1982) Baroreceptor reflex control of heart rate: A predictor of sudden death. Circulation 66:874–880

Billman GE, Schwartz PJ, Stone HL (1984) The effects of daily exercise on susceptibility to sudden cardiac death. Circulation 69: 1182–1189

Billman GE, McIlroy B, Johnson JD (1991) Elevated myocardial calcium and its role in sudden cardiac death. FASEB J 5: 2586–2592

Billman GE, Avendano CE, Halliwill JR, Burroughs JM (1993) The effects of the ATP-dependent potassium channel antagonist glyburide on coronary blood flow and susceptibility to ventricular fibrillation. J Cardiovasc Pharmacol 21:197–204

Billman GE, Castillo LC, Hensley J, Hohl CM, Altschuld RA (1997) β_2-adrenergic receptor antagonists protect against ventricular fibrillation: In vivo evidence and in vitro evidence for enhanced sensitivity to β_2-adrenergic stimulation in animals susceptible to sudden death. Circulation 96: 1914–1922

Billman GE, Englert HC, Schoelkens BA (1998) HMR 1883, a novel cardioselective inhibitor of the ATP-sensitive potassium channel; Part II: effects on susceptibility to ventricular fibrillation induced by myocardial ischemia in conscious dogs. J Pharmacol Exp Therap 286: 1465–1473

Collins MN, Billman GE (1989) Autonomic response to coronary occlusion in animals susceptible to ventricular fibrillation. Am J Physiol Heart Circ Physiol 257:H1886–H1894

Davis HT, Decamilla J, Bayer LW, Moss AJ (1979) Survivorship patterns in the post hospital phase of myocardial infarction. Circulation 64: 1252–1258

Gögelein H (2001) Inhibition of cardiac ATP-dependent potassium channels by sulfonylurea drugs. Curr Opin Invest Drugs 2: 71–80

Gögelein H, Hartung J, Englert HC, Scholkens BA (1998) HMR 1883, a novel cardioselective inhibitor of the ATP-sensitive potassium channel. Part I: effects on cardiomyocytes, coronary flow and pancreatic beta-cells. J Pharmacol Exp Ther 286: 1453–1464

Halliwill JR, Billman GE, Eckberg DL (1998) Effect of a vagomimetic atropine dose on canine cardiac vagal tone and susceptibility to sudden cardiac death. Clin Auton Res 8: 155–164

Houle MS, Billman GE (1999) Low-frequency component of the heart rate variability spectrum: a poor marker of sympathetic activity. Am J Physiol Heart Circ Physiol 267: H215–H223

Lappi MD, Billman GE (1993) The effect of ryanodine on ventricular fibrillation induced by myocardial ischemia. Cardiovasc Res 27: 2152–2159

La Rovere MT, Bigger JT Jr, Marcus FI, Mortara A, Schwartz PJ (1998) Baroreflex sensitivity and heart rate variability in prediction of total cardiac mortality after myocardial infarction. Lancet 351: 478–484

Schuster EH, Bulkley BH (1980) Ischemia at a distant site after myocardial infarction: a cause of early postinfarction angina. Circulation 62: 509–515

Schwartz PJ, Billman GE, Stone HL (1984) Autonomic mechanisms in VF due to acute myocardial ischemia during exercise in dogs with healed myocardial infarction: An experimental model for sudden cardiac death. Circulation 69: 790–800

Schwartz PJ, Vanoli E, Stramba-Badiale M, DeFerrari GM, Billman GE, Foreman RD (1988) Autonomic mechanisms and sudden death, new insight from the analysis of baroreceptor reflexes in conscious dogs with and without a myocardial infarction. Circulation 78: 969–979

Study Group on Experimental Arrhythmia Research of the Working Group on Arrhythmias of the European Society of Cardiology (1995) The role of basic arrhythmia research: the continued need for experiments in the intact heart and organism. Eur Heart J 16: 1469–1475

Task Force of the European Society of Cardiology and the North American Society of Pacing and Electrophysiology (1996) Heart rate variability: standards of measurement, physiological interpretation and clinical use. Circulation 93: 1043–1065

Trolese-Mongheal Y, Duchene-Marullaz P, Trolese J-F, Leinot M, Lamar J-C, Lacroix P (1985) Sudden death and experimental acute myocardial infarction. Am J Cardiol 56: 677–681

Zipes DP, Wellens HJ (1998) Sudden cardiac death. Circulation 98: 2334–2351

In-Vivo Models of Atrial Fibrillation

Ulrich Schotten, Yuri Blaauw and Maurits Allessie

Introduction

For decades the dominant interest of electrophysiologists has been arrhythmias of ventricular origin. Because of their life-threatening nature, diagnosis and treatment of ventricular arrhythmias always has been high on the list of important problems in basic and clinical electrophysiological research. For several reasons during the last decade atrial fibrillation (AF) has attracted the interest of an increasing number of cardiologists, physiologists and pharmacologists (Fig. 1). Firstly, both incidence and prevalence of AF are increasing. At present, the prevalence in the European Union approaches 1%. In elderly people (>75 years) the prevalence exceeds 8% (Benjamin et al. 1994) and with further ageing of our population it is expected to increase even further (Benjamin et al. 1998). Also, successful treatment of ventricular arrhythmias may have turned attention to the remaining challenges in arrhythmia management.

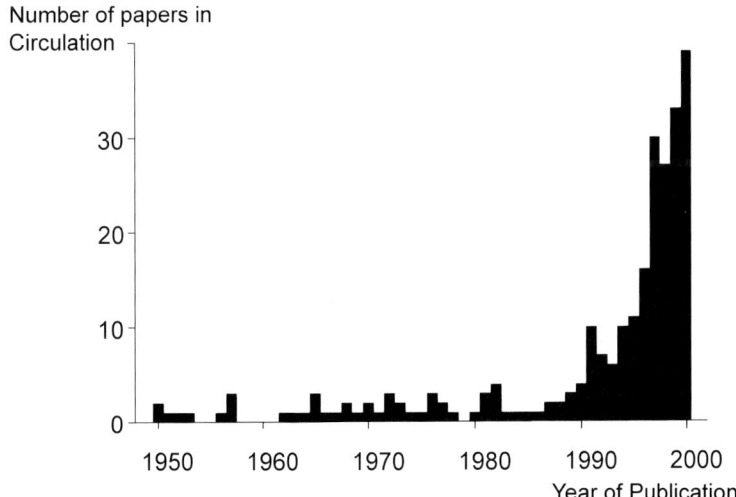

Figure 1
Number of papers on atrial fibrillation published in Circulation between 1950 and 2000. During the last decade, the interest in AF has increased exponentially. (From Duytschaever 2002, thesis, University Maastricht)

This book chapter gives an overview of the development of physiological and therapeutic concepts of AF during the past decades. Very often these achievements were closely related to the availability of appropriate animal models.

Historic Remarks

The first description of atrial fibrillation (AF) was given by McWilliam in 1887. He described patients with a "conspicuously irregular arterial pulse", which he attributed to "delirium of the heart" (McWilliam 1887). On examination, these patients suffered from palpitations, exercise intolerance, easy exhaustion, and a general feeling of ill health. The radial pulse revealed a totally disordered rhythm. The heart action was rapid and irregular, strong pulsations taking turns with runs of almost imperceptible beats, and the intervals between the beats varying markedly.

Although by that time it was already known that cardiac contractions are caused by electrical impulses (Sanderson 1879), the electrophysiology of the heart could not be properly investigated until 1903, when Einthoven invented the string galvanometer (Einthoven 1903). The first clinical electrocardiogram of AF was published in 1906 (Einthoven 1906). A few years later Rothberger and Winterberg (1909) and Lewis (1909) established uniform criteria for the diagnosis of AF, i.e. total irregularity of the ventricular cycle length (R-R-intervals), absence of discrete atrial activation (P waves) and irregular fast oscillations of the baseline.

Lewis supported the view that AF was caused by numerous electrical impulses in the atrial wall (Lewis 1909). Initially, he regarded it as a state in which many stimuli were generated at separate points, the uncoordination of the contraction of the atria being the result of multiple impulses that block locally. Although the known causes of ectopic impulses, like increased cardiac pressure, fibrosis, and ischemia, showed no consistent relationship with atrial fibrillation, Lewis regarded the arrhythmia initially as extra-systolic in nature. Later he changed his mind, after Mines demonstrated that under certain conditions, a continuous circus movement of the electrical impulse could be initiated in myocardial rings (Mines 1913, 1914): "... But if, on the other hand, the wave is slower and shorter (and it is made slower and shorter by the conditions which produce fibrillation) the excited state will have passed off at the region where the excitation started ... Under these circumstances, the wave of excitation may spread a second time over the same tract of tissue; once started in this way it will continue unless interfered by some external stimulus ...". Mines argued that the rate of beating is then controlled by three factors: the conduction velocity and the duration of the refractory period on the one hand, and the size of the circuit on the other (Allessie 1984). However, because of the irregular activity during AF it was difficult to prove any of the proposed mechanisms at that time, and it was not until 50 years later that Moe introduced his multiple wavelet hypothesis. Moe postulated that both ectopic activity and circus movement played a role in clinical atrial fibrillation (Allessie 1984). He assumed that if the spread of recovery is inhomogeneous, some fibers would already be excitable while nearby fibers would still be refractory. As a result "a grossly irregular wave front becomes fractionated as it divides about islets or strands of refractory tissue and each of the daughter wavelets may now be considered as independent offspring." Perpetuation of AF would then depend on the number of wavelets simultaneously present in the atria.

Experimental evaluation of the multiple wavelet hypothesis was made possible by the development of computer technology, enabling reconstruction of the activation patterns during AF by high density mapping. In experimental studies in isolated Langendorff-perfused canine hearts, episodes of atrial flutter and atrial fibrillation were induced by infusion of acetylcholine and rapid pacing (Allessie 1984). Endocardial mapping of both atria showed that during flutter a single fixed intra-atrial circuit existed, whereas during AF, multiple wandering and re-entering wave fronts were present. From these studies it was concluded that multiple re-entering wavelets played an important role in the genesis of AF.

Models of Tachycardia-induced Atrial Remodeling

In the 1990s several experimental investigations addressed the self-perpetuating and progressive nature of AF. In a dog model of prolonged rapid atrial pacing, Morillo et al. (1995a) found that the atrial refractory period was reduced by about 15%. In the goat, Wijffels et al. (1995). maintained AF by a fibrillation pacemaker. This custom-made device continuously analyzed a left atrial electrogram and automatically delivered a burst of stimuli (1 s, 50 Hz) as soon as sinus rhythm occurred (Fig. 2, upper panels). By this method AF could be maintained as long as desired. In this model, AF shortened atrial refractoriness from ~150 to ~80 ms (45%). More importantly, these two studies showed that long-term rapid atrial pacing or maintenance of AF led to a progressive increase in the stability of AF. After 6 weeks of rapid atrial pacing, episodes of AF lasting >15 min could be induced in 82% of the dogs (Morillo et al. 1995a).

In the goat, initially only short paroxysms of AF were induced by burst pacing (mean 6±3 s) but after 2 days of AF the paroxysms lasted several minutes and by that time AF had become sustained (>24 h) in 2 of 12 animals. After 2–3 weeks AF was persistent in 90% of the goats. This observation of tachycardia-induced electrical remodeling creating a background for persistent AF, led to the concept that "Atrial Fibrillation Begets Atrial Fibrillation" (Fig. 2, lower panel) (Wijffels et al. 1995). The longer duration of the AF episodes was explained by a shortening of the wavelength of the atrial impulse (Allessie 1998; Rensma et al. 1988) When the wavelength is short, small regions of intra-atrial conduction block may already serve as sites for initiation of re-entry, thus increasing the vulnerability for AF. A short wavelength is also expected to increase the stability of AF because it allows more re-entering wavelets to co-exist on the available surface area of the atria. A shortening of the atrial refractory period was also found in dogs undergoing prolonged rapid atrial pacing (42 days) (Fig. 3). In atrial cardiomyocytes of these animals I_{CaL} was found to be reduced by 70%, whereas repolarizing currents were less affected (Yue et al. 1997a). Inhibiting I_{CaL} of a control cell with nifedipine mimicked the action potential changes produced by atrial tachycardia, whereas increasing I_{CaL} with BayK8644 partly reversed action po-

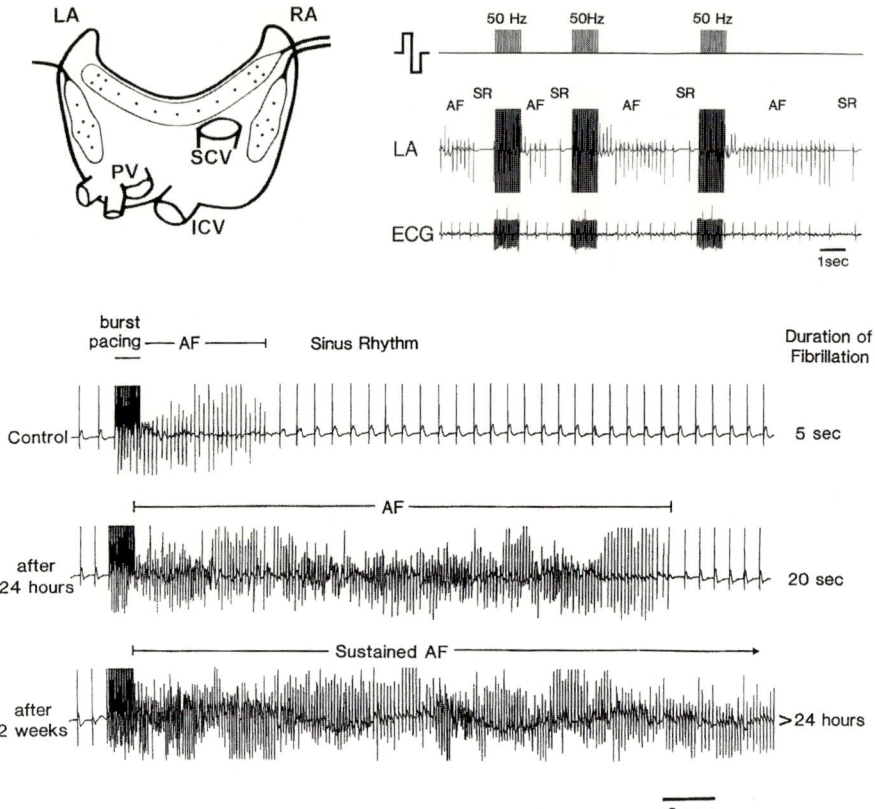

Figure 2
Upper left panel: Goats were chronically instrumented with 27 electrodes mounted on 3 silicon strips sutured on the atrial epicardium. One strip was placed along Bachmann's Bundle, the other two were fixed to the right and left atrial wall.
Upper right panel: A left atrial bipolar electrogram was continuously analyzed by the custom-made fibrillation pacemaker. As soon as sinus rhythm occurred, a burst of stimuli reinduced an episode of AF. By this technique AF could be maintained 24 h a day.
Lower panel: The duration of the AF episodes increased during the first days of AF. While AF was short-lasting under control conditions, it did not stop spontaneously after 2 weeks of artificially maintained AF. (From Wijffels et al. 1995)

tential alterations in tachycardia-remodeled cardiomyocytes. These results strongly suggest that a reduction of I_{CaL} indeed underlies the tachycardia-induced shortening of the refractory period.

However, there are reasons to believe that besides the shortening of refractoriness, other factors also play a role in the development of chronic AF. Already in the initial study in the goat model of AF, it was noted that the time course of the changes in atrial refractoriness did not run parallel with the increase in persistence of AF. Whereas the AF cycle length reached a new steady state within 3–5 days, it took an additional 1–2 weeks before AF became persistent (Wijffels et al. 1995). This led to the hypothesis that a so-called 'second factor' was involved in the development of persistent AF.

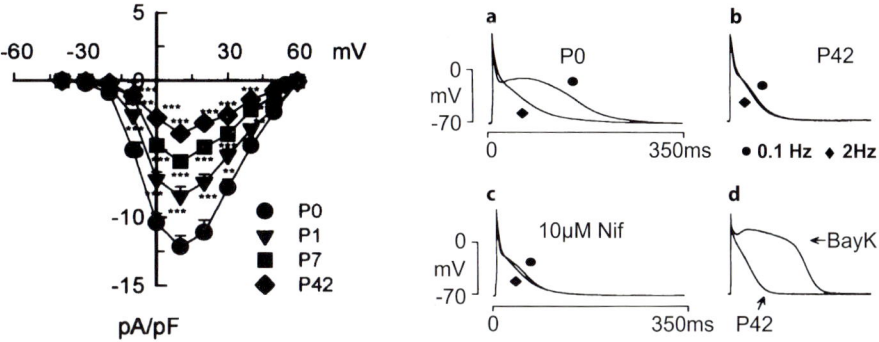

Figure 3
Left panel: Voltage current relationships of I_{Ca} during control (P0) and after 1, 7 and 42 days of rapid atrial pacing in the dog. The density of I_{Ca} was progressively reduced with the duration of rapid pacing. *Right panel:* Action potentials recorded at 0.1 (·) and 2 Hz (¨) in control atrial cells (P0) and after 42 days of rapid atrial pacing (P42). Addition of nifedipine (C) mimicked the effects of electrical remodeling, whereas the Ca-agonist BayK 8644 restored the plateau phase of the action potential (D) (from Yue et al. 1997)

We therefore recently suggested the existence of additional positive feedback mechanisms contributing to the self-perpetuating nature of AF (Allessie et al. 2002). Both changes in the mechanical properties as well as alterations in the ultrastructure of the atria might contribute to the domestication of the arrhythmia and increase the stability of AF.

The rapid and irregular atrial contractions during AF result in a depression of atrial transport function and contribute to the reduction in ventricular filling and cardiac output. Echocardiographic studies in patients have shown that not only during AF but also after cardioversion, the contractile function of the atria is impaired. Since I_{CaL} is also one of the most important regulators of the atrial contractile function, electrical remodeling is expected to follow the same time course after the onset of AF as the AF-induced atrial contractile dysfunction. To test this hypothesis goats were chronically instrumented with piezoelectric crystals positioned in the groove between auricle and aortic root and on the free atrial wall of each side (Fig. 4, upper panels) (Schotten et al. 2003). The crystals allowed the continuous recording of the right and the left atrial diameter. A pressure transducer was chronically implanted in the right atrium *via* one of the jugular veins. The atrial pressure was plotted against the atrial diameter and the area enclosed by this pressure diameter loop reflected the work performed by this atrial beat. During 5 days of artificially maintained AF, the refractory period shortened from ~140 ms to ~85 ms. In addition, the strength of the atrial contractions declined. Already after 2 days of AF, the open pressure-diameter loop became closed, i.e. the atrial contractile function was nearly completely abolished (Fig. 4, lower left panel). The atrial work index decreased from 16 mmx mmHg to 2 mmx mmHg and then remained constant until day 5. The reverse remodeling of the refractory period and the contractile function followed the same time course (Fig. 4, lower right panel). After 2 days of SR, the open pressure-diameter loop was completely recovered and the refractory period increased from 85 ms to 133 ms. Obviously, elec-

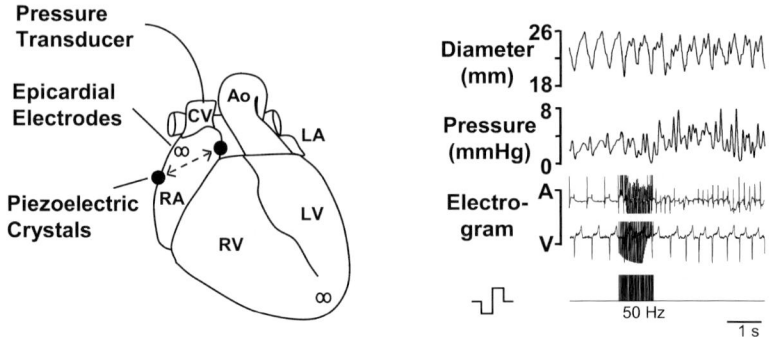

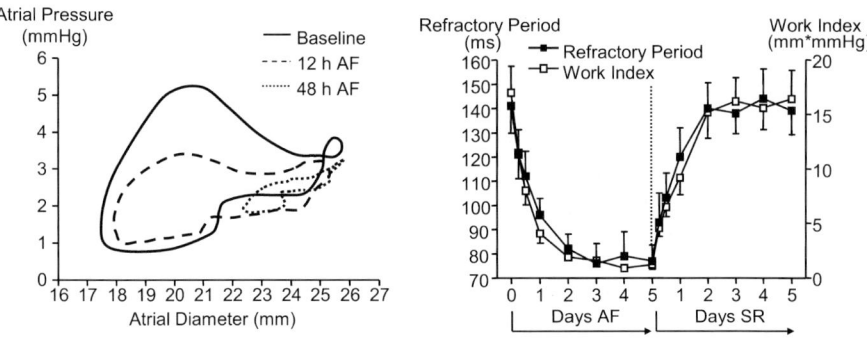

Figure 4
Upper left panel: Chronic instrumentation: Piezoelectric crystals were sutured to the right atrial epicardium. Right atrial pressure was measured with an implantable pressure transducer. *LA* left atrium, *RA* right atrium, *CV* superior caval vein, *Ao* Aorta.
Upper right panel: Simultaneous recording of the right atrial diameter and pressure. AF was induced by burst stimulation of the atria.
Lower panels: Time course of electrical and contractile remodeling during the first days of AF. Atrial contractile function and AERP were recorded 30 min after spontaneous cardioversion during atrial pacing at a cycle length of 400 ms. Left: Right atrial pressure and diameter recordings at baseline, after 12 h and after 48 h of AF. Right: Time course of electrical and contractile remodeling and reversibility in 7 goats. (From Schotten et al. 2003)

trical and contractile remodeling are very closely linked to each other and are probably due to the same underlying mechanism. Since the main cellular mechanism responsible for electrical remodeling is the reduction of I_{CaL}, it is reasonable to assume that the development of the atrial contractile dysfunction during the first 5 days of AF is mainly caused by the reduction of the Ca^{2+} inward current.

The first study showing that AF causes alterations in the ultrastructure of atrial myocytes was that of Morillo et al. (1995b). In dogs undergoing rapid atrial pacing for six weeks, electron microscopic investigation of the dilated atria showed an increase in size and number of mitochondria and disruption of the sarcoplasmic reticulum (Morillo et al. 1995a). In goats, Ausma et al. (1997a) maintained AF for 9–23 weeks.

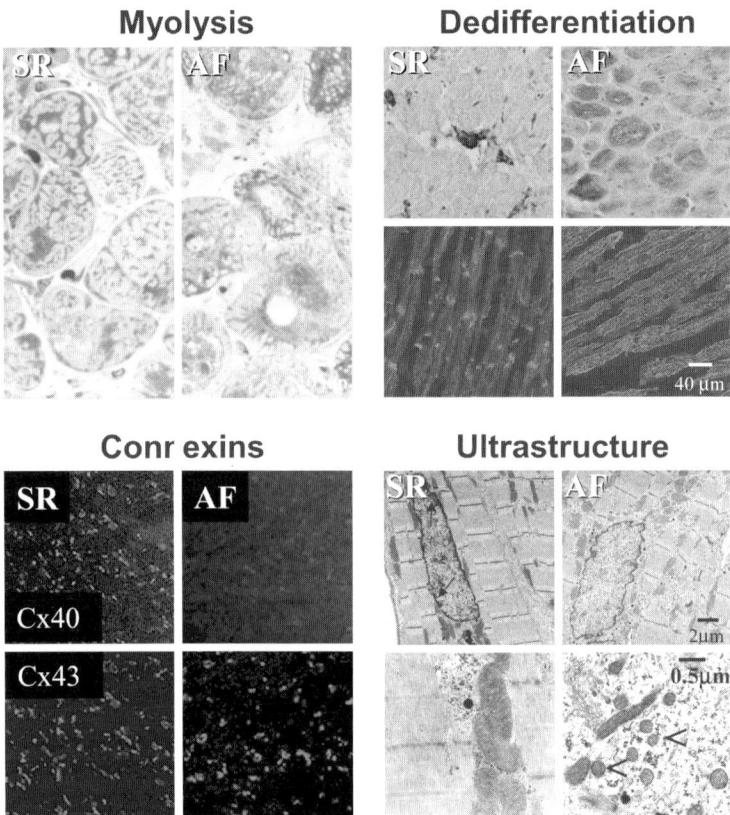

Figure 5
Structural remodeling of atrial myocytes after 4 months of AF in the goat. The *left-hand pictures* are taken from goats in sinus rhythm; the *right-hand photographs* are from goats in chronic AF. Light microscopy (*upper left panel*) shows cells with severe myolysis (loss of sarcomeres: blue staining) and accumulation of glycogen (red). Immunostaining of structural proteins (*right upper panel*) demonstrates the dedifferentiation of the atrial myocardium by a clear increase in fetal α-smooth muscle actin (red staining in *upper pictures*). In the *lower pictures* of this panel the myocytes are stained for desmin (red). The nuclei are stained by blue DAPI. During AF, desmin looses its cross-striated pattern in the cytoplasm and at the intercalated disks the intensified desmin staining is no longer present. In the *lower left panel* changes in gap-junctions are shown. Labeling of C×40 (green) and C×43 (red) revealed a clear reduction in C×40 and no change in C×43 expression. Electron microscopy (*lower right*) shows changes in the subcellular organization of the atrial myocytes. During AF, the atrial nuclei acquire a more homogeneous distribution of chromatin. For comparison the normal clustering of chromatin at the nuclear membrane is indicated by *arrows in the upper left panel*. During AF many small mitochondria can be found (*arrowheads right lower panel*). (From Ausma et al 1997a,b; Van der Velden et al. 2000). *For coloured version see appendix*

After this time, atrial myocytes showed marked changes in their cellular substructures, such as loss of myofibrils, accumulation of glycogen, changes in mitochondrial shape and size, fragmentation of sarcoplasmic reticulum, and dispersion of nuclear chromatin. Also, gap junctions became more heterogeneously distributed (Fig. 5).

These changes were accompanied by an increase in the size of atrial myocytes and closely resembled changes in ventricular myocytes due to chronic low flow ischemia (hibernation) (Borgers et al. 1993). This hibernation of fibrillating atrial myocardium is heterogeneously distributed, with some strongly affected cells next to virtually normal cells.

Although in general the different animal models show similar structural changes, some differences exist between different species and different models of atrial tachyarrhythmias. In the dog, a high atrial rate is associated with an increase in size of mitochondria (Morillo et al. 1995b), whereas in the goat model of AF numerous small mitochondria with longitudinally oriented cristae were found (Ausma et al. 1997b). Whereas in models with pure atrial tachyarrhythmias, the extracellular matrix was not changed (Morillo et al. 1995b; Ausma et al. 1997b), in canine atria subjected to a combination of rapid atrial pacing and mitral regurgitation, the volume of the intercellular space was increased (Everett et al. 2000).

In patients with AF, the degree of interstitial fibrosis, both between individual myocytes (endomysial) and atrial bundles (perimysial) is increased (Thiedemann et al. 1977; Wouters et al. 2001). It should be noted, however, that in fibrillating human atria, structural changes might differ significantly from the findings in animal models. Both in SR and AF, extensive tissue fibrosis and degenerative changes are very common and probably related to ageing and/or associated heart diseases (Bailey et al. 1968; Fenoglio et al. 1973, 1979; Pham et al. 1978; Mary et al. 1983; Kitzman et al. 1990; Schotten et al. 2001).

Vagal AF

In the 1970s evidence for a role of the parasympathetic nervous system was demonstrated in patients with AF. Coumel et al. (1978) reported that some cases of lone AF were associated with periods of enhanced vagal tone. These authors used the autonomic tone before the onset of AF to identify so-called vagal AF in humans. More recently, Chen et al. (1998) found in patients with paroxysmal supraventricular tachycardia that the baroreflex sensitivity and presumably parasympathetic tone was higher in patients who developed paroxysmal AF than in those without AF. These clinical observations emphasize the role of parasympathetic tone in modulation of atrial electrophysiology and propensity for AF.

Already in 1915 Rothberger and Winterberg had observed that AF could easily be induced in normal canine atria during vagal stimulation (Rothberger et al. 1915). These experiments provided the potential for testing new mechanistic hypotheses and new therapeutic strategies. In dogs, vagal stimulation shortens the refractory period (ERP) and the wavelength during AF (Rensma 1988). The increase in the number of coexisting wavelets makes AF less likely to self-terminate. The shortening of the refractory period during vagal stimulation has been shown to be heterogeneously distributed over the atria (Rensma et al. 1988; Alessi et al. 1959; Yue et al. 1997b). Induction of AF is most consistent when stimulation is performed in areas with shorter ERP. In such cases, block of premature beats in areas with longer ERP will result in slow propagation of the wave front around the area of long refractoriness with subsequent

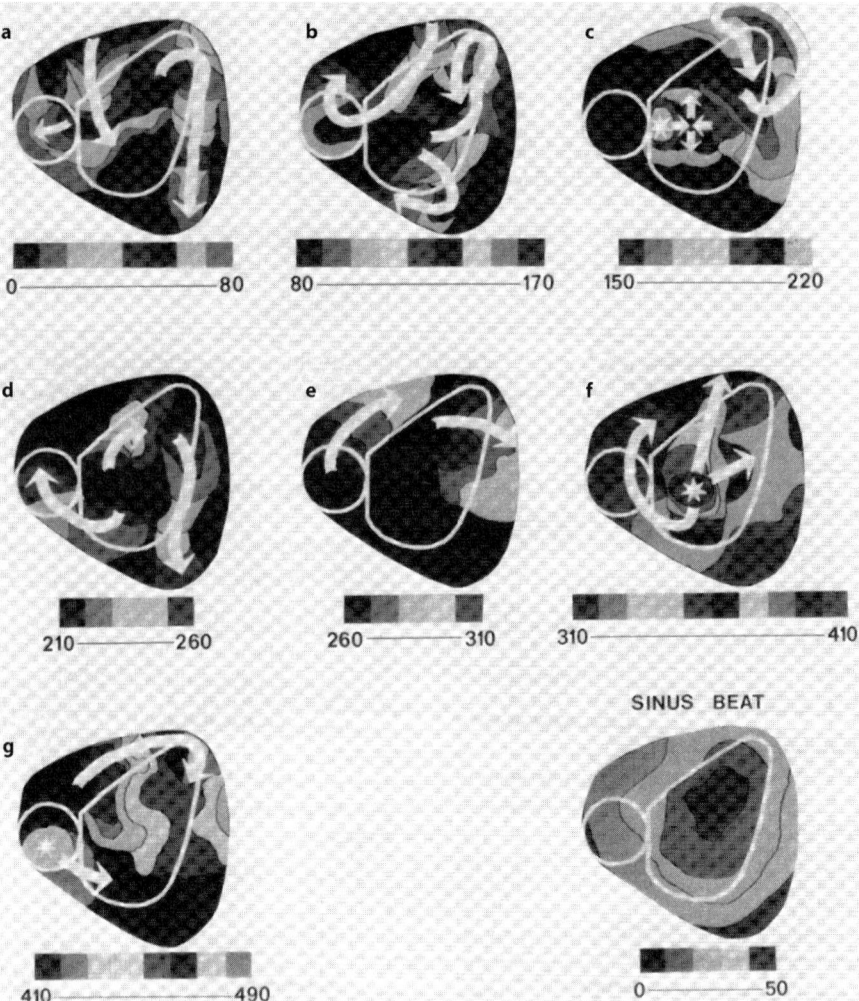

Figure 6
Spread of activation in the right atrium during 500 ms of stable AF in a Langendorff perfused canine heart (0.4 mg/l acetylcholine). Gray scale isochrones of 10 ms. Asterisks indicate impulses entering the right atrium from the left atrium. *Lower right corner:* Activation during sinus rhythm. (From Allessie et al. 1985)

reexcitation of previously depolarized sites. The more intense the vagal stimulation, the greater the dispersion of refractoriness and the likelihood of a premature beat to encounter refractory tissue (Wang et al. 1996).

The relative ease with which sustained AF can be induced in the presence of m-cholinergic stimulation was used by numerous investigators to unravel the fundamental electrophysiological mechanisms of AF. In 1985, Allessie et al. were able to map the spread of activation in canine atria during rapid-pacing induced AF in the presence of acetylcholine (Fig. 6) (Allessie et al. 1985). A custom-made high resolution mapping system allowed simultaneous recording of electrical activity from several hundred sites on the atrium. They demonstrated for the first time multiple propagating wave fronts during AF *in vivo* as had been postulated in Moe's multiple wavelet theory 30 years earlier.

Allessie et al. demonstrated that in their model a critical number of 4 to 6 wavelets are required to sustain AF. This idea was supported by the findings of Wang et al. (1993) who found in a similar model that termination of AF with class IC drugs was preceded by a decrease in the number of wavelets.

In 1992, Schuessler et al. (1992) demonstrated that in isolated canine atria, acetylcholine converted multiple reentrant circuits to one single rotating wave front with fibrillatory conduction in the periphery of the preparation. Under these conditions such 'rotors' (spiral waves) are stationary or travel slowly across the atrial wall until they are anchored to anatomical heterogeneities of the cardiac muscle. Schuessler et al. (1993) demonstrated discordant activation of the epicardium and the endocardium particularly in areas of the atrial wall thicker than 0.5 mm. The role of anatomical heterogeneities in the atrial activation pattern was further supported by Wu et al. (1998). These authors reported that in canine right atria, pectinate muscles could form a substrate for conduction block in the presence of acetylcholine allowing stationary re-entry.

It should be noted however, that this activation pattern does not necessarily reflect the electrical behavior of human atria. In general, reentry in the atria may be functional in nature (Allessie et al. 1973) and more recent mapping studies in human AF revealed no preferential sites of reentry. Also, spiral waves were only occasionally observed, were unstable, and tended to drift over the atria rather than being stationary (Konings et al. 1994).

Since vagal stimulation shortens the atrial refractory period and increases spatial dispersion of refractoriness, one might speculate that ablation of cardiac parasympathetic nerves might be beneficial, at least in patients with 'vagal AF'. The feasibility of selective atrial vagal denervation had been demonstrated by Randall and Ardell (1985). They identified two epicardial fat pads supplying fibers preferentially to the superior right atrium and the sinus node or to the AV-node and the left atrium, respectively.

Later a third fat pad was identified through which most efferent vagal fibers appeared to travel to the sinus node and the AV-node (Chiou et al. 1997). Ablation of all three fat pads was demonstrated to prevent vagally induced shortening of the refractory period and induction of AF during vagal stimulation. More recent studies showed that a selective ablation of atrial parasympathetic nerves is also possible using a transvascular approach and successfully abolished vagally mediated AF (Schauerte et al. 2000). This procedure provides an opportunity to study the usefulness of neural ablation in chronic animal models of AF and eventually in patients with AF and high vagal tone.

In summary, experimental models of vagal AF are relatively easy to establish and have certainly contributed to the development of antiarrhythmic drugs and some aspects of atrial electrophysiology during AF. However, one should be aware that disease states that promote atrial arrhythmias in humans differ widely. Mechanistic concepts and therapeutic approaches developed in these models might therefore fail in other causes of AF such as tachycardia-induced electrical remodeling or in dilated or structurally remodeled atria.

Sterile Pericarditis

In 1986 Waldo's group described a new model of atrial flutter (Page et al. 1986). During a thoracotomy both atria were dusted with sterile talc powder and additionally a single layer of gauze was put on both atria. Electrodes were sutured on multiple atrial sites and the chest was closed. During the first week after surgery, electrophysiological measurements were performed daily and the susceptibility for atrial arrhythmias was evaluated by various pacing protocols. The results clearly showed that atrial arrhythmias could easily be induced. In over 90% of the animals, atrial flutter was induced on at least 1 of the first 4 postoperative days. With time, the susceptibility for atrial arrhythmias decreased and 1 week after surgery flutter could be induced in only 1 out of 4 animals. The mechanism of the arrhythmia was unclear, both atrial refractoriness and conduction velocity were similar in susceptible and non-susceptible dogs.

It is of interest to note that the time-course of inducibility of atrial flutter in this model shows striking similarities with the appearance of atrial fibrillation in patients after cardiothoracic surgery. Thus it was concluded that the sterile pericarditis model could be very useful to study the mechanisms of postoperative atrial arrhythmias.

In subsequent studies the activation patterns during AF were studied. Kumagai et al. (1997) performed detailed multi-site mapping during induced AF and demonstrated that one to four circulating reentrant circuits with very short cycle lengths were responsible for maintenance of the arrhythmia. Unstable reentrant circuits involving the septum, the right atrial free wall, around the pulmonary veins and the inferior and superior vena cava were observed. In three of these reentrant circuits the wave front propagated along Bachman's bundle. Based on this, a subsequent study was designed to evaluate the possibility of terminating AF by interrupting this 'critical crossroad' with single-site radiofrequency catheter ablation. Indeed, catheter ablation of the Bachman bundle terminated and prevented the induction of AF by atrial pacing (Kumagai et al. 2000).

In a recent study from the same group, the anti-arrhythmic effects of steroids were evaluated (Goldstein et al. 2003). It was hypothesized that suppression of the inflammatory response with anti-inflammatory agents would reduce the occurrence of arrhythmias. Administration of oral prednisone completely prevented AF during the 4-day measurement period. Histological examination revealed that the degree of inflammation was indeed reduced in steroid-treated animals. Interestingly, in an earlier study Yared et al. (2000) showed that administration of a single dose of dexamethasone reduced the incidence of postoperative AF from 32.3 to 18.9% in patients undergoing elective coronary or valvular heart surgery. Although the underlying mechanisms were not addressed in that study, it supports a link between postoperative AF and an inflammatory response.

Heart Failure and Atrial Fibrillation

In clinical practice AF only occasionally develops in a background of tachycardia-induced electrical remodeling or inflammatory processes. In the majority of cases, AF is the end stage of long-term anatomical and histological changes induced by struc-

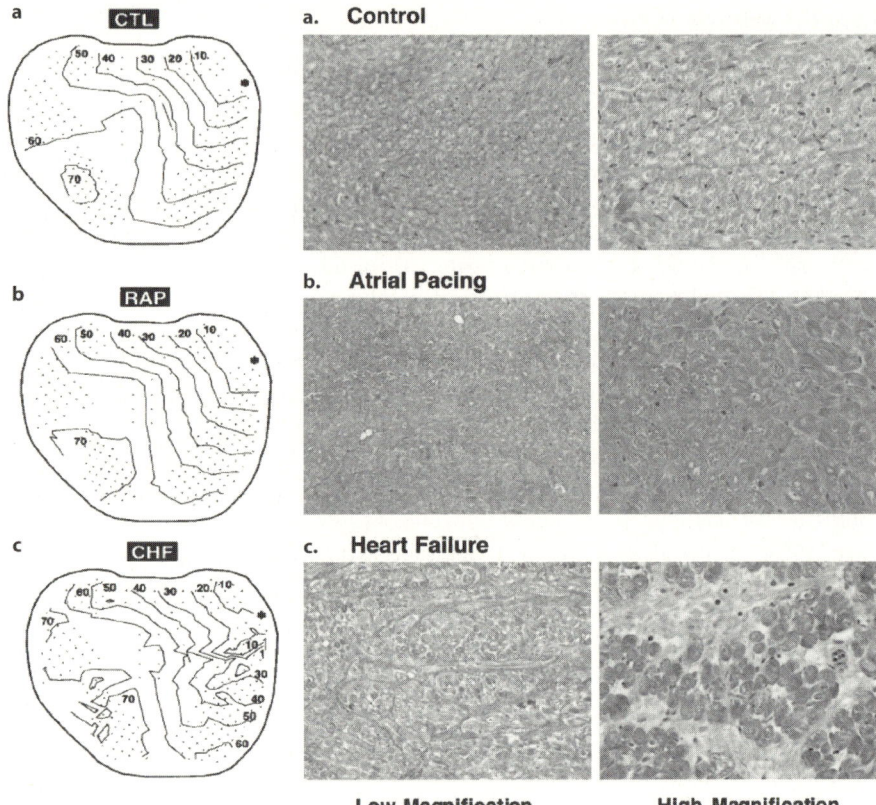

Low Magnification High Magnification

Figure 7a–c
Different kinds of atrial remodeling in canine atria. **a** Control. **b** Rapid atrial pacing for 6 weeks. **c** Tachycardiomyopathy produced by rapid ventricular pacing for 6 weeks. Both in rapid atrial pacing and in heart-failure dogs, the duration of electrically induced AF episodes was prolonged.
Left: Crowding of isochrones indicates local slowing of conduction only in the in the dog with heart failure. *Right:* Histological examination revealed severe tissue fibrosis in the heart-failure dog, whereas rapid atrial pacing had no significant effect on connective tissue formation.
The comparison shows that in the rapid atrial pacing model the stability of AF is related to shortening of the refractory period, whereas tachycardiomyopathy on the ventricular level creates a background for AF based on changes in the atrial ultrastructure with conduction disturbances. (Modified from Li et al. 1999). *For coloured version see appendix*

tural heart diseases such as valvular disorders, hypertension or heart failure. In 40% of all patients, the prevalence of AF is highest in severe heart failure. To elucidate how heart failure can promote vulnerability for AF, Nattel and co-workers (Li et al. 1999) studied the inducibility and stability of AF in a dog model of congestive heart failure. In these animals a pacing lead was inserted in the right ventricle and high rate ventricular pacing (220 to 240 bpm) was applied for a period of 3 weeks. As a consequence, the animals developed clinical and hemodynamic signs indicative of heart failure. After 3 weeks of pacing the stability of induced AF episodes had clearly increased. Sustained AF could be induced In 10 out of 18 dogs compared to none in the control dogs. AF was characterized by monomorphic electrograms and long AF cycle lengths. Mapping data suggested that the arrhythmia was maintained by only a small number of reentrant waves. Unlike the AF in the rapid atrial pacing model, the increased stability of AF was not based on a shortening of the atrial wavelength. No changes in refractoriness, conduction velocity or wavelength were noted. However, when local conduction properties were studied in more detail using high density mapping, discrete regions of slow conduction were observed. Histological analysis revealed a marked increase in fibrous tissue and this was assumed to be responsible for the local conduction disturbances (Fig. 7). Characterization of cellular electrophysiological changes revealed a decrease in I_{to}, I_{Ca} and I_{Ks}. In contrast, the Na^+/Ca^{2+} exchanger current was increased by 45% (Li et al. 2000). However, the resulting changes in shape and duration of the action potential seem to be less important than in tachycardia-induced atrial remodeling. Rather, increased atrial fibrosis leading to increased non-uniform tissue anisotropy and impaired conduction at a local level seemed to facilitate AF. Interestingly, the ultra-structural abnormalities show striking similarities with the histological findings observed in the elderly and in patients with underlying heart diseases such as rheumatic heart disease (Pham et al. 1982).

Recently, the ACE-inhibitor enalapril has been shown to attenuate atrial fibrosis and conduction disturbances in dogs with rapid pacing-induced heart failure (Li et al. 2001). This observation supports the hypothesis that the activation of the renin-angiotensin system is involved in the signaling cascade leading to atrial cell growth, proliferation of fibroblasts and atrial fibrosis. In clinical trials ACE-inhibitors proved to be effective against AF in patients with heart failure (Gurlek et al. 1994) or left ventricular dysfunction after myocardial infarction (Pedersen et al. 1999a). While this effect might be explained by an improvement in the patients' hemodynamics, a recent trial with the angiotensin receptor blocker irbesartan showed that blockade of the renin-angiotensin system can reduce the recurrence rate of AF in a heterogeneous patient population with less diseased hearts (Madrid et al. 2002).

Ischemia/Infarction and Atrial Fibrillation

Myocardial infarction is an independent risk factor for the development of atrial fibrillation. Up to 21% of the patients admitted for acute myocardial infarction will suffer from atrial fibrillation/flutter during the hospital stay (Pedersen et al. 1999b). The pathophysiological mechanism of how ischemia leads to AF is not well understood. The first experimental models examining the effects of coronary occlusion on the genesis of atrial arrhythmias have been developed only very recently. In a dog model, Jayachandran et al. observed an acute shortening of the atrial refractory period after occlusion of the proximal right coronary artery (RCA). In contrast, Sinno et al. (2003) found no effects on atrial refractoriness during the first hours after ligation of a branch of the RCA (right intermediate atrial artery). In the latter study, the duration of induced AF episodes was significantly increased 0.5 and 3 h after coronary occlusion (from seconds to minutes). In the ischemic atrial myocardium, the excitability threshold was increased and local conduction delays occurred. Miyauchi et al. (2003) investigated the long-term effects of occlusion of the left descending artery (below the first diagonal branch) on the susceptibility to AF in dogs. Eight weeks after LAD occlusion atrial electrophysiological measurements were performed. Both inducibility and stability of AF were increased after myocardial infarction (MI). The duration of induced episodes of AF was only 3 s in the control group whereas atrial fibrillation lasted 41 s in the MI dogs. Mapping of atrial activation during application of premature stimuli showed epicardial wavebreaks degenerating to AF. No difference in atrial action potential duration or refractoriness was found between MI and control dogs. However, at fast pacing rates, an increase in the dispersion of the monophasic action potential was seen in the MI dogs. Immunocytochemical staining for the atrial sympathetic nerves showed increased densities and marked regional heterogeneities at all atrial sites in MI as compared with control dogs. In addition a reduction and heterogeneous distribution of connexin 40 was observed (Ohara et al. 2002). It remains to be determined whether these changes are due to atrial ischemia or to other mechanisms. Histological studies revealed no signs of atrial ischemia or fibrosis in right or left atria. Thus, ventricular infarction itself might have created the atrial background for AF in this model. This may be related to nerve sprouting or to the effect of an impaired left ventricular function on the atria.

Atrial Dilatation

A relation between atrial size and AF was first described in 1955. Fraser and Turner (1955) showed that left and right atrial enlargement correlated with the incidence of AF in patients with mitral valve disease. More recently, large prospective trials established left atrial enlargement as an independent risk factor for the development of AF (Vasan et al. 1997; Vaziri et al. 1994).

In the Cardiovascular Health Study, increased left atrial size was a strong risk factor for new onset atrial fibrillation (Psaty et al. 1997). On the other hand, several studies imply that atrial enlargement is also a consequence of AF. Keren et al. (1987) showed that patients with mitral valve stenosis and sinus rhythm had normal right atrial dimensions but an increased left atrial size. In contrast, patients with mitral stenosis and AF, as well as patients with AF alone, showed significant enlargement of both right and left atria. In 1990, Sanfilippo et al. (1990) performed a small prospective echocardiographic study in patients with AF and normal atrial size at baseline and no cardiac abnormalities. After an average time of 20.6 months left and right atrial volume was significantly increased by ~50%.

In order to study the electrophysiological effects of atrial dilatation alone, several experimental models have been developed. The majority of these studies addressed the effects of acute atrial dilatation. In the Langendorff-perfused rabbit heart Ravelli et al. (1997) showed that an increase in atrial size was associated with a shortening of the atrial refractory period. In contrast, others have reported no changes (Wijffels et al. 1997) or a prolongation of atrial refractoriness (Satoh et al. 1996) after acute volume overload. However, in all studies both the vulnerability to and the stability of AF increased. In the isolated rabbit heart, Eijsbouts et al. (2003) found that with increasing atrial pressures, conduction velocity was slowed and the incidence of areas of slow conduction or block significantly increased. In the setting of a short atrial wavelength, lines of conduction block may serve as sites of wave break which can initiate AF.

Already in 1982 Boyden et al. (1982) evaluated the effects of chronic atrial dilatation on atrial electrophysiology in dogs. Right atrial dilatation was created by cutting part of the chordae tendineae of the tricuspid valve and constriction of the pulmonary artery. After a mean follow up of 93 days, the right atrial volume had increased by 39%. Susceptibility to arrhythmias had clearly increased and the proportion of induced episodes lasting >10 min was significantly increased. AF was, in general, of low rate and slow flutters were frequently observed. *In vitro* recorded atrial action potentials did not differ in duration from action potentials recorded from non-dilated atria. Instead, structural changes such as cellular hypertrophy and tissue fibrosis were found. Recently, Neuberger et al. (2002) investigated the relation between atrial dilatation and the stability of AF in goats with chronic AV block. Modified screw-in catheters with sonomicrometer ultrasound crystals were chronically implanted in the right atrium allowing simultaneous measurements of atrial electrophysiology and size. During the control period, electrically induced episodes of AF were generally short lasting (seconds). After His bundle ablation a progressive increase in atrial size was observed, due to the slow idioventricular rhythm. After 4 weeks atrial diameter had increased by 13%. The duration of AF episodes was assessed weekly. During the first 4 weeks of AV block the duration of AF paroxysms progressively increased from a few seconds to several hours (Fig. 8a). Consistent with the study of Boyden et al. (1982), no changes in refractoriness were observed. When AF was artificially maintained for 48 h by atrial burst pacing, atrial refractoriness clearly shortened. Surprisingly, this marked shortening of the refractory period was not associated with a shortening of the atrial fibrillation cycle length (Fig. 8b). This suggests that in dilated atria, AF is due to re-entry in anatomically fixed circuits. Chronic atrial dilatation may result in atrial conduction disturbances due to electrical isolation of muscle bundles or tissue fibrosis. Mapping of electrical activation during rapid atrial pacing indeed showed an increased spatial heterogeneity in conduction, which might explain the increased stability of AF in this model (Fig. 8c,d).

Computer Models of Atrial Fibrillation

In the early '60s the first computer model of AF was programmed by Moe and co-workers (1964). Using a two-dimensional 992-unit matrix, they predicted some key features of atrial fibrillation with surprising accuracy. Five states of different excitability were assigned to each unit as indicated in Fig. 9 (left panel). To introduce dispersion of refractoriness, the duration of the state with the lowest excitability differed from unit to unit. The "turbulent activity" of the matrix was sustained by irregular drifting wave fronts (Fig. 9, right panel) varying in position, number, and size. Prolongation of the refractory period resulted in arrest of activity. Reduction in the area of the model also favored self-termination, whereas the creation of internal obstacles resulted in a periodic circus movement flutter. The growing knowledge of atrial cel-

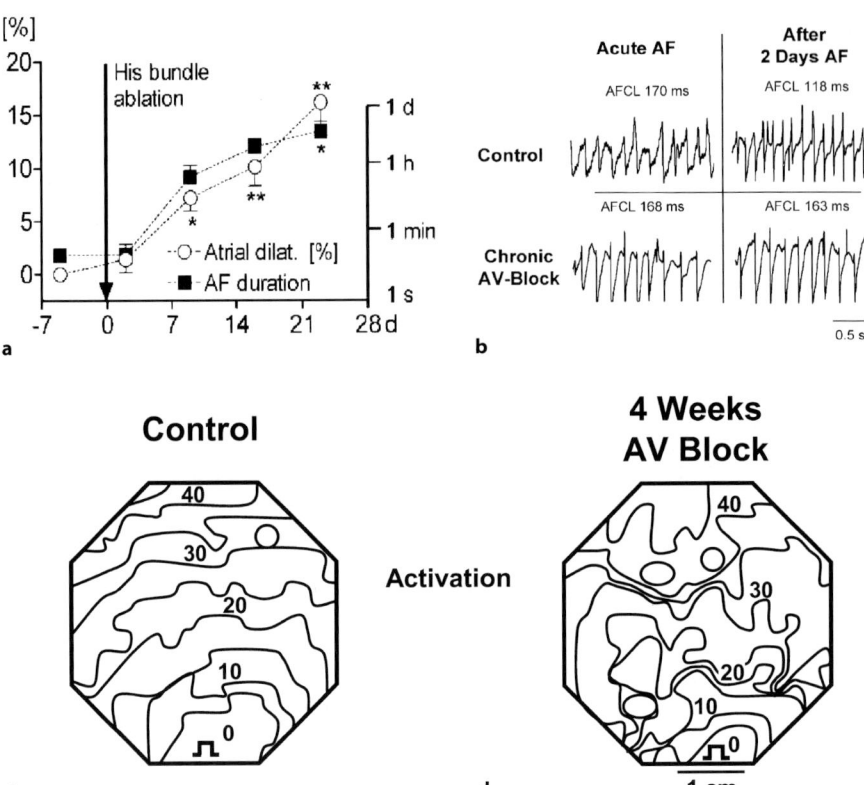

Figure 8a–d
Effect of atrial dilatation on the electrophysiological properties of dilated atria in goats with chronic AV-block. **a** Relative atrial dilatation and duration of induced AF episodes during control and 4 weeks of chronic complete AV block in 6 goats. (From Neuberger et al. 2002). **b** A representative example of unipolar endocardial atrial electrograms obtained from a goat after induction of AF by burst pacing. Under control conditions (conducting AV node, *upper panels*), the median AF interval and the AERP shorten during 2 days of AF. During chronic complete AV block (*lower panels*), AF maintenance during 2 days still reduces AERP, but AFCL keeps constant. This indicates a widening of the excitable gap during electrical remodeling in the AV block goat.
Lower panels: Right atrial activation maps during rapid atrial pacing (cycle length 200 ms) show an increased spatial heterogeneity in conduction in dilated atria

lular electrophysiology has allowed the design of more sophisticated computer simulations implementing ion currents, ion concentrations, subcellular compartments, membrane capacities and cell-cell coupling resistances. One example is the model proposed by Zou et al. (2002). These authors simulated cell grids of varying size in the presence of spatially distributed acetylcholine concentrations, providing different patterns of dispersion of refractoriness. In almost all cases, AF was sustained by a single spiral wave rotating around an area of a high acetylcholine concentration. When the grid became very small, AF was not sustained. However, above this critical size, the behavior of AF was qualitatively the same over an 11-fold range of atrial grid size, suggesting that the emphasis on tissue mass as an important determinant of AF

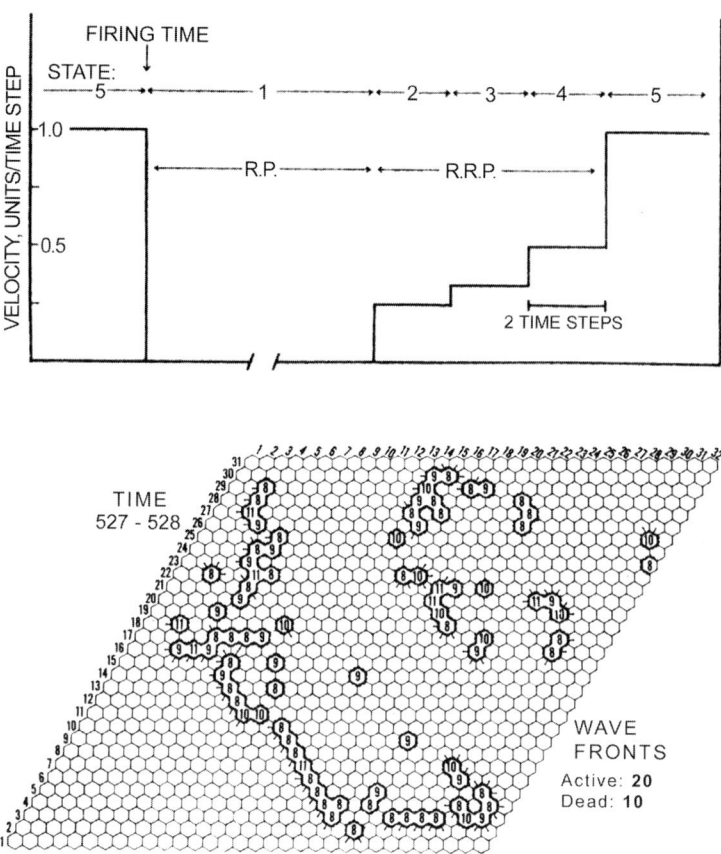

Figure 9
Moe's computer model of atrial fibrillation. *Upper panel:* Each unit of a 992-unit matrix was assigned to a state of excitability. State 1: absolutely refractory. State 2 to 4: relatively refractory with decreased conduction velocity in case of activation. State 5: fully recovered. *Lower panel:* Several simultaneously propagating wave fronts. They differ in location, size, and direction of propagation. *Arrows* indicate progress of wave fronts. (Modified from Moe et al. 1964)

stability might be overstated. Virag et al. (2002) developed a model of AF based on the anatomy of human atria. The three-dimensional surface was realistic in size and included obstacles corresponding to the location of major vessels and valves. However, anisotropy and variations in thickness of the atrial wall were not modeled. Up to 400 000 units were defined with a minimal distance of 200 µm.

Using standard personal computers (Pentium III, 933 MHz) 1 s of simulated time took 1 h of computation time. A 40 s episode of AF thus could be simulated within one weekend. The most interesting finding in this model was that single-site burst pacing of the atria could induce AF even in tissue with uniform membrane properties. As expected, shortening of the refractory period increased the duration of AF, emphasizing the crucial role of action potential duration in determining the duration of AF.

Troubleshooting

Due to the multifactorial nature of the pathophysiological mechanisms during AF, the time course with which AF becomes more stable with time varies a lot, depending on the background of the arrhythmia, the species and the way AF is induced. Also, interindividual differences within the same model are very pronounced, making group comparisons difficult. Studies focusing on effects on stability of AF therefore usually require large groups of animals with resulting consequences for funding and logistics. In such cases, paired comparisons are not always an option because AF in itself might change the stability of the arrhythmia and other parameters of interest.

Species differences are particularly important to consider. While AF can easily be induced and rapidly becomes sustained in goats, it is more difficult to induce and less stable in pigs and dogs. Therefore, the goat model is very suitable for studies focusing on the progressive increase of AF stability or mechanisms of cardioversion of AF, while effects on refractoriness, atrial contractility or conduction during slow atrial pacing can also be studied in dogs or pigs.

Finally, the existence of different time domains during AF must be taken into account. For example, minutes of AF already shorten atrial refractoriness due to adaptation of ion concentrations and ion pump activities. This shortening of the refractory period takes only minutes to recover and is therefore due to completely different mechanisms from the shortening of the refractory period during the first days of AF (=electrical remodeling) which also requires several days to recover. Thus, conclusions drawn from studies targeting the shortening of refractoriness during AF are only valid when the study was performed in the time domain of interest.

Concluding Remarks

From various animal models of AF developed during the past decade numerous physiological and therapeutic concepts have emerged which formed the basis of present knowledge of initiation, maintenance, and termination of AF. All these models, however, focused on specific etiologies and backgrounds that maintain AF. Even the most sophisticated model of AF does not mimic the diversity of etiologies and pathophysiological mechanisms in human AF. Nevertheless, the different experimental models have greatly enlarged our insight into the mechanisms operative during AF in patients. What we need most is development of clinical tools to diagnose the electrophysiological mechanisms and pathological backgrounds responsible for the occurrence and persistence of AF in individual patients.

References

Allessie MA (1998) Atrial electrophysiologic remodeling: another vicious circle? J Cardiovasc Electrophysiol 9: 1378–1393

Alessi R, Nusynowitz M, Abildskov J, Moe G (1959) Nonuniform distribution of vagal effects on the atrial refractory period. Am J Physiol 194: 406–410

Allessie MA, Bonke FI, Schopman FJ (1973) Circus movement in rabbit atrial muscle as a mechanism of trachycardia. Circ Res 33: 54–62

Allessie MA, Lammers WJ, Bonke IM, Hollen J (1984) Intra-atrial reentry as a mechanism for atrial flutter induced by acetylcholine and rapid pacing in the dog. Circulation 70: 123–135

Allessie M, Lammers WJ, Bonke FI, Hollen J (1985) Experimental evaluation of Moe's multiple wavelet hypothesis on atrial fibrillation. In: Zipes DP (ed) Cardiac electrophysiology and arrhythmias. Grune and Stratton, New York, p 265–275

Ausma J, Wijffels M, Thone F, Wouters L, Allessie M, Borgers M (1997) Structural changes of atrial myocardium due to sustained atrial fibrillation in the goat. Circulation 96: 3157–3163

Allessie MA, Ausma J, Schotten U (2002) Electrical, contractile and structural remodeling during atrial fibrillation. Cardiovasc Res 54: 230–246

Bailey GW, Braniff BA, Hancock EW, Cohn KE (1968) Relation of left atrial pathology to atrial fibrillation in mitral valvular disease. Ann Intern Med 69: 13–20

Benjamin EJ, Levy D, Vaziri SM, D'Agostino RB, Belanger AJ, Wolf PA (1994) Independent risk factors for atrial fibrillation in a population-based cohort. The Framingham Heart Study. JAMA 271: 840–844

Benjamin EJ, Wolf PA, D'Agostino RB, Silbershatz H, Kannel WB, Levy D (1998) Impact of atrial fibrillation on the risk of death: the Framingham Heart Study. Circulation 98: 946–952

Borgers M, Thone F, Wouters L, Ausma J, Shivalkar B, Flameng W (1993) Structural correlates of regional myocardial dysfunction in patients with critically coronary artery stenosis: Chronic hibernation? Cardiovasc Pathol 2: 237–245

Boyden PA, Tilley LP, Pham TD, Liu SK, Fenoglic JJJ, Wit AL (1982) Effects of left atrial enlargement on atrial transmembrane potentials and structure in dogs with mitral valve fibrosis. Am J Cardiol 49: 1896–1908

Chen YJ, Chen SA, Tai CT, Wen ZC, Feng AN, Ding YA, Chang MS (1998) Role of atrial electrophysiology and autonomic nervous system in patients with supraventricular tachycardia and paroxysmal atrial fibrillation. J Am Coll Cardiol 32: 732–738

Chiou CW, Eble JN, Zipes DP (1997) Efferent vagal innervation of the canine atria and sinus and atrioventricular nodes. The third fat pad. Circulation 95: 2573–2584

Coumel P, Attuel P, Lavallee J, Flammang D, Leclercq JF, Slama R (1978) The atrial arrhythmia syndrome of vagal origin. Arch Mal Coeur Vaiss 71: 645–656

Eijsbouts S, Majidi M, von Zandvoort M, Allessie M (2003) The effects of acute atrial dilatation on heterogeneity in conduction in the isolated rabbit heart. J Cardiovasc Electrophysiol (in press)

Einthoven W (1903) Ein neues Galvanometer. Ann Physik 4: 1059–1061

Einthoven W (1906) Le telecardiogramme. Arch Internat Physiol 4: 132–164

Everett TH, Li H, Mangrum JM, McRury ID, Mitchell MA, Redick JA, Haines DE (2000) Electrical, morphological, and ultrastructural remodeling and reverse remodeling in a canine model of chronic atrial fibrillation. Circulation 102: 1454–1460

Fenoglio JJ Jr, Wagner BM (1973) Studies in rheumatic fever. VI. Ultrastructure of chronic rheumatic heart disease. Am J Pathol 73: 623–640

Fenoglio JJ Jr, Pham TD, Hordof A, Edie RN, Wit AL (1979) Right atrial ultrastructure in congenital heart disease. II. Atrial septal defect: effects of volume overload. Am J Cardiol 43: 820–827

Fraser HRL, Turner RWD (1955) Auricular fibrillation with special reference to rheumatic heart disease. British Medical Journal 2: 1414–1418

Goldstein, RN, Khrestian, CM, Ryu, K, van Wagoner, D, Stambler, BS, Waldo AL (2003) Prevention of postoperative atrial fibrillation and flutter using steroids. PACE 26: 1068

Gurlek A, Erol C, Basesme E (1994) Antiarrhythmic effect of converting enzyme inhibitors in congestive heart failure. Int J Cardiol 43: 315–318

Keren G, Etzion T, Sherez J, Zelcer AA, Megidish R, Miller HI, Laniado S (1987) Atrial fibrillation and atrial enlargement in patients with mitral stenosis. Am Heart J 114: 1146–1155

Kitzman DW, Edwards WD (1990) Age-related changes in the anatomy of the normal human heart. J Gerontol 45: M33–M39

Konings KT, Kirchhof CJ, Smeets JR, Wellens HJ, Penn OC, Allessie MA (1994) High-density mapping of electrically induced atrial fibrillation in humans. Circulation 89: 1665–1680

Kumagai K, Khrestian C, Waldo AL (1997) Simultaneous multisite mapping studies during induced atrial fibrillation in the sterile pericarditis model. Insights into the mechanism of its maintenance. Circulation 95: 511–521

Kumagai K, Uno K, Khrestian C, Waldo AL (2000) Single site radiofrequency catheter ablation of atrial fibrillation: studies guided by simultaneous multisite mapping in the canine sterile pericarditis model. J Am Coll Cardiol 36: 917–923

Lewis T (1909) Auricular fibrillation and its relationship to clinical irregularity of the heart. Heart 1: 306–372

Li D, Fareh S, Leung TK, Nattel S (1999) Promotion of atrial fibrillation by heart failure in dogs: atrial remodeling of a different sort. Circulation 100: 87–95

Li D, Melnyk P, Feng J, Wang Z, Petrecca K, Shrier A, Nattel S (2000) Effects of experimental heart failure on atrial cellular and ionic electrophysiology. Circulation 101: 2631–2638

Li D, Shinagawa K, Pang L, Leung TK, Cardin S, Wang Z, Nattel S (2001) Effects of Angiotensin-converting enzyme inhibition on the development of the atrial fibrillation substrate in dogs with ventricular tachypacing-induced congestive heart failure. Circulation 104: 2608–2614

Madrid AH, Bueno MG, Rebollo JM, Marin I, Pena G, Bernal E, Rodriguez A, Cano L, Cano JM, Cabeza P, Moro C (2002) Use of irbesartan to maintain sinus rhythm in patients with long-lasting persistent atrial fibrillation: a prospective and randomized study. Circulation 106: 331–336

Mary RL, Albert A, Pham TD, Hordof A, Fenoglio-JJ J, Malm JR, Rosen MR (1983) The relationship of human atrial cellular electrophysiology to clinical function and ultrastructure. Circ Res 52: 188–199

McWilliam J (1887) Fibrillar contraction of the heart. J Physiol 8: 296–310

Mines G (1913) On dynamic equilibrium in the heart. J Physiol 46: 349–383

Mines G (1914) On circulating excitation in heart muscles and their possible relation to tachycardia and fibrillation. Trans Roy Soc Can 8: 43–52

Miyauchi Y, Zhou S, Okuyama Y, Miyauchi M, Hayashi H, Hamabe A, Fishbein MC, Mandel WJ, Chen LS, Chen PS, Karagueuzian HS (2003) Altered atrial electrical restitution and heterogeneous sympathetic hyperinnervation in hearts with chronic left ventricular myocardial infarction: implications for atrial fibrillation. Circulation 108: 360–366

Moe G, Rheinboldt W, Aboldskov J (1964) A computer model of atrial fibrillation. Am Heart J 67: 200–220

Morillo CA, Klein GJ, Jones DL, Guiraudon CM (1995) Chronic rapid atrial pacing. Structural, functional, and electrophysiological characteristics of a new model of sustained atrial fibrillation. Circulation 91: 1588–1595

Neuberger HR, Schotten U, Ausma J, Blaauw Y, Eijsbouts S, van Hunnik A, Allessie M (2002) Atrial remodeling in the goat due to chronic complete atrioventricular block. Eur Heart J 23: 138–138

Ohara K, Miyauchi Y, Ohara T, Fishbein MC, Zhou S, Lee MH, Mandel WJ, Chen PS, Karagueuzian HS (2002) Downregulation of immunodetectable atrial connexin40 in a canine model of chronic left ventricular myocardial infarction: implications to atrial fibrillation. J Cardiovasc Pharmacol Ther 7: 89–94

Page PL, Plumb VJ, Okumura K, Waldo AL (1986) A new animal model of atrial flutter. J Am Coll Cardiol 8: 872–879

Pedersen OD, Bagger H, Kober L, Torp-Pedersen C (1999) The occurrence and prognostic significance of atrial fibrillation/-flutter following acute myocardial infarction. TRACE Study group. TRAndolapril Cardiac Evalution. Eur Heart J 20: 748–754

Pedersen OD, Bagger H, Kober L, Torp-Pedersen C (1999) Trandolapril reduces the incidence of atrial fibrillation after acute myocardial infarction in patients with left ventricular dysfunction. Circulation 100: 376–380

Pham TD, Fenoglio-JJ (1982) Right atrial ultrastructure in chronic rheumatic heart disease. Int J Cardiol 1: 289–304

Pham TD, Wit AL, Hordof AJ, Malm JR, Fenoglio JJ (1978) Right atrial ultrastructure in congenital heart disease. I. Comparison of ventricular septal defect and endocardial cushion defect. Am J Cardiol 42: 973–982

Psaty BM, Manolio TA, Kuller LH, Kronmal RA, Cushman M, Fried LP, White R, Furberg CD, Rautaharju PM (1997) Incidence of and risk factors for atrial fibrillation in older adults. Circulation 96: 2455–2461

Randall WC, Ardell JL (1985) Selective parasympathectomy of automatic and conductile tissues of the canine heart. Am J Physiol 248: H61–H68

Ravelli F, Allessie M (1997) Effects of atrial dilatation on refractory period and vulnerability to atrial fibrillation in the isolated Langendorff-perfused rabbit heart. Circulation 95: 1686–1695

Rensma PL, Allessie MA, Lammers WJ, Bonke FI, Schalij MJ (1988) Length of excitation wave and susceptibility to reentrant atrial arrhythmias in normal conscious dogs. Circ Res 62: 395–410

Rothberger C, Winterberg H (1909) Vorhofflimmern und arrhythmia perpetua. Wien Klin Wochenschr 22: 839–844

Rothberger C, Winterberg H (1915) Archiv Ges Physiol 42

Sanderson J (1879) On the time-relations of the excitatory process in the ventricle of the heart of the frog. J Physiol 2: 384–435

Sanfilippo AJ, Abascal VM, Sheehan M, Oertel LB, Harrigan P, Hughes RA, Weyman AE (1990) Atrial enlargement as a consequence of atrial fibrillation. A prospective echocardiographic study. Circulation 82: 792–797

Satoh T, Zipes DP (1996) Unequal atrial stretch in dogs increases dispersion of refractoriness conducive to developing atrial fibrillation. J Cardiovasc Electrophysiol 7: 833–842

Schauerte P, Scherlag BJ, Pitha J, Scherlag MA, Reynolds D, Lazzara R, Jackman WM (2000) Catheter ablation of cardiac autonomic nerves for prevention of vagal atrial fibrillation. Circulation 102: 2774–2780

Schotten U, Ausma J, Stellbrink C, Sabatschus I, Vogel M, Frechen D, Schoendube F, Hanrath P, Allessie MA (2001) Cellular mechanisms of depressed atrial contractility in patients with chronic atrial fibrillation. Circulation 103: 691–698

Schotten U, Duytschaever M, Ausma J, Eijsbouts S, Neuberger HR, Allessie M (2003) Electrical and contractile remodeling during the first days of atrial fibrillation go hand in hand. Circulation 107: 1433–1439

Schuessler RB, Grayson TM, Bromberg BI, Cox JL, Boineau JP (1992) Cholinergically mediated tachyarrhythmias induced by a single extrastimulus in the isolated canine right atrium. Circ Res 71: 1254–1267

Schuessler RB, Kawamoto T, Hand DE, Mitsuno M, Bromberg BI, Cox JL, Boineau JP (1993) Simultaneous epicardial and endocardial activation sequence mapping in the isolated canine right atrium. Circulation 88: 250–263

Sinno H, Derakhchan K, Libersan D, Merhi Y, Leung TK, Nattel S (2003) Atrial ischemia promotes atrial fibrillation in dogs. Circulation 107: 1930–1936

Thiedemann K-U, Ferrans VJ (1977) Left atrial ultrastructure in mitral valvular disease. Am J Pathol 89: 575–594

Vasan RS, Larson MG, Levy D, Evans JC, Benjamin EJ (1997) Distribution and categorization of echocardiographic measurements in relation to reference limits: the Framingham Heart Study: formulation of a height- and sex-specific classification and its prospective validation. Circulation 96: 1863–1873

Vaziri SM, Larson MG, Benjamin EJ, Levy D (1994) Echocardiographic predictors of nonrheumatic atrial fibrillation. The Framingham Heart Study. Circulation 89: 724–730

Virag N, Jacquemet V, Henriquez CS, Zozor S, Blanc O, Vesin JM, Pruvot E, Kappenberger L (2002) Study of atrial arrhythmias in a computer model based on magnetic resonance images of human atria. Chaos 12: 754–763

Wang J, Bourne GW, Wang Z, Villemaire C, Talajic M, Nattel S (1993) Comparative mechanisms of antiarrhythmic drug action in experimental atrial fibrillation. Importance of use-dependent effects on refractoriness. Circulation 88: 1030–1044

Wang J, Liu L, Feng J, Nattel S (1996) Regional and functional factors determining induction and maintenance of atrial fibrillation in dogs. Am J Physiol 271: H148–H158

Wijffels MC, Kirchhof CJ, Dorland R, Allessie MA (1995) Atrial fibrillation begets atrial fibrillation. A study in awake chronically instrumented goats. Circulation 92: 1954–1968

Wijffels MCEF, Kirchhof CJHJ, Dorland R, Power J, Allessie MA (1997) Electrical remodeling due to atrial fibrillation in chronically instrumented conscious goats: roles of neurohumoral changes, ischemia, atrial stretch and high rate of electrical activation. Circulation 96: 3710–3720

Wouters L, Liu GS, Flameng W, Thijssen VL, Thone F, Borgers M (2001) Structural remodeling of atrial myocardium in patients with cardiac valve disease and atrial fibrillation. Exp Clin Cardiol 5: 158–163

Wu TJ, Yashima M, Xie F, Athill CA, Kim YH, Fishbein MC, Qu Z, Garfinkel A, Weiss JN, Karagueuzian HS, Chen PS (1998) Role of pectinate muscle bundles in the generation and maintenance of intra-atrial reentry: potential implications for the mechanism of conversion between atrial fibrillation and atrial flutter. Circ Res 83: 448–462

Yared JP, Starr NJ, Torres FK, Bashour CA, Bourdakos G, Piedmonte M, Michener JA, Davis JA, Rosenberger TE (2000) Effects of single dose, postinduction dexamethasone on recovery after cardiac surgery. Ann Thorac Surg 69: 1420–1424

Yue L, Feng J, Gaspo R, Li GR, Wang Z, Nattel S (1997) Ionic remodeling underlying action potential changes in a canine model of atrial fibrillation. Circ Res 81: 512–525

Zou R, Kneller J, Leon LJ, Nattel S (2002) Development of a computer algorithm for the detection of phase singularities and initial application to analyze simulations of atrial fibrillation. Chaos 12: 764–778

In-Vitro Techniques

2 Isolated Organs
— 153

3 Electrophysiological Techniques
— 213

4 Histological Techniques
— 455

5 Cell Culture Techniques
— 555

6 Biochemical and Analytical Techniques
— 659

2 Isolated Organs

- 2.1 **The Langendorff Heart** — 155
  Stefan Dhein

- 2.2 **The Working Heart** — 173
  Marc W. Merx and Jürgen Schrader

- 2.3 **Isolated Papillary Muscles** — 190
  Stefan Dhein

- 2.4 **Isolated Vessels** — 198
  Rudolf Schubert

The Langendorff Heart
Stefan Dhein

Introduction

It all began with the basic investigations of Oskar Langendorff who developed a method for investigation of the isolated heart (Langendorff, 1895). This was a major breakthrough in cardiovascular research. Oskar Langendorff was born on February 1, 1853 in Breslau. He studied in Breslau, Berlin, Freiburg and Königsberg, where he received his medical degree in 1875. In Königsberg he started his career as an assistant in the Physiological Institute and became a university lecturer in 1879, becoming a non-budgetary professor in Königsberg in 1884. Six years later he accepted an invitation to become chairman of the Institute of Physiology at the University of Rostock. There he wrote his famous work "Untersuchungen am überlebenden Säugetierherzen" which appeared in 1895 in Pflüger's Archiv ges Physiol. On May 10, 1908 he died after a short illness at the age of 55.

Langendorff's work has inspired generations of physiologists and cardiovascular researchers and made modern organ-orientated physiology possible for cardiovascular research. In the following paragraphs the preparation of an isolated heart according to Langendorff will be described in detail and two principle types of this technique, the pressure constant Langendorff heart and the constant flow Langendorff heart will be presented.

The basic principle is to maintain cardiac activity by perfusing the heart *via* the coronary arteries using an aortic cannula inserted into the ascending aorta. Perfusion solution is delivered to the heart in a retrograde manner *via* this cannula. This retrograde perfusion driven by a hydrostatic pressure (constant pressure model) or by a pump (constant flow model) closes the aortic valve and flows into the coronary arteries during diastole (Fig. 1). As under physiological conditions, during systole there is almost no coronary flow, since the intramural pressure is higher than the perfusion pressure (this has to be adjusted for the experimental model depending on the species under investigation). If the perfusion pressure is too high, cardiac tissue oedema will develop. After passing through the coronary circulation, the perfusate enters the right atrium via the coronary sinus and is driven out *via* the right ventricle and the pulmonary artery.

Two types of Langendorff heart preparations are in use (constant pressure and constant flow), which are based principally on consideration of the resistance of the coronary circulation.

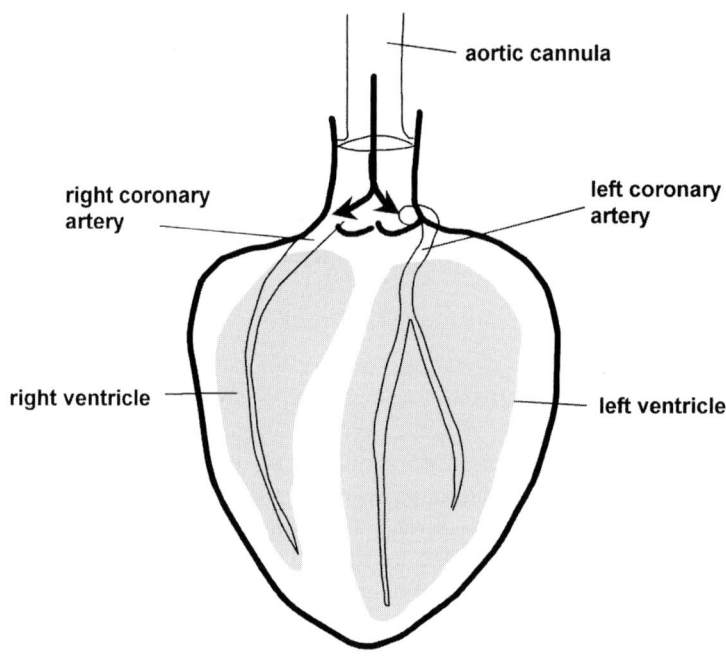

Figure 1
Scheme of the isolated perfused heart according to Langendorff. Perfusion solution is flowing retrogradely within the aorta and then orthogradely within the coronaries during diastole. A prerequisite is that the aortic valve is closed by the hydrostatic pressure of the perfusion solution

The resistance of the coronary circulation can be described in analogy to Ohms law as

$$R = \Delta P/\Phi$$

where ΔP = pressure difference (which is in the common Langendorff heart the perfusion pressure, since the outflow pressure is almost zero (this is different in working heart models, see there) and Φ = coronary flow. As a consequence for calculation of R either both variables have to be measured or only one if the other is kept constant. This has led to the development of the two forms of the Langendorff heart, the constant pressure model and the constant flow model. Since the flow resistance can be described according to Hagen-Poiseuille's law by the equation

$$R = 8\,\eta l/\pi\, r^4$$

where l = length of tube, η = viscosity of the solution and r = radius of the tube. A change in the diameter of the vessel caused by vasoconstriction or dilation leads to a change in the radius of the vessel and thereby to a change in resistance which is proportional to $1/r^4$. Thus, if pressure is kept constant, the term ΔP (= constant)$/\Phi$ is proportional to $1/r^4$ in a constant pressure Langendorff model and perfusion flow is the variable which can be measured as an indicator of $1/R$ or of r. On the other hand, if flow is kept constant the term DP/F (= constant) is proportional to $1/r^4$ and in that case the variable pressure has to be measured as an indicator of $1/r$ or R.

Description of Methods and Practical Approach
Setup and Preparation

The classical animals used for preparations according to the Langendorff technique are small animals such as rats, guinea pigs and rabbits. However, smaller animals such as mice and larger animals such as cats, dogs or even men have been used. The following description refers to the use of rats, guinea pigs or rabbits and has to be adapted if other animals are used. If large hearts are to be used, special care has to be taken of the heart, which in the case of small animal hearts hangs on the aortic cannula. In case of larger hearts, the heart is too heavy and therefore, requires additional suspension. This might be achieved by containing the heart in a saline filled reservoir, which would also maintain temperature and moisture (Table 1).

In preparation for the experiments solid food should be withdrawn from the animals 24 h prior to the experiment with no limitation in water supply. Shortly before sacrifice of the animal, heparin (500–1000 IU/kg) may be given intravenously (rabbits, rats) or intraperitoneally (guinea pigs) to prevent thrombosis. Since in guinea pigs blood coagulability is less than in other species, one may omit heparinization in these animals.

First the animal has to be anaesthetized. Normally, this is achieved by i.v. or intraperitoneal injection of thiopental or pentobarbital (rats, guinea pigs, rabbits). Alternatively, medetomidine and xylazine or fentanyl may be used (rabbits). These types of anaesthetics are normally washed out during perfusion and should not impair measurements. Volatile anaesthetics such as ethyl ether or halothane have to be applied *via* a vaporizer. Otherwise, the resulting concentrations may be too high and lead to

Table 1
Survey on the characteristics of several typical laboratory animals used for Langendorff heart preparations

Species	body weight [kg]	heart weight [g]	Coronary flow [ml/min]	Latex balloon [ml]
rat	0.1–0.2	0.8–1.0	6–8	0.03–0.06
guinea pig	0.3–0.5	1.3–1.9	7–14	0.1–0.2
rabbit	1.6	8–9	22–25	0.9
cat	3.5	17	27	4.7
dog	30	150	120	20

irreversible heart failure after transfer to the Langendorff apparatus. However, in some cases it might be necessary to avoid any additional drugs. In these cases the animal (up to 1500 g according to international guidelines) may be sacrificed by a sharp blow on the neck and subsequent exsanguination. However, in that case the following preparation has to be performed within 1 minute (until the insertion of the aortic cannula) to avoid ischemia and loss of high-energy phosphates. Thus, this can only be used by very experienced experimenters and should be restricted to those studies in which one fears an interaction between the anaesthetic and the drug to be investigated.

Before starting the experiment, the perfusion solution has to be equilibrated with the appropriate gas and to be warmed (typically to 38 °C, which is the physiological temperature of a rat or rabbit). Furthermore, we recommend the use of a second perfusion system which is nothing more than a bottle [filled with perfusion solution, gassed and equilibrated, room temperature (or even cooled)] with a tube connected to the aortic cannula *via* a three way stopcock. The bottle should be 60 to 70 cm above the level of the operating table to allow a sufficient hydrostatic pressure. All tubing to the aortic cannula in the auxiliary perfusion system and in the Langendorff apparatus has to be freed from air bubbles which might enter the coronary circulation and cause ischemia.

After anaesthesia the animal is fixed on an operating table and a cannula is inserted into the trachea for controlled ventilation with air. Thereafter, the skin is incised by a longitudinal cut starting at the throat and ending up in the middle of the abdomen. Subsequently, the abdomen is opened up to the thorax. Next the diaphragm is incised at the edges and is cut out from the ribs. Now there is an open view into the lower aperture of the thorax and the experimenter can see the pericardium if he gently lifts the sternum. The pericardium can now be incised from the bottom up to the top so that the ventral side of the heart is free from pericardium which helps during the following steps. Thereafter the thorax is opened by long cuts at the right and left side (as lateral as possible) so that the complete anterior thorax wall is turned upwards. Complete removal would produce excessive bleeding and therefore should be avoided. Now the rest of the pericardium should be removed, especially in the region of the ascending aorta. Next, the ascending aorta is separated gently from the pulmonary artery (using only forceps). Then the aorta is undermined by use of forceps (it is best to use the sinus transversus) and a thread is positioned around the aorta with a prepared surgical knot (Fig. 2). Similarly, the pulmonary artery is undermined and a thread positioned around the pulmonary artery. At this time one might wash the heart with cold saline solution which will cause bradycardia and reduce energy consumption. Prior to the next step in larger animals, occlusion of the inferior vena cava by a Diefenbach bulldog clamp is recommended to avoid excessive bleeding, which might impair surgical visibility. First the pulmonary artery is incised at the position where later on the pulmonary cannula will be inserted. This step is necessary to avoid overstretching of the right ventricle. Next, the aorta in incised transversely as far cranially as possible (but it should not be completely cut through) and the aortic cannula (3 mm outer diameter for rats and guinea pig; 4 mm outer diameter for small rabbbits) is inserted. Prior to insertion the stopcock of the perfusing system should be opened so that there is already some flow through the aortic cannula, which helps to avoid air bubbles entering the coronary arteries. This is the most critical step of the

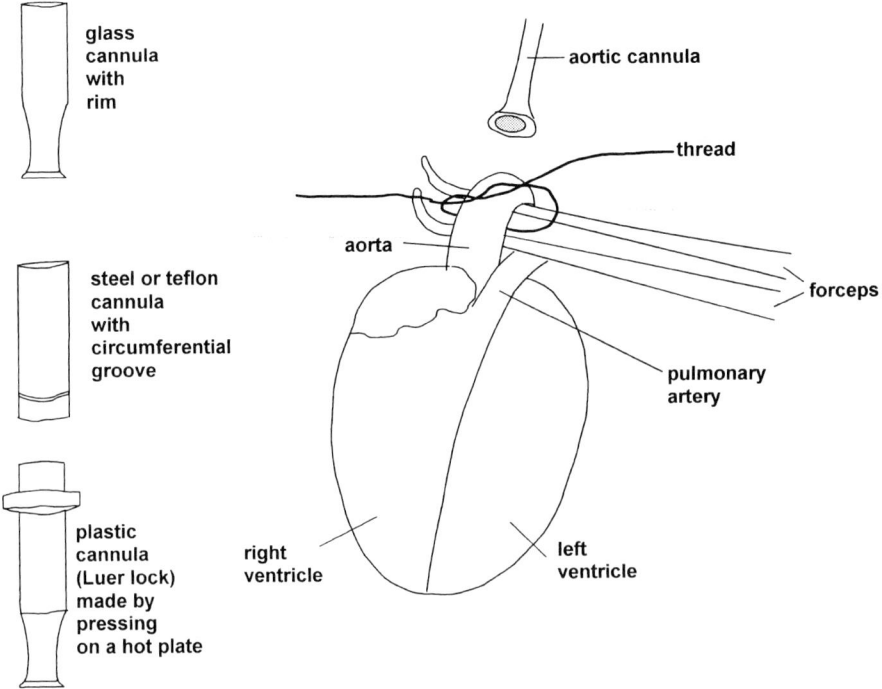

Figure 2
Preparation of the heart. The scheme shows the insertion of the aortic cannula. The scheme shows also various types of aortic cannula which may be made from glass, plastic (using a Luer lock cannula pressing the tube on a hot plate) or steel (ideally with an appertaining cable for electrical grounding)

entire procedure since it is necessary not to insert the cannula too deeply into the aorta in order to avoid obstruction of the orifices of the coronary arteries. After insertion, the knot has to be tightened and flow from the auxiliary perfusion system has to be completely opened. Now the heart is perfused at constant pressure (the hydrostatic pressure of the auxiliary perfusion system, 60 to 70 cm H_2O) and all remaining blood will be washed out.

Re-supply of oxygen starts at this point. Next, the pulmonary cannula is inserted into the pulmonary trunk, and the knot is tightened. At this point the experimenter should observe regular beating of the heart and considerable outflow of perfusion solution from the pulmonary cannula indicating correct coronary supply. Now the distal parts of the aorta and the pulmonary artery can be separated. Next the caval veins and pulmonary veins should be ligated. In small animals this might be performed in one single step with a global ligature of all dorsal vessels. However, this is critical because the sinus node which is in close vicinity to the estuary of the superior vena cava may be impaired by that kind of mass ligature. Therefore, a modified procedure may be recommended; after insertion of the aortic cannula and the resulting flow of perfusion medium, the heart is perfused and there is time to do the following steps carefully. The superior caval vein should be occluded far away from its estuary into the right atrium. The thread may be used after cutting through the superior caval vein to elevate the right atrium and the appertaining rest of the vein to avoid this area being impaired by the subsequent mass ligature. Next, in a similar way the inferior caval vein is ligated and cut through. Now, the heart can be gently moved and raised in order to allow the positioning of a thread around all the vessels (pulmonary veins) and tissue at the back of the heart. This mass ligature is then tightened and cut off and the heart can be removed. The heart is now isolated and perfused with saline solution *via* the aortic cannula connected to the auxiliary perfusion system. Next, the heart is transferred to the Langendorff apparatus and connected via the aortic cannula to the stopcock of the Langendorff apparatus.

Now, the remaining tissues such as excessive connective tissue, remains of vessels or fat can be removed. The pulmonary cannula is connected to an outflow tube. If measurement of force is intended, an isometric or isotonic force transducer is connected to the heart or, most commonly, a balloon for isovolumetric measurement of force is inserted *via* the left atrium into the cavity of the left ventricle. In the case of isometric or isotonic force transducers, a small hook is sutured to the heart surface (left wall) while the back wall and right wall are connected *via* sutures and holding threads to a mounting arch. A force transducer might instead be connected to the apex (as originally used in the first Langendorff preparations). However, the state of the art today is probably the use of an intraventricular latex balloon (size see Table 1; this balloon can be obtained commercially or made from condom or thin latex rubber) connected to a Statham force transducer and a Wheatstone bridge amplifier.

In the case of large hearts, it is not possible to hang the whole weight on the aortic cannula. In these cases, additional holding threads have to be attached. After connection to the desired measuring apparatus, a chamber has to be mounted around the heart in order to avoid heat loss and evaporation. This is normally achieved by a two-part moist chamber which can be opened at the front or a double-walled vessel which is connected in series to the thermostat of the Langendorff apparatus for thermo-constant perfusion. This vessel is open at the top and the bottom and can be easily positioned around the heart. Alternatively, a closed double walled vessel (open only at the top) filled with perfusion solution and kept at constant temperature may be used. If this preparation is used for epicardial mapping, such a covering is not possible due to the 256 wires. However, in this case the heart's surface is covered with the electrodes and plastic material (such as silicon) and is constantly rinsed with warm perfusion solution.

Measurements and Parameters

Three functional parameters are especially interesting when using isolated hearts, coronary flow or perfusion pressure, ventricular force and the electrocardiogram. First the assessment of coronary flow (for *constant pressure* Langendorff setup) or resistance should be described. In a simple way it is possible to count the drops flowing out from the pulmonary cannula and its tubing. This can be realized with a drop counter with either a photoelectrical cell or simply two electrodes which are connected with an electronic counter. If a drop connects the two electrodes with each other, current flows which activates the counter. However, this has the disadvantage of errors if the heart is moving and the drops do not exactly meet the electrodes.

Another more refined setup is the use of a Condon tipper (developed in 1913 by N.E. Condon), which is a kind of spoon for taking up the drops. This reservoir on a lever is mounted on a kind of balance which allows automatic emptying of the reservoir if a defined weight is reached. Movement of the tipper when emptying activates the electrical contacts of a counter.

Alternatively, the outflow is collected in a calibrated cylinder for measurement. In a modification of this method, the outflow can be collected in a funnel connected to an inclined tube which ends up in a T-connector. On the one side of the T-connector a Statham pressure transducer is mounted while the other side has a narrow opening to allow some outflow. The backward staunching within the inclined tube, which is proportional to the coronary outflow dropping into the funnel, results in a hydrostatic pressure which is measured *via* the transducer.

All these methods have some disadvantages, mainly that they are more or less discontinuous. The most advanced way to measure coronary flow is the use of an electromagnetic flow probe. The principle of the electromagnetic flow probe is based on Faraday's law of induction. A magnetic field is provided within the centre of the probe where the perfusion solution flows through. If the perfusion solution is an electrical conductor (as normally is the case) it will behave as if a metal conductor is moved in a magnetic field. In accordance with Faraday's law, a voltage is induced which depends on the flow rate and can be measured. This electromagnetic flow probe can be mounted around the aortic cannula or above it, or may be positioned around the pulmonary outflow tubing. This expensive method allows continuous registration of coronary flow which can be plotted together with the registration of the left ventricular pressure.

A problem with such a flow probe may arise from the fact that these are magnetohydrodynamic flow probes which may cause electrical noise and impair simultaneous ECG recording. This problem can be overcome if the flow probe is positioned around the pulmonary outflow tube outside the Faraday cage in which the Langendorff apparatus is positioned. In these cases the heart should be connected to electrical ground via a steel aortic cannula. In addition, it is sometimes necessary to ground the pulmonary tubing (before the flow probe; i.e. inside the Faraday cage) to electrical ground via a steel tube as well.

If a *flow constant* Langendorff setup is used, coronary flow is adjusted as required. The coronary resistance results in a certain perfusion pressure, which will be elevated if the coronary arteries contract and will decrease in case of vasorelaxation. In order to measure the perfusion pressure, a T-connector is mounted above the aortic cannula, which communicates with a Statham pressure transducer.

The problem with this constant flow setup, although it is very simple to handle, arises from the fact that the coronary flow will not be adjusted to varying energy demands. Moreover, if the perfusion pressure is too high this will result in cardiac oedema. Under physiological conditions there is a correlation between coronary flow (CF) and heart weight (HW) for all species which has been described by the equation

$$CF = 7.43 \times HW^{0.56}$$

(Döring and Dehnert 1988). This may be used when searching for the correct flow.

Regarding the measurement of force, there are, in principle, two possibilities. First, it is possible to use force transducers with a hook sutured to the heart's surface and a thread connected to the force transducer (Gottlieb and Magnus 1904; Beckett 1970). A second and third thread connect the heart with an immobile mounting arch. This allows "transverse" isometric measurement of force. However, this method and its modifications (e.g. the hook is inserted in the apex; "longitudinal" measurement of force) do not measure the developed force of the whole ventricle but only of a part.

Besides these methods, isovolumetric measurement of force is possible by insertion of a balloon into the left ventricle (see above) (introduced in 1904 by Gottlieb and Magnus). This has the advantage of giving an impression of the developed force of the whole left ventricle. The balloon size has to fit the size of the left ventricular cavity (see table 1 for a survey).

For rats and guinea pigs balloons with a diameter of 3 to 5 mm are used (filled, 0 mmHg pressure). In the balloon a small steel cannula is inserted with an attached tube which is connected to the Statham pressure transducer. The ligature of the balloon to the steel cannula is performed with a nylon thread. Care has to be taken, that the steel cannula is not inserted too deeply into the balloon, since if the orifice of the steel cannula comes into contact with the balloon membrane, measurement of pressure is impossible. The catheter tip must not press on the tissue of the apex. The balloon has to be evacuated before insertion into the ventricle and then has to be filled so that the desired end-diastolic pressure is achieved. For that purpose, the balloon pressure is increased in small steps of about 2 mmHg and the left ventricular developed force is recorded. It will be seen that as the balloon pressure increases the LVP also increases up to a certain point.

Further increase in balloon pressure now results in no more increase in LVP. The balloon pressure with the maximum developed force of the left ventricle indicates the optimal preload. In most cases an end-diastolic pressure (= preload) of 8–10 mmHg will be sufficient. Filling of the balloon (with distilled water or saline) is realized *via* a syringe connected *via* a three-way stopcock to the dome of the Statham pressure transducer. This dome is also filled with filling solution. At the bottom of the dome there is the membrane of the Statham pressure transducer which is connected to a Wheatstone bridge amplifier. It is necessary to adjust the bridge balance correctly and to calibrate the system at least once a week by applying definite pressures to the dome. When not in use, the balloon should be bathed in filling solution at zero pressure.

However, the balloon has to be replaced about every two weeks, since the latex material is subject to an ageing process and may become porous or inelastic. Moreover it is necessary to control the dome of the Statham for leakage. Sometimes greasing of the fitting helps. Another important step is to control the whole system (balloon, tubing and dome) for air bubbles. These have to be removed, since air is compressible and thus would affect and falsify the measurement.

The balloon now fills the cavity of the left ventricle and is compressed during systole. Since during diastole the aortic valve is closed and during systole the intraventricular pressure is higher than the hydrostatic pressure of the Langendorff apparatus, there is no fluid flow into the ventricular cavity. Intraventricular pressure measurement, however, may be impaired in case of aortic valve insufficiency.

Additional information on the cardiac mechanics and wall motion can be obtained from ultrasonic crystals sutured to the heart's surface. For this purpose piezoelectric ultrasonic transmitters with epoxy lenses are positioned on the left side wall (at the greatest transverse diameter of the heart) and the heart's base. The corresponding ultrasonic receivers are positioned in the cavity of the right ventricle and at the heart's apex. This system allows accurate continuous measurement of the longitudinal and transverse diameter during the whole cardiac cycle. This may be of special help if *local* disturbances of ventricular mechanics are induced e.g. by regional ischemia.

Often it is interesting to record an epicardial electrocardiogram (ECG) in parallel to LVP and CF. Measurement of ECG is achieved typically by using a bipolar circuit since this lowers electrical noise. One electrode is positioned at the left ventricle the other (reference) electrode at the right ventricle. A simple amplifier can be used for these recordings. AgCl electrodes are recommended for recording since they have lower polarization. The silver wire has to be chloride-coated after some experiments. The correct AgCl coat looks brownish and must be continuous. If one electrode is positioned at the right atrium it is also possible to record the atrioventricular conduction time. However, sometimes it is also possible to record a P-wave from the ventricle if the electrode is positioned near to the valvular plane. There is an interesting method described by Güttler et al. (1982), who used an intraventricular balloon for LVP recording and a hook and force transducer for recording atrial mechanics, so that they could also determine the mechanical atrioventricular delay.

Another possibility is to position one electrode on the front wall at the location of the septum (upper third of septum) and the second at the respective position on the back wall (at the upper third of septum). With a very high amplification of the resulting bipolar signal it is possible to record a His bundle electrogram in this manner as described by Stark and colleagues (Stark et al. 1987; Hofer et al. 1990). For electrical grounding of the heart it is best to use a steel aortic cannula connected to electrical ground as used in mapping experiments (see there). Alternatively it is possible to use a normal ECG recorder with Einthovens leads and to use three electrodes: one at the left ventricular wall, one at the right ventricular wall and the third at the apex. The aortic trunk is used for electrical ground. Thin cables which may also serve as springs for attaching the electrodes to the hearts surface are recommended. It is important that the pressure of these electrodes on the tissue is not too high so that the tissue is impaired. Such damage would be observed from alterations in the ST segment. Additionally, it is possible to record monophasic action potentials from the isolated Langendorff heart (see the respective chapter).

The classical parameters obtained from Langendorff experiments are heart rate (HR), left ventricular pressure (LVP), end-diastolic pressure (EDP), maximum contraction velocity (dP/dt_{max}), maximum relaxation velocity (dP/dt_{min}), atrioventricular conduction time, and the classical ECG parameters such as duration of QRS and QT, as well as either coronary flow or coronary perfusion pressure. Apropos the left ventricular force, it is necessary to distinguish between maximum left ventricular pressure, or developed left ventricular pressure (LVP) which is defined as maximum left ventricular pressure − EDP. The derived parameters contraction and relaxation velocity can be obtained if the LVP signal is also applied to the inputs of a differentiator. If inotropic effects of drugs are to be investigated, inotropy generally is measured as the increase in dP/dt_{max}.

If a spontaneously beating Langendorff heart is investigated, the parameter QT (duration of QT) should be normalized to heart rate and expressed as QT_c according to the formula:

$$QT_c = \frac{QT}{\sqrt{RR}}$$

with RR = RR interval (= 60/HR). Similarly, CF should also be normalized to the pressure rate product as

$$CF_c = CF/LVP \times HR.$$

Perfusion Solutions

As perfusion solutions for Langendorff experiments typical saline solutions such as Tyrode solution or Krebs Henseleit solution are used. They are usually buffered using $NaHCO_3$ and a phosphate buffer. For correct adjustment of pH it is necessary to equilibrate these solutions with CO_2. Moreover, O_2 has to be delivered in its physically solubilised form. Therefore rather high pO_2 values are needed. This is achieved by equilibrating the solution with 95% O_2 and 5% CO_2 resulting in pO_2 values of about 650 mmHg and (depending on the composition of the solution) a pH of 7.4. This mix of 95% O_2 and 5% CO_2 is called carbogen and can be obtained commercially. In our lab we use a modified K^+-rich Tyrode solution of the following composition: Na^+ 161.02, K^+ 5.36, Ca^{2+} 1.8, Mg^{2+} 1.05, Cl^- 147.86, HCO_3^- 23.8, PO_4^{2-} 0.42 and glucose 11.1 mmol/l, equilibrated with 95% O_2 and 5% CO_2, pH = 7.4). The enhanced K^+ concentration helps to minimize the incidence of arrhythmia. If induction of arrhythmia is to be investigated it is helpful to reduce K^+ to 2.5 or even 2.0 mM and to decrease Mg^{++} to 0.5 mM. If inotropic agents such as ouabain are to be investigated the inotropic effect can be better demonstrated if a Ca^{++}-deficient Tyrode solution is used with only 0.9 mM Ca^{++}.

The standard Tyrode solution is of the following composition: NaCl 136.9, KCl 2.68, $CaCl_2$ 1.8, $MgCl_2$ 1.05, $NaHCO_3$ 11.9, NaH_2PO_4 0.42, glucose 5.55 mM, equilibrated with 3% CO_2 and 97% O_2 resulting in a pH of 7.4 or 5% CO_2 and 95% O_2 and a pH of 6.8.

Others prefer the use of Krebs-Henseleit solution of the following composition: NaCl 118, KCl 4.50, $CaCl_2$ 2.52, $MgSO_4$ 1.66, $NaHCO_3$ 24.88, KH_2PO_4 01.18, glucose 5.55, Na-pyruvate 2.0 mM equilibrated with 5% CO_2 and 95% O_2 resulting in a pH of 7.4.

If the use of CO_2 must be avoided (for example in experiments investigating the role of the Na^+/HCO_3^- transporter in comparison to Na^+/H^+-transport), a bicarbonate-free buffer has to be chosen. For that purpose, a modified Ringer solution may be used of the following composition: NaCl 153.9, KCl 2.68, $CaCl_2$ 1.8 with a phosphate buffer. Phosphate buffer is composed from stock solution I: 1.432 g Na_2HPO_4 (* 12 H_2O)/100 ml H_2O and stock solution II: 1.56 g NaH_2PO_4 (*2 H_2O)/100 ml H_2O. 10 ml stock I and 1 ml stock II are added per litre modified Ringer solution.

The addition of 2 mM Na-pyruvate has been reported to result in higher creatine phosphate levels (Döring and Hauf 1977). If the high pO_2 should be avoided, a possibility is the use of fluorocarbons, such as perfluorotributylamine (Dixon and Holland 1975), although these solutions are very expensive and are therefore mostly used in recirculating setups.

Oxygenation

In many Langendorff setups oxygenation is achieved by use of a fritted glass plate fused to a glass pipe which is connected to a carbogen gas tank with a reduction valve (instead some labs use fritted glass stones normally used in aquaria). The fritted glass may be placed in the heat exchanger or in the bottle serving as reservoir for the perfusion solution. If in this system proteins have to be added to the perfusion solution, it is necessary to add these solutions *via* a T-connector directly to the pre-gassed perfusion solution at the level of the aortic cannula. Bubbling a solution containing proteins would otherwise produce large quantities of foam.

Alternatively, an oxygenator (according to Schuler) may be used for oxygenation of the perfusion solution. Oxygenation is not achieved by bubbling but by using the disc oxygenator of a heart-lung machine, giving a thin film in an O_2-rich atmosphere (commercially available). The perfusion solution passes the oxygenator before being delivered to the heart. This system has the advantage that fluids, such as blood or protein-containing solutions can be used without foaming.

Electrical Stimulation

In some cases it may be interesting to control heart rate. The right atrium may be paced using either a bipolar AgCl electrode (with two tips) placed near the insertion of the upper vena cava or a AgCl electrode in the centre of the outer ring electrode may be used (coaxial electrode, diameter about 2.5 mm, both parts may be made from V2A steel, however, it is necessary that both parts are made from identical material). The latter may be preferred since the area stimulated is restricted to the area of the outer ring electrode, while in the case of the bipolar electrode the electrical equipotential field lines with radial direction reach a large area (Fig. 3).

If heart rate is controlled by external stimulation, it is sometimes useful to eliminate the sinus node. This can be achieved by ligation of the right atrium near the insertion of the upper caval vein.

In a similar way, the ventricle can be stimulated to study for example longitudinal or transverse propagation of the activation (see chapter 3.3, "Epicardial Mapping in Isolated Hearts."). If a more regular area is required, the electrodes for ventricular stimulation may be positioned on the back wall. If ventricular stimulation is to mimic ventricular extra systoles, it might be useful to position the electrodes on the left wall.

Examples

Constant Pressure Langendorff Heart

There are in principle two different setups for use as a constant pressure Langendorff apparatus, one with a fixed perfusion pressure given by the length of the thermo-controlled perfusion tube (Fig. 4a) and the other with a adjustable hydrostatic pressure (Fig. 4).

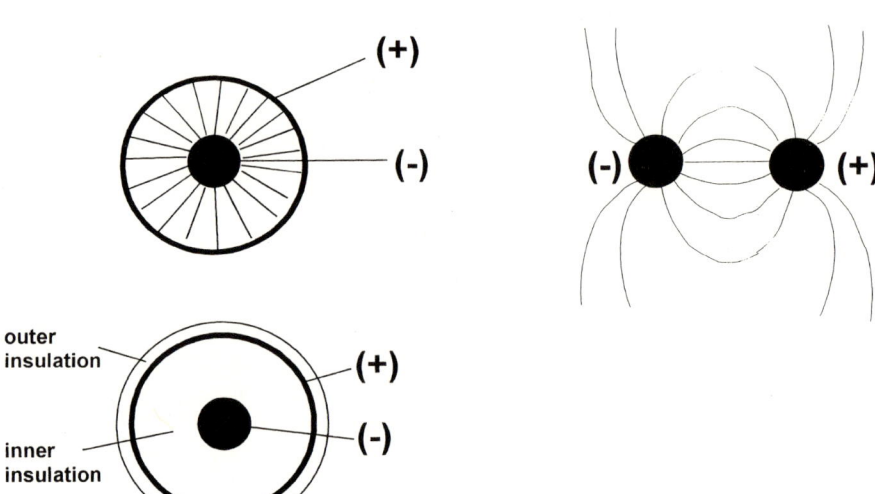

Figure 3
Electrodes for electrical stimulation. Coaxial electrode and bipolar electrode are shown with electrical equipotential field lines

In the first (simplest) case, a double-walled long glass tube is connected to a Boyle Marriott bottle which serves as a reservoir and is positioned on the top of the long tube. The double-walled tube is temperature controlled *via* a thermostat. The aortic cannula with the heart is fixed at the end of the tube. The perfusion pressure is kept constant by the use of the Boyle Marriott bottle and is as high as the hydrostatic pressure (length of cannula + length of tube + height of bottle) above the aortic valve.

An important issue is the selection of the correct hydrostatic pressure. If hydrostatic pressure is too high, cardiac oedema will occur. On the other hand, if hydrostatic pressure is too low, there will be hypoperfusion of the heart and ischemia, since the hydrostatic pressure is too low to overcome the resistance of the coronary circulation. Thus, for a rabbit heart about 75 cm H_2O (ca. 55 mmHg) is the correct constant hydrostatic perfusion pressure. For a rat heart 60–70 mmHg and for a guinea pig heart 50–60 mmHg seem appropriate.

Alternatively, an adjustment valve for setting the perfusion pressure, a so-called Gottlieb valve, may be used. This has the advantage, that the perfusion pressure may be adapted to various species. In this case, the perfusion solution is pumped to a double-walled heat exchanger and oxygenator chamber via a peristaltic pump. The perfusion solution is infused at the top of the chamber. At the bottom of the chamber, the solution accumulates and flows into the aortic cannula. The chamber has an inlet for carbogen, controlled by a reduction valve. In the upper half of the chamber, there is an outlet which is connected *via* a tube to the adjustment valve. This adjustment valve is simply a vertical pipe filled with water to the desired height of per-

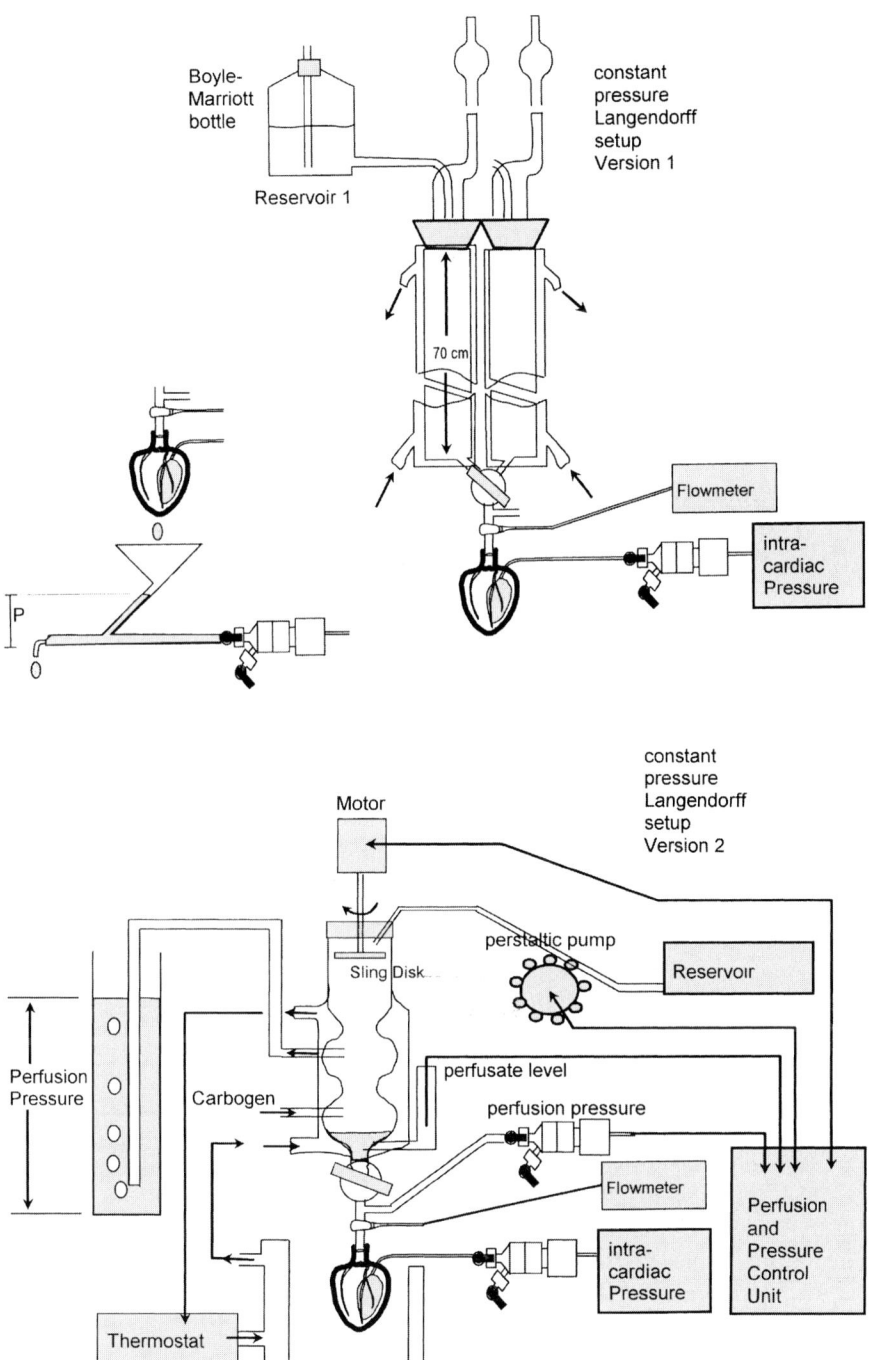

Figure 4
Two variants of a pressure constant Langendorff apparatus. **a** Variant A with long perfusion system (fixed perfusion pressure). **b** Variant B with adjustable perfusion pressure using a Gottlieb valve

fusion pressure and with the tube connected to the bottom of the pipe. Thus, the hydrostatic pressure increases the gas pressure within the chamber and thereby on the aortic valve at the bottom of the chamber. In this way, the hydrostatic pressure of the Gottlieb valve controls the perfusion pressure of the heart. Perfusion pressure may be changed to another value by altering the height of water filling the pipe. The double-walled chamber is heated and thermostated. Around the heart there is a second double walled chamber in the form of a cylinder which provides a warm and moisturised atmosphere around the heart.

At the beginning of an experiment it may be interesting to test the working myocardium by measurement of the Frank Starling mechanism. This can be easily done, if a balloon catheter for pressure measurement is used. For the first recording the dome of the Statham pressure transducer is left open so that the balloon pressure is equal to the atmospheric pressure. Next, the system is closed and balloon pressure is set to zero mmHg. One should now see considerably higher amplitudes of the LVP. In the next step, balloon pressure is set to 5, 10 and 15 mmHg up to 60 mmHg. If the working myocardium were not altered, the LVP would increase with the increase of the EDP (balloon pressure). However, increases above 10 mmHg only produce small increases in LVP until at higher balloon pressure LVP starts to drop.

The developed LVP (this is the maximum amplitude of LVP – end-diastolic pressure) is plotted as a function of the balloon pressure. The resulting curve should increase between 0 and about 15 mmHg and thereafter slowly decrease. The maximum of the curve indicates the optimum end-diastolic pressure for the experiment.

Constant Flow Langendorff Heart

As an alternative to the constant pressure setup, one may choose the constant flow experiment (see Fig. 5). In that case the heart is perfused at a constant flow rate, which has to be adjusted to the experimental requirements. The perfusion pressure is measured as an indicator of coronary resistance as outlined above. The correct coronary flow (under standard conditions) is a function of the heart weight. The correlation between coronary flow (CF) and heart weight (HW) for all species is described for physiological conditions by the equation

$$CF = 7.43 \times HW^{0.56}$$

(Döring and Dehnert 1988). This equation may be used for selection of the correct flow. The Langendorff apparatus consists of a perfusion solution bottle with an inlet and an outlet for carbogen (or other gas) connected to a peristaltic pump (10–50 ml/min; for rats, guinea pigs and rabbits) which transports the perfusion solution to a heat-exchanger chamber (normally a double walled cylinder connected to the thermostat) with the aortic cannula at its bottom. As described above, it is possible to use protein-containing solutions if, instead of bubbling, a rotating sling disk from a heart-lung machine is used at the top of the heat-exchange chamber. Alternatively, protein-containing solutions such as bovine serum albumin for maintaining a certain colloid osmotic pressure may be infused continuously *via* a T-connector at the level of the aortic cannula.

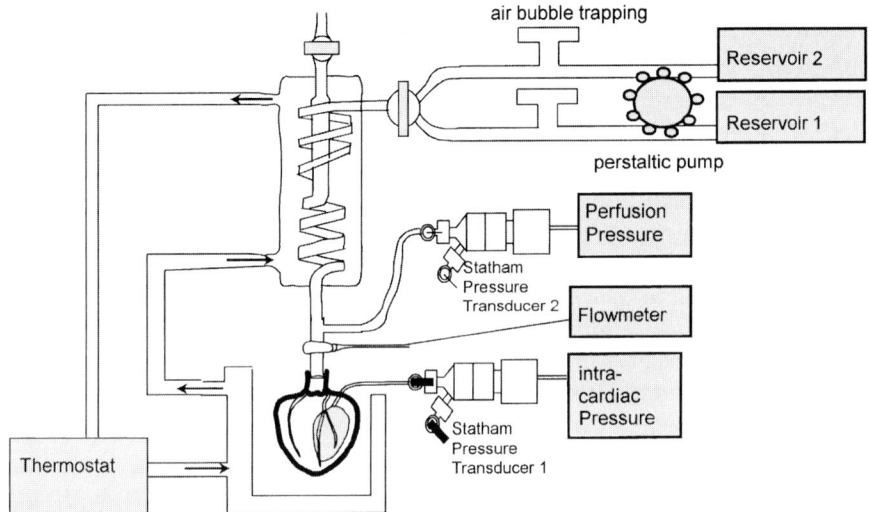

Figure 5
Flow constant Langendorff apparatus

The problem often encountered with this constant flow setup, although it is very simple to handle, is that the flow cannot be adapted to varying conditions e.g. during tachycardia or after administration of inotropic or chronotropic drugs which will enhance the energy and oxygen consumption and, *via* release of adenosine, decrease coronary resistance. This will be seen as a fall in perfusion pressure, however, since the flow rate is kept constant, there is no additional supply of oxygen or energy to the heart, which will result in relative ischemia.

Due to this consideration, the constant flow setup is probably best suited for the investigation of vasoactive drugs and may be less advantageous for the investigation of drugs influencing inotropy or heart rate and of complex situations such as ischemia and reperfusion.

The reactivity of the coronary vasculature may be tested at the beginning or the end of an experiment. Thus, it is possible to perfuse endothelin (1–100 nM) or angiotensin (1–100 nM) as vasoconstrictors, followed by a Ca^{++}-antagonist such as nifedipin (1–100 nM) as a typical vasodilator. Moreover, an endothelial dilatator such as acetylcholine, carbachol or bradykinin may be used. Such a test should be performed at the end of an experiment since it may be impossible to wash out the substances completely.

Alternatively, reactive hyperaemia may be used to test the vasomotion. For this purpose, coronary perfusion is stopped for a period of 10–60 seconds which will lead to the liberation of vasodilators such as NO or adenosine and will result in reduced perfusion pressure after switching on the perfusion again (or in a constant pressure setup increased CF). The endothelial component can be tested by repeating this test after a short infusion with collagenase-containing solution which will result in irreversible damage to the endothelial layer (Busse et al. 1983).

Coronary resistance (R) is calculated according to Ohm's law as

$$R = P/\Phi \; [\text{mmHg/ml/min}]$$

where P = perfusion pressure [mmHg] and Φ = coronary flow [ml/min].

Moreover, myogenic autoregulation (Bayliss effect) may be tested. For this purpose the coronary flow rate is increased suddenly or the perfusion pressure is enhanced abruptly (Schrader et al. 1977). This will immediately (as a first, very short response) passively stretch the vasculature; this is indicated by a sudden decrease in coronary resistance. This will be followed by a myogenic response consisting of vasoconstriction, which will enhance coronary resistance. In a constant pressure setup, a sudden increase in perfusion pressure will also cause a short transient positive inotropic response by passive stretching of the myocardium as a result of the enhanced filling of the coronaries, known as the "garden hose phenomenon". Myogenic autoregulation can be abolished by Ca^{++}-antagonists.

Fixation for Histology

At the end of an experiment it may be interesting to process the heart for histological examination. In that case the heart should be perfused with 4% p-formaldehyde for 10 min and then be cut free from the Langendorff apparatus. Subsequently, the heart (after removal of the balloon or other equipment) is transferred to a vessel containing 4% p-formaldehyde for 24 hours at 4 °C. Thereafter, the heart is incubated in 18% sucrose solution for another 24 h at 4 °C and then is wrapped in aluminium foil, covered with Tissue Tek and frozen at –80 °C.

Troubleshooting

With regard to coronary flow and its interpretation, it is necessary to keep in mind that saline solutions exhibit a lower viscosity and thus at the same perfusion pressure will exhibit a higher flow. Moreover, since coronary flow takes place during diastole, while during systole the enhanced tissue pressure impairs coronary flow, changes in the duration and strength of systolic action will affect coronary flow. At least it is important to remember that intramural and epicardial vessels will behave differently, since the epicardial arteries are not subject to systolic compression. This should be taken into account if vasoactive drugs are to be investigated.

When purely saline solutions are used, tissue oedema is caused by the lack of colloidal osmotic pressure. This is enhanced if perfusion pressure (constant pressure setup) or flow rate (constant flow setup) are too high. The oedema can be estimated if the heart is weighed after the experiment for wet weight and after drying for dry weight. Dry weight of guinea pig heart has been determined as 20–21% of wet weight *in situ* and may drop to 16% after 1 hour of saline perfusion (Döring and Dehnert 1988). Histologically, tissue oedema will cause separation of the fibres. The expansion of extracellular space can be prevented by perfusion with blood or by adding bovine serum albumin. On the other hand, the use of blood or protein solutions may cause various problems such as clotting, foaming, protein precipitation, erythrocyte aggregation and haemolysis with precipitation of erythrocyte remnants. Thus, other additives such as fluosol-43 (perfluorotributylamine in Pluronic F-68) and hydroxymethylstarch have been recommended. Others suggested the use of CMRL-1415 (Biochrom, Berlin) or of dextran (MW: 60,000 to 90,000; 3.6 g/100 ml). However, the results with these additives were controversial. McEwen (1956) suggested the use of a perfusion solution containing 0.45 g/100 ml saccharose which makes the perfusion solution hypertonic. This, however, may decrease the cardiac force of contraction. Another possibility is to enhance the tissues' pressure by immersing the heart in an organ bath or receptacle filled with the perfusion solution. Depending on the specific setup used, the setting of the parameters and the species and strain, cardiac tissue oedema may be more or less pronounced and should be determined for the setup used. In most cases, short experiments of a maximum duration of 120 minutes may be conducted without additives. However, if the experiments duration exceeds 120 minutes, enhancement of the colloidal osmotic pressure or of the tissue pressure is recommended.

Obstruction of the coronary orifices by the inserted aortic cannula may occur, and can be seen as a reduced coronary flow and signs of ischemia such as reduced LVP and elevated ST segments in the unipolar ECG. Care must be taken when inserting the aortic cannula not to obstruct the two coronary orifices by a too deep insertion.

Aortic valve insufficiency may be produced if during the preparation the aortic cannula is pushed through the valve. Care has to be taken during the preparation process. The failure can be seen, if the left ventricle and left atrium fill and overload with perfusion solution.

Arrhythmia may also be a problem found in Langendorff experiments. If these arrhythmias are present immediately after preparing the heart, they may be caused by stress to the animal prior to sacrifice and may be prevented by application of sedative drugs or by a more cautious handling of the animal. A short flick with the finger against the heart may stop fibrillation in the manner of a precordial stroke known from the clinic. In most cases the experiment has to be terminated if fibrillation occurs. Besides fibrillation, ventricular and supraventricular extra systoles may occur in the course of an experiment (this is found in many Langendorff experiments). It is necessary to evaluate all parameters during periods of stable rhythm of at least 5 minutes, since after an extra systole there is post-extra-systolic potentiation which would compromise LVP and CF measurements. The occurrence of extra systoles may be due to airflow to the heart's surface, if the heart is not kept in an organ receptacle, and may be overcome by shielding.

Sometimes, the recorded force may be too low. This might either be due to the preparation process, if the heart has become ischemic or may be caused by air bubbles which have entered the coronary circulation. On the other hand, the drugs used for anaesthesia may cause negative inotropy. In other cases the end-diastolic pressure is not optimal and should be checked. Moreover, the perfusion pressure may be too low. The pressure transducer has to be checked, including the balloon. The balloon material (latex) becomes porous after some weeks of use and should be changed weekly.

Other problems come from the coronary circulation. Thus, CF may be too low, which may be the results of embolization during preparation. This can be prevented by pre-treatment of the animal with heparin. Another cause of low flow is air bubbles entering the circulation. On the other hand, the coronary flow may be unusually high. Most often this is caused by omitting glucose from the perfusing solution. Another cause is reactive hyperaemia in response to a period of ischemia, most often during preparation. In the latter case, flow normalizes within a few minutes. However, in that case the preparation procedure has to be improved.

References

Beckett PR (1970) The isolated perfused heart preparation: two suggested improvements. J Pharm Pharmac 22: 818

Busse R, Pohl U, Kellner C, Klemm U (1983) Endothelial cells are involved in the vasodilatory response to hypoxia. Pflüger's Arch Ges Physiol 397: 78

Dixon DD, Holland DG (1975) Fluorocarbons: properties and synthesis. Fed Proc 34: 1444

Döring HJ, Dehnert H (1988) The isolated perfused warm-blooded heart according to Langendorff. Biomesstechnik Verlag March

Döring HJ, Hauf G (1977) Kontraktiliät sowie ATP- und Kreatinphosphat-Konzentrationen des Meerschweinchen-myokards bei Normoxie und verschiedenen Hypoxiegraden. Der Einfluß von Strophanthin, Isoproterenol und Kalziumchlorid. Herz/Kreislauf 9: 926

Gottlieb R, Magnus R (1904) Digitalis und Herzarbeit. Nach Versuchen am überlebenden Warmblüterherzen. Arch Exper Path Pharmakol 51: 30

Güttler K, Klaus W, Sander W, Valenta U (1982) The mechanical atrioventricular time of isolated hearts as a correlate of the atrioventricualr conduction time. In: Chasov, Smirnov, Dhalla (eds) Advances in myocardiology, vol. 3. Plenum Press

Hofer E, Stark U, Stark G, Tritthart HA (1990) Detection and continuous monitoring of intracardiac low-level potentials from the surface of the Langendorff-perfused heart. Basic Res Cardiol 85: 198–208

Langendorff O (1895) Untersuchungen am überlebenden Säugetierherzen. Pflüger's Arch Ges Physiol 61: 291–331

Schrader J, Haddy FJ, Gerlach E (1977) Release of adenosine, inosine and hypoxanthine from isolated guinea pig hearts during hypoxia, flow-autoregulation and reactive hyperemia. Pflüger's Arch Ges Physiol 369: 1

Stark G, Stark U, Tritthart HA (1987) Acute effects of amiodarone on the pacemaker- and conduction systems of the Langendorff perfused guinea pig heart. Z Kardiol 76 [Suppl 2]: 67

The Working Heart

Marc W. Merx and Jürgen Schrader

Introduction

Since the advent of genetically altered mice, a vast amount of fascinating cardiovascular phenotypes have been described with even more remaining to be explored (Doevendans et al. 1998; Gödecke and Schrader 2000). In addition to the many ways of assessing cardiac function in the intact animal through acute or chronic instrumentation or even non-invasively by echocardiography or MRI, the isolated, perfused heart remains a prominent investigative tool. This is because it offers a whole array of unique advantages:

The isolated heart provides a highly reproducible preparation that can be studied in a time and cost efficient manner. It allows a broad spectrum of biochemical, physiological, morphological and pharmacological indices to be measured, permitting detailed analysis of intrinsic ventricular mechanics, metabolism and coronary vascular responses. These measurements can be obtained without the confinements of systemic interference and side effects encountered in whole animal studies such as sympathetic and vagal stimulation, circulating neurohormonal factors and changes in substrate supply as well as alterations in systemic and pulmonary vascular resistance and left and right ventricular loading. Furthermore, experimental conditions such as ventricular pre- and after-load, perfusate oxygenation, substrate supply, coronary flow, heart rate and temperature, to name but a few, can be altered with ease and great precision to address the experimental question of interest. In addition, the measurement of physiological parameters is facilitated by the convenient exposure of the isolated heart, as is the application of pharmacological agents directly into the coronary circulation. The latter aspect also makes the working heart ideally suited for metabolic studies. Labelled precursors can be readily applied via the coronary system and their fate within the heart can be studied in a time-dependent manner. The preparation also readily allows the induction of whole heart or regional ischemia at various degrees of flow and at various degrees of oxygen deprivation. Thus, the isolated heart preparation is amenable to reperfusion or reoxygenation at various rates and with various reperfusate compositions, providing a powerful tool for assessing many aspects of ischemia- and reperfusion-induced injury.

The isolated, working heart preparation established under strict standards represents a functionally and metabolically stable system well suited for several hours of studies (Decking et al., 1997). However, as an *ex vivo* preparation, the isolated heart demands the application of appropriate precautions to maintain the organ's stability (see below). In addition, rigorous testing of the preparation must be performed and organs failing to live up to previously determined standards should be excluded from experimental analysis. These procedures should be repeated intermittently throughout the experimental course.

In principle two different isolated heart models exist:
- the isolated heart according to Langendorff (1895), in which hearts are supplied with coronary flow through retrograde perfusion (described in the previous chapter) and
- the working, fluid-ejecting heart, in which hearts are perfused via the left atrium and eject fluid through the left ventricle into the aorta thus perfusing their own coronaries.

The latter method was first described by Neely (Neely et al. 1967) and has since been adapted to a multitude of species including mice (Bardenheuer and Schrader 1986; Ng et al. 1991; Grupp et al. 1993; De Windt et al. 1999).

The working, fluid-ejecting heart performs pressure-volume work, an important distinction from its Langendorff counterpart, which performs energetically less demanding isovolumetric contractions. Because the left ventricle is filled with perfusate, left ventricular pressure and its derivative parameters can be obtained directly through the application of a pressure transducer. This eliminates the need for a balloon to be inserted into the left ventricle and thus avoids the confinements inherent to balloons such as: differences between ventricle and balloon geometry, compliance issues of balloon material, signal dampening due to minute air inclusions in the balloon system and the like.

With the working heart ejecting fluid, cardiac output, being the sum of aortic and coronary flow, can be measured continuously. Preload and afterload may be adjusted over a wide range of feasible loading conditions enabling detailed studies of ventricular function. Thus the isolated working heart adds functionally important parameters to the already broad arsenal provided by Langendorff preparations, while retaining ease of access to the organ and versatility in experimental design.

Description of Methods and Practical Approach

The Working Heart Apparatus

Since the first description of the working heart by Neely (Neely et al. 1967), this fascinating model has been eagerly welcomed by the scientific community and is thus found in many laboratories throughout the world. Numerous institutions use home-built apparatus enabling them to add modifications according to their individual research interests. In addition, several companies offer commercially available working heart setups (Experimetria, Hugo Sachs Elektronik/Harvard Apparatus for example). As it would be impossible to discuss all of these individual approaches to the working heart, we will concentrate on the model employed in our laboratories to illustrate essential components. The apparatus referred to is commercially available and produced by Hugo Sachs Elektronik/Harvard Apparatus. A diagram of the working heart setup and a photograph of the actual setup in our laboratories are given in Fig. 1a and b, respectively. A schematic diagram of the work-performing heart is given in Fig. 2a alongside a close up view of the heart in its actual experimental surrounding (Fig. 2b). An important advantage of this setup is that it facilitates seamless switching from Langendorff to working heart mode and, while in Langendorff mode, from constant pressure to constant flow perfusion. Furthermore, it is very compact and can easily be transferred from one location to another as all essential components are robustly mounted within the supportive structure. The whole apparatus is made of Plexiglas greatly reducing the risk of accidental damage as compared to glass constructions.

The components depicted in Fig. 1 include all necessary parts for the successful operation of a working heart model except for the thermostatic circulator and the measuring instruments. As the isolated heart is very vulnerable to temperature changes, every effort should be made to ensure constant and defined temperature conditions. To this end, the heart and all temperature sensitive components are installed inside a thermostated chamber (*15*) and (*16*).

The heart is connected to the apparatus by removable aortic (*2*) and atrial (*29*) cannulae. The cannulae can be made of glass or plastic but stainless steel is most commonly used. Cannula size is critical as, in contrast to Langendorff perfused hearts, total cardiac output, of which coronary flow is but a fragment, flows through both atrial and aortic cannulae. In addition, the cannulae are rigid, resulting in an energetically challenging resistance to left ventricular ejection in the case of the aortic cannula. The inner diameter of the cannula should therefore be at least the same as the aortic diameter and preferably as large as feasible. Due to the considerable elasticity of the aorta it is possible to stretch the aorta over a cannula with an outer diameter significantly larger than the original aortic diameter. The length of the cannula should be kept as short as possible for the same reasons (cannula design is discussed in elegant detail by De Windt et al. [1999]). Even if working with one species only, it is advisable to have several sizes of cannulae available in order to be able to employ the largest feasible for any given heart. For our mouse studies we use cannulae of 0.9 to 1.3 mm inner diameter in 0.1 mm graduations. These cover hearts ranging from approximately 100 mg to 600 mg wet weight and thus are applicable in mice as small as 18 g with no relevant upper weight/size limit. The same considerations hold true for the atrial cannula, although size constraints set by the individual heart studied pose less of a challenge in the atrium as the pulmonary vein orifice can easily be enlarged to accommodate a sufficiently sized cannula. Nevertheless, the cannula should present as little resistance to inflow as possible. In general, the atrial cannula should have a free flow (i.e. flow measured without the heart being attached to the cannula) of at least twice the flow expected to occur in the individual experimental setting. In our experience the maximum cardiac output generated by a working mouse heart (using high preload (25 mmHg) and low afterload (60 mmHg), see also experimental examples section below) lies between 20 and 25 ml/min. However, these high flows are only encountered in experimental designs where this unusual loading combination is of interest. The atrial cannula we are able to use in all but the smallest hearts, with an inner diameter of 1.3 mm is sufficient to permit a free flow of 70 ml/min at 12 mmHg preload.

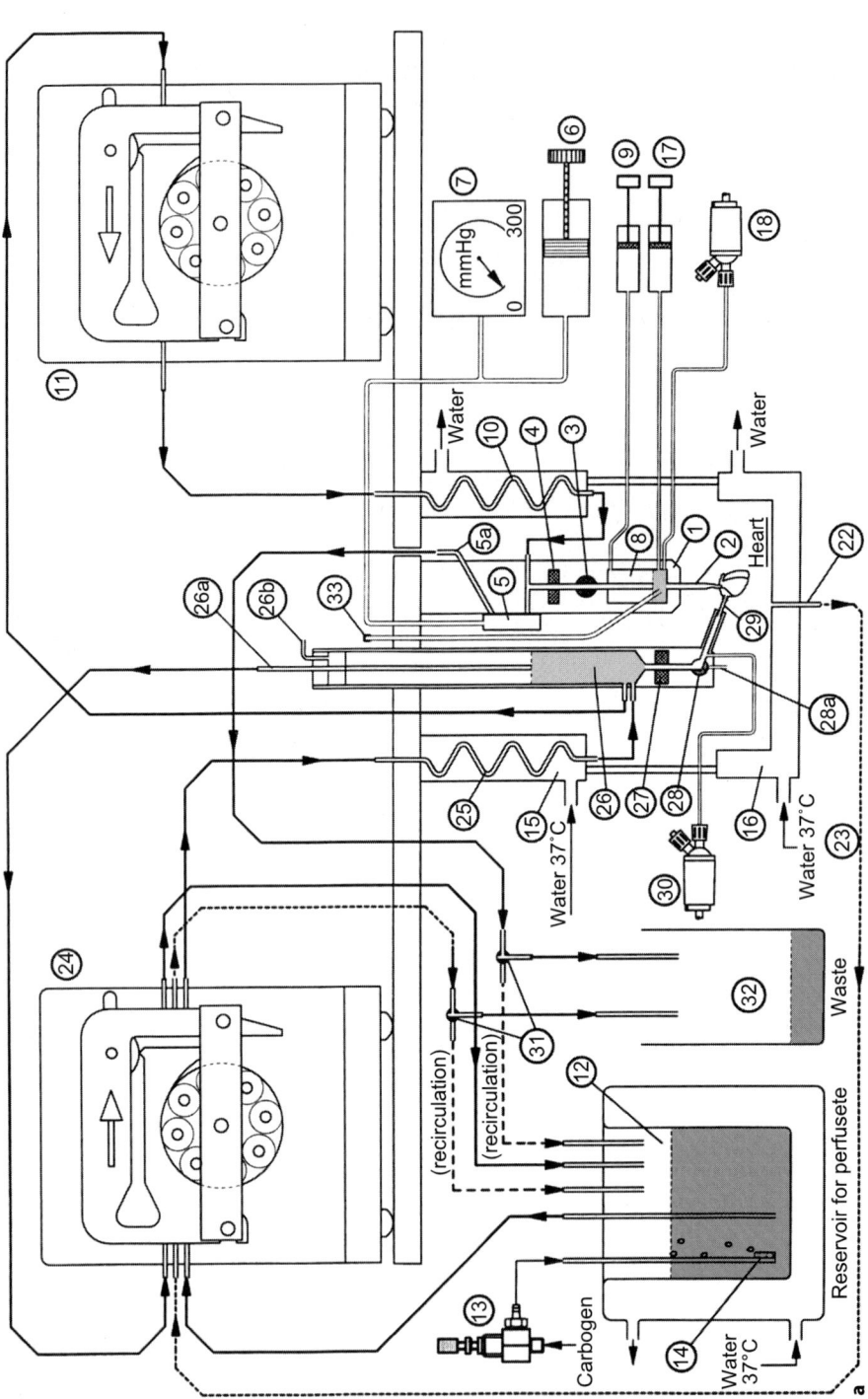

Figure 1a
Explanation see next page, part b

2.2 The Working Heart 177

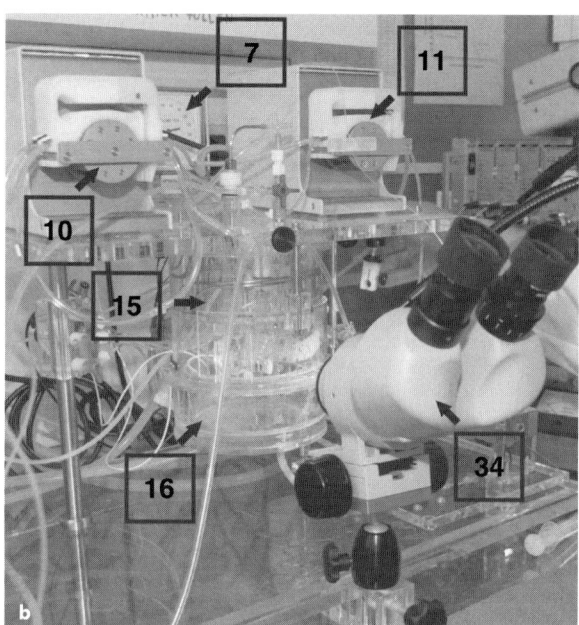

Figure 1a,b
Schematic diagram of (a) and actual (b) working-heart apparatus. Important components are marked and numbered as follows (see text for detailed explanation): *1* aortic block; *2* aortic cannula; *4* flow probe (coronary/aortic flow); *5* flow resistor; *6* rotary control pressure pump; *7* pressure gauge; *8* compliance chamber; *11* roller pump; *12* thermostated reservoir; *13* carbogen; *14* gassing filter; *15, 16* thermostated chambers; *18* pressure transducer (for perfusion pressure/afterload); *24* roller pump; *26* preload vessel; *26a* suction tube; *27* flow probe (atrial flow); *29* atrial cannula; *30* pressure transducer (preload measurement); *32* waste reservoir; *34* dissecting microscope

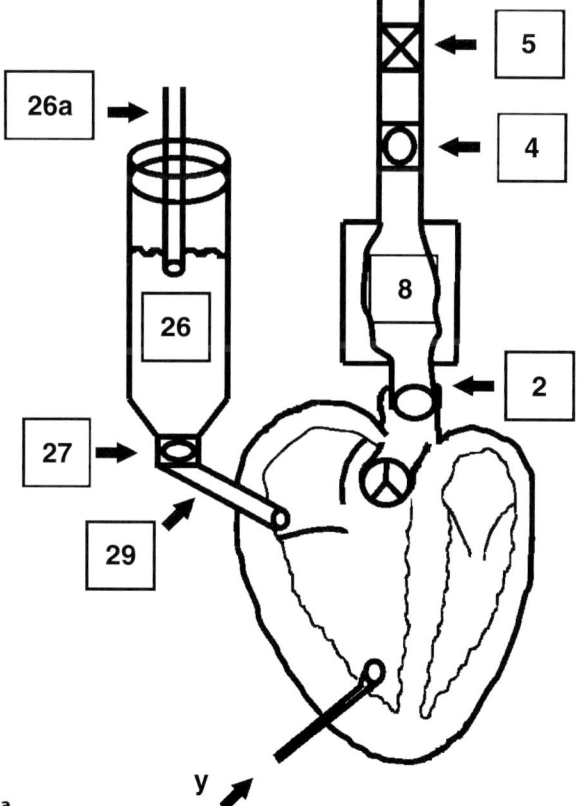

Figure 2a
Explanation see next page, part b

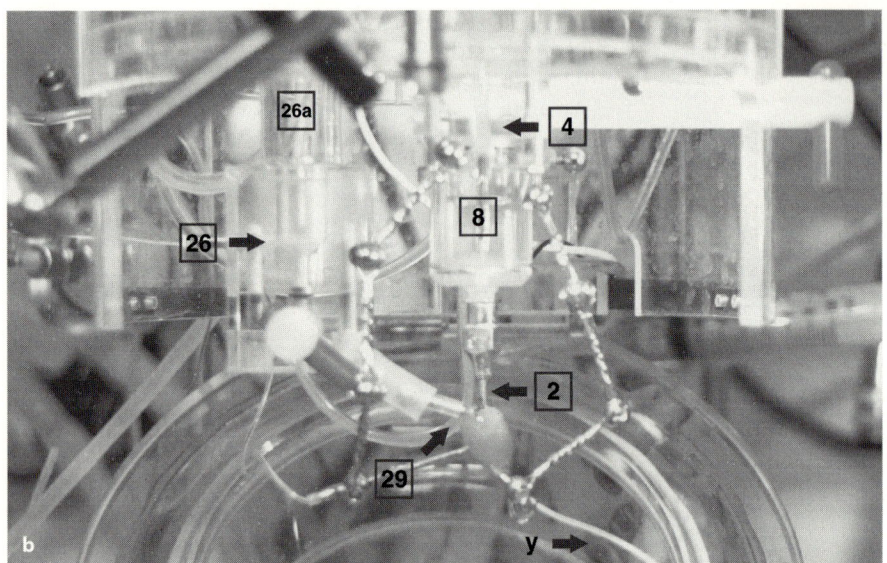

Figure 2a,b
Schematic diagram of (**a**) and actual (**b**) working-heart preparation. Important components are marked and numbered as follows (see text for detailed explanation): *2* aortic cannula; *4* flow probe (coronary/aortic flow); *5* flow resistor; *8* compliance chamber; *26* preload vessel; *26a* suction tube; *27* flow probe (atrial flow); *29* atrial cannula; PE-tubing connected to pressure transducer

The perfusate is oxygenised in a thermostated reservoir (*12*) by gassing through a glass filter (*14*) with carbogen (a gas blend of 95% oxygen and 5% carbon dioxide). Carbogen flow is regulated through a needle vent (*13*). If the perfusate employed is prone to foaming (see perfusate) a membrane oxygenator should be used instead.

Although the fluid-ejecting working heart is the aim, it is nevertheless necessary to perfuse the explanted heart in a retrograde fashion initially. Thus the apparatus is operated in Langendorff constant pressure mode (see also atrial cannulation and switch to working heart mode) with a roller pump (*11*; e.g. Reglo Digital ISM 834) supplying perfusate to the heart. To ensure constant pressure, the above-mentioned pump supplies more perfusate than actually required by the heart being perfused. The excess perfusate supplied by the pump and not required by the heart passes through a flow resistor (*5*) back to the reservoir (*12*) for oxygenation. It is thus possible to adjust the perfusion pressure by setting the flow resistor (*5*) to whichever perfusion pressure is desired, ensuring constant perfusion pressure over a wide range of flows. The flow resistor consists of a membrane to which perfusate is channelled from one side and pressure is applied from the other side, using a rotary control pressure pump (*6*) connected to a pressure gauge (*7*) indicating the actual perfusion pressure. In addition perfusion pressure is measured by a pressure transducer (*18*; e.g. ISOTEC single use, comparable-pressure transducers also available from Braun, COBE or Millar). The resulting coronary flow is measured with a flow probe (*4*; e.g. Transonic 1 N connected to T106, T206 or HSE-TTFM). After passing through the flow probe and a compliance chamber (8) doubling as bubble trap, the perfusate reaches the aortic cannula (2). A frequently used, albeit less versatile, setup consists of a pressurized water column with the height of the water column determining perfusion pressure.

If constant-flow perfusion should be required (this is not routinely recommended when initiating a working heart experiment), return flow of perfusate supplied by the pump (11) is prevented by setting the control (6) of the flow resistor (5) to a very high value (e.g. 250 mmHg) thus sealing the membrane of the flow restrictor. The required flow is then set on the pump (11). The resulting perfusion pressure is measured with the pressure transducer (18) and coronary flow rate is verified using the above mentioned flow probe (4).

In working-heart mode, the left atrium receives perfusate from the preload vessel (26) through the atrial cannula (29). Using a roller pump (24; e.g. Reglo Digital ISM 834) more perfusate is pumped into the preload vessel (26) than flows into the atrium. The preload vessel doubles as a bubble trap. The solution not required is pumped from the stainless steel suction tube (26a) back to the reservoir using one of the pump channels.

Preload is altered by vertical adjustment of the suction tube in much the same way as afterload would be adjusted in the case of a setup with a pressurized water column (although the pressure range being covered has to be much larger in the latter case; 26a). Preload is measured by a pressure transducer connected to the preload vessel (30) (e.g. ISOTEC P75). The resulting atrial flow (equalling cardiac output in the working-heart model) is measured continuously with a flow probe (27; transonic 1 N, see above).

The perfusate ejected by the left ventricle passes into the coronaries by way of the aortic root. Perfusate ejected by the heart but not required for coronary perfusion (which may be viewed as "effective cardiac output") flows into the aortic block (1) via the aortic cannula (2). Here it enters the compliance chamber which contains an adjustable amount of air (we recommend 1 ml) to provide elastic recoil (simulating the "Windkessel" characteristic of the aorta). The compliance chamber functions as a buffer against the low mechanical compliance of the setup as such. It lowers mechanical resistance to the ejecting heart and ensures coronary perfusion which occurs mainly during diastole in the work-performing heart. From the compliance chamber the perfusate runs through the adjustable flow resistance (5) that is now used to set afterload in the same way that it was previously used to adjust perfusion pressure. Via tubing (5a) connected to the flow resistor (5) the perfusate ejected by the heart is drained passively either to the oxygenating reservoir (12), providing recirculation of the perfusate, or alternatively to a waste reservoir (32). Afterload is now measured with the same pressure transducer previously used to measure perfusion pressure (18).

Aortic flow produced by the heart at any given afterload is measured continuously *via* flow probe (4). Again coronary flow is assessed with the same flow probe as in Langendorff mode. It is important to note that if the same flow probe is used for Langendorff and working-heart measurements, polarity has to be changed when switching from one mode to the other, as flow direction will change also (otherwise negative flow values will result). The difference between atrial flow (i.e. cardiac output) and aortic flow constitutes coronary flow in the working heart model. Depending on the data acquisition system preferred, the latter can be computed and displayed online (see below) or calculated after the experiment is completed. For calibration purposes, the coronary perfusate having passed through the coronaries, right atrium and ventricle can be collected form the pulmonary artery and its volume measured.

More importantly the perfusate collected from the pulmonary artery may be used to measure coronary venous P_{O_2}. For this purpose the pulmonary artery is cannulated with PE tubing and suctioned to a P_{O_2} electrode with constant flow (as P_{O_2} electrodes are very sensitive to flow alterations, e.g. ZABS PO1750). The rate at which the coronary venous perfusate is suctioned should always be well below the rate of coronary flow to avoid air being sucked into the P_{O_2} measuring chamber. Excess perfusate from the right ventricle is suctioned by a roller pump (24) through tubing (23) connected to a draining cannula (22) at the bottom of the thermostated chamber (16). It is than either recirculated to the oxygenation reservoir (12) or drained to the waste reservoir (32).

Left ventricular pressure is measured with a fluid filled catheter inserted into the left ventricle and connected to an additional pressure transducer (not shown in the diagram, e.g. ISOTEC MP15). Alternatively, a bespoke catheter with miniature pressure transducer mounted to its tip can be used for even truer pressure readings albeit at considerable cost (Millar, Radi).

Recently, an even more sophisticated (and costly) alternative has become available in the form of pressure volume catheters (Millar). In the latter case, a miniature pressure transducer at the catheter's tip is combined with induction coils at the catheter's distal end for volume measurements.

The electrocardiogram of the work-performing heart can easily be recorded by applying electrodes to the right atrium and ventricle. It is also possible to record the electrocardiogram *via* the atrial and aortic cannulae, although we have found the signal quality to be inferior to directly attached electrodes. If pacing of the heart is required in the experimental protocol, this can be achieved through the application of a, preferably bipolar, stimulation-electrode connected to a stimulator suitable for the high frequencies of up to 15 Hz required (e.g. Hugo Sachs Elektronik/Harvard Apparatus P105).

A further important consideration is the application of drugs to the heart to enable pharmacological studies. In principle, it is possible to add the agent directly to the perfusate (see also Perfusate). However, if different concentrations are to be studied or if several agents are of interest during the course of one experiment, it is more convenient to add the substance through a sidearm of the apparatus with a receptacle for one or more infusion lines. This sidearm should be as close to the atrial cannula as possible (or to the aortic cannula while in Langendorff mode). In the setup described here a sidearm is integrated directly proximal to both the atrial and aortic cannulae, thus enabling the precise application of even minute volumes through micro-infusion pumps (e.g. Precidor P104).

In addition to circumventing the need for several perfusate reservoirs with all the associated drawbacks (see perfusate), microinfusion through a proximal sidearm also avoids contamination of the whole setup wit the substance studied, which can be responsible for uncontrolled side effects due to prolonged wash out.

With the apparatus described here, preload can be set in the range of 0–30 mmHg and afterloads ranging from 0 to 300 mmHg are feasible. Atrial and retrograde flow (i.e. coronary flow in Langendorff) depend largely on the size of the cannulae and the pump and tubing employed. In our setup tailored to mice, atrial flows of up to 50 ml/min and retrograde flows of up to 25 ml/min are possible (using the cannula sizes mentioned above). Preload, afterload and left ventricular pressure as well as atrial (sometimes referred to as venous) and aortic (sometimes referred to as arterial) flows are measured continuously. Depending on the recording hard and software, a multitude of derivative parameters can be calculated online or after completion of the experiment.

Preparatory Steps

Prior to the first experiment of the day the working heart apparatus should be flushed with purified water (i.e. ultra-filtered water generated by e.g. a Millipore System). In general, letting the apparatus become dry should be avoided, as it is extremely tedious to eliminate small air bubbles adherent to the walls of the apparatus and tubing. If meticulous attention is not paid to keeping the setup free of air, air emboli can cause coronary occlusion in the isolated organ. It is thus advisable to keep the apparatus filled with purified water between experiments, unless it is decommissioned for long periods of time. Leaving the perfusate itself in place between experiments for more than a few minutes has the drawback of promoting crystallisation on apparatus and tubing walls. If the perfusate is left in place for hours, there is a risk of promoting microbial growth and thus colonization of the apparatus, a condition that is extremely difficult to treat and that may demand complete dismantling of the apparatus and replacement of significant parts. Along the same lines, the heating (and where applicable cooling) circuit of the apparatus should be kept as clean as possible by frequently replacing the purified water (i.e. ultra filtered water, see above) and by adding stabilizing antimicrobial agents.

Depending on the surrounding temperature it is necessary to initiate heating (and cooling) of the apparatus well before starting the experiment, as stable temperatures are essential to generate reproducible results. For mice the temperature of the perfusate provided at the tip of the aortic perfusion cannula should be 37 ± 0.5 °C. As the body temperature of rats and rabbits is slightly higher, 38 ± 0.5 °C should be aimed for in these species. The chamber surrounding the isolated heart should be heated to the same temperature. The chamber should also be as airtight as possible to avoid loss of humidity and minimize cooling of the isolated heart secondary to evaporation of perfusate from its surface. If heart preparation is performed in a cooled environment (see below) the heart should be held at a constant temperature of 4 ± 0.5 °C throughout preparation.

Perfusate

The perfusion solution should be prepared as close to the actual time of use as possible. In any case it is not recommended to store the substrate-containing perfusate for more than a few hours, as it is an excellent bacterial growth medium and bacterial contamination of the perfusate will thus readily occur.

The perfusate employed in isolated heart perfusion serves two main purposes providing (a) substrates and (b) oxygen to the heart while maintaining ionic and pH homeostasis. Because of the associated ease of use, saline solutions gassed with carbogen (95% O_2 + 5% CO_2, the latter to achieve the required pH of 7.4) and with glucose and pyruvate as substrates are employed most frequently. However, fatty acids are used in metabolic studies and albumin has been added to the perfusate to reduce the otherwise significant oedema associated with saline perfusion. If fatty acids or proteins are added to the perfusate, oxygenation should be carried out with membrane oxygenators as severe foaming will result from direct gassing.

Drugs or other agents may be added directly to any perfusate or, more elegantly, be injected through a side arm of the apparatus close to the atrial (or aortic) cannula. If the latter technique is employed, high concentrations of the agent must be used so that the injected volume remains minute (i.e. <1%) compared to the total flow of perfusate to the organ. Thus the amounts of substrates and oxygen delivered to the organ remain practically unaffected. However, especially with small hearts such as those encountered in murine studies precision pumps are necessary to apply the microliter-range volumes required (see above).

Turning to the second important function of the perfusate, the delivery of oxygen to the isolated heart, saline solutions are characterized by a relatively low oxygen carrying capacity. This poses a challenge, as continuous provision of oxygen in quantities sufficient to maintain normal metabolism and transmembrane gradients as well as to support aerobic ATP generation for contraction is essential for the survival of the isolated heart. The low oxygen carrying capacity of saline solutions can be counterbalanced by gassing with high partial pressures, as is the case with the application of carbogen.

Depending on ambient pressure O_2 partial pressures in excess of 650 mmHg are attained. Combined with the higher coronary flow observed in saline perfused hearts compared to sanguineous perfusion, this is sufficient to ensure adequate oxygenation. Furthermore, we were able to demonstrate that intracellular P_{O2} remains unaffected even if the saline perfusate is gassed with 70% oxygen, translating into a significant safety margin when working with carbogen (Merx 2001).

If, however, specific experimental questions require near normal coronary flow rates and/or higher oxygen transport capacity, donor blood or erythrocyte enriched aqueous solutions have been used successfully (Gamble et al. 1970; Qiu et al. 1993). It should be noted that because of the volumes required in most isolated heart setups, multiple donor animals are often required. Incompatibility of different species with respect to erythrocytes' ability to traverse the capillary bed of the recipient heart have to be taken into account. Here also gassing needs to be achieved through membrane oxygenators as direct gassing will cause excessive foaming and damage the erythrocytes and other cells in the case of whole blood perfusion. In the case of whole blood perfusion, sufficient anticoagulation is difficult to achieve given the prolonged exposure to all kinds of non-biocompatible materials.

As mentioned above, a saline perfusion solution based on the "physiological" solution first proposed by Krebs and Henseleit (1932) is adequate for the vast majority of isolated heart studies. The modified Krebs–Henseleit buffer used most commonly in our laboratories contains (in mM): 116 NaCl, 4.6 KCl, 1.1 $MgSO_4$, 24.9 Na HCO_3,

2.5 $CaCl_2$, 1.2 KH_2PO_4, 8.3 glucose and 2 pyruvate equilibrated with 95% O_2–5% CO_2 to yield a pH of 7.4. The chemicals used should be of high purity (at least pro analysis, "p.a." quality) and should be obtained from the same provider consistently (we use Sigma chemicals).

As the solution contains calcium and phosphate ions, the risk of calcium phosphate particles forming and precipitating should be avoided by ensuring that the pH of the bicarbonate buffered solution is lowered to 7.4 by gassing with carbogen and adding calcium as the last component thereafter. Finally, it is of great importance to filter the perfusate carefully (filter pore size 5 µm or smaller) as even the purest grade chemicals may contain enough debris to cause embolization especially in a vasculature as small as the murine.

Heart Explantation and Aortic Cannulation

Deep anaesthesia has to be induced in the animal prior to initiation of the required surgical procedure. In order to achieve optimal anaesthetic results with reproducible dosing, every effort should be made to minimize stress by keeping the animal in a quiet environment that the animal is accustomed to and by minimizing animal handling.

To prevent blood clotting in the excised heart, the animal should be sufficiently anticoagulated prior to the application of the anaesthetic agent. This is easily achieved by giving heparin by intravenous or intraperitoneal injection at a dose of 5 IU/g BW (because of its lipolytic properties heparin should be avoided in lipid or fatty acid metabolism studies). Anaesthesia is usually induced either by inhalation or by intravenous or intraperitoneal injection. Inhalative agents used in mice include ether, halothane, isoflurane, enflurane and methoxyflurane. Intravenous/intraperitoneal agents reported in mice include urethane, pentobarbitone, ketamine and propofol. Relaxing agents such as benzodiazepines and curonium-derivatives as well as analgetic substances such as morphine may be added.

The anaesthetic regime will depend largely on the purpose of the study and thus on considerations regarding the differing degree of cardio-depressant effects observed for the agents. In our labs we most commonly use a combination of ketamine (60 mg/kg body weight) and xylazine (10 mg/kg body weight). Anaesthesia will also be influenced by local animal welfare regulations. As substantial strain differences (and especially in mice and rats even differences between animals of the same strain but from different animal facilities) exist in the susceptibility to different anaesthetic agents, careful dose titration in preliminary experiments is mandatory.

After the animal is anaesthetized, the peritoneal aspect of the diaphragm is visualized by a transabdominal incision. While supporting the sternal apex the diaphragm is carefully incised so as not to damage any intrathoracic structure. While continuously supporting the sternal apex upward, the thorax is opened by bilateral incision at its dorsolateral edge. A sharp but sturdy (the ribs have to be cut in the process) pair of curved and blunt tipped scissors is usually well suited to perform the incision with minimal risk of damage to the heart or lungs. The now mobilized anterior half of the thoracic cage is subsequently deflected above the animal's head to give unhindered approach to the heart and lung. In larger species, the aorta, pulmonary vessels and cava can be cut directly, with some investigators even opting to cannulate the aorta *in situ*. Generally speaking, the procedure can be performed rapidly (well below 1 min) in larger species and does not pose a major challenge.

However, if mice are the species of interest it is more practical to extract the whole heart lung package out of the thorax. The most convenient approach in doing so is to grip the descending aorta with a pair of small forceps and cut the aorta below. Never letting go of the aorta, the vessel is deflected ventrally and the heart and lung dissected out of the thoracic cavity by a series of small incisions strictly parallel and as close as possible to the dorsal thoracic wall.

If the incisions are followed through cranially the heart and lung will be removed from the thoracic cavity by the forceps still holding the descending aorta. Heart and lung are immediately transferred to a bath containing cold, heparinised (5 IU of heparin/ml), modified Krebs–Henseleit solution (4°C, see above) and placed beneath a dissecting microscope.

Now the lungs, thymus, bronchi and oesophagus are dissected away taking great care to have full visualization of the intended cutting plane to avoid involuntary laceration of any cardiac structure. As soon as the aorta and its cranial branches are clearly visualized, the aorta is cut just below its first branch. The heart is then gently slipped on to the perfusion fluid-filled aortic cannula avoiding excessive strain and thus tearing of this delicate structure. A ligature is placed as above and correct location and sufficient tightness verified under the microscope.

The cannulated heart is transferred to the apparatus. The aortic connector for the cannula should be gently dripping with perfusate and the cannula approximated to the connector at an oblique angle to avoid air emboli at the time of heart attachment to the apparatus. After some practice it should be possible to perform the preparatory steps described above in less than 3 min.

Atrial Cannulation and Switch to Working-Heart Mode

With the heart now adequately perfused in the Langendorff mode and thus oxygenated, the further preparatory steps can be taken under a less rigid time constraint. Again a dissecting microscope (34) should be placed in front of the heart to facilitate clear visualization of the relevant structures (see Fig. 1b, in the case of species larger than mice the naked eye should suffice, but magnification is very helpful in training).

First any surplus tissue (thymus, fat, lung ...) is removed. To ensure unimpeded drainage of coronary venous perfusate the pulmonary artery should be incised. This is advisable as the close proximity of the pulmonary artery to the aorta and the connective tissue surrounding both vessels result in relatively frequent, inadvertent ligation or at least partial obstruction of the pulmonary artery. The incision also facilitates later cannulation of the pulmonary artery if arterial-venous differences in perfusate oxygen content are to be measured. Hereafter, the dorsal aspect of the left atrium is trimmed from surplus tissue, especially the pulmonary veins, taking care to leave the actual dorsal atrial wall intact. In mice two pulmonary veins drain into the left atrium, separated by a small trabecular structure. The latter is cut and the resulting combined orifice used for atrial cannulation. The atrial cannula should be dripping with perfusate when being inserted so that any air present in the left atrium or ventricle is removed. The cannula is then tied into the left atrial wall by securing the left atrial tissue surrounding the orifice above the flange at the distal end of the cannula with a suture.

If required, the pulmonary artery is cannulated next (i.e. to measure coronary venous P_{O2}). Electrodes for ECG recording or pacing are placed if desired. After instrumentation of the heart is completed (usually within 5 min after initiation of Langendorff perfusion, the heart is left for 20 min to equilibrate under retrograde perfusion (i.e. Langendorff mode, chapter 2.1) preferably under 100 mmHg constant perfusion pressure. It should be noted that there is no flow to the atrial cannula at this stage.

Thereafter, perfusion pressure is lowered to 60 mmHg and preload (i.e. atrial perfusion pressure) is set to 12 mmHg. After enabling flow through the aortic cannula, flow in the aorta should be reversed as the heart begins ejecting perfusate in an antegrade fashion and the aortic perfusion pressure becomes afterload. It is sometimes helpful to lower afterload further (to values as low as 20 mmHg) to facilitate the initiation of antegrade flow, but this should not be done for no more than a few seconds as afterload equals coronary perfusion pressure and cardiac hypoxia would result. After-load should then be increased to values between 80 and 100 mmHg and the heart left to equilibrate for another 10 min, after which the experimental protocol of choice may be started.

Data Acquisition

Afterload, preload, left ventricular pressure (LVP), atrial flow, aortic flow and if desired coronary venous P_{O2} as well as the electrocardiogram are measured continuously. The signals originating from the pressure transducers and flow meters as well as electrocardiogram and P_{O2} signals require amplification. This is usually performed by tailor-made amplifiers designed specifically for the signal in question that are often bundled with the respective probe or transducer. In our laboratories we use dedicated amplifiers by Hugo Sachs Elektronik/Harvard Apparatus (TAM-A for the pressure transducers, TTFM for the flow probes, ECGA for electrocardiogram and OPPM for coronary venous P_{O2}) slotted into a convenient single case (PLUGSYS).

Traditionally the amplifier output is plotted on a polygraph which allows the user to monitor and record the parameters studied. However, this implies often tedious manual evaluation after completion of the experiment. Analogue-digital converters connected to personal computers running specially designed software have the advantage of calculating derivative parameters online and displaying them together with the primary data in almost any fashion that suites the investigator.

In our laboratories we use an IBM-compatible personal computer with analogue-digital converter (Texas Instruments, 2000 Hz resolution) and specifically designed software (EMKA Technologies, Paris, France). The above-mentioned parameters as well as derivative parameters are displayed in real time and streamed onto hard disk (at a rate of approx. 30 Mb per hour). The derivative parameters we work with are:
a) coronary flow, being the difference between atrial and aortic flow;
b) the maximum rate of left ventricular pressure development (dP/dt_{max});

c) the maximum rate of relaxation (also referred to as minimum rate of pressure development; dP/dt_{min})
d) time to peak pressure (TPP), calculated as time from end diastolic pressure (EDP) to systolic pressure (SP);
e) relaxation halftime ($RT_{1/2}$), time from SP to DP/2).

B through e are all derived from left ventricular pressure curve analysis.

In addition to facilitating convenient display (we use a twin screen setup enabling us to monitor the real time signal curves as well as giving us a complete overview of all signal trends at any time) and storage of data, the software allows us to predefine or manually select time points in the course of the experiment during which data is written into an Excel table (Microsoft) in addition to and independent of the raw data being streamed to the hard disk. The fashion in which the data is written to the Excel table is freely chosen by the investigator e.g. coronary flow might be stored every 60 s with the value stored being the mean calculated over 30 s. In this way, through thoughtful design of the experiment and of the software storage functions, a large part of experiment evaluation can be automated.

Examples

The examples given here are taken from working heart experiments performed to analyse differences in cardiac function between myoglobin (Mb) knockout mice ($myo^{-/-}$) and their wild type counterparts. Weights of excised hearts ranged from 180–250 mg, with no significant differences between WT and $myo^{-/-}$. Left ventricular mass (including septum) as a percentage of whole heart wet weight was similar (64.7 ± 2.1% vs. 65.3 ± 2.7; WT vs. $myo^{-/-}$; p = n.s.).

Afterload was increased stepwise to simulate growing systemic resistance. As listed in Table 1, impaired contractility was demonstrated by slower contraction and relaxation reflected as time to peak pressure (TPP) and relaxation half-time ($RT_{1/2}$) in $myo^{-/-}$ hearts. As a further sign of decreased contractility, the rate of pressure development (dP/dt_{max}) was slower in $myo^{-/-}$ hearts at all afterloads studied. Intrinsic heart rate (HR), left ventricular developed pressure (LVDP) and pressure volume work (cardiac power) observed at the different degrees of afterload (pressure load) did not differ.

Figure 3a depicts the parallel coronary flow pattern observed in both groups at increasing afterloads. However, coronary flow in $myo^{-/-}$ hearts was almost twice as fast as that in WT hearts at the corresponding afterloads. As cardiac output (CO) was not increased in $myo^{-/-}$ hearts, resulting aortic flow was considerably smaller, even approaching zero at the highest afterload employed (120 mmHg).

Stepwise increase in preload was performed to analyze the influence of filling pressure on the given mouse hearts. Intrinsic HR, peak systolic left ventricular pressures (LVP) and pressure volume work (cardiac power) observed at the different degrees of preload (volume load) did not differ and rose only slightly with growing preload .

Table 1
Cardiac parameters of myo$^{-/-}$ and WT controls at selected afterloads

Afterload	50 mmHg	70 mmHg	90 mmHg	120 mmHg
WT				
Heart rate, bpm	470±27	481±21	491±17	503±18
LVDP, mmHg	72±2.8	93±2.9	113±3.8	142±6.4
Cardiac power, mmHgxml/min	2499±361	3313±545	3892±754	4396±630
dP/dt$_{max}$, mmHg/sec	4618±268	5359±168	6524±508	7542±535
TPP/mmHg, ms/mmHg	0.38±0.02	0.32±0.01	0.25±0.01	0.16±0.01
RT$_{1/2}$/mmHg, ms/mmHg	0.42±0.01	0.34±0.01	0.28±0.02	0.20±0.02
myo$^{-/-}$				
Heart rate, bpm	473±21	479±20	486±22	507±27
LVDP, mmHg	73±3.4	94±3.0	115±3.6	139±7.1
Cardiac power, mmHgxml/min	2628±465	3358±573	3882±584	4467±557
dP/dt$_{max}$, mmHg/sec	3883±351[b]	4789±526[b]	5782±640[b]	7243±733[a]
TPP/mmHg, ms/mmHg	0.49±0.02[c]	0.37±0.02[c]	0.31±0.02[c]	0.23±0.02[c]
RT$_{1/2}$/mmHg, ms/mmHg	0.52±0.02[c]	0.41±0.01[c]	0.33±0.02[c]	0.27±0.02[c]

Coronary flow remained stable at the various preloads studied (Fig. 3b) while being approximately 55% higher in myo$^{-/-}$ hearts compared to their WT counterparts, i.e. 20.2±2.0 mlxmin^{-1}xg^{-1} vs. 13.0 ± 1.9 mlxmin^{-1}xg^{-1} ($p<0.001$) at 5 mmHg preload. With CO being identical in both groups, aortic flow was significantly smaller in myo$^{-/-}$ hearts compared to WT hearts, i.e. 14.7±3.3 mlxmin^{-1}xg^{-1} vs. 23.4 ± 5.7 mlxmin^{-1}xg^{-1} ($p<0.005$) at 5 mmHg preload. The lower aortic flow values found for myo$^{-/-}$ hearts reflect the larger fraction of CO required to perfuse the coronaries of myo$^{-/-}$ hearts adequately (Fig. 3b).

Despite the absence of significant differences in LVDP and cardiac power between the two groups, a marked decrease in contractility was detected in myo$^{-/-}$ hearts at all preloads studied. This contractile impairment was especially pronounced at low preloads.

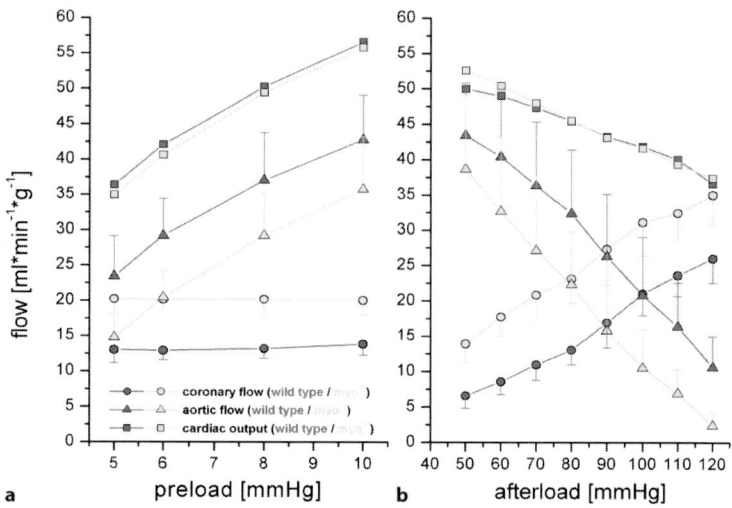

Figure 3a,b
Coronary and aortic flow per gram heart weight in the working heart setup for myo$^{-/-}$ and WT mice under a wide range of preloads (**a**) and afterloads (**b**). Cardiac output is calculated as sum of aortic and coronary flow (*p<0.05; **p<0.005; ***p<0.001). *For coloured version see appendix*

For example dP/dt$_{max}$ at 5 mmHg preload was 4688 ± 425 mmHg/sec in myo$^{-/-}$ hearts versus 5718 ± 435 mmHg/sec in wild type hearts (p<0.001) while at 10 mmHg preload the difference in dP/dt$_{max}$ between the respective hearts narrowed to 6001 ± 476 mmHg/sec *vs.* 6447 ± 547 mmHg/sec (p<0.05).

Troubleshooting

In general, meticulous attention should be paid to keeping every aspect of the apparatus clean and well calibrated. In addition, tubing should be replaced frequently. Although this is very time consuming and, in the case of tubing, costly, it should be kept in mind that contamination of the apparatus or a failure to calibrate the transducers, flow meters and other sensors used can easily ruin a whole experimental series. Furthermore, the complexity of the apparatus, connected electronics and software require the investigator to be as familiar as possible with his individual setup in order to gain the maximum information from any one experiment. Being familiar with the apparatus also allows the investigator to respond quickly and professionally to most problems that might occur during the experimental course and thus save an experiment that otherwise might have been lost.

- In our experience, the most common problems arising when using the working heart originate from small air bubbles. These can be entrapped in flow probes leading to a sudden interruption in flow measurement. Often these small bubbles will not pass through the flow probe and may have to be flushed out. While this manoeuvre is readily performed prior to the organ being hung in the apparatus, it can be a great nuisance during the experiment. Air bubbles can also significantly dampen the pressure signal if they find their way into PE catheters used for pressure measurements or even into the transducer domes. Because even minute air bubbles, which are extremely difficult to detect, can cause dP/dt values to fall by 30%, the whole apparatus should always be checked carefully for air bubbles and preferably not be allowed to become dry (see also preparatory steps).

- The isolated murine heart is very temperature sensitive. Drops in temperature due to opening of the heated chamber surrounding the heart, lead to a prompt decline in function and should be avoided whenever possible during the experiment.
- The chemicals from which the perfusate is made should be checked on a regular basis and they should be obtained from the same source whenever possible to eliminate alterations from delivery to delivery. The perfusate pH should always be controlled, as minute differences in pH greatly affect coronary flow and thus organ performance. In this context it should be noted that if working with perfusates being gassed by different gas mixtures, precisely 5% carbon dioxide should always be included in the mixture to ensure a pH of 7.4. In our experience this is only feasible through special, made to order, gas or by applying precision mass flow controllers.
- Finally, the animals studied should be in good health and rigorous monitoring routines should be in place at the local animal facility. This is especially important, as many murine infections are not accompanied by overt clinical symptoms.

References

Bardenheuer H, Schrader J (1986) Supply-to-demand ratio for oxygen determines formation of adenosine by the heart. Am J Physiol 250: H173–H180

De Windt LJ, Willems J, Reneman RS, Van der Vusse GJ, Arts T, Van Bilsen M (1999) An improved isolated, left ventricular ejecting, murine heart model. Functional and metabolic evaluation. Pflügers Arch 437: 182–190

Decking UKM, Arens S, Schlieper G, Schulze K, Schrader J (1997) Dissociation between adenosine release, MVO2, and energy status in working guinea pig hearts. American Journal of Physiology-Heart and Circulatory Physiology 41: H371–H381

Doevendans PA, Daemen J, de Muinck ED, Smits JF (1998) Cardiovascular phenotyping in mice. Cardiovascular Research 39: 34–49

Gamble WJ, Conn PA, Kumar AE, Plenge R, Monroe RG (1970) Myocardial oxygen consumption of blood-perfused, isolated, supported rat heart. Am J Physiol 219: 604–612

Godecke A, Schrader J (2000) Adaptive mechanisms of the cardiovascular system in transgenic-mice lessons from eNOS and myoglobin knockout mice. Basic Research in Cardiology 95: 492–498

Grupp IL, Subramaniam A, Hewett TE, Robbins J, Grupp G (1993) Comparison of normal, hypodynamic, and hyperdynamic mouse hearts using isolated work-performing heart preparations. Am J Physiol 265: 1401–10

Krebs HA, Henseleit K (1932) Untersuchungen über die Harnstoffbildung im Tierkörper. Hoppe-Seyler's Zeitschrift für Physiologische Chemie 210: 33–41

Langendorff O (1895) Untersuchungen am überlebenden Säugetierherzen. Pflügers Arch Ges. Physiologie 61: 291–332

Merx MW, Flogel U, Stumpe T, Godecke A, Decking UK, Schrader J (2001) Myoglobin facilitates oxygen diffusion. FASEB J 15: 1077–1079

Neely JR, Liebermeister H, Battersby EJ, Morgan HE (1967) Effect of pressure development on oxygen consumption by isolated rat heart. Am J Physiol 212: 804–814

Ng WA, Grupp IL, Subramaniam A, Robbins J (1991) Cardiac myosin heavy chain mRNA expression and myocardial function in the mouse heart. Circ Res 68: 1742–50

Qiu Y, Manche A, Hearse DJ (1993) Contractile and vascular consequences of blood versus crystalloid cardioplegia in the isolated blood-perfused rat heart. Eur J Cardiothoracic Surg 7: 137–145

Isolated Papillary Muscles

Stefan Dhein

Introduction

Isolated papillary muscles are among the standard experimental preparations in cardiovascular research. As early as 1861 Carl Ludwig developed an assay using a kymograph for recording muscular force, in the Institute of Physiology in Leipzig. Starting from these early experiments, the papillary muscle has become one of the most useful preparations for the investigation of pharmacological and physiological effects on mechanical force. This preparation is used for investigation of the mechanical properties of cardiac tissue such as inotropic or lusitropic effects or for the investigation of basic electrophysiological properties. For investigation of mechanical force, three setups are possible, the isotonic setup (i.e. the force is kept constant while the muscle is allowed to shorten), the isometric setup (i.e. the length of the muscle is kept constant while the force changes) and the auxotonic (both force and length are changing) (see Fig. 1).

To illustrate these forms of mechanical force one might imagine a man who lifts a heavy weight. First he lays his hands on the weight and starts to contract his muscles in order to lift the weight, but in the first phase of this contraction, the force of gravity is higher than the force of his muscles. Thus, during this phase the muscle develops force but does not change its length, which is an isometric contraction. Next, the force is steadily increased until it is higher than the force of gravity so that the weight is lifted. Now, there is a change in muscle length while the developed force will be maintained constant, which is an isotonic contraction.

The whole process comprising an isometric phase followed by an isotonic phase is called an auxotonic contraction. For a further detailed discussion see textbooks of physiology. Regarding the mechanical properties, it is possible to analyse force-time, length-time, force-length and velocity-force diagrams depending on the goal of the study.

If the muscle is stepwise stretched by enhancing the weight at its base, it is also possible to record the length of the muscle and to calculate the E-modulus (elasticity modulus) according to

$$E = K \times L/q \times \Delta L \; [N/cm^2]$$

where K is the force or the weight, L = initial length, ΔL = change in length and q = diameter. Thus, the E-modulus of a frog heart ranges from 1 to 10 N/cm^2.

For basic electrophysiology, intracellular action potential recordings are performed using sharp KCl-filled microelectrodes (20 M Ω). These are used to investigate, for example, drug effects on resting membrane potential, upstroke velocity (as a measure of the fast sodium channel) and action potential duration. Moreover, it is possible to determine the functional, relative and absolute refractory periods. In a more sophisticated setup it is also possible to measure conduction velocity in papillary muscles. This may be performed under experimental conditions simulating ischemia.

Description of Methods and Practical Approach

First of all the papillary muscle has to be prepared. The standard preparation is guinea pig or rat papillary muscle. Normally, the right ventricular papillary muscles are preferred for this preparation, since they are thinner and more elongated resulting in a better performance during the experiment. This is due to the fact that the papillary muscle in standard preparations is oxygenated and maintained by diffusion. In the case of a thick papillary muscle, the inner core will probably be ischemic. Therefore, the thinner right ventricular papillary muscle is preferred. A diameter exceeding 1 mm may be problematic. The critical radius R_{crit} can be calculated according to Hill (1938) as

$$R_{crit} = \sqrt{[(4 \times k \times y_0)/a]}$$

where k = Krogh's diffusion constant (in muscle 2×10^{-8} cm³/min × cm × mmHg), a = O_2 consumption (about 1.83×10^{-2} cm³/min × cm³) and y0 = P_{O2} at the border between tissue and solution (in the case of carbogen about 720 mmHg). With these values, the critical radius is 0.6 mm, i.e. the critical diameter is 1.2 mm. Alternatively to the method described above, (especially in larger animals) the papillary muscle can be prepared with a supplying coronary artery which can be perfused.

The animal (rat or guinea pig) is usually killed by a sharp blow on the neck with subsequent exsanguination. Then the heart is quickly removed, washed in cold Tyrode solution to remove remaining blood and transferred to a preparation bath filled with cold saline solution (e.g. Tyrode solution: Na⁺ 161.02, K⁺ 5.36, Ca²⁺ 1.8, Mg²⁺ 1.05, Cl⁻ 147.86, HCO₃⁻ 23.8, PO₄²⁻ 0.42 and glucose 11.1 mmol/l, pH 7.4, equilibrated with 95% O_2 and 5% CO_2). A bath which can be continuously gassed with 95% O_2 and 5% CO_2, to avoid hypoxia is highly recommended. Next the heart is opened with scissors along the septum from the anterior side of the heart, so that the right ventricle is opened (or the left, if it is necessary to investigate the left ventricular papillary muscle).

Now, the tricuspid valve with the appertaining papillary muscles can be seen. One should select a papillary muscle of the elongated type (without branches) and with a diameter of not more than 1 mm. First the appertaining part of the valve leaflet is cut out and then very carefully the base of the papillary muscle must be excised. It is absolutely necessary not to stretch the papillary muscle. Then the muscle is transferred to the organ bath.

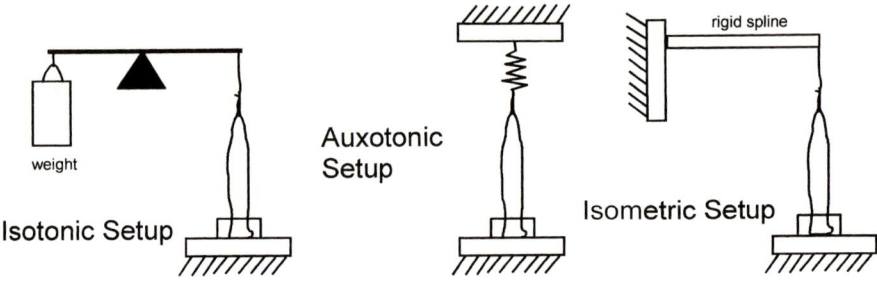

Figure 1
Principles of force recording

The organ bath differs depending on the measurements to be made. If force measurements are planned, a cylindrical double walled bath is normally used with an outer water-filled jacket for temperature control. At the bottom of the bath a small device for gassing the solution is provided. The papillary muscle is fixed with its base at the bottom of a long rod, while the tendon is connected to the force transducer (Fig. 2).

If electrophysiological measurements have to be performed, it is necessary to keep the papillary muscle in a horizontal position so that microelectrodes can be inserted. Normally a 10 ml temperature-controlled organ bath is used with an inflow and an outflow, so that the papillary muscle can be continuously superfused with fresh gassed Tyrode solution (usually at a rate of about 1 ml/min). It is not possible to gas in the bath since the bubbles would disturb the electrophysiological measurements due to mechanical dislocation of the microelectrodes.

In all cases it is necessary to stimulate the papillary muscles electrically. Since the solution which is used contains salts, it is possible that electrolytic processes may occur at the electrodes, which may polarize the electrodes or lead to the release of metals. To avoid this, non-polarizable electrodes are normally used. The standard is the Ag-AgCl electrode which can be easily prepared from silver wire, which is put into a 3 M KCl solution and connected to a battery overnight. Instead it is also possible to use Ag-AgI electrodes. These can be made by bathing the silver wire in Lugol's solution (or simply tincture of iodine) for at least 15 minutes (better overnight).

Examples

Isometric Force Recording

A setup is chosen in which the papillary muscle is pre-stretched so that there is no change in length when the muscle contracts, i.e. the muscle is fixed at both ends, one being connected to an isometric force transducer. For recording normally a curve of the isometric maxima is measured as illustrated in Fig. 3.

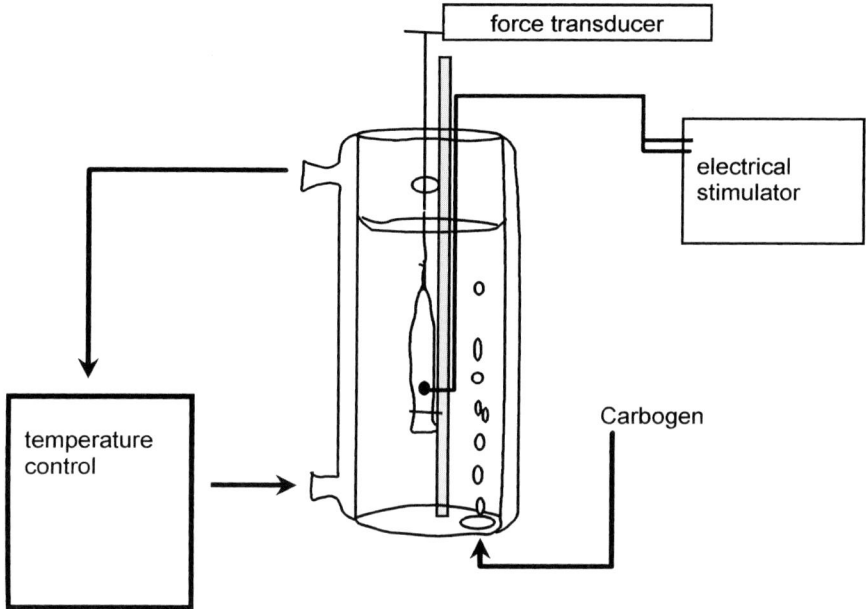

Figure 2
Setup for isometric force recording of an isolated papillary muscle paced at its base *via* 2 AgCl electrodes

The force under resting conditions is recorded at different pre-stretching values. Then a single electrical sti-mulus is applied and the developed force is recorded under isometric conditions. This gives a second point. This is repeated for different pre-stretches so that finally a curve results as shown in Fig. 3. At the end, the pre-stretch at which the maximum vertical shift of the curve was seen is determined and is defined as L_{max}.

Isotonic Force Recording

Similarly to the procedure described above, the muscle is fixed at one end while the other is connected to an isotonic force transducer. There are several different apparatuses commercially available. In principle there is movement when the muscle contracts (in contrast to isometric force recording) and this movement is recorded by some sort of transducer (see Fig. 1).

In order to obtain a force-length relationship and the curve of the isotonic maxima, the muscle is pre-stretched increasingly, the force is recorded, and a stimulus is given at a given pre-stretch which, in an isotonic setup, results in a horizontal shift of the point of the curve to the left, giving the isotonic contraction at a given pre-stretch.

After recording the relationship, the pre-stretch at which the maximum horizontal shift of the curve occurs is determined (Fig. 4). The corresponding length is defined as L_{max}.

Action Potential Recording

For action potential recording it is necessary to use sharp, high-resistance microelectrodes. In the author's lab, glass microelectrodes are normally used with a thin glass filament inside which helps to fill the microelectrode by capillary forces. The electrodes can simply be bathed in the filling solution. For intracellular recording using this type of electrode, 3 MKCl is normally used. The electrode is connected to an action potential amplifier or a patch clamp amplifier which allows a bridge mode. Another possibility is to use a current clamp to elicit an action potential by a short pulse (2–10 ms) and to record the resulting changes in voltage.

The papillary muscle is mounted in an organ bath which allows continuous superfusion of the muscle at a rate of about 1 ml/min with Tyrode solution (37 °C). The base of the muscle is fixed to the bottom of the bath by a clamp while the tendon is connected to a hook which communicates with an isometric force transducer. At both sides of the base of the muscle AgCl or AgI electrodes are located for pacing the muscle (Fig. 5). For pacing, rectangular pulses of 1–4 ms duration and 2-fold threshold are used, at a basal frequency of 1 Hz. Next the microelectrode is positioned above the papillary muscle using a micromanipulator. For recording, the electrode is manipulated into the papillary muscle. Since the muscle contracts, it is best to insert the pipette orthogonal to the long axis of the muscle to minimize motion artefacts.

Now the pipette is very slowly manipulated into the muscle until an action potential can be recorded. The optimal position is sought by small changes in the position, until an action potential with >100 mV amplitude and a resting membrane potential of about –80 mV is recorded.

For further investigation the refractory period has very often to be measured. This is achieved by a second stimulus which starts with a delay of about half the cycle length. The delay of the second stimulus is progressively shortened until the muscle no longer responds to the second stimulus. This delay gives the refractory period.

Another interesting test is to investigate the upstroke velocity under the influence of anti-arrhythmic agents. The sodium channel blockers suppress dU/dt_{max}. However, some of these drugs dissociate very early from the channel so that at low frequencies, there is no drug bound to the channel and, consequently, the effect is minimized (so called use-dependence of sodium channel blockers, typical drug: lidocaine), while others (such as flecainide) only dissociate from the channel very slowly, so that the effect on dU/dt_{max} can also be seen at low frequencies. Thus, if anti-arrhythmic drugs or drugs which may affect sodium channels are investigated, the drug effect is normally tested at different frequencies in order to evaluate use-dependence.

Thus, it is possible to distinguish between various actions on ionic channels using this simple setup. A sodium channel blocker would depress the action potential upstroke, and prolong the refractory period, a potassium channel blocker would lengthen the action potential duration thereby also prolonging the refractory period

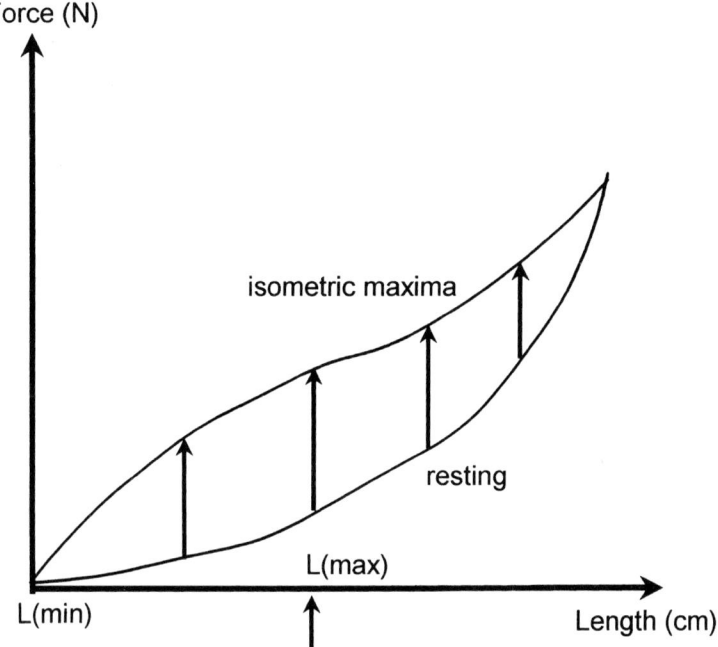

Figure 3
Curve of the isometric maxima of an isolated papillary muscle. For details see text

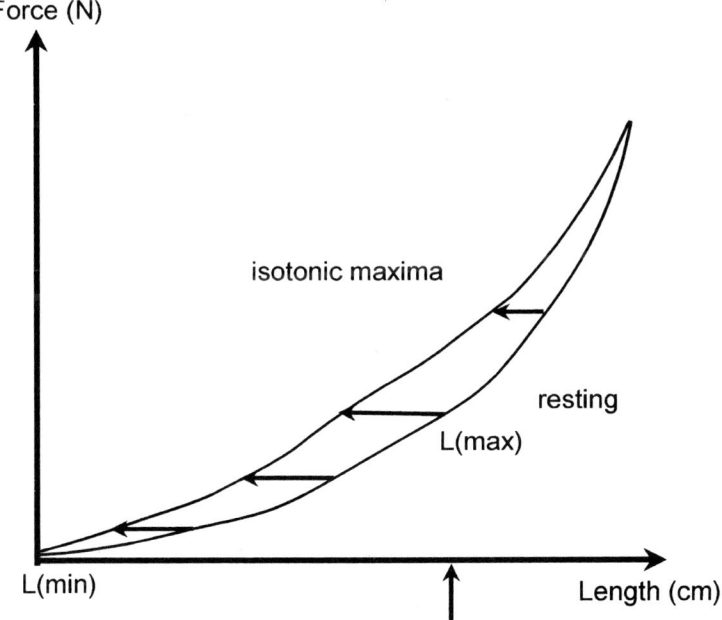

Figure 4
Curve of the isotonic maxima of an isolated papillary muscle. For details see text

(but without affecting dU/dt_{max}), while a calcium antagonist would exert a negative inotropic effect which might be accompanied by a shortening of the plateau phase of the action potential. However, the latter action depends on the portion of the calcium channel contributing to the action potential plateau.

Measurement of Conduction Velocity and Simulated Ischemia

A more sophisticated setup using two microelectrodes is needed if conduction velocity is to be recorded (alternatively optical mapping methods can be used, see there). The papillary muscle is stimulated electrically at its base and two electrodes are inserted at a chosen distance. The delay between the two action potentials is measured (see Fig. 5). It is necessary to choose a position well away from the stimulating electrodes in order to avoid stimulus artefacts.

Alternatively, if there is a long distance between the stimulating electrodes and the microelectrode, the stimulus-response delay may be measured. In that case, care has to be taken that the stimulus depolarizes only the base of the muscle and that the action potential really is a propagated action potential. If a bipolar electrode is used, artifacts may be produced by changes in the passive electrical properties. Thus, a ring electrode is recommended (as shown in chapter 2.1 "the Langendorff heart"). The use of an inner electrode with the reference electrode as a ring surrounding the inner electrode guarantees that only the tissue within the ring is depolarized, whereas the electromagnetic field around a bipolar electrode may also reach tissue outside the electrode pair.

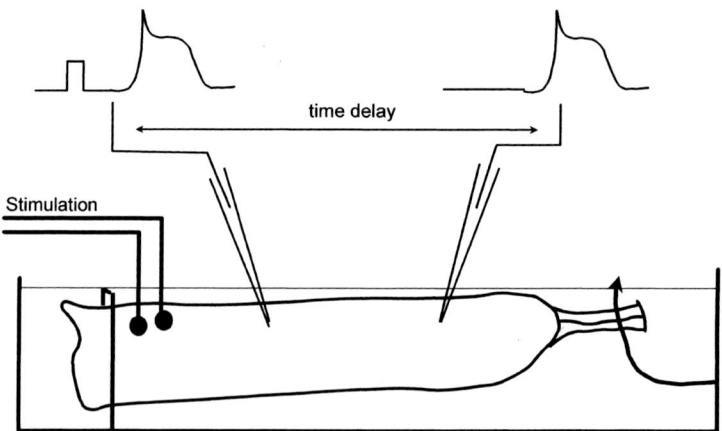

Figure 5
Setup for recording action potentials (1 or 2) from an isolated papillary muscle. This setup can be used with only 1 microelectrode if simply an action potential is to be recorded. Please note, that the distance between the pacing electrodes and the recording microelectrode has to be long enough to allow a proper distinction between the stimulus artifact and the action potential. For measurement of conduction velocity a second microelectrode is inserted at a given distance from the first and the delay between the two action potentials is measured

Often it is interesting to investigate the effect of a certain drug or manipulation on conduction velocity under ischemic conditions. There are two ways of inducing or simulating ischemia. First, it is possible to prepare the papillary muscle with a coronary artery for pressure- or flow-constant arterial perfusion (Dekker et al. 1996). Ischemia can then simply be induced by stopping the perfusion. Dekker and colleagues, in a very elegant study, found uncoupling of the papillary muscle after 14.5 min of ischemia under these conditions. The other possibility is to simulate ischemia by O_2- and glucose-free perfusion (Müller et al. 1997; Dhein et al. 1998). O_2 is replaced by N_2. CO_2 has to be maintained to buffer the pH. Under these conditions, Müller and co-workers (1997) found uncoupling after 12 min of simulated ischemia which is pretty similar to the findings of Dekker et al. (1996). Uncoupling can also be achieved by use of 50 mM sodium propionate, an organic acid, which reduces conduction velocity in the preparations (Dhein et al. 1998).

Troubleshooting

Sometimes the papillary muscle will not contract after preparation. This is the problem frequently encountered with this setup. In most cases this is due to the preparation technique and results from overstretching the muscle during preparation. Another common problem is the occurrence of arrhythmia, especially if bath solutions with low potassium and low magnesium are used. Sometimes it helps if the experimenter gently pinches the base of the papillary muscle with forceps. If this does not help, another papillary muscle has to be prepared.

References

Dekker LRC, Fiolet JWT, VanBavel E, Coronal R, Opthof T, Spartan JAE, Janse MJ (1996) Intracellular Ca^{2+}, intercellular electrical coupling and mechanical activity in ischemic rabbit papillary muscle. Circ Res 79: 237–246

Dhein S, Gottwald M, Schaefer T, Müller A, Tudyka T, Krüsemann K, Grover R (1998) Effects of an antiarrhythmic peptide on intercellular coupling via gap junctions. In: Werner R (ed) Gap junctions. IOS-Press, Amsterdam, pp 163–167

Hill AV (1938) The heat of shortening and the dynamic constants of muscle. Proc Royal Soc (London) B 126: 136–165

Müller A, Schaefer T, Linke W, Tudyka T, Gottwald M, Klaus W, Dhein S (1997) Actions of the antiarrhythmic peptide AAP10 on cellular coupling. Naunyn Schmiedeberg's Arch Pharmacol. 356: 76–82

Isolated Vessels

Rudolf Schubert

Introduction

Blood vessels play an important role in the regulation of blood pressure and blood flow distribution. In order to understand the mechanisms of these regulatory processes in health and disease, the *in vivo* behaviour of vessels and their interaction in vessel networks has to be known. However, under *in vivo* conditions, vessel responses depend on a complicated interaction between the different cell types of the vessel wall (smooth muscle cells, endothelial cells and various cells in the adventitia), factors released from nerve endings, metabolites originating from the surrounding tissue, hormones transported by the blood flow, mechanical factors like shear stress and transmural pressure and also the behaviour of proximal and distal vessel segments. The complexity of this system quite substantially limits the possibility of interpretation of experimental findings in mechanistic terms. Therefore, *in vitro* methods for the investigation of blood vessel function have been introduced, where many of these confounding factors can be controlled.

The first experiments performed to study the function of blood vessels employed large vessels. However, recent technical developments also allow experiments to be conducted on small arteries, arterioles and small veins from various vascular beds. In practice, vessel segments with a diameter in the range from about 20 µm to several millimeters and a length of about 0.1–10 mm are used. These vessel segments consist of endothelial cells in the tunica intima, smooth muscle cells in the tunica media and nerve endings, fat cells, fibroblasts etc. in the tunica adventitia. Investigations into the functioning of these vessel segments, i.e. of their reactions to the application of external stimuli such as vasoactive substances, pressure, etc., employ several different methods. In the past, spiral strip preparations were used. Since this procedure results in a relatively large number of damaged smooth muscle and endothelial cells and in disruption of the normal vascular architecture, the use of cylindrical vessel segments is now preferred. Two methods for the investigation of vessel segments have been developed. One method employs ring vessel segments threaded on to two hooks or wires and the other cannulated vessel segments fixed on two pipettes. In this chapter an overview of these two methods will be given.

Description of Methods and Practical Approach
Solutions

In *in vitro* experiments, vessels are studied after isolation from their normal environment. In order to simulate this environment, physiological saline solution is used and experiments are conducted at 37 °C. Here are some examples for the composition of the physiological saline solution reported in the literature (in mM):

- 120 NaCl, 4.5 KCl, 1.2 NaH_2PO_4, 1 $MgSO_4$, 1.6 $CaCl_2$, 0.025 EDTA, 5.5 Glucose, 26 $NaHCO_3$, 5 HEPES, pH 7.4.
- 145 NaCl, 4.7 KCl, 1.2 NaH_2PO_4, 1.2 $MgSO_4$, 2 $CaCl_2$, 0.02 EDTA, 5 Glucose, 2 Pyruvate, 18 $NaHCO_3$, pH 7.4.
- 145 NaCl, 4.7 KCl, 1.2 NaH_2PO_4, 1.17 $MgSO_4$, 1.5 $CaCl_2$, 0.02 EDTA, 5 Glucose, 2 Pyruvate, 3 MOPS, pH 7.4.

Obviously, there are differences in the compositions of the solutions used, but how critical are they?

The differences are smallest and most of them of only minor importance in the cases of the contents of Na^+, $H_2PO_4^-$, SO_2^-, HCO_3^-, Cl^-, Mg^{2+}, EDTA (used to chelate trace amounts of heavy metal ions), pyruvate and glucose. The same is true for K^+, but one should have in mind that addition or removal of just a few mM of K^+ has profound effects on the activity of the Na^+/K^+-pump and the activity of inward rectifier potassium channels, which have a considerable impact on the contractile state of small arteries (Zaritsky et al. 2000).

Ca^{2+} is an important ion, because it plays a central role in the molecular mechanism of contraction. The concentration of free calcium in blood plasma is around 1.5 mM. Therefore, a calcium concentration in this range should be used to simulate physiological conditions in the experimental solution.

H^+ is another important ion, especially for small arteries and arterioles, where small changes in pH induce considerable changes in diameter. The solution should therefore contain a pH-buffer. Often, $NaHCO_3$ is used as buffer, since this is the main physiological pH buffer in plasma. The protons and the bicarbonate ions establish equilibrium with CO_2 in the solution giving a P_{CO2} of about 35 mmHg. However, CO_2 leaves the solution into the surrounding air, where the CO_2 content is virtually zero. Thus, in order to stabilise the equilibrium, i.e. to control P_{CO2} and pH, solutions containing a bicarbonate buffer are commonly bubbled with carbogen, a gas mixture of 95% O_2 and 5% CO_2. Sometimes, an artificial pH buffer like HEPES is added in an attempt to further stabilise the pH. It should be mentioned however, that the use of carbogen will produce a P_{O2} in the range of 400–500 mmHg. This is an unphysiologically high value, which might be justified in large arteries in order to get a normal P_{O2} deep inside the thick vessel wall. However, it should be taken into account that O_2 affects vessel contractility directly. Thus, at least when studying small vessels, it is better to use a gas mixture of 75% N_2, 20% O_2 and 5% CO_2.

Sometimes the problems with the bicarbonate buffer have been avoided by using solutions without $NaHCO_3$, where only artificial pH buffers like HEPES or MOPS are used (see solution 3 above). Due to equilibration with the surrounding air, a P_{O2} of about 150 mmHg is achieved, which is still somewhat higher than physiological values. However, the P_{CO_2} is unphysiologically low under these conditions, which should be remembered in experiments on vessels sensitive to P_{CO_2}.

Vessel Isolation

An important issue for a successful experiment is the isolation of the vessel segments. Experiments on small vessels require an especially careful vessel preparation. Direct contact of the isolation instruments with the vessel and stretching of the vessel, especially in the longitudinal direction, should be avoided. In order to prevent hand tremor, special supports for the arms are helpful. Isolation of the vessels should be done with appropriate instruments. Often, fine forceps (Dumont No 5) and small scissors are used [for a very detailed discussion of practical aspects of the isolation procedure for small vessels see Duling et al. (1981)]. The isolation can be done in one of the solutions described above. If the solution contains $NaHCO_3$, the solution has to be gassed in order to ensure a physiological pH. Otherwise the pH will increase, which leads to contraction, particularly of small arteries. Such contracted vessels are very difficult to mount on the myograph (for mounting procedures see next paragraph) and are consequently prone to excessive damage. Since bubbling of the solution in the isolation chamber results in bad visibility, solutions without $NaHCO_3$ are often used. In addition, in order to prevent damage to the vessels, the solution used for vessel isolation may be kept at low temperature and may contain only a low calcium concentration. Thus, under appropriate conditions, the function of the smooth muscle cells as well as of the endothelium can be preserved in isolated, *in vitro* vessel preparations. It is common practice, and often even necessary for methodological reasons, for the adventitia to be more or less completely removed from the vessels. However, it should not be forgotten that the adventitia is an integral part of the vessel wall. Indeed, it has been shown that complete, careful removal of the adventitia without media damage leads to changes in some contractile and relaxant responses (Gonzalez et al. 2001).

Vessel Mounting

Ring Vessel Segments

This method is the classical, older approach, where ring segments are held on two hooks or similar devices or, in the case of resistance vessels, on two wires passed through their lumen (Bevan and Osher 1972; Mulvany and Halpern 1976, 1977; Mulvany et al. 1978). One of the hooks or wires is connected to a force transducer allowing wall force to be measured. These preparations can be investigated under isotonic conditions by adjusting the circumference during changes in activation in order to achieve a constant force (for example see Nilsson and Sjoblom 1985; Boels et al. 1990; Boonen and Demey 1994). In most cases, however, these preparations are used under isometric conditions, where the vessel circumference stays constant and changes in force during changes in activation are determined. The diameters of the hooks and wires have to be adapted to the diameter of the vessel under study in order not to damage the vessel due to undue stretching when inserting two hooks or wires into the vessel lumen. The use of wires as small as 14 µm has been reported (Bukoski et al. 2001). Nevertheless, there is a lower limit for the vessel diameter suitable for experiments on ring vessel segments. In addition, if tungsten wire is used, it has been observed that aged tungsten wire may undergo spontaneous surface oxidation, which resulted in altered vessel relaxant responses. Thus, it was concluded that gold or tungsten-free stainless steel wire should be used (Bukoski et al. 2001).

At the beginning of an experiment with ring vessel segments, the initial stretch, or preload, of the vessel has to be set in order to simulate its *in vivo* conditions. This procedure is important, because many vessel responses depend on the amount of initial stretch. Thus, noradrenaline sensitivity increased with increased stretch (Price et al. 1981; Nilsson and Sjoblom 1985). The maximum constriction to noradrenaline and to several other vasoconstrictors increased with increasing stretch and then decreased with further stretching resulting in a bell-shaped diameter–tension relationship (Nilsson and Sjoblom 1985; Boonen and Demey 1994). However, these diameter–tension relationships were different for different agonist and for different vessels (Boonen and Demey 1994). In addition, acetylcholine-induced membrane potential hyperpolarisation was larger in stretched compared to unstretched preparations and this difference was suggested to reflect the involvement of additional mechanisms (NO, PGI_2) in the stretched preparation (Parkington et al. 1993). The procedure of setting the initial stretch is known as "normalisation", because it allows the comparison of data from different vessels. To apply stretch to the vessel segment, the second hook or wire is connected to a micrometer. Thus, the distance between the hooks or wires, i.e. the vessel circumference, can be increased. A critical evaluation of common normalisation procedures by Halpern (Halpern 1991; Halpern and Kelley 1991) showed that some of them (stretch to a just detectable force, to a fixed force or to the *in situ* circumference) are not appropriate.

Often an initial stretch is selected, where the maximum of the active response to some agonist is achieved. This requires that the passive and the active force–circumference relationships be determined experimentally for the particular vessel and agonist desired. In practice, these data are available for a number of vessels and agonists in the literature. If documented in appropriate detail in order to understand how the values were obtained, one can use values of initial stretch reported previously. However, it should be taken into account that in many cases the maximum active response is achieved when the initial stretch, i.e. passive force, of the vessel is of the same order of magnitude as the total force. Hence, active force, the difference between total and passive force, is small and may be difficult to determine accurately. Thus, in many experiments a circumference 10 or 20% smaller than that at the maximum of the active response is used. Under these conditions the maximum active force is only slightly smaller but the passive force is considerably smaller compared to the situation at maximum active force, due to the steep exponential passive force-circumference relationship. Alternatively, an initial stretch corresponding to the *in vivo* pressure of the vessel (calculated using the La place relationship and the known circumference and passive stretch) may be chosen.

After the normalisation procedure, the performance of a viability test is recommended. Usually this includes 2–3 applications of an agonist at high concentration, sometimes combined with the addition of a high (120 mM) potassium solution. This procedure is necessary in order to observe stable contractile vessel responses after the vessel isolation and mounting procedure. However, the application of high agonist concentrations gives only first, rough information about the viability of the preparation. In addition, an agonist concentration about 100 times smaller than the saturating concentration should be tested. On top of this contraction an agonist able to activate the endothelium such as acetylcholine can be added in order to test the viability of the endothelium. In principle, a judgement about the viability of a vessel requires knowledge of the "normal" responses of the particular vessel under investigation. The level of these responses can be determined only experimentally. It is either already known from previous studies or, in the case of a not well-characterised vessel, has to be found during the course of a certain number of preliminary experiments on that vessel.

The investigation of ring vessel segments is performed most often using fixed supports for the hooks or wires, i.e. under isometric conditions. Vessel responses, i.e. levels of activation of the smooth muscle cells, are represented as changes in force (usually given in mN). However, in order to be able to compare responses of vessels with different lengths, wall tension, i.e. force per wall per unit of vessel length ($T = F/2L$, where T is tension, F is force and L is vessel length, given in mN/mm) is used. In addition, in order to be able to compare responses of vessels of different thicknesses, wall stress ($\sigma = T/w$, where σ is wall stress, T is tension and w is wall thickness, given in mN/mm^2) is employed. The latter requires the determination of vessel wall thickness. This can be done by microscopic observation of the vessel wall at the site of the hook or the wire using a calibrated eyepiece. It should be taken into account, however, that in this place the vessel wall is somewhat thinner than the upper and lower part of the vessel wall. This will result in a certain overestimation of wall stress.

Cannulated Vessel Segments

This method is a newer approach, in which vessel segments are fitted on to two cannulas and fixed using appropriate sutures (see inset in Fig. 1). The construction of the cannulas depends on the size of the vessel to be investigated. In most cases the outer diameter of the cannulas should be slightly smaller than the inner diameter of the isolated vessel, i.e. of the vessel without the distending influence of transmural pressure. Vessels down to a diameter of about 60–80 μm can be mounted on simple pipettes pulled from polyethylene tubing or from glass capillaries using a special micropipette puller (Halpern et al. 1984). Using these pipettes, the vessel is simply slipped on using fine forceps and secured by suture (see also inset in Fig. 1). For smaller vessels a double-barrel pipette system has proven useful (see Duling et al. 1981 for construction details). This is however difficult to prepare and to handle and has a high flow resistance in perfusion experiments. Mounting of the vessel is performed by pulling the vessel into the holding pipette by applying reduced pressure to the lumen of this pipette. Then a perfusion pipette is advanced into the lumen of the vessel, so that the vessel is fixed between the perfusion pipette and a constriction of the hold-

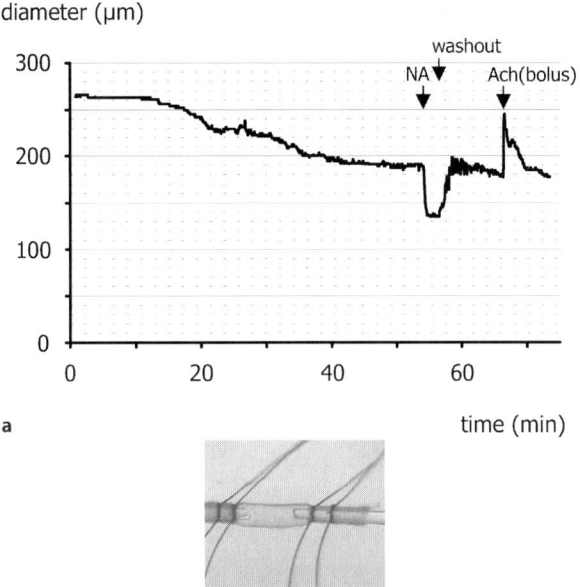

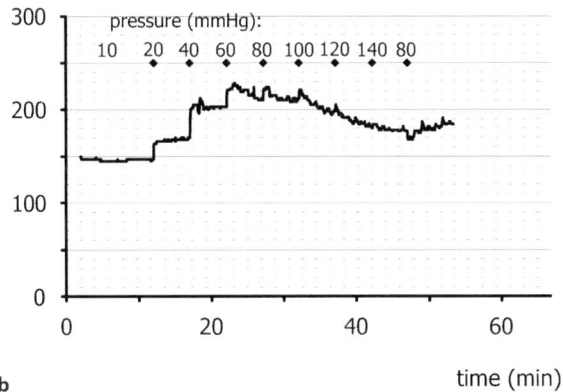

Figure 1
Cannulated vessel segments. An experiment on a rat skeletal muscle small artery (see inset) is presented showing the viability test with the development of a spontaneous myogenic tone and the application of noradrenaline (NA) at 10^{-7} M and, after washout, of a bolus of acetylcholine (Ach) at 10^{-6} M in **a** and the vessel response to different levels of transmural pressure in **b**. For more details refer to the text

ing pipette. An alternative double-barrelled pipette system consisting of two concentric micropipettes has been described by VanBavel et al. (1990) for small vessels with low flow resistance. One end of the vessel is sucked into the inner pipette and is held in place by applying sub-atmospheric pressure on the outer pipette. The inner pipette serves to apply pressure and flow to the vessel segment. Another method allowing physiological flows to be investigated and ensuring that the pressure drop across the cannula is much smaller than that over the vessel was developed by Hoogerwerf et al. (1992). Here the outer surface of a vessel is glued with fibrin glue to the inner side of a glass cannula with the aid of a smaller inner cannula, which is removed completely after the vessel is fixed.

For mounting, vessels are first secured on one cannula using appropriate sutures as mentioned in the previous paragraph. Then the vessel is flushed with saline to remove remaining blood. During this procedure the pressure applied should be low in order not to damage the vessel. Subsequently, the second end of the vessel is fixed on the second cannula. One of the cannulas is connected to either a reservoir, which can be elevated to a selected height, or a special pump producing the desired pressure. The other cannula can simply be closed in experiments without flow through the vessel lumen, or is connected to another reservoir or pump in experiments with flow. If non-flow conditions are selected, this condition should be controlled carefully during the course of the whole experiment.

After mounting, cannulated vessel segments are often subjected to a desired pressure in order to simulate *in vivo* conditions, a procedure similar to setting initial stretch in ring vessel segments. This leads to an increase in the length of the vessel (see for example Lew and Angus 1992), observed as a buckling of the vessel mounted between two fixed cannulas. Usually this buckle is removed by simply adjusting one of the cannulas connected to a micrometer. However, longitudinal stretch *in situ* has been shown to produce depolarisation in endothelium denuded preparations and depolarisation followed by hyperpolarisation at higher axial stretch in endothelium-intact preparations and to affect noradrenaline-evoked contractions (Monos et al. 1993, 2001). Therefore, longitudinal stretch may by an important parameter, which should be controlled for in experiments on cannulated vessel segments. Indeed, a study investigating the influence of longitudinal stretch on the contractile and relaxant responses of several small arteries *in vitro* showed that in some, but not all, vessels, responses to noradrenaline were optimised at longitudinal stretches larger than 20% (Coats and Hillier 1999). However, this was not observed for some other contractile agonists. Thus, if the effect of longitudinal stretch on the vessel response studied is unknown, it should be determined in preliminary experiments.

After pressurisation a viability test is recommended. This is of special importance for cannulated vessel segments, especially from resistance vessels, because pressure-induced vessel reactions have been shown to be especially sensitive to inappropriate handling during the vessel isolation procedure. The first indicator of viability is the development of a spontaneous myogenic tone after the pressure is increased and the temperature reaches 37 °C. In addition, the viability of the vessel, i.e. the reactivity to contractile and relaxing agents, including those acting *via* the endothelium, should be assessed (for an example see Fig. 1a). A judgement about the viability of a vessel requires knowledge of the "normal" responses of the particular vessel under investigation. These responses can be determined only experimentally. It is either already known from previous studies or, in the case of a not well-characterised vessel, has to be found during the course of a certain number of preliminary experiments on that vessel.

Responses of cannulated vessel segments are sometimes represented as changes in perfusion pressure during constant flow perfusion or as changes in perfusate flow rate during constant pressure perfusion (see as an example Machkov et al. 1998). However, in the majority of studies, responses of cannulated vessel segments are represented as diameter changes. These are best measured using optical techniques. This requires a microscope and appropriate tissue illumination in order to achieve an optimal visualisation of the vessel for precise diameter measurements. For large vessels (>400 µm), only the outer diameter can be determined, because the tissue is not transparent enough to find the inner edge of the vessel wall. For smaller vessels outer and inner diameter can be measured. In this case, inner, i.e. lumen diameter is the preferred readout, because this is the variable determining flow. Diameter can be measured manually by a micrometer eyepiece, an image splitting device or video scan lines. However, automatic methods based on video systems are more convenient (Halpern et al. 1984; Halpern 1991). These days, the vessel image is usually captured by a video camera attached to the microscope and presented on the computer monitor using a frame grabber card. There, special programs analyse the contrast profile produced by the vessel and find the outer and the inner diameter of the vessel using edge detection or pattern recognition algorithms (for example see Fischer et al. 1996 and references therein). Thus, an automatic tracking of vessel diameter changes is possible. Interaction from the user is only required when inner diameter changes need to be followed during strong contractions, where the contrast profile of the inner edge of the vessel wall may be too weak. An alternative approach is to fill the vessel lumen with FITC-labelled dextran and to determine the change in fluorescence emission, which reflects the mean cross-sectional area. Since cross-sectional area is proportional to the inner diameter, changes of the latter are easily derived from the recorded changes in cross-sectional area. This technique allows the determination of changes in inner diameter even in larger vessels which are not transparent enough for direct observation of the inner diameter (VanBavel et al. 1990).

In experiments on cannulated vessel segments, pressure and flow should be established at values close to the *in vivo* conditions for the vessel under investigation. Such data have been published for a number of vessels and should be taken from the literature. For orientation in small arteries with a diameter in the range from 50–200 µm, transmural pressure is in the range 40–100 mmHg and flow is in the range 6–15 µl/min (to get a physiological level of shear stress with saline, i.e. without the cellular components of blood). The control of transmural pressure and flow in this situation is based on the following basic principles (see also Halpern 1991). First, a pressure difference is established between the cannula at the proximal end of the vessel (P_1) and the cannula at the distal end of the vessel (P_2). Since the flow through the cannulas and the vessel segment is associated with some friction, pressure gradients may develop along this system. Thus, in order to control the pressure in the vessel segment, flow resistance should be estimated. This is based on the Poiseuille law for flow

$$Q = (P_1-P_2)\pi r^4/8\eta L$$

where P_1-P_2 is the pressure difference, r is the radius, η is the viscosity of the fluid and L is the length of the segment. Strictly speaking this equation holds only if certain limitations are met, but cannulated vessel segments do not critically violate these limitations. Thus, the criterion for laminar flow is met using vessel segments with a length about 3–4 times longer than the lumen diameter (see also Duling et al. 1981). In addition, flow is given by

$$Q = (P_1-P_2)/R$$

where R is flow resistance. Hence

$$R = (8\eta L)/\pi r^4$$

Taking for η a value of 6.92×10^{-3} poise (water at 37 °C – this is about one third of the value for whole blood, thus a three times larger flow as under physiological conditions will produce a physiological shear stress)

$$R = 3.5\times10^3 \; L/d^4 \; mmHg/\mu l/min$$

where the diameter (d) and the length (L) are expressed in µm. For example, a 450 µm long vessel segment with a lumen diameter of 150 µm has a R of 0.0031 mmHg/µl/min. Thus, a flow of 10 µl/min produces a pressure drop of 0.031 mmHg between the ends of the vessel. Such calculations can easily be performed for any other vessel size.

Flow may be measured by either weighing the effluent for a given interval of time (evaporation from these small volumes should be considered) or using a drop counter (uniform drop size should be obtained) or employing commercially available flow meters. In addition, flow can be estimated from the pressure difference (P_1-P_2) imposed when the flow resistances of the cannulas are much larger than that of the vessel, using $Q = (P_1-P_2)/R$. Under these conditions, the vessel flow resistance, which changes with altered diameter, can be neglected. However, in most situations, the flow resistance of the cannulas and of the vessel have similar values. Then, it is important to measure Q and P. A method of measuring the flow resistance of the cannulas is to insert them into a piece of polyethylene tubing of large diameter relative to the cannula and to measure perfusion pressure at various flows produced by a constant flow pump (for details see Halpern and Kelly 1991).

Pressure should also be known, because it has effects on vessel diameter itself and therefore, should often be kept constant in order to understand the effect of flow. The pressure in the vessel segment can be measured directly by using a servo-micropressure null measurement. However, for this to be accomplished the vessel has to be punctured, which may introduce too much damage to the vessel wall and release of vasoactive substances. An indirect approach is to use cannulas with the same flow resistance. At steady flow the pressure in the vessel segment will be the mean of P_1 and P_2. However, it should be noted that pressure transducers used in these studies should be carefully calibrated.

The investigation of cannulated vessel segments is often performed using a fixed transmural pressure. Because of the compliance of the tubing systems used to apply pressure, which accommodates the small volume changes during vessel diameter reactions, isobaric conditions are fulfilled during vessel reactions.

Comparison of Both Mounting Methods

A number of studies have shown that results obtained with the 2 mounting methods under the most commonly used conditions, i.e. ring vessel segments under isometric conditions and cannulated vessel segments under isobaric conditions, can be different. Thus, the sensitivity of ring segments to noradrenaline was higher than that of cannulated segments (Buus et al. 1994; VanBavel and Mulvany 1994). In addition, the depolarisation induced by a maximum concentration of noradrenaline was 2.6-fold larger in ring segments compared to cannulated segments (Schubert et al. 1996). Since wall tension increases in ring segments, but decreases in cannulated segments, these findings have been explained by assuming that part of the vasoconstrictor-induced responses are wall tension dependent. Thus, a clear understanding of the differences between the mounting methods is required in order to able to select the most appropriate method for the specific hypothesis to be tested.

Cannulated vessel segments are considered to be closer to *in vivo* conditions, because they (see also Halpern 1991):

- have a circular cross section. This is in sharp contrast to the two flat sheets of tissue when vessels are fixed on two hooks or wires.
- change their diameter in order to show alterations in the contractile state. This condition is also fulfilled in isotonic ring vessel segments, but not in the most often used isometric ring vessel segments.
- have an untouched endothelium. In contrast, the hooks and wires are in direct contact with the endothelium and may damage it during the mounting procedure in ring vessel preparations, especially in small vessels.
- are under the influence of a physiological stimulus, the transmural pressure, and develop spontaneous myogenic tone not usually seen with ring vessel preparations.
- are subjected to longitudinal elongation under pressurised conditions, which compensates for the retraction occurring during dissection. There is no elongation in ring vessel segments, which should be taken into account for morphological measurements. For example, in ring vessel segments larger wall-to-lumen ratios compared to cannulated vessel segments were observed. Thus, ring vessel segments are not a good estimate of *in vivo* wall-to-lumen ratio (for example see Lew and Angus 1992).
- allow agents to be superfused and/or perfused, enabling selective application from the luminal or the adventitial side of the vessel wall. Since receptors for vasoactive substances are often differentially expressed on endothelial and smooth muscle cells and the endothelium is a diffusion barrier for some, especially water-soluble substances applied from the vessel lumen, the route of application has to be taken into account. Indeed, different responses have been observed for phenylephrine and vasopressin, which were 10 to 100 time more potent when applied from the adventitial side (Lew and Angus 1992).

Examples

Ring Vessel Segments

A typical example of an experiment performed using a ring vessel segment is shown in Fig. 2. Here, changes in wall tension with time are shown. After mounting of the vessel, the myograph was heated to 37 °C during the first 20 min (Fig. 2a). Thereafter,

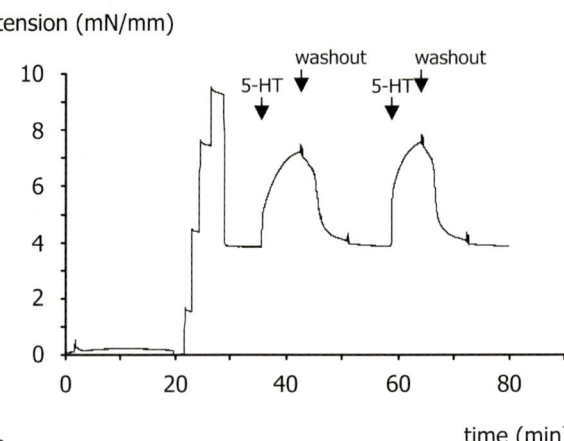

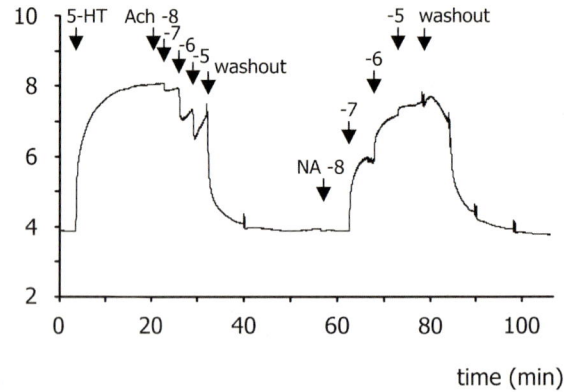

Figure 2a,b
Ring vessel segments. An experiment on a mouse aorta is presented showing the normalisation procedure and the viability test using serotonin (5-HT) at 10^{-5} M in **a** and the relaxation response to different concentrations of acetylcholine (Ach) and the contractile response to different concentrations of noradrenaline (NA) in **b**. For more details refer to the text

the normalisation procedure as described in detail above is shown, which ends with establishing the optimal vessel diameter corresponding to 90% of the passive diameter of the vessel at 100 mmHg. Subsequently, the vessel was exposed twice to serotonin at a concentration of 10^{-5} M during the viability test. The response of the vessel to serotonin at the second application was larger than that at the first application, demonstrating the need for the viability test in order to get stable vessel responses. Then, an experiment was performed (Fig. 2b), showing a relaxation induced by the application of 4 different concentrations of acetylcholine after preconstriction of the vessel with serotonin and, after appropriate washout, a constriction induced by the application of 4 different concentrations of noradrenaline.

Cannulated Vessel Segments

A typical example of an experiment performed using a cannulated vessel segment is shown in Fig. 1. The inset shows a vessel cannulated by two pipettes and fixed there using strands of suture. In this example, changes in inner vessel diameter with time are shown. After mounting of the vessel, the myograph was heated to 37 °C. During this period the vessel started to constrict, indicating the development of a spontaneous myogenic tone (Fig. 1a). Subsequently, the vessel was exposed to noradrenaline to test smooth muscle cell viability and, after washout, to acetylcholine in order to test endothelium viability. Then, an experiment was performed (Fig. 1b), showing the response of the vessel to consecutive pressure increases from 10 to 140 mmHg, i.e. the myogenic response, which is characterised by vessel dilations at lower pressure values and constrictions at pressures larger than 60 mmHg.

Troubleshooting

Solutions

Solutions should be prepared carefully; in particular the occurrence of calcium precipitates should be avoided. This is especially important in experiments where calcium concentrations up to 10 mM are used, for example to study the dependence of a certain response on extracellular calcium. At such high calcium concentrations, precipitates of calcium and the phosphate anion may occur. If this happens, phosphate should be eliminated from the solution.

Normalisation

As shown in Fig. 2, lengthening of the vessel during a normalisation step leads to a fast increase in wall tension, followed by a decrease in wall tension consisting of a quick and a slow phase. However, sometimes a different picture is seen. If the increase and the following decrease in tension are considerably slowed down, the mechanical connection between the hooks or wires used to mount the vessel and the force transducer should be checked for the ability to move freely. This is especially important under isometric conditions, where these movements are very small but essential for the measurement. In some small arteries, especially from the cerebral and the coronary circulation, another phenomenon is sometimes observed. There, the phase of decreasing tension may be followed by a spontaneous increase in tension, indicating the development of spontaneous active tone. Since the normalisation procedure requires the determination of the passive tension of the vessel, the appearance of active tone should be avoided. In order to fulfill this requirement, either a dilating agonist should be added or a solution containing a low calcium concentration should be used.

Viability test

In some experiments on ring segments of small arteries the first application of an agonist during the viability test may produce a response considerably smaller than expected from previous experiments suggesting poor viability of the vessel preparation. Before replacing such a vessel, a second or third application of the agonist should be performed, where normal responses are often observed. In experiments on cannulated small arteries the development of a spontaneous myogenic tone is sometimes not observed, suggesting poor viability of the vessel preparation. Before replacing such a vessel, a contractile agonist at a submaximal concentration should be added. After washout of the agonist, a stable partial constriction often remains, indicating the induction of a spontaneous myogenic tone. However, the vessel should be replaced if upon washout vessel diameter returns to the fully relaxed state, even if this process is very slow. Since experiments will usually last several hours, a stable spontaneous myogenic tone is essential.

Functional Antagonism

Two problems arise from the so-called functional antagonism. The first is the selection of the preconstriction level in relaxation experiments using ring vessel segments. Since these vessel preparations usually do not develop spontaneous tone, relaxation responses can only be studied after preconstriction. However, the increase in tension produced by the vasoconstrictor used for preconstriction is imposing a functional antagonism to the effect of the relaxant agent. Thus, the use of increasing concentrations of the preconstricting agent resulted in a considerable decrease of the maximum response and in some cases also of the sensitivity to several relaxant agents (Stork and Cocks 1994). A systematic study employing different levels of preconstriction revealed that functional antagonism could only be avoided using a concentration of the preconstricting agent producing not more than 40% of maximum constriction (Stork and Cocks 1994). The second problem arises in experiments aimed at comparing responses to a certain vasoactive substance in the absence and presence of a pharmacological inhibitor, which has an effect on the preconstriction level or the spontaneous myogenic tone. The change of the initial tone may induce enough functional antagonism to produce an altered response, which however may not be related to the specific action of the inhibitor. In this situation, control experiments evaluating the role of changes of the initial tone are absolutely required.

References

Bevan JA, Osher JV (1972) A direct method for recording tension changes in the wall of small blood vessels *in vitro*. Agents Actions 2: 257–260

Boels PJ, Claes VA, Brutsaert DL (1990) Mechanics of K(+)-induced isotonic and isometric contractions in isolated canine coronary microarteries. Am.J Physiol 258: C512–C523

Boonen HC, DeMey JGR (1994) Distension influences responses to agonists and potassium in several types of small artery. In: Halpern W, Bevan J, Brayden JE, Dustan H, Nelson MT, Osol G (eds) The resistance arteries. Humana Press, Totowa, p 13–21

Bukoski RD, Shearin S, Jackson WF, Pamarthi MF (2001) Inhibition of Ca2+-induced relaxation by oxidized tungsten wires and paratungstate. J Pharmacol Exp Ther. 299: 343–350

Buus NH, VanBavel E, Mulvany MJ (1994) Differences in sensitivity of rat mesenteric small arteries to agonists when studied as ring preparations or as cannulated preparations. Br J Pharmacol 112: 579–587

Coats P, Hillier C (1999) Determination of an optimal axial-length tension for the study of isolated resistance arteries on a pressure myograph. Exp Physiol 84: 1085–1094

Duling BR, Gore RW, Dacey jr RG, Damon DN (1981) Methods for isolation, cannulation, and *in vitro* study of single microvessels. Am J Physiol 241: H108–H116

Fischer JG, Mewes H, Hopp HH, Schubert R (1996) Analysis of pressurized resistance vessel diameter changes with a low cost digital image processing device. Comp Meth Prog Biomed 50: 23–30

Gonzalez MC, Arribas SM, Molero F, Fernandez-Alfonso MS (2001) Effect of removal of adventitia on vascular smooth muscle contraction and relaxation. Am J Physiol Heart Circ.Physiol 280: H2876–H2881

Halpern W (1991) Common *in vitro* investigative methods. In: Bevan J, Halpern W, Mulvany MJ (eds) The resistance vasculature. Humana Press, Totowa, pp 45–57

Halpern W, Kelley M (1991) *In vitro* methodology for resistance arteries. Blood Vessels 28: 245–251

Halpern W, Osol G, Coy GS (1984) Mechanical behavior of pressurized *in vitro* prearteriolar vessels determined with a video system. Ann Biomed Eng 12: 463–479

Hoogerwerf N, van der Linden PJ, Westerhof N, Sipkema P (1992) A new mounting technique for perfusion of isolated small arteries: the effects of flow and oxygen on diameter. Microvascular Research 44: 49–60

Lew MJ, Angus JA (1992) Wall thickness to lumen diameter ratios of arteries from SHR and WKY: comparison of pressurised and wire-mounted preparations. J Vasc Res 29: 435–442

Machkov VV, Vlasova MA, Tarasova OS, Mikhaleva LM, Koshelev VB, Timin EN, Rodionov IM (1998) Responses to noradrenaline of tail arteries in hypertensive, hypotensive and normotensive rats under different regimens of perfusion: role of the myogenic response. Acta Physiol Scand 163: 331–337

Monos E, Contney SJ, Dornyei G, Cowley AW, Stekiel WJ (1993) Hyperpolarization of in situ rat saphenous vein in response to axial stretch. Am J Physiol 265: H857–H861

Monos E, Raffai G, Contney SJ, Stekiel WJ, Cowley AW Jr. (2001) Axial stretching of extremity artery induces reversible hyperpolarization of smooth muscle cell membrane *in vivo*. Acta Physiol Hung 88: 197–206

Mulvany MJ, Halpern W (1976) Mechanical properties of vascular smooth muscle cells *in situ*. Nature 260: 617–619

Mulvany MJ, Halpern W (1977) Contractile properties of small arterial resistance vessels in spontaneously hypertensive and normotensive rats. Circ Res 41: 19–26

Mulvany MJ, Hansen OK, Aalkjaer C (1978) Direct evidence that the greater contractility of resistance vessels in spontaneously hypertensive rats is associated with a narrowed lumen, a thickened media, and an increased number of smooth muscle cell layers. Circ Res 43: 854–864

Nilsson H, Sjoblom N (1985) Distension-dependent changes in noradrenaline sensitivity in small arteries from the rat. Acta Physiol Scand 125: 429–435

Parkington HC, Tare M, Tonta MA, Coleman HA (1993) Stretch revealed three components in the hyperpolarization of guinea-pig coronary artery in response to acetylcholine. J Physiol 465: 459–476

Price JM, Davis DL, Knauss EB (1981) Length-dependent sensitivity in vascular smooth muscle. Am J Physiol 241: H557–H563

Schubert R, Wesselman JPM, Nilsson H, Mulvany MJ (1996) Noradrenaline-induced depolarization is smaller in isobaric compared to isometric preparations of rat mesenteric small arteries. Pflugers Arch Eur J Physiol 431: 794–796

Stork AP, Cocks TM (1994) Pharmacological reactivity of human epicardial coronary arteries: characterization of relaxation responses to endothelium-derived relaxing factor. Br J Pharmacol 113: 1099–1104

VanBavel E, Mooij T, Giezeman MJ, Spaan JA (1990) Cannulation and continuous cross-sectional area measurement of small blood vessels. J Pharmacol Methods 24: 219–227

VanBavel E, Mulvany MJ (1994) Role of wall tension in the vasoconstrictor response of cannulated rat mesenteric small arteries. J Physiol London 477: 103–115

Zaritsky JJ, Eckman DM, Wellman GC, Nelson MT, Schwarz TL (2000) Targeted disruption of Kir2.1 and Kir2.2 genes reveals the essential role of the inwardly rectifying K(+) current in K(+)-mediated vasodilation. Circ Res 87: 160–166

3 Electrophysiological Techniques

3.1 Optical Techniques for the Recording of Action Potentials — 215
Helmut A. Tritthart

3.2 Recording Action Potentials Using Voltage-Sensitive Dyes — 233
Vladimir G. Fast

3.3 Epicardial Mapping in Isolated Hearts –
Use in Safety Pharmacology, Analysis of Torsade de Pointes
Arrhythmia and Ischemia-Reperfusion-Related Arrhythmia — 256
Stefan Dhein

3.4 Voltage-Clamp and Patch-Clamp Techniques — 272
Hans Reiner Polder, Martin Weskamp, Klaus Linz and Rainer Meyer

3.5 L-Type Calcium Channel Recording — 324
Uta C. Hoppe, Mathias C. Brandt, Guido Michels and Michael Lindner

3.6 Recording Cardiac Potassium Currents
with the Whole-Cell Voltage Clamp Technique — 355
Erich Wettwer and Ursula Ravens

3.7 Recording the Pacemaker Current I_f — 381
Uta C. Hoppe, Fikret Er and Mathias C. Brandt

3.8 Recording Gap Junction Currents — 397
Ardawan J. Rastan and Stefan Dhein

3.9 Recording Monophasic Action Potentials — 417
Paulus Kirchhof, Larissa Fabritz and Michael R. Franz

3.10 Heart on a Chip – Extracellular Multielectrode Recordings
from Cardiac Myocytes in Vitro — 432
Ulrich Egert and Thomas Meyer

Optical Techniques for the Recording of Action Potentials

Helmut A. Tritthart

Introduction

Historical Perspective

Over the past years, fluorescence-based methods of investigation have become increasingly important in many different areas such as environmental analysis, biochemical analysis, diagnostics and also electrophysiology. Most of what we know regarding membrane potential changes in multicellular or cellular preparations comes from potential measurements made by impaling cells with glass pipette microelectrodes. In many experimental conditions, impalement stability and the likely damage to the cells limit the use of this method. Microelectrodes are not applicable to cells smaller than 3 µm diameter, in subcellular organelles and for monitoring on multiple sites simultaneously. For these and other reasons attempts were made in the late 1960s to develop new techniques to monitor membrane potential. In the search for a voltage-dependent optical signal of transmembrane potential with a good signal to noise ratio, more than 300 dyes were screened by Cohen et al. (1974). Most of them responded to potential changes through changes in absorption and fluorescence of up to 0.1% of the resting intensity during an action potential, with a signal to noise ration better than 10:1 in a single sweep. To function satisfactorily as a probe of membrane potential a dye must exhibit the following properties:
1. it must bind or interact with the plasma membrane to act as a sensor of membrane potential;
2. it should exhibit large fluorescence and/or absorption changes preferably linearly with changes in membrane potential;
3. its optical responses must be specifically related to potential changes and not to ion concentrations, transmembrane currents or membrane conductance;
4. staining of the heart with the dye should not result in pharmacological or toxic effects to the preparation;
5. the dye should be optically stable, e.g. not show photobleaching on exposure to intense light.

Table 1
Properties of selected potentiometric chromophores

Name	Chromophore	Description	ABS [nm]	EM [nm]	Structure
M-540	Merocyanine	One of the original and most thoroughly studied potentiometric dyes. First heart dye. Reorientation mechanism. T: ms; Time resolution: ms	555	578	
TMRE	Rhodamine	Rhodamine redistribution dye for single cell and mitochondrial potential measurements. T s – min; Time resolution: s – min	548	597	
Di-S-C3(5)	Cyanine	Very sensitive dye for cell suspensions. Can give 10-fold intensity changes by a redistribution/self-quench mechanism. T: s – min Time resolution: s – min	550	568	
Rhodamine-123	Rhodamine	Redistribution dye for mitochondrial staining. T: min	505	534	

Table 1
Continued

Name	Chromo-phore	Description	ABS [nm]	EM [nm]	Structure
DiBaC4(3)	Oxonol	Anionic on: off indicator. Also called "Bis-oxonol"; T: ms – s Time resolution: ms – s	493	516	
Di-4-ANEPPS	Naphthyl Styryl	Versatile fast styryl dye. Most common heart dye. Electrochromic mechanism. Dual wavelength ratio is an option. T: < μs Time resolution: better than ms	502	723	
RH155	Oxonol	Good choice for absorbance measurements: No fluorescence signals. T: ms Time resolution: ms	638		
RH795	Styryl	Good styryl dye for penetration into cortex; T: ms Time resolution: ms	530	712	

Mode of Action

Merocyanine, oxonol, styryl and rhodamine compounds exhibit voltage dependent responses in heart muscles and bind strongly to the cardiac membrane. A hydrophobic structure is advantageous for tight binding to the membrane as is a localised negatively charged group (SO_3^-) that prevents diffusion inside cells. All "fast response" dyes are of this type (see Table 1).

What are the mechanisms by which dyes can display spectral changes in response to changes in membrane potential?

On-Off Mechanism

The cyanines are positive dyes and the oxonols are negatively charged. A positively charged dye will have a greater binding constant to a polarised than to a depolarised membrane; the opposite holds for negative dyes. Therefore, the fluorescence of cyanine dyes that obey a pure on-off mechanism goes down upon depolarisation while that of oxonols goes up. Significant fluorescence enhancements are associated with a hydrophobic and viscous environment.

Redistribution

If a fluorescent membrane-permeant cation distributes between the extracellular medium and the cytosol, the ratio of fluorescence from inside and fluorescence from outside a cell is directly related to the membrane potential. Cyanine dyes show, in addition, a concentration-dependent aggregation of dye molecules Aggregates are non-fluorescent and not membrane permeant. Unfortunately, dyes using the redistribution mechanism are too slow to be useful for following cardiac action potential.

Reorientation

A change in the intramembrane electrical field can shift the balance *via* an electrostatic interaction with the dye dipole moment and thus, change orientation. Dyes oriented parallel to the incident light wave will be very poorly excited. Upon reorientation after depolarisation the geometry is appropriate for absorption of a photon and fluorescence emission. Merocyanine 540 is a fast optical dye for mapping of cardiac activity (see Table 1).

Electrochromism

Upon excitation, the negative electron cloud shifts from a density on the aniline side to the pyridinium side of the chromophore. In a polarised membrane, this coupling of the electrical field with the chromophore charge distribution will decrease the energy difference between the ground and excited states resulting in a red shift of both the excitation and emission spectra. Since the relative fluorescence change $\Delta F/F$, is being measured, it is best to choose a wavelength near the tails of the spectrum; the wavelength of maximum fluorescence should be avoided. Because electrochromism does not involve any molecular motion, a fast response to voltage changes is guaranteed (see di-4-ANEPPS in Table 1).

Description of Methods and Practical Approach
Methods

A good description of various methods used for optical mapping of cardiac excitation and arrhythmias can be found in the book of Rosenbaum and Jalife (2001). This method section will cover staining procedures, light sources, light collection, detectors, optics, signal processing and evaluation.

Dye solutions are typically prepared in ethanol or dimethyl sulphoxide or in saline solution. 1 to 1000 µmol/l are used for 10 to 30 min to stain heart muscles. Staining is superficial (less than 100 µm) and dye delivery through a coronary perfusate is often found to be superior, with lower dye concentrations needed and better signal to noise ratios. The important considerations for the selection of a dye are low rates of photobleaching, slow washout, minimal toxic, pharmacological or photodynamic effects and optimal efficacy for the preparation used, which depends on binding, penetration, persistence and solubility. Merocyanine, oxonol, styryl and pyridinium compounds (see Table 1) bind to heart muscle and exhibit voltage-dependent responses in heart muscle even after several hours of perfusion in dye-free solution. Due to their hydrophobic structure, they bind tightly to the cell membrane and exhibit "fast" voltage-dependent responses. Bleaching effects may cause signal drifts that cannot easily be distinguished from membrane potential changes. The most severe problem, however, is phototoxic side effects. To reduce these effects, the total exposure of a stained cell to light should be minimized. In single cardiac cells, phototoxicity of dyes is a problem when high light intensities are used and measurements are long lasting. Cells show action potential for prolongation, early after-depolarisations occur and finally arrhythmias, shrinking and hypercontracture are seen (Schaffer et al. 1994).

Three kinds of light sources have been used to measure optical action potentials in heart muscle, tungsten-halogen filament lamps, mercury/xenon arc lamps, and laser emissions. Tungsten-halogen lamps have the lowest intensity per unit area but also low noise and high intensity in the visible range and are stably running within seconds. Arc lamps provide a fine illumination spot with 2- to 3 times greater intensity than tungsten lamps and are particularly advantageous for small field examination (1–3 mm). The noise, however, is 10 times greater than with tungsten lamps. Laser emission provides high-intensity monochromatic light spots. Laser light is 10- to 50 times more noisy. The pure monochromatic light is often not the optimum to match the peak excitation wavelength of the dye molecule. The high intensity of laser per unit area is advantageous for narrow excitation beams (less than 1 mm). Argon ion, neodymium YAG, He-Ne and krypton lasers have mostly been used for illumination. The short duration of laser light emission is an additional advantage.

PDA (photodiode arrays): The signal to noise ratio is proportional to the number of measured photons and therefore an increase in either temporal or spatial resolution and a high quantum efficacy of the sensor is advantageous. Photodiode arrays were first introduced to simultaneously record electrical activity from multiple sites in cardiac muscle (Salama et al. 1987). A major advantage of photodiode array systems is the high temporal resolution achieved by the parallel readout of the diodes. With a large number of diodes a high spatial resolution is also possible. Data acquisition and analysis require sufficient computer hard and software support, but some systems are already commercially available. Fibre optic probes for laser illumination and photodiode detection *via* return fibres have also often been applied.

CCD arrays (charge-coupled device) differ from photodiodes in that photoexited charge carriers are collected within a single element (i.e. pixel) over a finite period (integration time). The magnitude of charge from each pixel is sequentially converted to an analog video signal and then passed to a frame grabber that digitises and stores each successive frame. Standard image processing software can be used to subtract background fluorescence and enhance contrast. Read-out time is a major factor, being dependent on pixel number and limiting the sampling rate of CCD systems. Since the total fluorescence measured consists mostly (90%) of background fluorescence, the lower dynamic range of CCDs as compared to photodiode detectors makes it difficult to capture large background fluorescence while providing adequate voltage resolution for the action potential.

Optical mapping requires the collection of fluorescent light at relatively low intensities. When a lens is used to magnify and focus the image on to a photodetector, the amount of light collected is directly proportional to the square of the numerical aperture which is an index of light gathering power and inversely proportional to the square of the magnification.

High-quality images can be acquired with either microscope or photography lenses. Fluorescence microscopes are commercially available with objective lens magnifications ranging from 4× to 100×, allowing for the mapping of preparations smaller than 4 mm^2. Microscope objectives are designed with high numerical apertures, ranging from 0.5 to 1.3. In fluorescence microscopy, the preparation is epi-illuminated; the preparation is efficiently and evenly illuminated. Microscope objectives have been optimised for observing small preparations at short working distances (i.e., distance from lens to preparation); however, the advantages of microscope objectives are not maintained at lower magnifications.

Photographic lenses are better suited for magnifications less than 10×, where they have numerical apertures ranging from 0.25 to 0.4. The working distance varies depending on the lens configuration and is on the order of 30 mm, much longer than the working distance of a microscope objective. The simplest way to use photographic lenses is to image a preparation with a single lens. The tandem lens configuration is a variation of the single lens design, and consists of two lenses aligned along an optical axis and separated by a distance. To implement the tandem lens configuration, two camera lenses are focused at infinity and are placed face to face. The preparation is placed at the focal plane of the first lens, and the image is formed at the focal plane of the second lens.

Theoretically, the frequency content of an optical action potential determines the minimum sampling rate required to reconstruct the action potential from digital samples accurately. Approximately 90% of the total energy of the action potential is contained below 150 Hz. Sampling theory requires a sampling rate to be at least 2×, better 3 to 5×, that of the highest frequency component (i.e. 750 Hz). Greater spatial resolution is required to accurately depict the complex wave fronts that occur during fibrillation, microreentry and arrhythmias or to investigate the discrete nature of propagation at the cellular level (Windisch et al. 1990). The effective number of recording sites for a CCD detector is greater than that of a PDA and, therefore CCD detectors are more appropriate for mapping larger areas at low magnification so that spatial resolutions of approximately 1 mm or less can be maintained. However, the high sampling rates and signal to noise ratio that can be achieved with PDAs make them ideal for high optical magnification when temporal resolution and signal fidelity are critical. When stored signals are processed, they are digitally filtered and the baseline drift resulting from dye bleaching needs to be eliminated. In a dual wavelength procedure, signals with and without membrane voltage changes can be obtained and the baseline drift eliminated. Optical signals can only reflect relative changes in the membrane potential, not the membrane potential itself, but calibration of the optical signal is possible.

Simultaneous microelectrode recordings or patch clamp techniques can be used for calibration of optical signals (Windisch 2001). Electrical test pulses of known field strength can also be used for calibration.

Examples and Troubleshooting

Single Cell Recordings

A significant advantage of optical recordings is the possibility of placing many photodiodes on one single cardiac cell or on a small group of interconnected cells to study conduction and to perform simultaneous action potential measurements over a large area of cardiac muscle (mapping). The long-lasting stability of these recordings is a further advantage but the distortion by mechanical activities of muscle cells is a disadvantage. The non-invasive approach to electrical signals by optical techniques is obviously superior to patch or microelectrode techniques as shown in Fig. 1. The rate of increase of the action potential is faster and earlier than that measured *via* a patch electrode with correct capacity compensation but the noise of the unfiltered optical signal is much stronger.

Figure 2 shows values of eleven photodiodes measuring the surface of a single cardiac cell stimulated by a patch electrode. The numbers given are the time needed in microseconds for the maximum rate of rise after the end of the stimulus. Surprisingly, excitation starts in the centre of the cell and not under the patch electrode and excitation velocity is much faster in the length axis of the muscle than at right angles to the axis.

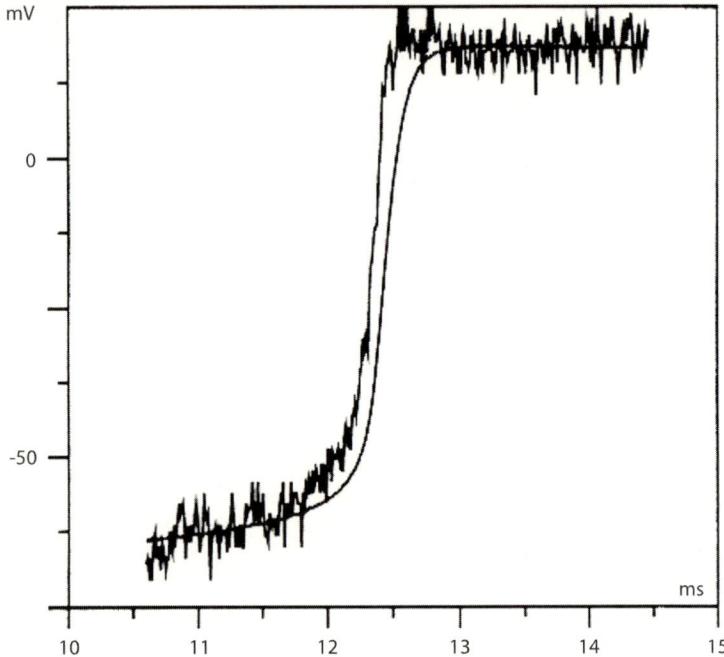

Figure 1
Comparison of an optical and a simultaneously obtained electrical signal. The optical signal (without any filtering) was normalized to the electrical signal, which was simultaneously recorded with a patch electrode. The optical signal occurred approx. 40 µs earlier and showed a steeper rising phase. (From Windisch 2001)

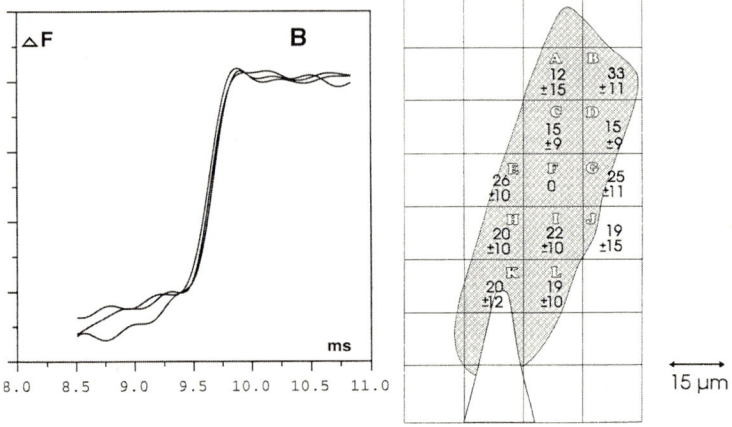

Figure 2
Values of eleven photodiodes measuring the surface of a single cardiac cell stimulated by a patch electrode. The numbers given are the time needed in microseconds for the maximum rate of rise after the end of the stimulus. Surprisingly, excitation starts in the centre of the cell and not under the patch electrode and excitation velocity is much faster in the length axis of the muscle than at right angles to the axis (see photodiode A as compared to E and G, with permission from Windisch 2001)

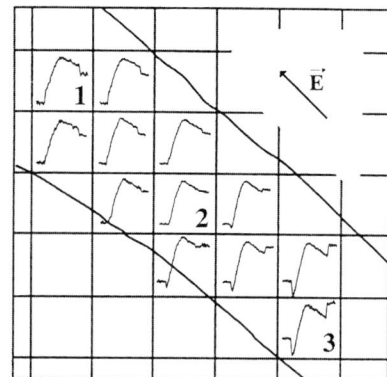

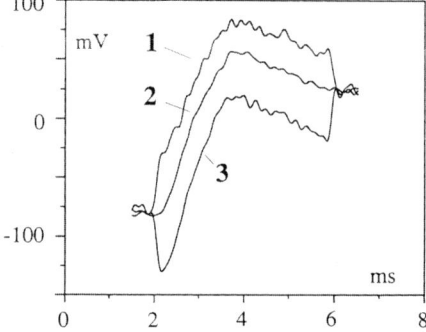

Figure 3
A 4 ms long stimulus was applied to one cardiac cell and the effects of field stimulation were studied (the *arrow* is the direction of the electrical field). In areas closer to the cathode, the stimulus caused a membrane depolarisation, in areas closer to the anode, a hyperpolarisation. This is best seen in the superimposed action potential rising phases of photodiodes 1, 2 and 3 (one measuring spot was 15×15 μm). (With permission from Windisch 2001)

In Fig. 3, a 4 ms long stimulus was applied to one cardiac cell and the effects of field stimulation were studied (the arrow is the direction of the electrical field). In areas closer to the cathode, the stimulus caused a membrane depolarisation, in areas closer to the anode, a hyperpolarisation. This is best seen in the superimposed action potential rising phases of photodiodes 1, 2 and 3 (one measuring spot was 15×15 μm).

Figure 4 shows the single cell response to uniform field stimulation along the long axis of a rat ventricular cell measured by 6 photodiodes. The response along the length of the cell is throughout linear and symmetric around zero when the field was reversed (filled circles) (Tung 2001). These recordings from single cells show that the field response consists of two components. The first is complete in less than 1 ms, has opposite signs at the two ends of the cell and varies linearly with field intensity. The second is much slower in time course, is governed by changes in the active membrane currents, and is relatively homogeneous across the cell.

Strands of cardiomyocyte one cell wide allow the measurement of intercellular propagation during normal gap-junction coupling. An example of such a measurement is shown in Fig. 5 (Rohr et al. 1992).

During action potential propagation from left to right, the simultaneously recorded action potential upstrokes revealed an activation gap between detectors 5 and 7, thus demonstrating that conduction was, as predicted, discontinuous at the cellular level. The intermediate timing of the action potential upstroke of detector 6 is ex-

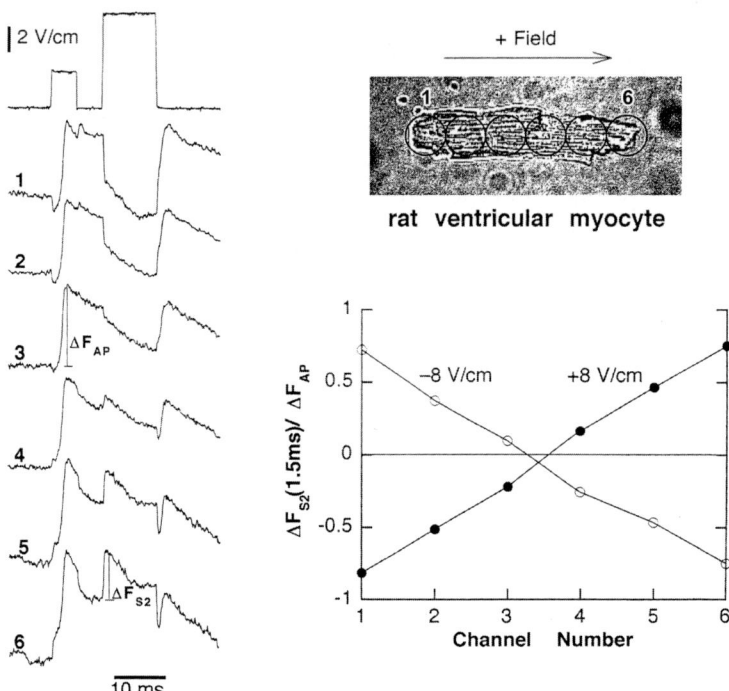

Figure 4
Single cell response to uniform field stimulation. Fluorescence from the cell was imaged *via* six optical fibres running to six photodetectors. After an action potential was elicited (ΔF AP left) a 14.5 V/cm field was applied (S$_2$) along the cell axis. The change in fluorescence (open circles) was measured 1.5 ms after the onset of the S2 pulse, and showed completely linear responses along the length of the cell. The responses were symmetric around zero when the field was reversed (filled circles). Unpublished data from V. Sharma, S. Lu, and L. Tung. (With permission of the author [Thung 2001])

plained by the circumstance that this detector received input simultaneously from the left and the right cell. Also in strands which are several cells wide as in Fig. 6 the spacing between isochrones is not homogeneous, but lateral gap-junctional coupling is likely to smooth out differences in local activation, as shown in a computer simulation study (Spach and Dolber 1986). Computer simulation studies have also indicated (Rudy and Quan 1991) that investigations of propagation at the cellular/subcellular level require a spatial resolution in the micrometer range and a temporal resolution with microsecond precision.

Mapping

In Fig. 7 spread of excitation in the surface of a papillary muscle was measured by a 16×16 grid of photodiodes (Müller et al. 1989). Maxima of inverted first time derivatives (−dF/dt) of the fluorescence signals were used to evaluate the arrival time of

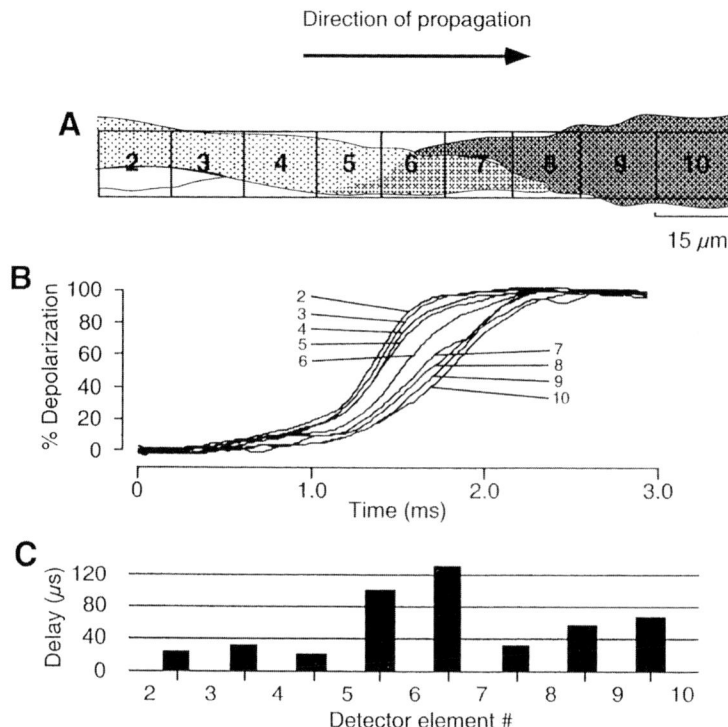

Figure 5a–c
Discontinuous conduction in "monolines" of cardiomyocytes. **a** Schematic drawing of the imaged region of the preparation consisting of two slightly overlapping cardio-myocytes (*light grey* and *dark grey*). The squares indicate the positions of individual photodetectors. **b** Action potential upstrokes recorded during propagation from left to right. Numbers correspond to the numbering of photodetectors in **a**. **c** Activation delays along the preparation. (With permission from Rohr and Salzburg 1992)

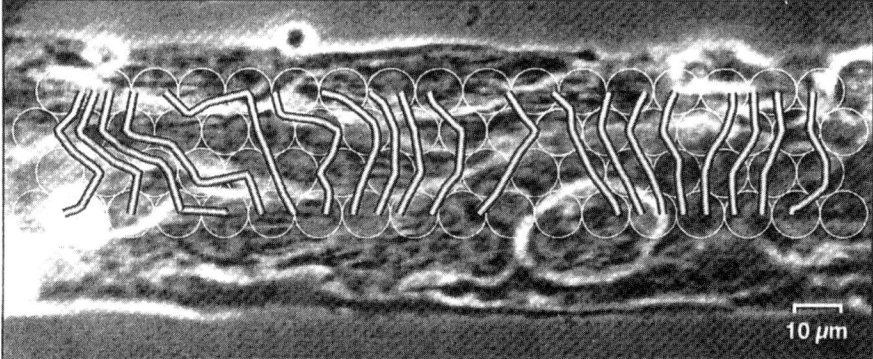

Figure 6
Microscopic impulse propagation in a several cell wide linear strand. Phase contrast picture of the preparation with overlaid white circles indicating the positions of the photodetectors and isochrones of activation (spacing: 20 μs) during impulse propagation from left to right. (Rohr and Kucera 2001)

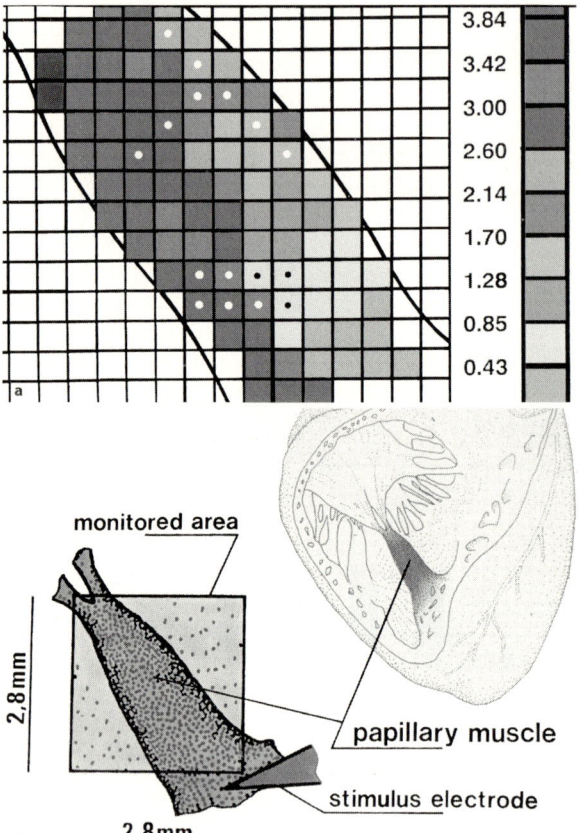

Figure 7
Fluorescence real-time monitoring of the microscopic exci-tation pattern (rat papillary muscle stained with di-4-ANEPS). The optically measured time of incidence of propagated excitation was depicted by the maximum rate of rise of the action potential (colour code in ms after stimulus 16×16 pixels, pixel size 180×180 µm^2). The conduction velocity measured in the above pixels was 0.9 m/s, discontinuous conduction was found in the lower blotted zone around pixel 187. *For coloured version see appendix*

propagated excitation for each pixel. Propagation proceeded with high velocity from the lower right side (close to the position of a stimulus electrode) in the longitudinal direction of the muscle fibres and much more slowly in the transverse direction. With cardiac impulse velocities of up to 1 m/s and small pixels (e.g. 10 µm diameter) a temporal resolution of about 10 µs is necessary. Beat to beat real time mapping with pixels of the size of cardiac muscle cells is of outstanding importance for investigations of irregular dynamics of the heart (e.g. Wenkebach phenomena, blocks, tachycardia, flutter and fibrillation).

The cardiac Arrhythmia Suppression Trial indicated a significant proarrhythmic effect of treatment with flecainide (Echt et al. 1991). We have shown that flecainide alters the cardiac microscopic activation pattern (Dhein et al. 1996) quite significantly. Figure 8 shows typical isochrones in the surface of a papillary muscle before and after treatment with flecainide (1.5 µmol/L). The activation pattern is significantly altered by flecainide in an inhomogeneous way, for instance in the right part of the preparation, conduction velocities are comparable (isochrones 0.57 to 2.85) but significantly reduced in the left part (isochrones 3.99 to 5.13) so that conduction velocity is only one fifth of that in the right part of the muscle. Another problem concerns

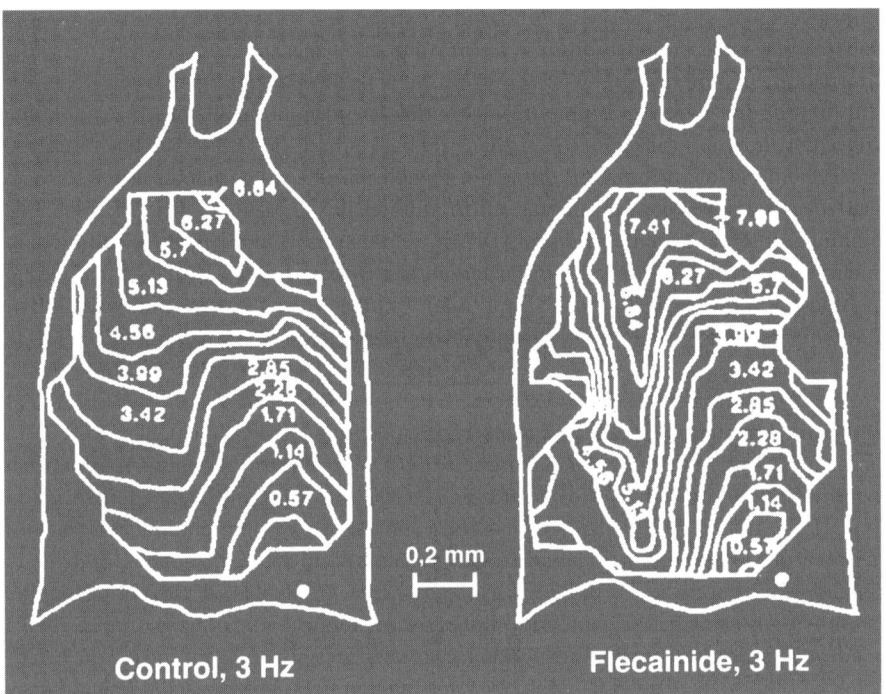

Figure 8
Isochrones (in ms) after activation of the first photodiode in the surface of a guinea pig papillary muscle (16×16 grid of photodiodes, spatial resolution 18 μm²). Results are shown under control conditions (*left panel*) or under the influence of 1.5 μmol/L flecainide (*right panel*). The position of the stimulation electrode is the black dot at the muscle base

the vector field similarity, a deviation of less than 5° was considered similar. Under control conditions at 3 Hz, 27.1% of the vectors of two activations 5 min apart were found to be similar according to the strict conditions above. After flecainide, the similarities of vectors were found to be reduced to 17.5%. Therefore the effects on conduction velocities and on activation patterns are not homogenously distributed, indicating influences other than simple sodium channel blockade by flecainide. These other factors may be anisotropic tissue properties, cellular gap junction coupling or passive electrical properties of the cell membrane (Arnsdorff 1990).

Studies focusing on the rate of rise of the action potential are much easier to perform than studies on de- and re-polarisation because repolarization is slower and significantly disturbed by mechanical activities modifying the optical signal. Windisch et al. (1987) have used a double beam technique, one beam with a wavelength not producing an optical signal. In this way, the mechanical distortion of the optical signal can be corrected. Mechanical fixation as well as pharmacological inhibition of contractility have also been used.

Figure 9 shows a nice example of mapping of de- and re-polarisation (wave front and wave tail) in the anterior and posterior surfaces of a rabbit heart. Pacing of the posterior epicardial surface of the left ventricle elicits a propagating wave front faster

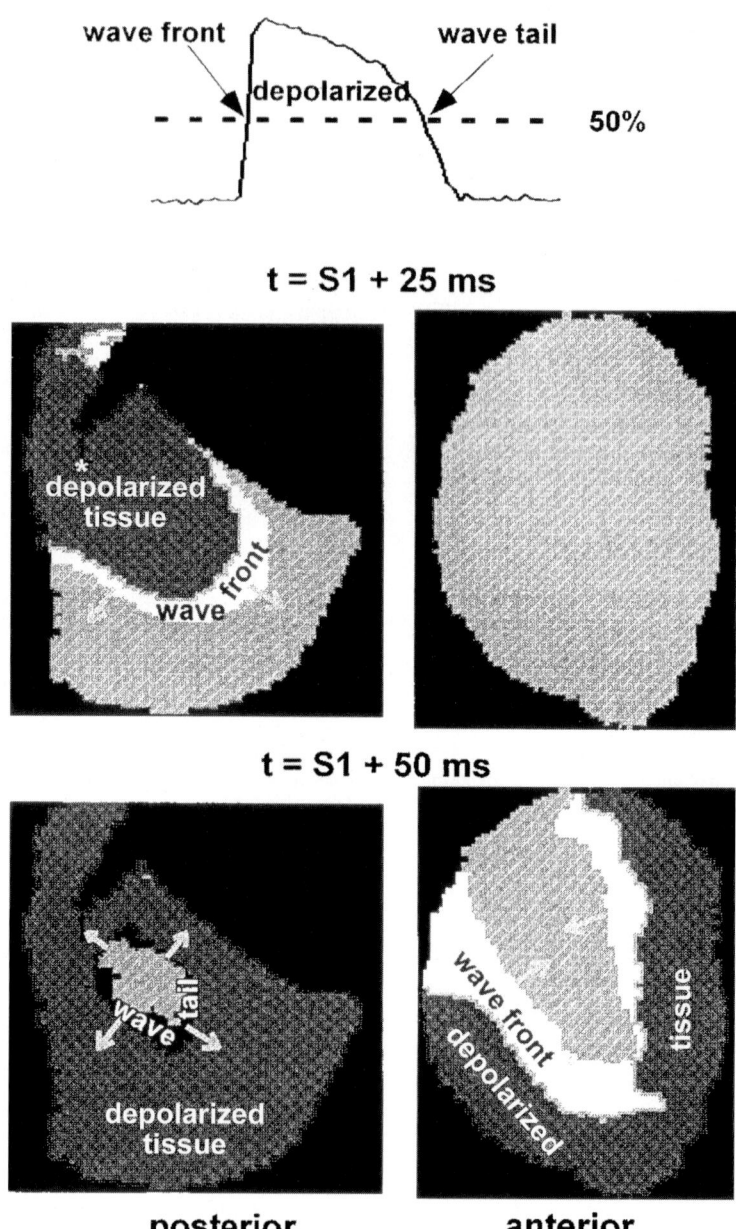

Figure 9
Wave front and wave tail (50% threshold) were mapped. About 20,000 pixels were measured in the posterior and anterior surfaces of a rabbit heart (spatial resolution 0.16 mm). Pacing the posterior epicardial surface elicits a wave front invading resting tissue (*grey*). The collision of the wave front occurs in the anterior surface in a "V shape". The wave tail (*lower right figure*) emerges and spreads similarly to the wave front. (With permission from Gray and Jalife 2001)

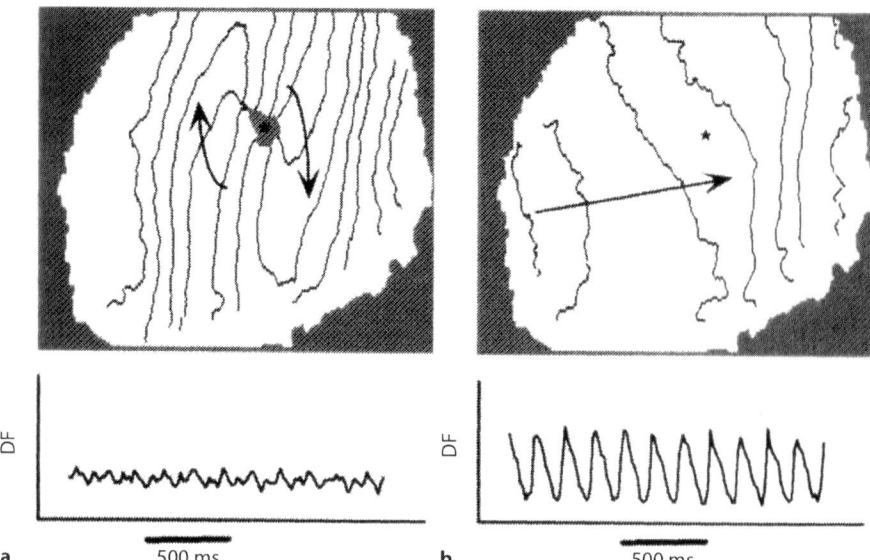

Figure 10
Stationary spiral waves of excitation in sheep epicardial muscle. Rotating around a core (*grey region*) 17 ms isochrones show the position of the wave front. Fluorescence changes (below, DF) measured in the core (*asterisk*) indicate a very low amplitude of activation. In B a planar wave (stimulating electrode left) is shown and the asterisk region is now excited (DF, below). (With permission from Baxter and Davidenko)

in fibre length axis and invading resting tissue (grey). Later the wave front reaches the anterior surface and collides in a "V shape". The wave tail spreads similarly to the wave front and starts near to the electrode. In this experiment the heart was constrained between two Plexiglas voids (Gray and Jalife 2001).

Figure 10 shows an isochronal map of a clockwise spiral wave rotating over the surface of a thin slice of sheep epicardial muscle (Baxter and Davidenko 2001). The isochrones are 16.7 ms apart, the rotation period is 150 ms, the core is delineated by the grey region near the centre. Within the core, at the point marked by the asterisk, there is very low amplitude activation indicating lack of regular excitation (DF, below). In part B the muscle was stimulated by a linear electrode along the left edge. Isochrones of planar waves (17 ms) show a regular pattern and indicate that the non-excited core (asterisk) of the preceding spiral wave is excitable tissue (DF, below) Drifting spiral waves are often found but are usually short-lived because heterogeneities or boundaries may prevent the core from moving.

This sequence of events is responsible for an electrocardiographic pattern characterized by the presence of a polymorphic tachycardia with varying QRS axis as well as irregular cycle length, followed by a monomorphic tachycardia with uniform QRS morphology and cycle length. Such transitions have also been described during the spontaneous initiation of ventricular tachycardias in humans (Bardy and Olson 1990).

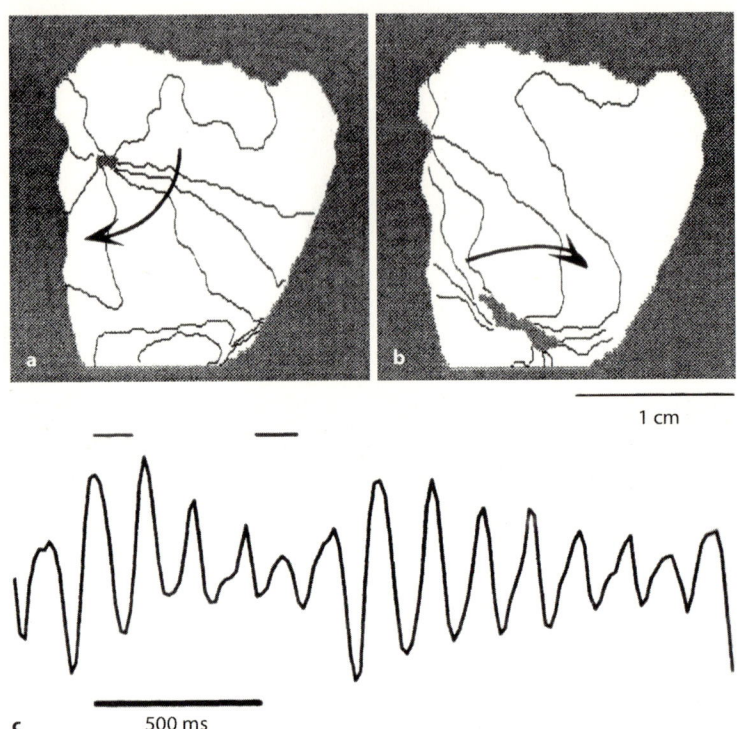

Figure 11a–c
Isochronal maps of two rotations in a sequence of non-stationary ventricular tachycardia in a rabbit heart. In **b** the rotor has drifted towards the apex 500 ms later. In **c** the pseudo-electrocardiogram is shown (bars above are tissues of the isochrone maps). (With permission of from Baxter and Davidenko)

Torsade-like patterns are seen in the ECG, when the drift velocities of spiral waves are approximately 10% of the propagation speed of excitation. If spiral waves moves more rapidly, 30% or more of wave speed, fibrillatory ECG patterns are likely. Figure 11 shows isochronal maps of two rotations in a sequence of non-stationary ventricular tachycardia. This rotor has drifted towards the apex 500 ms later with accompanying elongation of the core (b). Panel C shows the typical pattern of shifting axis in the pseudo-ECG generated during the entire episode.

Gray et al. (1995) have related the rotor's propagation speed and drift speed to the frequency spectrum of the ECG and their prediction showed excellent correspondence with the recorded ECG. They concluded that a single rapidly drifting rotor in the heart may underlie ventricular fibrillation. They have devised a method of quantifying spatial and temporal order during cardiac fibrillation and their analysis reveals an unexpected amount of organization during fibrillation (Gray 1998).

In Fig. 12 a defibrillation attempt is shown. The lower left map shows the spread of activation during the last beat of ventricular fibrillation before shock. Conduction was slow and emerged from several foci at the same time (white areas). Trace F (fluo-

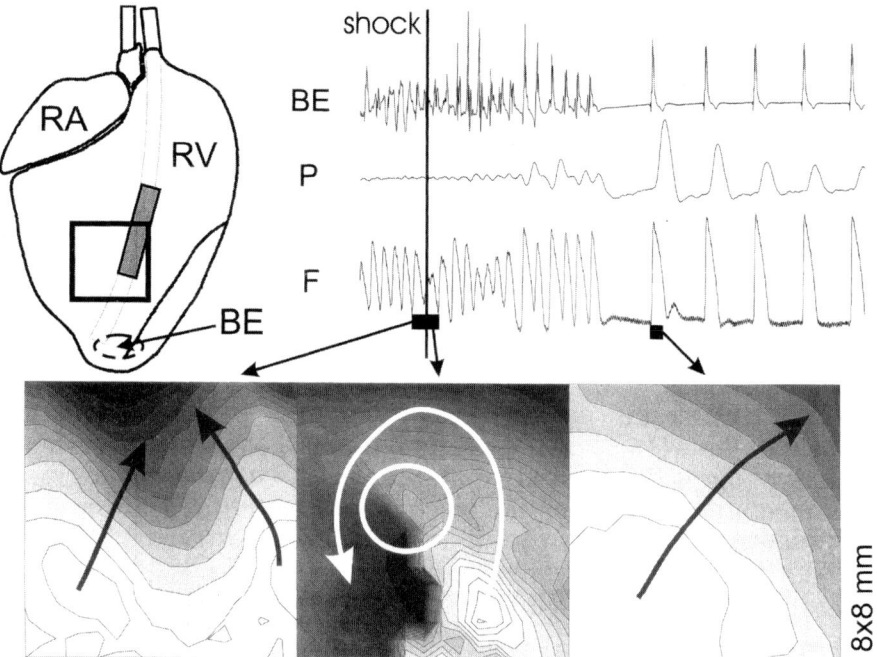

Figure 12
A phase singularity is produced during a failing defibrillation shock and later followed by restoration of sinus rhythm (*right*). The *top left panel* shows the field of view and the defibrillation electrode, the *top right panel* the bipolar electrogram (BE), aortic pressure (P) and fluorescent signal (F). The lower maps show 1 ms isochrones just before (*left*) immediately after shock (*middle*) and later (*right*). (With permission of Efimov and Cheng 2001)

rescence) shows that during fibrillatory electrical activity the transmembrane potential did not reach full overshoot or resting potential, and therefore there was no excitable gap. A cathodal monophasic shock (–15 V) showed that activation spread rapidly in the right half of the field of view near the electrode (middle activation map, isochrones 1 ms apart). Then it spread to the left in the upper half, while it was blocked in the lower half. Activation then spread downward, completing the re-entry cycle. The phase singularity is shown by a white circle. Phase singularities followed by re-entry were often found in unsuccessful defibrillation shocks (Efimov and Cheng 2001). The lower right map shows restoration of sinus rhythm. Before these types of experiments became possible, our knowledge of events occurring during and immediately after defibrillation was only based on indirect evidence, so the superiority of fluorescent methods is obvious.

In summary, fluorescent methods have some short-comings such as mechanical signal distortion, influencing predominantly repolarization, the noise of the light source and measuring errors due to the indirect detection of membrane potential, but they are a superior and new method opening many previously impossible approaches to fast and precise measurements of membrane potentials.

References

Arnsdorff MF (1990) Electrophysiological matrices, cardiac arrhythmias and antiarrhythmic drugs. In: Rosen MR, Janse MJ, Wit AL (eds) Cardiac electrophysiology. Futura Publishing, New York, pp 1063–1094

Bardy GH, Olson WH (1990) Clinical characteristics of spontaneous-onset sustained ventricular tachycardia and ventricular fibrillation in survivors of cardiac arrest. In: Zipes DP, Jalife J (eds) Cardiac Electrophysiology: From Cell to Bedside. W.B. Saunders, Philadelphia, pp 778–790

Baxter WT, Davidenko JM (2001) Video Mapping of Spiral Waves in the Heart. In: Rosenbaum S, Jalife J (eds) Optical mapping of cardiac excitation and arrhythmias. Futura Publishing, New York, pp 265–280

Cohen LB, Salzberg BM, Davila HV et al. (1974) Changes in axon fluorescence during activity: Molecular probes of membrane potential. J Membr Biol 19: 1–36

Dhein S, Hartbauer M, Müller W, Windisch H, Salameh A, Tritthart HA (1996) Flecainide alters the cardiac microscopic activation pattern. An *in vitro* study using voltage sensitive dyes. Pharmacological Research 33: 1–6

Echt DS et al. (1991) Mortality and morbidity in patients receiving encainide, flecainide or placebo. The cardiac arrhythmia suppression trial. New Engl J Med 324: 781–788

Efimov IR, Cheng Y (2001) Virtual electrode-induced wave fronts and phase singularities; mechanisms of success and failure of internal defibrillation. In: Rosenbaum S, Jalife J (eds) Optical mapping of cardiac excitation and arrhythmias. Futura Publishing, New York, pp 407–432

Gray RA, Jalife J (2001) Video Imaging of Cardiac Fibrillation. In: Rosenbaum S, Jalife J (eds) Optical mapping of cardiac excitation and arrhythmias. Futura Publishing, New York, pp 245–264

Gray RA, Pertsov AM, Jalife J (1998) Spatial and temporal organization during cardiac fibrillation. Nature 392: 75–78

Gray RS, Jalife J, Panfilov AV et al. (1995) Nonstationary vortexlike re-entrant activity as a mechanism of polymorphic ventricular tachycardia in the isolated rabbit heart. Circulation 91: 2454–2469

Müller W, Windisch H, Tritthart HA (1989) Fast optical monitoring of microscopic excitation patterns in cardiac muscle. Biophys J 56: 623–629

Thung L (2001) Responses of cardiac myocytes to electrica fields. In: Rosenbaum S, Jalife J (eds) Optical mapping of cardiac excitation and arrhythmias. Futura Publishing, New York, pp 313–334

Rohr S, Salzberg BM (1992) Discontinuities in action potential propagation along chains of single ventricular myocytes in culture: Multiple site optical recording of transmembrane voltage (MSORTV) suggests propagation delays at the junctional sites between cells. Biol Bull Mar Biol Lab 183: 342–343

Rosenbaum S, Jalife J (2001) (eds) Optical mapping of cardiac excitation and arrhythmias. Futura Publishing, New York

Rudy Y, Quan W (1991) Propagation delays across cardiac gap junctions and their reflection in extracellular potentials: A simulation study. J Cardiovasc Electronphysiol 2: 299–315

Salama G, Lombardi R, Elson J (1987) Maps of optical action potentials and NADH fluorescence in intact working hearts. Am J Physiol 252: H384–H394

Schaffer P, Ahammer H, Müller W et al. (1994) Di-4-ANEPPS causes photodynamic damage to isolated cardiomyocytes. Pfluegers Arch 426: 548–551

Spach MS, Dolber PC (1986) Relating extracellular potentials and their derivatives to anisotropic propagation at a microscopic level in human cardiac muscle. Evidence for electrical uncoupling of side-to-side fiber connections with increasing age. Circ Res 58: 356–371

Windisch H, Müller W, Tritthart HA (1987) A new method to overcome motion induced distortions in optically detected cardiac action potentials. 13th Canadian Medical and Biological Engineering Conference, Halifax, p 235–236

Windisch H (2001) Optical mapping of impulse propagation within cardiomyocytes. In: Rosenbaum S, Jalife J (eds) Optical mapping of cardiac excitation and arrhythmias. Futura Publishing, New York, pp 97–112

Recording Action Potentials Using Voltage-Sensitive Dyes

Vladimir G. Fast

Introduction

Synchronous contraction of the heart depends on regular propagation of the electrical impulse, which is maintained by generation of cellular action potentials and by flow of local electrical currents between excited and resting cells (Kleber et al. 2001). Alterations in the normal pattern of propagation lead to arrhythmias and loss of contractile function. Understanding the mechanisms of these arrhythmias has relied on visualization of activation spread using mapping techniques that involve measurements of electrophysiological parameters at multiple sites and reconstruction of their distribution patterns. Two main cardiac mapping methods are currently used.

The first mapping method introduced almost a hundred years ago and perfected in the last quarter of the 20th century involves registration of extracellular potentials using arrays of metal electrodes (Frazier et al. 1988). The main application of this method is measurement of local activation times and reconstruction of the activation sequence. In addition, it is used to measure distributions of extracellular potentials during application of defibrillation shocks (Wharton et al. 1992). Although there were attempts to extend this technique to mapping transmembrane potentials (V_m) using arrays of microelectrodes or suction electrodes, simultaneous registration of action potentials from more than several points proved to be difficult. For these reasons, more recent attempts to map transmembrane potential concentrated on optical approaches.

Optical mapping is based on staining cardiac tissue with voltage-sensitive dyes and registration of changes in optical dye properties using photodetectors. One of the important advantages of this approach is that it allows simultaneous non-contact registration of action potentials from multiple closely adjacent sites. In this way, patterns of repolarization can be monitored in addition to patterns of activation. The ability of optical mapping to report V_m changes is especially advantageous for studies of defibrillation where conventional electrical recordings are hampered by shock-induced artefacts.

Description of Methods and Practical Approach

Tissue Preparations

Optical mapping has been used to study cardiac excitation in a variety of preparations including whole hearts, isolated tissue preparations, cell cultures and single myocytes (Rosenbaum and Jalife 2001). Because blood strongly absorbs and scatters visible light, preparations are typically perfused or superfused with physiological solutions. The repolarization phase of optical action potentials is often distorted by motion artefacts caused by muscle contractions. If contractions are weak, tissue can be restrained mechanically (Choi et al. 2002; Girouard et al. 1996). More often, chemical agents that inhibit contractions are used. The most common agent is an electromechanical uncoupler 2,3-butanedione monoxime (BDM, Sigma), which reversibly inhibits contractions at a concentration of 15–20 mmol/L by blocking myosin ATPase activity and cross-bridge formation. It is known that BDM alters excitable properties of cardiac tissue (Selin and McArdle 1994), which should be taken into account in interpretation of experimental data. Another agent used in mapping studies is cytochalasin D (Sigma), an inhibitor of actin polymerization, which is effective at a concentration of 10–20 µmol/L (Wu et al. 1998). The effects of this drug are irreversible, it is toxic and should be handled with special care. The relative effects of two contraction inhibitors on excitable tissue properties are probably species-dependent. In canine cardiac preparations, it was reported that cytochalasin D affected excitable properties less than BDM (Biermann et al. 1998). In pig hearts, however, cytochalasin D was found to have stronger effects than BDM (Quin et al. 2003).

Voltage-Sensitive Dye Staining

Voltage-sensitive dyes bind to the cell membrane. Their optical properties such as light absorption or fluorescence are changed when membrane potential is altered. The fluorescent dyes are by far the most sensitive sensors of V_m, providing the highest signal-to-noise ratio (S/N). These dyes are very fast, responding to V_m changes with microsecond resolution, and linear within a range of at least ±400 mV. Direct comparison between optical traces and action potentials measured by intracellular micro-pipettes demonstrated that the shape of optical action potential upstrokes followed electrical traces with high precision (Fig. 1b; Fast and Kleber 1993).

Approximately ten fluorescent V_m-sensitive dyes are currently commercially available, mainly from Molecular Probes Inc. (Eugene, OR). In cardiac mapping, the two most popular dyes are di-4-ANEPPS and RH-237. Another dye, di-8-ANEPPS, which is a more lipophilic analog of di-4-ANEPPS, provides more stable optical recordings but it is more difficult to load and its application is limited to single cells and cell cultures.

Spectral properties of V_m-sensitive dyes strongly depend on the environment. When bound to a phospholipid bilayer membrane, di-4-ANEPPS has maximal absorption and emission at approximately 480 nm and 630 nm, respectively. For RH-237 dissolved in DMSO, the respective values are ~550 nm and ~800 nm (Fast and Ideker

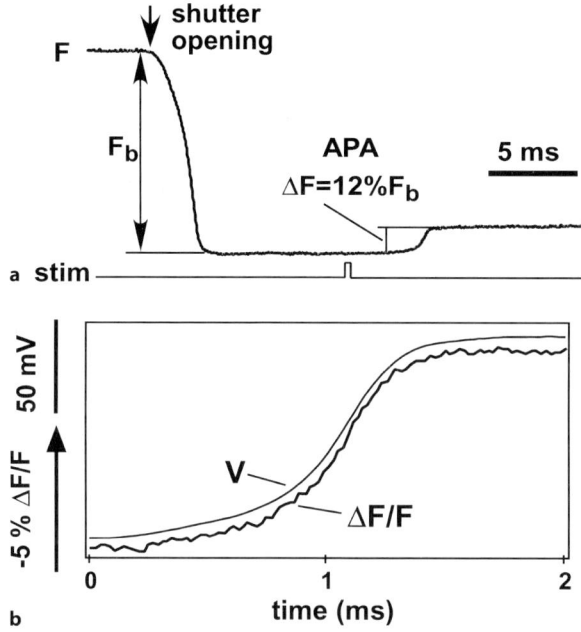

Figure 1a,b
a Optical recording of membrane potential using a voltage-sensitive dye. The recording was obtained using a photodiode in a cultured cell monolayer stained with dye RH-237. The first negative deflection of the signal corresponds to the opening of a shutter and start of illumination; the second deflection represents the upstroke of an action potential evoked by a stimulation pulse. The fractional change of fluorescence associated with the action potential was about 12% of the background level. (Reproduced with permission from (Fast et al. 1996). b Comparison of optical ($\Delta F/F$) and electrical recordings (V) of membrane potential obtained from closely adjacent membrane sites in a cultured myocyte. (Reproduced with permission from Fast and Kleber 1993).

2000); these wavelengths are expected to be shorter in a lipid membrane. Both dyes have broad absorption and emission spectra with a width at half-maximum of approximately 100 nm. They have similar levels of emitted fluorescence when excited near their absorption peaks, as well as similar levels of phototoxicity and photobleaching. Both dyes emit a significant amount of background fluorescence, which is insensitive to V_m. Figure 1a displays a fluorescent signal measured using the dye RH-237 in a cultured cell monolayer. The large negative deflection at the start of illumination corresponds to the background fluorescence. The next positive deflection corresponds to the upstroke of an action potential initiated by a stimulation pulse. The fractional change of fluorescence given by the ratio of the action potential amplitude and the background fluorescence depends on the preparation type as well as on the time elapsed after staining. The fractional change is the largest in isolated cells and cell cultures where it can reach 15% immediately after staining. It is smaller in the intact myocardium, about 5%, probably due to the contribution of non-myocyte cells to background fluorescence.

Di-4-ANEPPS and RH-237 are only weakly soluble in water and should be dissolved in an organic solvent such as ethanol or DMSO (dimethyl sulfoxide). It is convenient to prepare a 2–5 mmol/L stock solution of dye in DMSO in advance and store it in a deep freezer (–20 °C). In these conditions, the dissolved dye can be kept for at least 6 months without loosing its potency. Immediately before an experiment, the stock solution is thawed and dissolved in the perfusion solution at a concentration determined by the method of staining.

There are three main methods for dye staining:
1. by bolus injection,
2. by slow coronary perfusion and
3. by superfusion.

The first two methods are employed in experiments where a whole heart or an isolated tissue preparation is perfused through a coronary artery. In the bolus injection method, stock solution is dissolved to a concentration of 10–20 µmol/L and 2–4 ml of this solution are injected directly into the perfusion system, most often into the bubble trap. The dye solution should be filtered to avoid blockage of capillaries with small non-dissolved particles. This method is very quick, once the dye solution has passed through the heart, it is ready for optical measurements. In the coronary perfusion method, a lower-concentration (1–3 µmol/L) dye solution is perfused through the heart for 5–10 min.

In the third method, the dye is added to the superfusion solution at a higher concentration (up to 20 µmol/L) and staining lasts longer (up to 30 min) to allow for dye diffusion across the tissue surface.

After staining, dye molecules gradually leak out of the cell membrane into extracellular and intracellular spaces. In addition, membrane-bound dye molecules reorient themselves inside the membrane. Because of these effects, the total fluorescence level and the fractional V_m-sensitive change are reduced during the course of an experiment causing a decrease in the amplitude of optical signals at a rate of about 50% per hour (Fast and Ideker 2000). To offset this decrease, periodic additional dye staining or a continuous dye infusion at sub-micromolar concentrations can be performed.

In studies on cell cultures or isolated cells, staining by di-4-ANNEPS and RH-237 is easily achieved by superfusion with dye solution at a concentration of 2–4 µmol/L for 3–5 min. When di-8-ANEPPS is used, dye concentration should be higher, 80–150 µmol/L, and staining should last longer, 10–20 min.

To aid solubilization of the dye, Pluronic F-127 (Molecular Probes Inc.) should be added to the staining solution at a 0.05% concentration and the solution should be sonicated.

Optical Mapping System

Figure 2a shows the structure of a conventional optical mapping setup. The main elements of the setup are a light source, a set of optical filters, focusing optics, a photodetector with accompanying signal conditioning equipment and a specialized data acquisition hardware and software. Complete optical systems suitable for V_m-sensitive measurements in the heart are not commercially available. Therefore, all existing systems are custom built.

The main objective in designing such systems is to achieve the highest possible S/N while minimizing the adverse effects of optical measurements such as photobleaching and phototoxicity. Factors determining these parameters are considered below.

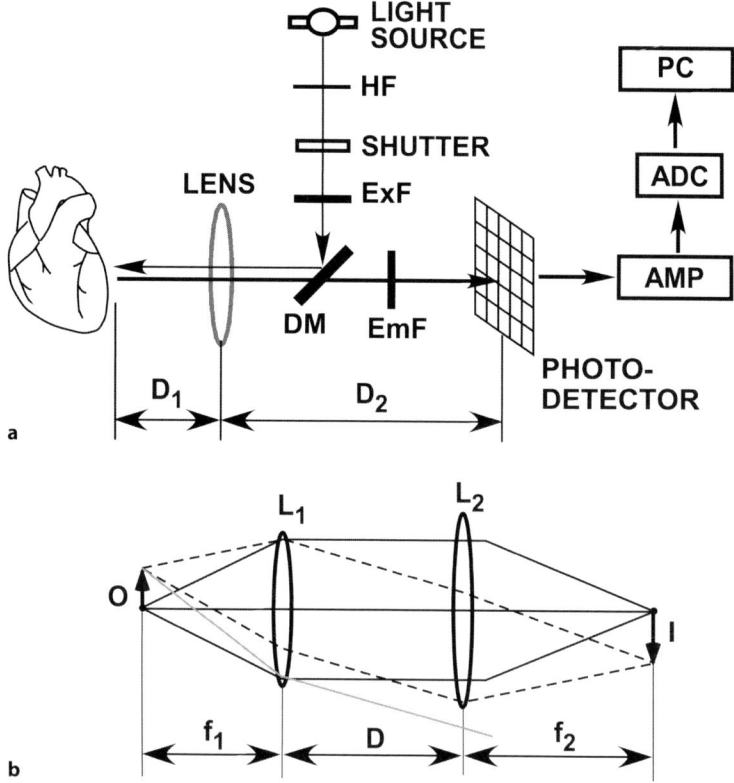

Figure 2a,b
a Schematic diagram of an optical mapping system. *HF* heat filter; *ExF* excitation filter; *DM* dichroic mirror; *EmF* emission filter; *AMP* amplifiers; *ADC* analog-to-digital converters. b Tandem lens configuration. *O* object; *I* image. Optical magnification is defined by the ratio of focal lengths of two lenses (f_2/f_1) and is not dependent on the lens separation, *D* Loss of marginal light rays (bottom dashed line) leads to vignetting

Signal-to-Noise Ratio

In cardiac mapping, the reference signal magnitude (S) is typically defined as the amplitude of optical action potential (APA). As mentioned above, it is proportional to the level of background fluorescence (F_b), APA = kF_b, where k is a fractional fluorescence change of about 5–15%. Signal noise has two main components, the noise of the fluorescent light (N_s) and the noise of the detection system (N_d). Since two sources of noise are independent, the total noise (rms) is given by

$$N = \sqrt{(N_s^2 + N_d^2)}$$

Assuming that emitted light has no periodic components due to, e.g. 60 Hz ripple, then N_s is determined by the "shot" noise, which is caused by statistical fluctuations in the photon flux.

For a given bandwidth, the shot noise is proportional to the square root of fluorescence intensity, which approximately equals

$$N_s = c\sqrt{F_b}$$

Thus, the total noise is

$$N = \sqrt{(c^2 F_b + N_d^2)} \quad \text{and} \quad \frac{S}{N} = \frac{kF_b}{\sqrt{(c^2 F_b + N_d^2)}}$$

Both shot noise and detector noise are proportional to the square root of the signal bandwidth, B. Therefore,

$$\frac{S}{N} \sim \frac{1}{\sqrt{B}}$$

The relationship for S/N can be simplified in two opposite situations:

1. when the shot noise is significantly larger than the detector noise (by a factor of 2 or more, $N_s > \sim 2N_d$), then S/N is proportional to the square-root of background fluorescence,

$$\frac{S}{N} = b\sqrt{F_b}$$

where b is a constant proportional to the fractional fluorescence change k;

2. when the detector noise is predominant ($N_d >\sim 2N_s$), S/N is proportional to F_b and inversely proportional to the detector noise,

$$S/N = kF_b/N_d.$$

For both cases, S/N is also scaled by $\frac{1}{\sqrt{B}}$

These relationships determine fundamental limits for signal quality. Signal quality is degraded if the excitation light contains additional noise besides the shot noise, for instance 60 Hz ripple.

Considerations given above suggest the following ways for improving the signal quality.
- Decreasing the noise of the light source up to the shot noise limit and decreasing the detector noise below the shot noise.
- Increasing the fluorescence intensity. This is achieved primarily by increasing the illumination intensity. It should be remembered, however, that this enhances adverse effects such as dye photobleaching and phototoxicity that limit the duration of optical recordings.
- Decreasing the recording bandwidth. Achieving these goals is the main task in designing an optical mapping system.

Light Source

Light source is one of the most important elements affecting signal quality in an optical system. Three types of light sources are currently used in optical mapping: tungsten-halogen lamps, short arc lamps and lasers. The light source should be selected according to the preparation type, the size of the imaging area, the desired signal-to-nose ratio and the cost.

Tungsten-Halogen Lamps. Tungsten-halogen (TH) lamps with a power of 100 or 250 W are the most common light sources. They have a moderate light intensity and a flat spectrum in the visible range providing a flexibility in choosing excitation wavelength. The 250 W bulb filament has dimensions of 7 by 3.5 mm, which makes it suitable for illumination of medium-sized preparations such as rabbit hearts (the filament image has to be de-focused on the preparation). Stronger TH lamps are available (up to 1000 W) but because of much larger filament dimensions, they provide insufficient illumination density. The TH bulbs have a long life-time, low cost and low noise level. In combination with a stabilized and relatively inexpensive (about $ 4000.–) DC power supply it is possible to achieve noise levels of ~0.01% rms (Table 1). Due to these characteristics, a TH lamp should be considered a first choice in a typical optical mapping application.

Arc Lamps. When the light intensity provided by a TH lamp is not sufficient, one of the arc lamps can be considered, a Xenon (Xe), a Mercury (Hg) or a mixed Hg/Xe lamp. Similar to a TH lamp, the Xe lamp has flat spectrum in the visible range. Most common Xe lamps used in optical mapping have power of 150 and 250 W. The Hg lamp has a line spectrum with two very bright lines at 540 and 580 nm making it the strongest lamp for exciting Vm-sensitive dye RH-237. Either 100 W or 200 W lamps of this type are typically used. The Hg/Xe lamp has the same spectrum as the Hg lamp but it is more stable and has a longer life-time. Both Xe and Hg lamps have relatively small arc dimensions, which makes them suitable for imaging small or medium-sized

Table 1
Noise characteristics of light sources

Light Source	Maximal Power	N_{1rms}	N_{2rms}
Tungsten-Halogen	250 W[a]	0.013%	0.010%
Xenon	150 W	0.015%	0.014%
Xenon	250 W	0.036%	0.034%
Mercury	100 W[b]	0.017%	0.016%
Mercury/Xenon	200 W	0.023%	0.020%

The Tungsten-Halogen lamp was tested with lamphouse 66181 and power supply 68831 from Oriel (Stratford, CT). All other lamps were tested with lamphouse 770U and power supply 1600 from Opti-Quip (Highland Mills, NY). N_{1rms} was measured using a photodiode and a digital Tektronix oscilloscope at a bandwidth of 10–20 MHz. N_{2rms} was measured using a photodiode and a data acquisition system described in Section 2 at a bandwidth of 0.02–2 kHz and a sampling rate of 4 kHz. [a]The actual power was set to 200 W. [b]Recordings with occasional spikes were excluded.

preparations. In general, arc lamps are more noisy than TH lamps but in combination with a high-quality stabilized DC power supply they can achieve comparable noise levels (see Table 1).

Lasers. The third type of light source is a laser that emits light at discreet wavelengths. There are several powerful lasers with emission lines at 488, 514 and 532 nm that can be used for exciting di-4-ANEPPS and RH-237. Among all light sources, lasers generate the highest illumination intensity. However, they typically have a significantly larger noise. Therefore, an increase in the light intensity causes a proportional increase in the noise level without improvement in the S/N. An exception is a new Verdi laser from Coherent Inc. (Santa Clara, CA). This is all-solid-state, diode-pumped, frequency-doubled Nd:YVO$_4$ laser providing single-frequency output at 532 nm with adjustable power of up to 6 W. The specified noise level of this laser is 0.02% rms, which is comparable with the best TH or arc lamps. Its disadvantage is a much higher cost ($ 55,000.–).

Exposure to strong light can cause dye bleaching and photodynamic tissue damage (phototoxicity). To minimize these effects, the duration of illumination should be limited to a necessary minimum. This is achieved by using an electromechanical shutter synchronized with the start of data acquisition. Shutters with different aperture diameters are available, which should be chosen according to the diameter of illumination beam. In a typical macroscopic application, a shutter with 35 mm aperture (Vincent Associates, Rochester, NY) can be used. For microscopic mapping, a lighter and faster 25 mm shutter is sufficient. If either a TH or an arc lamp is used as the light source, shutter blades will be exposed to intense heat radiated by the lamp, which can cause shutter malfunction. To prevent that, shutter blades should be made from a reflective material and a heat filter should be placed in front of the shutter.

Optical Filters

A typical optical mapping setup has at least two optical filters (Fig. 2b): an excitation filter (ExF) and an emission filter (EmF). The excitation filter serves to select the portion of light spectrum which is the most efficient for excitation of a V_m-sensitive dye. This filter is not necessary if a laser is used for illumination. The purpose of the emission filter is to separate the emitted fluorescence from the excitation light reflected on the heart surface, which is much brighter than the fluorescent light.

In addition to excitation and emission filters, a dichroic mirror (DM) can be used, which reflects a shorter-wavelength excitation light onto the preparation and transmits a longer-wavelength emission light to the photodetector. Using a DM allows excitation and emission beams to be sent along the same path with the same focusing optics, which improves illumination intensity and uniformity and enhances light collecting efficiency. An optical system incorporating a dichroic mirror is called "epi-fluorescent".

Filter characteristics are selected to match spectral properties of a V_m-sensitive dye. For di-4-ANEPPS, an excitation filter should be a band-pass filter centered near 500 nm with a width at half-maximum of approximately 50 nm (500/50 nm). The emission filter can be a long-pass filter with a cut-off wavelength of ≈620 nm. The dichroic mirror should have a cut-off wavelength somewhere in the middle, e.g. at 590 nm. For dye RH-237, the most efficient excitation is achieved using a band-pass filter at ≈540/50 nm, emission should be measured with a long-pass filter at >650 nm and the dichroic mirror can have a cut-off at ≈610 nm.

Both color-glass and interference filters can be used as EmF and ExF. The interference filters are more expensive but they provide sharper cut-offs, higher maximal light transmission and greater flexibility in choosing the transmission spectra. High-quality interference filters with desired spectral properties are supplied by Chroma Technology Corp. (Brattleboro, VT) and Omega Optical Inc. (Brattleboro, VT).

Focusing Optics

The purpose of the focusing optics is to project the excitation light onto a preparation as well as to collect and focus the emitted fluorescence on a photodetector. In an epi-fluorescent system, the same objective lens serves both purposes (Fig. 2). The preparation is placed at a certain distance D_1 from the lens and a photodetector is placed at a distance D_2 where the image is formed. D_1 and D_2 are determined by the lens focal length and desired optical magnification. Depending on optical magnification, lenses of three types can be used: microscope lenses, photographic 35 mm lenses and video lenses. The most important parameter of an objective lens is its numerical aperture (NA), which in photographic and video lenses is given by the stop F-number, which is equal to ≈1/(2NA). The number of photons collected by a lens is proportional to the square of NA. Because in an epi-fluorescent system both excitation and emission light pass through the same lens, the intensity of light reaching the photodetector is proportional to the fourth power of NA. Therefore, a lens with the highest numerical aperture (smallest F-number) should be used. For optical magnifications of 5× or higher, microscope lenses provide the best light collection efficiency (NA = 0.25–1.3). At these magnifications, it is convenient to employ a commercial microscope, which provides image-forming capabilities on a precise and rugged platform.

Although there are microscope lenses with optical magnifications of less than 5×, their NA is too low for V_m-sensitive recordings. At such magnifications, photographic or video-lenses provide much better light collection efficiency. The choice between the two depends on the size of a photodetector. Photographic lenses create a bigger image and are more suitable for large-area photodetectors such as photodiode arrays (dimensions of approximately 18×18 mm^2) whereas video lenses are used with video cameras (≈5×5 mm^2 or less). A wide range of lenses of both types is commercially available. The most popular photographic lenses used in optical mapping are 50 mm F/1.2 (NA = 0.42) or F/1.4 (NA = 0.36) and 85 mm F/1.4 or F/1.8 (Nikon or Pentax). Video-lenses can have F-number of up to 0.8, as in the 25 mm lens from Fujinon (F/0.85, NA = 0.58). To assemble a macroscopic optical setup and to precisely align its different components, it is convenient to use an optical bread-board, optical rails and other mounting equipment available from several manufacturers including Oriel (Stratford, CT) and Edmund Industrial Optics (Barrington, NJ)

The single-lens design described above is simple and convenient in providing the flexibility of gradual change of optical magnification. However, it might not be the most efficient for light collection and, because all distances are fixed, it places constraints on the inclusion of additional optical elements such as mirrors, beamsplitters or dichroic mirrors. These obstacles can be overcome by using the tandem-lens design (Laurita and Libbus 2001; Ratzlaff and Grinvald 1991). In such a system, two infinity-focused photographic lenses are placed face-to-face (Fig. 2b). The preparation is placed at the back-focal plane of the primary lens (L_1). Light emitted from a specimen is collected by this lens and formed into a parallel beam. The secondary lens (L_2) focuses this beam at its focal plane where a photodetector is placed. Optical magnification is given by the ratio of focal lengths of the two lenses, $M = f_2/f_1$. Changing magnification requires swapping one of the two lenses. It should be mentioned that this tandem-lens design is employed in all modern high-quality fluorescent microscopes where it is called "infinity corrected optics". The main advantage of this design is that magnification is not dependent on the distance (D) between the two lenses. Therefore, lenses can be moved apart to accommodate additional filters or dichroic mirrors allowing dual-wavelength recordings such as ratiometric V_m or simultaneous V_m and Ca_i^{2+} measurements. There are limitations, however, on how far apart the two lenses can be separated. Light coming from the edges of the object is collimated by the primary lens into a flux of parallel rays that propagate at an angle to the main optical axis (dashed lines in Fig. 2b). If the distance D is too large, some of the peripheral rays will not be captured by the secondary lens, which will lead to darkening of the image at the edges or, in extreme cases, a completely dark image; this effect is called "vignetting". Vignetting can be reduced by using a secondary lens with a larger entrance pupil diameter. It is difficult to predict the amount of vignetting for a particular lens combination and the distance between them; this should be established by trial and error.

Photodetectors, Conditioning Electronics and Data Acquisition Hardware

Presently, two types of photodetectors are the most common in optical mapping systems: photodiode arrays and CCD cameras. Photodetectors of both types consist of 2-dimensional arrays of silicon elements that transduce the energy of light photons into the energy of electrical charges.

Photodiode Arrays. In a photodiode, photogenerated charges immediately flow into an electrical circuit creating current with a strength proportional to the intensity of the incident light. The efficiency of conversion of photons to electrical current (quantum efficiency) by photodiodes at a wavelength of 600 nm, which is typical for optical mapping, is very high, about 90%. The photocurrent is converted to voltage by means of a current-to-voltage (I/V) converter. In the photodiode arrays (PDAs) used in mapping systems, each photodiode is individually wired to a separate I/V converter, which places constraints on the total number of photodiodes. As a result, although some experimental photodiode arrays can have as many as 50×50 elements, more common are arrays with several hundred photodiodes. These arrays can be made on a single piece of silicon or they can be assembled from separate photodiodes that are coupled by optical fibers.

The first single-chip 2-dimensional PDAs used for optical mapping were 10×10 and 12×12-element arrays from Centronic Ltd. (England). At the present time, one of the most popular PDAs is a 16×16-element array from Hamamatsu Photonics Corp.

(Japan), which is supplied with integrated I/V converters. Individual diodes in this array have dimensions of 0.95×0.95 mm^2; the center-to-center interdiode distance is 1.1 mm and the total array dimensions are 17.45×17.45 mm^2.

An I/V converter in the Hamamatsu array consists of an operational amplifier with a large feedback resistor in parallel with a capacitor (Fig. 3). The larger the feedback resistor, the higher the amplifier gain and the smaller the amplifier bandwidth. The array is available with a choice of three feedback resistors: 10, 50 and 100 MΩ. The corresponding bandwidth values are DC-10 kHz, DC-3 kHz and DC-1 kHz. Whereas it is possible to use the lower-gain I/V converters with additional amplification and filtration at later stages, it is generally advantageous to have the highest gain as close to the signal source as possible in order to achieve the best S/N. Taking into account that 1 kHz bandwidth is sufficient for faithful reproduction of action potentials in a majority of applications, the array with 100 MΩ feedback resistors is considered to be the best option. It should be noted that, whereas the signal frequency content is limited by the bandwidth specified above, the dark current noise has a much broader spectrum. This is because a portion of the dark noise is determined by the operational amplifier itself, which is not limited by the signal bandwidth. Therefore, in applications with relatively small signals where the dark noise is dominant, signals should be additionally low-pass filtered before digitizing to avoid aliasing (see below). The magnitude of the peak-to-peak dark current noise of the Hamamatsu array (100 MΩ feedback resistors) is approximately 0.8 mV and the corresponding rms value is ≈0.13 mV when measured with a bandwidth of 2 kHz at a sampling rate of 8 kHz. A two-fold lower noise was measured under similar conditions from a single photodiode (Hamamatsu) in combination with a custom-made I/V converter made from a low-noise operational amplifier OPA121 (Burr-Brown) and a 100 MΩ feedback resistor. This indicates that there is a room for significant improvements in the noise level of a PDA-based system using custom-made I/V converters.

Signal magnitude at the output of an I/V converter representing a typical action potential amplitude is on the order of 10 mV. This is comparable with the noise of a standard 12-bit analog-to-digital conversion (ADC) device. Therefore, signals need additional amplification by a factor of approximately 100 before digitizing. This is accomplished in second-stage amplifiers. Because the useful signal represents only a small fraction (5–15%) of the background fluorescence, amplification of the whole recording would saturate the ADC device. To avoid that, the second-stage amplifiers should include circuitry for subtraction of the background portion of signals before amplification. The subtracted and amplified signals should then be passed through anti-aliasing low-pass filters.

The second-stage amplifiers are typically custom made, which can take a large portion of the total development time. Recently, Dr. V. Fast and Dr. I. Efimov in collaboration with Innovative Technologies Inc. (Germantown, MD) developed amplifiers that are now available from Innovative Technologies. The amplifier circuit is schematically shown in Figure 3. The first stage of these amplifiers is a high-pass filter, which provides a choice between DC coupling (no filtration) and AC coupling with one out of three time constants: ≈20 sec (0.05 Hz), ≈3 sec (0.3 Hz) and <1 ms. Immediately after the start of illumination, the filter time constant is set to the lowest value causing a rapid (within 10 ms) drop of the signal to zero and, therefore, subtrac-

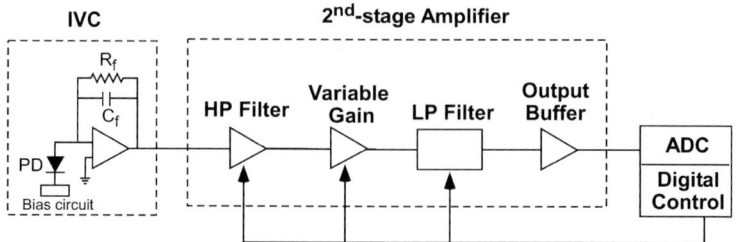

Figure 3
Schematic diagram of two stages of signal amplification in an optical system with a Hamamatsu photodiode array. *PD* photodiode; *IVC* current-to-voltage converter; R_f and C_f feedback resistance and capacitance; *HP* high-pass filter; *LP* low-pass filter; *ADC* analog-to-digital converter

tion of the background fluorescence. After subtraction, the time constant is set to a larger value (typically 20 sec) allowing the maintenance of a stable signal level. After that, signals are amplified with a gain of either 1, 10, 50 or 100. Amplified signals are passed through low-pass 4th order Bessel filters with continuously variable cut-off frequency. Because of the relatively slow roll-off of Bessel filters, the cut-off frequency should be at least 4 times lower than the sampling frequency to avoid aliasing. The last stage is a buffer amplifier whose purpose is to match impedances with the input amplifier of an ADC device. The amplifiers are assembled on printed-circuit boards with 64 channels per board that fit into a standard 6U rack. The input connectors on amplifier boards accept cables from the Hamamatsu array. Boards also provide DC power for the Hamamatsu array.

Signal sampling is performed by multi-channel ADC cards. The cards should be chosen according to a desired number of channels and sampling rate. In addition, the possibility of inter-channel multiplexing cross-talk should be considered. The multiplexing cross-talk may arise if the impedance of the input amplifier in the ADC card doesn't match the output impedance of the second-stage amplifier. This was the case for a combination of second-stage amplifiers from Argo Transdata Corp. (Clinton, CT) with the data acquisition cards from Microstar Laboratories Inc. (Bellevue, WA) (Fast and Kleber 2003).

Although the amplifier boards from Innovative Technologies can be interfaced with different data acquisition cards, they were specifically designed for two multifunction ADC cards, PCI-6071 E and PCI-6031 E from National Instruments Inc. (Austin, TX). Both cards have 64 analog input channels as well as digital, counter and analog output channels. The first card (PCI-6071 E) has a 12-bit resolution and a maximal aggregate sampling rate of 1.25 MHz, which translates into ≈19.5 kHz/channel. The second card (PCI-6031 E) has a higher resolution, 16 bit, but a lower sampling rate, 100 kHz (≈1.56 kHz/channel). Both cards are connector-compatible with the amplifier boards. The digital lines on the ADC cards can be used to control via software all amplifier settings including selection of time constants in high-pass filters, gains and cut-off frequency in low-pass filters. Extensive testing indicated that the inter-channel multiplexing cross-talk is negligible at sampling rates of up to ≈15 kHz/channel.

A total of four ADC cards is necessary for recording from one PDA, which requires four free PCI computer slots. Computers with up to five free PCI slots are available from major PC vendors. If more slots are needed, a 7-slot or 13-slot PCI expansion chassis (SBS Technologies Inc., St Paul, MN) can be used.

Alternatively, PXI analogs of the two ADC cards, PXI-6071 E and PXI-6031 E, can be used in a PXI chassis (National Instruments). The cost of the optical system including a Hamamatsu array, a set of second-stage amplifiers and data acquisition cards is approximately $ 30,000.

An array made from separate photodiodes coupled by optical fibers became recently available from RedShirtImaging (Fairfield, CT). It consists of 469 diodes coupled to optical fibers with a diameter of 0.75 mm that form a hexagonal bundle with a diameter of 20 mm at the image plane. The array is integrated in one box with I/V converters, second-stage amplifiers and a multiplexer. The I/V converter has a selectable feedback resistor of 5, 50 or 500 MΩ. The second-stage amplifiers provide gains of 1, 10, 50 and 500, fixed low-pass filtration at 0.8 kHz and a high-pass filter with a choice of time constants of 200 ms or 2 s. The array is interfaced with a 12-bit ADC card from Microstar Laboratories, Inc. (Bellevue, WA). The maximal sampling rate is 1.6 kHz/channel. The total cost of the array, amplifiers and the ADC card is approximately $ 67,000.

CCD Cameras. In a CCD ("charge coupled device") camera, photogenerated charges are integrated and stored locally in CCD elements for a certain period of time. After the integration time, the same CCD elements also serve as pipelines to transmit charges to a read-out amplifier, where they are sequentially converted to voltages and then digitized by a frame-grabber card. Typically, one read-out amplifier is used for the whole CCD array, which allows manufacturing arrays with a large number, up to several millions, of small (5–20 µm) photosensitive elements. CCD arrays are in the core of modern consumer video-cameras and they are used extensively in research cameras. As a result, a broad range of cameras and frame-grabbers is commercially available, which makes development of a CCD-based mapping system significantly faster than that of a PDA-based system. Quantum efficiency of the best CCD chips approaches 80%, which is comparable to photodiodes. The maximal amount of charge accumulated in individual pixel is limited by the CCD "full well capacity", which determines the camera saturation level and camera dynamic range (ratio between saturation level and noise level).

A standard CCD video-camera has 640×480 pixels, 30 frames/sec sampling rate and 8-bit resolution. Although such cameras were used in the early mapping studies, their grey-scale resolution and frame rate were too low for anything else besides a very rough mapping of activation spread. Both the resolution and the frame rate have to be substantially better for adequate monitoring of activation spread and especially for accurate recording of the action potential waveforms. This can be achieved in two ways: by increasing the data throughput rate and by recording from a smaller number of pixels.

The fastest cameras with a single read-out amplifier presently have a throughput rate about twice as high as standard cameras. Therefore, the main gains in speed and quality of video-recording come from reducing the number of pixels.

The minimal requirements for mapping activation spread are a 12-bit resolution and a frame rate of 100 frames/sec. To follow the time course of action potentials, the frame rate should be much higher, at least 1000 frames/sec. Video-cameras normally do not provide background subtraction before digitizing, as described above for the PDA-based systems. Therefore, to bring the ADC noise to an undetectable level, video-recording should have a 16-bit resolution. Cameras combining such speed and resolution are not currently available. One of the most advanced CCD cameras that approaches these requirements is a 14-bit camera with 80×80 pixels and a frame rate of 2000 frames/sec from RedShirtImaging (Fairfield, CT). The camera frame rate can be increased by decreasing the number of pixels or by reading from several pixels at once (binning). In a 3×3 binning mode (26×26 elements), this camera can run at 5000 frames/sec. Together with a frame-grabber this camera costs about $ 55,000.

Comparison between Photodiode Arrays and CCD Cameras. When comparing CCD cameras with photodiode arrays it is often noted that the former has higher spatial resolution whereas the latter has higher temporal resolution. This distinction is true with regard to standard video-cameras but it becomes blurred for specialized cameras which, with reduced number of pixels, can acquire data as fast as PDAs.

Besides speed and spatial resolution, the next most important parameter is signal quality, indicated by the S/N. Because of similar quantum efficiencies, signal amplitudes measured by CCD elements and photodiodes of the same dimensions would be nearly equal. With regard to the signal noise, two different situations should be considered:
1. when signal noise is dominated by the detector noise and
2. when it is dominated by the shot noise of the fluorescent light.

When the level of background fluorescence is relatively low, the signal noise is defined by the detector noise, which consists of thermal noise in the optical sensor itself and the noise of the accompanying electronics. Because photodiodes and CCDs employ the same photodetection principle, their thermal noise levels should be similar. The main difference between them is in how they process the photogenerated charges. In a CCD camera, charges from multiple elements are transferred along the same path. The transfer rate has to be very high to move all the charges between successive frames.

At such transfer rates errors can occur, hence increased noise. In addition, when charges arrive to the output of a CCD chip they are converted to voltages by a single read-out amplifier. To switch rapidly between sequential readings, the read-out amplifier must have a very small settling time and, therefore, a very wide bandwidth. The wider the bandwidth, the higher the noise level. The transfer noise and the amplifier noise together constitute so called read-out noise, which is the dominant noise in CCD cameras at standard video rates or higher. The read-out noise can only be reduced by slowing data transfer, which is achieved by decreasing number of pixels, reducing frame rate or both. This principle is employed in so called "slow-scan" cooled cameras that have very low noise

In contrast to CCD arrays, every element in a photodiode array has a direct connection to its own amplifier whose bandwidth can be adjusted to accommodate the frequency content of the recorded signal. Therefore, with all other conditions being equal, the detector noise of an optimized photodiode array is expected to be smaller than that of a CCD making the PDA a better choice for detector-noise limited applications. Taking into account that achieving a high level of emitted fluorescence is often difficult or, because of concomitant increase in phototoxicity and photobleaching, undesirable, cardiac mapping applications often fall into this category.

In the shot-noise limited applications with high intensities of emitted fluorescence, the detector noise is irrelevant and both PDAs and CCDs are expected to provide similar S/N. However, the range of light intensities where this requirement is fulfilled is expected to be smaller for CCDs in comparison to PDAs because of the lower CCD saturation level, which is limited by the CCD full-well capacity.

Thus, with all other conditions being equal, photodiode-based systems are expected to have a better S/N over a wide range of light intensities than CCD cameras. This makes photodiodes a better choice for applications where the fidelity of optical action potentials is critical. This requirement is less important for measuring patterns of activation spread. Also, measurements of this type can be carried out at a lower frame rate than the one necessary for action potential recordings. In such applications, a higher number of pixels and lower development time of CCD-based systems can make them a better choice.

Signal Analysis

Noise Removal

Optical signals typically exhibit a significant amount of high-frequency noise, especially in applications with low light levels. Although this noise can be decreased by anti-aliasing analog filters in second-stage amplifiers, the required signal bandwidth might not be known *a priori*. In addition, analog filtration is not the most efficient way for noise removal. Much better filters can be implemented in software and there is a flexibility of choosing optimal cut-off frequency suited for a particular signal. Therefore, it is often beneficial to record optical signals with a wider bandwidth and remove the extra noise later using a digital filter. Digital filters are provided by commercial software packages such as LabView (National Instruments Inc.) or MatLab (The MathWorks Inc, Natick, MA) or they can be relatively easily implemented in custom-made software. Because optical signals measured from the heart can have sharp fronts, filters with smooth, non-ringing step response should be used, such as moving average, Gaussian or Blackman filters.

Correction for Photobleaching

Photobleaching of a voltage-sensitive dye causes a reduction of fluorescence intensity seen as a drift of optical signals. When there is a significant amount of photobleaching, a correction algorithm can be employed to remove the drift. It should be remembered that, in general, photobleaching is an exponential process. Thus, its correction involves fitting a portion of a signal between action potentials with an exponential curve and a following subtraction of the fitted curve from the original signal. Because photobleaching rate can vary across a preparation, fitting curves should be calculated for each measuring spot independently. Signal noise strongly affects calculation of local photobleaching rates. Therefore, fitting should be carried out after signal filtration and it should employ a non-linear least-square fitting procedure. The correction procedure can be simplified for short recordings with a small degree of photobleaching, which can be approximated by a straight line.

Calculation of Activation and Repolarization Times

The most common measured parameters of optical action potentials are times of activation and repolarization. Activation times are typically defined using one of two methods: either as moments of maximal upstroke rate of rise, dV/dt_{max}, or as times when a specified signal level is reached, e.g. 50 of the upstroke amplitude, $V_{50\%}$. Both methods provide similar results in the case of smooth action potentials with a simple monophasic upstroke shape. When upstrokes are multiphasic such as during discontinuous conduction, the two methods can result in significant differences of activation times (Fast and Kleber 1995). Discrepancies can also be produced by signal noise, which especially affects activation times calculated by the dV/dt_{max}-based method. In these situations, the $V_{50\%}$ method is preferable.

The repolarization times are measured in a similar way, as a time when a specified level of repolarization, typically 50 or 80, is achieved during the repolarization phase of an action potential. The difference between local repolarization and activation times is taken as the action potential duration.

Measurement of V_m Changes

Optical signals reflect only relative changes of transmembrane potential. Their absolute values depend, in addition to V_m, on the density of dye staining, the degree of dye internalization and the local intensity of excitation light. Because all these parameters vary across the preparation, their combination results in a significant variability of fluorescence intensity, independently of the variation of V_m. The V_m-independent variability of optical signals can be somewhat reduced by measuring the fractional changes in fluorescence. This does not, however, eliminate the signal variability completely, because the fractional change of fluorescence itself can vary throughout the preparation.

Often it is necessary to compare V_m changes measured at different sites. To eliminate the V_m-independent variability, optical signals can be normalized using the portion, which represents the action potential amplitude (APA). In doing so, an assumption is made that APA does not vary throughout the imaged area. This assumption is likely to be true on a small scale, when the size of the imaged area is comparable to the length of the electrotonic constant. It might not hold true on a larger spatial scale or in pathologic conditions, such as ischemia, favoring non-uniform distribution of APA. This normalizing procedure is used extensively in analyzing tissue responses to defibrillation shocks.

Examples

Microscopic Mapping of Anisotropic Conduction in Cell Cultures

On the microscopic level, tissue structure is anisotropic and discontinuous due to elongated cell boundaries, discrete distribution of gap junctions and presence of resistive barriers such as connective tissue and blood vessels. Structural discontinuities become more pronounced with aging and in diseases including infarction and hypertrophy. It has long been known that tissue anisotropy causes directional differences in activation spread with faster conduction in a direction parallel to fiber orientation in comparison to a transverse direction. These differences were explained in the framework of continuous cable theory by directional dependence of the intracellular tissue resistance. Later, it was found that the maximal upstroke rate of rise (dV/dt_{max}) is also direction dependent, with higher values in the transverse than in the longitudinal direction (Spach et al. 1981). Moreover, premature impulses propagating in the longitudinal direction could be blocked, while they continued to propagate in the transverse direction giving rise to re-entry. Contrary to the conduction anisotropy, the directional dependence of dV/dt_{max} couldn't be explained by the continuous cable theory. Therefore, it was suggested that this effect is due to tissue discontinuities caused by cell borders (Spach et al. 1981). The direct assessment of this hypothesis was difficult because of the 3-dimensional complexity of myocardial structure and insufficient resolution of conventional multi-electrode mapping techniques but it became possible with the development of high-resolution optical mapping of V_m and its application in patterned cell cultures.

Microscopic optical mapping of V_m in cell cultures is technically one of the most challenging applications. This is because only two membrane layers contribute to optical signals in cell monolayers and light is collected from small areas only a few micrometers in diameter. The first setup for optical mapping in cell cultures (Fast et al. 1996) was built around an inverted epi-fluorescent microscope (Carl Zeiss, Germany). Cell monolayers were stained with V_m-sensitive dye RH-237. The excitation light was provided by a 100-W arc Hg lamp, which is the most efficient light source for exciting RH-237. The fluorescent filter set contained a band-pass excitation filter (530–585 nm), a dichroic mirror (600 nm) and a low-pass emission filter (615 nm). Light was collected using a high-NA objective lens and measured using a 10×10 photodiode array (Centronic) at a spatial resolution ranging of 5.6–56 µm/diode and a sampling rate of 5–10 kHz/channel. This technique was used to investigate the role of anisotropic structure in impulse conduction in cultured cell monolayers with anisotropic structure (Fig. 4) (Fast et al. 1996; Fast and Kleber 1994). Impulse conduction in these monolayers was anisotropic with the velocity ratio of ~2.5, which is similar to the degree of anisotropy in the intact ventricular myocardium. Nevertheless, optical mapping of action potentials at a resolution of 7 µm/diode revealed no directional differences in dV/dt_{max}. It was concluded that at a moderate degree of anisotropy cell borders do not create directional differences in dV/dt_{max} and suggested that other factors including large structural discontinuities (connective tissue septa and small vessels) and bidomain properties of ventricular myocardium may account for dV/dt_{max} anisotropy observed in the intact tissue.

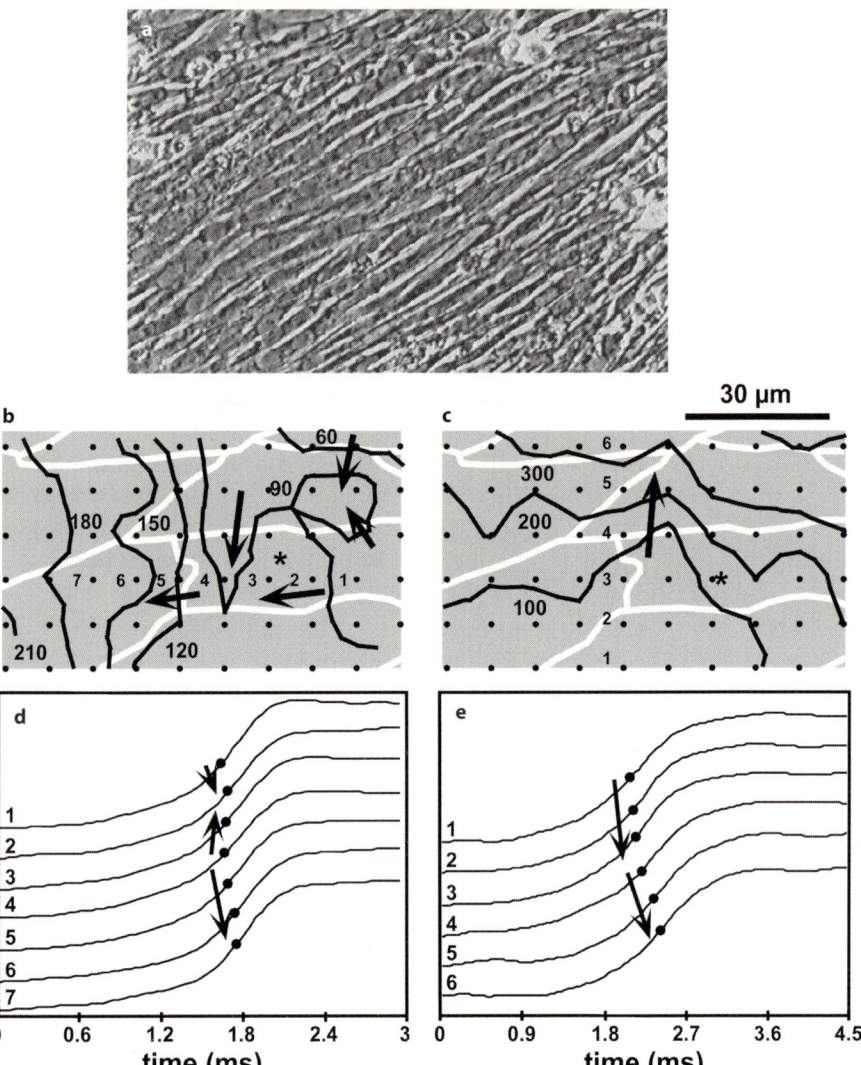

Figure 4a–e
Optical mapping of anisotropic activation spread in cell cultures. **a** Image of anisotropic cell monolayer. **b,c** Isochronal maps of longitudinal (**b**) and transverse (**c**) impulse propagation measured at a resolution of 7 μm/diode. White lines indicate cell boundaries. Points correspond to location of photodiodes. Large numbers depict activation times in μs. **e** Optical recordings of action potential upstrokes. (Reproduced with permission from Fast et al. 1996)

Mapping of V_m Changes During Defibrillation Shocks

Optical mapping proved to be very useful in investigation of the mechanisms of defibrillation (Efimov et al. 1998; Gillis et al. 1996; Knisley and Baynham 1997; Wikswo et al. 1995) During defibrillation, strong electrical shocks are applied to terminate a

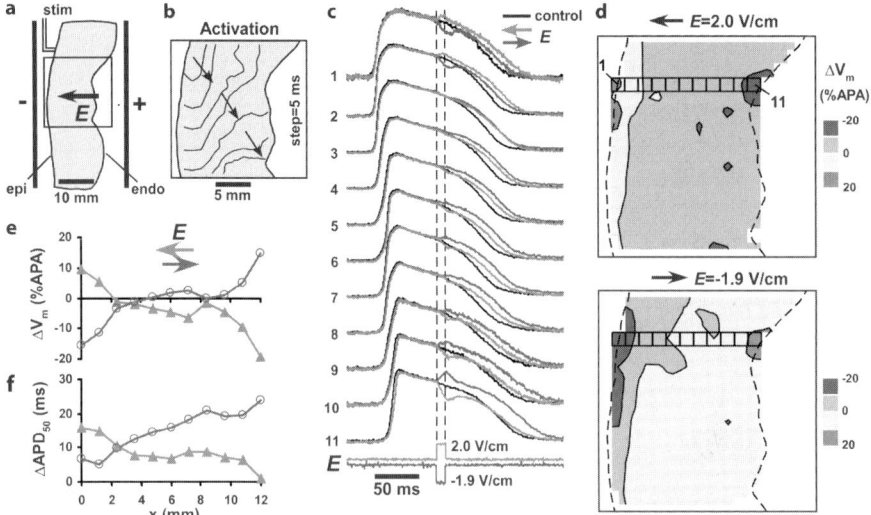

Figure 5a–f
Effects of electrical shocks on intramural V_m in left ventricular (LV) wall. **a** Outline of a transmural section of LV preparation and shock electrodes. **b** Isochronal map of transmural activation spread. **c** Optical recordings of V_m and shock (E) in control (black traces) and with two shocks of opposite polarity and strength E = 2 V/cm. The numbers correspond to the photodiodes indicated in Panel D. **d** Isopotential maps of ΔV_m distribution for two shocks at t = 9 ms after shock onset. **e** Spatial profiles of shock-induced ΔV_m and changes in action potential duration (ΔAPD_{50}). (Reproduced with permission from Fast et al. 2002). *For coloured version see appendix*

life-threatening cardiac arrhythmia. To be effective, shocks must induce changes of membrane potential (ΔV_m) in a critical mass of myocardium. However, the classical cable theory predicts that shock-induced ΔV_m decay rapidly with distance from electrodes or the tissue-bath interface so that no ΔV_m should be present beyond a few electrotonic space constants from the wall surface leaving intramural layers of left ventricle unaffected by a shock.

In a recent study, optical mapping was used to measure shock-induced V_m changes in the intramural layers of left ventricle (LV) (Fast et al. 2002). LV preparations were excised from porcine hearts and perfused through a coronary artery with Tyrode solution supplemented with BDM to suppress tissue motion. Preparations were immersed in a tissue bath containing a glass window for optical mapping. Rectangular shocks were applied across the LV wall via two large mesh electrodes located at the opposite sides of the bath. Preparations were stained with V_m-sensitive dye di-4-ANEPPS.

Fluorescence was excited at 540±10 nm using a 250 W tungsten-halogen lamp (Oriel). The emitted fluorescence was measured at >610 nm using a 50 mm F/1.4 photographic lens (Nikon), a 16×16 photodiode array and a multi-channel data acquisition system (see section 2) at a sampling rate of 5 kHz/ch and spatial resolution of 1.2 mm/diode.

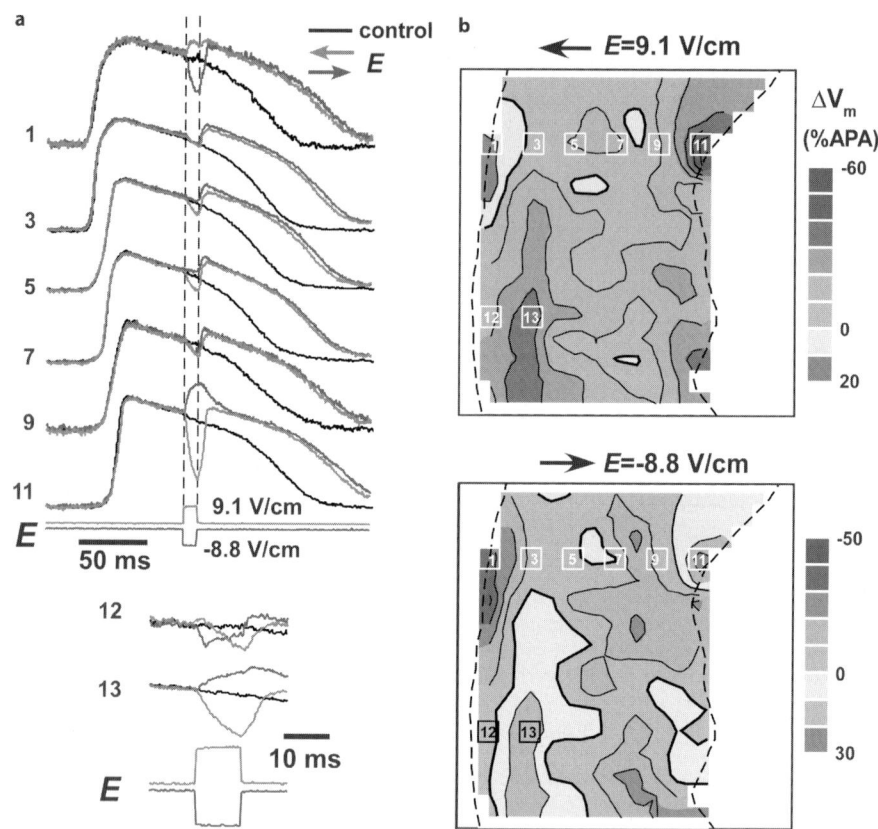

Figure 6a,b
Effects of strong shocks on intramural V_m. **a** V_m recordings in control and with 9.1 and -8.8 V/cm shocks. **b** Isopotential maps of shock-induced ΔV_m (Reproduced with permission from Fast et al. 2002). *For coloured version see appendix*

Figure 5 illustrates the effects of weak shocks on intramural V_m. These shocks induced positive ΔV_m at the tissue edge facing the cathode and negative ΔV_m at the edge facing the anode Fig. 5c and d). In both cases, maximal ΔV^+_m and ΔV^-_m were achieved at the wall edges and there was a relatively gradual transition in ΔV_m magnitude between the edges (Fig. 5e). Shocks caused prolongation in APD_{50} at sites of maximal ΔV^+_m whereas at sites of maximal ΔV^-_m the APD_{50} was either not changed or slightly prolonged (Fig. 5f).

Effects of stronger shocks (Fig. 6) were different in four main aspects:

1. These shocks produced localized increases of ΔV^+_m and ΔV^-_m inside the wall (Fig. 6b, bottom map). Such isolated polarizations indicated the presence of intramural ΔV_m not related to preparation boundaries, so-called "virtual electrodes".
2. ΔV_m induced by strong shocks were asymmetric with negative ΔV_m being much larger than positive ΔV_m at the same sites (Fig. 6a).
3. Negative ΔV_m extended towards the cathodal side of the preparation, such as in the lower part of the top map in Fig. 6b.

Stronger shocks prolonged APD at all sites across the wall for both ΔV^+_m and ΔV^-_m. Increasing the shock strength further caused predominantly negative ΔV_m across the wall. The degree of APD prolongation became similar for shocks of both polarities and it was not dependent on the local value of ΔV_m.

These results indicate that strong shocks indeed induce changes of V_m inside the ventricular wall supporting the long-standing hypothesis that defibrillation shocks must affect a critical mass of myocardium. The reasons for intramural V_m changes remain unclear at this time. The most plausible explanation for intramural ΔV_m is that they are caused by discontinuities in the tissue structure. Isolated areas of intramural polarizations were probably caused by relatively large-scale non-uniformities such as fiber rotation, variation in the surface-to-volume ratio or large blood vessels. As expected from ΔV_m produced by large non-uniformities, they changed their sign with changing shock polarity.

The other type of intramural polarizations, globally negative ΔV_m that did not change their sign with changing the shock polarity, were likely caused by microscopic discontinuities in the tissue structure such as collagen septa and blood vessels. High-resolution optical measurements indicate that shocks induce both positive and negative ΔV_m at the opposite sides of such structures (Fast et al. 2000). However, if these polarizations are measured on a macroscopic scale, which exceeds structure dimensions, then the negative and positive polarizations should be averaged out. In a system with a linear V_m response, the net result would be a zero or a negligible macroscopic polarization. This can explain the absence of detectable virtual electrodes during weak shocks when ΔV_m were nearly symmetric. Stronger shocks, however, induce non-linear ΔV_m with a strong negative bias ($\Delta V^-_m > \Delta V^+_m$) during the AP plateau. Because of this asymmetry, macroscopic measurements of ΔV_m produced by small discontinuities should yield only negative ΔV_m. This hypothesis for the microscopic nature of globally negative shock-induced polarizations needs further verification.

Troubleshooting

The most common problem in optical recordings is excessive noise, which results in a reduced signal-to-noise ratio. Two main types of noise in an optical mapping system are mechanical noise and electrical noise.

Mechanical Noise

Mechanical noise is caused by small displacements of either the preparation or photodetector relative to each other. These movements can be caused by vibrations of the floor transmitted via the optical table, vibrations of a shutter after its opening or by oscillations in the flow of the perfusion solution generated by peristaltic pumps. Typically, mechanical noise is less important in macroscopic measurements but it can be a dominant source of noise in microscopic recordings where even small preparation movements cause large changes in optical signals, especially in areas with strong gradients in fluorescent brightness, e.g., near the preparation border.

The best method to avoid the noise caused by floor vibrations is to mount the optical setup on an air-cushioned vibration-free table. Placing rubber cushions or air-filled rubber tubes under the table feet might also be sufficient.

Vibrations caused by a shutter last for a certain period of time after shutter opening. The easiest way to avoid this noise is to delay the start of optical recordings until oscillations become unnoticeable. This, however, prolongs the total exposure time, which might be undesirable in situations where photobleaching and phototoxicity are a concern. In this case, the shutter noise can be eliminated by detaching the shutter from both a microscope stand and a lamphouse. This can be achieved by installing a shutter cage between the microscope and the lamphouse and suspending the shutter in this cage on springs.

If peristaltic flow of perfusion solution causes oscillations in optical signals, they can be reduced by installing flow dampeners in the perfusion system. Alternatively, the peristaltic pump can be replaced by a gravity-flow perfusion system. In experiments with superfusion, fluctuations in light intensity can be caused by oscillations of the air-water interface. This can be prevented by using a water-immersion objective lens or by placing a glass coverslip on top of the solution.

Electrical Noise

Excessive electrical noise can be generated in different parts of an optical system including light source, photodiode array, I/V converters and 2nd stage amplifiers. To eliminate such noise, it is important first to localize its source. To do that, components of the optical system should be tested separately using noise-free equipment. For example, lamp output can be examined using a single photodiode and an oscilloscope. In a similar fashion, noise contributions from I/V converters and 2nd-stage amplifiers can be examined by providing noise-free test signals at the device inputs and measuring their outputs with an oscilloscope.

Among all components of a mapping system, perhaps the most frequent source of noise is the light source. In the case of the 250 W Tungsten-Halogen lamp from Oriel, the excessive noise in the form of 60 Hz ripple can be produced by the cooling fan built into the lamphouse. This fan has a separate power supply; it can be switched off for a short period of time during optical recording eliminating the ripple. With arc lamps, noise increases with bulb aging; in this case, replacing the bulb eliminates the problem. Another source of noise is the cable connecting a lamp power supply to the lamphouse. Electromagnetic radiation from this cable can create high-frequency noise in signal conditioning electronics. It can be reduced by moving the cables away and by folding cables and enclosing them in a grounded metallic screen such as aluminum foil. If all attempts to eliminate the excessive noise of the light source fail, it can be reduced by recording light intensity fluctuations directly from the light source using a reference photodetector and taking a ratio between the fluorescent and the reference signals.

As is often the case in electrophysiological measurements, a 60 Hz (50 Hz) ripple can appear in signals because of ground loops in electrical connections between different electrical devices. To eliminate noise of this kind, interconnections should be limited to a minimum and all ground leads should be connected at a single point. As with other periodic fluctuations, this noise can be reduced by band-pass digital signal filtration.

Other sources of noise include electrical or magnetic radiation from high frequency power supplies, power lines, computers and monitors. This noise can be reduced by moving the offending equipment away from sensitive circuitry.

References

Biermann M, Rubart M, Moreno A, Wu J, Josiah-Durant A, Zipes DP: Differential effects of cytochalasin D and 2,3 butanedione monoxime on isometric twitch force and transmembrane action potential in isolated ventricular muscle: implications for optical measurements of cardiac repolarization. J Cardiovasc Electrophysiol 9: 1348–1357, 1998

Choi BR, Nho W, Liu T, Salama G: Life span of ventricular fibrillation frequencies. Circ Res 91: 339–345, 2002

Efimov IR, Cheng Y, Van Wagoner DR, Mazgalev T, Tchou PJ: Virtual electrode-induced phase singularity. A basic mechanism of defibrillation failure. Circ Res 82: 918–925, 1998

Fast VG, Darrow BJ, Saffitz JE, Kleber AG: Anisotropic activation spread in heart cell monolayers assessed by high-resolution optical mapping: role of tissue discontinuities. Circ Res 79: 115–127, 1996

Fast VG, Ideker RE: Simultaneous optical mapping of transmembrane potential and intracellular calcium in myocyte cultures. J Cardiovasc Electrophysiol 11: 547–556, 2000

Fast VG, Kleber AG: Microscopic conduction in cultured strands of neonatal rat heart cells measured with voltage-sensitive dyes. Circ Res 73: 914–925, 1993

Fast VG, Kleber AG: Anisotropic conduction in monolayers of neonatal rat heart cells cultured on collagen substrate. Circ Res 75: 591–595, 1994

Fast VG, Kleber AG: Cardiac tissue geometry as a determinant of unidirectional conduction block: assessment of microscopic excitation spread by optical mapping in patterned cell cultures and in a computer model. Cardiovasc Res 29: 697–707, 1995

Fast VG, Kleber AG: Optical mapping of the effects of defibrillation shocks in cell monolayers. In: Shenasa M et al., editor. Cardiac Mapping. Futura, Armonk NY, pp 291–316, 2003

Fast VG, Rohr S, Ideker RE: Non-linear changes of transmembrane potential caused by defibrillation shocks in strands of cultured myocytes. Am J Physiol 278: H688-H697, 2000

Fast VG, Sharifov OF, Cheek ER, Newton J, Ideker RE: Intramural virtual electrodes during defibrillation shocks in left ventricular wall assessed by optical mapping of membrane potential. Circulation 106: 1007–1014, 2002

Frazier DW, Krassowska W, Chen P-S, Wolf PD, Daniely ND, Smith WM, Ideker RE: Transmural activations and stimulus potentials in three-dimensional anisotropic canine myocardium. Circ Res 63: 135–146, 1988

Gillis AM, Fast VG, Rohr S, Kleber AG: Effects of defibrillation shocks on the spatial distribution of the transmembrane potential in strands and monolayers of cultured neonatal rat ventricular myocytes. Circ Res 79: 676–690, 1996

Girouard S, Laurita K, Rosenbaum D: Unique properties of cardiac action potentials recorded with voltage-sensitive dyes. J Cardiovasc Electrophysiol 7: 1024–1038, 1996

Kleber AG, Janse MJ, Fast VG: Normal and abnormal conduction in the heart. Handbook of Physiology. Section 2: The Cardiovascular System: Oxford University Press pp 455–530, 2001

Knisley S, Baynham T: Line stimulation parallel to myofibers enhances regional uniformity of transmembrane voltage changes in rabbit hearts. Circ Res 81: 229–241, 1997

Laurita K, Libbus I: Optics and detectors used in optical mapping. In: Rosenbaum D, Jalife J, editors. Optical Mapping of Cardiac Excitation and Arrhythmias. Futura, Armonk, NY, pp 61–78, 2001

Qin H, Kay M, Chattipakorn N, Redden D, Ideker R, Rogers J: Effects of heart isolation, voltage-sensitive dye, and electromechanical uncoupling agents on ventricular fibrillation. Am J Physiol 284: H1818–H1826, 2003

Ratzlaff EH, Grinvald A: A tandem-lens epifluorescence macroscope: hundred-fold brightness advantage for wide-field imaging. J Neurosci Methods 36: 127–137, 1991

Rosenbaum DS, Jalife J, eds. Optical Mapping of Cardiac Excitation and Arrhythmias. Futura, Armonk, NY, p 458, 2001

Sellin LC, McArdle JJ: Multiple effects of 2,3-butanedione monoxime. Pharmacol & Toxicol 74: 305–313, 1994

Spach MS, Miller WTI, Gezelowitz DB, Barr RC, Kootsey JM, Johnson EA: The discontinuous nature of propagation in normal canine cardiac muscle. Evidence for recurrent discontinuties of intracellular resistance that affect the membrane currents. Circ Res 48: 39–54, 1981

Wharton JM, Wolf PD, Smith WM, Chen PS, Frazier DW, Yabe S, Danieley N, Ideker RE: Cardiac potential and potential gradient fields generated by single, combined, and sequential shocks during ventricular defibrillation. Circulation 85:1510–1523, 1992

Wikswo JP, Lin S-F, Abbas RA: Virtual electrode effect in cardiac tissue: a common mechanism for anodal and cathodal stimulation. Biophys J 69: 2195–2210, 1995

Wu J, Biermann M, Rubart M, Zipes DP: Cytochalasin D as excitation-contraction uncoupler for optically mapping action potentials in wedges of ventricular myocardium. J Cardiovasc Electrophysiol 9: 1336–1347, 1998

Epicardial Mapping in Isolated Hearts – Use in Safety Pharmacology, Analysis of Torsade de Pointes Arrhythmia and Ischemia-Reperfusion-Related Arrhythmia

Stefan Dhein

Introduction

Epicardial multielectrode mapping is a technique which allows the analysis of the spreading of action potentials on the epicardial surface and the velocities along and transverse to the fiber axis (Dhein et al. 1999; Spach and Dolber 1985). Moreover, it allows the detection of local dispersion and inhomogeneities in repolarization (Kleber et al. 1978; Kuo et al. 1983; Lesh et al. 1989; Dhein et al. 1993). This technique can be employed in safety pharmacological analysis of drugs with regard to action potential prolonging effects (e.g. Dhein and Perlitz 2002; Carlsson et al. 1990), inhomogeneous effects on action potentials, elicitation of arrhythmia and treatment of arrhythmia, thereby allowing the assessment of the pro-arrhythmic activity of drugs (e.g. Dhein et al. 1993; Brugada and Wellens 1988). Moreover, it is possible to analyze certain forms of arrhythmia with regard to the pathways of a given arrhythmia (Allessie et al. 1977; Janse et al. 1980).

Thus, this method can be used for analysis of ischemia-reperfusion-induced arrhythmia. In this setting it is possible to analyze the causes for the elicitation of an arrhythmia and this can be related to the location of the ischemic area, which can be detected by the area of ST-elevation (in unipolar potentials ischemia leads to ST-elevation; Coronel et al. 1988; Gottwald et al. 1998). In addition, activation velocity of the propagating wave front can be assessed longitudinal and transversal to the fibre direction, by delivery of a rectangular depolarizing pulse within the mapping matrix using a pair of mapping electrodes as stimulating electrodes for the assessment of anisotropy (Hindricks et al. 1993; Spach and Dolber 1985; Dhein et al. 1999).

In the following a description of a computer-aided automated 256 channel multielectrode mapping system is given, with emphasis on its use for safety pharmacology.

Description of Methods and Practical Approach

For our experiments we use the mapping systems HAL 3 and HAL 4, which are both commercially available (Ing.-Büro Peter Rutten, Bussestr. 10, 22299 Hamburg). The mapping systems are used in the classical pressure-constant Langendorff technique of isolated perfused hearts (see chapter 2.1).

Male white New Zealand rabbits (conventional, normally fed *ad libitum*, 1500 to 1800 g) are treated with 1000 IU/kg heparin i.v. 5 min before they are stunned by a sharp blow on the neck and rapidly killed by subsequent exsanguination. The heart is excised, prepared and perfused according to the Langendorff technique at constant pressure (70 cm H_2O; this is important since only if perfusion pressure exceeds 65 mmHg will it be high enough to allow complete coronary perfusion) with Tyrode's solution of the following composition: Na^+ 161.02, K^+ 5.36, Ca^{2+} 1.8, Mg^{2+} 1.05, Cl^- 147.86, HCO_3^- 23.8, PO_4^{2-} 0.42 and glucose 11.1 mmol/l, equilibrated with 95% O_2 and 5% CO_2. The surface temperature of the heart is 37 °C. The hearts are connected to a 256 channel mapping system HAL3 (temporal resolution: 4 kHz/channel; amplitude resolution: 0.04 mV, inter-channel coupling <-60 dB; bandwidth of the system: 0.5 Hz–20 kHz, data were not filtered) or HAL 4 (temporal resolution: 20 kHz/channel) as described previously (Dhein et al. 1988). 256 AgCl electrodes are cast in 4 polyester plates (in 8×8 orthogonal matrices with 1 mm inter-electrodes distance), which are attached to the heart surface in an elastic manner, so that they can follow the heart movements easily without dislocation, covering the right, front, left and back ventricular walls. The cables of the electrodes are used as elastic springs. The hearts are spontaneously beating during the entire experimental protocol. As a variation, the heart can be paced supraventricularly at the right atrium using a conventional stimulator. In this case, it is necessary to use an isolator between the stimulator and the pacing electrodes. However, care has to be taken of grounding loops. All electrical groundings have to be performed in the manner of a star grounding. The electrical grounding of the heart is achieved *via* the aortic cannula, which is made from steel and is connected to electrical ground, so that the Tyrode solution perfusing the heart is grounded.

Subsequently three kinds of experiments are described:
1. safety investigation of a drug and elicitation of torsade de pointes arrhythmia;
2. investigation of ischemia-reperfusion-arrhythmia;
3. assessment of anisotropy.

Drugs can be easily administered in increasing concentrations intracoronarily by infusion *via* a three-way side-connection to the aortic cannula. Infusion velocity in rabbits' hearts should be as low as 1 ml/min and the concentration of the drug solution has to be adjusted to the coronary flow (concentration in the perfusion syringe × 1 ml/min/coronary flow = desired end concentration)

Ischemia can be induced by ligature of a side branch of the lateral descending coronary artery. For this purpose, two threads for ligature have to be placed and a knot (using the first thread) has to be made on a small short steel wire (0.5 mm diameter) inserted under the knot without occluding the vessel, before the mapping electrodes are attached to the heart. At the desired time point, the ligature is tightened without dislocation of the electrode plates. It can be easily released by removing the steel wire from the knot.

For equilibration a period of 45–60 min should be allowed. Thereafter, the experiment starts. In drug experiments each concentration should be administered for about 5–20 min (depending on the drug kinetics). The entire set of experiments should not exceed 180 min since after that time oedema may occur (or one may adjust for the colloid osmotic pressure with an adequate amount of bovine serum albumin).

In ischemia experiments, ischemia is induced by tightening the first thread. Be careful not to dislocate the electrodes during this step. At the end of the ischemia period, the occlusion is opened by cutting the thread, and reperfusion starts. At the end of an ischemia-reperfusion experiment, a second occlusion at the same location is achieved by using the second thread. Evans blue is injected into the coronary circulation, so that the occluded zone can be seen as the non-stained area. The location of the electrodes is marked by injection of ink at the edges of the electrode plate. Thereafter, the electrodes are removed and the heart is disconnected from the Langendorff apparatus. After weighing the whole heart, the occluded zone is excised and weighted and after cutting into small cubes of 0.5 mm length incubated in 0.5% nitro blue tetrazolium for 30 min. All tissue samples which are stained yellowish after this incubation are weighed again giving the infarct size, which is expressed as the percentage of the occluded zone. Alternatively, the heart is processed for classical histology, which then permits correlation of the mapping data with the underlying histology.

Ischemia is confirmed during the experiment by (a) the reduction in coronary flow, (b) the area of the ventricle, in which ST-elevation is observed, (c) the intensity of ST-elevation, (d) the reduction in left ventricular pressure and, after the experiment, by the infarct size.

In addition, functional parameters such as maximum systolic left ventricular pressure (LVP), end-diastolic LVP (EDP), heart rate (HR) and coronary flow (CF) are assessed continuously as described (Dhein et al. 1993) (see chapter 2.1).

Epicardial potential mapping is either performed in each experimental phase during periods of constant cycle length of at least 4 min, in order to make it possible to compare the activation patterns (of single heart beats) or their alterations (if the influence of a drug on the activation pattern is to be analyzed), or during the entire arrhythmia (if initiation, maintenance and termination of arrhythmia are to be analyzed).

For evaluation of the mapping data the activation time points at each electrode were determined as $t(dU/dt_{min})$ (Spach and Dolber 1986; Dhein et al. 1993; Durrer and Van der Tweel 1954). The morphology of the QRS complex in these unipolar potentials is a function of the waves approaching and leaving the electrode (Burgess et al. 1988).

Next, the repolarization time points were determined as $t(dU/dt_{max})$ during the T-wave (Dhein et al. 1993; Millar et al. 1985). After automatic determination, activation and repolarization time points have to be verified (or corrected if necessary) manually by the experimenter. From these data for each electrode, an activation–recovery interval (ARI) is calculated as the difference between the time point of activation and the time point of repolarization, indicating the epicardial action potential duration. Activation-recovery intervals are only calculated if the QRS complex showed both a positive and a negative component and if there was a well-defined T-wave, as published for analysis of activation-recovery intervals in ischemic tissue by Gottwald et al. (1998) and in accordance with Janse and coworkers (1993).

Activation-recovery intervals are determined for each region of the heart (right, front, left and back wall) as well as (if appropriate) for the ischemic centre and border zone. Centre and border can be determined from ST-elevation and dye injection, which gives the localization of the occluded zone. In addition, the distribution of the activation-recovery intervals is analyzed for each area of the heart, (i.e. front, left, right or back wall) calculating the standard deviation of the activation-recovery intervals at 64 electrodes, and expressed as dispersion of the activation-recovery intervals (ARI-dispersion). Alternatively, homogeneity of ARI can be calculated as the percentage of electrodes which exhibit an ARI not deviating more than ±5 ms from the mean ARI. Dispersion is increased if cellular uncoupling occurs (Lesh et al. 1989; Dhein et al. 1999) or in the course of ischemia between border and centre zone (Dhein et al. 2000).

From the activation time points, an activation sequence is determined. We determine those electrodes which were activated before any of the neighboring ones and define them as "breakthrough-points" (BTP) which can be considered as the origins of epicardial activation (Arisi et al. 1983). These breakthrough-points are determined for heartbeats under control conditions and for heartbeats under treatment. Heartbeats in the various phases of ischemia and reperfusion are compared to those under control conditions by calculating the percentage of breakthrough-points with identical location to their location under control conditions (identical = deviating not more than 1 mm from their location under control conditions). Similarly, the beat-to-beat variability can be assessed. That means, that two identical heartbeats should reveal a similarity in breakthrough-point location of 100%. It is, however known from previous studies, that identical heartbeats only occur rarely and that arrhythmogenic stimuli can reduce breakthrough-point similarity (Dhein et al. 1988, 1993). Decreasing values for this breakthrough-point similarity indicate progressive deviation from the initial (control) activation pattern and, together with other alterations, may mean pro-arrhythmic activity.

In a similar way the spread of epicardial excitation is analyzed. In order to allow a quantitative and comparative description of the activation process for each electrode, an activation vector is calculated from the activation times and the locations of the surrounding electrodes which were activated after the central electrode (i.e. a maximum number of 8 single vectors, Fig. 1), as described by Müller et al. (1991). These vectors then are summed up giving one resulting vector which gives direction and apparent velocity of local activation at the electrode under investigation. This is repeated for all electrodes. The percentage of similar vectors (VEC) between heartbeats in the various experimental phases compared with those under control conditions is determined (vectors deviating not more than 5° from their original direction are considered to be similar). The critical value beneath which arrhythmia often occurs (see above) for VEC-similarity is 10% as determined in previous studies (Dhein et al. 1988, 1993).

Taken together, the parameters BTP and VEC characterize the geometry of the epicardial activation process, and represent the beat similarity of the cardiac impulse as compared to heartbeats under control conditions. Thus, decreasing values for BTP or VEC indicate progressive deviation from the initial (control) activation pattern.

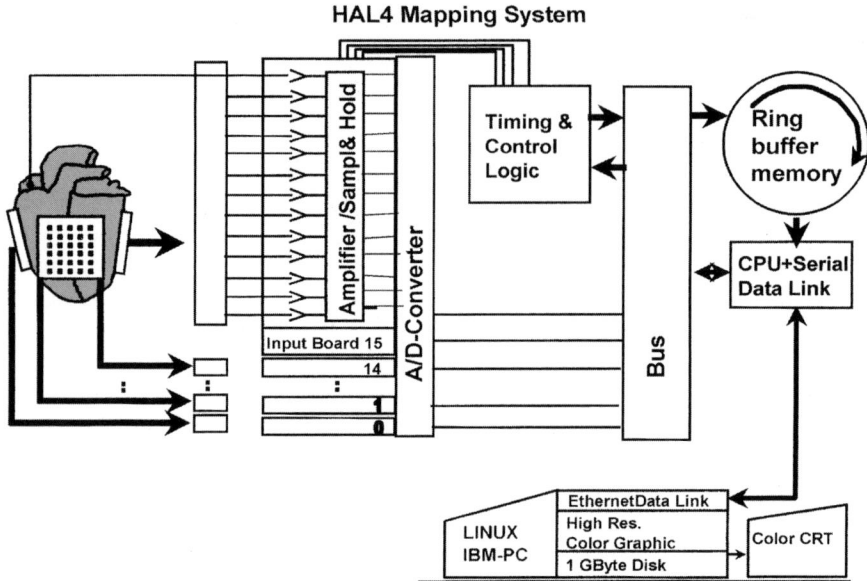

Figure 1
Setup for 256 channel mapping

In addition, the ST-segments of the 256 ECGs are analyzed. We sum up all deviations from the isoelectrical level at the time point 50% of mean activation-recovery interval and calculate the total ST-deviation of 256 leads in arbitrary units [a.u.]. An increase in that parameter points to an increase in efflux of positively charged ions during the action potential and is indicative of ischemic regions (Coronel et al. 1988; Gottwald et al. 1998).

In addition, it is possible to assess cardiac anisotropy with this method by delivering depolarizing stimuli *via* a pair of electrodes within the mapping area. The isochrones around the stimulating pulse are constructed and, later on, compared with the underlying histology. The fibre's longitudinal and transversal axes are determined and velocity along and transverse to the fibre can be calculated from the isochrones (Fig. 2). The ratio V_L/V_T is defined as anisotropy. Table 1 gives a survey of the parameters under control conditions.

Figure 2
Anisotropy

Parameter	Mean ± SEM
ARI left (ms)	125.9 ± 6.4
ARI right (ms)	142.7 ± 8.5
Dispersion (ms)	12.2 ± 1.3
TAT (ms)	10.7 ± 0.9
QRS (ms)	20.4 ± 0.4
PQ (ms)	58 ± 2
VEC (%)	34.2 ± 5.3
BTP (%)	75 ± 34
VL (m/s)	0.56 ± 0.1
VT (m/s)	0.26 ± 0.1
LVP (mm Hg)	102 ± 6
CF (ml/min)	27.8 ± 2

Table 1
Parameters of epicardial mapping. Normal values for rabbit hearts

ARI activation recovery interval; *TAT* total activation time; *QRS* duration of QRS complex; *PQ* atrioventricular conduction time; *VEC* vector field similarity of two succeeding heart beats; *BTP* breakthrough point similarity of two succeeding heart beats; V_L longitudinal ventricular propagation velocity; V_T transverse ventricular propagation velocity; *LVP* left ventricular pressure; *CF* coronary flow.

Examples (Torsade de Pointes; Ischemia-Reperfusion Arrhythmia; V_L/V_T)

In the following, examples will be given which illustrate the use of such a mapping system. The first example elucidates its use in investigation of drug-induced arrhythmia; the second shows how to use the system for evaluation of ischemia-reperfusion alterations and arrhythmia. Finally an example will be given of how to assess the anisotropic properties of the tissue.

Drug-Induced Arrhythmia

A typical drug-induced arrhythmia is the torsade de pointes arrhythmia which can be elicited by action potential-prolonging drugs such as class III antiarrhythmics, several antihistaminic drugs, certain antibiotics and some neuroleptic drugs (Dhein 2000). Risk factors for this type of arrhythmia are hypokalemia, bradycardia, action potential prolongation, dispersion, low magnesium and female gender. In order to investigate whether a certain drug, in the example we will use haloperidol, can elicit torsade de pointes arrhythmia, these risk factors have to be modelled as well. Thus, we used female rabbits and perfused the isolated heart according to the Langendorff technique with a modified Tyrode solution containing only 2.5 mM K$^+$ and 0.5 mM Mg^{2+}. An

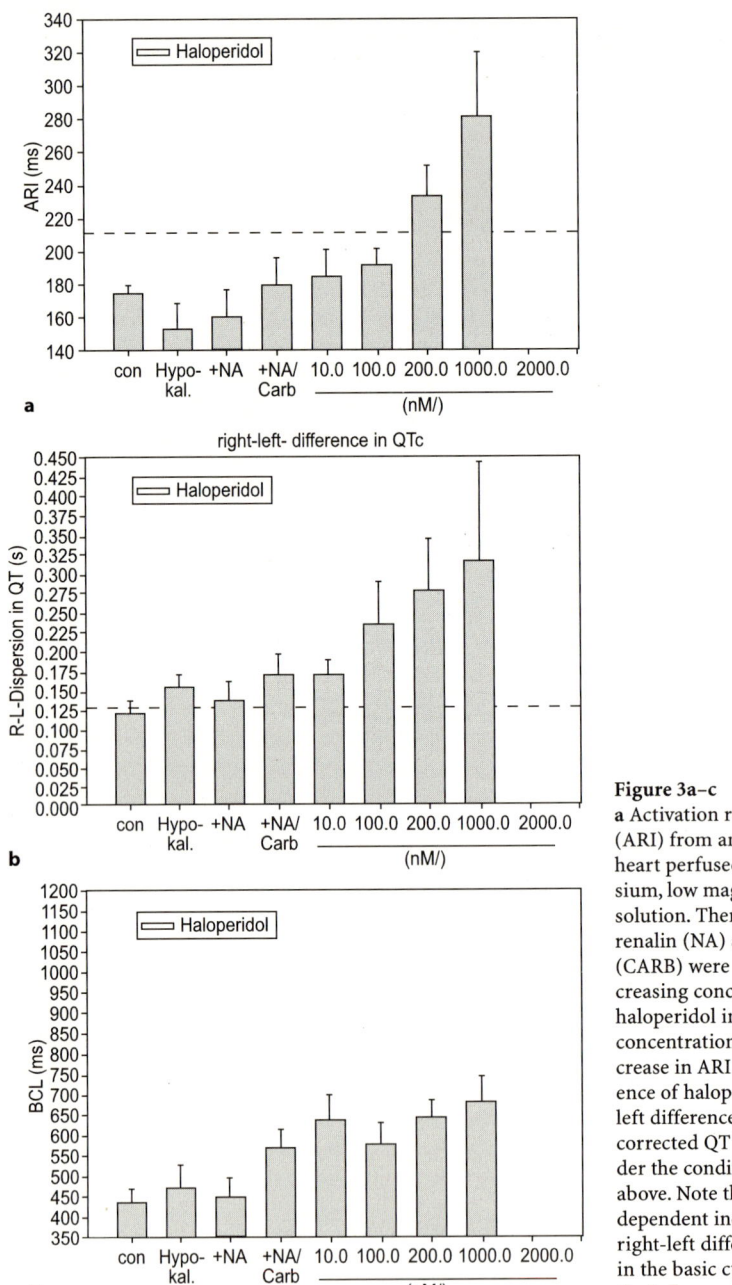

Figure 3a–c
a Activation recovery intervals (ARI) from an isolated rabbit heart perfused with low potassium, low magnesium Tyrode solution. Thereafter, noradrenalin (NA) and carbachol (CARB) were applied and increasing concentrations of haloperidol infused. Note the concentration-dependent increase in ARI under the influence of haloperidol. b Right-left difference of the frequency corrected QT time QTc under the conditions described above. Note the concentration-dependent increase in the right-left difference. c Increase in the basic cycle length under the influence of haloperidol

autonomous tone was modeled by infusing 0.1 μM noradrenaline and 1 μM carbachol resulting in a slight bradycardia. Both autonomic transmitters were given to allow detection of sympatholytic and parasympatholytic effects of a given drug. After

15 min equilibration under these conditions, haloperidol was infused intracoronarily in increasing concentrations (10–1000 nM) for 10 min/concentration step. Under these conditions epicardial potential mapping was performed.

We observed a concentration-dependent increase in the activation-recovery intervals (Fig. 3a), with longer potentials at the right wall as compared to the left, so that the right-left difference in QTc (frequency corrected QT time) was concentration-dependently increased (Fig. 3b). Concomitantly there was a slight increase in the basic cycle length (BCL) (Fig. 3c), while the other parameters such as left ventricular pressure, coronary flow, total activation time and QRS duration did not change.

We found Torsade de pointes (TdP) arrhythmia in 3/6 hearts under the influence of haloperidol (>0.1 µM) and in 0/6 control hearts treated with vehicle. Each TdP was preceded by an R on T extra systole and a highly inhomogeneous repolarization pattern of the previous action. R on T extra systoles were found in 3/6 hearts under haloperidol (>0.1 µM). Initiation of TdP occurred at the location where the R on T extra systole was observed if, in the rest of the heart, long ARI (151–190 ms) with high dispersion (29.8–38.8 ms) were detected. The activation pattern of the TdP was complex and exhibited a long wave running several times around the heart (Fig. 4). Typically, TdP was self-terminated after splitting the activation wave into two waves which then collided thereby extinguishing the ongoing TdP. Thus, it was possible to define a TdP risk for haloperidol in concentrations >0.1 µM which was related to an increase in the right-left difference of QTc and a prolongation of ARI with concomitant slowing of the heart rate.

Ischemia-Reperfusion Arrhythmia

Another arrhythmia which is often investigated is ischemia-reperfusion-induced arrhythmia. Ischemia is usually induced by occlusion of a coronary artery, typically of a branch of the left descending coronary artery. A problem arises from the fact that it is necessary to record activation maps prior to occlusion, during occlusion and after the release of the ligature without dislocating the electrodes. Therefore, in our group we use the following technique: a branch of the coronary artery is undermined with a double thread. One thread is knotted with a small steel rod under the knot prior to positioning the electrode plates. It has to be checked that there is no ST elevation in the area of choice after this preparation. After 45 min of equilibration the coronary artery is occluded and mapping is performed. After 30 min or 60 min of ischemia the occlusion is released by careful removal of the steel rod or by cutting the knot. After 30 to 60 min of reperfusion with continuous mapping, the experiment is terminated and finally the area at risk and infarct size are determined as described above.

For analysis it is necessary to evaluate each individual potential since the signals often exhibit unusual forms arising from the marked ST elevation, the depolarisation of the fibers and slowing of conduction. Monophasic extracellular unipolar potentials often do not represent activation but may be interpreted as electrotonic potentials. If there is a clear intrinsic deflection, an activation time point may be determined (see below). We found in such experiments during phases of rhythmic beating that the total activation time in the ischemic area is considerably prolonged and that the propa-

202
5 mV
500 ms
last action of torsade de pointes
wave collision
block zone
&wave collision
wave splitting
right
front
left
back

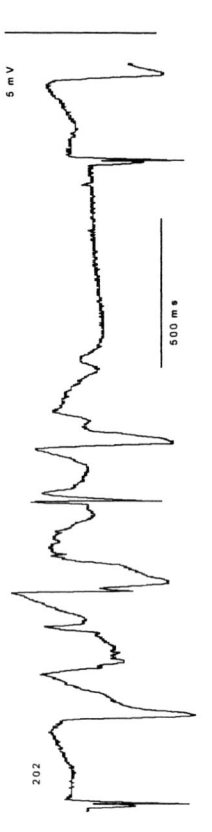

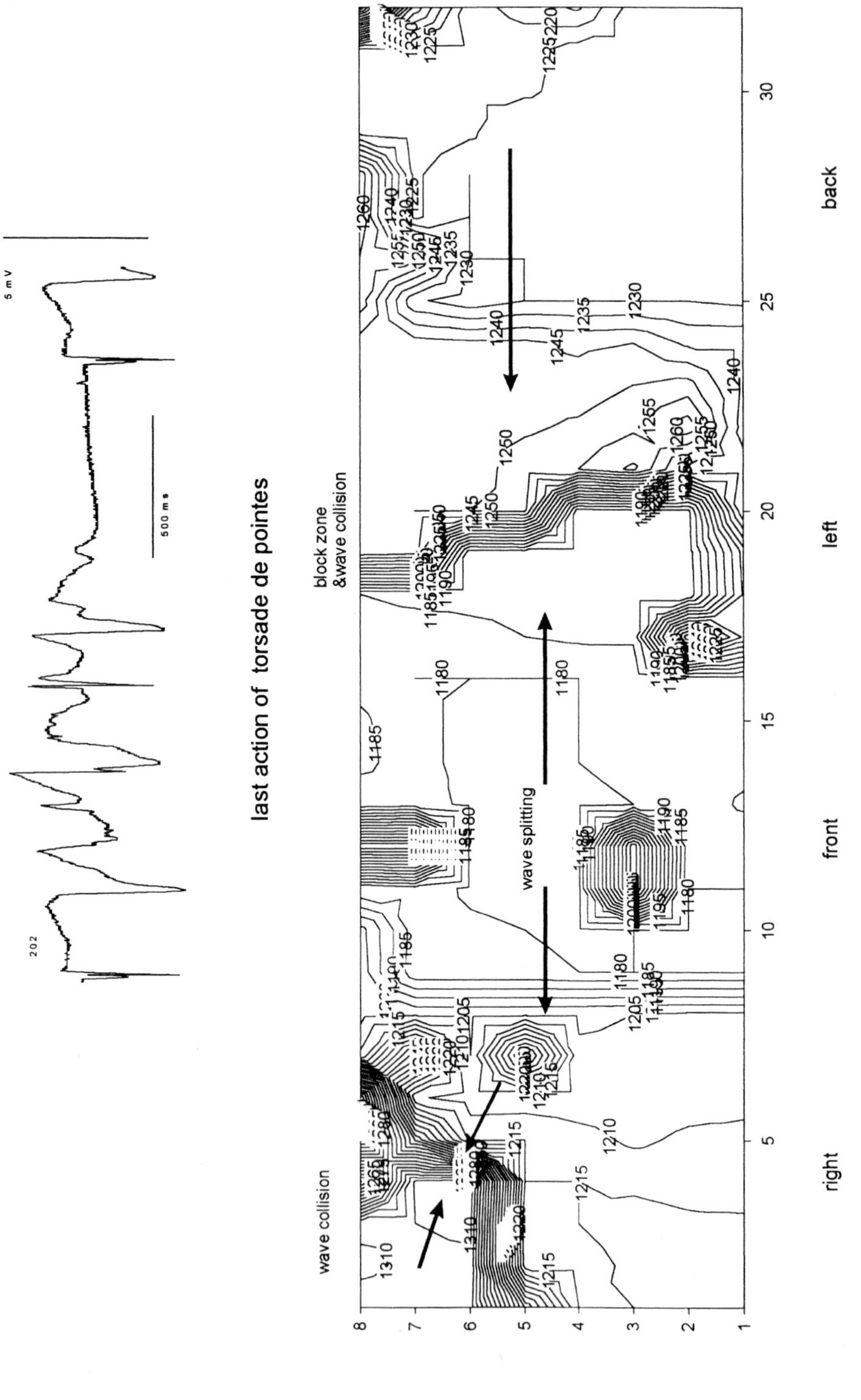

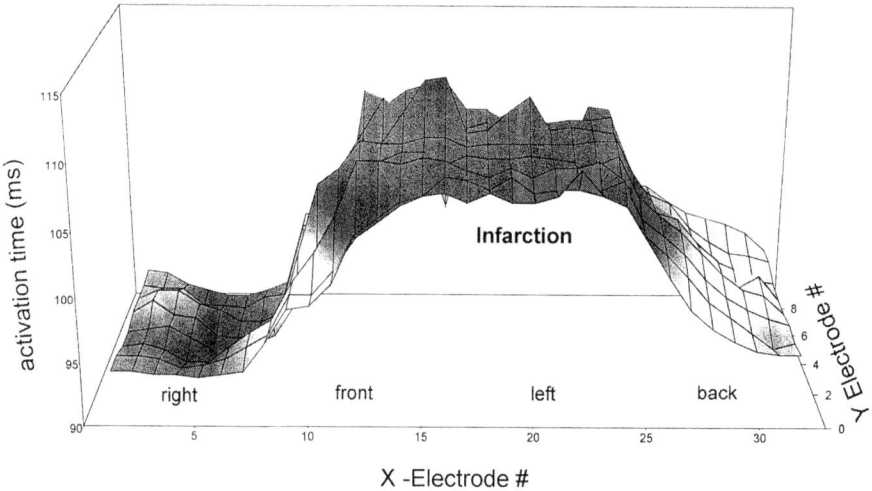

Figure 5
Activation time points on the ventricular surface during ischemia. The position of the right, front, left and back wall is indicated. The Y-axis gives the activation time point. Note the later activation of the ischemic area

gation velocity of activation is markedly slowed (Gottwald et al. 1998; Dhein et al. 1998). This can be seen if activation time points are plotted as a function of the X,Y-position (Fig. 5). Thus, activation propagation is slowed locally (Fig. 5), 15 to 20 min after occlusion (Kleber et al. 1986) and is due to progressive depolarisation of the myocytes, thereby reducing sodium channel availability and uncoupling the gap junctional coupling (Dekker et al. 1996). A consequence of this slowing is that for discrimination of wave fronts it is necessary to use a small inter-electrode distance (Janse 1993). This slowing may elicit arrhythmia. It is generally accepted that slowing of conduction is among the prerequisites for the initiation of reentrant arrhythmia. For analysis sinus rhythmic beats and arrhythmic beats have to be carefully distinguished. In order to see drug effects on ischemia-induced alteration of electrophysiology, it is necessary to evaluate rhythmic beats. Sometimes, however, the initiation of arrhythmia and the ongoing arrhythmia may be of interest. A consequence of this slowing is that for discrimination of wave fronts it is necessary to use a small inter-electrode distance.

The area of ischemia can be assessed by the area showing ST-elevation (Coronal et al. 1988; Dhein et al. 1998; Gottwald et al. 1998). This can be integrated giving a quantitative parameter which can be assessed online. Regarding the repolarization pattern, we found a reduction in the duration of the activation recovery intervals.

◀ **Figure 4**
Isochrones of a Torsade de pointes arrhythmia. Note the long activation wave running around the hearts surface. The picture shows the whole ventricular surface with from left to right: right-front-left-back wall. The X-axis represents electrode number. The inter-electrode distance was 1 mm. The Y axis gives the electrode position in mm from cranial to caudal

However, it should be noted that it is often very difficult, or in some cases impossible, to determine the repolarization time point. It can only be estimated correctly if there is an intrinsic deflection indicating activation followed by a clear positive wave which can be considered a T-wave. Only in these cases can the time point of the steepest increase during the T-wave be assessed. We found a reduction in the activation recovery intervals of the order of 50% after 25 min of ischemia. After several minutes of ischemia, there is normally no activation in the central ischemic zone. Thus, it is necessary to differentiate between the center and the border zones of ischemia (Dhein et al. 2000). Due to the graded reduction in the duration of the activation repolarization intervals between the normal, the border and the center zone, there is high inhomogeneity of the activation recovery intervals. This can be measured as the standard deviation of the activation recovery intervals at a given number of electrodes. This parameter is defined as dispersion. Moreover, it is possible to determine the maximum difference in the activation recovery intervals between the border and center zone. This is, for example, reduced if an $I_{K,ATP}$ inhibitor is administered prior to ischemia (Dhein et al. 2000). Such an increase in dispersion is another factor involved in the initiation of reentrant arrhythmia (Kuo et al. 1983). Moreover, between the ischemic area and the normal zone there is a so-called flow of injury current which may depolarize fibres, thereby eliciting arrhythmia (Janse et al. 1980). This arrhythmia may be further promoted by dispersion and slowing of conduction.

Finally, it is necessary to monitor the type of arrhythmia. We use a scheme for classifying arrhythmias during ischemia. We count the incidence of single monotopic ventricular extra systoles, of polytopic ventricular extra systoles, of pairs, or triplets and of runs of ventricular extra systoles. The latter can be subdivided into monomorphic and polymorphic ventricular tachycardia. Moreover, the occurrence of reentrant arrhythmia is analyzed. These incidences can be compared between hearts treated with vehicle and those treated with the drug of interest. Each arrhythmia can also be analyzed by the mapping technique. We therefore analyse the point of origin of the arrhythmia by the earliest activation time point of the extra systole, which in our experiments was mostly located in the border zone of ischemia.

Assessing the Anisotropic Ratio

With regard to the safety factor of action potential propagation, a basic feature of cardiac tissue is the anisotropy of cardiac tissue (Spach et al. 1987). The longitudinal resistance of cardiac tissue is lower than the transverse resistance. *Vice versa*, the capacitance is higher in the longitudinal than in the transverse direction. These directional differences have an independent role in determining the shape of the upstroke and τ_{Foot} depending on the direction of propagation in relation to the orientation of the fibres. Thus, fast upstrokes were observed with low propagation velocities (transverse to the fibre axis). Interestingly, propagation with low velocity has been found to be more resistant to disturbances. It is necessary to suppose, that if membrane capacitance is lower, a smaller amount of the depolarizing current I_{Na} is needed to charge the membrane. Another feature arising from these directional differences is that sodium channel-blocking drugs such as quinidine show higher binding in the case of longitudinal propagation since more I_{Na} is in the appropriate state (Spach et al. 1987).

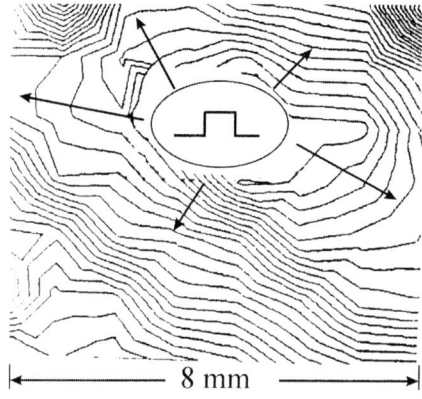

Figure 6
Assessment of anisotropy. Note the elliptical form of the isochrones. The velocities were 0.56±0.05 m/s in the longitudinal direction and 0.26±0.05 m/s in the transverse direction

Thus, sometimes the assessment of the biophysical properties may be interesting. For that purpose the activation propagation velocities along and transverse to the fibre axis have to be evaluated. For assessing the longitudinal (V_L) and transverse (V_T) velocities of propagation an extra stimulus has to be delivered at the ventricles. We use an electrode matrix with two electrodes in the middle of the plate, which are connected to a stimulator. Rectangular pulses are delivered to the ventricular back wall. First, we determine the threshold for capturing the stimulus and thereafter deliver pulses of twice the threshold amplitude and 2 ms duration. During stimulation, the resulting activation is mapped. This is repeated in the presence of the drug (or intervention), which is being investigated. At the end of the experiment, the position of the electrode plates on the ventricular surface is marked by ink injection. Thereafter, the macroscopic fibre orientation is noted. The next step is to determine all activation time points and to construct an isochrone plot (an isochrone surrounds all electrodes which are activated within a certain time interval). This isochrone plot is then compared with the fibre orientation in that area and V_L and V_T can easily be determined from the isochrone plot (Fig. 6).

The longitudinal velocity is mainly dependent on the availability of the fast sodium current (Buchanan et al. 1985) due to the long membrane length, while the transverse propagation is more sensitive to gap junctional uncoupling (Delmar et al. 1987; Dhein et al. 1999).

Testing the Preparation

There are some simple tests which may be performed on a preparation at the end of an experiment. First, if an electrically paced heart is used, the response to an increase in heart rate should be tested. Normally, an increase in heart rate results in a decrease in QT or ARI, and within certain limits in a positive inotropic response (rat heart, 200–400 beats/min, guinea pig and rabbit heart, 60–100 bpm). At higher rates, a negative inotropic response is found. Furthermore, the β-adrenergic agonist isoproterenol (10–500 nM) may be applied, which should result in an increase in heart rate, inotropy and a decrease in QT or ARI. Concomitantly, the atrioventricular conduction time should be decreased. In addition, carbachol (100–1000 nM) may be applied. This should result in a bradycardic response with increased atrioventricular conduction time but without alteration in the ventricular parameters.

Another test is the application of a known antiarrhythmic agent such as quinidine (0.1 to 5 μM), which blocks I_{Na} and to a certain degree repolarizing currents and, thus leads to slowing of conduction and prolongation of the action potential. Accordingly, after application of quinidine, total activation time should be prolonged as the duration of the QRS complex. This is accompanied by a prolongation of ARI (Dhein et al. 1993). Regarding tests for Frank-Starling mechanism or the coronary circulation and myogenic autoregulation, please see the chapter on the Langendorff heart.

Troubleshooting

There are several problems often encountered in epicardial mapping. The first possible problem is an electrode problem coming from the polarisation of the metal electrodes kept in saline solution. The experimenter observes a drift in the zero voltage line. There are two possible ways to circumvent this problem. First the use of AgCl electrodes instead of Ag is recommended. Secondly, it is possible to use so-called chopper amplifiers as input amplifiers. These amplifiers possess 2 inputs and switch between inputs 1 and 2. While input 1 is read, input 2 is set to zero (electrical ground) again.

Another big problem using mapping setups comes from electrical noise, which can be detected as a 50 Hz signal overlaying the ECG. Sometimes higher frequency noise may also be present. The high frequency components may come from the laboratory lamps if neon lamps are used. The 50 Hz noise is usually a result of insufficient or inadequate grounding. Most frequently grounding loops are used. To give an example, the heart is connected to ground *via* the aortic cannula thereby also connecting the perfusing solution to ground. If there is an additional grounded electrode in the perfusing system also connected to electrical ground, then a loop ground-heart-Tyrode-ground is produced, which can evoke noise due to its resistance. To avoid such problems, usage of a so-called star ground is recommended. Each part of the setup is grounded individually by only one cable to one common ground, which may take the form of a big metal block which is connected to the electrical zero of the institute. At the beginning of an experiment, the electrodes have to be connected to the heart's surface. This may influence the heart's mechanical properties due to the attachment pressure of the electrode plates or the elastic properties of a silicon sock electrode. Artifacts due to attachment of electrodes can be detected if the left ventricular pressure, the end-diastolic pressure and the coronary flow are continuously measured before, during and after the attachment of the electrodes. If the attachment pressure is too high, one may notice an increase in the end-diastolic pressure and a concomitant decrease in coronary flow. In addition, the ST segments of the unipolar ECGs measured in the area of increased pressure are elevated as a sign of relative ischemia.

A typical problem during analysis of a mapping experiment is to decide which is the activation time point. Normally, the activation time point is defined as the time point of the steepest intrinsic deflection (Durrer and van der Tweel 1954). However, in rare cases the QRS complex may be fractionated (this is often observed in aged

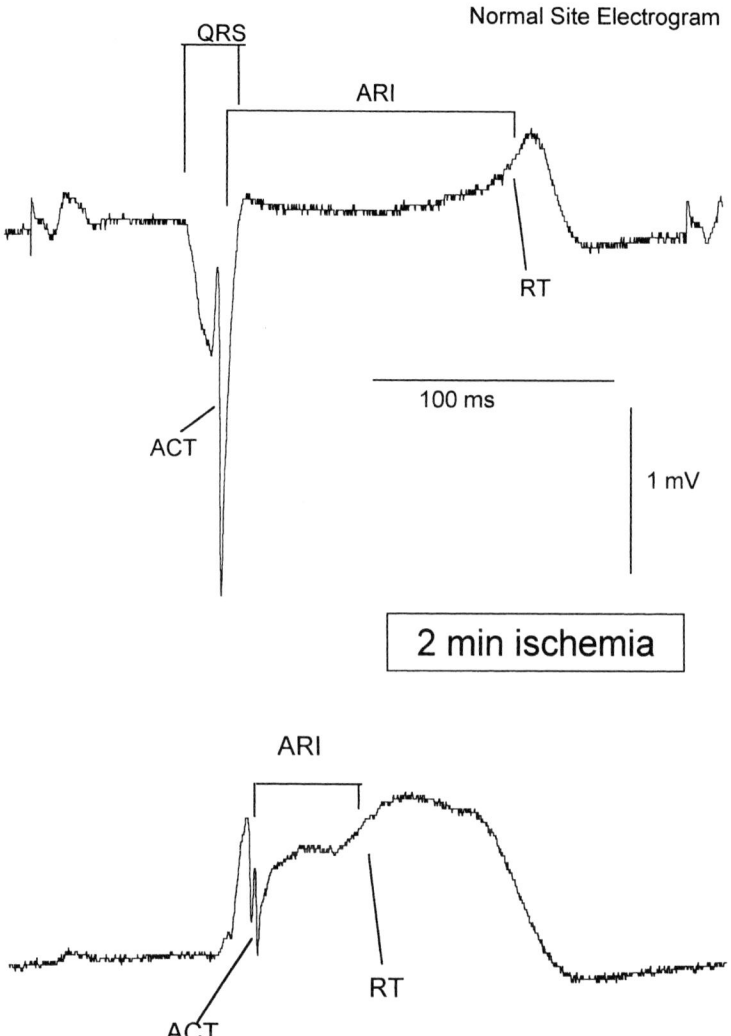

Figure 7
Electrograms from a normal and an ischemic site. The arrows indicate the activation and repolarization time points. Note that in the monophasic extracellular potential no activation time point can be determined

hearts) so that there may be two or three deflections which all exhibit the same steepness. In such a case, one can take the time point of the steepest deflection within the main portion of negative movement of the signal, i.e. within the main deflection. Looking at the QRS complexes of the neighboring electrodes, which might have similar but clearer signals is a help. Another possibility is to construct isochrones of that area and see whether the electrode with the time point of activation in question forms a line with the other electrodes thus forming an activation wave. However, in a given case this decision may be very difficult.

Another problem often encountered in epicardial mapping is the determination of the repolarization time point, if there is some noise within the T-wave. Typically this is a problem in T-wave analysis since the T-wave is a rather slow signal with low amplitude. As with the activation time points one may look at the neighboring electrodes or construct isochrones of repolarization. On the other hand, it may be helpful to filter the T-wave digitally using a gliding mean algorithm over 3 or 5 samples.

The biggest problems arise from ischemic potentials which are often very difficult to evaluate, since there is a considerable ST-elevation in the ischemic area (Fig. 7). Due to the depolarisation of the tissue, sometimes only monophasic electrotonic responses can be recorded, which do not allow the determination of an activation time point. First it has to be decided whether there really is an active response beneath the electrode.

One criterion for an active response is the occurrence of a steep negative deflection. Sometimes one observes only a more or less monophasic wave at electrodes from the ischemic center. These signals cannot be evaluated. In the other cases the activation time point may be determined as the time point of the steepest negative deflection as usual. This deflection is often directly followed by a positive T-wave due to the action potential shortening. The time point of the maximum increase can be determined as the repolarization time point, if a clear T-wave can be found (for further details see Gottwald et al. 1998 and Janse 1993).

During the experiment, dislocation of electrodes may occur either due to instrumentation of the heart (e.g. if ischemia or reperfusion is induced) or due to changes in the heart's movements as may occur if highly positive or negative inotropic drugs are administered. Such a dislocation of electrodes can be detected by the experimenter by a sudden change in the morphology of the QRS complex. It is therefore necessary to have 8 or more ECGs from various heart regions online on the monitor. The change in the QRS morphology if the electrode is dislocated is due to the fact that QRS morphology is mainly influenced by the direction and velocity of the propagating activation wave in the close vicinity beneath the electrode.

Another problem related to the Langendorff heart preparation perfused with saline solution is the development of oedema. In our hands there is no serious oedema formation within 120–180 min. This can be checked by weighing the hearts wet and dry and measuring the heart wet weight/dry weight ratio. If there is oedema, development due to the extended duration of the experiments one might try to overcome the problem by adding bovine serum albumin to the perfusate. However, this should be infused directly into the aortic root (*via* the cannula) and cannot be added to the Tyrode solution to avoid foaming.

For troubles caused by the isolated heart model, please see the chapter on isolated heart Langendorff model.

References

Allessie MA, Bonke FIM, Schopman FJG (1977) Circus movement in rabbit atrial muscle as a mechanism of tachycardia III. The leading circle concept. Circ Res 41: 9–18

Arisi G, Macchi E, Baruffi S, Spaggiari S, Taccardi B (1983) Potential field on the ventricular surface of the exposed dog heart during normal excitation. Circ Res 52: 706–715

Brugada P, Wellens HJJ (1988) Arrhythmogenesis of antiarrhythmic drugs. Am J Cardiol 61: 1108–1111

Buchanan JW, Saito T, Gettes LS (1985) The effects of antiarrhythmic drugs, stimulation frequency and potassium induced resting membrane potential changes on conduction velocity and dV/dt_{max} in guinea pig myocardium. Circ Res 56: 696–703

Burgess MJ, Steinhaus BM, Spiker KW, Ershler PR (1988) Nonuniform epicardial activation and repolarization properties of in vivo canine pulmonary conus. Circ Res 62: 233–246

Carlsson L, Almgren O, Duker G (1990) QTU-prolongation and torsade de pointes induced by putative class III antiarrhythmic agents in the rabbit: etiology and interventions. J Cardiovasc Pharmacol 16: 276–285

Coronel R, Fiolet JWT, Wilms-Schopman FJG, Schaapherder AFM, Johnson TA, Gettes LS, Janse MJ (1988) Distribution of extracellular potassium and its relation to electrophysiologic changes during acute myocardial ischemia in the isolated perfused porcine heart. Circulation 77: 1125–1138

Dekker LRC, Fiolet JWT, Van Bavel E, Coronel R, Opthof T, Spaan JAE, Janse MJ (1996) Intracellular Ca^{++}, intercellular electrical coupling, and mechanical activity in ischemic rabbit papillary muscle. Effects of preconditioning and metabolic blockade. Circ Res 79: 237–246

Delmar M, Michaels DC, Johnson T, Jalife J (1987) Effects of increasing intercellular resistance on transverse and longitudinal propagation in sheep epicardial muscle. Circ Res 60: 780–785

Dhein S, Rutten P, Klaus W (1988) A new method for analysing the geometry and timecourse of epicardial potential spreading. Int J Biomed Computing 23: 201–207

Dhein S, Krüsemann K, Schaefer T (1999) Effects of the gap junction uncoupler palmitoleic acid on activation and repolarization pattern in isolated rabbit hearts. A mapping study. Br J Pharmacol 128: 1375–1384

Dhein S, Müller A, Gerwin R, Klaus W (1993) Comparative study on the proarrhythmic effects of some antiarrhythmic agents. Circulation 87: 617–630

Dhein S, Krüsemann K, Engelmann F, Gottwald M (1998) Effects of type 1 Na^+/H^+-exchange inhibitor cariporide (HOE 642) on cardiac tissue. Naunyn Schmiedeberg's Arch Pharmacol 357: 662–670

Dhein S, Pejman P, Krüsemann K (2000) Effects of the IK.ATP-blockers glibenclamide and HMR 1883 on cardiac electrophysiology during regional ischemia and reperfusion. Eur J Pharmacol 398: 273–284

Dhein S, Perlitz F (2002) Haloperidol induces Torsade de Pointes Arrhythmia in an isolated rabbit heart model. A mapping study. Naunyn Schmiedeberg's Arch Pharmacol 365 [Suppl]: R98

Durrer D, Van der Tweel LH (1954) Spread of activation in the left ventricular wall of the dog. Activation conditions at the epicardial surface. Am Heart J 47: 192–203

Gottwald E Gottwald M Dhein S (1998) Enhanced dispersion of epicardial activation-recovery intervals at sites of histological inhomogeneity during regional ischaemia and reperfusion. Heart 79: 474–480

Hindricks G, Kottkamp H, Vogt B, Haverkamp W, Shenasa M, Borggrefe M, Breithardt G (1993) Mapping of anisotropic conduction in myocardial infarction. In: Shenasa M, Borggrefe M, Breithardt G (eds) Cardiac mapping. Futura Publishing Company Inc, Mount Kisco, NY, pp 225–235

Janse MJ (1993) Mapping in acutely ischemic myocardium. In: Shenasa M, Borggrefe M, Breithardt G (eds) Cardiac mapping. Futura Publishing Company Inc, Mount Kisco, NY, pp 115–123

Janse MJ, van Capelle FJL, Morsink H, Kleber AG, Wilms-Schopman F, Cardinal R, Naumann dÁlnoncourt C, Durrer D (1980) Flow of "injury cirrent" and patterns of excitation during early ventricular arrhythmias in acute myocardial ischemia in isolated porcine and canine hearts. Circ Res 47: 151–165

Kléber AG, Janse MJ, van Capelle FJL, Durrer D (1978) Mechanism and time course of ST and TQ segment changes during acute regional myocardial ischemia in the pig heart determined by extracellular and intracellular recordings. Circ Res 42: 603–613

Kléber AG, Janse MJ, Wilms-Schopman FJG et al. (1986) Changes in conduction velocity during acute ischemia in ventricular myocardium of the isolated porcine heart. Circulation 73: 189–198

Kuo CS, Munakata K, Reddy CP, Surawicz B (1983) Characteristics and possible mechanism of ventricular arrhythmia dependent on the dispersion of action potential durations. Circulation 67: 1356–1367

Lesh MD, Pring M, Spear JF (1989) Cellular uncoupling can unmask dispersion of action potential duration in ventricular myocardium. Circ Res 65: 1426–1440

Millar CK, Kralios FA, Lux RL (1985). Correlation between refractory periods and activation recovery intervals from electrograms: effects of rate and adrenergic interventions. Circulation 72: 1372–1379

Müller A, Klaus W, Dhein S (1991) Heterogeneously distributed sensitivities to potassium as a cause of hypocalemic arrhythmias in isolated rabbit hearts. J Cardiovasc Electrophysiol 2: 145–155

Spach MS, Dolber PC, Heidlage JF, Kootsey JM, Johnson EA (1987) Propagating depolarization in anisotropic human and canine cardiac muscle: apparent directional differences in membrane capacitance. Circ Res 60: 206–219

Spach MS, Dolber PC (1986) Relating extracellular potentials and their derivatives to anisotropic propagation at a microscopic level in human cardiac muscle. Circ Res 58: 356–371

Spach MS, Dolber PC (1985) The relation between discontinuous propagation in anisotropic cardiac muscle and the "vulnerable period of reentry". In: Zipes DP, Jalife J (eds) Cardiac Electrophysiology and Arrhythmias. Grune and Statton, New York, NY, pp 241–252

Voltage-Clamp and Patch-Clamp Techniques

Hans Reiner Polder, Martin Weskamp, Klaus Linz, Rainer Meyer

Introduction

History of Membrane Potential and Current Recordings in Cardiac Tissue

This chapter describes various methods of analysis of the electrical behaviour of excitable cells using microelectrodes. Since their introduction in the 1920's, microelectrodes have become the "workhorses" of electrophysiology, and a comprehensive number of publications exist about this topic. Here, we give a consolidated overview of the most important methods of investigation at single cell level, however, high throughput methods and automated recording procedures are not discussed. There is a reference list (Further Reading) at the end of this chapter, detailing some of the most important books published in recent decades.

Since the nineteenth century, it has been well known that excitable cells are able to produce electrical signals. However, until the invention of the first glass microelectrodes, by Ling and Gerard in 1949, the origin of these electrical signals could not be proven. For the first time, these glass micropipettes allowed the detection of the membrane potential of a cell, as their tips were small enough to penetrate the cell membrane without destroying the cells, and their high electrical resistance avoided shunting the membrane potential (see chapter Principles of Electrodes). These microelectrodes were connected to the high resistance input of a voltage amplifier. The monitoring of the membrane potential, delivered the base of our actual understanding of electrical events inside the heart.

In 1951, the first experiments on mammalian heart muscle tissue using these electrodes were published (Draper and Weidmann 1951). During their experiments, the negative membrane potential of around –80 mV and the cardiac action potential (AP), in its typical shape and with its real amplitude, could be recorded. Application of the voltage clamp technique (Cole 1949; Hodgkin et al. 1952), adapted to cardiac tissue (Deck et al. 1964), revealed the different current components of the cardiac action potential, which are described in chapter Membrane Currents During the Action Potential. A further leap in progress for cardiac physiology was gained by the development of techniques to isolate single living cardiac myocytes in the late 1970's (Dow et al. 1981). At the same time, the patch clamp technique was invented (Hamill et al. 1981). Some small changes in the geometry of the electrodes, as well as the development of new amplifiers (patch and single electrode clamp amplifiers), opened a completely new field as the recording of current through single channels became possible. In addition, monitoring of membrane potential, as well as currents, was highly simplified. This allowed the description of new membrane currents and detailed analysis of their molecular basis, a process that still continues today.

Description of Methods and Practical Approach
Membrane Currents During the Action Potential

The basic ionic currents during the AP were discovered by means of voltage clamp experiments on multicellular cardiac tissue preparations. Depolarisation, is caused by a voltage dependent sodium inward current, I_{Na}. Depolarisation, in turn, leads to a drop in K$^+$ conductance, and the opening of voltage gated Ca^{2+} channels giving rise to an inward-calcium current, I_{Ca}. I_{Ca} lasts for less than twenty up to two hundred milliseconds, depending on the species and thus AP- duration, e.g. murine AP-duration is around 40 ms (own unpublished observations) whereas the guinea-pig AP lasts for about 400 ms (Linz and Meyer, 1998a). The interplay of low K$^+$ conductance and I_{Ca} keeps the membrane potential depolarised, and thus forms the plateau of the cardiac AP. During the plateau phase, the K$^+$ conductance gradually re-increases, the I_{Ca} finally inactivates, and outward potassium currents repolarise the membrane. A detailed overview of cardiac excitation contraction coupling is presented in Bers (2002).

As mentioned above, isolation of living cells and the invention of the patch clamp technique simplified experiments on cardiac myocytes, thus our knowledge of cellular electrical events in the heart has blown up in the last twenty years. Therefore, some more details have to be added to the concept mentioned above. The role of the depolarising I_{Na} remains unchanged. As a family of Ca^{2+} currents in many different cells has been discovered, it has become clear that the most important current in cardiac myocytes is the L-type current, $I_{Ca,L}$ (see chapter 3.5). In addition, a so-called high voltage activated Ca^{2+} current, the T-type current, is expressed in cardiac myocytes. The concept of K$^+$ currents has become relatively complicated in recent years. Differences in AP shape between species and cardiac tissues like pacemaker cells, cells of conductive tissue, atrial and ventricular myocytes, depend mainly on the expression of different types of K$^+$ channels. As the diversity of K$^+$ currents is not the topic of this report, only a few aspects will be mentioned here (for a more detailed review see chapter 3.5). In many species a transient outward current I_{to} is activated very rapidly. This current induces an initial repolarisation after the peak of the AP. The amplitude of I_{to} determines the potential at which the plateau starts, and thereby I_{to} also determines duration and shape of the AP. The final repolarisation is brought about by two slowly activating K$^+$ current components, I_{Kr} and I_{Ks}. At potentials negative of –50 mV, I_{K1} becomes the dominating K$^+$ current, determining the resting potential.

Principles of Electrodes

Since the invention of glass microelectrodes, different forms have been developed, however, all follow the same principles as described in this chapter. "Microelectrodes" are micropipettes made of glass, filled with electrolytic solutions, with an electric connection to the recording amplifier. The microelectrode is in direct contact with the cell interior, either by penetration of the cell membrane ("sharp microelectrode recordings"), or by rupturing the membrane inside a suction electrode sealed to the surface of the cell (whole cell patch configuration). In case of a "perforated patch", some pore forming agents are used in the pipette solution to give access to the cell interior (see chapter Perforated Patch). Microelectrodes consist of the stem, the shoulder, the taper and the tip (Fig. 1). The stem with the constant diameter is the longest part of the microelectrode, followed by the shoulder and then the taper that has a continuously decreasing diameter. The taper ends in a fine tip. Depending on the diameter of the tip, microelectrodes are termed "sharp" (0.5 µm or less) or "patch" electrodes (typically 1 to 3 µm, fire polished). Microelectrodes are filled with electrolyte solution (see below). Normally, an Ag-AgCl wire is immersed into the electrolyte, connecting the electrode to the recording amplifier. Thus, the microelectrode converts ionic current in solution, into an electron current in wires, according to the following reversible reaction:

$$Cl^- + Ag \rightleftharpoons AgCl + e^-$$

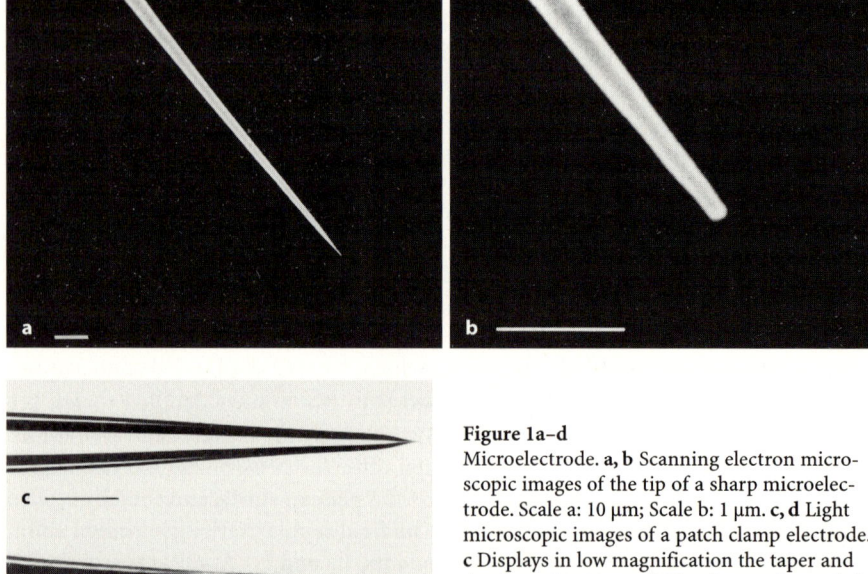

Figure 1a–d
Microelectrode. **a, b** Scanning electron microscopic images of the tip of a sharp microelectrode. Scale a: 10 µm; Scale b: 1 µm. **c, d** Light microscopic images of a patch clamp electrode. **c** Displays in low magnification the taper and the tip, scale 500 µm. **d** Tip of same electrode in higher magnification, scale 10 µm. Filled with 135 K^+, Na^+, 135 Cl^- 10 HEPES, 0.5 EGTA, all in mM, the electrode had a resistance of 4 MΩ

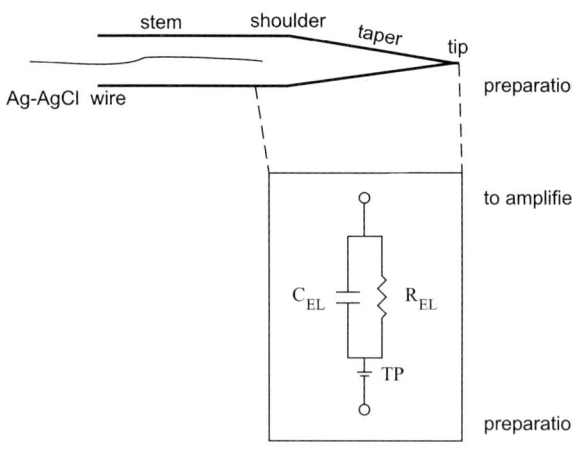

Figure 2
Equivalent circuit microelectrode (ME). Terminology and equivalent circuit of a microelectrode. C_{EL} electrode capacity, R_{EL} electrode resistance, TP tip potential

Chloriding of silver wires can easily be done by electrolysis. Many available microelectrode holders have built-in Ag-AgCl pellets, which are a good but more expensive alternative to chlorided silver wires. In terms of electrochemistry, only this part is an "electrode". In electrophysiology, the terms "microelectrode", "patch" or "suction electrode", are used for the glass micropipette and the electrochemical electrode.

In most cases, the reference ("ground signal") for the measurement is the bath surrounding the cell. The electrical connection is also made via chlorided silver wire or an Ag-AgCl pellet. This reduces a part of the occurring offset potentials. Offset potential compensation is a very important procedure, and can be done prior to an experiment if all offsets are constant. In case of solution changes, offset potentials will also change and therefore correction procedures may be necessary (Neher 1995).

Electrical Properties

From an electrical point of view, microelectrodes are RC-elements (Fig. 2) with a battery. The resistance (R), capacitance (C), and electrode potential are mostly non-linear and spread along the thin part of the microelectrode. The most unpleasant non-linearity is often called "rectification", this is because the microelectrode resistance varies depending on the direction of current flow. Beside mechanical sensitivity, these factors are serious limitations, which require sophisticated recording electronics. A simplified equivalent circuit diagram shows a resistor in parallel to a capacitor and in series to a source of voltage, the tip potential. Microelectrodes are selected carefully to have linear electrical properties in the range of operation. Therefore, the non-linear electrical properties (rectification of electrodes) are usually of minor practical importance and are omitted.

The microelectrode resistance R_{el} is basically dependent on the glass species, the diameter and length of the tip, the concentration of the electrolyte inside the microelectrode, and the concentration of the solution into which the microelectrode is immersed. The lower the concentration of the filling solution and the finer the diameter of the tip, generally, the higher the microelectrode resistance. The tip length is proportional to the microelectrode resistance, whereas the tip diameter is inversely proportional to the resistance. Filling the microelectrode with highly concentrated salt solution (2–4 M) reduces the microelectrode resistance.

The microelectrode capacitance C_m results from the electrolytes inside and outside of the electrodes representing electrical conductors, and the glass wall representing the dielectric. Since the capacitance of a capacitor is inversely proportional to the diameter of the dielectric, thin-wall electrodes have a higher capacitance than thick-wall electrodes. Furthermore, the capacitance is proportional to the depth of immersion in the bath solution. The deeper the microelectrode is immersed, the higher the capacitance (typically 1 pF/mm). In addition, the pipette holder also introduces a capacity of 1–2 pF, and the input amplifier adds another 2–10 pF, resulting in a total stray capacitance of 10–15 pF (Sigworth, 1995). A highly concentrated filling solution further reduces microelectrode capacitance. Another useful method in reducing the electrode stray capacitance is coating the tip with a layer of Sylgard (Corning), or to use thick walled glass. If these measures are still not sufficient, electronic measures can be applied, such as the use of driven shields (see chapter Capacity Compensation and Driven Shield Configuration). Sometimes, electrodes and holders are covered with conductive paint, and this layer is also connected to the "driven shield" signal. Since all these measures are tedious, it is very important to select the correct glass and pulling protocol to obtain the best possible electrodes for a given experiment.

The battery shown in Fig. 2 is usually non-linear and depends on several factors, such as glass species, solutions, temperature etc. It is an offset potential, composed of the liquid junction potential and the tip potential. Both are dependent on several factors. The liquid junction potential develops whenever two solutions of different concentrations and mobility of anions and cations get in contact; here, typically 3 M KCl inside the microelectrode and 0.1 M KCl in the bath solution. Other parameters determining the tip potential are the surface charge of the glass, which can be reduced by using borosilicate glass, and the pH of the solutions inside the microelectrode and the bath. The latter is of minor importance with a pH of between 6 and 8. The tip diameter is also an important factor, as when the tip is enlarged, the tip potential is substantially reduced.

In practice, a compromise has to be found between a fine tip, that will not harm the cell and that prevents the highly concentrated electrolyte flowing into the cell, and the better electrical properties of electrodes with a larger tip diameter.

Usually, the tip potential represents the offset of the microelectrode, and is compensated by the amplifier. Offset compensation is done by performing a test measurement prior to cell penetration and cancelling the offset with the amplifier's offset control.

In whole-cell patch clamp experiments, the electrolyte inside the pipette is from the same osmolarity as the cytoplasm. This results in a liquid junction potential in the bath solution that is cancelled during offset correction of the microelectrode. When going into whole-cell configuration this liquid junction potential disappears, resulting in a wrong offset compensation prior to the experiment. Thus in whole-cell mode experiments, the results should be corrected by the liquid junction potential (Neher

1995). In experiments with sharp microelectrodes, correction for liquid junction potentials is done by bathing the microelectrode in a cytoplasm-like solution after the experiment, and correcting the offset accordingly.

Due to the electrical properties of the microelectrode, the measured signals are low-pass filtered. For instance, a microelectrode with 10 MΩ resistance and 4–5 pF capacitance has a high-frequency limit of 3–4 kHz. Taking into account the pipette holder and amplifier input capacitance of 10 pF the frequency response is only around 1 kHz. If electronic capacity compensation is used, the frequency is boosted by a factor of 2–10, yielding an acceptable bandwidth for recording fast potential changes (see chapter Capacity Compensation and Driven Shield Configuration). For the application of the time-sharing recording technique (see chapter Single Electrode Clamp) an even higher bandwidth is required, which can be obtained by using supercharging protocols (Armstrong and Chow 1987; Müller et al. 1999; Polder and Swandulla 2001).

Amplifiers

Recording of Electrical Signals, General Principles, Ion Sensitive Amplifiers

The general configuration, in recording electrical signals from living tissues, is an electrode that transfers biological phenomena into an electrical signal and a sensitive amplifier. The amplifier must have high input impedance, low noise, a high gain with an appropriate bandwidth and some facilities to compensate for distorting signals (e.g. offsets, stray capacities, common mode noise etc.).

If recordings are made on a cellular basis, one usually employs a microelectrode as the signal-transducing element (see chapter Principles of electrodes). The recording devices are FET operational amplifiers that have a very high input impedance (10^{12}–10^{15} Ω), low noise in the mV range and sufficient bandwidth at high gains. Such amplifiers are often called "buffer" or "electrometer" amplifiers. Sometimes two buffer amplifiers are used, which are connected to a differential amplifier with a very high common mode rejection. Such a configuration eliminates common mode signals (e.g. noise pickup in ECG recordings), and is also used for some special microelectrode configurations (e.g. ion sensitive electrodes or two electrode voltage clamps for high currents. (See Fig. 3 and chapter Introduction to Two Electrode Voltage Clamp).

AC/DC Amplifier, Offset

Very often electrophysiological amplifiers are so-called AC amplifiers, i.e. they are not capable of recording DC potentials. This is helpful in many cases where only changes of the signal are of interest, whereas the steady-state signal is of minor importance. Such amplifiers are used e.g. in ECG recordings. They automatically suppress DC electrode potentials.

If DC recordings are required, an offset compensation circuit must compensate for the electrode potential. This is usually a ten-turn control with mV resolution or an automatic compensation circuit.

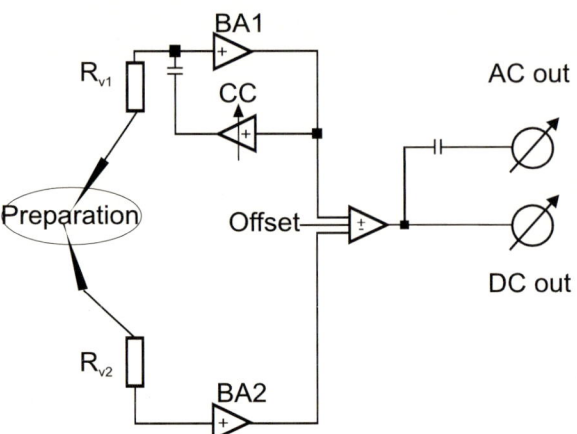

Figure 3
Differential amplifier. Basic microelectrode recording circuit. The differential recording mode reduces the effect of common mode disturbance signals. This amplifier can be used for DC recordings of very small signals, e.g. from ionsensitive microelectrodes. If common mode signals are small (e.g. in an in vitro recording chamber) the negative input can be grounded and the buffer amplifier is not needed. *BA* buffer amplifier, *CC* capacity compensation

Capacity Compensation and Driven Shield Configuration

Biological signals cover a frequency range from DC to a few kHz. Very often, microelectrodes have frequency characteristics that are below this required range for good recordings, due to the high resistance shunted by the stray capacity (see chapter Principles of Electrodes). To reduce this effect, one possibility is the use of a capacity compensation circuit ("negative" capacity, generated by a so-called negative impedance converter (NIC) circuit). A high-speed amplifier forms the compensation circuit, with a variable gain connected to a small capacitor that injects a well-defined amount of charge into the electrode, so that the stray capacity is charged from this low impedance source. The signal bandwidth is increased (3–5 fold in practice); at the same time the noise is also increased. Such a circuit is a closed loop system with positive feedback. Therefore, if a certain gain is reached, the system will oscillate. A special version of this circuit is the so-called "driven shield" approach. It is a capacity compensation circuit with gain one. All the components, between electrode and recording amplifier (pipette holder, cable, even the headstage enclosure), are NOT connected to ground but to the output of the buffer amplifier that typically will have a gain of one. The capacity, formed for example by the inner core of the electrode cable and the shield, will be omitted since the shield and the core are isopotential in this configuration. A driven shield increases the bandwidth considerably, without the risk of oscillations. As before, the noise will also increase.

Current Clamp Recordings and Bridge Amplifiers

Adding a current injection device to an electrometer amplifier will give a current clamp instrument. With such a device, one can inject a certain amount of current and observe the membrane potential change. Current clamps are basically intracellular amplifiers, i.e. they must have direct access to the interior of the cell. The simplest way to perform well-defined current injections is to use a high value resistor connected to a battery. To give an error <1%, the value of this resistor must be a hundred fold

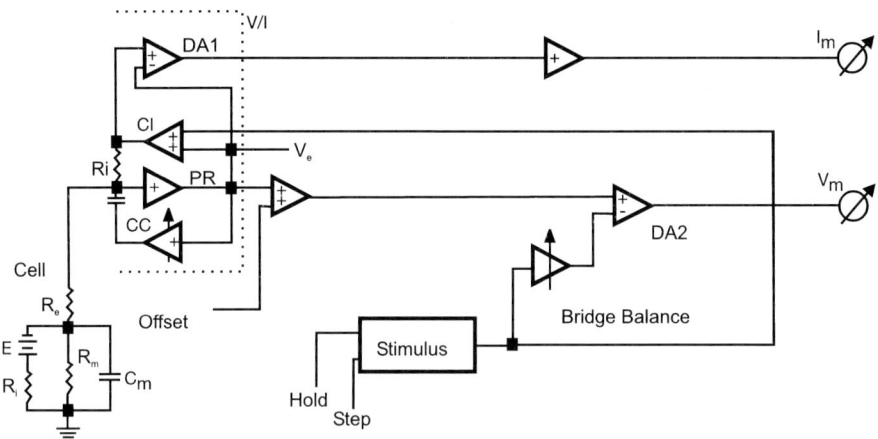

Figure 4
Bridge amplifier. The bridge amplifier is used for intracellular recordings in current clamp mode. It can inject current into the cell by using an electronic circuit called "voltage controlled current source". The voltage deflection caused by the current flow is compensated by subtracting a current proportional signal ("bridge balancing") and one can record the membrane potential accurately. *DA* differential amplifier, *CI* current injection, *CC* capacity compensation, *PR* potential recording

higher than the value of the recording microelectrode. This leads to very high resistance values and the use of voltages of a few hundred Volts is necessary, which in practice is not useful. Therefore, one uses an electronic circuit called a "voltage controlled current source" (Fig. 4). Such a circuit uses feedback to generate a well-defined current, regardless of the load resistance. In the case of microelectrodes, one needs currents from pA to µA. Thus, generally low voltage operational amplifiers are used. An exception to this rule, is the two-electrode voltage clamp (see chapter Introduction to Two-Electrode Voltage Clamp), where large currents are sometimes required that demand the use of high voltage techniques (e.g. clamping large cells such as *Xenopus* oocytes).

Even small amounts of current flowing through a microelectrode will cause a voltage deflection that in general cannot be ignored. There are three solutions to this problem:
1. Using separate microelectrodes for potential recording and current injection. For example: Two electrode clamp systems (see chapter Introduction to Two Electrode Voltage Clamp).
2. Interruption of current flow during potential recording. For example: Time-sharing (switching) amplifiers, (SEVC) (see Single Electrode Clamp).
3. Electronic compensation of the electrode artefact. For example: bridge amplifiers, Rs compensation in patch clamp amplifiers (see Introduction to Patch Clamp).

In a bridge amplifier, a current proportional amount is subtracted from the recorded potential. In this way, the voltage deflection caused by the current flow is compensated ("bridge balancing"), and one can record the membrane potential accurately. It is clear that the microelectrode must have linear behaviour (no "rectification", see chapter Principles of Electrodes). The equivalent circuit is shown in Fig. 4.

Electrical Stimulation

Electrical stimulation plays an important role in cardiac electrophysiology, since bioelectrical relations determine most of the phenomena under investigation. This is a very old investigation method (e.g. the famous experiment on frog muscles performed by L. Galvani (1791), and there are two basic methods used:
1. Stimulation using stimulus isolators
2. Stimulation from the recording amplifier

Stimulus isolators are used in conjunction with bipolar electrodes to elicit a signal locally, in remote parts of the preparation, which is transferred to the recording site (example: recording action potentials from Purkinje fibres or papillary muscle preparations).

With this method, large populations of cells are usually stimulated. To avoid artefacts due to current flow through the tissue, one uses an isolation unit that produces a local electric field, which is strong enough to depolarise cells that then produces action potentials. These are transferred to other cells in a similar manner as intrinsically produced signals. In this way, one can investigate, for example, action potentials in the presence of drugs in a well-defined manner.

Stimulus electrodes are small, e.g. two insulated twisted Platinum wires (diameters in the range of 100 μm), and have resistances of several hundred kΩ up to MΩ. Due to this high resistance, one usually needs rather high voltages, in the range of tens of Volts, to obtain an adequate stimulus. Stimuli are short (μs to ms) and do not normally deteriorate the recording. Some amplifiers have a "blank" circuit, which suppresses the stimulus artefact.

Internal electrical stimulation is used on single cells, e.g. by injecting a certain amount of current through the recording electrode. One can use this method both in voltage clamp (VC) and current clamp (CC) mode. In general, the artefact caused by the stimulus deteriorates the measurement, and must be compensated (see chapter Current Clamp Recordings and Bridge Amplifiers).

Current Recordings from Single Cells

Introduction to Voltage Clamp

In a voltage clamp (VC) experiment, the membrane potential of a cell is controlled from an external device (the VC amplifier), with the goal of measuring the ionic currents that flow through the channels in the cell membrane at this given command potential. This requires an active compensation of the current flow across the membrane. The membrane potential is measured and compared to the command signal; the VC amplifier compensates by active charge injection the deviation to keep the error as small as possible. The quality of the current recording is mainly determined by this error signal.

In practice, the performance of a given VC system is limited by the following three factors:

1. The non-ideal geometry of the cell (space clamp error). An ideal performance (isopotentiality independent of the location) from a microelectrode based VC system can only be obtained in a perfectly spherical cell with the tip of the current injecting microelectrode exactly in the centre. With real cells, there will always be local deviations of the membrane potential. This problem will not be treated in this chapter, since mainly technical aspects of the amplifiers are described here. For details please see references Ferreira and Marshall (1985), Hille (1992), and Jack et al. (1975) in further reading at the end of this chapter.
2. The electrical properties of the recording microelectrodes (see chapters Principles of Electrodes and Amplifiers)
3. The electric resistance Rs of the intracellular structures located between the tip of the recording electrodes and the cell membrane (series resistance error, see chapters Single Electrode Clamp and Introduction to Patch Clamp).

In cardiac electrophysiology, mainly single electrode systems are used. For completeness, the two-electrode clamp technique is also described, especially since it is widely used in *Xenopus* oocyte expression systems.

VC instruments (except patch clamp amplifiers) are closed-loop control systems based on electronic feedback. Such feedback systems can be described in the framework of control theory. Since control theory and control technology are used in nearly all branches of engineering to design feedback systems, a large variety of "ready-made" solutions for optimising control loops is available.

Control Loop Analysis and Optimisation

Fortunately, VC systems are composed only of elements that react with a retardation to a change (delay elements). The time constants of these individual delay elements fall into two categories: one is basically determined by the cell, is in the range of milliseconds and dedicated as a "large" time constant. The other (basically the recording microelectrode and amplifier) is clearly in the sub-millisecond range and defined as "small" time constants. These "small" time constants can be summed yielding an equivalent time constant. The performance of such control systems can be optimised by "modulus hugging", a standard method in engineering based on the adequate shaping of the frequency response magnitude of the control loop. This procedure yields optimised systems with respect to speed of response and clamp accuracy.

Choice of Controller

The ideal controller for this kind of feedback loop is the "proportional-integral" (P-I) controller. "Proportional" means an amplifier with high gain ("gain" knob of the VC instrument). This amplifier will react instantaneously to a change, but it needs a steady input to have an output signal. Therefore, it always produces a constant clamp error.

This error is avoided by using the "integral" part, which is basically an operational amplifier with a capacitor as a feedback circuit. This device will cause a constant output if the input is zero, i.e. it will supply the steady state signal needed to keep the membrane potential constant. As soon as there is a change (i.e. error signal not zero), it will follow this signal with a certain delay defined by the integrator time constant, until the input (error signal) becomes zero again. So it generates a zero clamp error, but it is slower than the proportional amplifier. One can show that the gain of the proportional amplifier and the time constant of the integrator are determined solely by the two basic time constants of the feedback loop described above.

An empirical procedure can be derived from this theoretical approach, which allows the optimal tuning of VC instruments based on PI controllers, while running an experiment (Polder and Swandulla 2001).

Criteria for Setting Up a Controller

Proper tuning of the VC instrument is very important for electrophysiologists. Described most in the literature is the "setting with no overshoot", but if one applies control theory as depicted before, one can demonstrate that this will lead to false results. This method is the "weakest" of the three methods recommended for the setting of PI control units.

Linear Optimum (LO) Method

With this method, the step response of the controlled variable to a reference step change shows a slow approach to the final value without any overshoot, i.e. the step response corresponds to the aperiodic limiting case. This method does not require a PI controller; a simple amplifier with variable gain is sufficient. This setting is known as "critical damping" in the voltage clamp literature, and is normally the recommended tuning procedure. Clamps tuned in this way react slowly and achieve only a poor fidelity; clamp accuracy is a maximum of 90–97%, which is not sufficient for most applications (for an overview see Smith et al. 1985).

Modulus or Absolute Value Optimum (AVO)

This method provides a response that is twice as steep a step command input as that obtained with the LO method, but there will be a small overshoot of approx. 4% before the magnitude of the step is reached. It requires a PI-controller and provides the fastest transition to a new command level (Hofmeier and Lux 1981). It is applied if the maximum speed of a response to a command step is desirable, e.g., if large voltage-activated currents are investigated (e.g. see Hofmeier and Lux 1981; Müller et al. 1999).

Symmetrical Optimum (SO)

The SO method is the standard procedure used in engineering. It optimises the performance of the control system with respect to a disturbance, in the case of a VC system, to a change in the measured membrane potential. The response to a command step shows a very steep rising phase followed by a considerable overshoot of 43%. This overshoot can be prevented, by adequate filtering of the command signal (see below).

The SO method is favourable wherever the maximum precision for membrane potential control is required (e.g. to record currents from electrically coupled cells, Müller et al. 1999).

Speed of Response of Optimised Systems

The speed of response of an ideal clamp system is determined only by the cell capacity and the amount of charge that can be injected. The theoretically possible rise time of a clamp system can be estimated from the charge/voltage relation of the membrane capacitance:

$$dV/dt = I/C \ [\text{V/s}]$$

Combining this formula with Ohm's Law and the essential parameters of the VC system (R_{el} resistance of the current injecting microelectrode, U_{out} maximum output voltage of the VC instrument, C_m membrane capacitance, ΔV applied voltage command step, Δt rise time), the maximum speed of response of a given VC system under ideal conditions can be calculated:

$$I_{max} = U_{out}/R_{el} \text{ and } dV/dt = U_{out}/(R_{el}*C_m)$$

For a given command step ΔV the theoretically shortest duration can be calculated as:

$$\Delta t = \Delta V * R_{el} * C_w/U_{out}$$

The real (optimised) clamp system will always react more slowly than an idealized VC system, in practice 2–3 times slower. The settling time of the real clamp system is determined mostly by the sum of "small" time constants. Therefore, the higher the bandwidth of the microelectrode/clamp amplifier system, the faster the clamp will react (see Polder and Swandulla, 2001 for details).

Tuning of VC Systems with PI Controllers During an Experiment

During an experiment, the parameters of the control chain are not known in most cases. Fortunately, it is possible to tune the clamp controller, by optimising the response to test pulses applied to the command input. The AVO and SO methods, are both derived from a mathematical "modulus hugging" procedure, and behave in a similar manner. It is self-evident that the SO method, which provides the tightest control, will be the most sensitive to parameter settings. Of course, the transitions between the optimisation methods are blurred, and the tuning procedure is adapted, to the experimental requirements.

In practice, of course, all parameters that influence clamp performance (microelectrode offsets, capacity compensation, etc.) must be optimally tuned before starting the PI controller tuning procedure.

The tuning procedure involves three steps:

1. Tuning of the proportional gain: The integral part of the PI controller is disconnected (e.g. by a switch). The reference input is used without smoothing, and adequate command pulses are applied (e.g. small hyperpolarizing pulses). The gain is tuned to the desired value, i.e. until the overshoot according to the selected tuning method appears (0% with the LO method and ca. 4% with the AVO and with the SO methods). Since the integral part of the controller is disconnected, a steady state error in the range of a few percent will be present.
2. Integrator tuning: The integrator is reconnected to form the complete PI controller. Again adequate test pulses are applied without filtering. The integrator time constant is adjusted to achieve the overshoot of the selected optimisation method (4% with the AVO method and 43% with the SO method). Now the steady-state error must disappear.
3. Tuning of the reference smoothing circuit (low-pass filter): If necessary, especially when using the SO method, the reference input has to be filtered by an adequate low pass system. The tuning is performed by again applying adequate step commands, and setting of the time constant, until the overshoot is reduced to the desired value.

Introduction to Two-Electrode Voltage Clamp

Two (or double) electrode clamp (TEVC) systems have been used since the late 1940's. In 1949, Cole described the first voltage clamp system. The equivalent circuit of the two-electrode VC system is given in Fig. 5. The membrane potential is recorded differentially to compensate for extracellular series resistances. Intracellular series resis-

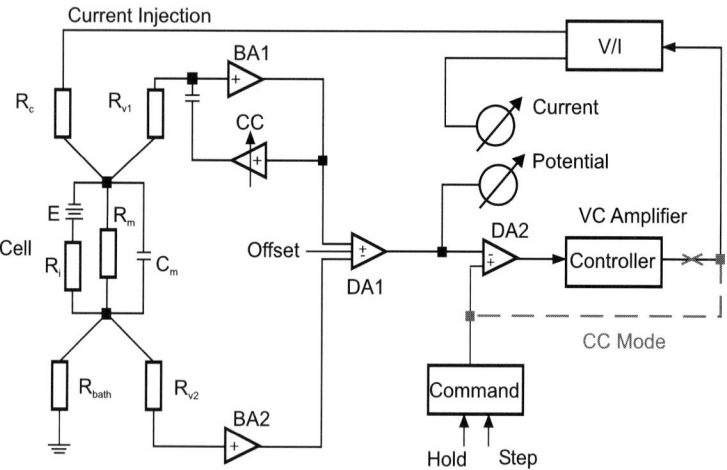

Figure 5
Double electrode VC. Equivalent circuit of a double electrode voltage clamp system. The cell is described by a passive network and an active current source that represents membrane currents. The electrodes are represented as resistances that are connected to the electronic controller via high impedance buffers. All elements have low-pass character (delay elements). Dashed shaded lines represent current clamp mode, black lines are voltage clamp mode. *DA* differential amplifier, *CC* capacity compensation, *V/I* voltage to current converter

tance is not discussed in this chapter since it is only of importance if very large membrane currents are recorded, e.g. in *Xenopus* oocytes. The treatment of this intracellular series resistance is discussed elsewhere (Greeff and Kühn 2000). In order to enhance the speed of response of the potential recording circuit (i.e. to reduce the sum of "small time constants" T_e), a conventional capacity compensation circuit with positive feedback and driven shield arrangement is used. When optimal compensation is achieved, this circuit can be considered as a first-order delay element with the equivalent time constant T_e (see Polder and Swandulla 2001). For the compensation of tip potentials etc. a DC offset compensation circuit is used.

The membrane potential signal obtained in this way is then subtracted from the command signal by means of a differential amplifier giving the error signal, which is the input signal of the controller. The output of the controller is connected to a voltage to current conversion circuit, which can be a high voltage amplifier connected to the current injecting microelectrode (TEVC A). In this case, the ohmic resistance of the electrode performs the conversion of the controller output signal to the injected current, which in general is non-linear and unstable, thus influencing the clamp performance considerably. Therefore, a better approach is to use an electronic voltage to current converter (voltage controlled current source (VCCS), TEVC B). In this way, the influence of the electrode can be largely reduced (Polder and Swandulla 2001; Kordas et al. 1989).

In the first case (TEVC A), the membrane current is recorded with a virtual ground circuit, while in the second case (TEVC B), the current is measured differentially in the voltage to current converter. The type of the output circuit has considerable effects on the performance of the clamp circuit. The TEVC A system is characterized by the time constant, introduced by the current injecting electrode in parallel with the membrane resistance (R_m) and the cell capacity. This time constant is in the range of milliseconds to seconds (e.g. in *Xenopus* oocytes), and therefore considerably limits the performance of the clamp system. The performance is dependent on both the membrane resistance and the electrode resistance. Note that both resistances are non-linear and change with time, sometimes by orders of magnitude (e.g. if voltage activated channels open). The transfer function is dimensionless (V/V) (see Polder and Swandulla 2001). With this approach, current clamping will need a closed feedback loop.

The performance of the TEVC B System is no longer dependent on the time constant, and is therefore independent of the resistance of the current injecting electrode (as long as the current source is not saturated), since the system output is a current that is injected into the cell. The current can be measured directly in the VCCS device, which is the major advantage compared to the TEVC A system. The transfer function has the dimension of a conductance (A/V). The clamp performance is dependent mainly on the membrane capacity, which is a constant, and the maximum amount of current available, which is dependent on the output voltage of the VCCS circuit. One major advantage of this approach is that current clamping can be achieved easily by simply opening the feedback loop, and applying an input signal directly to the VCCS circuit. A disadvantage of the TEVC B system is that this approach is dependent on stray capacities at the VCCS output. These stray capacities determine to a large degree the "small" time constant T_e, and therefore define the maximum gain and speed of response of the system. In addition, the current needed to charge these stray capacities is added to the membrane current. These stray capacities must be minimized, e.g. by using driven shield arrangements or electronic capacity compensation circuits (Polder and Swandulla 2001).

Single Electrode Clamp

The Principle and the Amplifier

Time-sharing single electrode clamp systems (Fig. 5) are characterized by the discontinuous mode of operation: for a period of time T_I current is passed through the recording electrode while potential registration is suppressed, during the following period T_V, no current will be passed and the potential registration is activated. In 1971, Brennecke and Lindemann described the first time-sharing (switched) amplifier. Their goal was to avoid series resistance errors by turning off current injection during potential recording. Based on this approach, in 1975 the first single electrode clamp (SEVC) amplifier was described by Wilson and Goldner (for details see Brennecke and Lindemann 1974; Polder and Swandulla 2001). The principle of this operation yields major advantages:
- One can do current and voltage clamping in deep layers ("blind" recording).
- The membrane potential is measured without current flow through the microelectrode, i.e. without any deterioration from series resistances.
- The amplifier measures membrane potential and membrane current in each cycle.
- Recordings can be performed with all kinds of configurations: sharp microelectrode, perforated and tight seal patch clamp (whole cell configuration).

The discontinuous action is described mathematically by the switching frequency f_{sw} and the duty cycle D:

$$f_{sw} = 1/(T_I + T_V); \qquad D = T_I/(T_I + T_V) \qquad T_{S/H} = 1/f_{sw}$$

The selection of an adequate switching frequency and duty cycle is crucial for the correct application of SEVC systems. The error (ripple of the resulting membrane potential caused by the discontinuous current injection) is proportional to the injected amount of current, and the reciprocal of the membrane capacity. It also depends on the switching frequency and the duty cycle. SEVC systems can be considered as linear systems if this error is below 1 mV (Polder and Swandulla 2001). In this case, the dead time caused by the discontinuous mode of operation can be approximated by a first order delay with a time constant $T_{S/H}$ related to the switching frequency (Polder and Swandulla 2001).

This time constant will be added to the sum of the "small" time constants of the control loop, and will contribute mainly to the resulting equivalent time constant. This equivalent time constant must be kept in the range of microseconds in order to achieve good clamp accuracy and a fast clamp response (see chapters Criteria for setting up a controller and Speed of response of optimised systems), which means that high switching frequencies (10–40 kHz) must be used. This can be achieved with a properly designed voltage/current converter (VCCS device), with an electronic compensation for the electrode time constant at the recording site (see Polder and Swandulla 2001 for details). This allows almost complete cancellation of any stray capacitance around the electrode, so that the electrode behaves as a pure ohmic resistor. The relation of switching frequency, electrode time constant, capacity compen-sation and bandwidth of the recording microelectrode, filter setting, and data acquisition sampling rate has been analysed experimentally and leads to the "switching frequency formula" (Weckström et. al. 1992; Juusola 1994):

$$f_e > 3f_{sw}, f_{sw} > 2f_s, f_s > 2f_f > f_m$$

Where f_e is the upper cut off frequency of the microelectrode, f_{sw} switching frequency of the dSEVC, f_s sampling frequency of the data acquisition system, f_f upper cut off frequency of the low pass filter for current recording, and f_m upper cut off frequency of the membrane (see Müller et al. 1999 for an example). With the time constant of 1–3 µs recorded for the electrode resistances used in this study (Müller et al. 1999) f_e is 80–160 kHz, the switching frequency of the dSEVC was selected 30–50kHz (calculated range is 25–53 kHz), data were sampled at 10 kHz and the current signals have been filtered at 5 kHz. These settings are currently used for recordings in many labs (Müller et al. 1999; Lalley et al. 1999).

The switching protocol induces a delay in the control loop that is proportional to the reciprocal of the switching frequency. Therefore, the dynamics of SEVC systems are basically determined by the cell capacity and the switching frequency. If the previously described optimisation is performed, the parameters of the VC amplifier can

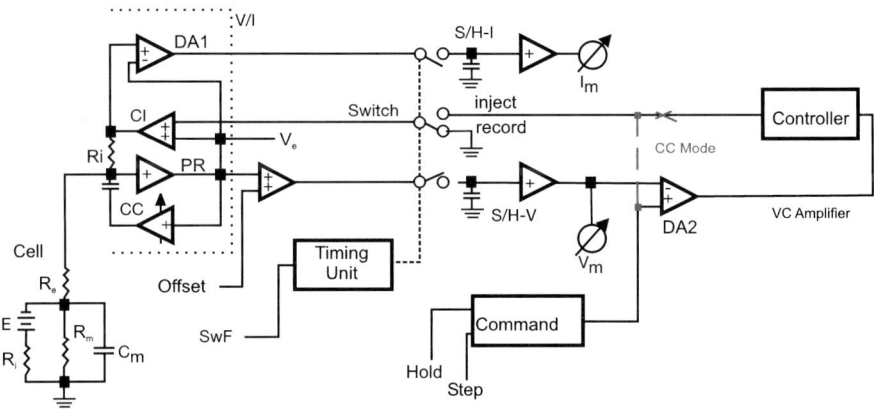

Figure 6
Single electrode VC. Block diagram of time-sharing single electrode voltage clamp system. The dashed lines point to those elements related to the time-sharing operation. Since with high switching frequencies the system can be considered linear, these units can be split into independent blocks. The time sharing operation is considered by a dead time which can be substituted by a delay element with a time constant related to the reciprocal of the switching frequency. Dashed shaded lines represent current clamp mode, black lines are voltage clamp mode. See text for details. *SwF* switching frequency, *DA* differential amplifier, *CI* current injection, *CC* capacity compensation, *PR* potential recording, *S/H* sample-and-hold, *V/I* voltage to current converter

be calculated from the relation between short time constant (delay caused by the switching frequency) and the cell capacity (see Polder and Swandulla 2001 for details). After proper selection of a switching frequency, a SEVC amplifier can be considered in both current and voltage clamp modes as an idealized TEVC (TEVC B) with a virtual second electrode (see Müller et al. 1999 for an example of proper tuning). Current clamp recordings can be obtained in a similar manner, as with the TEVC B configuration, by simply opening the feedback loop and applying an input signal directly to the VCCS circuit. Due to the switching operation, one obtains accurate values both of the injected current and the resulting membrane potential.

Measures to Improve Clamp Stability

- Output current limiter: VC systems with voltage/current converter outputs (TEVC B, SEVC) are designed, based on the assumption, that the converter suppresses the influence of the electrode and the included stray capacity compensation circuits. Microelectrodes have a strong tendency to increase their resistance during current passage (electrode block), which can lead to saturation of the voltage/current converter. In this case, an input change causes no output change, i.e. the control loop is distorted and the system will oscillate. This unstable state can be avoided by including an electronic limiter circuit, which limits the output current to a safe level (i.e. to the level at which the electrode does not block). If strong limiting is necessary (e.g. with high resistance microelectrodes), the speed of response of the clamp is affected (see chapter Principles of Electrodes).
- Electrode shielding, driven shield arrangements: In our control models of different voltage clamp systems, possible couplings between electrodes (TEVC) and the environment (stray capacity effects, etc.) have not been considered in a detailed manner, since our aim was to show the basic principles of clamp loop optimisation. Coupling between electrodes in TEVC systems, and capacitive charging of the electrode in SEVC systems, basically contribute to the instabilities of clamp systems. These effects can be diminished, by correct positioning of the electrodes, shielding (Smith et al. 1985) or coating (Juusola et al. 1997). Since the accuracy and speed of response of all described systems is determined by the equivalent time constant T_e, the use of driven shields (Smith et al. 1985; Ogden 1994) rather than grounded electrode shields is recommended.

Introduction to Patch Clamp

The Principle and the Amplifier

Patch clamp recordings are the basis of modern electrophysiology, and their importance to related research fields cannot be underestimated. Patch clamp recordings are based on the use of blunt, fire polished microelectrodes that form a so-called "gigaseal" with the cell membrane. The invention of the gigaseal, and development of the various patch methods in the late 1970's by Erwin Neher, Bert Sakmann and their colleagues were rewarded with the Nobel Prize in 1991.

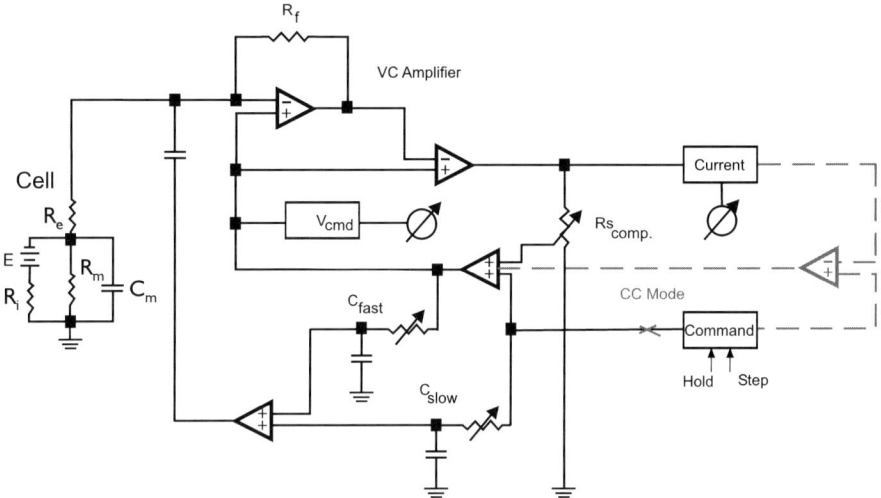

Figure 7
Patch clamp. Equivalent circuit of a resistive feedback patch clamp amplifier in the whole cell recording configuration. Dashed shaded lines represent current clamp mode, black lines are voltage clamp mode. See text for details

Originally the term "patch clamp" referred to voltage clamp recordings of currents through individual ionic channels from an isolated patch of membrane. This isolation is obtained starting with the "cell attached configuration". If a fire polished microelectrode with an opening of 1–2 µm is used, a chemically and electrically stable connection between the cell membrane is formed, which due to its high electrical resistance in the GΩ range, was called "gigaseal". This enables the recording of currents in the pA range with low background noise.

Various arrangements are known, one of the most important being the "whole cell" configuration, which corresponds to the intracellular recording situation described in previous paragraphs. In this recording approach, which is very important in heart physiology, the membrane is ruptured inside the pipette and a stable connection to the cell interior is formed. The access resistance to the cell interior in the "whole cell" configuration is in the MΩ range. The patch clamp configurations will be described in detail at the end of this chapter (see Patch Clamp Configurations and Whole-Cell Configuration).

The equivalent circuit of a patch clamp amplifier (whole cell configuration) is shown in Fig. 7. Patch clamp amplifiers are based on a current-to-voltage converter circuit, which transfers the pipette current into an equivalent output voltage. Therefore, they cannot measure membrane potentials directly. In voltage clamp mode, the command signal is imposed in a "feed forward" manner, whereas, for current clamping a closed loop feedback system is needed (dashed shaded lines).

For recording currents in the pA range, a high value feedback resistor R_f is needed (up to 50 GΩ). In this case the voltage drop across the pipette resistance can be neglected. Large resistors have several disadvantages, and are serious sources of noise.

Another approach used for high-resolution recording is the "capacitive feedback" technique (also called integrating headstage). Here, a capacitor replaces the feedback resistor and the headstage circuit becomes an integrator. The output signal is a ramp; the slope corresponding to the current signal. If this signal is passed through a differentiator, the output voltage will be proportional to the current signal. This approach has a superior noise performance compared to the resistive feedback, as long as the input (stray) capacitance can be kept low (clearly below 10 pF).

In the whole cell configuration, larger currents are needed (in the nA range), therefore, the feedback resistor is in the range of a few ten MΩ. In this case, the voltage deflection across the pipette cannot be ignored, and needs to be compensated electronically.

If a command step is applied to the pipette, the stray capacity must be charged. This causes large transient currents to flow, which will saturate the I/V converter circuit. Therefore, adequate amounts of charge are injected through a small capacitor (C_{fast} compensation). Also, the charge for the membrane capacity is supplied from a compensation circuit (C_{slow}). So far, the speed of the system has not improved. At this point, series resistance compensation can be applied by adding a current proportional fraction to the command signal. This is a closed loop system with positive feedback that will become unstable at a certain point. With this technique, compensation levels of up to 70% can be obtained (theoretically 90%, for details see Sigworth 1995). For small cells, the remaining error becomes tolerable, however, if large cells are investigated, series resistance errors become significant (see Müller et al. 1999 for details).

To enable current clamp recordings, the current flow across the pipette must be under control of the investigator. Therefore, a closed loop system is used which sets the command signal so that the current is constant. Such a system works fine for slow signals, but in the case of fast transient signals (e.g. action potentials), considerable errors are induced (see Magistretti et al. 1996 for details). In CC mode, series resistance compensation is not effective, therefore the voltage decay, due to the current flow, must be considered. Also, the correct setting of C_{fast} compensation is important to avoid dynamic errors induced by the uncompensated stray capacitance.

Patch clamp amplifiers are ideal for recording small currents (pA...nA range). In whole cell configuration, the fraction of uncompensated series resistance, as well as the fact that these amplifiers do not record potentials directly, limits their use.

Patch Clamp Configurations

Originally, "patch clamp" referred to voltage clamp recordings of currents through individual ionic channels from an isolated small patch of membrane. This isolation is obtained starting with the "cell attached configuration". The first step is when an electrode approaches a cell. Gentle positive pressure is applied to the interior of the electrode. This leads to a slow, but steady, stream of solution out of the electrode, which protects the tip of the electrode against contamination. A clean electrode tip is the prerequisite for the formation of the gigaseal. The second step begins when the tip of the electrode touches the cell membrane at the outer surface, and gentle negative pressure is applied to the electrode interior. This sucks the membrane tightly to the edges

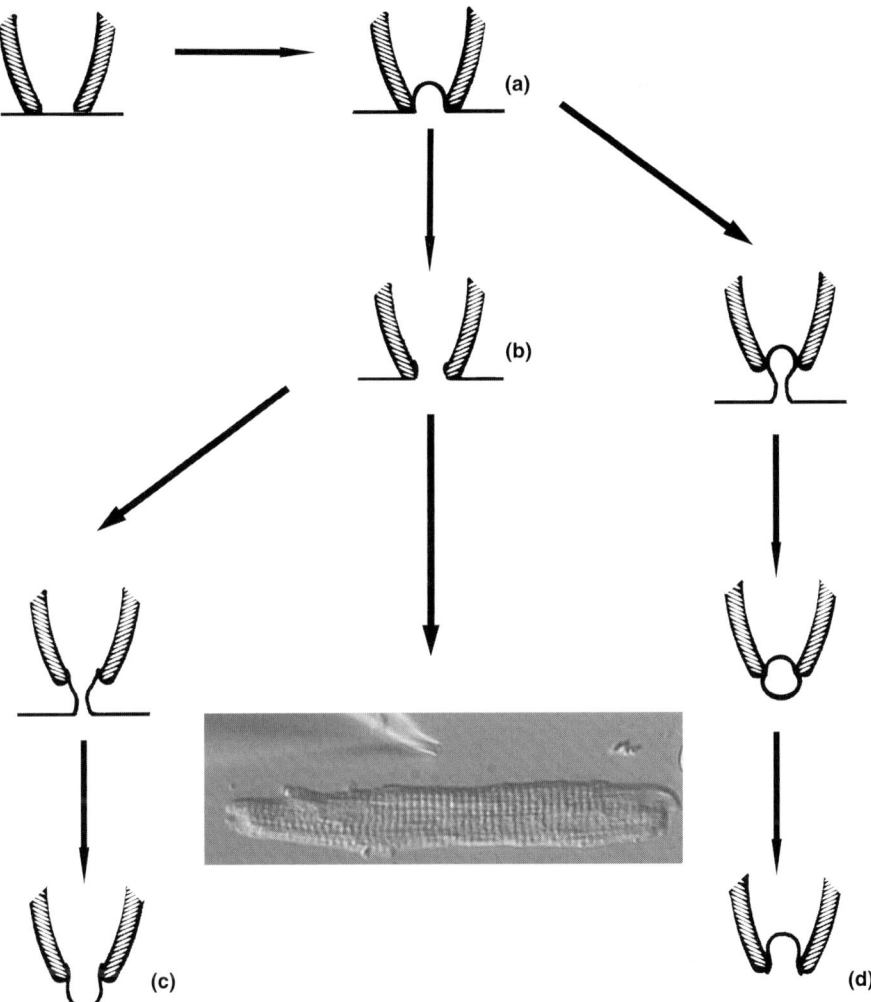

Figure 8a–d
Patch clamp configurations. Different recording configurations with patch clamp electrodes. Illustrated is the tip of the electrode together with the surface membrane of the cell. After attaching the electrode to the cell surface suction is applied and the gigaseal develops in the "cell-attached configuration" (a). Starting from this configuration additional suction ruptures the membrane and the whole-cell configuration is established (b). Retracting the electrode in whole-cell configuration from the cell leads to an outside-out patch (c). An inside-out patch can be established by retracting the electrode in the cell-attached configuration and destroying the outer half of the membrane vesicle (d)

of the electrode tip, which will induce the formation of the gigaseal. This configuration is called "cell attached" (see Fig. 8a). The development of the gigaseal can be controlled easily, if a train of rectangular test pulses is applied to the electrode. These pulses will induce a current flow through the patch clamp electrode to the reference electrode. The resistance of the electrode is in the range of 1–5 MΩ. According to Ohm's law, the current flow depends mainly on the electrode resistance. As soon as the electrode is attached to the membrane, the current has to flow through the gigaseal or membrane into the cytoplasm, and through the membrane again. Both ways have resistances, which are some orders of magnitude higher than that of the electrode, therefore, the current flow decreases after the formation of the gigaseal.

Starting with the cell-attached configuration, different measuring configurations can be reached. In the "cell-attached mode", single channel currents already within the membrane patch, inside the electrode, can be recorded. A second suction pulse will cause a rupture of the membrane patch inside the electrode. In this situation, there is an open connection between the electrolyte solution in the "patch-clamp" electrode and the cytoplasm. This configuration is called "whole-cell mode" (Fig. 8b). Whole-cell mode is the recording configuration that allows the recording of membrane potential and membrane currents of a cell, in a way that is comparable to a sharp microelectrode.

After establishing the whole-cell mode, the patch-clamp electrode can be retracted from the cell. As the membrane sticks very well to the glass of the electrode, a tube of membrane is pulled from the cell surface. The walls of the tube will approach, and finally join into, a membrane patch. The former outer surface of the membrane forms the outside of the patch, and the side that points to the electrode lumen, is the former cytoplasmic surface of the membrane. This configuration is called "outside-out" mode (Fig. 8c), a measuring configuration that is also used for recording single channel currents.

Starting with the cell-attached configuration, a retraction of the electrode from the cell leads to the formation of a membrane vesicle. This vesicle is again "outside out". However, manipulations like exposing the electrode air for a short time, or to a solution with low calcium content, can destroy the outer hemisphere of the vesicle. Finally, the inner hemisphere of the vesicle remains, exposing the former membrane inside to the external solution. This configuration is thus called "inside-out" mode (Fig. 8d), and is also used for single channel recordings. The configurations for single channel current recording will not be discussed here in detail, because single channel recording is not specific in cardiac cells, i.e. single channel currents can be recorded with the same protocols as in other excitable cells.

Whole-Cell Configuration

Whole-cell configuration is used in nearly every electrophysiological recording of cardiac cells today. Therefore, we want to discuss this configuration in more detail. One of the most important advantages of this recording mode is the relatively low access resistance to the cell. This is the major prerequisite, if a standard patch clamp amplifier (as described in The Principle and the Amplifier, this chapter) is used, and allows a simplified voltage-clamp set up. The resistance of the patch-clamp electrode is in series with the cell-membrane resistance, but the cell resistance is much higher than the electrode resistance. If a voltage clamp signal is applied to such a circuit, voltage will drop along the circuit in proportion to the resistances, i.e. if the resistance of the electrode amounts to 10% of the cell-membrane resistance, 10% of the voltage will drop at the electrode and 90% at the cell membrane. In the case of application of a voltage-clamp pulse to the electrode, the distribution of resistances in the circuit will induce a voltage in the cell that is in proportional to its contribution to the total resistance in the circuit. In the example of 10% resistance in the electrode and 90% in the cell, a voltage-clamp pulse from –80 mV to 20 mV (100 mV amplitude) would clamp the cell to 10 mV. However, this voltage deviation can be reduced by a series resistance compensation, which is incorporated in all actual patch clamp amplifiers. The series resistance compensation increases the voltage pulse by the amount of the expected deviation. It is a positive feedback loop that increases noise and jeopardizes stability. Clearly, full compensation is not possible, however, compensation of about 80% of the series resistance is practically achievable. Higher compensation often induces instability (ringing) of the voltage clamp signal. In the discussed example, a voltage deviation of 2 mV will finally result. If a high conductance current system like I_{Na} is activated rapidly, the membrane resistance will drop dramatically and this may induce more important voltage deviations.

Alternatively, the use of a discontinuous amplifier (SEVC), as described in chapter Single Electrode Clamp, will avoid series resistance effects completely. This is important for the recording of large currents, or error-free recording of gap conductance in electrically coupled cells (see chapter Dhein – Recording Gap Junction Currents, Dhein 1998 and Müller et al. 1999 for details). In addition, this type of amplifier avoids current clamp errors, since membrane potential is recorded at zero current (see Magistretti et al. 1996). SEVC amplifiers can also be used in the "perforated patch" configuration (see chapter Perforated Patch) or with sharp microelectrodes, allowing the free selection of recording method.

Patch-clamp electrodes, with their relatively wide tip, exchange substances by diffusion with the cytoplasm. This allows application of membrane impermeable molecules directly from the electrode into the cytoplasm (internal perfusion, see chapter Internal Perfusion). However, exchange of substances between the electrode and the cytoplasm may also lead to a loss of important metabolites, limiting the lifetime of cells in whole-cell recording mode. Some channels, like those of the L-type Ca^{2+}, are sensitive to this phenomenon. They exhibit a so-called "run down", i.e. the current amplitude decreases with time. This can be prevented by limiting the exchange between the electrode and the cytoplasm, e.g. by using electrodes with relatively high resistances that will then lead to inferior voltage control, or by switching to voltage-clamp techniques with sharp microelectrodes, e.g. using a time-sharing single electrode clamp amplifier (see Single Electrode Clamp, this chapter). Another opportunity to overcome the problem of "run down" is the perforated patch method, which is described in chapter Perforated Patch of this article.

Experimental Concepts

Protocols for AP-Recordings

Action potentials (APs) are typically recorded in current clamp mode, and can be elicited by current injection or field stimulation with external electrodes. In the case of external stimulation with a pair of gold wires, we found the duration of 0.4 ms and amplitude of 30 V was usually sufficient. However, the stimulus amplitude depends

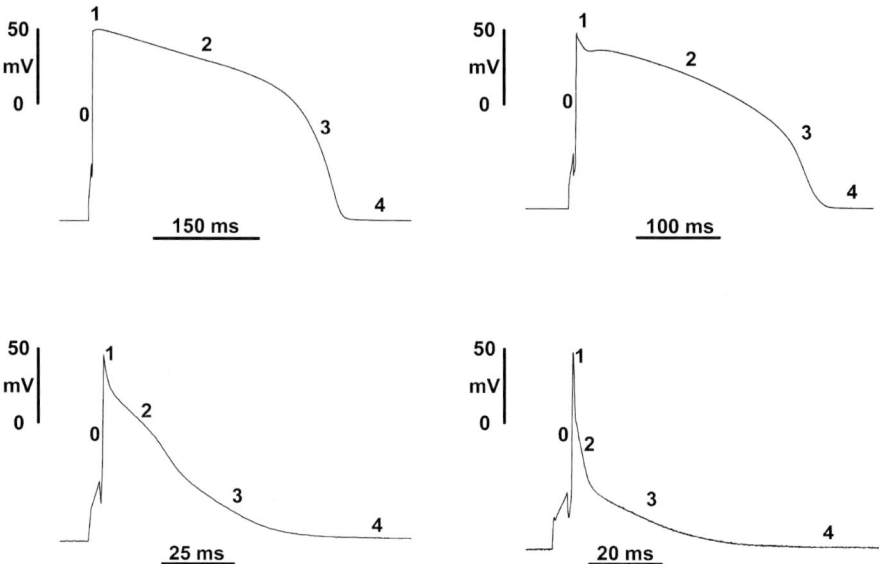

Figure 9
AP recordings from different species. Ventricular APs of guinea pig (*upper left*), rabbit (*upper right*), rat (*lower left*) and mouse (*lower right*). The time scale is different in all plots. Different phases are marked: 0 depolarisation, 1 initial repolarisation, 2 plateau, 3 repolarisation, 4 resting potential. The initial repolarisation depends on I_{to} and determines the plateau phase and the APD. Guinea pig is devoid of I_{to}, rabbit ventricular myocytes show a modest I_{to}, and in rat and murine ventricular myocytes I_{to} has a high amplitude leading to a short plateau phase and thus APD

very much on the distance of the electrodes and the position of the cell relative to the electrodes, as the electrical field is not homogeneous near the electrodes. In order to record APs, an electrode has to have access to the cytoplasm, either a sharp microelectrode or a patch clamp electrode. In this case, it is also feasible to use this electrode for the application of the stimulus. The depolarisation must reach the threshold, but should not exceed this to a high extent. This allows a clear separation between the stimulus and the depolarisation phase of the AP. The size of the stimulus depends very much on the series resistance of the electrode and the size of the cell (see Fig. 9 Murine AP). We found it very useful to insert an amplifier with variable amplification between the "analog out" of the computer and the "stimulus in" of the amplifier, allowing adjustment of the stimulus amplitude to each cell by turning a knob. Stimulus duration was 2 ms in our experiments.

Usually APs are recorded in steady state at a constant frequency. We found that in most species 20 beats are sufficient to reach a steady state in AP-duration. Relevant stimulation frequencies depend very much on the heart rate of the species from which the cells were isolated. Only a few shall be mentioned here (Table 1).

AP-recordings are usually carried out in physiological solutions. The external Tyrode's solution, which we used for the APs in Fig. 9, was composed of (in mM): NaCl 135, KCl 4, $MgCl_2$ 1, $CaCl_2$ 1.8, HEPES 2, Glucose 10 at a pH of 7.4. The pipette solution consisted of (in mM): NaCl 5, KCl 90, KOH 35, MgATP 2.5, EGTA 1, HEPES 5 at a pH of 7.4. Although a stimulation rate of 1 Hz is not within the physiological range of the

Table 1
Protocols for AP-recordings

Species	Heart rate	Frequencies of interest
Guinea pig	200–320	3.3– 5.3
Human	40–180	0.5– 3.0
Mouse	380–750	6.0– 12.5
Rabbit	120–280	2.0– 4.6
Rat	250–400	4.0– 6.7

heart rate in species like mouse, it is often applied in experiments to allow comparison between different species. APs are usually recorded in the current-clamp mode of the amplifier, or with a so-called "bridge" amplifier (see Current Clamp Recordings and Bridge Amplifiers, this chapter). In current-clamp mode, the current flow through the electrode is kept constant at preset values. If the preset value is "zero current", the amplifier acts as a voltage follower and will measure the actual membrane potential. The use of patch clamp amplifiers is problematic (see The Principle and the Amplifier, this chapter), due to errors induced by transient signals (Magestretti et al. 1996). In contrast, SEVC amplifiers have no series resistance artefacts and can be used with both patch and sharp microelectrodes.

After a stimulation pause, heart cells develop a Bowditch staircase, i.e. contractile force or shortening amplitude increases with each beat (positive staircase, guinea pig) or decreases with each beat (negative staircase, rat). Some species, like rat and mouse, clearly exhibit elevated contractile amplitude of the first beat after the pause (post-rest contraction). In some experiments it is of interest to investigate the AP eliciting the post-rest contraction. In such cases, pulse trains of twenty pulses are applied after varying pauses, e.g. trains of 20 pulses are divided by a variable period of rest: 1st rest 2 s; 2nd rest 5 s; 3rd rest 10 s; 4th rest 30 s; 5th rest 60 s; 7th rest 120 s; 8th rest 240 s.

AP-Analysis

A cardiac AP gives information on different electrical parameters of the cell, and analysis of the AP tries to extract as much information as possible. In Fig. 9, APs of guinea pig, rabbit, rat and mouse are shown. They can be divided into five phases, 0: depolarisation; 1: early repolarisation; 2: plateau; 3: final repolarisation; 4: resting potential. Resting membrane potential, and peak amplitude of the action potential are important voltages. The steepness of the depolarisation (dV/dt) can be taken as an estimate of the I_{Na}. The AP duration is usually calculated at 50% and 90% repolarisation, called APD_{50} and APD_{90}. The first characterizes the duration of the plateau, and the second the end of the repolarisation. The 50% value is useful if the AP has a clear plateau, like those from guinea pig or rabbit. APD_{50} depends on the inward currents flowing during the plateau phase, like $I_{Ca,L}$, persisting Na$^+$, $I_{Na,P}$ and Na$^+$/Ca^{2+} exchanger current, but also on the size of the outward potassium currents. APs from rats or mice are not very well described by APD_{50}, because these show a very fast initial repolarisation, due to the activation of I_{to}. The final repolarisation is mainly carried by the potassium currents $I_{K,r}$ and $I_{K,s}$. APD_{90} can, therefore, be used to describe these current systems. The ratio of APD_{50}/APD_{90} is useful to describe the shape of repolarisation.

Protocols for Ionic Currents

The membrane currents underlying the action potential are measured in the VC configuration of the recording amplifier. When the membrane potential is forced to a new level by a voltage clamp step, several different channel types will be activated in a voltage and time dependent manner, comparable to an AP. For example, a voltage clamp pulse depolarising the membrane for 500 ms, from –80 mV to –10 mV will, in the case of guinea pig ventricular cardiomyocytes, first activate the I_{Na}, then $I_{Ca,L}$, later I_{Kr} and I_{Ks} are the dominating ionic currents. In addition to these ionic currents running through the channels, are the currents generated by electrogenic transporters like the Na^+/Ca^{2+} exchanger. In the case of atrial cardiomyocytes, or other species like mouse, the same pulse will activate additional current components. The recorded current flow is a sum of all these different currents. Usually, the aim of a voltage clamp experiment is the identification of the voltage and time dependency of a single ionic current. A precondition for the investigation of a single current is the separation of this current from the overlapping current components. There are different techniques to differentiate between various current components all activated by the same pulse. Concepts on how to measure these will be described in the next chapter.

Concepts to Characterise Current Components

Separation of Different Ionic Currents

There are different ways to separate one single ionic current from overlapping currents. At first glimpse, the easiest way is to block all overlapping currents by pharmacological blockers. An example of this, is to measure $I_{Ca,L}$ in guinea pig ventricular cardiomyocytes after block of the I_{Na} by tetrodotoxin, and after block of I_{Kr}, I_{Ks}, and I_{K1} by substituting CsCl for KCl. However, this concept has some shortcomings. Block of all overlapping currents is only possible if they are known, and if selective blockers exist for these ionic currents.

Another problem is that a block of a current component may influence the current of interest, i.e. block of the I_{Na} may lead to a decreased intracellular sodium concentration, which in turn will influence the Na^+/Ca^{2+} exchanger. A reduced Na^+/Ca^{2+} exchanger may result in an increased cytoplasmic Ca^{2+} concentration, $[Ca^{2+}]_i$, which in turn may influence $I_{Ca,L}$. Intracellular Ca^{2+} buffering with 10 mM BAPTA can minimize the influence of the Na^+/Ca^{2+} exchanger. However, this changes $I_{Ca,L}$ inactivation, and is thus not suited for the recording of this current. Another important shortcoming of the block of all overlapping conductances, is that many events of excitation-contraction coupling will be influenced, and it is therefore impossible to combine such current recordings with measurement of contractility or $[Ca^{2+}]_i$.

Another concept is the selective block of the current component of interest. In the case of $I_{Ca,L}$, this means recording the sum of all membrane currents during a voltage clamp step, then block the $I_{Ca,L}$ by a specific calcium antagonist, and apply the same voltage step again. This will now activate all currents without the blocked $I_{Ca,L}$. Finally, the difference between both currents is calculated point by point, and the resulting current represents the $I_{Ca,L}$. Theoretically, this seems to be a very good way to measure $I_{Ca,L}$. However, this method also has its shortcomings: the current of interest has to be blocked exclusively and all others have to remain unchanged. Na^+/Ca^{2+} exchanger current depends on the $[Ca^{2+}]_i$ and this depends on the $I_{Ca,L}$. Thus, a change in Na^+/Ca^{2+} exchanger will be induced, which in turn causes a corresponding error in the calculation of $I_{Ca,i}$. Block of the Na^+/Ca^{2+} exchanger during such experiments is complicated, as a selective pharmacological blocker exists only for reverse mode (Dipla et al. 1999). The main advantage of this type of recording is that, during the first recording, all events of excitation-contraction coupling can be monitored under physiological conditions.

A third approach to separate ionic currents is selective activation. If currents have different thresholds, they are activated to different potentials by voltage clamp steps. This allows the separate activation of currents. This method is very helpful if the I_{Na}, the $I_{Ca,T}$ or the I_{to} are to be separated from other currents, as these currents have relatively negative thresholds, < −35 mV. A pre-clamp to −35 mV before the test clamp will activate these currents. Therefore, this is a widely used approach in heart physiology. Again, this method has its specific shortcomings. Activation of I_{Na} sometimes leads to a loss in voltage control, then $I_{Ca,L}$ is partly activated, and in extreme situations contractions can even be seen. The L-type Ca^{2+} channels, which have been activated during the pre-clamp, become inactivated like the Na^+ channels. This will lead to an underestimation of the $I_{Ca,L}$. Some people do not use a pre-clamp, but simply shift the holding potential from −80 mV to −40 mV to avoid the loss of voltage control. This has the disadvantage that the Na^+/Ca^{2+} exchanger is less effective, and the $[Ca^{2+}]_i$ or the Ca^{2+} content of the sarcoplasmic reticulum may increase.

Determination of Current Characteristics

To characterize a single ionic current, it is not sufficient to isolate it from overlapping conductances, different parameters determining the current flow have to be recorded. To achieve this, various voltage-clamp patterns have been designed.

The simplest voltage-clamp pattern is the application of square pulses. Square pulses are often applied as a graded series to increasing potentials, e.g. with an increment of 5 mV from −70 to −20 mV to elicit the current-voltage relation of I_{Na} (Fig. 10). Square pulses can be used as a series with constant potential and frequency to test the effect of a pharmacological substance on the current amplitude. Variations of the frequency of square pulses can help to demonstrate the influence of the stimulation frequency on the current amplitude. This can be demonstrated by clamping the membrane to a constant potential with increasing interruptions, i.e. a square pulse to +10 mV for 400 ms activates $I_{Ca,L}$. After clamping back to holding potential $I_{Ca,L}$ recovers from inactivation. The time course of recovery from inactivation can be tested by

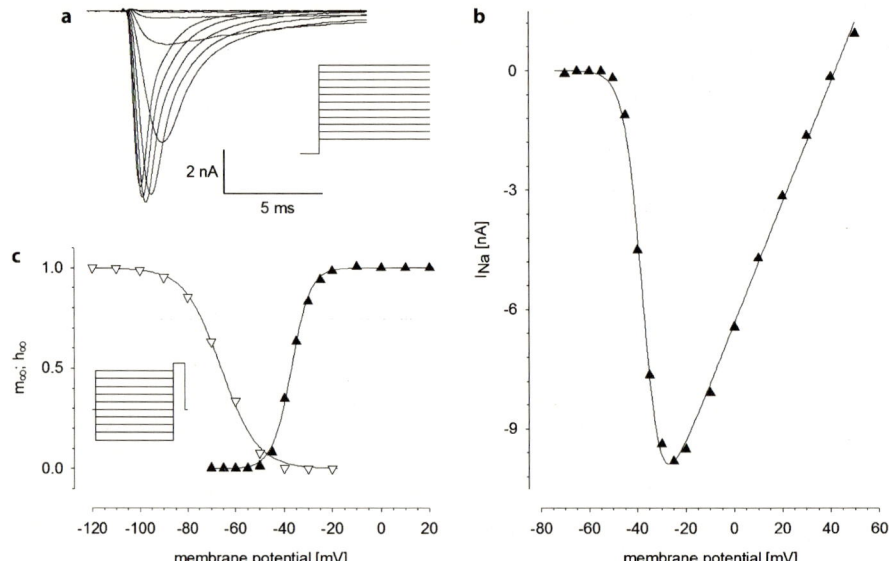

Figure 10a–c
Na⁺ current. I_{Na} of a guinea pig ventricular cell is characterised by rectangular voltage-clamp pulses from a holding potential of -80 mV at a stimulation rate of 0.5 Hz. **a** Original current records elicited by clamp pulses of 20 ms duration (inset) to stepwise increasing potentials between -70 and -20 mV (5 mV step-width). **b** Current voltage relation of I_{Na}. **c** The voltage dependence and the steady-state activation (m_∞; filled triangles) and of the steady-state inactivation (h_∞; open triangles). Inset double-pulse protocol combining a conditioning clamp to increasing potentials between -120 and -10 mV (duration: 130 ms; 10 mV step-width) and a subsequent test-clamp to -20 mV (duration: 20 ms). The pipette solution consisted of (in mM): 120 CsCl, 4 $MgCl_2$, 4 Na_2ATP, 10 EGTA and 10 HEPES; pH 7.2 with CsOH. The superfusion solution contained (in mM): 30 NaCl, 107 CsCl, 0.5 $CaCl_2$, 2.5 $MgCl_2$, 0.001 nifedipine 10 HEPES, 10 glucose; pH 7.4 with CsOH/NaOH (3:1)

application of a series of pairs of square pulses, the first clamp has a potential that activates the peak current, and is long enough to achieve complete inactivation. This clamp pulse is followed after a very short time, e.g. 10 ms, by a second clamp. The next pair has a higher distance, e.g. 20 ms, and the following have increasing distances.

If a first square pulse is followed directly by a second pulse, two different situations can be distinguished:
1. Preceded by a fixed pre-clamp, the variable test clamp separates the investigated current from overlapping ones (see Separation of Different Ionic Currents in this chapter).
2. The first variable clamp, here called the conditioning clamp, is followed by a second fixed test clamp, and both elicit the same current system. The currents elicited by this second pulse are called tail currents. The principle is to demonstrate the channels that are still open at the end of the first clamp by changing the driving force. Such tail currents are utilized for monitoring the degree of inactivation in I_{Na} and I_{Ca} (see Na-Current and Ca^{2+} Currents, this chapter), and also to record K⁺ currents (see Potassium Currents, this chapter).

Besides square pulses, ramp clamps are also applied to elicit time independent currents like I_{K1}. Ramp clamps have the advantage that a complete current-voltage relation can be achieved during one clamp without further evaluation (see Potassium Currents).

In some cases, if the time course of a current system during an AP is to be directly demonstrated then digitised AP are used as a command voltage. This method is called AP-clamp, and is explained in detail in chapter Action Potential Clamp.

Na Current

I_{Na} is the first current in the atrial and ventricular AP, and its activation causes the depolarisation. The threshold of the I_{Na} in ventricular cells lies between −55 and −40 mV, this relatively negative activation potential allows activation of I_{Na} by simple voltage clamp patterns. A jump from −80 mV holding potential to any potential positive of the threshold will activate I_{Na} instantaneously. The size of the current depends on the conductance and driving force. The conductance is proportional to the number of open channels, which are determined by the position of the activation gate m and the inactivation gate h.

The equations describing I_{Na} are:

$$g_{Na} = \overline{g_{Na}} * m^3 * h \times j$$

$\overline{g_{Na}}$ Is the peak conductance. m, h and j are variables that can vary between 0 and 1. They characterise the open probability of the two classical gates of the Na^+ channel, the activation gate m and the inactivation gate h. An additional gate, j, has been added describing slow inactivation (Luo and Rudy 1994).

$$g_{Na} = I_{Na}/(V - E_{Na})$$

V actual membrane potential, E_{Na} reversal potential of I_{Na}, $V - E_{Na}$ driving force

Thus:
$$I_{Na} = \overline{g_{Na}} * m^3 * h * j (V - E_{Na})$$

In order to characterise I_{Na} by a voltage-clamp experiment, the command voltage pattern should be designed to monitor these parameters of the current without interference of other ionic currents. Overlapping currents that may interfere with the I_{Na} are mainly $I_{Ca,T}$, $I_{Ca,L}$, I_{to}, and I_{K1}; other K^+ currents like I_{Ks} and I_{Kr} activate too slowly. If I_{Na} shall be recorded directly, these currents have to be blocked. An example for an I_{Na} monitoring in guinea pig ventricular cells is given in Fig. 10.

The superfusion solution contained 1 mM Nifedipine to block $I_{Ca,L}$, and K^+ was substituted for Cs^+ in both pipette and external solution to prevent current flow through K^+ channels. I_{Na} was characterised by applying rectangular voltage-clamp pulses from a holding potential of −80 mV at a stimulation rate of 0.5 Hz. Single clamp pulses of 20 ms duration to stepwise increasing potentials between −70 and +50 mV (5 mV step-width at potentials ≤−20 mV and 10 mV step-width at potentials > −20 mV) were used to determine the voltage dependence and the steady-state activation (m_∞) of I_{Na}. The current activates rapidly and increases until maximal amplitude is reached after 1–2 ms, however, it decays again within a few ms (Fig. 10A). I_{Na} was calculated as the difference between the peak current and the current at the end of the clamp pulse. The current voltage relation is then constructed by plotting peak currents as a function of the clamp potential (Fig. 10b). Between −50 and −25 mV I_{Na} amplitude increases with increasing clamp potential. Positive of −25 mV, clamp potential current amplitude decreases with increasing clamp potential. Current direction reverses at +40 mV in the example in Fig. 10b. The points were fitted by the function of I_{Na} printed above.

The steady-state activation (m_∞) can be calculated from the records used for the current-voltage relation by calculating g_{Na} for each potential and standardising these to the highest peak conductance, which is set to "1" (Fig. 10c). These values are plotted as a function of the clamp potential and fitted by a Boltzmann function:

$$m_\infty(V) = 1/[1 + e^{(V_{1/2}-V)/k}]$$

The steady-state inactivation (h_∞) was determined by a double-pulse protocol combining a conditioning clamp to increasing potentials between −120 and −10 mV (duration: 130 ms; 10 mV step-width) and a subsequent test clamp to −20 mV (duration: 20 ms). According to the nomenclature introduced above, the test clamp elicits tail currents.

The idea of this protocol is to set the h-gates to their potential dependent value by the conditioning clamp, then to clamp the membrane to a constant potential at which the activation value is one. Under these conditions, the inactivation variable is the only parameter that determines the tail-current amplitude. Therefore the values for h_∞ can be directly deduced from the peak current amplitude during the second clamp step. The highest peak-current amplitude is set to "1" and the tail-current amplitudes elicited after other conditioning clamps are standardised to this value. These values are plotted as a function of the conditioning clamp (Fig. 10c) and fitted by the following Boltzmann function:

$$h_\infty(V) = 1/[1 + e^{(V-V_{1/2})/k}]$$

I_{Na} activates very fast and has high amplitudes. This may lead to a loss of voltage control and thus to incorrect results. To overcome this problem several precautions have to be taken when recording I_{Na}. One should keep I_{Na} small and thus within the secure range of the voltage clamp circuit.

Recordings are usually performed at room temperature and with reduced external Na^+ concentration; in the example in Fig. 10, 30 mM NaCl was present. The patch-clamp electrodes should have a relatively low tip resistance (between 1 and 2 MΩ is recommended) and small cells should be chosen to gain small surface areas with a small number of Na^+ channels.

If the I_{Na} shall be recorded as residual current or if the I_{Na} shall be blocked to isolate other currents, this can be done by substitution of NaCl in the external solution by choline chloride or by Tris, by addition of local anaesthetics like lidocaine or novocaine or by addition of tetrodotoxin.

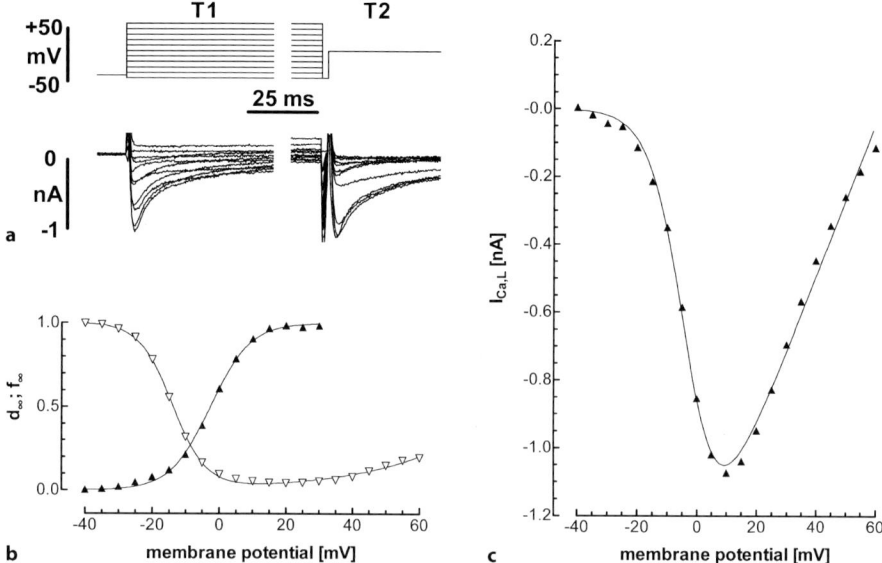

Figure 11a–c
Ca²⁺ current. $I_{Ca,L}$ of a guinea pig ventricular cell is elicited by rectangular voltage-clamp pulses from a holding potential of -80 mV at a stimulation rate of 0.5 Hz.
a *Upper panel:* Clamp pattern consisting of a four pulse protocol. First step is a prepulse from -80 mV to -40 mV for 200 ms, to inactivate T-type Ca²⁺ current and Na⁺ current (not shown completely), the preclamp is followed by the first testclamp (T1) to stepwise increasing potentials between -40 mV and 60 mV (5 mV step-width) for 400 ms duration. T1 is separated from the second testclamp (T2) to -10 mV by a 2 ms pulse to -40 mV to reset the d-gate. *Lower panel:* Original current records elicited by clamp pulses.
b Current voltage relation of $I_{Ca,L}$. **c** The voltage dependence the steady-state activation (d_∞; filled triangles) and of the steady-state inactivation (f_∞; open triangles). The pipette solution consisted of (in mM): 120 CsCl, 4 MgCl₂, 4 Na₂ATP, 10 EGTA, and 10 HEPES, pH 7.4 with CsOH. The superfusion solution contained (in mM): 135 NaCl, 3 CsCl, 1 KCl, 1.8 CaCl₂, 1 MgCl₂, 10 HEPES, 10 glucose; pH 7.4 NaOH

Ca²⁺ Currents

Two types of Ca²⁺ currents (Review: McDonald et al. 1994) are found in ventricular cardiac myocytes the T-type (Bean et al. 1985) and the L-type current. The T-type current, $I_{Ca,T}$, is activated at potentials > -50 mV, it inactivates more rapidly, and its amplitude is smaller than that of $I_{Ca,L}$. The current voltage relation has its peak around -40 mV or even at more negative potentials, it is less sensitive to Cd²⁺ and more sensitive to Ni²⁺ than the L-type current, and it is insensitive to β adrenergic stimulation. A selective pharmacological blocker of the T-type current is mibefradil. Some calcium antagonists, block L-type current selectively, and some block both L- and T-type (De Paoli et al. 2002). The T-type current will not be demonstrated further in this article, as an example for Ca²⁺ currents, the recording of $I_{Ca,L}$ will be described here.

$I_{Ca,L}$ can in many aspects be described analogous to the I_{Na} by two gates called d and f (Reuter 1967). However, the L-type current is activated at more positive potentials than I_{Na} and $I_{Ca,T}$ around -40 mV. This allows inactivation of these two currents by a pre-clamp from -80 to -40 mV.

$I_{Ca,L}$ inactivates voltage- and $[Ca^{2+}]_i$-dependent (see also chapter 3.6). This requires a voltage-clamp pattern different to that presented for I_{Na}. In the example in Fig. 11, clamp pulses were applied at a frequency of 0.5 Hz to guinea pig ventricular cells. The clamp pulses consisted of a pre-clamp to –40 mV of 200 ms duration to inactivate I_{Na} and $I_{Ca,T}$, a testclamp of 400 ms duration increasing stepwise (10 mV step-width) from –40 to +60 mV, then the membrane was always clamped back to –40 mV for 2 ms to reset the d-gate and finally tail currents were elicited by a clamp pulse to +10 mV. During the test-clamp the current activates rapidly and increases within 3 to 5 ms to a maximal amplitude. Decay is slower than that of I_{Na}. Nearly complete inactivation of $I_{Ca,L}$ takes place within about 100 ms. If K$^+$ currents have been blocked completely the peak current amplitude can calculated as absolute inward current. If the block is incomplete, the peak current amplitude has often been calculated as the difference between the maximal current and the current at 100 ms. A current voltage relation can be plotted in the same way as described for I_{Na}. However, the voltage dependence of $I_{Ca,L}$ differs from that of I_{Na}. $I_{Ca,L}$ starts to activate at potentials > –40 mV, reaches its maximum between 0 and 10 mV, and reverses around 60 mV.

Usually the current-voltage relation is fitted by the following equation:

$$I_{Ca,L} = g_{Ca} (V-E_{Ca}) / 1 + e^{(V_{1/2}-V)/k}$$

V actual membrane potential, E_{Ca} reversal potential of $I_{Ca,L}$, g_{Ca} actual conductance V–E_{Ca} driving force, $V_{1/2}$ potential of 50% activation

The steady-state activation (d_∞) can be calculated from the records used for the current-voltage relation by calculating g_{Ca} for each potential, and standardising these to highest peak conductance, which is set to "1". The procedure is similar to that used for calculation of steady state activation of I_{Na}, and the values are fitted by the same Boltzmann function.

The steady-state inactivation (f_∞) was determined by evaluating the tail currents. The theory has already been described in the chapter regarding the steady-state inactivation of I_{Na}. Similar to h_∞, the values for f_∞ can be directly deduced from the peak current amplitude during the tail current. The highest peak-current amplitude is set to "1", and the tail-current amplitudes elicited, after other conditioning clamps are standardised to this value. These values are plotted as a function of the conditioning clamp (Fig. 11c) and fitted by the sum of two Boltzmann functions (Luo and Rudy 1994).

$$f_\infty = 1 / (1 + e^{(V-V'_{1/2})/k'}) + a / (1 + e^{(V''_{1/2}-V)/k''})$$

V actual membrane potential, $V'_{1/2}$ and respectively $V''_{1/2}$ potential of 50% inactivation of the 1st and the 2nd Boltzmann function, k´ and respectively k" slope of the 1st and the 2nd Boltzmann function, a scaling factor

This short methodological introduction to $I_{Ca,L}$ explains only how to record $I_{Ca,L}$. Many more details and findings about this current are gathered in Hoppe – Recording L-type Ca^{++}-current of this book.

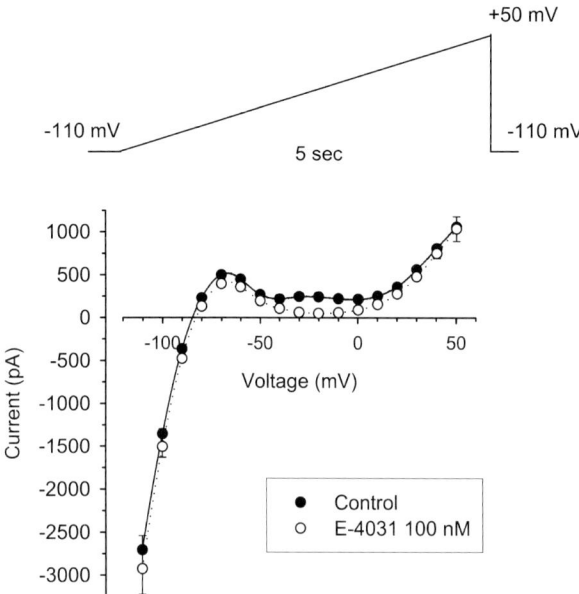

Figure 12
K+ current. Ramp clamp for the determination of K+ conductances. The voltage clamp pulse is plotted in the upper trace. A ramp with a slope of 32 mV/s and 160 mV amplitude reveals a steady-state current-voltage relation. The pipette solution consisted of (in mM): NaCl 5, KCl 90, KOH 35, MgATP 2.5, EGTA 1, HEPES 5 at a pH of 7.4. The superfusing solution, was composed of (in mM): NaCl 135, KCl 4, $MgCl_2$ 1, $CaCl_2$ 1.8, HEPES 2, glucose 10 at a pH of 7.4. $I_{Ca,L}$ was blocked by 10 μM nifedipine in the external solution. Current data are mean ± SEM, n=5

Potassium Currents

In cardiac cells, potassium currents are mainly responsible for the maintenance of the resting potential and the repolarisation of the AP. The electrophysiologically recorded K+ current systems found in myocardium exhibit a wide divergence. This is based on an extended family of membrane channels, depending on the expression of a wide variety of genes. The divergence of AP shapes among different species (Fig. 9), relies mainly on differences in the expression of K+ channel genes. As K+ currents play an important role in excitation-contraction coupling of the heart, a separate chapter of this book presents their recording and function (see chapter 3.6). Therefore, K+ current recording will be employed here only for the introduction of a further voltage clamp pattern, the ramp clamp.

During a ramp clamp, the membrane potential is shifted continuously from an initial potential to final value, i.e. a ramp from −110 to 50 mV (32 mV/s) can be applied to record a current voltage relation of a membrane (see Fig. 12). Ramp clamps are not suited to activate current systems that depend on a rapid shift of the membrane potential across a threshold like the I_{Na}. However, steep depolarising ramps are sometimes applied for the monitoring of $I_{Ca,L}$, but continuous shifts of the voltage are mainly used to record K+ currents, as these are in part time independent or slowly activating. An example of the recording of K+ currents by a ramp clamp in a guinea-pig ventricular myocyte is shown in Fig. 12. $I_{Ca,L}$ is blocked by addition of 1 mM nifedipine to the superfusing solution, thus neither the I_{Na} nor $I_{Ca,L}$ contribute to the recorded current. The shape of the current-voltage relation is determined by the activation of at least three K+ currents, I_{K1}, I_{Kr}, and I_{Ks}, where I_{K1} is the dominating current < −40 mV. Between −40 and 10 mV I_{Kr} is responsible for most of the current, and

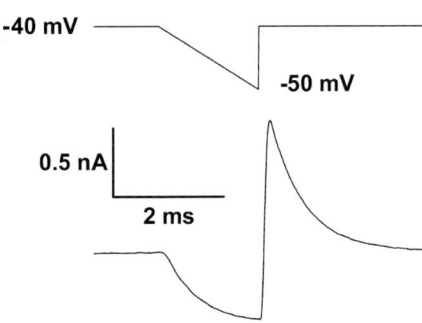

Figure 13
Membrane capacity determination. Ramp clamp for the determination of the membrane capacity. Part of the voltage clamp pulse is plotted in the upper trace. A ramp with a slope of 5.5 mV/ms and –10 mV amplitude elicits a saturating current. From the peak current during the ramp clamp the cell capacity can be calculated. The current is the average of five successive identical ramps. The capacitance of this cell was calculated to be 91 pF

positive of 10 mV I_{Ks} conducts the highest portion of K⁺. Addition of E-4031 to the superfusing solution blocks selectively I_{Kr}, and thus abolishes the current plateau between –50 and 10 mV.

Protocols for Recording Membrane Capacitance

Ventricular cardiac myocytes of common experimental animals and humans are between 100 and 150 µm long, between 10 and 15 µm wide, and 5 to 10 µm high. If one regards the cells as a cuboid, the surface amounts to 3000 µm² for small cells, or to 7500 µm² for big cells. The surface membrane is additionally enlarged by T-tubules and caveolae. The area of the cell membrane is an important determinant for the size of current, as it determines the number of channels. Each activated channel contributes its conductivity to the whole cell current, as this is the sum of all single channel currents. Therefore, most whole cell currents are in proportion to the surface area of the membrane. For comparison of membrane currents among different cells, it is thus necessary to standardise the current amplitude to the membrane area. Measuring the cell capacitance can achieve this, since the capacitance of a cell follows the membrane area by 1 µF/cm. The averaged cell capacitance of ventricular cardiac myocytes of the guinea pig is around 120 pF, which corresponds to a surface area of approximately 12000 µm². The calculated surface area of a cardiac myocyte, based on the microscopic image, is usually 30 to 50% smaller than that gained by recording the membrane capacitance, due to the enlargement of the cell membrane by folds, T-tubules and caveolae.

Theoretically, the membrane capacitance can be calculated from the time course of a change in membrane potential induced by application of a rectangular current pulse. The observed delay of membrane polarisation is due to the charging of the membrane capacitance. In practice, this way of determining cell capacitance is not very precise. Therefore, another protocol has been established and is applied by most groups today.

The electrical capacitance of the cell membrane can be determined prior to membrane capacitance compensation ("τ slow"), by applying a fast voltage ramp from –40 to –50 mV (see Fig. 13). This method is also applicable if a SEVC amplifier is used. In order to record mainly capacitive currents, the ramp is applied in the repolarising direction and covers a potential range in which only few current systems are activated. The overlapping I_{Na} can be inactivated by a pre-clamp or by holding the cell at –40 mV. To gain a reproducible signal, we apply this voltage clamp pattern successively 5× and average the current records. The current saturates, and the peak current is taken for the calculation of the membrane capacitance.

The membrane capacitance is then calculated off-line according to:

$$C_m = Q/V = (I \times dt)/dV$$

C_m membrane capacitance, Q charge, V voltage, I peak current at the end of the ramp, dt duration of the ramp, dV voltage amplitude of the ramp.

Practical Guide to Intracellular Recordings

Fabrication of Microelectrodes

The fabrication of good and reliable microelectrodes is very important, since their properties affect the quality of the recording. This topic has plenty of publications dedicated to it, and therefore we will only describe a few basic aspects here.

Microelectrode Glass

There are three different parameters of glass to be considered: the type of glass, the inner and outer diameter of the tubing (Penner 1995).

Most investigators today use borosilicate glass. It has good electrical properties (relatively low surface charges, low noise), can be pulled with almost every puller, is available in a variety of diameters and is not too expensive. If the tubing is not the right length, it can be easily cut using a commercial diamond glasscutter. No special cleaning is usually necessary, but the microelectrode glass should be kept dust-free.

Quartz glass has very good electrical properties and is used for the lowest noise recordings, e.g. single channels with low conductance. However, it is very expensive, and because of its high melting point, it can only be pulled with laser pullers, which are also very expensive.

Inner and outer diameters of the glass tubing also determine mechanical, geometric and electrical properties of the microelectrode (Sakmann and Neher 1995). Borosilicate glass is commonly used with a 1.5 mm outer diameter and about 0.9 mm inner diameter with a filament. The filament considerably facilitates backfilling of the microelectrode, and is highly recommended. This glass can be used for sharp and patch microelectrodes.

Puller

Generally, two types of pullers are currently available. In vertical pullers, the microelectrode is oriented vertically during the pulling process, and usually only one part of the microelectrode is moved. In horizontal pullers, the microelectrode is oriented horizontally during the pulling process and both parts are moved, resulting in two identical microelectrodes. Because smaller tips can be achieved with horizontal pullers, they should be used for sharp, intracellular microelectrodes, whereas vertical pullers can also be used to fabricate patch electrodes.

As mentioned above, pullers using a laser for heating the glass tubing, have to be used for pulling quartz glass.

Care should be taken in adjusting the heating filament of a puller. The glass should be exactly in the middle, i.e. the distance of the filament to the glass tubing should be maintained the same. The width of the filament influences the form of the taper, generally, the smaller the width of the filament, the shorter the taper. Also, the distance of the glass tubing from the filament, determines the overall length of the tip. A shorter distance results in shorter tips.

Most pullers have several settings to enable modification of the final form and properties of the microelectrode. Usually, pulling velocity, heat and pulling time can be adjusted. Unfortunately, it is not possible to exactly predict the effect of changing a pull parameter. It is a good idea to start with generally applicable parameters, which are described in the puller manual. As a rule, increasing heat results in smaller tips, longer taper and higher resistance. Increasing pulling velocity gives smaller tips, and increasing pulling time results in a shorter taper. It is very important to change only one parameter at a time.

Some pullers allow the microelectrode to be pulled in two or more steps, including short pulling intervals where heating of the filament stops, or a little puff of air is applied to cool down the filament. Then, the second pull starts with it's own pull parameters. The more the filament cools, down the shorter the taper and the lower the resistance (Brown and Flaming 1977).

Additional Procedures

Depending on the type of microelectrode, sharp or patch, additional fabrication steps can be accomplished to achieve microelectrodes with improved parameters.

Bevellers

For easy penetration of the cell membrane, it is necessary to use very fine microelectrode tips, with the drawback that due to their small diameter these tips are rather noisy.

One possible method of solving this problem is to pull microelectrodes with a much higher resistance than required, and break the tip afterwards. This is done using a micromanipulator mounted on a microscope. A more elegant but also more expensive method is bevelling. Bevelling of the microelectrode at a steep angle is a possibility in reducing the noise, because bevelling enlarges the opening of the microelectrode.

Most commercially available bevellers have a plane rotating plate coated with a suspension of alumina or diamond dust. The microelectrode is then lowered with a micromanipulator until it touches the rotating plate. The desired form is achieved by monitoring the microelectrode resistance or by visual inspection.

Microforges

Patch microelectrodes get their finish by heat (fire) polishing with a microforge, as they have to form a "gigaseal". This is an electrically and mechanically stable connection with the membrane of the cell (see Introduction to Patch Clamp). Therefore, the tip of these electrodes needs special processing (heat polishing), and must be kept very clean until the recording starts. The procedure, which was established by Erwin Neher after the discovery of the gigaseal in the 1970's, is done with a special instrument called microforge. Heat (fire) polishing removes imperfections of the tip surface, which may lead to damage of tiny membranes and facilitates seal formation. A microforge consists of an inverted microscope, a heating filament and a manipulator to move the microelectrode. For polishing, the microelectrode is moved towards the glowing filament until the tip shrinks a little bit.

Many investigators coat their microelectrodes in order to improve the electrical properties. Sylgard #184 from Dow Corning (Midland, MI) is very hydrophobic, and prevents the bathing solution from creeping up the wall of the microelectrode, which limits a source of noise.

Filling of Microelectrodes

After fabrication, microelectrodes have to be filled with electrolyte. Sharp electrodes are usually filled with 1 M to 3 M KCl or K-acetate. For experiments in whole-cell or outside-out configuration, patch microelectrodes are filled with a solution mimicking the intracellular milieu, e.g. in mM: 140 KCl, 8 NaCl, 1 $CaCl_2$, 10 EGTA, 2 Na_2ATP, 3 MgATP, 0.1 Na_2GTP, and 10 HEPES, pH adjusted to 7.2 with KOH. ATP- and GTP compounds are used to prevent fast run-down of ion channels. The solution should be filtered in order to remove dirt, which can lead to clogging of the microelectrode.

Microelectrodes are usually back-filled with a long cannula (e.g. from Hamilton) mounted on a small syringe. If capillaries with filament are used, the tip of the microelectrode is filled because of the capillary force. Air bubbles can be removed by tapping against the electrode.

Testing of Microelectrodes

Before recording, microelectrodes should be checked for their electrical properties. Connect the microelectrode to the recording amplifier, immerse the microelectrode into the bath as deep as necessary for the experiment, and measure the microelectrode resistance. This can be done using either the built-in electrode resistance test mode of the amplifier, or by application of rectangular current pulses to the microelectrode. Record the resulting voltage deflection and apply Ohm's law to get the resistance. Use the microelectrode capacitance compensation of the amplifier to eliminate capacitive artefacts caused by the microelectrode capacitance. The voltage deflection should be as square as possible.

In particular, sharp microelectrodes with high resistances show a non-linear behaviour called rectification, i.e. they alter their resistance and sometimes also their offset potential, if current flows through the microelectrode. Rectification can be tested by application of differing amplitude current pulses to the microelectrode. The amplitude range of the tests should be the same as in the experiment. The measured microelectrode resistance and offset must always be the same.

Experimental Set Ups

Electrophysiological recordings of cardiac cells are mainly performed on isolated cells. Therefore, a set up designed for the monitoring of isolated cells will be described here.

It mainly consists of the following components:
- An inverted microscope with the experimental chamber.
- A temperature control maintaining a preset temperature.
- A perfusion system allowing controlled flow of the bathing solution.
- The electrode mounted to a micromanipulator and connected to the amplifier.
- The amplifier connected to a stimulus generator and components for signal storage and visualization.
- A vibration isolation table that carries the microscope and a Faraday's cage.

Microscopy and Experimental Chamber

In research on isolated cells as well as on cultured cells, the central part of a set up is an inverted microscope. An inverted microscope is constructed in order that the objective is located below the specimen and the illumination is above. The distance between the illumination and the specimen can be in the range of 2 to 5 cm, which allows a relatively free access of electrodes and other tools to the cells. If the bottom of the experimental chamber consists of a coverslip, objectives of high numerical aperture can be used, because the distance between the front lens of the objective and the cell can be kept below 200 µm.

However, the disadvantage of this construction is that only cells that are located on the bottom of the experimental chamber can be clearly visualised. If the specimen consists of several layers of cells, like a tissue section, only the layer on the bottom is visible at good quality. An electrode has to penetrate all the cell layers on top until it reaches the visible part. This would contaminate the electrode tip and thus prevent patch clamp recordings. Therefore, upright microscopes are preferred for experiments on tissue sections. The experimental chamber mounted on the stage of the microscope should offer the ability for permanent perfusion with fresh solution and temperature control, as experiments on isolated cardiac cells should be performed at body temperature.

Isolated cardiac myocytes are large cells that can be easily visualised by bright field microscopy in transmitted light. If only electrical recordings are planned, phase contrast or other ways of contrast enhancement are usually not required. The most challenging step is the attachment of the electrode to the cell. For this, the magnification of a 40× or 63× objective is sufficient. These objectives can be obtained without requiring oil or glycerol immersion. The use of dry objectives is very practical, as the desired cell is chosen at low magnification e.g. with a 10× objective, that operates without immersion. If one switches from an immersion to a dry objective, the bottom of the experimental chamber has to be cleaned. This will happen each time a new cell is tested, and will slow the speed of the experiments remarkably.

In advanced set ups, so many different components are often mounted to the microscope that a manual change of the objective becomes impossible, and the use of motorized objective changers is then indispensable. However, electrical components delivered by the microscope producers are usually powered by alternating current, which may add 50/60 Hz noise to the recordings. This has to be checked separately in every case, e.g., we do not use transformers for the bright field illumination, which are integrated into the microscope, our transformer is mounted outside the Faraday's cage and the lamp is powered by direct current.

Inverted microscopes can be equipped with many different stages. The chosen stage is very much influenced by the shape of the experimental chamber, and the necessary additional components like fast perfusion, micromanipulators etc. For whole cell patch clamp recordings in conjunction with monitoring of cell shortening and cytoplasmic calcium concentration, a sliding stage, which glides on an oil film, is often sufficient. This type of stage has two advantages, it is the cheapest type of stage available, the experimental chamber is movable in X/Y directions, and can be rotated.

However, there are some disadvantages too, the sliding stage has to be moved manually, and therefore it is difficult to move it to defined places repetitively. As the stage is only fixed by adhesion, it does not withstand mechanical force, and therefore all tubes and cables connected to the experimental chamber have to be mechanically uncoupled. This is also advisable if other types of stages are used, to avoid the transfer of vibrations to the specimen. If defined reproducible movement of the specimen is necessary, a stage with X/Y adjustment is required. These are available with manual and motorized actuation. Motorized stages are very helpful if there is not enough space for the hand.

Some of the motorized types allow programmed movement, which helps to switch between several cells. There are numerous highly specialized stages available from several companies. Some of them are mounted at a vertical aluminium shape together with the head of the micromanipulator. They do not have any mechanical connection to the microscope avoiding the transfer of vibrations from the microscope to the specimen and the electrode. This is advantageous if finest vibrations have to be avoided.

Experimental chambers have been constructed in many different ways. It is difficult to propose an ideal one, as the shape and construction depends very much on the type of stage of the inverted microscope. If motorized stages or stages with X/Y adjustment are used, the experimental chamber has to fit into the mounting of the stage, which is usually designed for object slides. Therefore, only the basic requirements will be mentioned here. For the application of objectives with high apertures, the bottom has to be made of a coverslip. The bigger the coverslip, the more fragile it becomes, therefore it is not advisable to use experimental chambers, which are relatively spacious. A solution inlet and outlet has to be integrated, to allow a permanent perfusion of external solution (see chapter Perfusion). A switch to a different external solution requires an exchange of the complete volume, which can be gained more quickly in chambers with small volume. A reference electrode has to be incorporated. Facilities for heating have to be provided (see below).

Temperature Control

The easiest way to control temperature is to heat the solution, which perfuses the experimental chamber. The heating circuit should pre-warm the perfusing solution, and also keep the temperature inside the experimental chamber at the desired temperature. A simple solution is to mount a small chamber connected to the heating circuit near the experimental chamber. The perfusing solution passes through this chamber in silicone tubing before it reaches the experimental chamber. The solution is pre-warmed to the desired temperature before it reaches the specimen. To avoid cooling of the solution, it is sufficient to connect the experimental chamber itself to the heating circuit. One way of achieving this, is to use annular heating foils that are glued to the bottom of the chamber.

In our experiments, warm water flows around the experimental chamber, and a battery powered temperature gauge monitors the temperature inside. In most cases, using simple methods of temperature control is sufficient, however, such simple systems may cause problems. Very often, the frequency of the alternating current of the electricity network is present in the water flowing in the heating circuit. This may induce 50/60 Hz noise in the electrophysiological recordings. It is important to connect the water in the heating circuit to the ground, to minimize this phenomenon. It also helps to use distilled water with low conductivity. Some people use oil in the heating circuit to prevent noise, which is efficient to prevent noise, but small leakages in the heating circuit may cause oily contaminations on the set up. If objectives with high aperture are applied, it is important to connect the front lens to the coverslip by immersion oil or glycerol. This connection will conduct heat from the specimen to the objective, which may cause a non-uniform temperature distribution within the experimental chamber, and thus a loss of temperature control. In these cases it is important to heat the objective, which can be done by connecting the heating circuit to the objective, e.g. silicone tubing, through which warm water is pumped, is wrapped around the objective or by using commercially available objective heaters.

Such a simple system is only feasible if a preset temperature can be stabilized, and the perfusion with solution has a constant flow. If the flow of the perfusion changes, the temperature will also change. To avoid such temperature fluctuations, the temperature gauge in the experimental chamber has to be connected with the water bath by a feedback loop. Many commercially available temperature control devices are especially designed for electrophysiology avoiding 50/60 Hz noise. They consist mainly of Peltier elements, which are able to control temperature by fast heating or cooling. If temperature profiles during an experiment are planned, such devices are essential.

Another relatively complicated system may be useful, if the air above the experimental chamber has to have a controlled composition. Microscope producers offer hoods, which incorporate temperature control and control of the gas inside the hood. These hoods fit exactly to some microscopes and are designed for cell culture on the table of the microscope. There is a problem with these hoods, in that the electrode holder and connection to the amplifier and micromanipulator have to be placed inside. Each time the electrode has to be changed the hood has to be opened, and mounting the electrode inside such a hood may be complicated.

Perfusion

External Perfusion. A control of the external solution around cells is important in many experiments, e.g. if the influence of different drugs shall be tested. Such a control can be gained by a permanent perfusion system. Not only is a perfusion system necessary in the case of solution changes, but also if the temperature of the solution inside the experimental chamber is higher than the ambient temperature. This temperature gradient favours evaporation of water from the chamber, thereby increasing the concentration of salts in the external solution, which may influence the cells. Therefore, a perfusion system has to be used in nearly all experiments.

Perfusion systems consist of two different parts, the inwardly and the outwardly directed flow. Depending on the desired exchange rate of the bathing solution, these systems are of a different complexity. Slow perfusion of the experimental chamber means a complete exchange of the solution around the investigated cell in around 10–30 s. This can be performed by relatively simple components. If the exact time course of the influence of a substance is to be tested, solution change has to be at least 10× faster than the expected time course of the effect, and in this instance, so called fast perfusion systems are mounted.

In some experiments, not only control of the external solution, but also of the internal solution is desirable. In this case, the solution inside a patch-clamp electrode has to be changed during the recording, which is termed internal perfusion. The three different perfusion systems for whole cell experiments are described below.

In most perfusion systems, the inwardly directed flow is simply driven by gravity. Stock containers of solution are usually 50 or 100 ml syringes mounted 30–40 cm above the experimental chamber. The flow rate is adjusted by means of a tap, usually found in drip sets, for the infusion of patients. Higher accuracy and reproducibility is achievable by electronically controlled droppers, which count droplets photoelectrically, and adjust the diameter of the solution providing silicone tubing in a feedback loop. Application of various solutions can be achieved by mounting more parallel channels, which converge to one end near the experimental chamber. This forms the solution inlet of the chamber. Solution switch is obtained in very simple systems using manual taps. In the case of cheap solutions, it is advantageous to use three-way taps.

All solutions flow constantly into a waste receptacle, only the actual one is connected to the specimen. The waste receptacle should be mounted at the same height near the experimental chamber, in order to achieve similar pressure in the unused channels as well as the one connected to the specimen. In such a system, solution switches can be performed with minimal disturbance of the flow rate. If an automatic solution change is required, magnetic valves compress the inwardly directed tubes. One valve is required for each channel. Such systems are commercially available, and can easily be synchronized to computer controlled voltage clamp programs. Small disturbances in flow rate may appear during solution switch. One problem in these gravity driven systems is to gain an equal flow rate in all channels. Equal flow rates have to be adjusted manually before the experiment, because diverse flow rates in the different channels will cause problems as soon as a solution switch is performed. The monitored cells may be moved and thereby loose the contact to the electrode. Alternatively, a pressurised system can be used. In this case, the solution flow is not controlled by gravity but by pressure. In several commercially available systems, this pressure can be adjusted to get the desired flow rate.

Another alternative is the use of peristaltic pumps, which are sometimes used for the inwardly directed flow. Peristaltic pumps have the advantage that the flow rate can be easily controlled, because a change in the rotation speed of the pump influences the flow rate in all channels equally. However, peristaltic pumps can only be used together with the described three-way valves. If solution flow in an unused channel were to stop, it would cause an increase in pressure in this channel. In the case of a solution switch, the elevated pressure would be released as a solution wave, spoiling most recordings. Therefore, it is difficult to combine peristaltic pumps with automatic solution changers. The main disadvantage of peristaltic pumps is that the solution flow varies to a small extent, due to the peristaltic waves.

An important problem in most perfusion systems is that the external solution is directly connected to the monitored cell and reference electrode. Therefore, precautions have to be taken to avoid 50/60 Hz noise, which may couple into the solution filled tubes of the system.

Gravity-driven systems can be mounted completely inside the Faraday's cage, which will prevent these problems. Systems with a peristaltic pump cannot be used inside the cage, because the electric and magnetic fields of the pump might interfere with the recordings. The peristaltic pump should be located outside the Faraday's cage. If the fields of the power network influence the solution filled tubes, it is helpful to include a dropper in the system inside the Faraday's cage. This prevents the conduction of noise into the experimental chamber.

The same amount of solution, which flows into the experimental chamber, has to be sucked out of it. It is important to achieve this without producing waves or changing solution levels inside the chamber. In theory, this seems very easy, but in reality suction causes many problems. It is not possible to suck the solution from the bottom of the experimental chamber, because small differences between solution inflow and outflow could lead to a complete removal of solution from the chamber. Therefore, solution has to be sucked from the surface. As soon as the solution surface reaches the level of the suction pipette, liquid is sucked out of the chamber. If the solution level sinks below the level of the suction pipette, outflow should sever. However, this very often does not happen, because adhesion of water is stronger than the weight of a small droplet hanging to the tip of the suction pipette, and subsequently all of the solution can be sucked out of the chamber.

This problem can be overcome by the use of glass tubing with a very small tip, inducing frequent siphoning off of solution. The suction pipette can be made of microelectrode glass, which can be pulled to the desired tip diameter. We found this easy to do by hand, by heating in the flame of a small alcohol powered lamp. After the desired tip has been produced, it is bent into a rectangular angle by heating one side of the glass tube. If an electrode beveller (see Bevellers, this chapter) exists in the lab, the tip of the suction pipette can be bevelled into a steep angle. Bevelling of the tip of the suction pipette can also be done by hand with a diamond dust coated file, as this tip is large compared to an electrode tip.

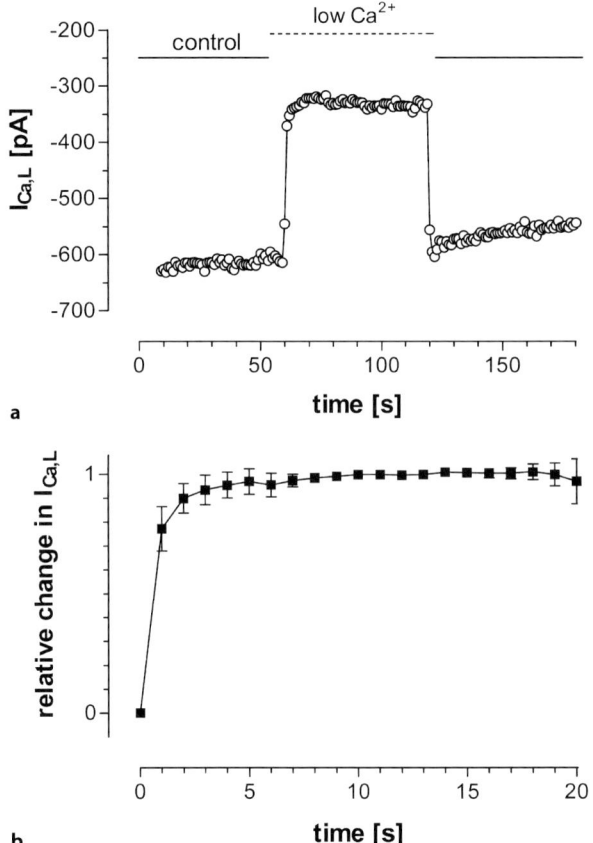

Figure 14a,b
Fast external perfusion. Effect and time course of the fast external perfusion. A ventricular cardiac myocyte of a guinea pig was clamped from −40 to 10 mV, each clamp was preceded by a preclamp from −80 to −40 mV, to inactivate I_{Na} and $I_{Ca,T}$. **a** Inward current peak plotted as function of time, during "low Ca" $CaCl_2$ concentration in the external solution was reduced from 1.8 to 0.9 mM. $I_{Ca,L}$ amplitude decreases from about 600 to 300 pA and recovers again after reintroduction of the control Ca concentration. **b** Standardised plot of the first $I_{Ca,L}$ amplitudes after reduction of external calcium concentration. Within three seconds more than 90% of the current reduction is reached

Negative pressure has to be connected to the suction pipette. The easiest way to do this is to use a pump that gases water in an aquarium. The suction side of this pump is connected to a filter flask, from which a tube leads to the suction pipette. To adjust the pressure in the bottle, a second inlet has to be installed, consisting of a tube with an adjustable clamp to compress it. The amount of air that enters the bottle via this shunt regulates the pressure in the whole system. The bottle should be located inside the Faraday's cage.

External Fast Perfusion. It is sometimes important to exchange the solution around a cell very quickly, e.g. if the time course of the effect of a substance has to be monitored. Many fast perfusion systems have been developed for different cells and purposes. In research on cardiac cells, very fast perfusion systems are not required, because it is not sufficient to exchange the solution around the cell. To gain a full effect, solution inside the T-tubule also has to be changed. According to our experience, this takes about 3 s (Fig. 14). Therefore, exchanging the external solution in 10 ms instead of 100 ms will not improve the quality of the recording significantly, unless the T-tubules are not contributing to the investigated effect.

Fast perfusion systems applied in research on cardiac cells are basically constructed along the same principles described in chapter External Perfusion, and usually driven by gravity. The solution outlet is a micropipette, which is positioned with its tip near the investigated cell. It is necessary for the different channels to end as near as possible to the investigated cell. In some systems, this is realized by a multibarrel pipette, alternatively all different channels end inside the pipette near the shoulder. This has the disadvantage that the volume of the taper has to be exchanged before the new solution reaches the tip of the pipette, i.e. systems with single tip pipettes are somewhat slower than those with multibarrel pipettes. However, this is not important in cardiac cells as exchange times of about 40 ms can be achieved with single tip pipettes (Meyer et al. 1998). The main shortcoming of most commercially available fast perfusion systems is that they are not heated. As it is desirable to work with 36 °C, these systems are not suited for cardiac cell experiments. At first glimpse, it appears simple to heat the tubes of the fast perfusion system near the pipette, and therefore the solutions are warm before they reach the cell. However, this will not work, as the increasing temperatures lead to a decreased solubility of gases in the solutions.

Heating the solution near the pipette might induce small bubbles in the perfusing solutions, which will interrupt the solution flow as soon as it reaches the tip of the pipette. Therefore, the system has to be heated to its highest temperature in the stock containers to degas them to a higher degree than at 36 °C. In our system, we installed a decreasing temperature gradient inside the fast perfusion system. Solution switches are performed by magnetic valves, which press the tubes.

The fast perfusion system is usually used in addition to the slow perfusion of the whole experimental chamber. Both solutions are sucked out of the experimental chamber via the normal solution outlet. At the beginning of the experiment, the same external solution, usually normal Tyrode's solution, comes out of both systems.

During the experiment, a fast perfusion system has various advantages. Solution switches can be programmed into the voltage clamp software. The point in time, at which the solution reaches the cell, is well defined. Different solutions can be applied in short intervals. As the application of solution is local, cells which are located upstream of the perfusion pipette have not been touched by the test solutions, which subsequently allows the use of more than one cell inside the experimental chamber. We found it very helpful to use long experimental chambers in combination with a fast perfusing system, to have a clear upstream region. These obvious advantages are combined with some shortcomings. It is necessary to glue the cells to the bottom of the experimental chamber, to avoid their dislocation into the solution stream. This can be achieved by laminin coating of the glass surface. But laminin adhesion is an additional procedure, which takes time and makes experiments more complicated. In addition, the filling and use of the fast perfusion is also time consuming. Even if one handles the system very thoroughly, small bubbles will occasionally block a channel. As this is not foreseeable, an otherwise successful recording may be spoiled. When all is taken into account, the use of fast perfusion makes experiments more complicated. Therefore, it is advisable to apply such a system only if fast and defined solution changes are really required.

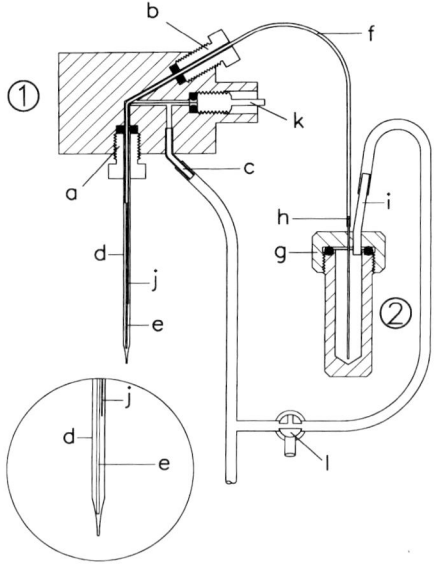

Figure 15
Pipette perfusion. Schematic drawing of a closed pipette perfusion system. *1* Pipette holder with: patch pipette d, Ag/AgCl wire j, perfusion pipette e, connection to the preamplifier k, connection to the pressure system c, seals a, b. Inset exhibits the patch electrode in higher magnification. *2* Vessel for perfusion solution with: connection to the perfusion pipette f, h, connection to the pressure system; valve l, seal g

Internal Perfusion. As the filling solution of the patch clamp electrode has access to the cytoplasm of the attached cell, it is possible to bring substances via the electrode directly into the cardiomyocyte, i.e. substances that are in the electrode filling solution will diffuse into the cytoplasm. If the filling solution of the electrode is varied during the experiment, the new contents will also enter the cytoplasm. Apparatus to vary the contents of the electrode filling solution is called an internal perfusion system. The first internal perfusion systems were custom made, but today are also commercially available, based on the ideas of Tang et al. (1990, 1992).

The system consists of a vacuum generator connected to the patch electrode and a thin quartz-glass pipette, which is inserted into the patch pipette. Its tip is about 75 µm behind the tip of the patch electrode. The quartz-glass pipette is connected to a small vessel containing the second perfusion solution. By applying negative pressure, solution is sucked into the patch electrode via the quartz-glass pipette. The quartz-glass pipette is pulled by hand (gravity) from polyamide coated quartz-glass capillaries (outer diameter 245 µm; inner diameter 100 µm). After the pull, burned residues of the coating have to be removed using a scalpel, and the taper has to be shortened to gain an inner tip diameter of 10–20 µm. An advantage of this glass is its extreme flexibility. A shortcoming of this system is that during seal formation, negative pressure is applied to the patch pipette, which will suck solution from the vessel into the pipette, and the pressure drop may not be sufficient for the formation of a good seal.

Therefore, the system created by Tang and co-workers, was further developed from an open system into a closed one (Linz and Meyer 1997). In a closed system, positive or negative pressure is always applied to both the patch electrode and the perfusion

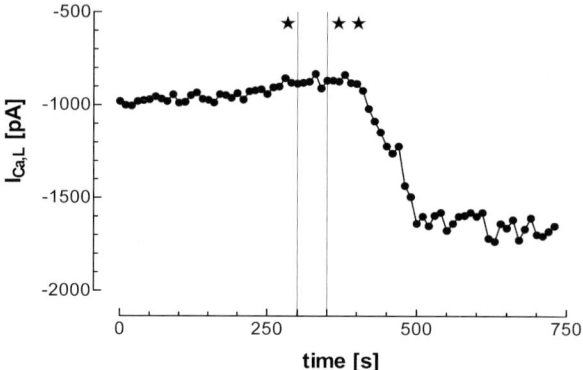

Figure 16
Time course of pipette perfusion. Time course of internal perfusion. Voltage clamp steps from −40 mV to +10 mV are applied at 0.1 Hz. $I_{Ca,L}$ amplitude is plotted as function of time. At * suction starts, at ** solution with 10^{-6} M cAMP appears at the taper of the patch pipette. From this time point it takes 120 s until a new steady state of $I_{Ca,L}$ is reached

pipette (Fig. 15). This construction improves formation of the "gigaseal", and avoids uncontrolled solution changes during the recording. Only in the case of intentional solution changes different pressures are applied. For optical control of the perfusion process, the second solution can be indicated by 0.5 mM phenol red, which does not produce obvious changes in membrane currents. In a closed system, negative pressure of 26–33 kPa can be applied continuously throughout the measurements, to avoid changes in series resistance due to variations in pressure.

The efficiency of internal cell dialysis could be determined in ventricular cardiomyocytes of the guinea pig as a shift in the reversal potential of the I_{K1}, after changing the K⁺ concentration of the pipette solution. Upon an increase in K⁺ from 130 mM to 150 or 170 mM, the reversal potential of I_{K1} was shifted by −4.5 ± 1.3 mV (n=4) or −7.2 ± 0.7 mV (n=21), respectively. These values are in correct agreement with the shifts in K⁺ equilibrium potential calculated by the Nernst equation. The time course of the internal perfusion is demonstrated in an experiment in Fig. 16. A ventricular cardiomyocyte of the guinea pig was repetitively clamped from −40 mV to +10 mV at 0.1 Hz. 10^{-6} M cAMP was sucked into the patch pipette. cAMP will increase the $I_{Ca,L}$ via activation of the cAMP dependent protein kinase A, which phosphorylates the L-type channels. After appearance of the phenol red at the tip of the patch pipette, it took 120 s until the $I_{Ca,L}$ had increased by about 50% and reached a new steady state. However, the time course of internal perfusion will vary with the diameter of the patch pipette and the size of the cell, and may often be somewhat slower than in the demonstrated example.

Changes in the internal solution of the patch pipette may also artificially affect an experiment, i.e. variations of the internal Cl⁻ concentration can cause changes in the surface potential at the chlorided silver wire connecting the patch pipette to the preamplifier, or changes in the ion concentration in the pipette may influence the pipette access resistance.

Manipulators

Electrical recordings from living cells require the approach of an electrode to a cell to be made by controlled movements in the μm range. For this purpose, so-called micromanipulators have been designed. The type of recording determines the properties of the manipulator used. For intracellular recordings with sharp microelectrodes, one needs a high acceleration to be able to penetrate the membrane of the cell. Therefore, such manipulators can move in small, well-defined steps in the nm- to μm range with high velocity. Such a high velocity can be obtained by a stepper motor with adequate mechanics or by a piezo stepper.

Patch recordings require smooth movement of the electrode tip, because the electrode should not injure the cell membrane. An intact membrane is a precondition for the formation of a stable gigaseal. Movements have to be smooth when a cell is approached, but also when the electrode is withdrawn from the cell, e.g. to obtain an excised patch. Three types of micromanipulators are used for patch clamp:
- Hydraulic systems
- Motor driven systems
- Piezoelectric system

Hydraulic systems move softly and are electrically noise free. The head of the manipulator is small and can be mounted on most set ups. As it is usually connected to the main part by thin tubes, mechanical uncoupling is relatively simple. Manipulators are cheaper than motor driven systems and piezo manipulators. We found these manipulators to be very suitable for use with cardiomyocytes. However, they do have one disadvantage; in the case of long-term recordings they have a tendency to drift. Sometimes, this can be overcome by lifting the cell at the tip of the electrode a few micrometers. A drift of the manipulator will then not spoil the gigaseal.

Motor driven systems have a very comfortable handling due to the development of digital electronics. They are of a big advantage if the same region is to be approached several times. However, they do produce high magnetic and electric fields and also heat up, which may lead to drift. Compared to hydraulic manipulators, they are more stable.

Piezo manipulators are different from piezo steppers because they move softly. They are electrically noise free, since they need a pure DC voltage. They do not warm up (no current flows through the piezo electric crystal), and their resolution is in the atomic range. They are also small and light. They are ideal tools for patch clamping, and are recommended whenever precise movement of the patch pipette and drift-free operation over long periods of time is required.

Vibration Isolation Table

To avoid the conduction of vibrations from the building in which the lab is located, it is necessary to install the microscope on a vibration isolation table. The principle of these tables is simple. A very heavy tabletop made of metal, concrete or granite is mechanically inert and does not follow high frequent vibrations easily. This tabletop is usually carried by rubber buffers, which uncouple it mechanically from the table legs. Many different types of vibration isolation tables are commercially available. Some have buffers, which can be adjusted by filling them with compressed air; some even use an air bearing to carry the tabletop. The required quality of the vibration isolation table depends very much on the situation of the building. Sometimes, very easy constructions with simple rubber buffers are sufficient, however, constructions with adjustable buffers are suitable in most cases for cardiac electrophysiology.

Stimulus Generator

Stimulus generation is done today using a computer program. These programs usually perform data acquisition and generate stimulus patterns. In the case of extracellular stimulation, the stimuli are fed into a stimulus isolator that is connected to the stimulating electrode. For intracellular recording, the computer is connected to the amplifier that applies the stimuli intracellularly. There are many computer programs for data acquisition and stimulation on the market, ranging from free to expensive programs with a large amount of capabilities.

To list these programs would go beyond the scope of this chapter and thus, we refer to specialised literature in this field.

Amplifier

The amplifier of choice depends on the kind of experiments one wants to perform. For intracellular current clamp recording, a bridge amplifier is sufficient (see Current Clamp Recordings and Bridge Amplifiers, this chapter). If the voltage of the cell needs to be controlled for recording membrane currents, a voltage (see Electrode Voltage Clamp and Single Electrode Clamp, this chapter) or patch clamp amplifier (see Introduction to Patch Clamp, this chapter) is used. Two-electrode voltage clamps can be used whenever the cells are big and easy enough to penetrate with two electrodes. Patch clamp amplifiers are recommended in culture cells, and are a must for single channel recordings. Switched single electrode amplifiers can be used with sharp microelectrodes and patch pipettes, and are recommended for use in tissue preparation and the recording of gap junction currents (see chapter 3.8).

Advantages and disadvantages of the respective amplifiers are described in more detail in the respective chapters.

Data Acquisition

As is the case for stimulation (see Stimulus Generator), computers are used today for data acquisition. Many systems are available which differ in acquisition speed (sample rate), resolution, capability of further data processing and price. For most experiments sample rates of 5 to 10 kHz with 12-bit or 16-bit resolution is sufficient. Some researchers prefer to use different programs for data acquisition and processing, which gives more flexibility for specific needs. Again, to list all these programs would go beyond the scope of this chapter and thus, we refer to specialised literature in this field.

Specific Electrical Methods

Action Potential Clamp

The described whole cell voltage clamp protocols are based on square pulses. This is a simple concept, which allows the calculation of membrane conductivity from the two known parameters, voltage and current. As conductivity very often changes as a function of time, a constant voltage is necessary to reveal this relationship. However, neither cardiac nor nerve APs can be reflected by a square pulse, therefore, the use of an AP as a voltage clamp pulse seems to be more realistic. Theoretically, the use of an AP as a voltage clamp signal should lead to zero current, because the AP is the result of all time and voltage dependent conductance changes of the cell. This works if an AP is used together with the exciting stimulus is recorded from a cell and thereafter played back to the same cell (Doerr et al. 1989, 1990).

The current recorded after the block of one component, is an inverted compensatory current of the size and time course of the blocked current. The different current components during the cardiac AP could be demonstrated thus for the first time.

An easier approach to the AP clamp is to apply a standard AP as a voltage pulse (Arreola et al. 1991). If this voltage pulse is devoid of the preceding stimulus, zero current flow will not be achieved, as the depolarising part of the AP will activate the Na^+ current just like a square pulse, and also the following current components will be activated afterwards in the same way. The advantage of this method lies in the use of prepared clamp patterns, however, this is also the disadvantage, as the standard AP may differ somewhat from the real AP shape of the recorded cell, thus elicited currents are not completely identical to currents during an AP of this cell. However, currents elicited by standard APs, can be taken as a good measure of the real currents during an AP. If a standard AP is applied, isolation of currents can be obtained by the same methods described above (see Protocols for Ionic Currents, this chapter).

I_{Na}, $I_{Ca,T}$ and possibly also I_{to} can be inactivated by a pre-clamp to -35 mV (Linz and Meyer 1998a,b). Pharmacological block of all current components, except the desired one, reveals its time course (Linz and Meyer 1998a). Alternatively, in a first step the sum of all currents is recorded under control conditions. In a second step the current of interest is selectively blocked by appropriate pharmacological treatment, i.e. $I_{Ca,L}$ by 100 mM Cd^{2+} (Linz and Meyer 1998a,b), and the remaining current components are recorded by means of the same voltage clamp pattern. The current of interest is then calculated as the difference in current between both recordings.

Perforated Patch

As already mentioned the section on Internal Perfusion, the filling solution in a patch clamp electrode and the cytoplasm exchange substances, via diffusion. This may be advantageous, if substances are to be brought directly into the cytoplasm, but it is disadvantageous, as the cell loses contents into the electrode, which may cause run down of current components (see The Principle and the Amplifier). Therefore, it is often helpful to avoid diffusion of bigger molecules between the cytoplasm and the cell. One way to avoid diffusion is the use of sharp electrodes in conjunction with a switch amplifier (see Single Electrode Clamp, this chapter). Another method that can be applied in combination with a conventional patch clamp amplifier is the perforated patch configuration. The principle of this method is rather simple. The cell-attached configuration is established. An ionophore is dissolved in the pipette filling solution. After a few minutes, the ionophore will incorporate into the membrane patch, and the access resistance to the cell decreases gradually. This technique was first invented in neuronal cells with the ionophore nystatin (Horn and Marty 1988); also, later on, amphotericin B (Rae et al. 1991) and gramicidin (Tajima et al. 1996) were introduced for this technique. Gramicidin has the advantage of being cation-selective, i.e. the cytoplasmic Cl⁻ concentration is not influenced. When applying amphotericin B for recordings of $I_{Ca,L}$, we found a concentration of 200 µg/ml added from a stock solution of 60 mg/ml in DMSO to a filling solution of 90 KCl, 40 KOH, 5 NaOH, 10 Hepes, 10 EGTA, 20 TEA, 2.5 Mg-ATP (all in mM), pH 7.2 very effective. This was used in combination with an external solution of (in mM) 135 choline chloride, 4 KCl, 1.8 $CaCl_2$, 2 $BaCl_2$, 2 4-AP, 2 Hepes, 10 glucose, pH 7.2 (Meyer et al. 1998). The perforated patch-clamp technique has two main shortcomings. The first being that one has to wait for about 10 min until a sufficient amount of ionophore has incorporated into the membrane patch before one knows whether a good recording is possible or not. This will reduce the rate of successful recordings per time. Secondly, the access resistance will always be much higher than in the case of conventional patch clamp recordings. Therefore, the voltage control is inferior in perforated patch recordings using patch clamp amplifiers, however, series resistance problems can be avoided using a switch amplifier (see Single Electrode Clamp).

Combined Methods

Electrophysiological recordings of cardiac myocytes are very often combined with the monitoring of other physiological parameters, like shortening and/or intracellular ionic concentrations; mostly cytoplasmic calcium, $[Ca^{2+}]_i$. Such combinations have been widely used since the introduction of fura-2 as an indicator dye for $[Ca^{2+}]_i$ (Grynkiewicz et al. 1985). As fluorescence dyes like fura-2 can be monitored by photometry or by imaging systems, both have been combined with electrophysiological recordings. From the technical viewpoint this is not very complicated, as inverted microscopes usually offer a port to mount a video camera. This port can also be used to adapt an intensified camera for fluorescence microscopy, a photomultiplier or photodiode based fluorescence detector. Confocal microscopy has also been combined with electrophysiological recordings of cardiac myocytes, using confocal microscopes based on inverted microscopes (Lipp and Niggli 1994).

Simultaneous recording of unloaded shortening with electrophysiological recordings can be performed in a comparably simple manner, if they are based on video signals. Even electron microscopy has been combined with electrophysiological recordings of isolated cardiac cells (Wendt-Gallitelli and Isenberg 1989; Gallitelli et al. 1999). The aim of these experiments is the ultrastructural localization of elements, taken as a measure for the corresponding ions, in conjunction with differences in activation of membrane currents.

Another fascinating approach is to measure ionic currents in a cell and then monitor the expression of specific channel encoding genes by reverse transciptase-polymerase chain reaction in the same cell (single cell RT-PCR; Schultz et al. 2001). This allows a check as to whether expression of a specific gene is correlated with the appearance of an electrically identifiable membrane current or not, e.g. Kv2.1 expression was not correlated with the size of I_K in rat cardiac myocytes (Schultz et al. 2001).

Besides simultaneously measuring different parameters, additional stimuli have been applied to isolated cardiac myocytes while recording membrane currents. Cells have been stretched in order to open stretch activated membrane channels. This is done by attaching a pair of carbon fibres to the myocyte of interest, in addition to a centrally located patch-clamp electrode (Cooper et al. 2000). These experiments are very complex to perform and have thus been only rarely carried out. Another very rarely applied method is the use of alternative stimuli, such as high frequency electromagnetic fields, to simulate the influence of the emission of cellular phones on membrane currents (Linz et al. 1999).

Summary and Conclusions

Microelectrode and patch recordings from cardiac cells have provided considerable information about their individual behaviours, functions, and coherences within the different cardiac tissues. In this chapter, we have deliberately focused on protocols developed for recordings from individual cells. Such recordings are the basis for further investigations. In other chapters of this book, modern electrophysiological and optical techniques reveal functional and structural properties of larger tissues and complete organs. Hopefully, many of the techniques and information from this chapter will be utilized as the basis for such studies.

Acknowledgement. The authors would like to thank Dr N. Best for critically reading the manuscript.

References

Armstrong CM, Chow RH (1987) Supercharging: A Method for Improving Patch-Clamp Performance. Biophys. J. 52:133–136
Arreola J, Dirksen RT, Shieh RC, Williford DJ, Sheu SS (1991) Ca^{2+} Current and Ca^{2+} Transients Under Action Potential Clamp in Guinea Pig Ventricular Myocytes. Am. J. Physiol. 261:C393–397
Bean BP (1985) Two Kinds of Calcium Channels in Canine Cardiac Atrial Cells: Differences Kinetics, Selectivity, and Pharmacology. J. Gen. Physiol. 86:1–30
Bers DM (2002) Cardiac Excitation Contraction Coupling. Nature 415:198–205
Brennecke R, Lindemann, B (1974) Theory of a Membrane-Voltage Clamp with Discontinuous Feedback Through a Pulsed Current Clamp. Rev. Sci Instrum. 45:184–188
Brown KT, Flaming DG (1977) New Microelectrode Techniques for Intracellular Work in Small Cells. Neuroscience 2:813–827
Cole KS (1949) Dynamic Electrical Characteristics of the Squid Axon Membrane. Arch. Sci. Physiol. 3:253–258
Cole KS (1968) Membranes, Ions and Impulses. University of California Press, Berkley and Los Angeles
Cooper PJ, Lei M, Cheng L-X, Kohl P (2000) Axial Stretch Increases Spontaneous Pacemaker Activity in Rabbit Isolated Sinoatrial Node Cells. J. Appl. Physiol. 89:2099–2104
De Paoli P, Cerbai E, Koidl B, Kirchengast M, Sartiani L, Mugelli A (2002) Selectivity of Different Calcium Antagonists on T- and L-Type Calcium Currents in Guinea Pig Ventricular Myocytes. Pharmacol. Res. 46:491–497
Deck KA, Kern R, Trautwein W (1964) Voltage Clamp Technique in Mammalian Cardiac Fibres. Pflügers Arch. 280:63–80
Dhein S (1998) Cardiac Gap Junction Channels, Physiology, Regulation, Patophysiology and Pharmacology, Karger, Basel
Dipla K, Mattiello JA, Margulies KB, Jeevanandam V, Houser SR (1999) The Sarcoplasmic Reticulum and the Na^+/Ca^{2+} Exchanger Both Contribute to the Ca^{2+} Transient of Failing Human Ventricular Myocytes. Circ. Res. 84:435–444
Doerr T, Denger R, Trautwein W (1989) Calcium Currents in Single SA Nodal Cells of the Rabbit Heart Studied with Action Potential Clamp. Pflügers Arch. 413:599–603

Doerr T, Denger R, Doerr A, Trautwein W (1990) Ionic Currents Contributing to the Action Potential in Single Ventricular Myocytes of the Guinea Pig Studied with Action Potential Clamp. Pflügers Arch. 416:230–237

Dow JW, Harding NGL, Powell T (1981) Isolated Cardiac Myocytes. I. Preparation of Adult Myocytes and their Homology with the Intact Tissue. Cardiovasc. Res. 15:483–514

Draper MH, Weidmann S (1951) Cardiac Resting and Action Potentials Recorded with an Intracellular Electrode. J. Physiol. 115:74–94

Finkel AS, Gage PW (1985) Conventional Voltage Clamping with Two Intracellular Microelectrodes. In: Smith, TG, Lecar H, Redman SJ, Gage PW, (eds): Voltage and Patch Clamping with Microelectrodes, Chapter 4. The William and Wilkins Company, Baltimore, p 47

Gallitelli MF, Schultz M, Isenberg G, Rudolf F (1999) Twitch-Potentiation Increases Calcium in Peripheral More than in Central Mitochondria of Guinea Pig Ventricular Myocytes. J. Physiol. 518: 433–447

Galvani, L: De viribus electricitatis in motu muscularis. Commentarius. Proc.Academia Bologna, 7, 363–418, 1791

Greeff K., Kühn F (2000) Variable Ratio of Permeability to Gating Charge of rBIIA Sodium Channels and Sodium Influx in *Xenopus* Oocytes, Biophys. J. 79: 2434–2453

Grynkiewicz G, Ponie M, Tsien RY (1985) A New Generation of Ca^{2+} Indicators with Greatly Improved Fluorescence Properties. J. Biol. Chem. 260: 3440–3450

Halliwell J, Whitaker M, Ogden D (1994) Using Microelectrodes. In: Ogden D (ed) Microelectrode Techniques. The Plymouth Workshop Handbook, Second Edition: The Company of Biologists Limited, Cambridge, p 1–16

Hamill OP, Marty A, Neher E, Sakmann B, Sigworth FJ (1981) Improved Patch-Clamp Techniques for High-Resolution Current Recording from Cells and Cell-Free Membrane Patches. Pflügers Arch. 391: 85–100

Hodgkin AL, Huxley AF, Katz B (1952) Measurement of Current-Voltage Relations in the Membrane of the Giant Axon of *Loligo*. J. Physiol. 116: 424–448

Hofmeier G, Lux HD (1981) The Time Course of Intracellular Free Calcium and Related Electrical Effects after Injection of $CaCl_2$ into Neurons of the Snail *Helix Pomatia*. Pflügers Arch. 391: 242–251

Horn R, Marty A (1988) Muscarinic Activation of Ionic Currents by a New Whole-Cell Recording Method. J. Gen. Physiol. 92: 145–159

Juusola M (1994) Measuring Complex Admittance and Receptor Current by Single Electrode Voltage-Clamp. J. Neurosci. Meth. 53: 1–6

Kordas M, Melik Z, Peterc D, Zorec R (1989) The Voltage-Clamp Apparatus Assisted by a "Current Pump", J. Neurosci. Meth. 26: 229–232

Lalley PM., AK Moschovakis, Windhorst U (1999) Electrical Activity of Individual Neurons *in Situ*: Extra- and Intracellular Recording, in: Windhorst U, Johansson H (eds) Modern Techniques in Neuroscience Research, Springer, Berlin, New York

Ling G, Gerard RW (1949) The Normal Membrane Potential of Frog Sartorius Fibres. J. Comp. Physiol. 34: 127–156

Linz KW, Meyer R (1998a) Control of L-Type Calcium Current During the Action Potential of Guinea Pig Ventricular Myocytes. J. Physiol. 513: 425–442

Linz KW, Meyer R (1997) Modulation of L-Type Calcium Current by Internal Potassium in Guinea Pig Ventricular Myocytes. Cardiovasc. Res. 33: 110–122

Linz KW, Meyer R (1998b) The Late Component of L-Type Calcium Current During Guinea Pig Action Potential and its Contribution to Contraction. Pflügers Arch. 436: 679–688

Linz KW, Westphalen C v, Streckert J, Hansen V, Meyer R (1999) Membrane Potential and Membrane Currents of Isolated Heart Muscle Cells Exposed to Pulsed High-Frequency Electromagnetic Fields. Bioelectromagnetics, 20: 497–511

Lipp P, Niggli E (1994) Sodium Current-Induced Calcium Signals in Isolated Guinea Pig Ventricular Myocytes. J. Physiol. 474: 439–446

Luo CH, Rudy Y (1994) A Dynamic Model of the Cardiac Action Potential: Simulations of Ionic Currents and Concentration Changes. Circ. Res. 74: 1071–1096

Magistretti, J., Mantegazza, M, Guatteo, E., Wanke, E (1996) Action Potentials Recorded with Patch-Clamp Amplifiers: Are they Genuine? Trends Neurosci. 19: 530–534

McDonald TF, Pelzer S, Trautwein W., Pelzer DJ (1994) Regulation and Modulation of Calcium Channels in Cardiac, Skeletal and Smooth Muscle Cells. Physiol. Rev. 74: 365–507

Meyer R, Linz KW, Surges R, Meinardus S, Vees J, Hoffmann A, Windholz O, Grohé C (1998) Rapid Modulation of L-Type Calcium Current by Acutely Applied Oestrogens in Isolated Cardiac Myocytes from Human, Guinea Pig, and Rat. Experimental Physiol. 83: 305–321

Müller A, Lauven M, Berkels R, Dhein S, Polder HR, Klaus W (1999) Switched Single-Electrode Voltage-Clamp Amplifiers Allow Precise Measurement of Gap Junction Conductance. Am. J. Physiol 276: C980–C987

Müller CM (1992) Intracellular Microelectrodes. In: Kettenmann H, Grantyn R (eds) Practical Elektrophysiological Methods. Wiley-Liss, New York, p 183–188

Neher E (1995) Voltage Offsets in Patch-Clamp Experiments. In: Sakmann B, Neher, E (eds) Single-Channel Recording. Second Edition. Plenum Press, New York, London, p 17–20

Ogden DC (1994) Microelectrode electronics. In: Ogden D.C. (ed.) Microelectrode techniques. The Plymouth Workshop Handbook, Second Edition: The Company of Biologists Limited, Cambridge

Penner R (1995) A Practical Guide to Patch Clamping. Pipette Fabrication. In: Sakmann B, Neher, E (eds) Single-Channel Recording. Second Edition. Plenum Press, New York, London, p 17–20

Polder HR, Swandulla D (2001) The Use of Control Theory for the Design of Voltage Clamp Systems: A Simple and Standardized Procedure for Evaluating System Parameters. J. Neurosci. Meth. 109: 97–109

Rae J, Cooper K, Gates P, Watsky M (1991) Low Access Resistance Perforated Patch Recordings using Amphotericin B. J. Neurosci. Meth. 37: 15–26

Reuter H (1967) The Dependence of the Slow Inward Current in Purkinje Fibres on the Extracellular Calcium-Concentration. J. Physiol. 192: 479–492

Richter DW, Pierrefiche O, Lalley PM, Polder HR (1996) Voltage-Clamp Analysis of Neurons Within Deep Layers of the Brain. J. Neurosci. Meth. 67: 121–131

Sakmann B, Neher E (1995) Geometric Parameters of Pipettes and Membrane Patches. In: Sakmann B, Neher, E (eds) Single-Channel Recording. Second Edition. Plenum Press, New York, London, p 17–20

Schanne OF, Lavalle M, Laprade R, Gagn S (1968) Electrical Properties of Glass Microelectrodes. Proc. IEEE, 56: 1072–1082

Schultz J-H, Volk T, Ehmke H (2001) Heterogeneity of Kv2.1 mRNA Expression and Delayed Rectifier Current in Single Isolated Myocytes from Rat Left Ventricle. Circ. Res. 88:483–490

Sigworth FJ (1995) Electronic Design of the Patch Clamp. In: Sakmann B, Neher E (eds) Single-Channel Recording. Second Edition. Plenum Press, New York, London, p 95–126

Smith TG, Lecar H, Redman SJ, Gage PW (ed) (1985) Voltage and Patch Clamping With Microelectrodes. The William and Wilkins Company, Baltimore

Tajima Y, Ono K, Akaike N (1996) Perforated Patch-Clamp Recording in Cardiac Myocytes using Cation-Selective Ionophore Gramicidin. Am. J. Physiol. 271: C524–532

Tang JM, Wang J, Eisenberg RS (1992) Perfusing Patch Pipettes. Methods Enzymol. 207: 176–181

Tang JM, Wang J, Quandt FN, Eisenberg RS (1990) Perfusing Pipettes. Pflügers Arch. 416: 347–350

Van Rijen HVM, Wilders R, Van Ginneken ACG, Jongsma HJ (1998) Quantitative Analysis of Dual Whole-Cell Voltage Clamp Determination of Gap Junctional Conductance. Pfluegers Arch. 436: 141–151

Veenstra, RD, Brink PR (1992) Patch-Clamp Analysis of Gap Junctional Currents. In: Cell-Cell Interactions, edited by Stevenson BR, Gallin WJ & Paul DL. Oxford: Oxford University Press, p 167–201

Weckström M, Kouvaleinen E., Juusola M (1992) Measurement of Cell Impedance in Frequency Domain using Discontinuous Current Clamp and White-Noise Modulated Current Injection. Pflügers Arch. 421: 469–472

Wendt-Gallitelli MF, Isenberg G (1989) X-ray Microanalysis of Single Cardiac Myocytes Frozen Under Voltage Clamp Conditions. Am. J. Physiol. 256: H574–583

Further reading

Boulton AA, Baker G, Walz W (eds) (1995) Patch Clamp Applications and Protocols, Humana Press, Totowa, New Jersey

Conn MP (ed.)(1998) Ion Channels (Part B), Meth. In Enzymology, Vol. 293, Academic Press, San Diego

Conn MP (ed.)(1998) Ion Channels (Part C), Meth. In Enzymology, Vol. 294, Academic Press, San Diego

Dhein S (1998) Cardiac Gap Junction Channels, Physiology, Regulation, Pathophysiology and Pharmacology, Karger, Basel

Ferreira HG, Marshall MW (1985) The Biophysical Basis of Excitability, Cambridge University Press

Hille B (1992) Ionic Channels of Excitable Membranes, Second Edition, Sinauer Associates Inc. Sunderland, Mass.

Jack JJB, Noble D, Tsien RW (1975) Electric Current Flow in Excitable Cells. Claredon Press, Oxford

Kettenmann H, Grantyn R (eds)(1992) Practical Elektrophysiological Methods. Wiley-Liss, New York

Numberger M, Draguhn A (eds)(1996) Patch-Clamp Technik (in German), Spektrum Akademischer Verlag. Heidelberg

Ogden DC (ed.)(1994) Microelectrode Techniques. The Plymouth Workshop Handbook, Second Edition: The Company of Biologists Limited, Cambridge

Rudy B, LE Iverson (eds)(1992) Ion Channels, Meth. In Enzymology, Vol. 207, Academic Press, San Diego

Sakmann B, Neher E (eds)(1995) Single-Channel Recording. Second Edition. Plenum Press, New York, London

Smith TG, Lecar H, Redman SJ, Gage PW. (eds)(1985) Voltage and Patch Clamping with Microelectrodes. Chapter 4. The William and Wilkins Company, Baltimore

Walz W, Boulton AA, Baker GB. (eds)(2002) Patch-Clamp Analysis. Humana Press, Totowa, New Jersey

Weiss TF (1997) Cellular Biophysics, Vol. 1 Transport. The MIT Press, Cambridge, Mass.

Weiss TF (1997) Cellular Biophysics, Vol. 2 Electrical Properties. The MIT Press, Cambridge, Mass.

Windhorst U, Johansson H (eds) (1999) Modern Techniques in Neuroscience Research. Springer, Berlin, New York

L-Type Calcium Channel Recording

Uta C. Hoppe, Mathias C. Brandt, Guido Michels and Michael Lindner

Introduction

Calcium channels constitute a large family of voltage- and ligand-operated ion-channels. They share several structural similarities with voltage-gated Na$^+$- and K$^+$-channels. All three channel populations appear to originate from the same gene superfamily. Ca^{2+} channels are ubiquitous, they can be found in almost any type of excitable and most unexcitable cells in a wide variety of species.

Their key functional role is to transduce membrane depolarization to an entry of Ca^{2+}-ions into the cell. This important physiological trigger serves as a uniform effector of a vast number of functions in different cells. The specific physiological consequence of Ca^{2+} entry into the cytoplasm depends on the corresponding cell type. An increase in [Ca^{2+}]$_i$ initiates transmitter secretion in nerve terminals and intracellular Ca^{2+} release and sarcomere shortening in skeletal and cardiac myocytes, generates the action potential in cardiac pacemaker cells and regulates gene expression in neurons. When considering the regulation of these processes, it is important to remember the voltage-dependence of most types of Ca^{2+} channels. Due to the voltage-dependence of Ca^{2+} entry, these functionally related and primarily Ca^{2+}-dependent processes acquire a secondary voltage-dependence. In this context, Ca^{2+} ions serve as an intracellular second messenger (Hille 2001).

In cardiac myocytes, at least four types of calcium channels have been discovered, the L-type and T-type Ca^{2+} channels coexisting on the cell surface and the ryanodine receptor and IP$_3$-receptor on intracellular membranes.

Molecular Diversity of Voltage-Gated Calcium Channels

All voltage-gated Ca^{2+} channels characterized at the molecular level up to now show a similar subunit composition, illustrated in Fig. 1. They consist of five specific subunits: α_1, α_2, linked to δ *via* disulfide bindings, β, located intracellularly, and γ (Hoffmann et al. 1999). The skeletal muscle calcium channel was the first to be characterized at the molecular level. The subunit composition of calcium channel complexes from other tissue types do not exactly resemble those from skeletal muscle.

High threshold Ca^{2+}-channels (HVA, high voltage-activated, non-L-type and L-type channels) activate at more positive membrane potentials, whereas low-voltage activated channels (LVA or T-type, transient, tiny current) require relatively low mem-

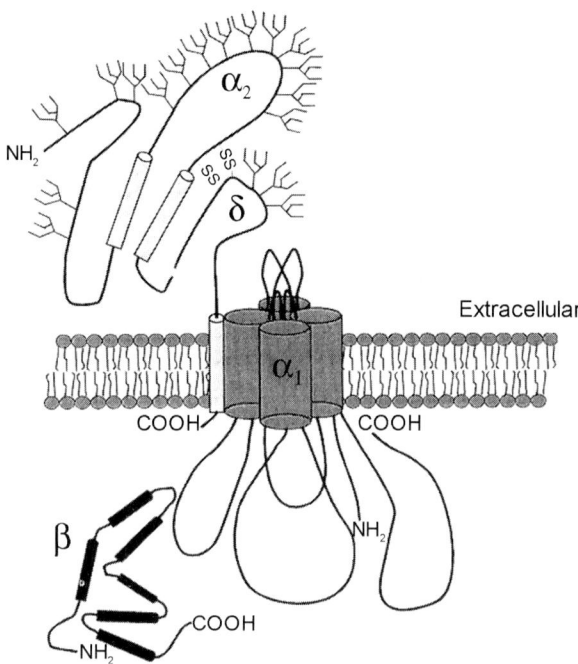

Figure 1
Overview and subunit composition of voltage-gated Ca^{2+} channels. The main structural components are the pore-forming α_1-subunit, accessory α_2 subunit, closely linked to the α_1-subunit *via* the δ-subunit, and the intracellular β-subunit (adapted from Gurnett et al. 1996)

brane potentials for activation. (Fig. 2, Ertel et al. 2000). LVA Ca^{2+} channels comprise $Ca_v3.1$–$Ca_v3.3$ (α_1G, α_1H, α_1I). L-type (long lasting channels) or DHP-sensitive channels are subdivided into four classes according to their α_1-subunit, $Ca_v1.1$ (α_1S, skeletal muscle), $Ca_v1.2$ (α_1C), $Ca_v1.3$ (α_1D, neuronal, pancreas, kidney, endocrine cells) and $Ca_v1.4$ (α_1F, retina). The $Ca_v1.2$ (α_1C)-subunit has several splice-variants, $Ca_v1.2a$ in heart, $Ca_v1.2b$ in smooth muscle and lung and $Ca_v1.2c$ in neurons and heart. Non-L-type or DHP-insensitive channels are encoded by $Ca_v2.1$–$Ca_v2.3$, corresponding to α_1A or P (Purkinje-cell)/Q-type, α_1B or N (neuron)-type and α_1 E or R-type. Distinct recordings of HVA and LVA channels were first made in canine atrial cardiomyocytes (Bean et al. 1985) and guinea pig ventricular myocytes. The estimated density of functional L-type Ca^{2+} channels (1–5/µm^2) is about 10–20 times greater than that of T-type channels.

The pore-forming α_1-subunit (175–275 kD, Fig. 3) is the largest component and determines the characteristic functional and pharmacological properties of every Ca^{2+} channel. It contains the voltage-sensor, the ion-conducting pore, the selectivity filter, binding sites for channel blockers and interaction sites for other subunits. The core α_1-subunit is divided into four homologous repeats or domains (DI-DIV), each consisting of six predicted membrane-spanning segments, S1 to S6, and two short segments, SS1 and SS2, located between S5 and S6. The channel pore is formed by a conformation of S1 to S4, where the linker-connection between the segments S5 and S6, the P(pore)-region, is directed to the inner side of the channel in each of the four repeats. The P-regions from each of the four repeats contain a short SS2 segment with glutamic acid residues of high negative charge density directed to the inner side of the pore, which determine the basis of ion selectivity. Mutations in the amino-acid se-

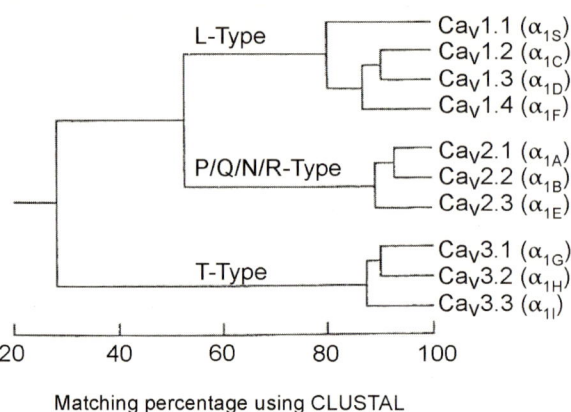

Figure 2
Phylogenetic relationship of voltage gated Ca^{2+} channel subunits illustrated by sequence identities within the membrane-spanning domains of the α_1-subunit. Three large families of Ca^{2+} channels with 80% intra-family sequence identities can be distinguished: L-type channels ($Ca_v1.1$ to $Ca_v1.4$), non-L-type, comprising P/Q,N and R-Type ($Ca_v2.1$ to $Ca_v2.3$) and T-type ($Ca_v3.1$ to $Ca_v3.3$). The corresponding nomenclature of α_1-subunit isoforms is indicated in brackets. (Adapted from Ertel et al. 2000)

quence of this selectivity filter to neutral or positive charges cause alterations in the Ca^{2+} channel affinity for Ca^{2+}, in single-channel conductance and in sensitivity to block by divalent cations. The binding site for pharmacological channel blockers is also located within the P-region of the α_1-subunit. The extracellular mouth of the pore is lined by SS1 and SS2 segments.

The S4-segment contains the voltage-sensor. Like other voltage-gated ion channels, every third residue within the S4-segment of the Ca^{2+} channel contains positively charged domains of arginine or lysine. Depolarization causes a translocation of the S4-segment with positive charge movements across the cell membrane (gating currents), leading to a conformational change in the channel protein from the closed to the open state. Mutations within repeats I and III of the S4 sequence to neutral or negative residues lead to a reduction of gating charge and a reduced sensitivity to membrane depolarization.

While the α_1-subunit alone is sufficient for the expression of functional Ca channels, the other subunits have important regulatory functions for activation, inactivation, gating, and opening probability of the channel pore.

The β-subunit (50–70 kD) is entirely located intracellularly and has several potential phosphorylation sites for cAMP-dependent protein kinases, phosphokinase-C (PKC), and cGMP-dependent kinases. The subunits are not glycosylated and do not co-purify with membranes. β-subunits modulate several parameters of α_1 activity, including the level of channel expression, threshold of activation, rate of inactivation, and steady-state inactivation (Walker and De Waard 1998). The molecular diversity of the β-subunit is caused not only by the expression of four different genes, but also by differential splicing. Four different isoforms, $β_1$ to $β_4$, have been identified and are expressed, like the α_2-subunit, in a tissue-specific pattern. $β_{1a}$ is expressed in skeletal muscle, $β_{1b}$ in the brain and $β_2$ predominantly in cardiac tissue and, to a lesser extent, in aorta, trachea, lung and brain (Biel et al. 1990). The $β_3$ and $β_4$ variants are also present in different regions of the brain. Except for the brain $β_2$-subunit of the rat, the

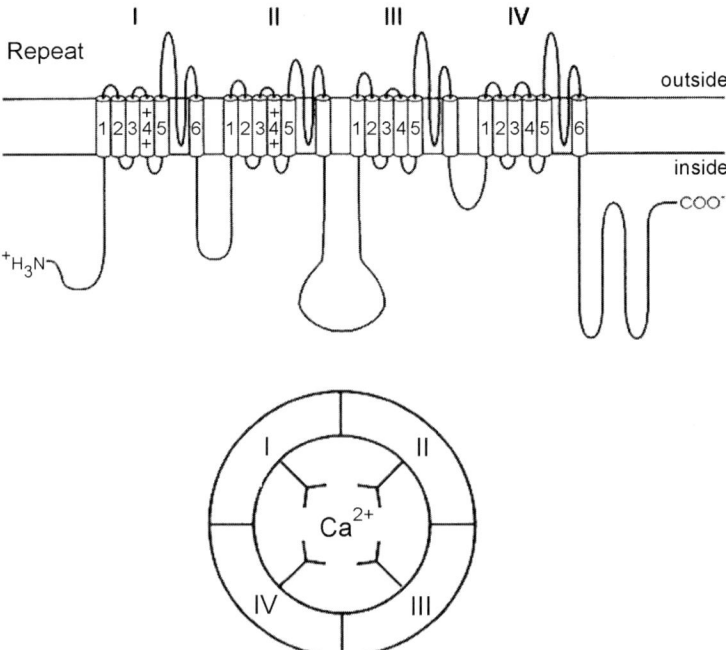

Figure 3
Schematic representation of the α_1-subunit of voltage-gated Ca^{2+} channels. The a_1-subunit consists of four homologous domains, DI to DIV, each consisting of six predicted transmembrane segments, S1 to S6. As illustrated in the inset, a conformation of S1 to S4 in each domain forms the channel pore, with the linker connections between S5 and S6 of domains DI to DIV directed to the inner side of the channel, to form the selectivity filter. (Adapted from Melzer et al., Biochem Biophys Acta 1995; 1241: 59–116)

co-expression of β-subunits with different α_1-subunits facilitates channel pore opening, and results in an increase in the peak-current amplitude. The interaction between α_1 and β-subunits is governed primarily by highly conserved domains in each subunit (α_1- and β-subunit interaction domains; Walker and De Waard 1998).

The disulfide-linked α_2-δ subunit (143 kD and 27 kD) of the voltage-operated calcium channel was the first isolated as a co-precipitate of immunoprecipitated rabbit skeletal muscle DHP receptors. cDNA cloning subsequently revealed that the two subunits are the product of a single gene, being translated from one mRNA and then processed into two proteins of 935 amino acids (α_2-subunit) and 144 amino acids (δ-subunit; Hoffmann et al. 1999). Hydropathy analyses suggest that the δ-subunit has one transmembrane spanning segment with an intracellular C- and an extracellular N-terminus. The α_2-subunit is anchored to the α_1-subunit by this transmembrane domain of the δ-subunit. Different splice variants of the α_2δ-complex with tissue specific expression have been identified. α_2δ-1 is found ubiquitously, α_2δ-2 is expressed in heart, intestinal organs, skeletal muscle and brain and α_2δ-3 is primarily expressed in different parts of the brain (Klugbauer et al. 1999). From electrophysiological studies in different cell types, it can be deduced that co-expression of α_2δ-with α_1- and β-subunits results in a shift of the current-voltage curve to more positive potentials, an increase in the maximal channel conductance and acceleration of activation and inactivation in α_{1C}- (Bangalore et al. 1996) and α_1 E-type (Quin et al. 1998) calcium channels. This effect appears to be mediated by interaction with the α_{1C}-subunit.

The γ-subunit (25–35 kD) consists of four transmembrane domains and contains two extracellular loops with potential glycosylation sites. Up to now, four tissue-specific isoforms, $γ_1$ to $γ_4$ have been identified. The $γ_1$-subunit is found in skeletal muscle only ($Ca_v1.1 \times β \times α_2δ \times γ_1$; Eberst et al. 1997), the neuronal $γ_2$-(stargazin), $γ_3$- and $γ_4$-subunits in the central nervous system and the $γ_5$-subunit in liver, kidney, heart and lung (Klugbauer et al. 1999, 2000). Furthermore, results from Klugbauer et al. (2000) suggest that $γ_2$-, $γ_3$- and $γ_4$-subunits can associate with $α_1A$, $α_1B$ and $α_1$ E channels. The $γ_5$-subunit could be an auxiliary subunit of T-type channels. In rat cardiomyocytes, coexpression of the γ-subunit with the cardiac calcium channel complex leads to a shift in the inactivation curve to more negative potentials and accelerated inactivation, without affecting other voltage-dependent channel properties. Similar results were obtained from co-expression of the γ-subunit with $α_1$-, β-, and $α_2δ$-subunits in oocytes.

Biophysical Properties

The basic electrophysiological properties of voltage-dependent L-type calcium channels ($Ca_v1.1$–$Ca_v1.4$) can be characterized by their ion conductance and voltage dependence of activation and inactivation. Important biophysical characteristics are the steep voltage-dependence of activation and inactivation, slow inactivation kinetics and high values for slope conductance. Ca^{2+}-channels activate at membrane potentials around -30 mV and reach their peak whole-cell current amplitude at +10 mV. With further depolarization $I_{Ca,L}$ decreases again, due to a reduction in the electrochemical driving force.

Conductance and Calcium-Permeation

Calcium flow through single L-type Ca^{2+} channels occurs at a rate of ~10^6 ions/s, with an error rate of about ~1 ion in 10^4. Under physiological conditions, calcium channels transport calcium ions and monovalent cations with high selectivity. Even in the presence of other cations, Ca^{2+} is transported almost exclusively.

The kinetics of ion channel transport through the calcium channels differs from free diffusion, even when following the electrochemical gradient. The size of the inward Ca^{2+} current does not increase linearly with $[Ca^{2+}]_o$, but shows the shape of a saturation function. This effect is due to the fact that the permeating Ca^{2+} ions do not pass independently, but compete for the same binding site. Similar results were established for other cations (see Examples).

A major distinguishing feature that has favoured multi-ion occupancy in calcium-channels is the anomalous mole fraction effect (AMFE) between calcium and barium. In the presence of a solution containing equimolar concentrations of Ca^{2+} and Ba^{2+}, the overall channel conductance is smaller than in pure solutions containing either ion. The AMFE was not found in cardiac L-type calcium channels at single channel level (Yue und Marban 1990), and the validity of the AMFE as an indicator of multiple occupancy has been severely questioned by other authors. Kuo and Hess (1993) proposed that the calcium channel was a multi-ion pore ('two or more site model') that contains two sets of binding sites, one composed of high-affinity sites and located near the external pore mouth, and another composed of low-affinity sites and placed intracellularly.

Kinetics of L-type Calcium Channels

The activation of voltage-dependent ion channels is the result of multiple conformational changes involving positively charged, transmembrane polypeptide regions. Displacement of these charge-bearing intramolecular domains, in response to changes in the transmembrane electric field, produces gating currents. Gating currents, generated by the movement of the channel voltage sensors, are considered to be the primary events in signal transduction for all cellular processes involving voltage-dependent ion channels.

Calcium currents are rapidly activated by depolarisation, reaching a peak in ~2–7 ms, depending on temperature and membrane-potential (E_m). Calcium channel activation appears to depend primarily on E_m, but, as for most voltage-sensitive ion channels, is also sensitive to changes in surface potential. The magnitude of the current across the membrane depends on the density of channels, the conductance of the open channel, and how often the channel is in its open position or its open probability. A possible mechanism is that a change in the membrane potential results in a reorientation of dipoles or an actual charge movement within the membrane field that produces a conformational change in the channel molecule, which in turn results in favouring the open or closed state of the pore.

Activation

Domain I of the ion-conducting α_1-subunit is responsible for calcium channel activation and inactivation (Zhang et al. 1994). The amino acid composition of the S3 and S4 segments within domain I and within the linker connecting between S3 and S4 is critical for the difference in activation kinetics between cardiac and skeletal muscle L-type calcium channels. Activation kinetics, however, are not determined by the IS3 segment and the IS3-IS4 linker alone. The rate of activation is also affected by the current density. On membrane depolarisation, a stretch of S4 moves outward and initiates a number of conformational changes leading to channel opening. The voltage-activated channels seem to open by movement of the inner parts of the S6 α-helices. Conserved proline residues are in the middle of the S4-voltage-sensor of domains I and III in voltage-dependent calcium channels.

As the presence of proline introduces a kink into a helical protein structure, these residues might have an intrinsic function within the voltage sensor ('intrinsic channel agonist'). Yamaguchi et al. (1999) reported that the removal of S4 prolines resulted in a dramatic shortening of channel open time whereas the introduction of extra prolines to the corresponding positions in motif IIS4 and IVS4 increased channel open-time.

Inactivation

L-type calcium channels display calcium-sensitive inactivation, a biological feedback mechanism in which elevation of intracellular calcium concentration speeds up channel inactivation. During sustained depolarisation, voltage-gated calcium channels progressively undergo a transition to a non-conducting, inactivated state, preventing calcium overload of the intracellular space. This transition is triggered by the entry of calcium (calcium-dependent inactivation) and by the membrane potential (voltage-dependent inactivation). Inactivation of L-type calcium channels occurs in two phases, an initial fast phase that depends on a calcium-calmodulin complex binding to the cytoplasmic side of the channel protein and a slower second phase that is voltage-dependent. Both mechanisms act to induce a conformational change in the channel protein, resulting in pore closure.

Calcium-dependent inactivation is only recorded in L-type calcium-channels and is an important regulatory factor for calcium-activated intracellular processes such as excitation-contraction coupling, secretion and gene expression. Calcium ions entering the cell through calcium channels can bind to a specific site located close to the inner mouth of the channel and promote its inactivation. This type of inactivation, as opposed to voltage-dependent inactivation, is not recorded when Ba^{2+} or Sr^{2+} are used as charge carriers (Findlay 2002; see Examples, Fig. 4). Ba^{2+} ions permeate calcium channels even better than Ca^{2+} without producing inactivation.

While voltage-dependent inactivation has been found in all types of calcium channels, the calcium-dependent inactivation seems to be specific for DHP-sensitive L-type calcium channels and has been suggested to arise from a completely different mechanism. The influence of the auxiliary β-subunit on the calcium-dependent inactivation has been tested and it has been suggested that the same molecular determinants affect both voltage- and calcium-dependent inactivation. Up to now, calcium-dependent inactivation of the L-type calcium channel has been considered to be a property of the $α_1$C-subunit ($Ca_v1.2$), with additional influences from the β- and $α_2δ$-subunits.

Other types of non-skeletal L-type calcium channels, which are involved in synaptic transmission (P/Q-, R- and N-types), do not show substantial calcium-induced inactivation. Accordingly, different sequences of the $α_1$C-subunit ($Ca_v1.2$), including a putative EF-hand calcium-binding site, have been shown to be essential for calcium-dependent inactivation (Soldatov et al. 1997). These sequences are located at the carboxy-terminal end of the $α_1$C-subunit ($Ca_v1.2$) and their transposition to other $α_1$-subunits transferred calcium-dependent inactivation to channels that do not usually display this type of inactivation. Peterson et al. (1999) showed that calmodulin was necessary for calcium-dependent inactivation and was pre-bound to the C-terminus of the calcium channel. Calcium ions entering as a result of channel opening bound to the tethered calmodulin and led to its interaction with the IQ motif, thereby producing channel inactivation. P/Q-channels have also been shown to be modulated by calmodulin (Lee et al. 1999). The binding mode of calmodulin depends on the free calcium concentration and calcium-binding to calmodulin itself. Other studies suggest that the IQ-motif may not be the only determinant necessary for calcium-dependent inactivation of these channel types.

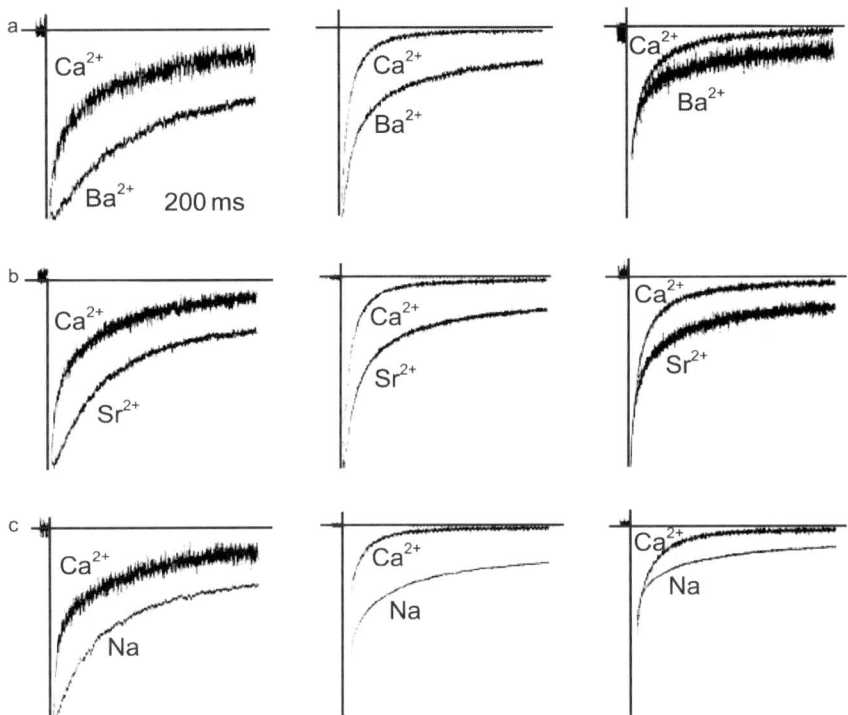

Figure 4
Inactivation kinetics of L-type Ca^{2+} channel current due to different charge carriers. Normalized whole-cell currents elicited by depolarization steps to −20 mV (*left column*), 0 mV (*middle column*) and +20 mV (*right column*). The superimposed normalized recordings were performed with Ba^{2+} (A), Sr^{2+} (B) and Na^+ (C) as the main positive charge carrier, compared to recordings with Ca^{2+}. In all three sets of experiments, inactivation was markedly slower when Ca^{2+} was replaced by other ions (Findlay 2002)

L-type Ca^{2+} channels do not inactivate exclusively in a Ca^{2+}-dependent fashion. Voltage-dependent inactivation was distinguished from calcium-dependent inactivation by replacing extracellular calcium with magnesium and recording outward currents through calcium channels.

Inactivation due to voltage has been considered to play a minor role in the decay of L-type calcium current in cardiac myocytes following β-adrenergic stimulation (Findlay 2002). β-adrenergic stimulation slows the voltage-dependent inactivation kinetics of native cardiac L-type calcium channels. The apparent reduction in the voltage-dependent decay of calcium currents induced by isoproterenol (isoprenaline) seems to be due to a conversion of channels from a rapidly inactivating to a slowly inactivating kinetic form. Conversely, Findlay (2002) showed that voltage-dependent inactivation played a major role in the decay of native L-type calcium channels under basal conditions (see Examples). With increasing holding potentials from −20 to +20 mV, a step depolarisation to a fixed pulse potential results in faster inactivation kinetics (Fig. 5). Other investigators (Hirano et al. 1999) showed that strong de-

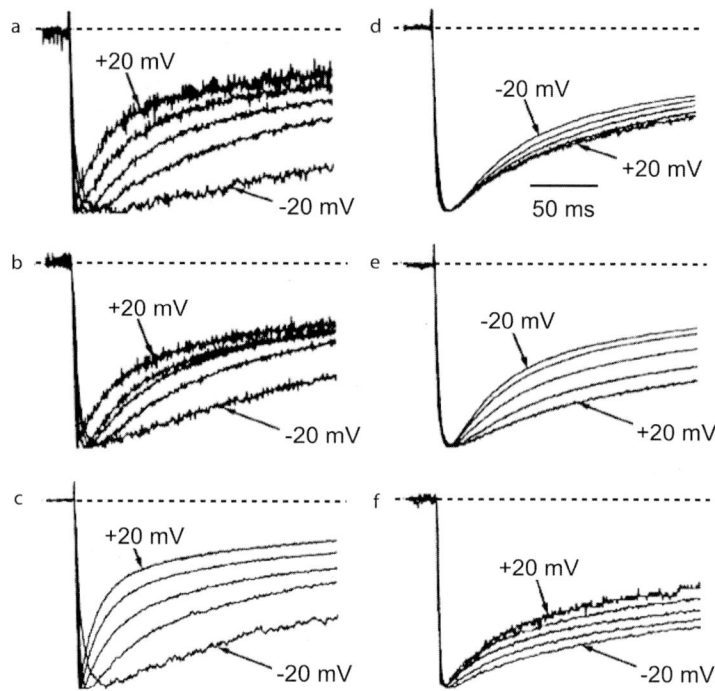

Figure 5
Inactivation kinetics of L-type Ca^{2+} current in relation to different holding potentials and charge carriers. Normalized superimposed whole-cell Ca^{2+} current carried by Ba^{2+} (A), Sr^{2+} (B) and Na^+ (C) elicited by depolarisation steps to –20 mV, –10 mV, 0 mV, +10 mV and +20 mV. Consistently with all three charge carriers, the channel inactivation was markedly increased with increasing levels of depolarisation, indicating voltage-dependent inactivation. The *right column* (D, E, F) shows the results of the same experiments in the presence of 100 nM isoproterenol (Findlay 2002)

polarisation could evoke 'mode 2' type behaviour in single cardiac L-type calcium channels, this process has also been shown to be enhanced by β-adrenergic stimulation (Yue et al. 1990). It is therefore possible that voltage-dependent potentiation of the L-type calcium current results from the loss of voltage-dependent inactivation. Single amino acids in segments IIIS6 and IVS6 have been identified as determinants of voltage-dependent inactivation. Furthermore, previous studies showed that a segment in IVS5 of the human α_1C ($Ca_v 1.2$) subunit is critically involved in inactivation of the channel (Bodi et al. 2002).

Modulation of L-type Calcium Channels

Second messenger-activated protein kinase phosphorylation is a crucial physiological regulative mechanism for the calcium channel protein. cAMP-activated protein kinase A (PKA) increases $I_{Ca(L)}$ whereas the cGMP-activated kinase (PKG) decreases it. Calcium channels can also be regulated directly by G proteins (Gbγ-subunits).

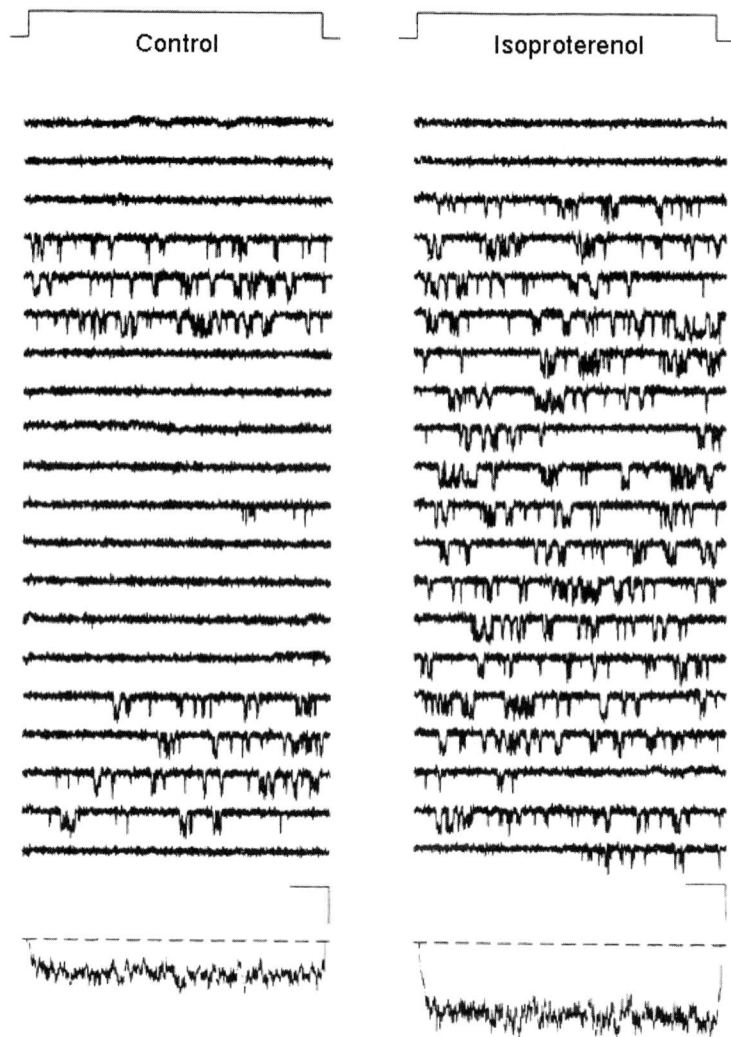

Figure 6
Effect of isoproterenol on Ba^{2+} currents through single L-type Ca^{2+} channels. *Upper part:* Pulse protocol with voltage steps from -100 mV to +20 mV. *Middle:* Unitary current recordings before (*left*) and after (*right*) application of 0.1 mM isoproterenol. *Bottom:* ensemble average current of control (300 sweeps) and isoproterenol (420 sweeps) experiments (Schröder and Herzig 1999)

GTP-binding proteins (G-proteins) exist as heterotrimeric complexes, composed of a Gα-subunit and a Gβγ-dimer. On activation of a G-protein-coupled receptor, the heterotrimer dissociates into free Gα-GTP and Gβγ-dimer. These free Gβγ-subunits are thought to be responsible for fast, membrane-delimited, voltage-dependent G-protein inhibition of certain neuronal voltage-dependent channels. Voltage-dependent modulation of calcium channels by G-proteins causes a decrease in whole-cell current, a depolarizing shift in the current voltage (I–V) relationship and slowed activation kinetics.

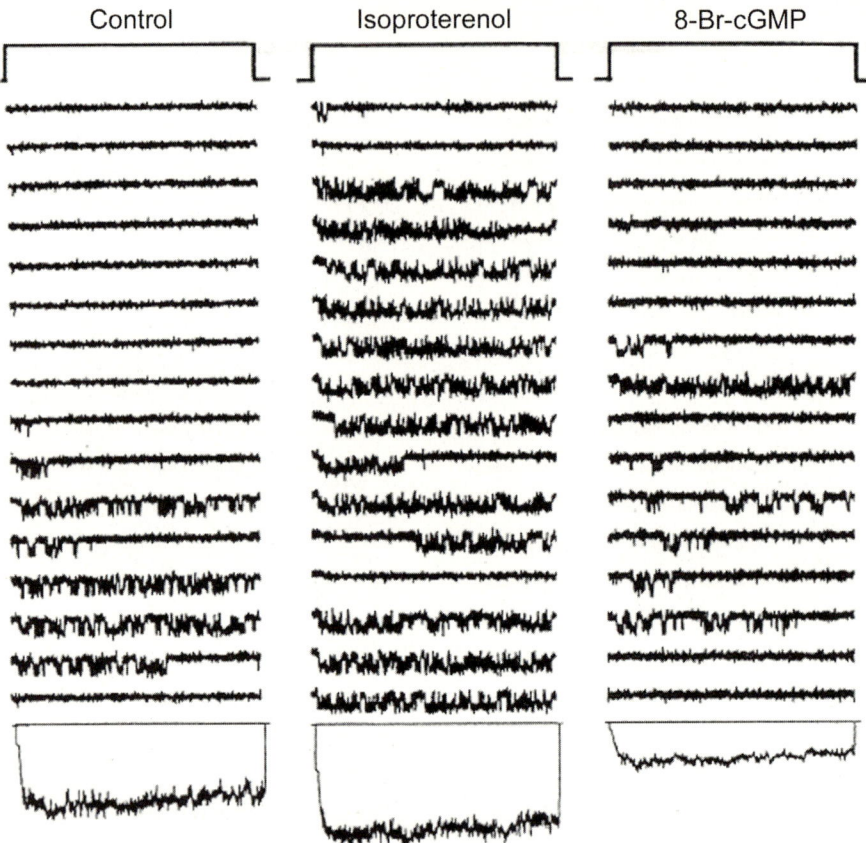

Figure 7
Ba^{2+} currents through single channel L-type Ca^{2+} channels measured in the presence of isoproterenol and 8-Br-cGMP. *Upper part:* Pulse protocol with voltage steps from −100 mV to +20 mV. *Middle:* Unitary current recordings in with added isoproterenol (*left*) and additional 8-Br-cGMP. *Bottom:* ensemble average current of isoproterenol (600 sweeps) and 8-Br-cGMP (600 sweeps) experiments. The scale bars indicate 20 ms (horizontal), 2 pA (unitary current traces) and 50 fA (ensemble average current), respectively (Klein et al. 2000).

Another characteristic is the loss of G-protein modulation with large depolarisations. Consequently, a large depolarizing prepulse immediately preceding a test pulse transiently removes inhibition, and activation is accelerated, a phenomenon referred to as prepulse facilitation (Bean 1989). Native cardiac L-type channels have long been known to exhibit G-protein-induced stimulation *via* the $G\alpha_s$- and cAMP-dependent protein kinase pathway. Viard et al. (1999) demonstrated stimulation of smooth-muscle L-type currents by $G\beta\gamma$ *via* a phosphoinositide 3-kinase pathway. Inhibition *via* activation of $G\alpha_{i/o}$, and subsequent inhibition of adenylate cyclase, is another modulatory G-protein path that regulates cardiac L-type channels.

Several studies have shown that the $\alpha_1 C$-subunit is a substrate for PKA *in vitro*, and Ser1928 has been identified as a potential PKA target. Channel phosphorylation leads to an increase in channel activity. The target protein of PKA is a sub-membrane protein, called AKAP79 (A-kinase anchoring protein). Mutations of Ser1928 to alanine in the C-terminus of the α_1C-subunit resulted in a complete loss of cAMP-mediated phosphorylation and a loss of channel regulation.

Stimulation of the β-adrenergic receptor with zinterol or isoproterenol has been shown to increase Ca^{2+} single channel currents (Schröder and Herzig 1999; Fig. 6). In mouse ventricular myocytes 8-Br-cGMP reverses all isoproterenol-induced changes in L-type calcium channel gating (Klein et al. 2000; Fig. 7).

Pharmacology

Pharmacological modulation of the L-type Ca^{2+} current and its molecular basis have been the subject of extensive experimental studies in the past decades. Although most Ca^{2+} channel agonists and antagonists are not completely selective for different Ca^{2+} channel subtypes, the application of specific channel blockers has been an extensively used criterion to distinguish between different types of Ca^{2+} channels. The ability of different compounds to block or enhance L-type calcium current depends on substance-specific properties and their ability to interact with particular binding sites on the channel complex.

Binding Sites

Although the auxiliary subunits have important regulatory influences, all essential pharmacological and biophysical properties of L-type Ca^{2+} channels are determined by the α_1-subunit. All major compounds with the ability to alter L-type Ca^{2+} current properties interact here. The high sensitivity of L-type Ca^{2+} channels towards different classes of antagonists is unique among other Ca^{2+} channel isoforms.

The principal chemical classes of Ca^{2+} channel inhibitors are 1,4-dihydropyridines (DHP), phenylalkylamines (PAA) and benzothiazepines (BTZ). From initial experimental studies, it was proposed that distinct binding sites exist in the α_1-subunit of the L-type Ca^{2+} channel for each of the three substance groups. Antagonists from each group are able to affect each others' binding abilities in a non-competitive manner, leading to an "allosteric" model of Ca^{2+} antagonist binding (Fig. 8). Glossmann et al. (1983) showed that verapamil, gallopamil, and the inorganic Ca^{2+} channel antagonist La^{3+} inhibited diltiazem binding non-competitively in a temperature-dependent manner. DHP binding was inhibited by verapamil binding but stimulated by (+)cis-diltiazem. The affinity to isradipine, a DHP compound, was increased by diltiazem at 37 °C, but incompletely inhibited at 2 °C (Glossmann et al. 1983). Other investigators confirmed a temperature-dependent potentiation of diltiazem Ca^{2+} channel block in hamster cardiomyocytes by nitrendipine, which in itself did not have a blocking effect. PAAs competitively inhibited BTZ binding in rabbit skeletal muscle with a slope factor of about 1.

These and other observations of a direct antagonism between PAA and BTZ binding have led to the assumption that the binding domains of the two calcium antagonists are identical. However, PAA binding increases the dissociation rate of BTZ from the Ca^{2+} channel, which is not the case between different BTZ compounds (Hagiwara

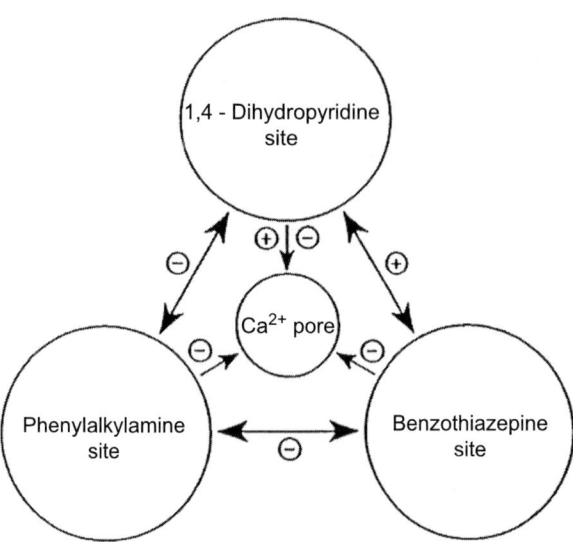

Figure 8
Allosteric model of Ca^{2+} antagonist interaction sites on the α_1-subunit of L-type Ca^{2+} channels. Dihydropyridines (DHP), phenylalkylamines (PAA) and benzothiazepines (BTZ) influence each others' binding properties to the α_1-subunit. This has been attributed to allosteric interaction between the three closely related binding sites. (Adapted from Triggle, J Cardiovasc Pharmacol 1996; 27 (Suppl A): S11–S16)

et al. 1997). In contrast to the allosteric model, Mitterdorfer et al. (1998) propose an "amphiphilic multisubsite domain" with the assumption of a single pore-associated site, accommodating different chemical classes of drugs.

The three major classes of Ca^{2+} antagonists bind to the channel α_1-subunit in close proximity to each other near the channel pore and close to the Ca^{2+} binding site. The domains III and IV in S6 and III in S5 form a pocket that serves as a "hot spot" for drug binding and drug action.

More precise structural information on the binding site for DHP and other Ca^{2+} antagonists was obtained from photoaffinity labelling studies using photoreactive DHP and PAA molecules. Glossmann et al. (1987) incorporated 1,4-dihydropyridine (azidopine) and other compounds into purified skeletal L-type Ca^{2+} channels and identified the site of labelling by proteolysis and immunoprecipitation of the α_1-subunit.

With these initial and other experiments, high-affinity Ca^{2+} antagonist-binding determinants were identified within the S6 segments in repeats III and IV and the extracellular portion of linker connection IIIS5-S6. As both segments are located in the centre of the channel molecule, these mapping results suggested that the drug-binding domains were located close to the ion-conducting pathway. Information on specific amino acids required for Ca^{2+} antagonist binding were obtained from various mutational analyses, mostly involving modifications of the α_1-subunit. These included alanine-scanning experiments where individual amino acid residues which differed between L-type and non L-type channels were systematically replaced by alanine. The novel α_1-subunits were expressed in mammalian cells with other subunits to determine their drug-binding properties. Peterson et al. (1997) showed that mutation of four residues in IIIS6 (Tyr-1152, Ile-1153, Ile-1156 and Met-1161) and one in IVS6 (Asn-1472) reduced DHP binding affinity more than five-fold. In a "gain-of-function" approach, specific photoaffinity-labelled regions of antagonist-sensitive L-type Ca^{2+} channels were transferred to homologous regions of the α_1-subunit in non-L-type channels.

Interaction with Ca^{2+}

The drug-binding properties of Ca^{2+} channels are modulated substantially by the presence of channel-bound Ca^{2+} ions. The great selectivity of calcium channels for Ca^{2+} ions depends on the selectivity filter that contains a highly specific Ca^{2+} binding site. It is constituted of 4 glutamate residues conserved throughout all Ca^{2+} channels located in the pore-forming S5-S6 linker helices. At this site, one Ca^{2+} ion is bound with a K_D of 0.7 µM and blocks the channel pore (non-conducting state). The second Ca^{2+} ion is bound with a K_D of about 100 mM and allows permeation of the previous ion.

In the absence of extracellular Ca^{2+}, the sensitivity of L-type Ca^{2+} channels to Ca^{2+} antagonists is markedly decreased. In a different approach, it could be shown that mutation of the high-affinity Ca^{2+} binding selectivity filter also decreased DHP binding. This indicates that Ca^{2+} ions must occupy a high-affinity Ca^{2+} binding site in order to stabilize high-affinity DHP binding. Peterson and Catterall (1995) considered a possible allosteric mechanism of interaction between Ca^{2+} and the DHP binding site. When the glutamate residues in the S5-S6 domain were replaced by glutamine in a_1C (Mitterdorfer et al. 1995, 1996) or a_1S (Peterson et al. 1995) calcium channels, there was an 11- to 35-fold decrease in the Ca^{2+} binding affinity. The sensitivity to DHPs was also reduced.

Only when a higher extracellular Ca^{2+} concentration was applied, could DHP sensitivity be restored, indicating the importance of Ca^{2+} ions in stabilizing the binding of DHP to its binding site in the channel. Two Ca^{2+} ions bound to the Ca^{2+} channel α_1-subunit, on the other hand, destabilize the binding of all classes of Ca^{2+} antagonists.

Ca^{2+} Channel Agonists and Antagonists

The three 'classic' groups of calcium channel blockers contain derivates of the chemically unrelated dihydropyridines (nifedipine), phenylalkylamines (verapamil) and benzothiazepines (diltiazem), that had originally been developed as coronary vasodilators in the early 1960s.

Even before voltage-clamp experiments were performed, the observation that their inhibitory influence on skeletal muscle contraction force and cardiac contractility could be reduced by increasing the level of extracellular Ca^{2+} led to their definition as 'Ca^{2+} antagonists'. Higher (millimolar) concentrations of divalent cations inhibited drug binding to all domains. Therefore one or more Ca^{2+} binding sites allosterically coupled to the drug-binding domains were included into the allosteric model.

Despite their high affinity to individual binding sites within the a_1-subunit, calcium antagonists do not bind exclusively to L-type calcium channels. All types of calcium antagonists have been reported to bind with lower affinity to various other membrane proteins including T-type Ca^{2+}-channels, Na^+-channels, K^+-channels and membrane transporters.

Dihydropyridines

1,4-Dihydropyridines (DHP) are very selective modulators of L-type Ca^{2+} channels (Ca_v1-family, namely $\alpha_1S, \alpha_1C, \alpha_1D, \alpha_1F$ or $Ca_v1.1, Ca_v1.2, Ca_v1.3, Ca_v1.4$). The different members of this pharmacological group can be divided into Ca^{2+} channel agonists and antagonists. Classic compounds among DHP calcium antagonists are nifedipine, nitrendipine, amlodipine, felodipine and isradipine. The highly lipophilic DHP derivates access the calcium channel protein through the lipid phase of the membrane (lipophilic path). Because of their very poor water solubility, it is unlikely that the drugs enter into the channel from the cytoplasmic side. Therefore, the DHPs appear to bind to the channel at or near the channel/lipid interface behind the P loop. Antagonists showed non-polar interactions with the residues at the crossing of domains III and IV S6 helices at the bottom of the crevice that could prevent helical movements involved in activation by stabilizing the closed state. Agonists in this conformation were not able to interact with the hydrophobic crossing residues and lead to a destabilizing of the closed state (Lipkind and Fozzard 2003).

The preferential effect on different parts of the vascular bed is determined by the chemical structure of the different types of DHP compounds. The first generation DHP, nifedipine, primarily acts on the peripheral vasculature and coronary arteries, reducing the peripheral vascular resistance and thus lowering blood pressure. Amlodipine, felodipine and isradipine are more potent blockers of Ca^{2+} channels in peripheral vascular smooth muscle. Nimodipine acts more selectively in cerebral vascular smooth muscle cells. This remarkable tissue sensitivity is caused by the different blocking properties of these DHP compounds.

Like the other classes of Ca^{2+} antagonists, DHP binding to the α_1-subunit of the L-type Ca^{2+} channel depends on the transmembrane segments IIIS6, IVS6 and the S5-S6 linker in repeats III and IV of the channel protein. Amino acids responsible for DHP or PAA interaction in transmembrane segments IIIS6 and IVS6 were identified by systemic replacement with alanine or non-L-type α_1 (α_1E, α_1B) sequences. Results from photoaffinity labelling studies have shown that further residues in the transmembrane segment IIIS5 are crucial for DHP interaction. In addition to the two IIIS5 residues, at least eleven additional amino acids, seven in IIIS6, participate in the formation of the binding pocket for DHPs. Additional binding sites with specific importance for DHP were identified in repeat I and repeat III of the α_1-subunit. In IIIS5, nine amino acid residues differ between L-type and non-L-type Ca^{2+} channels. A part of the DHP interaction domain already exists in non-L-type calcium channels, but is not sufficient for high-affinity DHP sensitivity. The co-expression of β-subunits dramatically enhanced L-type α_1-subunit-associated high-affinity DHP binding. β-subunit association seems to cause a conformational change in α_1-subunits, similar to the action of Ca^{2+}, which converts the DHP binding domain to a high-affinity state. This can be summarised as low-affinity (β-subunit deficient) and high-affinity (β-subunit present).

Dihydropyridines exert voltage-, enantioselective- and use-dependent block of L-type calcium channels. The state-dependent interaction (voltage- and use-dependent action) has been demonstrated in terms of the well-accepted modulated-receptor hypothesis. The extent of the DHP block of L-type calcium channels depends on the holding potential and increases with more depolarizing membrane potentials at which the channels start to inactivate. Hydrophobic molecules like nifedipine and nitrendipine preferentially bind to the inactivated state of the calcium channel at depolarized membrane potentials. At holding potentials of -80 mV, where L-type Ca^{2+} channels are in the resting state, DHP block is much weaker. These findings explain why vascular smooth muscle cells (membrane potential about -50 mV) are blocked more effectively by first generation Ca^{2+} antagonists like nifedipine than ventricular cardiomyocytes (membrane potential about -80 mV; Adachi-Akahane 2000).

By construction of chimeric α_1 subunits and pharmacological characterization after coexpression with $\alpha_2\delta$- and β_{1a}-subunits in Xenopus oocytes, Mitterdorfer et al. (1996) identified Thr1066 and Gln1070 as necessary for DHP antagonist (isradipine) and agonist (−)Bay K 8644) actions. While isradipine required only Thr1066, and the presence of Gln1070 only increased the channel sensitivity to the DHP antagonist, DHP agonist modulation by Bay K 8644 depended on the additional presence of Gln1070.

Like other classes of calcium antagonists, the newer DHPs do not bind to L-type Ca^{2+}-channels alone. In rat hippocampal neurones, nicardipine, nifedipine and nimodipine block T-type Ca^{2+}-channels in a use-dependent way. Nicardipine blocks voltage-gated K^+-channels in cerebellar neurons. Like tertiary amine local anaesthetics, nifedipine blocked Na^+ currents in rat ventricular neonatal cardiomyocytes in a dose-dependent fashion; Na^+ current restitution was achieved by additional application of Bay K 8644.

DHP Ca^{2+} Agonists

DPH-derivates like S(−)Bay K 8644, CGP 28–392, (+)S202–791 and YC-170, the benzoylpyrrole FPL 64176 and the benzodiazocine CGP 48506 are known to act as Ca^{2+} channel agonists. They have been developed as scientific tools but are not used therapeutically. The chemical differences between agonist and antagonist 1,4-dihydropyridines lies in their chemical structure – DHP-calcium channel blockers have two freely rotating ester groups whereas the agonists have only one. Agonist activity is produced only by substitution of small polar groups in the ester group on the left side (Lipkind and Fozzard 2003). Bay K 8644 modulates L-type Ca^{2+} channels in two ways: one enantiomer (+)Bay K 8644 acts as a Ca^{2+} antagonist, the stereoisomer (−)Bay K 8644 shows agonistic effects (Adachi-Akahane et al. 2000). In the presence of Bay K 8644, Ca^{2+} influx through the L-type Ca^{2+} channel during depolarization is increased by interaction with the open state of the channel. In contrast to DHP-antagonists, 1,4-dihydropyridine activator interactions are significantly less voltage-dependent.

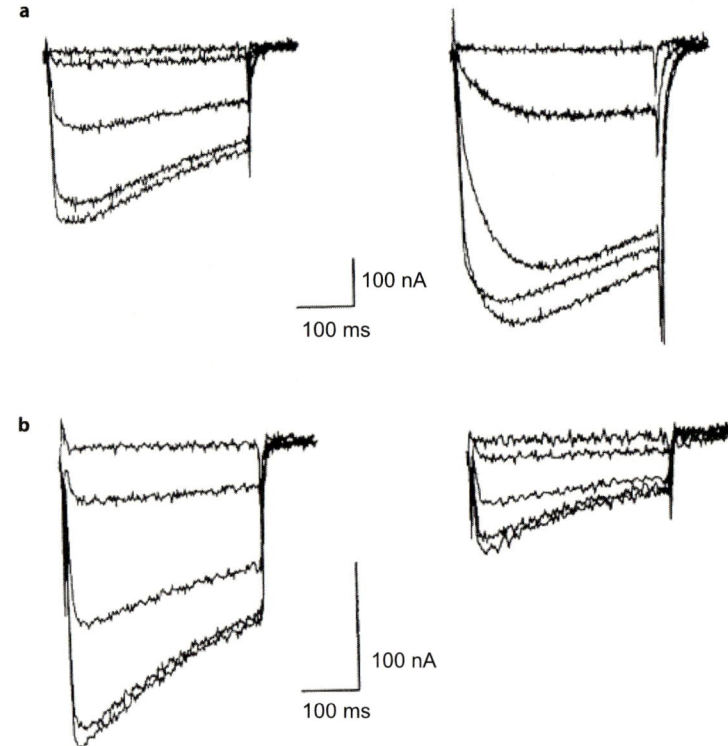

Figure 9a,b
Modulation of Ba^{2+} current through chimeric L-type Ca^{2+} channels by Bay K 8644 (**a**) and isradipine (**b**). Experiments were performed in the presence of 40 mM Ba^{2+} at test potentials from -30 mV to +10 mV (Grabner et al. 1996)

Kokubun et al. (1984) demonstrated this by whole-cell and single-channel studies with Ba^{2+} as charge carrier. The whole-cell current amplitude in neonatal rat cardiomyocytes increased in a concentration-dependent fashion up to 3.5-fold in the presence of 10^{-7} M Bay K, consistent with an increase in the single-channel slope-conductance from 18.3 pS to 24.0 pS. This could be related to an increase in the number of available open channels with long channel openings and a marked prolongation of the channel mean open time in the presence of Bay K 8644. These effects were independent of intracellular cAMP levels, indicating that phosphorylation steps of channel subunits were not involved. Similar effects of BayK with an increase in whole cell current and longer openings in single-channel measurements were obtained by Grabner et al. (1996) and Michels et al. (2002, see Examples). Both DHP compounds bind to a common binding site in the calcium channel protein.

Sanguinetti et al. (1986) reported that the influence of Bay K 8644 on Ca^{2+} channel gating properties in calf Purkinje fibres is not unanimously agonistic but, as for other DHPs, shows voltage-dependent, frequency-dependent and concentration-dependent variations. When hyperpolarizing membrane potentials (-60 mV) were applied as conditioning prepulse, the peak Ca^{2+} current was enhanced, due to a shift of the I-V

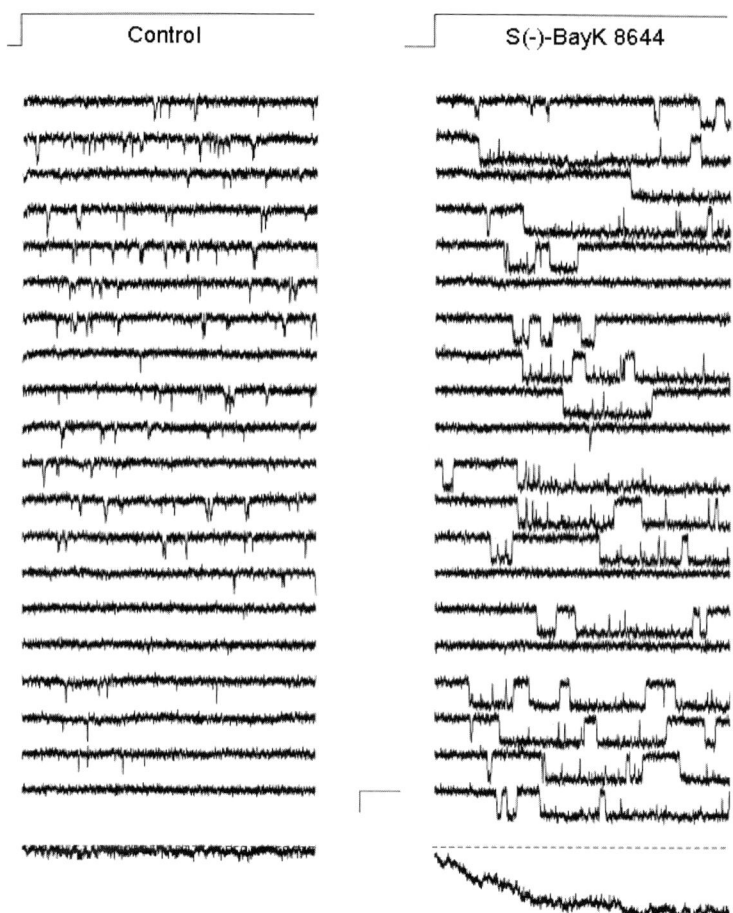

Figure 10
Effect of S (–)Bay K 8644 on L-type Ca^{2+} channels. Upper part: Voltage-protocol at a holding potential of –90 mV and test potential of +10 mV. Middle: original single channel sweeps recorded at a pulse duration of 150 ms. Below: Ensemble average current from 117 sweeps (control) and 179 sweeps (0.1 mM Bay K 8644). The scale angle indicates 15 ms (*horizontal*) and 1 pA (*vertical*) for single channel traces, 0.075 pA for ensemble average current (Michels et al. 2002)

curve in the hyperpolarizing direction and faster rates of inactivation over a wide range of test potentials. At depolarizing prepulses (20 mV) the current amplitude was decreased. The agonistic effect on inward current was also diminished in the presence of high pulse-frequencies. These effects could be attributed to modulation of Ca^{2+} channel gating currents by Bay K 8644, caused by a drug-induced slowing of the transition of the Ca^{2+} channel from the open to the closed channel. The effect of BayK 8644 application on whole-cell Ca^{2+} current through chimeric Ca^{2+} channels is demonstrated in Fig. 9. Single L-type Ca^{2+} channel recordings from human hMT cells in the presence of 0.1 mM BayK 8644 are demonstrated in Fig. 10 (see Examples).

Phenylalkylamines

Beside verapamil, the classic phenylalkylamine (PAA), two other compounds from this group have been extensively studied: methoxyverapamil (D600/gallopamil) and desmethoxyverapamil (D888/devapamil). The only PAA currently in clinical use is verapamil, a potent drug for slowing AV-nodal transmission, which is used in the treatment of supraventricular tachycardias.

As the binding sites for PAAs, DHPs and BTZs are located close to each other, with possible allosteric interaction at the α_1-subunit, PAA binding interferes with channel block by compounds from both other substance groups. The affinity of Ca^{2+} channels for PAAs is higher than those for DHP and BTZs. Within the PAAs, the binding affinity to L-type Ca^{2+} channels is in the order desmethoxyverapamil > methoxyverapamil > verapamil. All PAA compounds have a chiral centre and exist as levorotatory (–) and dextrorotatory (+) enantiomers, where the (–) enantiomers are the more potent calcium antagonists.

Like DHPs, Ca^{2+} channel block by phenylalkylamines is voltage- and state-dependent, as the different conducting states of Ca^{2+} channels, resting, open or inactivated, have different affinities to PAAs. The affinity to PAA block is greatest when a major proportion of the Ca^{2+} channels is in the inactivated, non-conducting state, and lowest at membrane potentials near -70 mV, when the most of the channels are in the resting state. Drug binding and electrophysiological studies indicate that this preference can be explained by a conformational change within the PAA binding site on the α_1-subunit caused by membrane depolarisation. In contrast to dihydropyridines, PAA block of Ca^{2+} channels also shows marked use-dependence. Verapamil and diltiazem have prominent frequency-(use-)dependent antagonisms and nifedipin exhibits prominent voltage-dependent block. This explains the antiarrhythmic and cardiac depressant properties of verapamil and diltiazem and the general vascular selectivity of 1,4-dihydropyridines.

Several authors have shown that rapid trains of depolarisations cause an increased fraction of drug binding to inactivated channels, with progressive reduction of whole cell current. The extent of use-dependent calcium current block increases with higher stimulation frequencies and increasing pulse durations – and differs markedly between different classes of calcium antagonists.

As pointed out by Kanaya et al. (1983), high affinity drug binding to the inactivated state slows the transition of the channel protein to the resting state and thereby stabilizes channel inactivation. Consistently, the time constant of recovery from block at -70 mV is longer for PAAs ($\tau 2 = 2.4$ min; McDonald et al. 1984) compared to DHPs ($\tau_1 = 1.5$ s, $t_2 = 30$ s; Sanguinetti and Kass 1984). This characteristic is of clinical importance for PAA Ca^{2+} antagonists as antiarrhythmics. Frequency-dependent block with prolonged recovery from the inactivated state slows down transmission of excitation at the AV-node and reduces the ventricular rate in supraventricular tachyarrhythmias.

The PAA binding site at the Ca^{2+} channel α_1-subunit has been characterized by similar experimental methods to those used in studies of the DHP binding site, including photoaffinity labelling, alanine scanning experiments and expression of genetic constructs. Amino-acid residues with PAA binding function were identified in segments IIIS6 and IVS6. The IVS6 residues and Ile1153 from segment IIIS6 are specific for L-type Ca^{2+} channels. These amino acid residues are not present in non-L-type Ca^{2+} channels and may therefore be responsible for their low PAA sensitivity. The two residues (Phe1164 and Val1165), which are very close to the intracellular C-terminal end of IIIS6 and are uninvolved in DHP-binding, showed a ~10-fold decrease in affinity for D888 upon alanine substitution. Individual mutation of any of these residues to alanine or glutamine decreased PAA sensitivity 10- to 60-fold.

Benzothiazepines

The most relevant compound and the only one in clinical use from the group of benzothiazepine (BTZ) calcium antagonists is diltiazem. Other compounds are SQ32,910, which has a higher affinity for L-type Ca^{2+} channels than diltiazem, and (+)cis-azidodiltiazem, which is used for photoaffinity labelling experiments. The properties of BTZs are intermediate between those of DHPs and PAAs in a number of chemical and pharmacological respects. Their potency as peripheral vasodilators is weaker than that of nifedipine or nitrendipine. Compared to verapamil, they have a weaker negative chronotropic effect on the SA- and AV-node, and only a modest negative inotropic effect on the ventricular myocardium. BTZs are moderately selective for L-type Ca^{2+} channels in vascular smooth muscle cells. As for the other groups of calcium antagonists, diltiazem blocks other types of ion channels at higher concentrations (40 µM and above), including N-, R- and P/Q-type Ca^{2+} channels in neurons (Diochot et al. 1995).

All BTZ compounds have two chiral centres and exist in four possible diastereoisomers, where the corresponding (+) isomers are more potent Ca^{2+} channel blockers. As for DHPs and PAAs, BTZ binding alters the binding properties of the other classes of calcium antagonists to their binding sites, showing a temperature-dependent effect. At 25 and 37 °C, nitrendipine binding was enhanced to 140% and 200% of control respectively in the presence of 10 µM diltiazem. At 0 °C however, nitrendipine binding was reduced to 68%, indicating allosteric modulation of the spatially closely related binding sites of BTZs and PAAs.

The properties of BTZ binding to L-type Ca^{2+} channels also indicate an intermediate place between DHPs and PAAs. Diltiazem binding causes more resting block than verapamil but less than nitrendipine. The same applies to the question of frequency dependence. In a train of depolarizations, diltiazem reaches the maximum level of blockade more slowly than nitrendipine, where use-dependent block is virtually absent, but faster than verapamil, which shows marked use-dependence. These findings are consistent with time constants for channel recovery from diltiazem block ($\tau=2$ s) being intermediate between those for nitrendipine ($\tau=0.5$ s) and verapamil ($\tau=15$ s).

Bodi et al. (2002) showed that a segment in IVS5 of the human α_1C ($Ca_v 1.2$) subunit is critically involved in inactivation of the channel. Mutants constructed in this region lost the characteristic use-dependent block by PAA and BTZ and recovered from inactivation significantly faster after drug block compared with the wild type Ca^{2+}-channel.

The BTZ binding side of the L-type Ca^{2+}-channel is formed by amino acid residues in segments IIIS6 und IVS6, located in close proximity to the PAA binding site. PAA and BTZ share residues Tyr1463, Ala1467, and Ile1470 in segment IVS6 as common binding motifs.

PAAs and BTZs possess a distinct structure-activity relationship for blocking but access their binding domains from opposite sides (PAAs, the cytoplasmic side, BTZs, the extracellular side) of the channel. To investigate the access of BTZs to their binding site on the α_1-subunit, comparative studies were performed with SQ32,910, a tertiary BTZ, and SQ32,428, its quaternary derivate, which supported the theory that BTZ Ca^{2+}-antagonists access their binding site from the extracellular side of the cell membrane.

Description of Methods and Practical Approach

Recording Techniques

Whole Cell Recording

The study of calcium channel function in whole cell configuration depends to a great extent on the patch clamp method, using single myocytes. Various methods of dissociation of myocardial and non-myocardial myocytes have been published in the past. In whole-cell experiments, a thin pipette with tip resistances, depending on the experimental settings, around 3–5 MΩ is placed at the front of a head stage connected with a patch clamp amplifier and a computer unit to control holding- and test-pulse potentials. The head stage is connected with a syringe used to generate negative pressure at the tip of the patch pipette. The pipette is filled with electrolyte solution equivalent to intracellular ion concentrations.

Electrolyte Solutions

When recording native Ca^{2+} channels in cardiomyocytes, the typical extracellular solution contains about the following [mM]: TEA 126, CsCl 5.4, $CaCl_2$ 2, $MgCl_2$ 1, NaH_2PO_4 0.33, dextrose 10, and HEPES 10. The pH is adjusted to 7.4 with CsOH. The pipette solution replaces the intracellular medium of the cell once the whole-cell configuration is achieved. A typical composition is [mM]: Cs-aspartate 110, CsCl 20, $MgCl_2$ 1, EGTA 10, GTP 0.1, Mg-ATP 5, HEPES 10 and Na_2-phosphocreatinine 5. The pH is adjusted to 7.4 with CsOH. Ca^{2+} ions are replaced by equimolar amounts of Ba^{2+} or other charge carriers if desired.

Pipette Preparation

Patch pipettes with a tip resistance, depending on the experimental settings, around 2–4 MΩ, are pulled from borosilicate glass capillaries, filled with intracellular solution and placed into the head stage for experiments without delay.

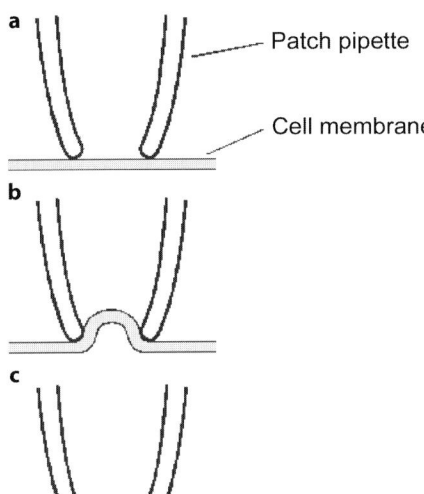

Figure 11a–c
Sequence of pipette configurations during whole-cell patch-clamp experiments: After positioning of the pipette on top of the cell membrane (**a**), gentle vacuum suction is applied to the pipette tip by a syringe attached to the pipette holder to establish a high resistance connection (Giga-ohm seal) between pipette tip and membrane in the cell-attached configuration (**b**). With additional suction, the membrane patch underneath the pipette opening is ruptured (whole-cell configuration, **c**)

Experimental Protocol

The whole cell patch-clamp configuration is established by a sequence of pipette manoeuvres: At the beginning of the experimental procedure, a few disaggregated myocytes are placed in extracellular solution within a recording chamber mounted on an inverted microscope. By use of a micromanipulator, the patch pipette is positioned above a myocyte in the bath solution. At first the pipette filled with intracellular solution is lowered into the recording chamber. Slight positive pressure is applied to the pipette holder to prevent clotting of the pipette tip. At this stage, the amplifier indicates the pipette resistance and the offset of the amplifier has to be calibrated to 0 mV, which requires the calculation of the junction potential between intracellular and extracellular solution. While the pipette is placed next to a potential cell for recordings, the patch-clamp amplifier is set to voltage-clamp mode and the computer generates a rectangular pulse of about 5 mV. The patch pipette is placed on the cell membrane (see Fig. 11a) and gentle suction is applied to the pipette holder by an external vacuum syringe to facilitate the formation of a high-resistance seal between pipette tip and cell membrane (Giga-ohm seal, Fig. 11b). After giga-seal formation, further suction is applied (break-in) to rupture the membrane patch underneath the patch pipette and establish a whole-cell configuration for current recordings. The break in manoeuvre removes the barrier between intracellular medium and intracellular solution in the pipette. At this stage, changes in the holding potential will result in net ion fluxes across the entire cell membrane that can be recorded as whole cell currents.

The pulse protocol used for stimulation of the calcium channels under study depends on the aim of the experiment and the cells used. As stated before, different cell types differ in their electrophysiological properties, e.g. their resting membrane potential (Fig. 12).

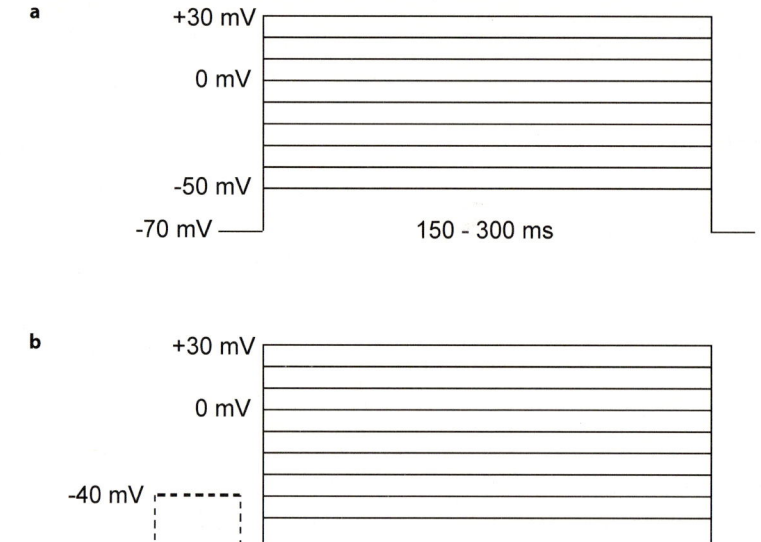

Figure 12a,b
Typical pulse protocol for whole-cell calcium current recordings. From a holding potential of −70 to −50 mV, depending on the cell type studied, depolarization steps to +30 mV in 10 mV increments are administered. If the Na$^+$ current is not blocked by pharmacological means (**a**), a depolarizing prepulse to −40 mV must be added to the protocol (**b**)

Single Channel Recording

In this approach to patch clamp recording, a small heat-polished glass pipette is pressed against the cell membrane forming an electrical seal. The method was first introduced by Neher and Sakmann. They electrically isolated small patches of membrane on frog muscle fibres by enzymatically cleaning them and then pressing the small glass pipette against them.

It was observed that tight pipette-membrane seals, with resistances of 10–100 GΩ, can be obtained when suction is applied to the pipette interior ("Giga-seal"). Giga-seals are mechanically very stable, so that if the pipette is withdrawn, the seal usually remains intact and the membrane patch is excised from the cell (Hamill et al. 1981). The high resistance, in parallel with the greatly reduced capacitance of a membrane patch having an area of only a few square micrometers, allows resolution of the microscopic ionic currents (pA-range, depending on test- and holding-potentials) that intermittently flow through any channels that happen to have been trapped in the membrane patch.

The high resistance of a "giga-seal" reduces the background noise of the recordings by an order of magnitude, and allows a patch of membrane to be voltage-clamped without the use of microelectrodes. Here are some helpful rules to produce a giga-seal. Avoid dirt on the pipette, using a fresh pipette for each seal. Each pipette should be used only after positive pressure has been relieved. Following enzyme treatment of muscle preparations, the surface of the bathing solution is frequently covered with debris with readily adheres to the pipette tip, preventing giga-seal formation. HEPES-buffered pipette solutions should be used when calcium is present in the pipette solution. Filtered solutions should be used in the bath as well in the pipette. When a slight negative pressure of 20–30 cm H_2O was applied the resistance increased within a few seconds to ~20–80 GΩ. In some cases giga-seals develop spontaneously without suction. In other cases suction has to be applied for periods of 10–60 s, or a seal may develop only after suction has been released.

Recording Solutions

When a pipette is sealed tightly on to a cell it separates the total cell surface membrane into two parts: the area covered by the pipette (the patch area) and the rest of the cell. Solutions used to fill the pipette or to bathe cells will dependent on the currents and the type of cells to be studied. The solution mimics the normal and extracellular environments of mammalian cells. A typical patch pipette (usually borosilicate glass) is filled with pipette solution (first "tip filling" and then "back filling" with 110 mM $BaCl_2$, 10 mM HEPES, pH 7.4 – adjusted with tetraethylammonium hydroxide) and sealed against the surface membrane. Single channel experiments were performed in an external bath solution containing 120 mM K^+-glutamate, 25 mM KCl, 2 mM $MgCl_2$, 10 mM HEPES, 2 mM EGTA, 1 mM $CaCl_2$, 1 mM Na-ATP, and 10 mM dextrose, pH 7.4.

Pipette Fabrication

Borosilicate pipettes are pulled in two stages using a vertical microelectrode puller and the standard heating coils supplied with it. The capillary is thinned over a length of ~10 mm to obtain a minimum diameter of 200 µm. The glass is then recentred with respect to the heating coil and in the second pull the thinned part breaks, producing two pipettes. In order to reduce the pipette-bath capacitance and to form a hydrophobic surface, pipette shanks are coated with Sylgard to within 50 µm of the tip. Polishing of the glass wall at the pipette tip is done on a microforge shortly after Sylgard coating. We use pipettes with resistance values in the range 67 MΩ. These have openings diameters between 0.5 and 1 µm.

Recording calcium channels in the cell-attached configuration, the pulse protocol can be changed in different electrophysiological experiments (activation experiments, different depolarizing test pulses –10 to +30 mV and constant holding potentials –90 mV (Fig. 13), inactivation experiments, constant depolarizing test pulses and different holding potentials). Ba^{2+} currents were elicited by depolarization test pulses delivered at 0.5 Hz, recorded at 10 kHz and filtered at 2 kHz (–3 dB, four-pole Bessel) using an Axopatch 1 D or Axopatch 200 A (Axon Instruments).

Data-Analysis

Linear leak and capacity currents were digitally subtracted using the average currents of non-active sweeps (Fig. 14).

Openings and closures were identified using the half-criterion (pClamp 6.0). Data were further analyzed by histogram analysis (open-time and closed-time histograms). Closed time analysis was restricted to patches where only one channel was present. NP_o (the product of the number of channels in the patch times their individual open

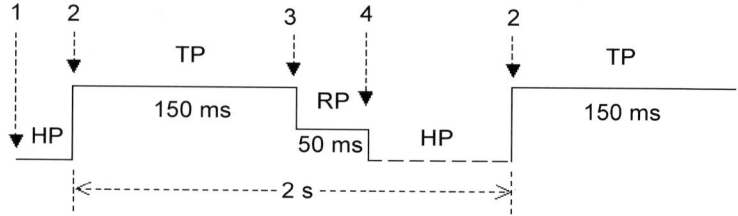

Figure 13
Typical pulse protocol for Ca^{2+} single-channel recording: *1* beginning of rest potential, *2* beginning of depolarization step, *3* end of depolarization step and beginning of repolarization, *4* end of repolarization, *HP* holding potential, *TP* test potential, *RP* repolarization potential, duration of all repetitive pulses 2 s (0.5 Hz), duration of depolarization 150 ms

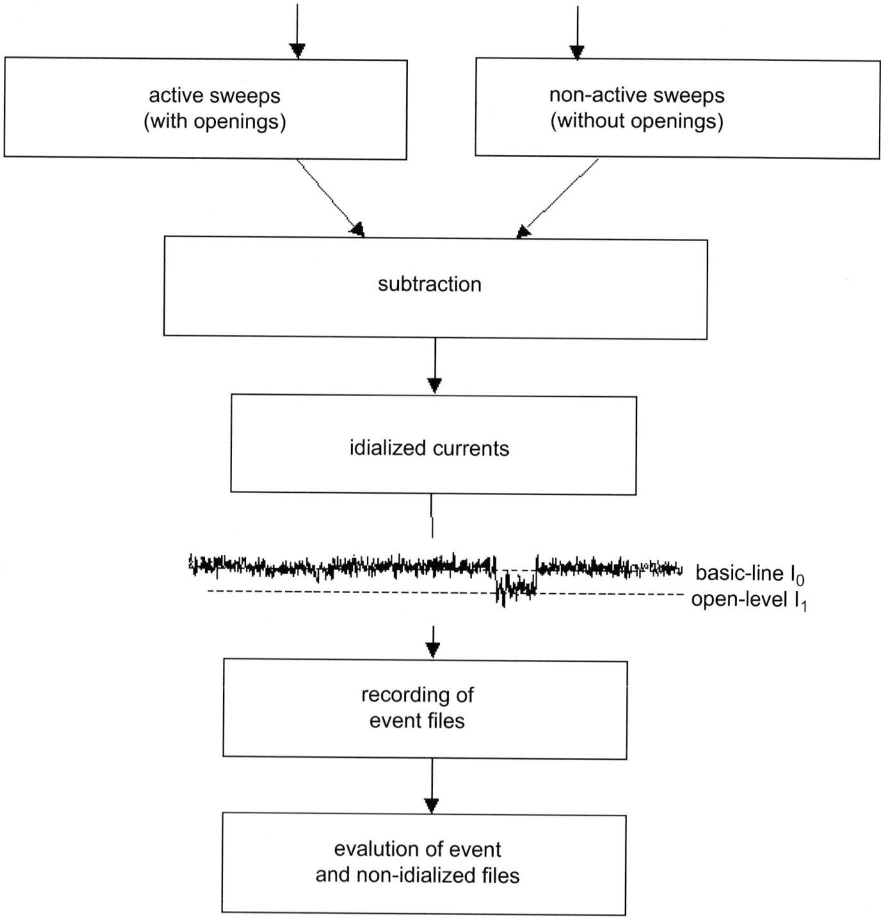

Figure 14
Algorithm of data analysis for single channel recordings

probability) was calculated as the ratio between total open time and the total recording time at the test potential. P_o (the single channel probability) was calculated as the ratio of the total open time and the total time recorded at the test potential, divided by the number of channels in the patch (N) where necessary and possible.

Activation and inactivation data were fitted to a Boltzmann-type function according to the following equation: $y = y_{max} \, 1/(1 \exp [(V_{0.5} - V)/k])$, where y ($y_{max}$) is the (maximum) availability of channels, V is the membrane potential, $V_{0.5}$ is the potential at which activation or inactivation is half-maximal, and k is the slope factor describing the steepness of the curve at $V_{0.5.}$ (for detailed data-analysis, see Michels et al. 2002).

Examples

Basic Current Properties

A typical whole-cell L-type Ca^{2+} channel recording from guinea pig ventricular myocytes is shown in Fig. 15. Similar test potentials were applied in single-channel measurements of L-type Ca^{2+} channels in guinea ventricular myocytes demonstrated in Fig. 16.

Inactivation Kinetics in the Presence of Different Charge Carriers

According to reversal potential measurements estimated under bi-ionic conditions, the relative permeability sequence for divalent cations is $Ca^{2+} > Sr^{2+} > Ba^{2+}$, and $Li^+ > Na^+ > K^+ > Cs^+$ for monovalent cations. Under normal conditions monovalent cations are much less permeant than divalent ions. In the absence of external calcium however, calcium channels become highly permeable to monovalent ions. Hagiwara et al. (1974) concluded that this effect was caused by the fact that both ions compete for a common binding site at the channel pore, which has a weaker affinity for sodium. Figures 4 and 5 show Ba^{2+}, Sr^{2+} and Na^+ current measurements through the L-type Ca^{2+} channel in the absence of extracellular Ca^{2+}.

Obviously, in the presence of extracellular Ca^{2+} ions, at least one calcium ion is bound within the channel at all times, excluding monovalent ions from entering the channel pore (Hille 2001). Other divalent cations, such as Zn^{2+}, Co^{2+}, and Ni^{2+}, competing for the same binding site block L-type Ca^{2+} channels at concentrations of 10 µM to 20 µM.

Figure 4 shows the effect of different charge carriers (Ba^{2+}, Sr^{2+} and Na^+) on L-type Ca^{2+} current amplitude and current inactivation kinetics compared to recordings with Ca^{2+}. It is obvious that (1) in the absence of extracellular Ca^{2+} the channel becomes permeant for the cations studied, (2) increasing levels of depolarization accelerate current inactivation, and (3) that, as with all depolarization steps, inactivation is markedly slowed in the absence of extracellular Ca^{2+}. The last finding can be explained by an absence of calcium-dependent inactivation of the Ca^{2+} channel.

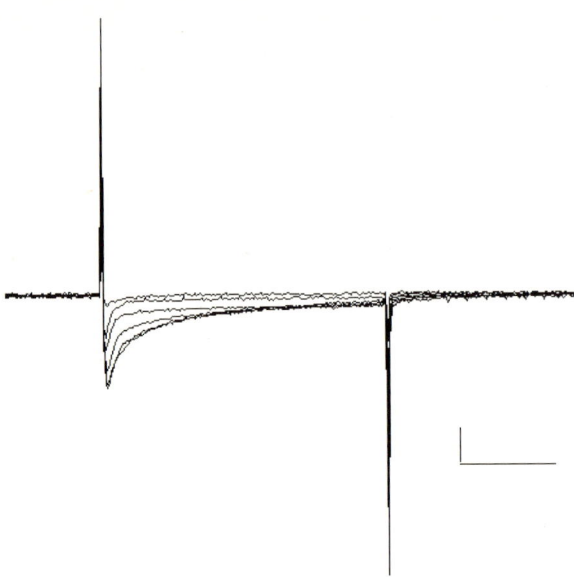

Figure 15
Typical L-type Ca^{2+} whole cell current elicited by step depolarizations of 300 ms duration from 30 mV to 20 mV. The current was recorded in guinea pig ventricular myocytes. The scale bars indicate 50 ms (horizontally) and 2.5 nA

Voltage-Dependent Inactivation

As discussed before, Ca^{2+} current inactivation is also affected by voltage. Findlay et al. (2002, see Fig. 5) showed that with increasing holding potentials from -20 to +20 mV, a step depolarisation to a fixed pulse potential resulted in faster inactivation kinetics. This was demonstrated with recordings where Ca^{2+} was replaced by Ba^{2+} (A and D), Sr^{2+} (B and E) and Na$^+$ (C and F, see Fig. 5).

This characteristic is markedly reduced in the presence of 100 nM isoproterenol (D, E, F). As a result of β-adrenergic stimulation by isoproterenol, inactivation kinetics are slowed, due to a conversion of channels from a rapidly inactivating to a slowly inactivating kinetic form. With increasing holding potentials from –20to +20 mV, a step depolarisation to a fixed pulse potential results in faster inactivation kinetics. This effect is consistent between measurements with Ba^{2+}, Sr^{2+} and Na$^+$ as charge carrier and does not therefore seem to be influenced by the charge carrier.

Modulation by DHP Ca^{2+} Agonists and Antagonists

Dihydropyridines comprise the two classes of agonistic and antagonistic Ca^{2+} channel modulators. Grabner et al. (1996) tested dihydropyridine sensitivity in chimeric Ca^{2+} channels generated with DHP-sensitive motifs transferred from L-type to originally DHP-insensitive brain calcium channels (see Fig. 9). In the presence of 10 µM BayK 8644, the total current amplitude was markedly increased, as opposed to recordings with isradipine.

Michels et al. (2002, see Fig. 10) showed similar results from single-channel measurements of single L-type Ca^{2+} channels in the presence of 0.1 mM BayK 8644. Due to the DHP Ca^{2+}-agonist, the single channel amplitude was increased from

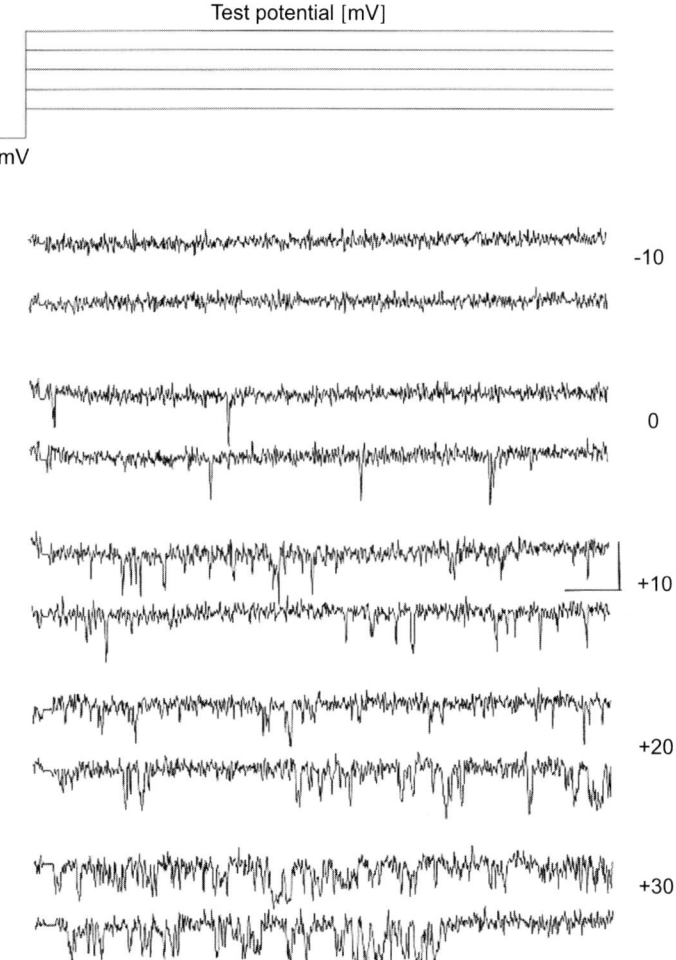

Figure 16
Single channel registration of L-type Ca^{2+} channel current at different test potentials (TP). The scale angle indicates 1 pA (*vertical*) and 15 ms (*horizontal*)

0.89 ± 0.04 pA to 1.13±0.09 pA and the average open-times were prolonged consistently.

Modulation by β-Adrenergic Activation

Under β-adrenergic stimulation, an increase in the Ca^{2+} current can be observed with further reduction of current inactivation. On a single-channel level, Schröder and Herzig (1999, see Fig. 6) showed an increase in channel availability with a larger number of openings and a markedly increased ensemble average current in the presence of 0.1 mM isoproterenol.

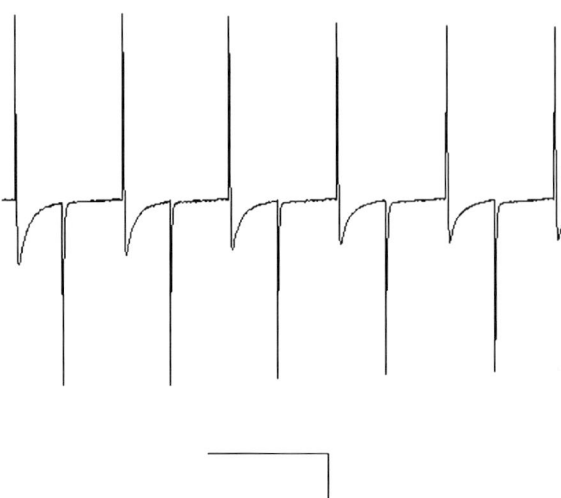

Figure 17
Ca^{2+} channel run-down elicited by repetitive depolarization to +10 mV in non-failing human ventricular cardiomyocytes at a frequency of 1 Hz. With an increasing number of stimulations, the current amplitude decreases steadily. The scale bars indicate 1000 ms (*horizontally*) and 0.1 nA (*vertically*)

Troubleshooting

Run-Down

Early investigators had already noticed that Ca^{2+} currents in various cell types tended to inactivate during long recordings under certain conditions, a phenomenon known as "run-down". Especially in whole cell recordings, dialysis of the intracellular medium by the intracellular solution in the tip of the patch pipette resulted in a steady decline in the current amplitude (Kostyuk et al. 1981). Similar results were seen in excised patch recordings where the membrane patch was immersed in an artificial intracellular solution (Nilius et al. 1985). This observation was independent of the charge carrier used, when extracellular Ca^{2+} was replaced by Ba^{2+}, run-down was not affected. Markwardt and Nilius (1990) showed that not only the total current amplitude but also current inactivation time constants decreased during calcium channel run-down in guinea-pig ventricular myocytes. From the work of a number of authors, various factors influencing the time-course of run-down have been identified. In the presence of Ca^{2+}-chelating agents (EDTA), Mg^{2+}ATP, cAMP and phosphodiesterase inhibitors, run-down could be prevented or even reversed. The same effect was observed when the catalytic subunit of protein kinase A (PKA) was added to the extracellular medium, indicating that Ca^{2+}-dependent phosphorylation and dephosphorylation of the Ca^{2+} channel are involved in run-down. Hao et al. (1999) separated the intracellular cytoplasmic extract into different fractions by gel filtration and found that a combination of an intracellular protein of >300 kD, called calpastatin and ATP restored the initial current amplitude by 87%. An example of Ca^{2+} whole cell current run-down by repetitive stimulation at a frequency of 1 Hz is demonstrated in Fig. 17.

Apart from adding Mg^{2+}ATP and EDTA to the pipette solution, run-down can be prevented by minimizing dialysis of the intracellular medium making use of the perforated patch method.

References

Adachi-Akanane S, Nagao T (2000) Ca^{2+} channel antagonists and agonists. In: Endo M, Kurachi Y, Mishina M. Pharmacology of ionic channel function. Activators and inhibitors. Springer, Berlin Heidelberg New York Tokyo

Bangalore R, Mehrke G, Gingrich D, Hofmann F, Kass RS (1996) Influence of L-type Ca channel alpha 2/delta-subunit on ionic and gating current in transiently transfected HEK 293 cells. Am J Physiol 270:H1521–H1528

Bean BP (1989) Neurotransmitter inhibition of neuronal calcium currents by changes in channel voltage-dependence. Nature 340: 153–155

Biel M, Ruth P, Bosse E, Hullin R, Stühmer W, Flockerzi V, Hofmann F (1990) Primary culture and functional expression of a high voltage activated calcium channel from rabbit lung. FEBS Letters 269: 409–412

Bodi I, Koch SE, Yamaguchi H, Szigeti GP, Schwartz A, Varadi G (2002) The role of region IVS5 of the human cardiac calcium channel in establishing inactivated channel conformation. J Biol Chem 277: 20651–20659

Diochot S, Richard S, Baldy-Moulinier M, Nargeot J, Valmier J (1995) Dihydropyridines, phenylalkylamines and benzothiazepines block N-, P/Q- and R-type calcium currents. Pflügers Arch 431: 10–19

Eberst R, Dai S, Klugbauer N, Hofmann F (1997) Identification and functional characterization of a calcium channel γ subunit. Pflügers Arch 433: 633–637

Ertel EA, Campbell KP, Harpold MM, Hofmann F, Mori Y, Perez-Reyes E, Schwartz A, Snutch TP, Tanabe T, Birnbaumer L, Tsien RW, Catterall WA (2000) Nomenclature of voltage-gated calcium channels. Neuron 25: 533–535

Findlay I (2002) Voltage- and cation-dependent inactivation of L-type Ca^{2+} currents in guinea-pig ventricular myocytes. J Physiol 541: 731–740

Fischmeister R, Hartzell HC (1986) Mechanism of action of acetylcholine on calcium currents in single cells from frog ventricle. J Physiol (Lond) 376: 183–202

Glossmann H, Ferry D, Striessnig J, Goll A, Moosburger K (1987) Resolving the structure of the Ca^{2+} channel by photoaffinity labelling. Trends Pharmacol Sci 8: 95–100

Glossmann H, Linn T, Rombusch M, Ferry DR (1983) Temperature-dependent regulation of d-cis[3H]diltiazem binding to Ca^{2+} channels by 1,4-dihydropyridine channel agonists and antagonists. FEBS Letters 160: 226–232

Grabner M, Wang Z, Hering S, Striessnig J, Glossmann H (1996) Transfer of 1,4-Dihydropyridine sensitivity from L-type to class-A (BI) calcium channels. Neuron 16: 207–218

Gurnett CA, DeWaard M, Campbell KP (1996) Dual function of the voltage-dependent Ca2+ channel alpha(2)delta subunit in current stimulation and subunit interaction. Neuron 1996; 16: 431–440

Hagiwara M, Adachi-Akahane S, Nagao T (1997) High-affinity binding of DTZ323, a novel derivate of diltiazem, to rabbit skeletal muscle L-type Ca^{2+} channels. J Pharmacol Exp Ther 281: 173–179

Hao L-Y, Kameyama A, Kameyama M (1999) A cytoplasmic factor, calpastatin and ATP together reverse run-down of Ca^{2+} channel activity in guinea-pig heart. J Physiol 514: 687–699

Hille B (2001) Ion channels of excitable membranes. Third Edition. Sinauer

Hirano Y, Yoshinaga T, Murata M, Hiraoka M (1999) Prepulse-induced mode 2 gating behaviour with and without β-adrenergic stimulation in cardiac L-type calcium channels. Am J Physiol 276: C1338–1345

Hoffmann F, Lacinová L, Klugbauer N (1999) Voltage-dependent calcium channels: From structure to function. Rev Physiol Biochem Pharmacol 139: 33–87

Kanaya S, Arlock P, Katzung BG, Hondeghem LM (1983) Diltiazem and verapamil preferentially block inactivated cardiac calcium channels. J Mol Cell Cardiol 15: 145–148

Klein G, Drexler H, Schröder F (2000) Protein kinase G reverses all isoproterenol induced changes of cardiac single L-type calcium channel gating. Cardiovasc Res 48: 367–374

Klugbauer N, Lacinová L, Marais E, Hobom M, Hofmann F (1999) Molecular diversity of the calcium channel $\alpha_2\delta$-subunit. J Neurosci 19: 684–691

Klugbauer N, Dai S, Specht V, Lacinova L, Marais E, Bohn G, Hofmann F (2000) A family of γ-like calcium channel subunits. FEBS Lett 470: 189–197

Kokubun S, Reuter H (1984) Dihydropyridine derivates prolong the open state of Ca channels in cultured cardiac cells. Proc Natl Acad Sci USA (Cell Biology) 81: 4824–4827

Kostyuk PG, Veselovsky NS, Fedulova SA (1981) Ionic currents in the somatic membrane of rat dorsal root ganglion neurons. II. Calcium currents. Neuroscience 7: 2431–2437

Kuo CC, Hess P (1993) Characterization of the high-affinity Ca^{2+} binding sites in the L-type Ca^{2+} channel pore in rat phaechromocytoma cells. J Physiol London 466: 657–682

Lee A, Wong ST, Gallagher D, Li B, Storm DR, Scheuer T, Catterall WA (1999) Ca^{2+}/calmodulin binds to and modulates P/Q-type calcium channel. Nature 399: 155–159

Lipkind GM, Fozzard HA (2003) Molecular modeling of interactions of dihydropyridines and phenylalkylamines with the inner pore of the L-type Ca^{2+} channel. Mol Pharmacol 63: 499–511

Markwardt F, Nilius B (1990) Changes of calcium channel inactivation during run-down. J Gen Physiol 9: 209–218

McDonald TF, Pelzer D, Trautwein W (1984) Cat ventricular muscle treated with D600: characteristics of calcium channel block and unblock. J Physiol 353: 217–241

Michels G, Matthes J, Handrock R, Kuchinke U, Groner F, Cribbs LL, Pereverzev A, Schneider T, Perez-Reyes E, Herzig S (2002) Single-channel pharmacology of mibefradil in human native T-type and recombinant Ca$_v$3.2 calcium channels. Mol Pharmacol 61: 682–694

Melzer W, Herrmann-Frank A, Lüttgau H C (1995) The role of Ca2+ ions in excitation-contraction coupling of skeletal muscle fibres. Biochimica et Biophysica Acta 1241: 59–116

Mitterdorfer J, Sinnegger MJ, Grabner M, Striessnig J, Glossmann H (1995) Coordination of Ca^{2+} by the pore region glutamates is essential for high-affinity dihydropyridine binding to the cardiac Ca^{2+} channel alpha 1 subunit. Biochmistry 34: 9350–9355

Mitterdorfer J, Wang Z, Sinnegger MJ, Hering S, Striessnig J, Grabner M, Glossmann H (1996) Two amino acid residues in the IIIS5 segment of L-type Ca^{2+} channels differentially contribute to 1,4-Dihydropyridine sensitivity. J Biol Chem 271: 30330–30335

Mitterdorfer J, Grabner M, Kraus RL, Hering S, Prinz H, Glossmann H, Striessnig J (1998) Molecular basis of drug interaction with L-type Ca2+ channels. J Bioenerg Biomembr 30: 319–334

Peterson BZ, Catterall WA (1995) Calcium binding in the pore of L-type calcium channels modulates high affinity dihydropyridine binding. J Biol Chem 270: 18201–18204

Peterson BZ, DeMaria CD, Adelman JP, Yue DT (1999) Calmodulin is the Ca^{2+} sensor for Ca^{2+} dependent inactivation of L-type calcium channels. Neuron 22: 549–558

Peterson BZ, Johnson BD, Hockerman GH, Acheson M, Scheuer T, Catterall WA (1997) Analysis of the dihydropyridine receptor site of L-type calcium channels by alanine scanning mutagenesis. J Biol Chem 272: 18752–18758

Quin N, Olcese R, Stefani E, Birnbaumer L (1998) Modulation of human neuronal a_{1E}-type calcium channel by $\alpha_2\delta$-subunit. Am J Physiol 274: C1324–C1331

Sanguinetti MC, Kass RS (1984) Voltage-dependent block of calcium channel current in calf cardiac Purkinje fiber by dihydropyridine calcium channel antagonists. Circ Res 55: 336–348

Sanguinetti MC, Krafte DS, Kass RS (1986) Voltage-dependent modulation of Ca channel current in heart cells by Bay K8644. J Gen Physiol 88: 369–392

Schramm M, ThomasG, Towart R, Franckowiak G (1983) Novel dihydropyridines with positive inotropic action through activation of Ca^{2+} channels. Nature 303: 535–537

Schröder F, Herzig S (1999) Effects of β_2-adrenergic stimulation on single-channel gating of rat cardiac L-type Ca^{2+} channels. Am J Physiol 276:H834–H843

Soldatov NM, Zühlke RD, Bouron A, Reuter H (1997) Molecular Structures Involved in L-type Calcium Channel Inactivation. Role of the carboxyl-terminal region encoded by exons 40–42 in a1C subunit in the kinetics and Ca^{2+} dependence of inactivation. J Biol Chem 272: 3560–3566

Triggle DJ (1996). The classification of calcium antagonists. J Cardiovasc Pharmacol. 27 (Suppl A):S11–S16

Viard P, Exner T, Maier U, Mironneau J, Nurnberg B, Macrez N (1999) Gbγ dimers stimulate vascular L-type Ca^{2+} channels via phosphoinositide 3-kinase. FASEB J 13: 685–694

Walker D, De Waard M (1998) Subunit interaction sites in voltage-dependent Ca^{2+} channels: role in channel function. Trends Neurosi 21: 148–154

Yamaguchi H, Muth J, Varadi M, Schwartz A, Varadi G (1999) Critical role of conserved proline residues in the transmembrane segment 4 voltage sensor function and in the gating of L-type calcium channels. PNAS 96: 1357–1362

Yue DJ, Backx PH, Imredy JP (1990a) Calcium sensitive inactivation in the gating single calcium channel. Science 250: 1735–1738

Yue DJ, Marban E (1990b) Permeation in the dihydropyridine-sensitivity calcium channel: multiple occupany but no anomalous mole-fraction effect between Ba^{2+} and Ca^{2+}. J Gen Physiol 95: 911–939

Zhang JF, Ellinor PT, Aldrich RW, Tsien RW (1994) Molecular determinants of voltage dependent inactivation in calcium channels. Nature 327: 97–100

Recording Cardiac Potassium Currents with the Whole-Cell Voltage Clamp Technique

Erich Wettwer and Ursula Ravens

Introduction

Potassium channels are the most diverse group of ion channels. Until now, about 200 K^+-channel genes have been identified, with more than 20 different channels in the cardiovascular system. In the heart, K^+-channels control resting membrane potential and action potential repolarization (Tables 1 and 2).

The major common property of all K^+-channels is their high selectivity for permeation of K^+. In contrast, specific electrophysiological characteristics exhibit large variations. K^+-channels can be divided into four groups: The first group consists of the voltage gated channels that are activated by membrane potential; the second group comprises Ca^{2+}-activated K^+-channels which open upon a rise in intracellular Ca^{2+}-concentration; the third group contains the inward rectifier K^+-channels, i.e. favouring K^+-flux in inward over outward direction. Channels activated by G-protein coupled receptors, e.g. $I_{K,ACh}$, or channels regulated by ATP, e.g. $I_{K,ATP}$, belong to this group. The fourth group are the background or leak channels, which behave like K^+-selective holes in the membrane and are regulated by pH, metabolites or the redox status of the cell.

Table 1
Pore forming α-subunits of potassium channels and currents in the mammalian heart (cf Coetzee et al. 1999; Shieh et al. 2000; Nerbonne 2001)

Group		Gens	Currents
Voltage-gated	6TM1P	KCND4, ERG, KCNQ1, KCNA5	I_{to}, I_{Kr}, I_{Ks}, I_{Kur}
Ca^{2+} activated	6TM1P	KCNN1,2	BK_{Ca}
Inward rectifiers	2TM1P	KCNJ-family	I_{K1}, $I_{K,ACh}$, $I_{K,ATP}$
Background channels	4TM2P	KCNK-family (TWIK, TREK)	I_{Kp}, I_{Kb}

Table 2
Accessory β-subunits modulating potassium channel function

	Name	Type	Modulation of	Effect
KChiP	K^+ channel interacting protein	Cytoplasmic	$I_{to,f}$ (Kv4.2,3)	Functional expression ↑, Inactivation kinetics slowed
MiRPs (KCNE1-5)	Min-K-related protein	1TM domain	I_{to}, Herg, I_{Ks}, I_{Kr}	Functional expression ↑, kinetics altered
KChAP	K^+ channel accessory protein	Cytoplasmic	I_{to}	Functional expression ↑, kinetics unaltered
Kvb	K^+ channel beta subunit	Cytoplasmic	I_{Kur}, $I_{K,DR}$ (Kv2.1) $I_{to,s}$ (Kv1.4)	Functional expression ↑, kinetics altered
DPPX	Dipeptidyl-peptidase-like-protein	1TM domain	I_{to} (?)	Functional expression ↑, inactivation kinetics accelerated

Constituent	Concentration	Bath
KCl	40.0	5.4
K-aspartate	100.0	–
NaCl	8.0	150.0
$CaCl_2$	2.0	1.8
EGTA	5.0	–
HEPES	10.0	10.0
MgATP	5.0	–
$MgCl_2$		2.0
GTP-Tris	0.1	–
pH 7.4, adaptation with KOH	~30.0	pH 7.4, adaptation with NaOH

Table 3
Composition of a typical electrode and bath solution for measuring K^+-currents (concentration in mmol/l)

The overall K^+-concentration is set to about 150 mM. The osmolarity is about 330 mosmol. It has to be noted, that even more K^+ is added when adjusting the pH with KOH. This may amount up to 30 mM! The free Ca^{2+} concentration is set by the Ca-buffering system Ca^{2+}/Ca-EGTA. With 2 mM of total Ca^{2+} and 5 mM of EGTA, the free Ca^{2+}-concentration is calculated to be 43 nM and the free Mg^{2+} concentration is 586 µM at 20°C and pH 7.4. At physiological temperature the respective values are 35 nM Ca^{2+} and 372 µM Mg^{2+}. At this low intracellular Ca^{2+} concentration contraction of cardiomyocytes is inhibited, and other Ca^{2+}-dependent processes should be largely reduced. The liquid junction potential of this pipette solution is calculated with JPCALCW (Barry and Lynch, 1991) and has a value of +12 mV. The true membrane potential (V_m), under voltage clamp conditions, will therefore deviate to negative values from the pipette potential (V_p) by the liquid junction potential (V_L): $V_m = V_p - V_L$.

The different groups of K⁺-channels vary substantially in structure. The pore containing moiety of voltage-gated channels is a tetramer consisting of four α-subunits. Each of these subunits has 6 transmembrane spanning segments. The linker between segment 5 and 6 dips back into the membrane and forms the lining of the pore. Thus, the α-subunit of voltage-gated channels consists of 6 transmembrane domains and 1 pore forming linker (6TM1P). Inward rectifiers also have 4 α-subunits, each with two transmembrane domains and 1 pore region (2TM1P). α-subunits of background channels have 4 transmembrane domains, but two pore regions (4TM2P), and therefore two α-subunits are sufficient for a functional channel.

The diversity of K⁺-channels is multiplied by the formation of heteromultimers of different α-subunits. In addition, various splice variants are known. The functional complexity is further increased by accessory or β-subunits co-assembling with the α-subunits, and substantially modulating their electrophysiological characteristics. Channel function is further diversified by different associated proteins such as regulatory enzymes or cytoskeletal proteins (Table 3). The reader is also referred to the excellent reviews of K⁺-channel nomenclature, structure and function (Snyders 1999; Coetzee et al. 1999; Yellen 2002; Nerbonne 2000, 2001).

In this chapter, we will focus on methodological details in the measurement of those voltage-dependent potassium currents, which are major contributors to the cardiac action potential, e.g. the transient outward current I_{to}; the rapid and slow activating outward rectifiers, I_{Kr} and I_{Ks}; the ultra rapid delayed rectifier I_{Kur}; and the inward rectifiers I_{K1} and $I_{K,ACh}$.

Description of Methods and Practical Approach

K⁺-currents are studied in native cells or in expression systems with patch electrodes (Chapter 3.11), by means of the voltage clamp technique (Chapter 3.5). Native cells are enzymatically dissociated from the hearts of different mammalian species, e.g. rat, mouse, guinea pig, ferret, cat, dog or man. Both expression systems and native cells have special advantages as well as drawbacks. Native cells allow K⁺-channels to be studied in their physiological environment, providing all necessary sub-units and cellular factors for physiological activity. Major draw backs are

- exposure to enzymes which may also be aggressive to proteins required for channel function;
- necessity for fresh cell isolation, because adult cardiac myocytes cannot be kept in primary culture without profound alterations in electrophysiological and morphological properties;
- other contaminating currents must be suppressed.

The latter is achieved by adjusting the ion composition of the extracellular and intracellular (pipette) solution, by blocking unwanted components or by using elaborate voltage protocols (see below).

Expression systems facilitate electrophysiological channel characterization, because they express only the channel under investigation, and are easily cultivated.

To overcome these difficulties, K^+-currents are often studied in heterologous expression systems, where the channel genes are transiently or permanently expressed in cells that can be easily cultured. The most popular cell systems are mammalian cell lines like HEK (Human embryonic kidney cells), CHO (Chinese hamster ovary cells), COS cells (kidney cells from the monkey *Cercopithecus* aethiops) and fibroblasts. These cell lines are primarily used for screening purposes where a large number of substances have to be studied. They are also used in new high throughput patch clamp techniques that have been developed recently to measure several cells in parallel. Preferred by researchers, *Xenopus* oocytes are easily transfected, and as they are large cells (1 mm diameter), can be accurately voltage clamped.

A disadvantage is that the surrounding of the channels may not be the same as in native cells hence channel properties may differ profoundly, if the native regulatory proteins or β-subunits are absent. Channel sensitivity to toxins or drugs may also vary between expression systems and native cells.

Electrophysiological Characteristics of K^+-Channels

Several parameters are used to classify and characterize ion channels in general, and K^+ channels in particular.

Selectivity

Channel selectivity is used for classification of channel families. It can be tested by measuring current amplitude with various ions as charge carrier under otherwise identical conditions. Since the osmolality of the solutions has to be kept constant, increasing extracellular concentrations of K^+ will have to be compensated by reducing Na^+. Moreover, some cations exert interfering effects, and relative concentrations have to be taken into account ("mole fraction").

I-V Curve (amplitude)

The simplest way of studying potential dependence of an ion channel is to measure the current-voltage relation. Current amplitudes provide some information about the abundance of channels and/or their conductance.

Reversal Potential

By definition, the I-V curve reverses direction at the reversal potential. By comparison, by using the Nernst potential on various ions, the reversal potential allows some conclusion about the major conducting ion.

Kinetics – Activation and Inactivation

The rising current amplitude upon a depolarising voltage step is considered to reflect the transition of closed channels into their open state (activation). Many K^+ channels close again, despite persisting depolarising clamp potential (inactivation).

The time courses of activation and inactivation allow conclusions about the kinetics of the K⁺ channel under investigation.

Recovery from Inactivation

The transition of a channel from the inactivated state back to a state from which it is re-available for activation requires time, and is greatly facilitated by strongly negative potentials. The kinetics of this process are characterised by measuring the recovery from inactivation.

Pharmacology – Use-Dependent Action of Drugs

Pharmacological agents can bind to resting, activated or inactivated channels. Since membrane potential is a major determinant of the activation state of the channel, drug binding and hence also drug efficacy become potential dependent, if the agents exhibit preferential selectivity for any one of the channel's states. Moreover, onset of block, and recovery from block, are important parameters to be evaluated.

Examples

The Major Cardiac K⁺ Currents

The Transient Outward Current I_{to}

General Description. Mammalian cardiomyocytes possess two types of transient outward currents, which are distinguished on the basis of specific kinetic parameters: $I_{to,f}$ recovers rapidly ("f" for "fast") whereas $I_{to,s}$ recovers slowly ("s") from inactivation. $I_{to,f}$ is found to be present in the hearts of many mammalian species including man (atria and ventricles). The K⁺ channel protein for $I_{to,f}$ is encoded by the KCND3 (Kv4.3) gene. The current activates and subsequently inactivates rapidly upon depolarisation. The kinetics of recovery from inactivation is fast. In contrast, $I_{to,s}$ has been described in rabbit ventricle only. The respective channel is encoded by the gene KCNA4 (Kv1.4), its kinetics of recovery from inactivation is slow. Some species like the guinea pig, do not express any I_{to} at all.

Current Separation. To explore whether a cardiomyocyte under investigation possess any $I_{to,f}$, it suffices to measure an I-V curve with rectangular voltage clamp steps, to increasingly positive membrane potentials. The rapid increase and decline of outward current amplitude during a single clamp step is already characteristic for the transient outward current, since the peak of $I_{to,f}$ is reached within a few ms upon membrane depolarisation. Other currents with a similarly fast activation, e.g. sodium current I_{Na} and L-type calcium current $I_{Ca,L}$, may overlap. Because of their inward direction they oppose outward current, and hence, may lead to false (too small) estimation current amplitude. With increasingly positive potentials, however, the contribution of I_{Na} to the whole cell current is reduced as I_{Na} approaches its reversal potential.

To clearly separate $I_{to,f}$ from interfering I_{Na} and $I_{Ca,L}$, these currents have to be minimized, either using a prepulse in the voltage clamp protocol to inactivate I_{Na}, or by using Na⁺-free bath solutions where Na⁺ is substituted by NMDG (N-metyhl-D-glucamine) or choline. An alternative is to block the cardiac sodium channel with tetrodotoxin. However, large concentrations (>10 µM) are needed, since the tetrodotoxin sensitivity of cardiac sodium channels is low compared to the sensitivity of neuronal sodium channels. A prepulse from the holding potential of −100 or −80 mV to −40 mV for 25 ms would be sufficient to quickly activate and inactivate the fast sodium current. With the subsequent depolarizing clamp step to positive membrane potentials, only the $I_{to,f}$ is activated. $I_{Ca,L}$ interferes with $I_{to,f}$ more substantially, since the peak activation of $I_{Ca,L}$ is reached at 0 mV, while $I_{to,f}$ activation begins at −20 mV. $I_{Ca,L}$ cannot be inactivated by a prepulse without also inactivating $I_{to,f}$. Therefore, $I_{Ca,L}$ has to be inhibited using blockers and/or reducing the extracellular Ca²⁺-concentration ($[Ca^{2+}]_o$).

The Ca²⁺ channel blocker nisoldipine (1–5 µM) is a suitable tool to reduce $I_{Ca,L}$. In addition, $[Ca^{2+}]_o$ can be lowered to 0.5 mM to further reduce residual I_{Ca}, without having an effect on membrane stability. In the example of isolated rat ventricular myocytes (Fig. 1a,b), I_{Na} was inactivated by a 25 ms prepulse, and $I_{Ca,L}$ was inhibited with 0.1 mM of Cd²⁺ in the presence of 0.5 mM $[Ca^{2+}]_o$. However, it should be noted, that any blocker of contaminating current could also affect the current under investigation (Hatano et al. 2003). Cd²⁺ is known to alter the kinetics of I_{to} and change the voltage dependence of steady-state activation and inactivation (Wettwer et al. 1993). Even a prepulse for inactivation of I_{Na} may induce inactivation of the I_{to}. Therefore, no method of current separation is ideal, and when comparing results from different labs, the recording conditions have to be carefully analysed.

Current-Voltage Relation, Steady-State Activation and Inactivation Curve, Recovery from Inactivation

Current Voltage Relation

The voltage dependency of the $I_{to,f}$ current is constructed from the current recordings at each tested membrane potential, i.e. the peak amplitude of the current is plotted versus the potential of the test step (Fig. 1c). The current amplitude of $I_{to,f}$ increases monotonously with membrane depolarisation. To compare $I_{to,f}$ from cells which differ in size, and are therefore expected to differ in the number of active ion channels and whole cell current, the whole current may be normalized to the cell size. Since the cell surface is proportional to the electrical capacitance C_M of the cell measured in pF, $I_{to,f}$ can be normalized to C_M and expressed as current density in pA/pF (Fig. 1c).

Activation and Inactivation

The terms activation and inactivation describe the time course of current increase to its maximum value, and the subsequent time-dependent decrease. $I_{to,f}$ is a very fast activating and inactivating current. At a potential of +60 mV, the maximum current

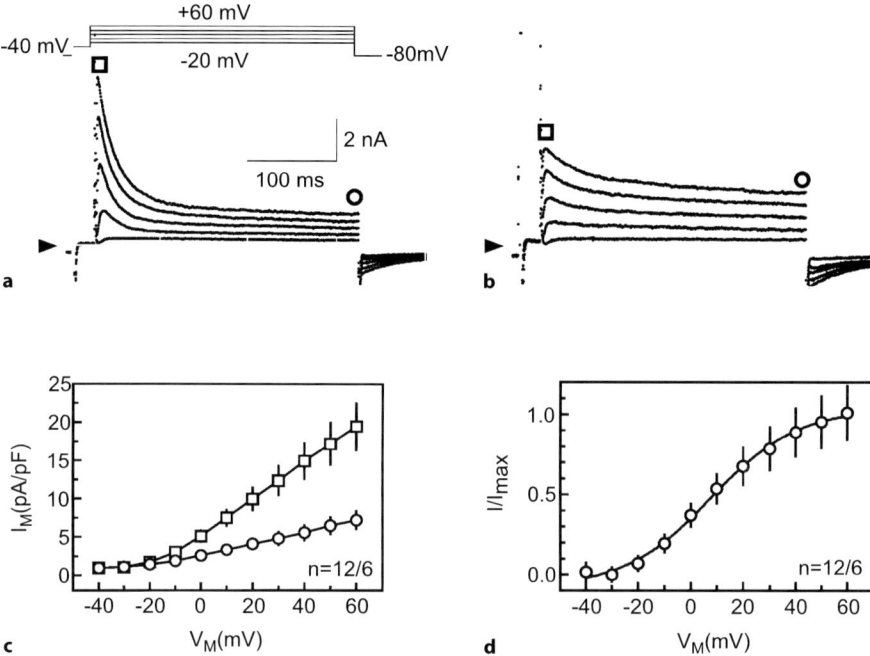

Figure 1a–d
Current records of I_{to} in isolated ventricular myocytes of the rat heart. **a** Example of a prominent transient outward current component. Holding potential –80 mV; 25 ms prepulse to –40 mV to inactivate I_{Na}. Depolarizations to –20, 0, +20, +40 and +60 mV, pulse frequency 0.2 s⁻¹, duration 300 ms. **b** Example of small transient current component but large steady-state component probably from different region of the ventricle. Both cells are from the same heart. **c** Current-voltage relation of the peak □ and late current amplitudes ○ expressed as current density (pA/pF) (mean values ± SEM). **d** Activation curve constructed from peak current amplitudes divided by the driving voltage (V_M–E_{rev}) with E_{rev} of –65 mV. Fitting Boltzmann curves to the data resulted in a $V_{0.5}$ of 10.7 ± 3.5 mV and a slope factor k of 12.5 ± 3.5 mV. T, 22°C. (Data from Wettwer 1997)

amplitude is reached within 5 ms. Inactivation starts early and is largely completed within 100 ms (Fig. 1a). Activation and inactivation are often temperature dependent, as shown for $I_{to,f}$ from human ventricular myocytes in Fig. 2. At the physiological temperature of 37 °C, activation at +60 mV is complete after only 3 ms, and inactivation is even more accelerated with time constants of less than 10 ms. The speed of the time dependency, may limit the accuracy of the current measurements. The activation phase may coincide with the decay of the capacitive transient, and cannot be separated from the latter. This is especially valid for large cells such as myocytes. In these cases, it may be appropriate to decrease the temperature to a level where activation and decay of capacitive transient can be separated. The decay of the capacitive transient can be accelerated using large electrodes with reduced resistance and good access to the cell, so that the access resistance is as low as possible. Therefore, great care has to be taken if I_{to} measurements are to be done at physiological temperature.

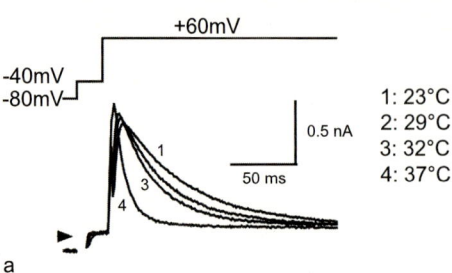
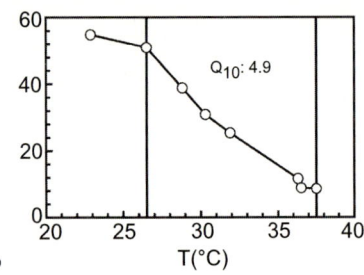
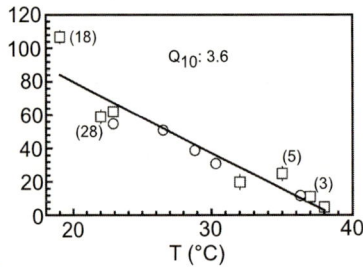

Figure 2a–c
Temperature dependency of I_{to} inactivation in isolated human ventricular myocytes. **a** Current records of I_{to} at four different temperatures between 23 °C and 37 °C. Holding potential −80 mV, 20 ms prepulse to −40 mV. Membrane depolarisation to +60 mV, 300 ms, 0.2 s^{-1}. The current records were fitted with exponential equations $Y = A \times exp(-t/\tau_f) + B$. **b** Temperature dependency of the inactivation time constant τ. From the same cell as in (**a**). Calculation of Q_{10} according to: $Q_{10} = exp\,[\{10/(T_2-T_1)\}\,\ln(\tau_1/\tau_2)]$ (Kiyosue et al. 1993). In the temperature range indicated by vertical lines the Q_{10} was determined to be 4.9. **c** Temperature dependency of τ in different cells. The steepness of the regressions line was −43 ms/10°C. Q_{10} was calculated to be 3.6. (Data from Wettwer 1997)

In order to quantify time courses of activation and inactivation, fitting procedures are performed. From the fits of the current traces, time constants of activation and inactivation are extracted. These time constants have important current characteristics that may differ largely between species, or with pharmacological intervention.

Steady State Activation Curve

The steady-state activation curve determines the proportion of channels open at a certain membrane potential. The term "steady-state" refers to the fact that the time dependent process of opening is completed and inactivation has not yet begun. The degree of activation, i.e. the fraction of open channels, is experimentally determined at a single appropriate clamp potential that follows activation at various test steps. During the first test step, channels open in a voltage-dependent manner. The membrane is then clamped back to a potential at which the channels are normally closed. The decay of current, gives rise to the so-called "tail current", and reflects the process of channel closing. The maximum amplitude of the tail current, immediately following the test pulse, is proportional to the number of open channels. The potential at which tail currents are to be detected has to be sufficiently negative for channel clo-

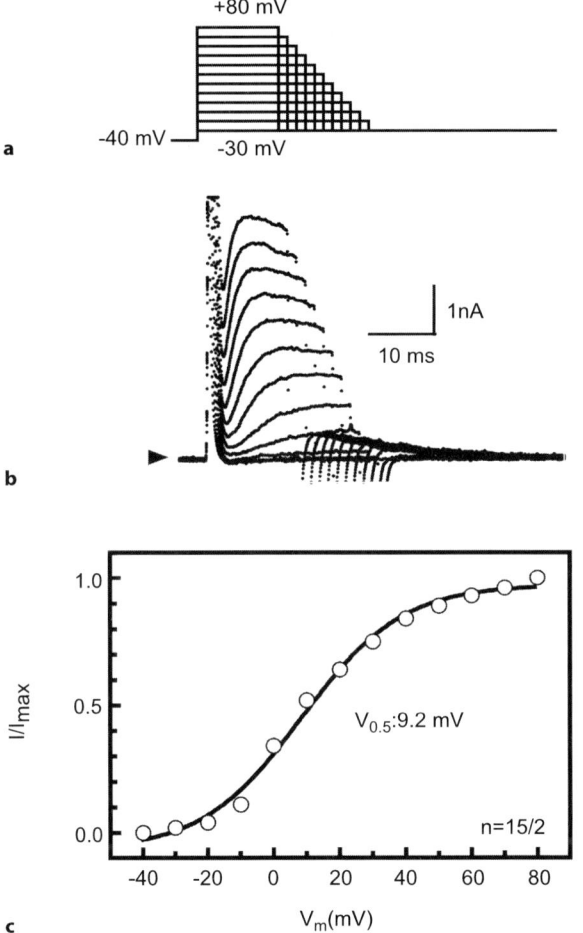

Fig. 3a–c
Activation curve of I_{to} in sub-epicardial myocytes of the human ventricle. a,b Current records of I_{to}. a Clamp protocol, holding potential: –80 mV, 25 ms prepulse to –40 mV to inactivate I_{Na}. Depolarisations between –30 and +80 mV in 10 mV increments, 0.2 s^{-1}. The pulse duration was continuously diminished from 25 ms to 10 ms. Return to –30 mV to determine tail current amplitudes. c Normalized activation curve (I/I_{max}) of peak tail current amplitudes. Mean $V_{0,5}$ value determined from individually fitted activation curves was +9,2 ± 1,8 mV with a slope factor k +13,0 ± 0,6 mV (n = 15/2), T, 22 °C. (Data from Wettwer 1997)

sure, yet sufficiently different from the reversal potential in order to provide the driving force for K$^+$, so that the current is large enough to be measured accurately. For $I_{to,f}$, which has a reversal potential of about –60 mV (see below), an appropriate potential is –30 mV (Fig. 3a). The amplitudes of the tail currents are normalized to the peak tail current and plotted against membrane potential (Fig. 3b). This activation curve can be fitted with a Boltzmann equation from which two characteristic values are derived:
- the potential of half maximum activation $V_{0.5}$, in our example +9.5 mV and
- the slope factor k of the curve which in this case was 13 mV.

The activation curve of I_{to} is experimentally difficult to obtain, because the current starts to inactivate very soon after activation. An example of how this problem can be overcome is given in Fig. 3: once the current has reached its maximum, or shortly thereafter, the membrane is clamped back to the potential that has been chosen for measuring tail current. In this protocol, the duration of the test step becomes shorter with more depolarised membrane potential.

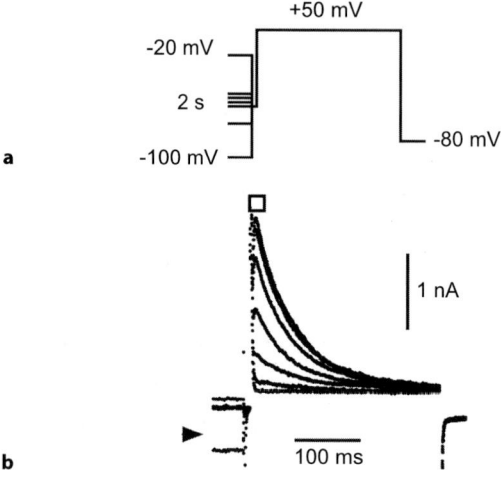

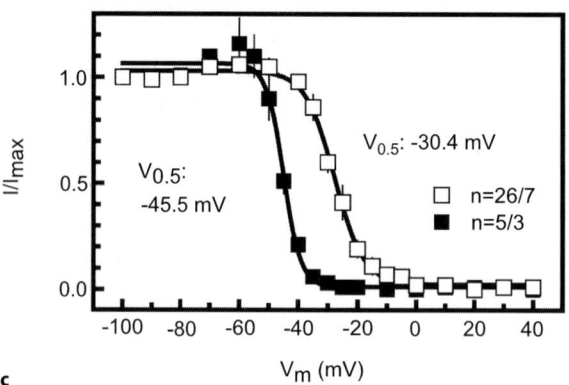

Figure 4a–c
Steady-state inactivation of I_{to} in supepicardial human ventricular myocytes. **a** Voltage clamp protocol: Holding potential –80 mV, conditioning prepulse of 2 s to potentials between –100 and +20 mV (prepulse only partially shown), in steps of 10 mV, 5 mV in the potential range –40 and 0 mV, 0.2 s^{-1}. Short 15 ms intermediate pulse to –40 mV to inactivate I_{Na}. Test pulse to +50 mV, 300 ms, in order to estimate the non-inactivated part of I_{to}. **b** Current traces of the test pulse to +50 mV following conditioning prepulses to –100, –60, –40, –35, –30, –25 and +20 mV. Peak current amplitude (o). **c** Steady-state inactivation curve of I_{to}. *Ordinate:* Normalized portion of the peak current amplitude (I/I_{max}). *Abscissa:* Potential of conditioning prepulses V_M. For normalization peak current amplitude following a prepulse of –100 mV was set to 1, and set to zero after a prepulse to +20 mV. (o) Inactivation curve in presence of Cd^{2+} (0.1 mM), (n) in presence of nifedipine (1µM). Fitting the normalized data of single experiments with a Boltzmann equation led to $V_{0.5}$ of –30.4 ± 1.2 mV and a slope factor k of –4.5 ± 0.2 mV (n=26/7) in presence of Cd^{2+} and $V_{0.5}$ was –45.5 ± 1.2 mV and k –4.6 ± 0.8 mV (5/3) in presence of nifedipine. Curve fitting to the mean values $V0,5$ and k were –27.4 mV and –5.3 mV in presence of Cd^{2+} and –44.9 mV and –3.0 mV in presence of nifedipine. (Data from Wettwer 1997)

Steady-State Inactivation

I_{to} channels can only be activated by depolarisation if the membrane potential has been sufficiently negative prior to activation. With less negative membrane potentials, fewer channels will open, until eventually all channels are in an inactivated state and no longer open at all. The potential dependence of this process is investigated with the steady-state inactivation protocol, which provides information about the availability of I_{to} channels at a given membrane potential. In an initial voltage step, the cell is polarized for rather a long time (1–2 s) to a conditioning potential (–100 up to +20 mV for I_{to}). This step is followed by a test pulse, at which the current will normally be fully activated (+50 mV for I_{to}). A brief (15 ms) intermediate pulse to −40 mV may be necessary to inactivate I_{Na}, and to provide a constant capacitive current transient. The peak amplitude of I_{to}, elicited by the constant test step, is analysed and plotted versus the conditioning potential. The resulting inactivation curve can be fitted with a sigmoidal Boltzmann function providing the $V_{0.5}$ of inactivation (−45 mV). The slope factor is −5 mV (Fig. 4). Steady-state inactivation may be substantially altered by the recording conditions. Blockers for $I_{Ca,L}$, which interfere with the I_{to} in native cells, may influence $V_{0.5}$ of steady-state inactivation. In the example shown in Fig. 4c, the $V_{0.5}$ values obtained for inactivation in the presence of Cd^{2+} and nifedipine differ by about 15 mV.

Recovery from Inactivation

I_{to} current inactivates at positive potentials. The membrane potential must return to negative voltages in order to allow the channels to recover from inactivation, so that they can activate again upon depolarisation. How much time does this process take and how is it influenced by membrane potential? It is studied using the "recovery from inactivation" protocol. During a first depolarising pulse to +20 mV, I_{to} activates and also rapidly inactivates. In order to allow the channels to recover from inactivation, the membrane potential is stepped back to the holding potential of −80 mV for intervals of increasing duration, i.e. from 5 to 6000 ms. Thereafter, I_{to} is activated again by a test pulse to +20 mV. I_{to} recovers from inactivation with an exponential time course, reaching the full current amplitude after 200 ms of recovery. Interestingly, recovery from inactivation exhibited an overshoot for $I_{to,f}$ in human ventricular myocytes (Wettwer et al. 1994). Recovery from inactivation is also potential dependent. It takes more time for I_{to} to recover from inactivation at a more positive recovery potential. The analysis is as follows: The normalized I_{to} amplitude is plotted against the duration of the recovery interval. The data points may be fitted using exponential equations, and a time constant of recovery calculated. In the case of I_{to}, the time constant was 25 ms at −100 mV, but 80 ms at −60 mV (Fig. 5a,b).

Reversal Potential

The reversal potential E_{rev}, is defined as the membrane potential at which the current flow through K^+-channel is zero. Positive to E_{rev} K^+ currents are outwardly directed negative to E_{rev} inwardly directed. For a purely K^+ selective channel, E_{rev} is identical to the Nernst' potential for K^+-ions, which is determined by the ratio of logarithms of intra- and extracellular K^+ concentrations (strictly speaking of the K^+ activities). In cardiomyocytes, E_K is about −100 mV. With the pulse protocol to determine E_{rev}, the K^+-current (I_{to} in our case) is activated to a potential where all channels are active (+50 mV). On return to −30 mV, where channels would be closed, we observe the deactivating tail current. At −30 mV, this current is still outward directed. With more negative membrane potentials, the outward directed tail current gets smaller and reverses to inward directed tail currents, negative to the reversal potential. The reversal potential is defined as the potential of no tail current, i.e. no net current flow. For I_{to},

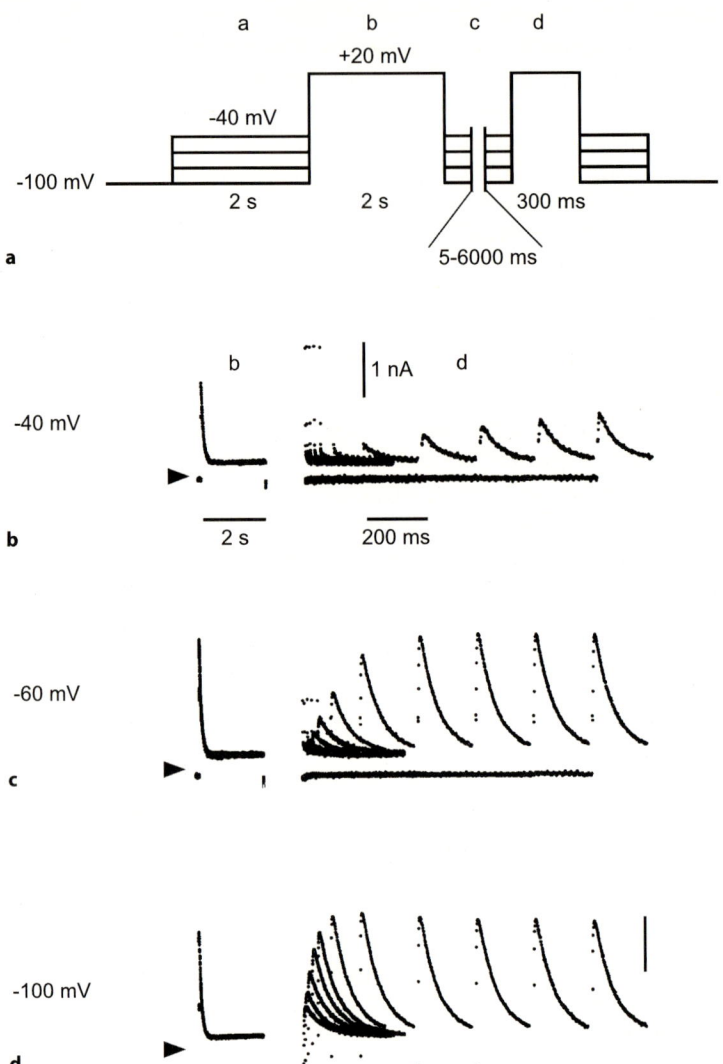

Figure 5a–d
Recovery from inactivation of I_{to} in human ventricular myocytes. **a** Clamp protocol, holding potential –100 mV. **a** Conditioning clamp step to –100, –80, –60 and –40 mV, duration 2 s. **b** Step to +20 mV, 2 s, to activate and inactivate I_{to}. **c** Recovery interval at –100, –80, –60 or –40 mV durations between 5 and 6000 ms. **d** Test pulse to +20 mV, 300 ms, to determine recovery from inactivation. **b–d** Original recordings show the superimposed traces during clamp step (**b**) and with a gap and at higher time resolution during recovery step (**c**) and test step (**d**) after recovery intervals of 5, 10, 20, 35, 55, 100, 200, 400, 600, 800 und 1000 ms. The potential of the recovery interval is depicted on the left, *arrows* point to the zero current level. (Data from Wettwer 1997)

E_{rev} is about –60 mV, which means that this channel is not completely selective for K^+ but also selective for other ions (Na^+, Ca^{2+}), the reversal potential is therefore more positive.

Examples of a careful and comprehensive characterisation of the transient outward current in mammalian cardiac myocytes can be found in the papers by Franqueza et al. 1999; Kong et al. 1998, and in the review by Nerbonne 2000.

Blockers of I_{to}

There are no selective blockers of I_{to} presently available. Like many other K$^+$-channels I_{to} is blocked by 4-aminopyridine in millimolar concentrations (IC$_{50}$ ≈1 mM, Amos et al. 1996). Tarantula toxins, selective for Kv4.x channels (especially for the cardiac Kv4.2 and Kv4.3 I_{to} channels) have recently been discovered and investigated (Sanguinetti et al. 1997; Diochot et al. 1999; Escoubas et al. 2002). Some of these venoms inhibit I_{to} channels in the low nM range.

Pharmacological block of ion channels needs to be considered in several aspects. The degree of current inhibition may be *potential dependent*, and may increase with membrane depolarisation, but can also show a reduced effect or even relief from block. The block may be *state dependent*, i.e. a compound may preferentially bind to closed, inactivated or activated channels. If a compound binds preferentially to either activated or inactivated channels, the block may become frequency-dependent, because the more often the channels pass through these stages, the more drugs are able to bind.

Such block patterns will produce "*use-dependency*" of block, indicating that block may be enhanced with increased "use" of the channels. Therefore, membrane potential, duration and frequency of voltage clamp pulses will substantially affect the block pattern.

Figure 6 demonstrates the effect of the class III antiarrhythmic agent tedisamil on I_{to} in human ventricular myocytes. The drug inhibits open channels. The block is use dependent and develops faster with higher rates of channel activation. The current recovers from block at negative membrane potentials. The recovery from block lasts much longer than the recovery from inactivation. It has to be noted, however, that tedisamil is by no means a selective I_{to} blocker, but also inhibits other cardiac K$^+$-currents (Faivre et al. 1995). Other examples of a comprehensive investigation into channel drug interactions can be found in Spector et al. 1996; Dumaine et al. 1998; Walker et al. 1999.

Questions to be kept in mind

- Is interference from other membrane currents to be expected?
- Which separation method is suitable? Does a prepulse for inactivation of I_{Na} influence the current under investigation?
- Does the temperature allow full fidelity of current measurement?
- Is there any indication that the blocker of $I_{Ca,L}$ affects the current under investigation?
- Can the recording conditions be optimised? Electrode solution, bath solution with appropriate blockers. Electrode resistance, access resistance cell dimensions?

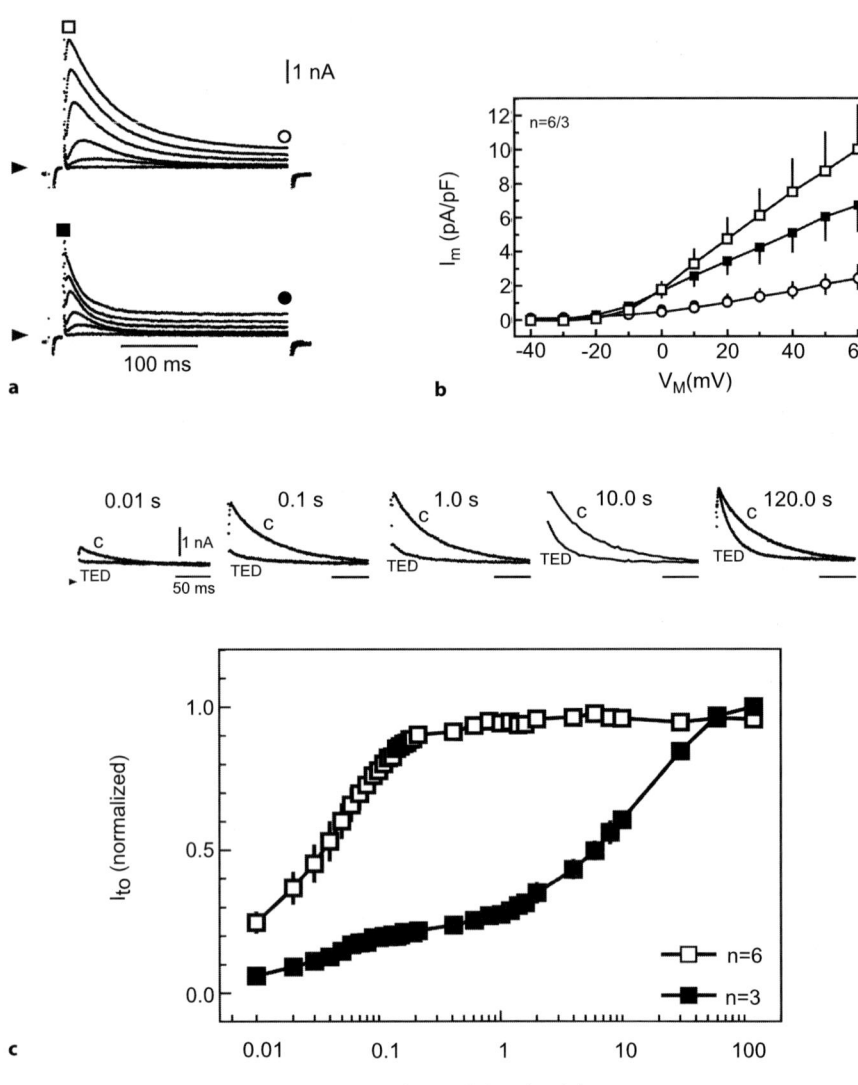

Figure 6a–c
Effect of tedisamil on I_{to} in human ventricular myocytes. **a** Control registration of I_{to} with clamp steps between −20 and +60 mV (*top*) and 5 min after addition of tedisamil (10 µM, *below*). Tedisamil accelerates inactivation of I_{to} with little effect on the peak current amplitude. **b** Current voltage relation of peak (□■) and late (○●, superimposed) current amplitudes. **c** I_{to} recovery of inactivation (□) and recovery from block (■) after addition of 10 µM tedisamil. Tedisamil retards the recovery process. Only with 100 s long recovery intervals the full current amplitude is obtained compared to 200 ms without drug. Original tracings at selected recovery intervals are depicted above the graph. (Data from Wettwer et al. 1998)

Good advice is to repeat classical experiments from a good paper on a standard preparation. After the experimenter has gained enough confidence with the measurements, he or she can turn to the object of interest. As an example of a comprehensive investigation into current characteristics of I_{to} in ferret myocytes, the reader could study the paper by Campbell et al. (1993), species differences are shown by Wettwer et al. (1993). Many more references can be found, in the review on potassium currents, in mammalian heart by Nerbonne (2001).

The Rapid Outward Rectifier I_{Kr}

General Description

The rapidly activating I_{Kr} potassium outward current is associated with the HERG channel (human ether a-go-go related gene channel), and is found in the myocytes of many mammalian species. Rabbit cardiac myocytes are well suited for analysis of the current's properties, because the overlapping I_{Ks} is small in these cells (Veldkamp et al. 1993). In the human heart I_{Kr} is detected in atrial and ventricular myocytes. Common expression systems for the HERG channel are HEK cells or fibroblasts. Several splice variants of HERG have been identified, and therefore electrophysiological characteristics of I_{Kr} may differ between expressed and endogenous channels (compare Snyders 1999).

The special molecular structure of the HERG channel allows numerous drugs to bind, and hence block-channel function. Inhibition of I_{Kr} prolongs the cardiac action potential, and therefore may contribute to cardiac arrhythmias (LQT-syndrome). Since the channel is a target for a large number of agents, I_{Kr} current has raised enormous interest, especially for pharmaceutical companies.

Current Separation

Current-Voltage Relation, Steady-State Activation and Inactivation Curve, Recovery from Inactivation

Examples of individual current traces, and the current voltage relation of I_{Kr} from an expression system, is shown in Fig. 7a–c. The kinetics of I_{Kr} are unusual in many aspects: The current rapidly activates with depolarising membrane potentials, and increases in amplitude up to 0 mV, but then decreases again with more positive potentials. This property of I_{Kr} is also called "inward rectification", because current amplitude is reduced at positive membrane potentials, just like the inward rectifier potassium currents. The reason for the reduction in current amplitude with depolarisation is the very fast process of channel closing (inactivation) at positive membrane potentials. There is a second peculiar feature of this current. When the membrane potential is repolarised from a positive value to a negative potential where I_{Kr} channels would normally close, a large tail current is observed (Fig. 7a,b). Channels that are inactivated at positive potentials, very rapidly recover from inactivation into an open state at the negative potential, giving rise to substantial current flow. However, the current amplitude decays as the channels change into the closed state characteristic for the chosen membrane potential. This deactivating current is also called "tail current". As shown previously for I_{to}, the amplitude of the deactivating tail current can

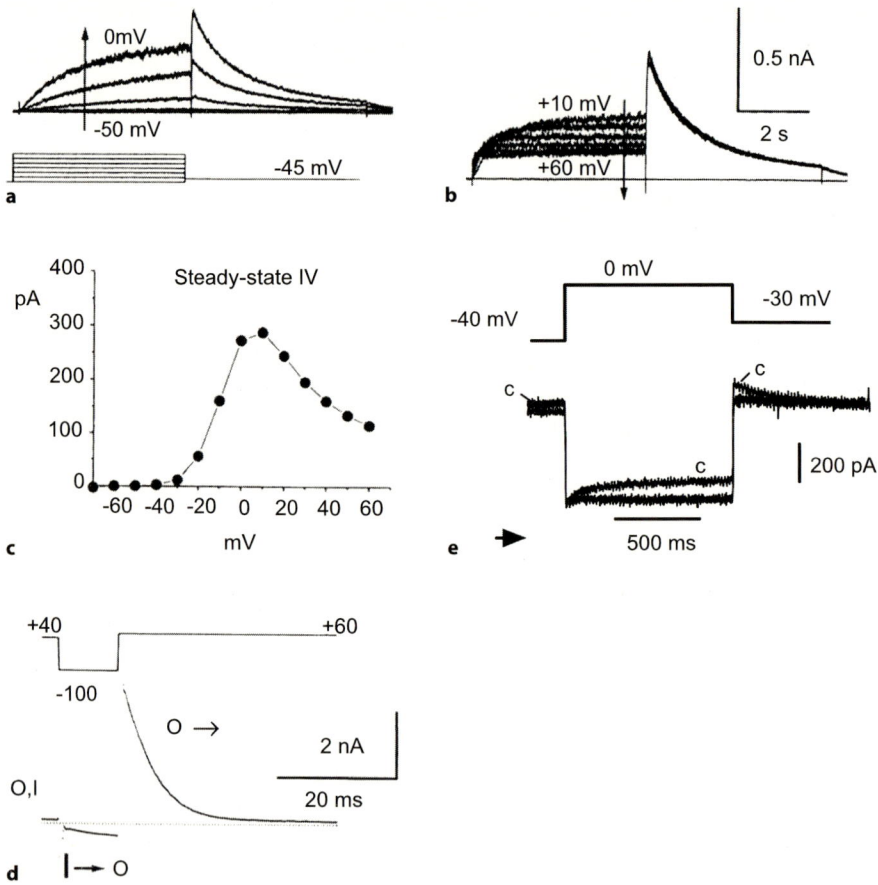

Figure 7a–e
I_{Kr} (HERG) currents in an heterologous expression system. **a,b** with increasing membrane depolarisation, current amplitude increases in the potential range between –50 and 0 mV (**a**) but decreases with more positive depolarisation +10 to +60 mV (**b**). **c** The current voltage (IV) of the steady-state current measured at the end of the test pulse displays "inward rectification" at potentials positive to 0 mV. **d** Inward rectification is due to fast inactivation of HERG channels at positive potentials. A large deactivating tail current develops (compare **a** and **b**) when returning to a negative membrane potential (–45 mV, **a**), because channels convert from the open into the closed state (deactivation). At –100 mV channels recover very rapidly from inactivation. At +60 mV the large initial current with rapid decline in amplitude indicates the fast transition from the open to the inactivated state (inactivation). Redrawn from Snyders (1999). **e** Effect of haloperidol (0.3 µM) on outward currents in a guinea-pig ventricular myocyte. I_{Kr} is activated from a holding potential of –40 mV to 0 mV. The activating I_{Kr} is small compared to the large I_{K1} measured at the holding potential (zero current level is indicated by *arrow*). Returning to –30 mV a tail current decays. In presence of haloperidol I_{Kr} (activating and tail current) is completely inhibited. (Data from: Wettwer et al. 2003)

be plotted against the test voltage, to yield an activation curve with the characteristic $V_{0.5}$ of –20 mV (Fig. 8). Drug effects on I_{Kr} are often determined as effects on I_{Kr} tail currents. The effect of the neuroleptic haloperidol is chosen as an example of a drug-induced block of I_{Kr} (Fig. 7d).

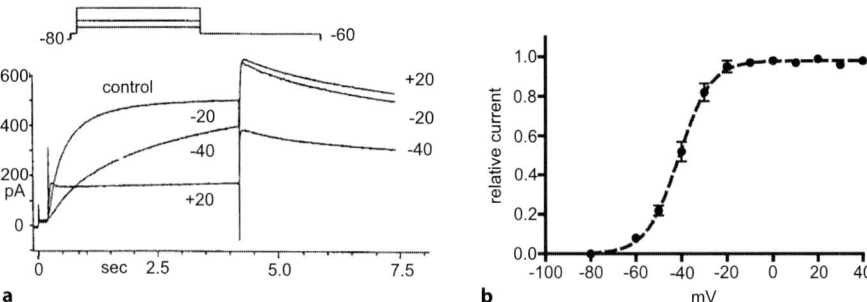

Figure 8a,b
I_{Kr} current recordings in xenopus oocytes expressing HERG. **a** Current tracings of I_{Kr} following depolarisation to −40, −20 and +20 mV. **b** Activation curve obtained from the analysis of tail currents. $V_{0.5}$ of activation was −40 mV, substantially more negative compared to I_{Ks} (redrawn from Spector et al. 1996). In native cells $V_{0.5}$ for I_{Kr} was at more positive potentials (−21 mV, Sanguinetti and Jurkiewicz 1990).

Figure 7e shows a clamp protocol for studying the fast inactivation process. At −100 mV, all channels recover from inactivation within 20 ms, whereas at +60 mV, the channels activate and immediately start to inactivate. Therefore, the fast decay of the outward current at +60 mV reflects the time course of inactivation.

In native cells, the activating current of I_{Kr} is sometimes very small, compared to all other currents. Therefore, I_{Kr} is best analysed in expression systems for HERG channels.

However, it must be kept in mind, that in native cells the HERG channel protein is associated with additional β-subunits, as for instance the MIRP related proteins (MiRP1 or KCNE2) which alter the current kinetics and also the sensitivity to drugs (for review see Tseng 2001). Therefore, not only I_{Kr} properties in native cells and expression systems (especially when *Xenopus* oocytes are used) may vary, but also sensitivity to drugs may be substantially different. Figure 8 depicts I_{Kr} tracings from transfected Xenopus oocytes. In this example, $V_{0.5}$ of activation was substantially more negative (−40 mV) when compared with native cells (Sanguinetti and Jurkievicz 1990).

Another drawback is that, deactivating tail currents are produced by several outward currents, which may interfere with the tail currents of I_{Kr}.

I_{Kr} shows an unexpected dependence on extracellular K^+, $[K^+]_o$. If $[K^+]_o$ is reduced, the current amplitude decreases, although the driving force for K^+ increases. Elevation of $[K^+]_o$ on the other hand increases the amplitude of I_{Kr} (see experiments by Sanguinetti and Jurkiewicz 1992). This property may be used to separate I_{Kr} from I_{Ks} since the latter current does not show this anomalous K^+ dependence. Decrease in extracellular K^+ would reduce I_{Kr} and enhance I_{Ks}, elevation of K^+ should increase I_{Kr} and reduce I_{Ks}.

By 1990, Sanguinetti and Jurkiewicz had first detected I_{Kr} in guinea pig heart. Examples for drug effects on I_{Kr} in expression systems of HERG can be found in the papers of Walker et al. (1999) and Dumaine et al. (1998). Tseng (2001) gives an excellent review on the I_{Kr} current.

The Slowly Activating Outward Rectifiers I_{Ks}

General Description

The I_{Ks} current is a very slowly activating outward current, first described in ventricular myocytes of the guinea pig heart. I_{Ks} channels are constructed by at least two different proteins, the pore forming KvLQT1 (KCNQ1) and the minK protein (KCNE1). Only the association of the two proteins gives rise to the characteristic slow current kinetics. I_{Ks}, has been found in many mammalian myocytes, including human atrial and ventricular cells.

In guinea pig, I_{Ks} has a slow time constant of deactivation which is thought to cause accumulation of outward current at high frequencies, thus contributing to the frequency-dependent shortening in action potential duration (Lu et al. 2001). However, this mechanism may not work in other species. In human ventricular myocytes, the time course of I_{Ks} deactivation is reported to be fast (Virag et al. 2001). I_{Ks} is modulated by phosphorylation, β-adrenoceptor stimulation, for instance, activates the current (at least in guinea pig, Yazawa and Kameyama 1990). Sometimes this property is used to enhance I_{Ks} current amplitude.

Current Separation

Since I_{Ks} is difficult to separate from other outward currents in cardiac cells, expression systems are often used for detailed study. There are some selective blockers of I_{Ks} available, which allow the dissection of a blocker-sensitive current component from total current, which is then defined as I_{Ks}. The most potent selective blocker of I_{Ks} is the chromanol derivative HMR 1556 (overview by Gerlach 2001).

Current-Voltage Relation, Steady-State Activation, Lack of Inactivation

I_{Ks} activates with time constants in the range of 200 ms, maximum amplitude is only reached after several seconds (Fig. 9a). With more positive potentials, the current increases monotonously in amplitude. A typical I-V curve of I_{Ks} is shown in Fig. 9b. On returning to the holding potential, or a potential clearly positive of the reversal potential, I_{Ks} currents deactivate with an exponential time course. Plotting the peak amplitude of tail current versus test potential results in a sigmoidal curve, which reflects the steady-state activation curve.

Again, the potential for half maximum activation is an important value characteristic of I_{Ks} (Fig. 9c,d). Since this current does not inactivate during membrane depolarisation, a steady-state inactivation curve cannot be constructed. I_{Ks} is quite temperature dependent.

Separation of I_{Kr} and I_{Ks} by the "Envelop-of-Tails" Test

The envelop-of-tails test is a classical clamp protocol to separate current components in sheep Purkinje fibres. The idea is, that with a single current species, the time dependent increase in maximum current amplitude and deactivating tail current amplitude

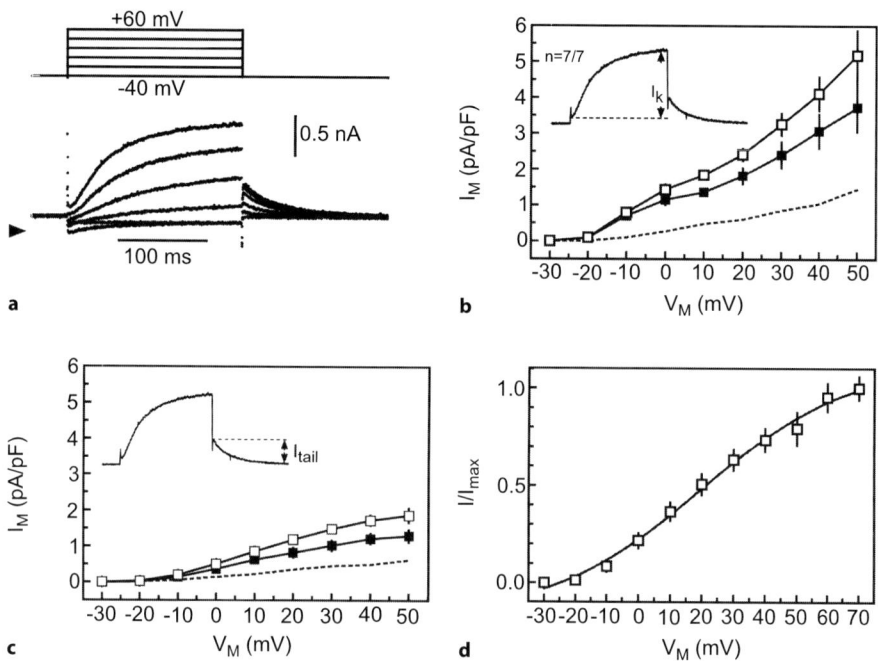

Figure 9a–d
Outward currents in guinea pig ventricular myocytes (mainly I_{Ks}). **a** Clamp protocol and current recordings of slowly activating outward current. **b** I-V curve of outward current I_K, directly after access to cell (□) and 5 min later (■). **c** I-V curve of tail current immediately after access to cell (○) and 5 min later (●). The *dotted lines* in (b) and (c) depict the fraction of spontaneous current reduction. **d** Activation curve for outward current I_K, $V_{0.5}$ was determined with 19.7 mV. The tail current included both I_{Kr} and I_{Ks}. $V_{0.5}$ of I_K is nearly identical with $V_{0.5}$ of I_{Ks} (compare Sanguinetti and Jurkiewicz 1991). (Data from Wettwer 1997)

should be identical. In guinea pig myocytes this is not the case, because two current components, I_{Kr} and I_{Ks}, contribute to the activating current and deactivating tail current. With short clamp pulses, the activating outward current is small. The tail current, however, is considerably larger due to the fast recovery from inactivation of the I_{Kr} component, so that the quotient of tail and activating current is larger than 1, but decreases with longer clamp pulses. For a genuine current, this quotient should be constant and independent of the pulse duration, and should be determined by the driving force of the respective ion species (~0.4 in case of I_{Ks}). In guinea pig myocytes, this can be accomplished by blocking I_{Kr} with E-4031, a selective I_{Kr} blocker. The envelop-of-tails-test was frequently used to show the presence of I_{Kr} component in many mammalian cardiac preparations. An example of the envelop-of-tail-test in guinea pig ventricular myocytes is shown in Fig. 10.

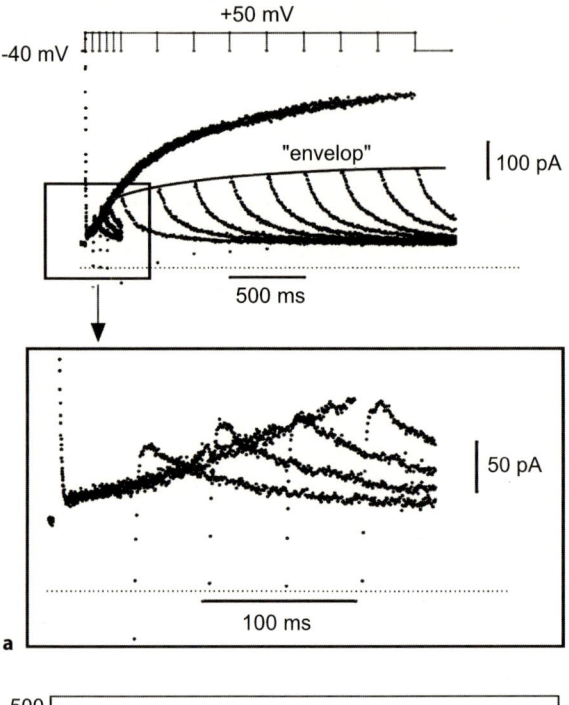
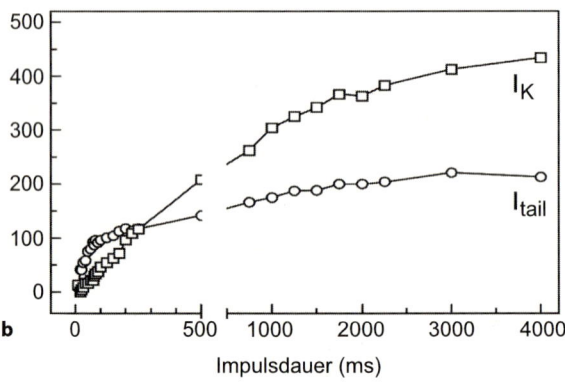
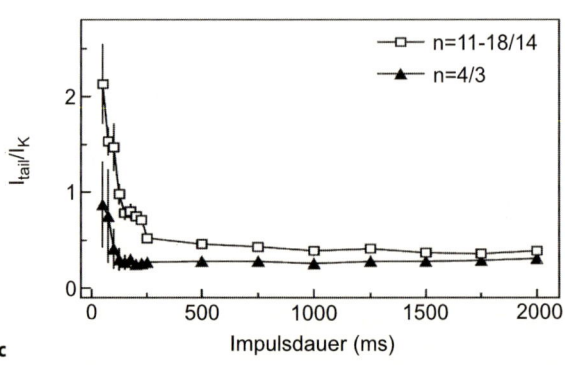

Fig. 10a–c "Envelop-of-tails" test. Two outward current components in guinea pig ventricular myocytes. **a** *Top:* Pulse protocol to activate outward currents. Holding potential –40 mV, depolarisation to +50 mV with pulse durations between 50 and 4000 ms (only shown up to 2500 ms) and current recordings of slowly activating outward currents shown in magnification for pulse durations up to 200 ms below. **b** Plot of the activating current (□) and tail current (○) against the duration of voltage clamp steps. **c** Quotient of tail current (I_{tail}) and activated current (I_K) as a function of pulse duration for control (□) and after addi-tion of the I_{Kr} blocker almo-kalant (3 μM, ▲). With pulses durations longer than 250 ms the quotient is constant (~0.4). With the I_{Kr} blocker the quotient is constant almost at all pulse durations indication that only one current component is left. (Data from Wettwer 1997)

The Ultra Rapid Outward Rectifier I_{Kur}

General Description

For the ultra-rapidly activating outward current I_{Kur}, the channel is encoded by the Kv1.5 gene. I_{Kur} is predominantly expressed in atrial myocytes, and I_{Kur} plays an important role in action potential repolarization in these cells. Therefore, it has been regarded as a potential target for the therapy of atrial arrhythmias, since inhibition of I_{Kur} should prolong the action potential duration and refractory period. In smooth muscle cells, I_{Kur} contributes to regulation of vascular tone (Clément-Chomienne et al. 1999).

Current Separation

In atrial myocytes, I_{Kur} and I_{to} activate in an overlapping time window and potential range. Since no specific I_{to} blockers are available it is difficult to separate both currents. I_{Kur} inactivates less than I_{to}, at room temperature the inactivation is minor (Amos et al. 1996). The more negative $V_{0.5}$ of steady-state inactivation of I_{to} (−37 mV) than that for I_{Kur} (−9 mV, in human atrial myocytes), may be employed for current separation. I_{to} can be inactivated by using a positive holding potential of −20 mV (Amos et al. 1996), or by using a prepulse to positive potentials (Wang et al. 1993). I_{Kur} is also analysed in expression systems without interference from other membrane currents. A comprehensive investigation of I_{Kur}, expressed in mouse fibroblast, is given by Snyders et al. (1993).

Current-Voltage Relation, Steady-State Activation and Inactivation Curve, Recovery from Inactivation

The current voltage relation of I_{Kur} is monotonous, with no signs of inward rectification, as seen with I_{Kr}. Activation of I_{Kur} becomes faster with stronger membrane depolarisation (Fig. 11a). The steady-state activation curve, constructed from the deactivating tail currents, (measured at −20 mV) yields a $V_{0.5}$ of +4 mV in human atrial myocytes but −16 mV in a mouse fibroblast expression system (Fig. 11d). I_{Kur} is quite sensitive to temperature. At 37 °C the initial current amplitude is much larger than at 22 °C, and the time constant of inactivation is faster (Fig. 11b,d; Amos et al. 1996; Rich and Snyders 1998). Thus, I_{Kur}, is an often cited example of how optimisation of recording conditions (room temperature) may give results, that lead to misinterpretation of the physiological role of the current for the shape of the action potential in a native cell. At physiological temperature, I_{Kur} is most similar to a transient outward current than to a non-inactivating constant outward current component. Steady-state inactivation also varies with experimental conditions. In human atrial myocytes, $V_{0.5}$ is −9 mV in the fibroblast expression system and −30 mV at 37 °C. Since the inactivation time constant is rather slow compared to I_{to}, long conditioning prepulses of 5 s are needed to reach a steady state. Recovery from inactivation is biexponential in the expression system, as one fraction of inactivating current only recovers slowly from inactivation. Therefore, the interval between successive pulses has to be sufficiently long (10 s, 0.1 Hz) in order to obtain a full recovery of current.

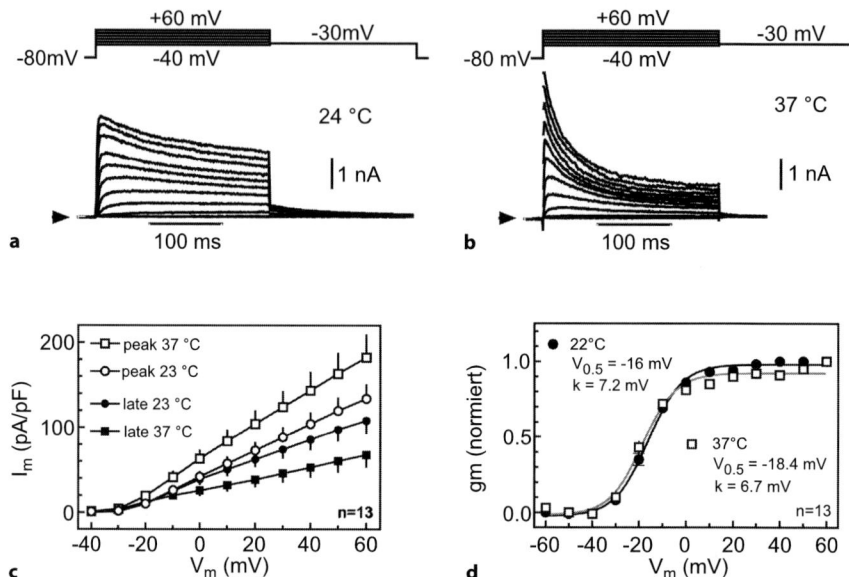

Figure 11a–d
a,b Current registrations of I_{Kur} expressed in mouse fibroblast at 24 °C (a) and 37 °C (b). Holding potential –80 mV, clamp steps from –40 to +60 mV, tail currents measured at –30 mV. c Current voltage relations for peak (□○) and currents at the end of the clamp step (late, ●■) at 24 °C and 37 °C. d Activation curves constructed from tail currents at both temperatures. (Data from Gerwe 1999)

Pharmacology

4-aminopyridine in low concentrations (10–100 µM) is a selective blocker of I_{Kur}. In native cells, I_{Kur} is blocked with an IC_{50} value of 6 µM, while the respective value for blockade of I_{to} is 1 mM (Amos et al. 1996; Yue et al. 1996). Selective blockers of I_{Kur} are developed currently by the pharmaceutical industry for tentative use in atrial fibrillation.

Rectifiers (I_{K1}, $I_{K,ACh}$)

I_{K1}. Inward rectifiers conduct current flow of K⁺ more easily in the inward than outward direction (see above). The channels are permanently open at the resting membrane potential, which is therefore largely determined by the permeability of I_{K1} channels. The inward rectifier I_{K1} is large in ventricular myocytes and much smaller in atrial cells. With membrane depolarisation I_{K1} channels close, but open again during action potential repolarization. I_{K1} therefore plays an important role in the final repolarization process of the cardiac action potential. I_{K1} can be studied with a ramp protocol, during which the membrane potential is continuously changed from negative to positive potentials (i.e., from –100 mV up to +50 mV). The idea is to depolarise the membrane at a sufficiently slow rate to allow all rapidly activating inward currents (I_{Na} and I_{Ca}) to inactivate, before further currents activate during the following poten-

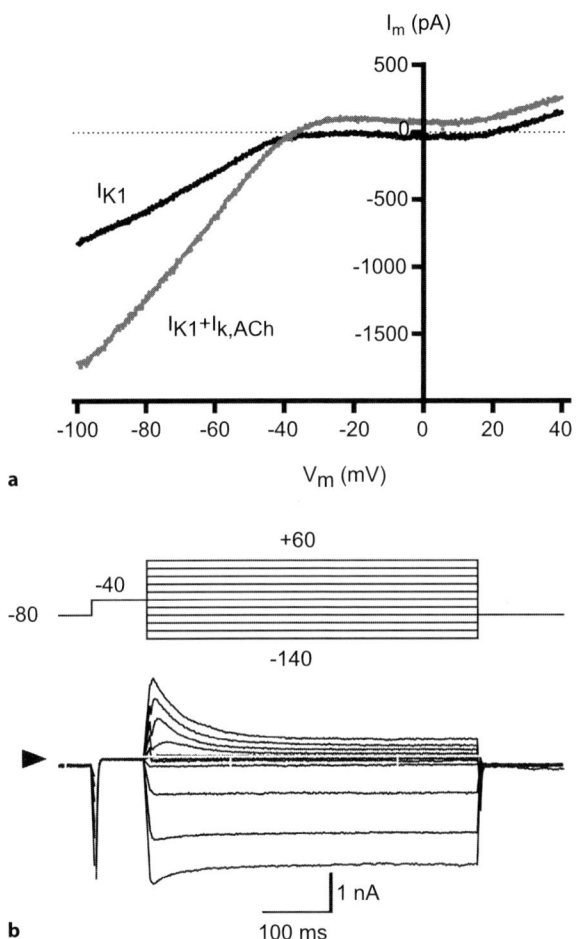

Figure 12
Inward rectifiers, registrations of I_{K1} and $I_{K,Ach}$. **a** Original recordings of total membrane currents with a ramp protocol from –100 to +40 mV in a human atrial myocyte, duration 1250 ms. With stimulation of muscarinic receptors by carbachol (2 µM) $I_{K,ACh}$ develops. Measurements were performed in solutions with 20 mM extracellular potassium to get larger membrane currents at negative membrane potentials. The reversal potential is therefore close to –40 mV. **b** Registrations of total membrane currents in a hu-man ventricular myocyte with regular rectangular clamp steps from –140 to +60 mV. Holding potential –80 mV, prepulse of 80 ms to –40 mV to inactivate I_{Na}. At potentials positive to +20 mV the transient outward current is activated. (Data from Wettwer 1997)

tial increment. If the incline of this ramp is set properly (~100 mV/s) I_{Na} and I_{Ca} will not contribute, and the resulting membrane current only represents I_{K1}. To be more precise, it consists of nearly instantaneously active currents, and only so called background or "leak currents" could contribute to the ramp current (compare Crumb et al. 1995 for non-selective currents in human atrial myocytes). With a ramp protocol, any fast activating and slowly inactivating current will be detected. Therefore, in human atrial myocytes, the fast activating I_{Kur} contributes to the outwardly directed currents, detectable with a ramp protocol (Fig. 12a), which are not apparent in ventricular myocytes where I_{Kur} is not present. The time course of activation and inactivation can only be studied with rectangular pulse protocols. As depicted in Fig. 12b, I_{K1} also shows time dependent inactivation, which is especially pronounced at strongly negative membrane potentials (Biermans et al. 1987; for a review of inward rectifiers see Vandenberg 1994 and Nichols and Lopatin 1997).

$I_{K,ACh}$: $I_{K,ACh}$ is an example of a G-protein coupled ion channel. Binding of acetylcholine to muscarinic receptors activates the heterotrimeric G-protein, leading to dissociation of βγ- and α-subunits. The βγ-subunit binds to the ion channel and enhances its open probability. Thus, $I_{K,ACh}$ is activated by a receptor-mediated process, but nevertheless has the characteristic of an inward rectifier. $I_{K,ACh}$ is frequently used for functional studies of G-protein controlled processes (compare Dobrev et al. 2001).

Since current amplitude is larger in the inward than in the outward direction, I_{K1} is often studied with test pulses negative to the resting membrane potential. If I_{K1} is small, as in atrial cells, the resting membrane potential may be shifted to positive values by elevating extracellular $[K^+]_o$ (i.e., 20 mM) to obtain larger inward currents. Since only the outward directed currents through inward rectifiers contribute to action potential repolarization, it is often important to evaluate these outward currents, although the current amplitude is much smaller due to the inward rectification of the channel.

Selective blockers for I_{K1} are not available. Both I_{K1} and $I_{K,ACh}$ are inhibited by μM concentrations of Ba^{2+} ions (Alagem et al. 2001). $I_{K,ACh}$ channels are selectively inhibited by nM concentrations of the bee venom tertiapin (Kitamura et al. 2000).

If I_{K1} currents are very large, due to high potassium conductance, as in ventricular myocytes of many mammalian species, measurement artefacts may arise (see also below, "Troubleshooting"). Large currents may saturate the patch-clamp amplifier and lead to large voltage errors of the clamp potential, due to the current flow over the series resistance. In guinea pig myocytes, I_{K1} measured with a two-electrode voltage clamp technique reached –10 nA at –120 mV (Biermans et al. 1987).

Troubleshooting

Most of the technical problems arising from electrical or mechanical noise will be discussed in this book. You will find good advice in Chapter 5 of the Axon Guide from the Axon Company (www.axon.com), or in the handbook by Sakmann and Neher. When membrane currents are large (>1 nA), which may easily be the case if expression systems are used, substantial voltage error can occur due to a voltage drop across the series resistance. Therefore, the best possible access to the cell should always be retained, by using the largest possible electrodes. Capacity and series re-sistance should be carefully compensated. The access should also be checked within an experiment. Series and capacity compensation may, however, produce artefacts that pretend to be real membrane currents. Acquaint yourself with possible artefacts by running the same voltage protocol with and without compensation.

Careful consideration should be taken of the experimental conditions, especially the checking of extracellular and electrode solutions, for composition and also osmolarity. If K^+-currents are measured very often, the intracellular Ca^{2+}-concentration is buffered using an $EGTA/Ca^{2+}$ buffering system. Computer programs help with calculating the concentrations needed. The blockers to be used should be carefully checked for "unwanted effects" on systems other than ion channels (receptors, Ca-release etc. enzymes).

In most cases, physiological temperature is desirable as an experimental temperature. However, temperature has to be controlled and checked carefully, since the current in question may be very temperature sensitive. In addition, may be experienced due to physiological temperature, as the current kinetics is too fast and current activation cannot be separated from the capacity transients. In these cases, start your investigation at room temperature. The most serious problem one has to face in native cells is the identification of a current component.

References

Alagem N, Dvir M, Reuveny E. Mechanism of Ba^{2+} Block of a Mouse Inwardly Rectifying K^+ Channel: Differential Contribution by Two Discrete Residues. J Physiol (Lond) 2001; 534: 381–393

Amos GJ, Wettwer E, Metzger F, Li Q, Himmel HM, Ravens U: Differences Between Outward Currents of Human Atrial and Subepicardial Ventricular Myocytes. J Physiol (Lond) 1996; 491: 31–50

Barry PH, Lynch JW. Liquid Junction Potentials and Small Cell Effects in Patch Clamp Analysis. J Membr Biol 1991; 121: 101–117

Biermans G, Vereecke J, Carmeliet E. The mechnism of the inactivation of the inward-rectifying K current during hyperpolarizing steps in guinea-pig ventricular myocytes. Pflüger's Arch 1987; 410: 604–613

Campbell DL, Rasmusson RL, Qu Y, Strauss HC : The Calcium-Independent Transient Outward Potassium Current in Isolated Ferret Right Ventricular Myocytes. I. Basic Characterization and Kinetic Analysis. J Gen Physiol. 1993; 101: 571–601

Clement-Chomienne O, Ishii K, Walsh MP, Cole WC : Identification, Cloning and Expression of Rabbit Vascular Smooth Muscle Kv1.5 and Comparison with Native Delayed Rectifier K^+ Durrent. J Physiol (Lond) 1999; 515: 653–667

Coetzee WA, Amarillo Y, Chiu J, Chow A, Lau D, McCormack T, Moreno H, Nadal MS, Ozaita A, Pountney D, Saganich M, Vega-Saenz de Miera E, Rudy B: Molecular Diversity of K^+ Channels. Ann N Y Acad Sci. 1999; 868: 233–285

Crumb WJ, Pigott JD, Clarkson CW: Description of a Nonselective Cation Current in Human Atrium. Circ Res 1995; 77: 950–956

Diochot S, Drici MD, Moinier D, Fink M, Lazdunski M: Effects of Phrixotoxins on the Kv4 Family of Potassium Channels and Implications for the Role of $I_{to,1}$ in Cardiac Electrogenesis. Br J Pharmacol 1999; 126: 251–263

Dobrev D, Graf E, Wettwer E, Himmel HM, Hala O, Doerfel C, Christ T, Schuler S, Ravens U: Molecular Basis of Downregulation of G-Protein-Coupled Inward Rectifying K^+ Current $I_{(K,ACh)}$ in Chronic Human Atrial Fibrillation: Decrease in GIRK4 mRNA Correlates with Reduced $I_{(K,ACh)}$ and Muscarinic Receptor-Mediated Shortening of Action Potentials. Circulation 2001; 104: 2551–2557

Dumaine R, Roy ML, Brown AM: Blockade of HERG and Kv1.5 by Ketoconazole. Pharmacol Exp Ther. 1998; 286: 727–735

Escoubas P, Diochot S, Celerier ML, Nakajima T, Lazdunski M: Novel Tarantula Toxins for Subtypes of Voltage-Dependent Potassium Channels in the Kv2 and Kv4 Subfamilies. Mol Pharmacol. 2002; 62: 48–57

Faivre J-F, Gout B, Bril A : Tedisamil. Cardiovasc Drug Rev. 1995; 13: 33–50

Franqueza L Valenzuela C, Eck J, Tamkun MM, Tamargo J, Snyders DJ. Functional expression of an activating potassium channel (Kv4.3) in a mammalian cell line. Cardiovasc Res 1999; 41: 212–219

Gerlach U. I_{Ks} Channel Blockers: Potent Antiarrhythmic Agents. Drugs of the Future 2001; 26: 473–484

Gerwe M: Charakterisierung des Kv1.5, ein Kaliumkanal des Menschlichen Herzens, Exprimiert in Fibroblasten der Maus. Inaugural-Dissertation, Medizinische Fakultät der Universität – Gesamthochschule Essen, 1999

Hatano N, Ohya S, Muraki K, Giles W, Imaizumi Y: Dihydropyridine Ca^{2+} Channel Antagonists and Agonists Block Kv4.2, Kv4.3 and Kv1.4 K^+ Channels Expressed in HEK293 Cells. Br J Pharmacol 2003; 139: 533–544

Kitamura H, Yokoyama M, Akita H, Matsushita K, Kurachi Y, Yamada M: Tertiapin Potently and Selectively Blocks Muscarinic K (+) Channels in Rabbit Cardiac Myocytes. J Pharmacol Exp Ther 2000; 293: 196–205

Kong W, Po S, Yamagishi T, Ashen MD, Steffen G, Tomaselli GF. Isolation and characterization of the human gene encoding Ito: further diversity by alternative mRNA splicing. Am J Physiol 1998; 275: H1963–H1970

Lu Z, Kamiya K, Opthof T, Yasui K, Kodama I: Density and Kinetics of I_{Kr} and I_{Ks} in Guinea Pig and Rabbit Ventricular Myocytes Explain Different Efficacy of I_{Ks} Blockade at High Heart Rate in Guinea Pig and Rabbit: Implications for Arrhythmogenesis in Humans. Circulation 2001; 104: 951–956

Nerbonne JM : Molecular Basis of Functional Voltage-Gated K^+ Channel Diversity in the Mammalian Myocardium. J Physiol (Lond) 2000; 525: 285–298

Nerbonne, JM: Molecular Analysis of Voltage-Gated K^+ Channel Diversity and Functioning in the Mammalian Heart. In Handbook of Physiology, Section 2: The Cardiovalscular System. Oxford University Press 2001, pp 569–594

Nichols CG, Lopatin AN: Inward Rectifier Potassium Channels. Annu Rev Physiol. 1997; 59: 171–191

Rich TC, Snyders DJ: Evidence for Multiple Open and Inactivated States of the hKv1.5 Delayed Rectifier. Biophys J 1998; 75: 183–195

Sakmann B, Neher E: Single-Channel Recording. Ed: Bert Sakmann, Erwin Neher. Plenum Press, New York, 2nd edition, 1995

Sanguinetti MC, Jurkiewicz NK: Two Components of Cardiac Delayed Rectifier K⁺ Current. J Gen Physiol 1990; 96: 195–215

Sanguinetti MC, Jurkiewicz NK: Role of Externa Ca^{2+} and K⁺ in Gating of Cardiac Delayed Rectifier K⁺ Currents. Pflügers Arch 1992; 420: 180–186

Sanguinetti MC, Johnson JH, Hammerland LG, Kelbaugh PR, Volkmann RA, Saccomano NA, Mueller AL: Heteropodatoxins: Peptides Isolated from Spider Venom that Block Kv4.2 Potassium Channels. Mol Pharmacol 1997; 51: 491–498

Shieh CC, Coghlan M, Sullivan JP, Gopalakrishnan M: Potassium Channels: Molecular Defects, Diseases, and Therapeutic Opportunities. Pharmacological Rev 2000; 52: 557–593

Snyders DJ, Tamkun MM, Bennett PB: A rapidly Activating and Slowly Inactivating Potassium Channel Cloned from Human Heart. J Gen Physiol 1993;101: 513–543

Snyders DJ: Structure and Function of Cardiac Potassium Channels. Cardiovasc Res. 1999; 42: 377–390

Spector PS, Curran ME, Zou A, Keating MT, Sanguinetti MC: Fast Inactivation Causes Rectification of the I_{Kr} Channel. J Gen Physiol 1996;107: 611–619

Tseng G-N. I_{Kr}: The hERG Channel. J Mol Cell Cardiol 2001; 33: 835–849

Vandenberg CA: Cardiac Inward Rectifier Potassium Channel. In: Ion Channels in the Cardiovascular System: Function and Disfunction. PM Spooner, AM Brown, WA Catteral, GJ Kaczorowski, HC Strauss (eds.) Futura Publications, Armonk, New York, pp. 145–167 (1994)

Virag L, Iost N, Opincariu M, Szolnoky J, Szecsi J, Bogats G, Szenohradszky P, Varro A, Papp JG: The Slow Component of the Delayed Rectifier Potassium Current in Undiseased Human Ventricular Myocytes. Cardiovasc Res 2001; 49: 790–797

Veldkamp MW, van Ginneken AC, Bouman LN: Single Delayed Rectifier Channels in the Membrane of Rabbit Ventricular Myocytes. Circ Res. 1993; 72: 865–878

Walker BD, Singleton CB, Bursill JA, Wyse KR, Valenzuela SM, Qiu MR, Breit SN, Campbell TJ: Inhibition of the Human Ether-A-Go-Go-Related Gene (HERG) Potassium Channel by Cisapride: Affinity for Open and Inactivated States. Br J Pharmacol 1999; 128:444–450

Wang Z, Fermini B, Nattel S: Sustained Depolarisation-Induced Outward Current in Human Atrial Myocytes. Circ Res 1993; 73: 1061–1076

Wettwer E, Dobrev D, Christ T, Ravens U: Physiology of Cardiac K⁺ Channels: New Aspects of Channel Regulation. In: Atrial Fibrillation, ed, J.G.Papp, M. Straub and D. Ziegler. IOS Press/Ohmsha, Amsterdam, Tokio, 2003, pp 13–26

Wettwer E, Amos G, Gath J, Zerkowski HR, Reidemeister JC, Ravens U. Transient outward current in human and rat ventricular myocytes. Cardiovasc Res 1993; 27:1662–1669

Wettwer E, Amos GJ, Posival H, Ravens U: Transient Outward Current in Human Ventricular Myocytes of Subepicardial and Subendocardial Origin. Circ Res. 1994; 75:473–482

Wettwer E: Charakterisierung Spannungsabhängiger Kalium-Ströme an Menschlichen Herzmuskelzellen. Habilitationsschrift, Medizinische Einrichtungen der Universität – Gesamthochschule Essen, 1997

Wettwer E, Himmel HM, Amos GJ, Li Q, Metzger F, Ravens U: Mechanism of Block by Tedisamil of Transient Outward Current in Human Ventricular Subepicardial Myocytes. Br J Pharmacol 1998; 125: 659–666

Wettwer E, Kaiser M, Schmiedl S, Ravens U: Aktionspotential Verlängernde Wirkung der Neuroleptika Haloperidol und Sertindol an Herzmuskelpräparaten des Meerschweinchenherzens. Herzschr Elektrophys 2003; 14: 50–60

Yazawa K, Kameyama M: Mechanism of Receptor-Mediated Modulation of the Delayed Outward Potassium Current in Guinea Pig Ventricular Myocytes. J Physiol (Lond) 1990; 421: 135–150

Yellen G: The Voltage-Gated Potassium Channels and their Relatives. Nature 2002; 419: 35–42

Yue L, Feng J, Li G-R, Nattel S: Characterization of an Ultrarapid Delayed Rectifier Potassium Channel Involved in Canine Atrial Repolarization. J Physiol (Lond) 1996; 496: 647–662

Recording the Pacemaker Current I_f

Uta C. Hoppe, Fikret Er and Mathias C. Brandt

Introduction

A key feature of specialized cardiac and neuronal tissues is their ability to generate spontaneous action potentials. During the last phase of an action potential, in phase 4, a slow depolarizing inward current increases the membrane potential to less negative values until the threshold to initiate a new action potential by rapid depolarization is reached, thus producing repetitive activity. This characteristic with continuous regular depolarizations defines cardiac and neuronal pacemaker cells. During the diastolic depolarization in phase 4, there is a balance between the currents underlying this pacemaker mechanism, the delayed rectifier (I_K), inward rectifier (I_{K1}), Na$^+$-Ca^{2+} exchanger and hyperpolarization-activated inward currents (Fig. 1).

The hyperpolarization-activated inward current, also termed the pacemaker current, is activated by membrane hyperpolarization. Due to this unusual property, the pacemaker current is referred to as I_f ("funny"), I_h ("hyperpolarization") or I_q ("queer"). By convention, the pacemaker current is preferentially named I_f when considering cardiac tissue, and I_h or I_q in cells of the central or peripheral nervous system. I_f is an unselective monovalent cation current, permeable for potassium and sodium ions under physiological conditions. Ratios of K$^+$ to Na$^+$ permeability of the channel, $P_K:P_{Na}$, from 3:1 to 5:1 have been reported in different tissues. Divalent cations neither permeate nor block the channel.

The I_f-current consists of a small variable instantaneous component and a major time-dependent part. The exact significance of the instantaneous current has not yet been fully resolved. The I_f current size is voltage-dependent with increasing amplitudes at more negative test potentials. Activation kinetics get faster at more hyper-

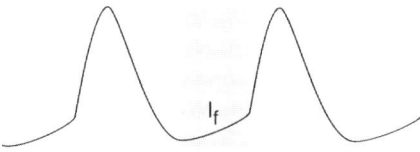

Figure 1
Action potentials of a sino-atrial node cell. A new action potential is generated due to spontaneous diastolic depolarisation; the membrane potential slowly becomes more positive until the threshold for a new action potential is reached. During this phase the I_f current is activated

polarising voltages. Another characteristic of I_f is its modulation by cyclic nucleotides (cAMP, cGMP). In cardiac myocytes β-adrenergic stimulation raises the intracellular cAMP level *via* activation of adenylyl cyclase. This function is of physiological importance as changes in internal cAMP are a key process in acceleration of the heartbeat during sympathetic stimulation. Experimental sympathetic stimulation increases I_f current size at the mid-activation potential by shifting the activation curve to more positive voltages, while the maximum current size remains unchanged. Conversely, parasympathetic activation shifts the activation curve to more negative potentials.

At least four physiological roles have been postulated for I_f:
1. triggering of spontaneous activity,
2. control of the resting membrane potential,
3. control of membrane resistance and dendritic integration,
4. regulation of synaptic transmission.

I_f and HCN-Channels

The hyperpolarization-activated inward current was initially identified in cardiac myocytes and reptile retinal photoreceptors (Bader et al. 1979; Brown and Difrancesco 1980). I_f plays a role in maintaining the resting membrane potential. In addition contributions of I_f have been suggested in cardiac and neuronal rhythmogenesis, shaping of synaptic potentials and controlling synaptic transmitter release (Chen et al. 2001). First current activation and current kinetics of I_f vary between different tissue types.

Recently, four mammalian genes have been cloned which produce an I_f-like current in heterologous expression systems. These 4 genes were named hyperpolarisation-activated cyclic nucleotide-gated cation channels (HCN1–4) (Ludwig et al. 1998; Santoro et al. 1997).

The putative structure of HCN channels is similar to that of voltage-gated potassium channels (Kv-channels, Fig. 2). HCN channel subunits are composed of six transmembrane helices (S1-S6). Four of these α-subunits are believed to coassemble and form a functional tetrameric channel complex. A loop between segments S5 and S6 forms part of the pore region. The pore region contains a glycin-tyrosin-glycin (GYG) signature which is thought to be responsible for ion selectivity. The voltage sensor is located in a specific region within the S4 segment of high positive charge density. The cyclic nucleotide-binding domain (CNBD) is localized at the C-terminal end.

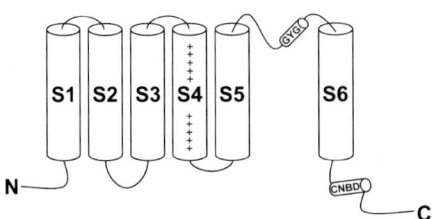

Figure 2
Structure of HCN-channels: 6 transmembrane helices (S1–S6). Positively charged S4 region. The pore region is localized between segments S5 and S6 with the GYG motif. *C* C-terminus; *N* N-terminus

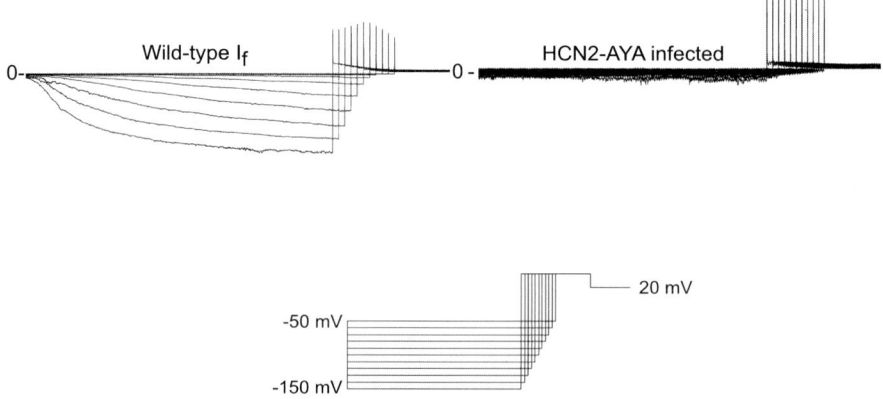

Figure 3
Neonate ventricular myocyte. Left: recording of native (wild type) I_f. Right: suppressed I_f current size after infection with a dominant-negative HCN2-mutant

Adenoviral-mediated gene transfer of an HCN2-AYA pore mutant suppressed wild type I_f in neonate ventricular myocytes (Er et al. 2003) (Fig. 3). This indicates that HCN genes are the major molecular correlate of native I_f. By functional interference, it has been proposed that different HCN isoforms can coassemble to form heteromultimeric channel complexes. Coexpression of HCN1 and HCN2 in *Xenopus laevis* oocytes resulted in an inward current, that differed from the original channel properties in its kinetics, steady-state voltage-dependence, and cAMP dose–response curve and that could not be explained as a linear sum of independent populations of HCN1 and HCN2 homomers (Chen et al. 2001). Further evidence for functional heteromerization of HCN1 and HCN2 channels has been provided by use of a concatenated cDNA construct encoding two connected subunits expressed in *Xenopus laevis* oocytes (Ulens and Tytgat 2001). In addition, an HCN2-pore mutant was demonstrated to suppress HCN4 in a dominant-negative fashion when coexpressed in CHO cells (Er et al. 2003). The heteromultimerization of different HCN subtypes provides a potential explanation and molecular basis for the heterogeneity of I_f among different cell types.

As a result of cDNA injection in *Xenopus* oocytes and immunoprecipitation experiments, it has been proposed that HCN channels form the α-subunit of a possible larger structure. Co-expression of the MinK-related peptide 1 (MiRP1) and HCN accelerated protein expression and altered the activation kinetics of HCN channels. These results indicate, that MiRP1 is a potential β-subunit of HCN-channels (Yu et al. 2001). All known members of the HCN channel family are expressed in the brain. In the heart HCN1, 2 and 4 have been identified to date.

I_h and Brain

I_h plays an important role in shaping the autonomic rhythm of neurons. All known HCN-genes (HCN1–4) were found in the brain (Ludwig et al. 1998). HCN1 is mainly expressed in the neocortex, the CA1 region of the hippocampus, the superior colliculus, and the molecular cell layer of the cerebellum (Ludwig et al. 1998; Moosmang et al. 1999). HCN2 is found throughout the brain, however it is predominantly expressed in the olfactory bulb, cerebral cortex, hippocampus, thalamus, amygdalae, superior and inferior colliculi, cerebellum, and brainstem (of mice brains) (Moosmang et al. 1999). HCN3 is weakly expressed in the brain with slightly higher expression rates in the olfactory bulb (Moosmang et al. 1999). The highest expression of HCN4 was demonstrated in the olfactory bulb, habenula, thalamus and substantia nigra (Moosmang et al. 1999; Seifert et al. 1999).

Most electrophysiological information has been obtained by examinations of the thalamus (for review see Gauss and Seifert 2000). The thalamus is the "interface" between afferent sensory input and the cerebral cortex. It is the first area where incoming signals can be modulated. By interaction of low-threshold T-type Ca^{2+} channels and HCN channels the autonomic rhythm input is carried towards thalamocortical relay cells. Activation of Ca^{2+} channels leads to a steep rise in the intracellular Ca^{2+} concentration, the equivalent of Ca^{2+} sparks in confocal experiments, and high-frequency firing of Na^+/K^+ action potentials.

When Ca^{2+} channels are inactivated, Ca^{2+} sparks are terminated and the membrane potential hyperpolarizes followed by activation of I_h. A persistent activation of I_h during the spindle wave epoch shifts the membrane potential by up to 5 mV to more positive values.

This afterdepolarisation, based on I_h activity, stops the oscillation and therefore modifies the "communication" between neurons of the thalamus and the cortex (Bal and Mccormick 1996). Recent experiments on HCN2-deficient mice demonstrated spontaneous absence seizures during an increased susceptibility to oscillations (Ludwig et al. 2003).

I_f and the Heart

In the heart, I_f was primarily identified in sino-atrial node (SAN) cells. In addition to primary and secondary pacemaker cells (SAN, AV-node and Purkinje fibres), I_f could be recorded in the working myocardium of atrium and ventricle (Yu et al. 1993). I_f currents recorded in myocytes from different species and different regions vary in their first activation potentials and kinetics. In pacemaker cells, first activation occurs at voltages of about −40 mV to −50 mV (Kokubun et al. 1982; Vassalle et al. 1995; Yanagihara and Irisawa 1980). First activation of I_f in human atrial and ventricular myocytes is more negative, at potentials of approximately −60 mV to −80 mV (Hoppe and Beuckelmann 1998; Hoppe et al. 1998).

In the rabbit SA node, the dominant HCN transcript is HCN4, representing approximately 80% of the total HCN message. HCN1 is also expressed in SA nodal cells at a lower level. Rabbit Purkinje fibres contain almost equal amounts of HCN1 and HCN4 transcripts with low levels of HCN2 (Shi et al. 1999). In ventricular myocardium, HCN2 is predominantly expressed. In addition low mRNA levels of the HCN4 isoform were detected. Ventricular expression of HCN channels appears to be age-dependent. The ratio HCN2:HCN4 increases from 5:1 in neonate rat ventricle to 13:1 in adult rat ventricle.

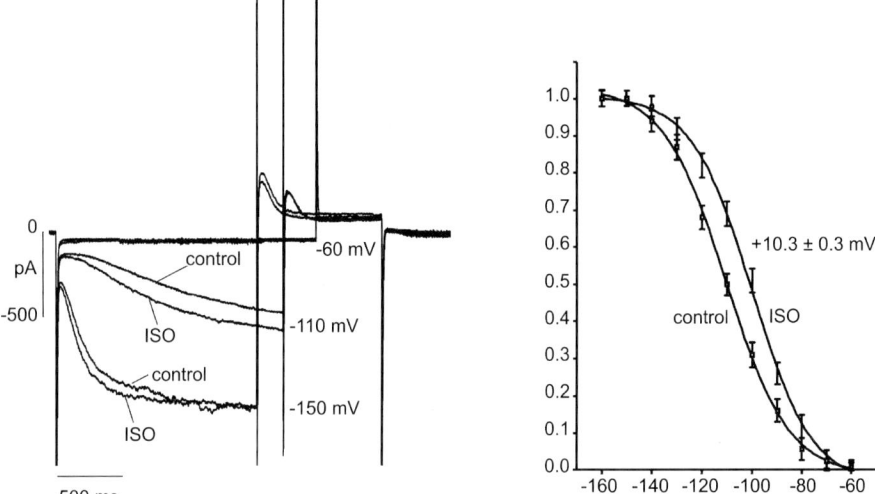

Figure 4
Effect of β-adrenergic stimulation. Human ventricular myocyte (perforated patch) in standard Tyrode's solution (control) and the same solution with addition of isoproterenol 10^{-5} mol/L (ISO). Activation curves calculated by Boltzmann fits show that isoproterenol shifts the half maximal activation by approximately +10 mV in the positive direction

A typical characteristic of I_f is its regulation by cyclic nucleotides. Elevation of intracellular cAMP levels, e.g. by sympathetic stimulation, shifts the mid-activation voltage of the I_f-current to more positive potentials, typically by about 5–15 mV (Fig. 4). Experiments with inside-out patches demonstrated that cAMP binds directly to the channel at its CNB-domain. Deletion of CNBD mimics the effect of cAMP by shifting the voltage dependence of HCN gating to more positive values by an amount similar to the maximal shift seen with saturated concentrations of cAMP. Conversely, cholinergic stimulation shifts the mid-activation voltage back to more negative potentials.

Recently a mutation of the HCN4 gene has been identified in a patient with sinus node dysfunction (Schulze-Bahr et al. 2003). Transient transfection of this HCN4-mutant (HCN4–573X) in COS-7 cells exhibited a dominant-negative effect on the wild type current. These data indicate a possible link between inherited sinus node dysfunction and mutations of HCN genes.

In diseased ventricular myocardium, the expression level of I_f is altered compared to normal myocardium. Increased current densities of I_f have been demonstrated in hypertrophy and heart failure in animal models and humans (Cerbai et al. 1994; Hoppe et al. 1998). Some authors report differences in I_f expression between ischemic and dilated cardiomyopathy. The relevance of I_f overexpression for arrhythmogenesis in the failing human heart is currently not fully understood.

In spontaneously beating neonate rat ventricular myocytes, overexpression of HCN2 and HCN4 using adenovirus-mediated gene transfer accelerated the beating rate from 80 bpm in controls to approximately 240 bpm in infected myocytes. This

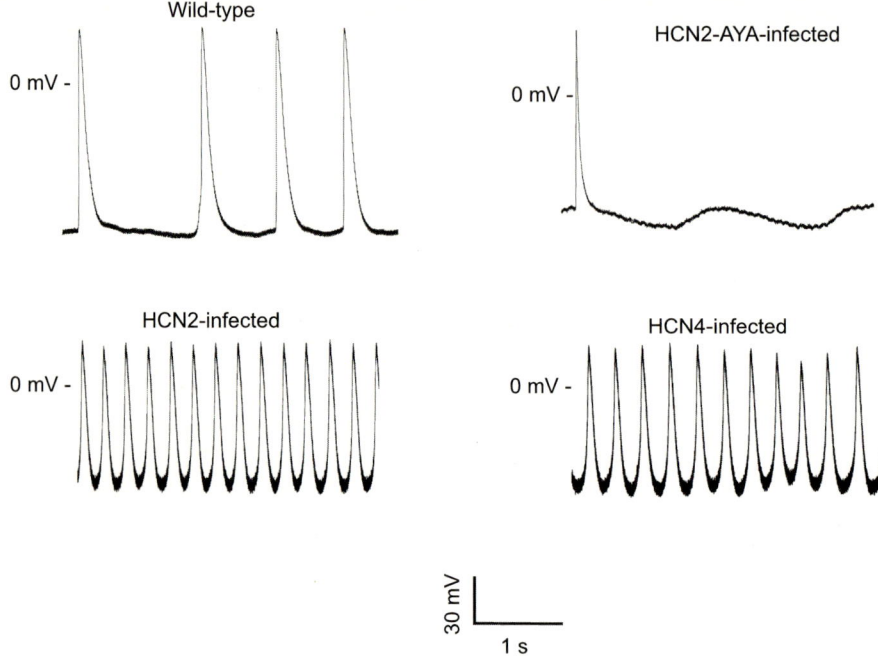

Figure 5
Effects of HCN overexpression and dominant-negative suppression on spontaneous activity of neonatal ventricular myocytes. Infection with HCN2 and HCN4 accelerates the beating rate. Conversely, infection with the dominant-negative construct HCN2-AYA, completely undermines spontaneous beating activity; the single action potential in HCN2-AYA-infected myocytes is artificially induced with a short depolarisation pulse

demonstrates an important role of HCN channels in heart rate regulation. More importantly, dominant-negative suppression of I_f undermined spontaneous beating completely (Er et al. 2003). This indicates an essential role of I_f in the generation of spontaneous heartbeats at least in neonate rat cardiomyocytes (Fig. 5).

Description of Methods and Practical Approach

I_f is generally recorded in the whole-cell configuration using the ruptured patch technique. The perforated patch method can be advantageous for experiments evaluating channel regulation and to avoid current run-down. The pulse protocol and the extra- and intra-cellular solutions differ between recordings of wild type I_f in isolated cells and experiments in heterologous expression systems.

Solutions

Generally the extracellular (bath) solution contains physiological ion concentrations, e.g. in mmol/L, NaCl 135, KCl 5, $CaCl_2$ 2 and $MgCl_2$ 1 (glucose 10 and HEPES 10 are regularly added). Recordings in native cells often require additional blockers for interfering currents. Cd or Ni is added to the extracellular solution to block the L-type calcium channel. Barium can be used to block the inward rectifier potassium current (I_{K1}), which activates in the same voltage range as I_f. 4-aminopyridine is regularly added to block the transient outward current I_{to}, which may cause interference with the tail currents of I_f.

Under physiological conditions I_f is mainly carried by potassium ions. Therefore, the current density depends on the extracellular potassium concentration. Generally K^+ concentrations used are about 5, 25, 50 and 100 mmol/L and Na^+ is adjusted to obtain equimolar concentrations. In native cells, which physiologically have small I_f current densities, it is advisable to use high external K^+ concentrations to increase current size.

The intracellular or pipette solution contains ions in physiological concentrations, e.g. in mmol/L, KCl 140, NaCl 5, $MgCl_2$ 1 (and Hepes 10). After Mg^{2+}-ATP has been added to the pipette solution (5 mM), it should be stored on ice (even during experiments). Some investigators prefer using intracellular K-glutamate or K-aspartate instead of KCl. This will lead to a appreciable liquid junction potential which has to be corrected in all measurements. The pH has to be adjusted to physiological values. The pH of the intracellular solution is adjusted with KOH to approximately 7.2 and the pH of the extracellular solution to approximately 7.4 with NaOH. For perforated patch recordings the pipette solution should contain amphotericin-B or nystatin.

Pulse Protocol

Most authors use a holding potential close to the resting membrane potential of the target cell type or close to the reversal potential of the current. In myocytes expressing a fast Na^+ current, a prepulse of about −40 mV with a length of 20–100 ms is useful to inactivate this current. Otherwise a Na^+-channel blocker like tetrodotoxin (TTX) has to be added to the bath solution.

Hyperpolarizing steps activate the I_f-current. The duration of the hyperpolarizing voltage steps should be long enough to achieve full current activation. At less negative potentials this might be difficult due to slow activation kinetics. The duration of the hyperpolarization step should be adjusted accordingly. However, even after 5 s, full current activation may not be possible close to the first activation potential. To obtain maximal current activation, hyperpolarization up to −120 mV to −150 mV is required in most tissues.

For fast current deactivation, hyperpolarization steps can be followed by a depolarization step (i.e. +20 mV). Alternatively, tail currents may be obtained by a final step to the maximal hyperpolarization potential. Finally, the voltage is stepped back to the holding potential (Fig. 6).

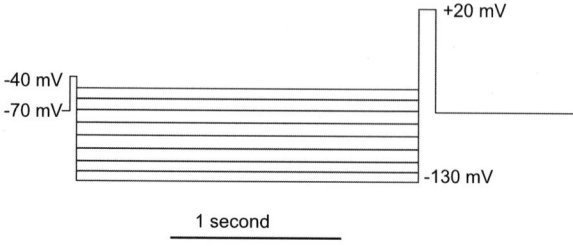

Figure 6
Example of a pulse protocol for recording in myocytes: holding potential at –70 mV, prepulse of –40 mV, hyperpolarization steps from –50 mV to –130 mV in 10 mV increments, depolarization step to +20 mV and final holding potential

I_f Registration and Current Density Measurement

The size of the hyperpolarization-activated inward current can be measured as the difference between the instantaneous current at the beginning of the hyperpolarisation step and the steady-state current at the end of hyperpolarization (Fig. 7). Alternatively, tail current amplitudes can be used to determine current size.

Current amplitudes should be normalized to the membrane capacitance to calculate current densities. The specific conductance of If can be determined for each cell according to the equation $g = I/(V_m - V_{rev})$, where g is the conductance calculated at the membrane potential Vm, I is the current amplitude and Vrev is the reversal potential which can be calculated from the analysis of tail currents. In the example given above, V_m is –100 mV and V_{rev} is –16.7 mV. I is calculated as –1435 pA– (–67 pA) = –1368 pA. The current density (membrane capacitance 30 pF) is 1368 pA/30 pF –45.6 pA/pF. The specific conductance in the example can be calculated as g = 45.6 pA/pF/(–100 mV+16.7 mV).

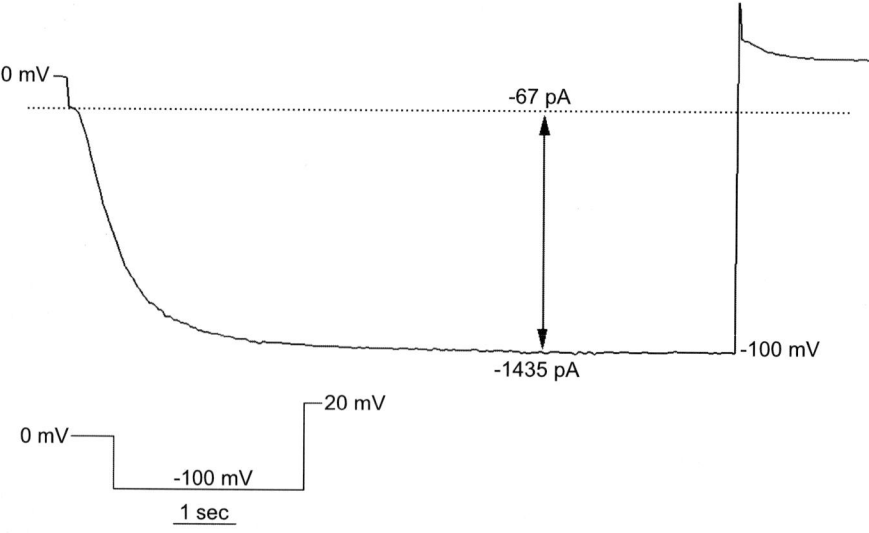

Figure 7
Measurement of the absolute current amplitude at hyperpolarization to –100 mV: difference between the steady state and instantaneous current [–1435 pA– (–67 pA)]

The voltage dependence of I_f activation is usually assessed by the activation curve, in which the conductance is plotted as a function of the hyperpolarization step used to activate the current. Typically, these activation curves show an S-shaped dependence on hyperpolarization voltages and can be fitted well by a Boltzmann function, $g/g_{max} = 1/\{1+\exp[(V_{1/2}-V_m)/S]\}$, where V_m is the membrane voltage, $V_{1/2}$ the voltage at half-maximal activation and S a slope factor at $V_m = V_{1/2}$

Current Reversal Potential

The reversal potential (V_{rev}) is the potential at which the electrochemical gradients for inward and outward currents across the cell membrane are equal. It depends on the intra- and extra-cellular concentrations of the traversing ions. A pure potassium-selective channel should have a reversal potential closed to the equilibrium potential for potassium. I_f shows reversal potentials of more positive values, indicating an additional permeability for ions other than potassium. The other physiological ion permeating the I_f channel is sodium; therefore the reversal potential of the I_f-current is more positive than expected for a strictly potassium-selective channel. The effects of different extracellular concentrations of potassium and additional ions other than sodium are shown in Table 1.

Current reversal in the presence of extracellular Li^+ indicates permeability for this cation in addition to potassium. Permeability for rubidium (Rb^+) has also been shown (Maruoka et al. 1994), whereas no evidence exists for a permeability of choline.

Interestingly, the sodium conductance of I_f depends on the presence of extracellular potassium. Without external potassium the permeability for sodium decreases dramatically.

Figure 8a shows an original recording of I_f current reversal in a human atrial myocyte $[K^+]_o$ 25 mmol/L. To open the I_f channels the cell membrane was hyperpolarized to –120 mV for 1 s. Tail currents were obtained by depolarization steps from +20 mV to –50 mV in 10 mV increments. The tail current size was measured as the difference between the positive or negative peak at the beginning of the depolarization step and

Table 1
Effects of extracellular cations on current reversal in Na^+-free solutions

$[K^+]_o$ [mmol/L]	$[choline]_o$ [mmol/L]	$[Li^+]_o$ [mmol/L]	Vrev [mV]
140	–	–	2.3±0.1
25	115	–	–44.6±1.2
50	90	–	–25.5±1.2
50	90+1 µmol/L atropine	–	–24.9±1.9
25	–	115	–34.5±1.1
50	–	90	–21.1±1.7

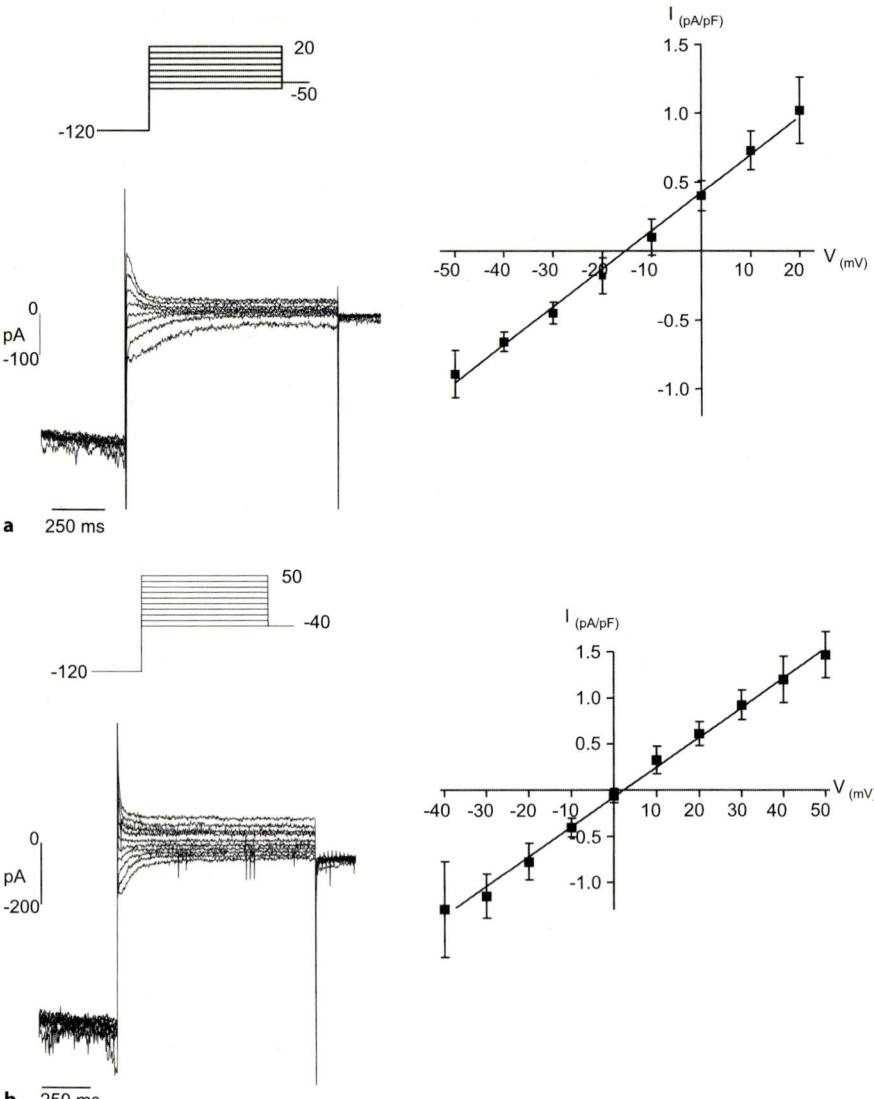

Figure 8
Effect of the extracellular potassium concentration on the reversal potential of I_f in human atrial myocytes. Original current recordings and I–V relations indicate a reversal potential of −15.3 mV at $[K^+]_o$ 25 mmol/L (A) and 2.3 mV at $[K^+]_o$ 140 mmol/L (B) respectively

the steady-state current at the end of depolarization. The tail current amplitudes were normalized to the membrane capacitance. For easier identification of the reversal potential, tail current densities were plotted as a function of the depolarization voltage s. The reversal potential is the voltage where the current density is 0 pA/pF. Best fit through data points gave a linear relationship with a reversal potential of

−15.3±0.3 mV (K_o 25 mmol/L). This reversal potential was more positive than would be expected for a pure potassium conductance. The relative permeability of potassium and sodium ($P_{Na/K}$) was estimated by fitting the Goldmann-Hodgkin-Katz equation. The $P_{Na/K}$ ratio calculated for a $[Na^+]_i$ range of 1–10 mmol/L was 0.45–0.47. Figure 8b shows I_f current reversal in an external solution containing a potassium concentration of 140 mmol/L and no sodium. The calculated reversal potential after fitting was 2.3±0.1 mV, close to the predicted pure potassium conductance.

I_f Blocking

Several blockers of the hyperpolarization-activated current have been characterized. The most frequently used blockers are discussed below.

The "classic" I_f-blocker is probably caesium (Cs^+, Fig. 9). Low concentrations of Cs^+ (0.1–5 mM) reduce the time-dependent inward current voltage-dependently and reversibly. As for all reversible blockers, it is useful to apply caesium by a perfusion system, which also allows a washout. Cs^+ blocks the channel from the extracellular (out)side. It has been proposed, that Cs^+ ions enter the channel pore for a fraction of the electrical distance (~71% from outside) before binding to the blocking side (Difrancesco 1982).

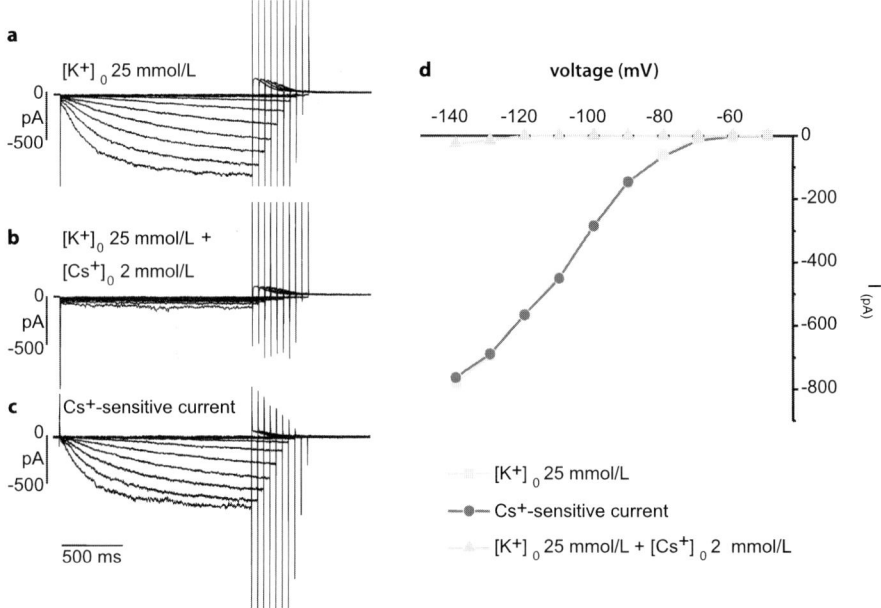

Figure 9a–d
Human ventricular myocyte. Effect of external Cs^+ on the hyperpolarization-activated inward current. Current traces of a single cell hyperpolarized in standard Tyrode's solution before (**a**) and during (**b**) the addition of 2 mmol/L external Cs^+. **c** Cs^+-sensitive current. **d** I-V relations in presence and absence of Cs^+. *For coloured version see appendix*

Falipamil, which has been developed by structural modification of the calcium-antagonist verapamil by replacement of the lipophilic alpha-isopropylacetonitrile moiety by various heterocyclic ring systems, blocks I_f in micromolar concentrations (Van Bogaert and Goethals 1987). UL-FS49 a modified derivate of falipamil gives more specific blocks at similar concentrations. Block of I_f by UL-FS49 takes effect from the intracellular side of the channel and decreases at more negative potentials (Difrancesco 1994). In addition to I_f-blockade, UL-FS49 reduces the current sizes of I_K, I_{CaL} and I_{CaT}.

For clinical applications the most promising blocking agent at present is ivabradine. Recently, ivabradine was introduced successfully in a clinical trial (Borer et al. 2003). In a double-blind placebo-controlled study, ivabradine improved exercise tolerance and increased the time until the first development of ischemia during exercise in patients with coronary heart disease (Borer et al. 2003). This effect is presumably due to a reduction in the heart rate and thus a decrease in myocardial oxygen demand. In cell-attached and in inside-out macro-patch configurations, it could be demonstrated that ivabradine interacts with I_f channels from the intracellular side of the channel complex (Bois et al. 1996). Ivabradine blocks I_f channels at concentrations of about 3 µM. Ivabradine is an open channel blocker (Bucchi et al. 2002).

Examples

I_f Recording Solutions

The composition of intra- and extracellular solutions suitable for I_f recording have been described. Figure 10 shows the effect of varying extracellular potassium concentrations on native I_f in a single human atrial myocytes.

The extracellular solution with a physiological potassium concentration contained (in mmol/L), NaCl 140, KCl 5, $CaCl_2$ 2, glucose 10, $MgCl_2$ 1 and HEPES 10.

The potassium concentration was decreased/increased to 0 mmol/L, 5 mmol/L, 25 mmol/L, and 140 mmol/L. NaCl was adjusted equimolarly. Since the recordings were performed in an atrial myocyte, the interfering currents I_{CaL}, I_{K1} and I_{to} were blocked by the addition of Cd^{2+} (100 µmol/L), Ba^{2+} (5 mmol/L) and 4-aminopyridine (4 mmol/L), respectively. Ba^{2+} also reduced the I_f current (Fig. 11). Therefore, the concentration of Ba^{2+} should not exceed the minimal concentration necessary to block the inward rectifier current. With high potassium concentrations the maximum current size and activation speed increased. The micropipette electrode solution used for these measurements contained (in mmol/L), K-glutamate 130, KCl 15, NaCl 5, $MgCl_2$ 1, HEPES 10, Mg-ATP 5 and EGTA 5.

The extracellular and intracellular solutions used in this experiment lead to a liquid junction potential of approximately –10 mV, mainly due to the high internal K-glutamate concentration.

The pH was adjusted to 7.2 with KOH. EGTA was added to the pipette solution to buffer internal Ca^{2+}, which may be helpful in patch clamp experiments on vulnerable cardiomyocytes.

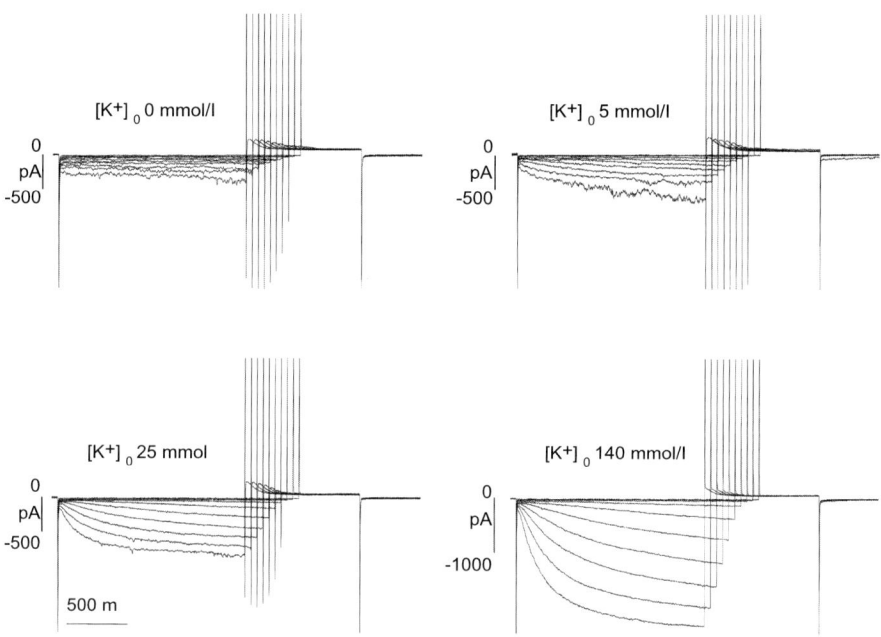

Figure 10
Effect of the extracellular potassium concentration on I_f current size. Current recordings of a single human atrial myocyte superfused with 0 mmol/L, 5 mmol/L, 25 mmol/L and 140 mmol/L $[K^+]_o$

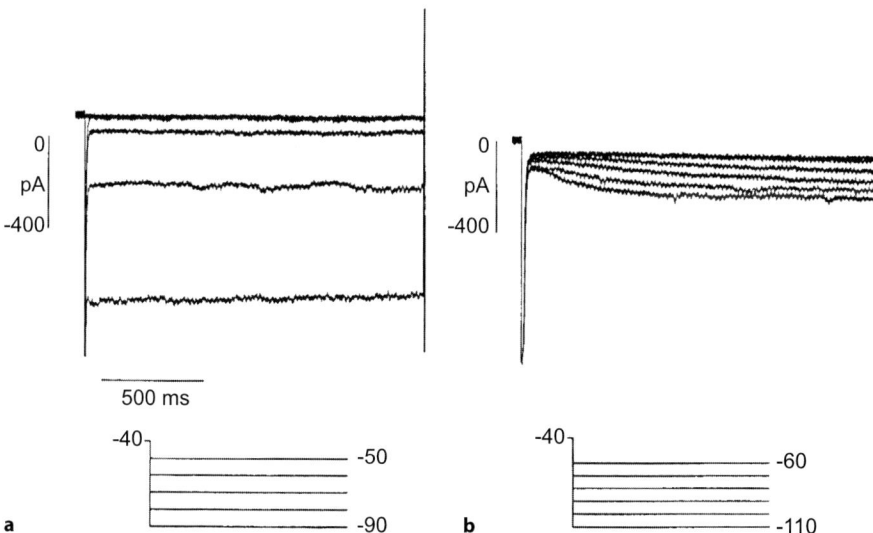

Figure 11a,b
Human ventricular myocyte. Current recordings in the absence (a) and presence (b) of 5 mmol/L extracellular Ba^{2+}. **a** The I_f current is overlapped by a large I_{K1} current

Troubleshooting

Failing I_f Registration

A cell has been patched in whole-cell configuration using the ruptured-patch technique. The capacitance could be measured without any relevant leak, however no typical I_f current can be recorded.

Choose a pulse protocol with a single hyperpolarization step to a very negative potential where full current activation is expected, preferentially between –120 mV and –150 mV.

The Software Settings are Correct but There is Still No Measurable I_f. Check the intra- and extra-cellular solutions. In native cells it is necessary to block interfering currents. This is particularly important for the inward rectifier I_{K1}, which activates in the same voltage range as I_f and may be blocked by external Ba^{2+}. On the other hand Ba^{2+} itself decreases the I_f current size (see Fig. 11). Therefore, the external Ba^{2+} concentration should be reduced to the minimal concentration which is necessary to block I_{K1} effectively. In addition, elevation of the external potassium concentration may be helpful, especially in cells with low native I_f current densities. In working myocardium, an extracellular potassium concentration of 25 mmol/L has been used preferentially.

Remember that the pipette solution should be stored on ice, since Mg^{2+}ATP degenerates at room temperature.

If I_f current can still not be recorded, check whether I_f has been recorded before in the chosen cell type. In some cells, such as rabbit ventricular myocytes, no I_f current has been detected so far.

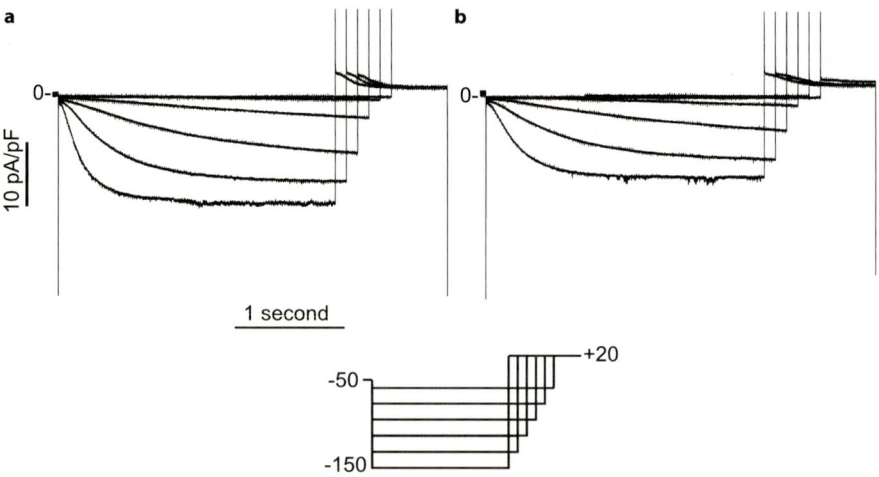

Figure 12a,b
HCN4 infected neonate cardiomyocyte. Original current recordings performed immediately after rupturing the membrane (**a**) and 10 min later (**b**) demonstrate a marked current run-down

Time-dependent current run-down may reduce I_f current size and may make I_f virtually undetectable. To check whether or not the current exists in the chosen cell type, try to start the recordings as fast as possible after rupturing the cell membrane or use the perforated-patch technique (Fig. 12).

Another possible reason for recordings without any I_f current may be the cell isolation technique. Macroscopically well-shaped and striated cells do not always guarantee electrophysiologically competent cells.

Finally in every error search the hardware setup should be included, e.g. using a hardware cell model.

Beta-Adrenergic Stimulation Does not Show Any Effects. In experiments using the ruptured-patch technique, current run-down might interfere with current increase at mid-activation potentials by β-adrenergic stimulation. To avoid current run-down and obtain the expected shift of the activation curve, experiments should be performed using the perforated-patch technique.

An Assumed I_f Blocker Does not Show Any Effect. Remember that some blockers like ivabradine are open channel blockers. Thus, channels have to be opened by hyperpolarisation for the blocker to interact with the ion channel subunits.

References

Bader CR, Macleish PR, Schwartz EA (1979) A voltage-clamp study of the light response in solitary rods of the tiger salamander. J Physiol 296: 1–26

Bal T, McCormick DA (1996) What stops synchronized thalamocortical oscillations? Neuron 17: 297–308

Bois P, Bescond J, Renaudon B, Lenfant J (1996) Mode of action of bradycardic agent, S 16257, on ionic currents of rabbit sinoatrial node cells. Br J Pharmacol 118: 1051–1057

Borer JS, Fox K, Jaillon P, Lerebours G (2003) Antianginal and antiischemic effects of ivabradine, an I(f) inhibitor, in stable angina: a randomized, double-blind, multicentered, placebo-controlled trial. Circulation 107: 817–823

Brown H, Difrancesco D (1980) Voltage-clamp investigations of membrane currents underlying pace-maker activity in rabbit sino-atrial node. J Physiol 308: 331–351

Bucchi A, Baruscotti M, DiFrancesco D (2002) Current-dependent block of rabbit sino-atrial node I(f) channels by ivabradine. J Gen Physiol 120: 1–13

Cerbai E, Barbieri M, Mugelli A (1994) Characterization of the hyperpolarization-activated current, I(f), in ventricular myocytes isolated from hypertensive rats. J Physiol 481 (Pt 3): 585–591

Chen S, Wang J, Siegelbaum SA (2001) Properties of hyperpolarization-activated pacemaker current defined by coassembly of HCN1 and HCN2 subunits and basal modulation by cyclic nucleotide. J Gen Physiol 117: 491–504

DiFrancesco D (1982) Block and activation of the pace-maker channel in calf purkinje fibres: effects of potassium, caesium and rubidium. J Physiol 329: 485–507

DiFrancesco D (1994) Some properties of the UL-FS 49 block of the hyperpolarization-activated current (i(f)) in sino-atrial node myocytes. Pflugers Arch 427: 64–70

Er F, Larbig R, Ludwig A, Biel M, Hofmann F, Beuckelmann DJ, Hoppe UC (2003) Dominant-negative suppression of HCN channels markedly reduces the native pacemaker current I(f) and undermines spontaneous beating of neonatal cardiomyocytes. Circulation 107: 485–489

Gauss R, Seifert R (2000) Pacemaker oscillations in heart and brain: a key role for hyperpolarization-activated cation channels. Chronobiol Int 17: 453–469

Hoppe UC, Beuckelmann DJ (1998) Characterization of the hyperpolarization-activated inward current in isolated human atrial myocytes. Cardiovasc Res 38: 788–801

Hoppe UC, Jansen E, Sudkamp M, Beuckelmann DJ (1998) Hyperpolarization-activated inward current in ventricular myocytes from normal and failing human hearts. Circulation 97: 55–65

Kokubun S, Nishimura M, Noma A and Irisawa H (1982) Membrane currents in the rabbit atrioventricular node cell. Pflugers Arch 393: 15–22

Ludwig A, Budde T, Stieber J et al. (2003) Absence epilepsy and sinus dysrhythmia in mice lacking the pacemaker channel HCN2. Embo J 22: 216–224

Ludwig A, Zong X, Jeglitsch M, Hofmann F, Biel M (1998) A family of hyperpolarization-activated mammalian cation channels. Nature 393: 587–591

Maruoka F, Nakashima Y, Takano M, Ono K, Noma A (1994) Cation-dependent gating of the hyperpolarization-activated cation current in the rabbit sino-atrial node cells. J Physiol 477 (Pt 3): 423–435

Moosmang S, Biel M, Hofmann F, Ludwig A (1999) Differential distribution of four hyperpolarization-activated cation channels in mouse brain. Biol Chem 380: 975–980

Santoro B, Grant SG, Bartsch D, Kandel ER (1997) Interactive cloning with the SH3 domain of N-src identifies a new brain specific ion channel protein, with homology to eag and cyclic nucleotide-gated channels. Proc Natl Acad Sci USA 94: 14815–14820

Schulze-Bahr E, Neu A, Friederich P, Kaupp UB, Breithardt G, Pongs O, Isbrandt D (2003) Pacemaker channel dysfunction in a patient with sinus node disease. J Clin Invest 111: 1537–1545

Seifert R, Scholten A, Gauss R, Mincheva A, Lichter P, Kaupp UB (1999) Molecular characterization of a slowly gating human hyperpolarization-activated channel predominantly expressed in thalamus, heart, and testis. Proc Natl Acad Sci USA 96: 9391–9396

Shi W, Wymore R, Yu H, Wu J, Wymore RT, Pan Z, Robinson RB, Dixon JE, McKinnon D, Cohen IS (1999) Distribution and prevalence of hyperpolarization-activated cation channel (HCN) mRNA expression in cardiac tissues. Circ Res 85: e1–6

Ulens C, Tytgat J (2001) Functional heteromerization of HCN1 and HCN2 pacemaker channels. J Biol Chem 276: 6069–6072

Van Bogaert PP, Goethals M (1987) Pharmacological influence of specific bradycardic agents on the pacemaker current of sheep cardiac Purkinje fibres. A comparison between three different molecules. Eur Heart J 8 [Suppl L]: 35–42

Vassalle M, Yu H, Cohen IS (1995) The pacemaker current in cardiac Purkinje myocytes. J Gen Physiol 106: 559–578

Yanagihara K, Irisawa H (1980) Inward current activated during hyperpolarization in the rabbit sinoatrial node cell. Pflugers Arch 385: 11–19

Yu H, Chang F, Cohen IS (1993) Pacemaker current exists in ventricular myocytes. Circ Res 72: 232–236

Yu H, Wu J, Potapova I et al. (2001) MinK-related peptide 1: A beta subunit for the HCN ion channel subunit family enhances expression and speeds activation. Circ Res 88: E84–87

Recording Gap Junction Currents

Ardawan J. Rastan and Stefan Dhein

Introduction

The heart acts as a functional syncytium that allows coordinated contraction and ejection of blood. The prerequisite of this behaviour is successful propagation of the action potential from cell to cell. There is broad consensus, that the transfer of an action potential from cell to cell is realized *via* gap junction channels. These channels can be considered to be low resistance pathways that allow current, ions, and small molecules (molecules <1000 D or with an ionic radius <0.8–1.0 nm; there is a slightly higher conductivity for cations over anions) to pass from one cell to the next. Gap junction channels (approx. length 100–150 Å, approx. pore width 12.5 Å, bridging the 20 Å gap between the cells) are dodecamers composed from proteins that are termed connexins. Each of the neighbouring cells provides a hexameric hemi-channel, a connexon consisting of 6 connexins. Two of these connexons dock to each other *via* their extracellular loops thereby forming the complete gap junction channel. There exist a number of isoforms of the connexins, which all belong to one protein family comprising two groups (group I: Cx26, Cx30, Cx30.3, Cx31, Cx31.1, Cx32; group II: Cx33, Cx37, Cx38, Cx40, Cx42, Cx43, Cx45, Cx50, Cx56; for details see: Bennett et al. 1995; Bruzzone 2001). A connexin consists of an intracellular N-terminal, 4 transmembrane domains, 2 extracellular and 1 intracellular loops and an intracellular C-terminal. The C-terminal is the most variable part of a connexin and differs in length and amino acid sequence between the various connexin isoforms. Connexins are defined by their molecular weight, i.e. Cx43 means a connexin of 43 kD molecular weight. The C-terminal is the most variable part of a connexin and contains consensus sequences that can be phosphorylated by protein kinases (for detailed information and species variability see Dhein 1998). Such phosphorylation reactions have been shown to play a role in regulation of channel conductance and of its degradation. In the heart muscle there are mainly three subtypes of connexins, Cx40, Cx43 and Cx45. Cx43 is the most abundant connexin, while Cx40 is mainly found in atrial tissue and in the conduction system. Cx45 has been detected predominantly during early development of the heart (for more details see Dhein 1998, 1998a).

As stated above, the dominant function of these channels in the heart is to allow propagation of the action potential from cell to cell. The normal and directed propagation of the activation wavefront is related to the subcellular distribution of the gap junction channels, which are more or less confined to the cell poles in the intercalated disks (which are referred to in older light microscopy as "Glanzstreifen") with only small amounts of the protein usually found at the lateral borders of the cell. Together with the geometry of a cardiac cell, this ensures that the action potential propagates faster along a fibre and that there is only a small propagation transverse to the fibre axis. Thus there is a directional difference between the longitudinal and transverse propagation velocities and the tissue's electrical resistance (with respect to direction), a biophysical property that is called anisotropy. Changes in this parameter, for example by incorporation of connective tissue between the fibres, are often arrhythmogenic. Moreover it has been found that atrial fibrillation may alter anisotropy (Polontchouk et al. 2001).

While classical transmembrane ionic channels typically exhibit a closed state and one open state with a certain conductivity, gap junction channels do not exhibit only one conductance state but can switch between various substates, which seem (at least in some cases) to depend on the phosphorylation state of the connexins. However, there is still a controversy about the role of the substates in regulation of channel conductance because the latter is dependent on the portion a certain substate represents (for details see Christ and Brink 1999; readers interested in these introductory remarks are referred to Dhein 1998, for a more complete review on cardiac gap junction channels).

In principle, the channel conductance can be regulated by (a) the number of channels as well as (b) by the mean open time and the mean closed time and (c) the substate of single channel conductance. The number of channels depends on the rate of synthesis of connexins, which can be influenced by a variety of stimuli (including cAMP, angiotensin and endothelin). Furthermore, the density of channels in the membrane is regulated by the transport of the subunits from the sarcoplasmic reticulum to the trans-Golgi network (where they are assembled into connexons; Musil and Goodenough 1993) and their integration into the membrane, as well as by the rate of degradation (Brink 1998). The half-life time of these channels is 1–5 hours (in the case of Cx43, 90 minutes has been measured) rather short for integral membrane proteins (Fallon and Goodenough 1981; Laird 1996).

There are several mechanisms that have been shown to affect gap junctional conductance acutely. First of all, ions passing the channels such as Na^+, H^+, Ca^{++} and Mg^{++} can reduce gap junctional coupling. Moreover, protein kinases that can phosphorylate the C-terminus of certain connexins such as PKC, PKG and PKA as well as MAPK may influence channel conductance. Since various receptors are linked to these pathways or may alter intracellular ionic homeostasis, it is interesting to study the effects of cardiac receptor stimulation on gap junctional communication. Moreover, many drugs act on these receptors or may interfere with intracellular ionic concentrations. Thus, pharmacological interventions might also influence cardiac gap junction conductance. To study such effects it is necessary to measure the intercellular current before and after receptor stimulation or any other intervention of interest. The method of choice is the double cell voltage clamp technique, which will be described in the following paragraphs.

Description of Methods and Practical Approach

The double cell voltage clamp method is based on the classical voltage clamp (see these chapters, i.e. 3.5, 3.6, 3.7 and 3.8). However, there are two cells to be clamped. The method can be used with cultivated cells, e.g. neonatal rat cardiomyocytes (see chapter 5.2), cultivated endothelial or smooth muscle cells, or freshly isolated cells (see below). The basic principle is to control (clamp) the potential of both cells that are interconnected *via* gap junction channels thereby establishing a transjunctional potential difference. In consequence a current flows across the intercellular channels that can be measured.

Double Cell Voltage Clamp

The basic functional property of gap junction channels is their conductance and intercellular coupling. Thus, it is very often desirable to measure the conductance of gap junctional channels. In principle, there are two possibilities: one can measure the single channel conductance or the total conductance between two cells. It is important to make this choice before establishing the experimental setup, since different amplifiers or at least head stages may be used for these two kinds of investigation. A serious problem that is often encountered with gap junction voltage clamp recordings is the serial resistance (e.g. of the pipettes, see below for more details) that may disturb accurate measurements of the total resistance between two cells. The problem arises from the change in potential before and after the pipette (which serves as a serial resistor) during current injection *via* this serial resistance. According to a highly interesting paper by Wilders and Jongsma (1992) the series resistance resulting from the pipette and from the cytoplasm can make it difficult or even impossible to measure the voltage dependence of gap junctions accurately.

This series resistance problem can be, at least partially, avoided or minimized by the use of discontinuous single electrode voltage clamp amplifiers (dSEVC) or switch clamp amplifiers. These amplifiers switch between voltage measurement and current injection thereby avoiding artefacts due to the resistance of the pipettes (Fig. 1). Thus, the command voltage in the cell is held by injection of current. This is so far the normal principle of a patch clamp amplifier. However, in many cases the clamp current is continuously injected. In contrast, discontinuous single electrode voltage clamp amplifiers alternate between current injection and voltage measurement at frequencies of up to 50 kHz. Thus, during voltage measurement in dSEVC amplifiers there is no current flowing and consequently serial resistance problems are reduced (Müller et al. 1999). However, the tuning process of these amplifiers is very critical and care has to be taken to adjust the bridge balance, the proportional integral circuit, the gains and the capacity compensation correctly and to tune the command signal. The use of switch clamp amplifiers from the present point of view can be recommended for the measurement of the total conductance between two cells. However, it should be noted that the use of these amplifiers is a bit more complicated than that of normal patch clamp or voltage clamp amplifiers, since the switching frequency, gain, duty cycle and capacity compensation have to be adjusted very accurately. Since voltage should be

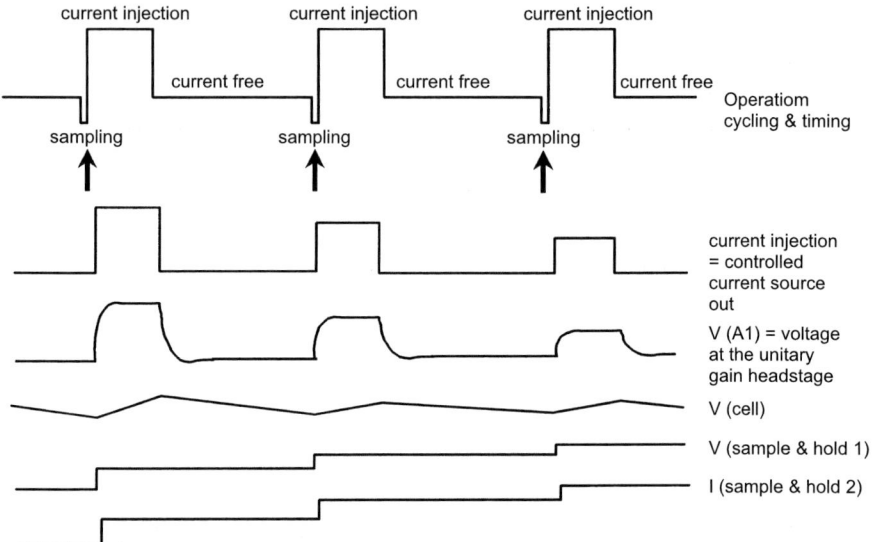

Figure 1
Working principle of a discontinuous single electrode voltage clamp amplifiers (dSEVC). Note that there is no current flowing during the sampling of the voltage

measured after the injection of current, it is necessary to adjust the system in such a way that the voltage developed on the microelectrode resistance and capacitance by the injected current is decayed prior to voltage sampling. Figure1 shows the working principle of a dSEVC. With accurate capacity compensation it is possible to measure the membrane potential at a time when no current passes through the recording electrode. However, switch clamp amplifiers are more problematic if single channel conductance is to be measured, although it is accurately possible, as was shown previously (Müller et al. 1999). Some can be used for that purpose with specially designed headstages. A disadvantage of dSEVC for single channel recording is a higher noise level. Most investigators use classic patch clamp amplifiers for measurement of single channel events.

In the authors' lab, gap junction conductance between two cells is measured using the double cell voltage clamp method with two switch clamp amplifiers (SEC-05, NPI-electronic, Tamm, Germany) in a double whole cell patch configuration. An example of the procedure is described in the following paragraph.

The double cell voltage clamp setup (as used in the authors' lab) consists of the following components:
- 2 dSEVC amplifiers (SEC 05, npi electronic, Tamm, Germany);
- 1 inverted fluorescence microscope (Zeiss, Jena, Germany) (objectives 10×, 20×, 40×, all long-working distance with correction for the thickness of the glass base of the bath; eyepiece: 10×; phase contrast);
- 2 three axis micromanipulators with electronic remote command (Luigs and Neumann, Ratingen, Germany);

- 1 break-out box (for connection of the amplifiers to the computer);
- 1 PC-system equipped with a A/D-converter;
- software (Cellworks, npi-electronic, Tamm, Germany) for controlling the SEVC amplifiers (make sure that your software can control two amplifiers; it is preferable if the software can record 2 voltage and 2 current traces). Moreover, it is necessary that the amplifiers are synchronized;
- a table protected against vibrations (pneumatic attenuation);
- bath with inlet and outlet (it is recommended to use a bath with temperature control);
- roller pump;
- tubing;
- ground;
- Faraday cage;
- pipette puller;
- microforge (optional).

It is absolutely necessary to provide a proper grounding of all components in the set-up. The microscope, the manipulators and the bath have to be shielded by a Faraday cage. The amplifiers, the PC-system, oscilloscopes and roller pump are located outside the cage. All components of the setup have to be connected to a star point (but be careful to connect each part only once to the star point!). The star point is often represented by a solid copper bar with banana jacks. No component must be coupled (directly or indirectly) more than once to the star point. Otherwise, so-called grounding loops will be created which cause noise. The star point itself is connected to the electrical ground of the Institute.

Problems often arise from the saline-filled tubes. Ingoing and outgoing tubes should be interrupted by some sort of an air-filled dropper as used with common infusion tubings.

The next point to be considered is a mechanical one. It is necessary to use a table that attenuates all vibrations, since otherwise the two cells might move against each other so that the seal might be lost. Moreover, it is necessary to use highly exact micromanipulators with electrical drives and remote control.

To establish a double cell voltage clamp, it is necessary to clamp both cells synchronously. Therefore, isolated or cultured cells are used (according to the protocols given below). Pull pipettes of 2–5 MΩ resistance, fire-polish in a microforge or treat with Sylgard. Prepare the following solutions (according to Müller et al. 1997):

Extracellular solution:
- NaCl   135.0 mmol/l
- KCl   4.0 mmol/l
- $CaCl_2$ 2.0 mmol/l
- $MgCl_2$ 1.0 mmol/l
- NaH_2PO_4 0.33 mmol/l
- HEPES   10.0 mmol/l
- glucose   10.0 mmol/l
- pH   7.4

Pipette solution (= "intracellular solution")
- CsCl   125.0 mmol/l
- NaCl   8.0 mmol/l
- $CaCl_2$ 1.0 mmol/l
- EGTA   10.0 mmol/l
- Na_2ATP 2.0 mmol/l
- MgATP   3.0 mmol/l
- Na_2GTP 0.1 mmol/l
- HEPES   10.0 mmol/l
- pH   7.2 (with CsOH)

This solution should be filtered through a sterile filter before use. It should be mentioned that the kinetics of gap junction currents (voltage dependent inactivation) are sensitive to the pipette solution used (Valiunas et al. 2000). The solutions given above are one example, but may be modified according to the demands of the experiment that is planned. Thus, others have used KCl, or tetraethylammonium aspartate (TEA-aspartate) or Cs aspartate as main charge carriers. Noise from non-junctional channels may be suppressed by adding 6 mM $NiCl_2$, 2 mM CsCl and 1 mM $BaCl_2$ to the external bath solution (Verheule et al. 1997).

Other authors (Polontchouk et al. 2002) replaced chloride by aspartate and used the following intracellular solution.
- Cs-aspartate 120.0 mmol/l
- NaCl   10.0 mmol/l
- MgATP   3.0 mmol/l
- $MgCl_2$ 1.0 mmol/l
- $CaCl_2$ 1.0 mmol/l
- EGTA (pCa=8) 10.0 mmol/l
- HEPES   5.0 mmol/l
- pH   7.2

and for superfusion
- NaCl   140.0 mmol/l
- KCl   4.0 mmol/l
- $CaCl_2$ 2.0 mmol/l
- $MgCl_2$ 1.0 mmol/l
- glucose   5.0 mmol/l
- pyruvate   2.0 mmol/l
- HEPES   5.0 mmol/l
- pH   7.4

For whole cell recordings it is also possible to use the following intracellular solution, which allows control of cytoplasmic pH, if a HEPES buffered saline (HEPES 100 mM, $CaCl_2$ 1 mM, $MgCl_2$ 1 mM, 52.5–74.25 mM K-gluconate, 7.5–0.5 mM $(NH_4)_2SO_4$) is used for extra-cellular superfusion (Grinstein et al. 1994)
- K-gluconate 100.0 mM
- KOH   8.0 mM

- MgCl$_2$ 1.0 mM
- Na$_2$ATP   5.0 mM
- PIPES   5.0 mM
- BAPTA   0.5 mM
- (NH$_4$)$_2$SO$_4$ 25.0 mM
- pH   7.0

For more details see Van Rijen et al. (2001). Transfer an aliquot of cell containing solution to the bath that is positioned on the stage of an inverted microscope or use coverslips with cells grown on top in the bath. Perfuse the bath at a constant rate of 1 or 2 ml/min at either room temperature (21–24 °C) or at 37 °C as desired. Seek for a cell pair (use a 40× objective with 10× eyepieces and phase contrast) and position electrodes in the direct vicinity of the cells. For approaching the cell we apply a small pressure to the electrode. Adjust the amplifiers and compensate for series resistance or capacity. If dSEVC amplifiers are used adjust the switching frequency to values of about 25–40 kHz. Make sure that the command potential is reached within 3–5 ms with an accuracy of <5 mV (better <1 mV) even when large currents are recorded. When the electrode is in close vicinity to the cell, the amplifier is switched to bridge mode and bridge balance and offset have to be adjusted to zero. Electrode resistance is also determined at this moment. Then a 1 nA/v 30 ms pulse is applied and bridge balance is adjusted again so that there is a zero line in the voltage signal. Thereafter, the amplifier is switched to the current clamp mode and a holding current of +150 nA is applied at a low switching frequency (<5 kHz). Then, capacity has to be compensated so that correct rectangular pulses can be seen. It is necessary that the switched signal (i.e. the output of the amplifier) shows correct rectangular pulses. Thereafter, switching frequency is enhanced to about 35 kHz and tuning has to be repeated until rectangular switched pulses can again be seen. This is then repeated for the second electrode with the other amplifier. For patching the neighbouring cell a position of the pipette should be sought which ensures that no torque is applied. Next, the amplifier of cell 1 is switched to voltage clamp mode, gain is set to zero and a 10 mV/20 ms pulse is applied while the pipette is slowly approaching the cell surface. Then gain is enhanced until the signal shows a 10 nA amplitude. Next the pipette is brought closer to the cell until the signal starts to diminish and reaches about 1/3 or 1/4 of its initial value. When the tip is near the cell, one may see a small dent on the cell surface ("dimpling") in phase contrast microscopy. Now the pressure is released from the pipette and a little suction is applied. The signal now starts to oscillate, which is terminated by reducing the gain to zero again. Now the cell-attached configuration is achieved. Negative pressure should now be released. Then seal resistance is determined and afterwards holding potential is set to –40 mV. Next, pulses of suction are applied while a –80/–40, 50 ms pulse is applied until a break-in is achieved, which can be seen from the activated sodium current signal and a larger and broadened capacity artifact. The current filter is adjusted to about 2 kHz (from initially 20 kHz).

Thereafter the gain of the proportional integral controller is enhanced until the signal starts to oscillate, and is then diminished until oscillation stops. Then the time integrator constant is enhanced until the signal shows optimal rectangular shape. It is necessary that a gigaseal (seal resistance should exceed 5 GW) should have been

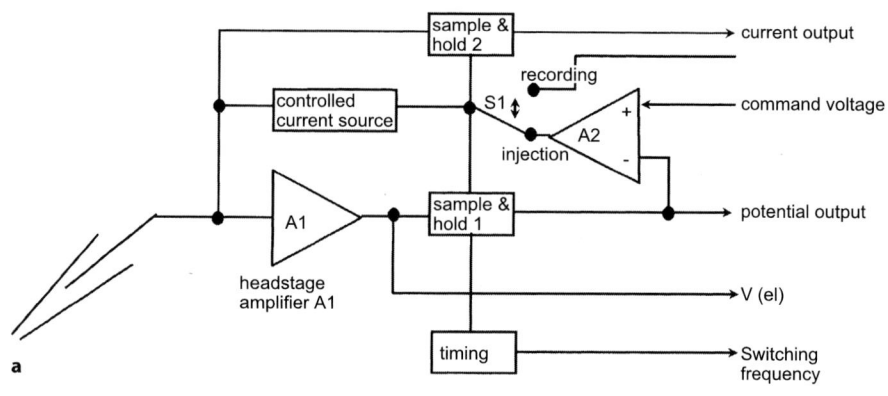

Figure 2
Schematic drawing of the experimental arrangement for a dual voltage clamp

achieved. The procedure is then repeated for cell 2. At the end a 10 mV hyperpolarizing pulse (−80/−90, 20 ms) is applied to determine membrane resistance. The holding potential is set to −40 mV.

Thereafter the cells are allowed to equilibrate with the pipette solution for about 3–5 min. 3–5 min after establishing the whole cell configuration the experiments is started. Sampling frequency is adjusted to 10 kHz and the signal obtained is low-pass filtered at 1 kHz using a Bessel filter. During the recordings 1 mmol/l $BaCl_2$ should be added to the external solution. It is important that the seal resistance is high enough and that it is equal on both sides. Any leak currents would adulterate or distort the measurements.

For dSEVCs we found the following relationships between the upper cut-off frequency (−3 dB frequency) of the electrode, f_e, the f_{sw} of the dSEVC, the sampling frequency f_s of the data acquisition system, the filter frequency f_f, and the cut-off frequency of the membrane f_m (Müller et al. 1999):

- $f_e > 3f_{sw}$,
- $f_{sw} > 2f_s$,
- $f_s > 2f_f > f_m$.

A dual voltage clamp configuration has now been established as depicted in Fig. 2. The standard method for gap junction current recording is the double cell voltage clamp technique (Spray et al. 1981, 1985; Weingart 1986) carried out as a double whole cell patch as described by Giaume (1991). The principle is that a transjunctional voltage difference (by clamping the two cells to different potentials) is applied for a short time to a pair of coupled cells and the current necessary for maintenance of the voltage difference is measured.

In order to achieve such an experimental setup, two voltage clamp amplifiers are connected *via* a patch clamp pipette to either cell (see Fig. 2). While in one cell the membrane potential is kept at, for example –40 mV, (in order to inactivate the sodium current) the membrane potential of the other cell is set to –30 mV thereby applying a transcellular voltage of 10 mV. In a similar way transjunctional voltages ranging from –50 mV to +50 mV are applied. Symmetry is controlled by alterations in the cell being kept at –40 mV. Since current can flow across the cell membrane and across the junction between both cells, the current in cell 1 I_1 can be described under these conditions by the equation

$$I_1 = (V_1/r_{m1}) + [(V_1-V_2)/r_j]$$

and accordingly the current in cell 2 by

$$I_2 = (V_2/r_{m2}) + [(V_2-V_1)/r_j]$$

with V_1 and V_2 being the voltage relative to the holding potential V_H (e.g. –40 mV in order to inactivate the sodium current) and r_{m1} and r_{m2} the membrane resistances in cells 1 and 2, respectively. If cell 2 is kept at V_H the currents I_1 and I_2 can be described as

$$I_1 = (V_1/r_{m1}) + (V_1/r_j)$$
$$I_2 = V_1/r_j$$

so that I_2 is a direct measure of the current flowing across the junctional membrane.

The gap junction conductance g_j can be described as

$$g_j = I_1/(V_1-V_2)$$

for cell 1, if cell 1 is kept at V_H and

$$g_j = -I_2/(V_1-V_2)$$

for cell 2, if cell 2 is the non-stepped cell.

A problem arises if junctional resistance is significantly lower than serial resistance or if series resistance is appreciably high (if dSEVC are not used). In that case a numerical correction for series resistance is required:

$$g_j = I_1/(V_1 - I_1 \times R_{S1}) - (V_2 - I_2 \times R_{S2})$$

for cell 1, if cell 1 is kept at V_H and

$$g_j = -I_2/(V_1 - I_1 \times R_{S1}) - (V_2 - I_2 \times R_{S2})$$

for cell 2, if cell 2 is the non-stepped cell.

The serial resistances have to be determined. If the membrane resistance is also low, this has to be taken into consideration as well and in this condition the equations have to be reformulated as:

$$g_j = I_1 - [(V_1 + I_1 \times R_{S1})/R_{m1}]/[(V_1 - I_1 \times R_{S1}) - (V_2 - I_2 \times R_{S2})]$$

for cell 1, if cell 1 is kept at V_H and

$$g_j = -I_2 + [(V_2 + I_2 \times R_{S2})/R_{m2}]/[(V_1 - I_1 \times R_{S1}) - (V_2 - I_2 \times R_{S2})]$$

for cell 2, if cell 2 is the non-stepped cell (see Van Rijen et al. 2001 for a detailed discussion).

Problems may arise from the series resistance of the pipettes and, in some preparations, eventually from the cytosolic resistance or from the ratio between these different resistances (for a more detailed discussion see Wilders and Jongsma 1992). The current measured is then plotted against the transcellular voltage V_j (see Fig. 3). Linear regression reveals the total intercellular resistance. However, at that point one has to be careful, since gap junction current can exhibit the phenomenon of voltage-dependent inactivation (see below). Thus, at higher transjunctional voltages the gap junctional current inactivates and it is necessary to distinguish between the instantaneous current and the steady state current. Thus, the linear regression is only correct for a certain transjunctional voltage range and should refer to the instantaneous current. Otherwise the analysis is more complex and both instantaneous and steady state conductances have to be considered (see below). It should also be noted that voltage-dependent inactivation has only been detected in cells which were only weakly coupled, i.e. if gap junction conductance was of the order of 10 nS or below (detailed discussion: Wilders and Jongsma 1992).

By addition of the currents flowing in the resting and the pulsed cell the sarcolemmal current in the pulsed cell can be calculated as a current-voltage relationship (Weingart 1986) and the input resistance can be estimated from the chord conductance between −80 and −40 mV. Measurements should be done in both cells alternately.

The gap junctional conductance g_j follows the equation

$$g_j = N\gamma_j P_o$$

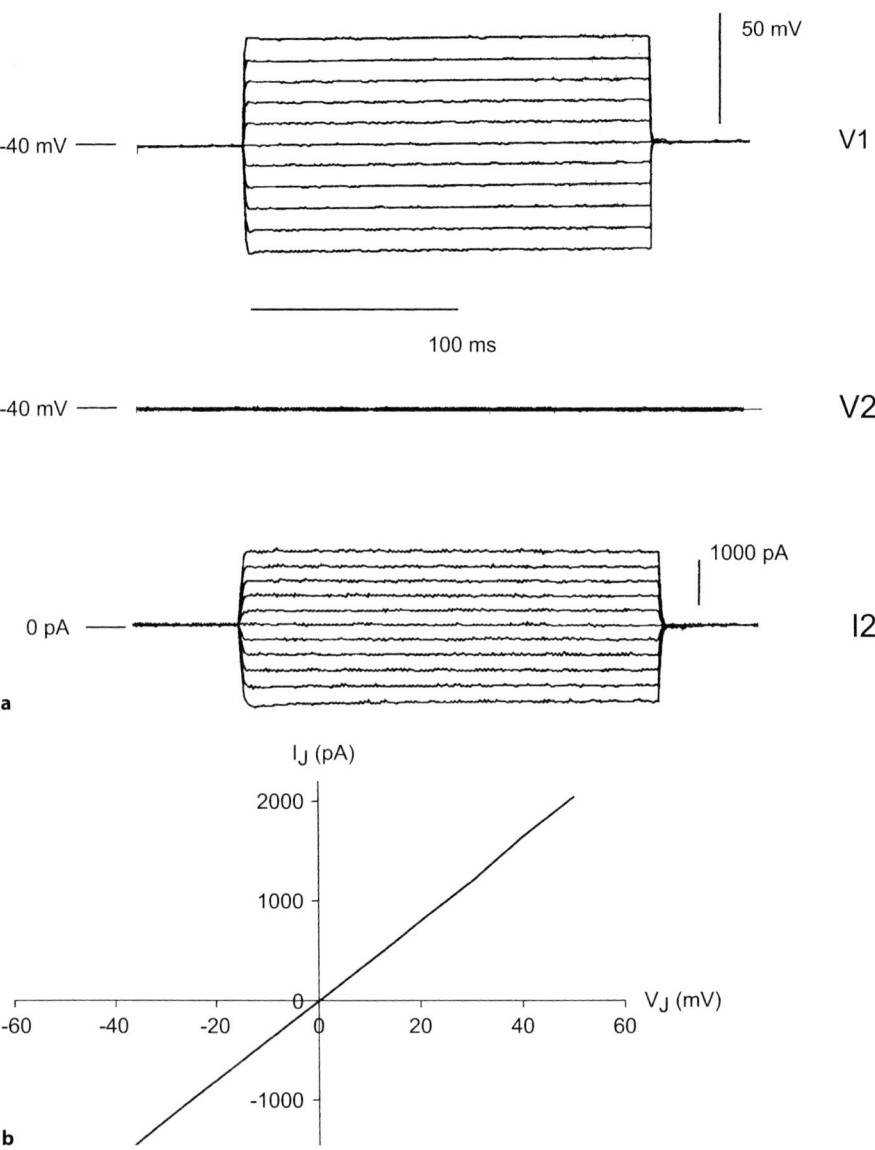

Figure 3a,b
a Family of I_j signals elicited by dual cell voltage clamp with transjunctional voltage gradients (V_j) of variable amplitude and polarity. Cell 1 was clamped to potentials ranging from −90 mV to +10 mV (pulse duration: 200 ms) while cell 2 was kept at −40 mV so that transjunctional voltages of -50 to +50 mV were applied. I_j was recorded in cell 2 as described in the text

where N is number of channels capable of opening and closing, P_o is the open probability and γ_j the single channel conductance. If under the experimental conditions described above cells are progressively uncoupled by application of e.g. heptanol or halothane, some types of amplifiers allow observation of single channel openings shortly before total uncoupling occurs. Alternatively gap junction channels can be reconstituted in lipid bilayers for observation of single channel conductances.

Voltage-Dependent Inactivation of Gap Junction Currents Using the Double Cell Voltage Clamp

Looking at the current measured using such a protocol with a pulse duration of about 2 s in weakly coupled cells, one can distinguish two components of the junctional current: (a) the instantaneous component and (b) the steady state component. Plotting the instantaneous current I_j versus V_j may reveal a linear relationship as shown by Veenstra et al. (1993) which means that the instantaneous gap junctional conductance is constant, i.e. $g_j = I_j/V_j$ = constant. A linear current voltage relationship under such conditions means that the junctional channel behaves like an ohmic resistor with a constant resistance that is insensitive to the transjunctional voltage.

If it is desired to investigate the phenomenon of voltage-dependent inactivation, it is necessary to work with weakly coupled cells which are coupled by a gap junction conductance of about 10 nS or less (Wilders and Jongsma 1992) and to use long pulses of 2 or 5 seconds length so that a stable steady state current can be recorded. Moreover, it should be kept in mind that below transjunctional voltages of 50 mV there is only weak voltage-dependent inactivation, so that it is necessary to apply high transjunctional voltage gradients ranging from –130 mV to +130 mV. For further analysis the steady state conductance $g_{j.ss}$ is normalized to the instantaneous conductance $g_{j.Inst}$. Investigation of the steady state current and the steady state conductance is normally carried out by fitting the normalised $g_{j.ss}/V_j$ relationships with the two state Boltzmann distribution which follows the function

$$G_j = g_{j.ss}/g_{j.Inst} = \{(g_{max} - g_{min})/(1+\exp[A (V_j - V_0)]\} + g_{min}$$

according to Spray et al. (1981) and Veenstra et al. (1993) with g_{max} being the maximum conductance (= 1, normalised to instantaneous $g_{j.Inst}$) and g_{min} the minimum conductance. V_0 is the half inactivation voltage where g_j is between g_{min} and g_{max} and $A = zq/kT$ (z = number of equivalent electron charges, q = voltage sensor, k = Boltzmann constant, T = temperature).

One can use either a symmetrical or an asymmetrical protocol (for details see Banach and Weingart 1996). For the asymmetrical protocol both cells are clamped to –40 mV holding potential in order to inactivate sodium current. Thereafter, one cell is clamped to potentials ranging from –140 mV to +60 mV for 2 or 5 seconds. Thereby, a transcellular voltage difference of ±100 mV can be applied and the current measured in the non-pulsed cell can be taken as the gap junctional current (Spray et al. 1981; Weingart 1986). Gap junction conductance can be calculated as the slope of the current-voltage relationship by linear regression analysis of the instantaneous current, if the relationship is linear (see above).

For each transjunctional voltage $g_{j.Inst}$ and $g_{j.ss}$ have to be calculated. Next the values for $g_{j.ss}/g_{j.Inst}$ are plotted versus transjunctional voltage V_j and the data are fitted using the Boltzmann equation given above. Figure 3.8-4 gives an example. From this

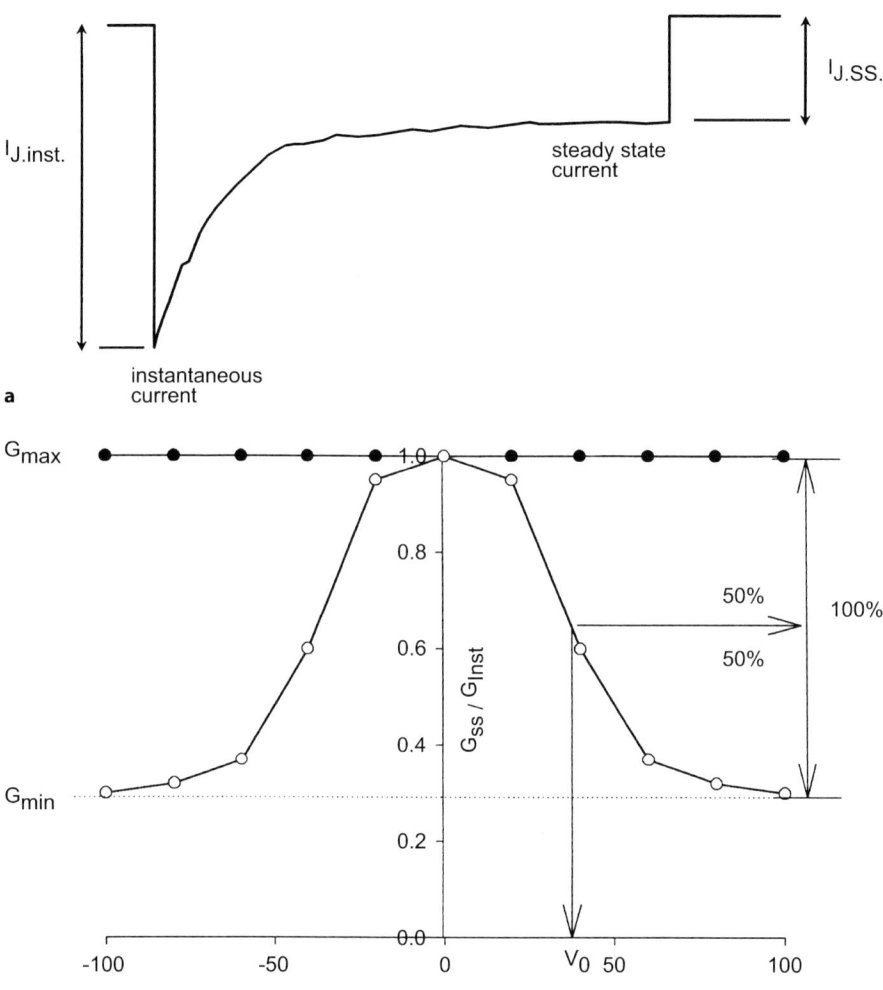

Figure 4
Example of voltage-dependent inactivation. The upper part shows a transjunctional current which shows clear voltage-dependent inactivation. The lower part shows the Boltzmann fit for a complete experiment and gives the $g_{j.SS}/g_{j.Inst}$ ratio

fit the half-inactivation voltage V_0 is calculated as well as G_{min} and the slope factor. If an asymmetrical protocol is used, it is necessary to give V_0 for negative and for positive transjunctional voltages separately.

For a symmetrical protocol both cells are clamped to the common holding potential of −40 mV. Thereafter, both cells are pulsed equally but with opposite polarity. Thus, cell 1 is clamped to −10 mV relative to the holding potential (i.e. to −50 mV in absolute terms) and cell 2 to +10 mV relative to the holding potential (i.e to −30 mV in absolute terms), then to −60 mV and −20 mV, respectively, and so forth. As was described by Banach and Weingart (1996) with the symmetrical protocol, half-maximum voltage-dependent inactivation is equal in both polarities (while it is not if an asymmetrical protocol is used).

If cells are progressively uncoupled by heptanol it is possible to observe single channel conductance, if the head stages used allow measurements in the respective current range (e.g. Müller et al. 1999). A detailed description of the methods for single channel analysis would be out of the scope of this chapter. Readers interested in single channel analysis are referred to the literature (Van Rijen et al. 2001).

Preparing the Cells for Double Cell Voltage Clamp

Isolation of Pairs of Cardiomyocytes from Biopsies

For cell pair isolation we use in principle a protocol which we learnt in the lab of Prof. Ravens and Dr. Wettwer (Dresden, Germany) and which we have slightly adapted to our needs. Directly after taking the biopsy the tissue is bathed in 100 ml 10°C Ca^{++}-free solution with 30 mM 2,3 butane dione monoxime. Thereafter the tissue is transferred to a Petri dish and carefully cut into small pieces of 1 mm³. These tissue pieces are then washed 3 times for 3 min with 20 ml Ca^{++}-free solution and gassed with O_2. Next the solution is removed and replaced by 20 ml collagenase/protease solution for 5 minutes with constant O_2 and stirred (30 °C). After 5 minutes 40 µl 10 mM $CaCl_2$ (= 20 µM) are added and the solution is constantly stirred for another 5–10 minutes (atrial tissue: 37 °C; ventricular tissue: 30 °C). Thereafter, the collagenase/protease solution is quickly removed and replaced by collagenase solution. Immediately 40 µl 10 mM $CaCl_2$ (= 20 µM) are added. The solution is constantly stirred (30 °C) and gassed with O_2 until cell pairs and isolated striated rod shaped cells become visible. To stop the digestion, the supernatant is removed and centrifuged (170×g, 5 min). The tissue remnants are immersed in Feng medium and minced using forceps. This supernatant is also centrifuged at 170×g for 5 min. After centrifugation, the supernatant is quickly removed. The resulting pellets are resuspended in 4 ml Feng medium. Thereafter the Ca^{++} concentration is enhanced stepwise. First 80 µl 10 mM $CaCl_2$ are added; after 15 minutes another 40 µl 10 mM $CaCl_2$ are added. After 15 minutes another 80 µl 10 mM $CaCl_2$ are added so that a final extracellular Ca^{++} concentration of 0.5 mM is reached.

Solutions:
1. Ca^{++} free solution
    - NaCl   100.0 mM
    - KCl   10.0 mM
    - KH_2PO_4 1.2 mM
    - $MgSO_4$ 5.0 mM
    - Taurine   50.0 mM
    - MOPS   5.0 mM
    - Glucose   10.0 mM (should be added immediately before use)
    - pH   7.2 (with 1 M NaOH)

2. Feng medium
   - KCl   20.0 mM
   - KH_2PO_4 10.0 mM
   - Glucose   10.0 mM
   - Glutamic acid   70.0 mM
   - β-OH-butyrate   10.0 mM
   - Taurine   20.0 mM
   - EGTA   10.0 mM
   - Albumin   1.0%
   - pH   7.4 (with KOH)
3. Collagenase/protease solution
   - Ca^{++}-free solution   20.0 ml
   - Collagenase (type I, Worthington)
     (254 U/mg)   22.5 mg
   - Protease XXIV
     (8.8 U/mg)   11.5 mg
4. Collagenase solution
   - Ca^{++}-free solution   20.0 ml
   - Collagenase (type I)
     (254 U/mg, Worthington) 22.5 mg

The isolation procedure described was successfully applied in our lab to rabbit, pig, sheep, and human atrial and ventricular tissue.

Isolation of Cardiomyocytes from a Guinea Pig Heart Using the Langendorff Technique

If adult cardiomyocytes are used for double cell voltage clamp it is desirable to produce a large number of cell pairs. Therefore, protocols using proteases such as trypsin should not be used, because proteases may enhance separation of the cells and disrupt or destroy the gap junctions. Similarly, protocols using proteases are critical if ion channels or receptors with large extracellular protein domains are to be investigated in freshly isolated cells. In the authors' lab a collagenase protocol, which is described in the following paragraphs, is commonly used for isolation of adult guinea pig cardiomyocyte-pairs. It should be noted that this is assuredly not the "only true" protocol, but it is a suitable one. First of all the following solutions have to be prepared.

1. Solution A
   - 3 mol/l NaCl   21.0 ml
   - 3 mol/l KCl   783.0 µl
   - 0.1 mol/l KH_2PO_4 6.0 ml
   - 0.1 mol/l $MgSO_4$ 12.5 ml
   - V0.4 mol/l $NaHCO_3$ 31.1 ml
   - 0.5 mol/l HEPES/Na   5.0 ml
   - glucose   0.54 g
   - H_2O to 500.0 ml
2. Solution B
   - pyrovate   44.0 mg

- bovine serum albumin 200.0 mg
- solution A   to 200.0 ml
- equilibrate with 95% O_2 and 5% CO_2
3. Solution C
   - 1 vial collagenase Worthington type II 100.0 U/ml
   - 12.5 µl 0.1 mol/l $CaCl_2$
   - solution B to 10 ml
4. Solution D
   - solution B   20 ml
   - 0.1 mol/l $CaCl_2$ 10 ml
   - equilibrate with 95% O_2 and 5% CO_2
5. Solution E (only for short-time culture of the cells)
   - foetal calf serum 10% 1 ml
   - penicillin 2.4 mg (or 100 IU/ml)
   - streptomycin 4.0 mg (100 IU/ml)
   - glutamine 200 mmol/l 100 µl
   - M 199 to 20.0 ml

After the guinea pig (250–350 g) is killed, the heart is prepared according to the Langendorff technique, transferred to a Langendorff apparatus and perfused at 37 °C for 10 minutes with solution B (i.e. Ca^{++}-free saline). Thereafter, the heart is perfused with solution C in a recirculating mode for about 30 minutes. It is important to make sure that the solutions do not get mixed. While perfusing with the collagenase solution, the heart becomes "slimy" and a little transparent. During that phase the perfusion rate often has to be reduced. At the end of this period the heart is removed from the apparatus, the atria are removed and the remaining heart is cut into small pieces using two scalpels. The tissue is transferred to a glass test-tube and treated with the rest of the collagenase solution, slightly gassed with 95% O_2 and 5% CO_2 at 37 °C.

Next, the suspension containing the tissue is filtered through a 200 µm mesh-size gauze and centrifuged for 1 minute at about 600 rpm (ca. 62×g). After removing the supernatant, the pellet is resuspended in 10 ml solution D (37 °C; do not gas the solution). Again the suspension is centrifuged for 1 minute at 600 rpm (ca. 62×g) and the pellet resuspended in solution D. After 1 minute the calcium concentration in the suspension is gradually increased (this is a critical phase for the cells, since during this procedure many cells are impaired) by adding 5 µl 0.1 mol/l $CaCl_2$, 7.5 µl after another minute, 7.5 µl after the next minute and 10 µl and 15 µl in the following two minutes, thereby adjusting the calcium concentration finally to about 0.45 mmol/l.

Following these steps, the solution is centrifuged a last time for 1 minute at 600 rpm and the resulting pellet is either resuspended in 20 ml solution B (with additional Ca^{++}) or in Tyrode solution if the cells are to be used immediately for an experiment, or the pellet is resuspended in solution E to culture the cells. For this purpose 2 ml of the cell-containing solution are mixed with 5 ml solution E in Petri dishes (3 cm diameter) and kept in the incubator for a maximum of 3 days. However, it should be noted that the content of cell pairs gradually declines with time and is maximal shortly after isolation.

Troubleshooting

Asymmetrical Signals

Sometimes one may see asymmetry in the signals. Thus, it may be possible that voltage-dependent inactivation is not symmetrical if positive or negative transjunctional voltages are applied. This is normal if an asymmetrical protocol is used and was first shown by Banach and Weingart (1996). However, the underlying mechanism is still a matter of discussion and investigation. On the other hand, it might be that using the asymmetrical protocol but with short pulses not exceeding $V_j = \pm 50$ mV some asymmetry is also found. This might indicate that there is leak current in one cell. In that case the recording cannot be used.

Another cause for asymmetric behaviour in the analysis of macroscopic gap junction conductance and voltage-dependent inactivation is the presence of different connexins as discussed by Polontchouk et al. (2002). It cannot be excluded that heteromeric channels may exist which could produce asymmetric signals during voltage-dependent inactivation. For more details see Polontchouk et al. (2002).

Series Resistance and Related Problems

The Problem of Series Resistance

Suppose the membrane resistance is very high (or infinite) then the current measured in the non-stepped cell 1 can be described as

$$I_1 = I_j = (V_1 - V_2)/(R_{S1} + R_{j} + R_{S2})$$

If R_j becomes low or if serial resistance is increasing, significant error can occur if there is no compensation. If dSEVC are used, serial resistance is avoided, as pointed out above (for a detailed discussion and detailed investigation of the accuracy of dSEVC for double cell patch clamp see Müller et al. 1999). Otherwise, a correction should be calculated. The series resistance leads to a voltage drop across the series resistance and thus minimizes the voltage drop across R_j. In that respect the ratio of R_j/R_S is very important. Thus, the truly applied voltage gradient may differ from the difference between the two command voltages.

Thus, according to Van Rijen et al. (1998) the true gap junctional conductance $g_{j.t}$ is related to the measured $g_{j.m}$ by the equation:

$$F_j = g_{j.m}/g_{j.t}$$

where

$$F_j = 1/[1+(R_{S2}/R_{m2})]$$

and

$$R_j = V_1 - I_1 \times R_{S1} - (V_2 - I_2 \times R_{S2})/[I_1 + \{(I_1 \times R_{s1})/R_{m1}\} - (V_1/R_{m1})]$$

Readers interested in a detailed discussion are referred to the paper by Van Rijen and colleagues (1998). For well coupled cells in which R_j approaches the range of R_s, Rook and colleagues (1988) have developed a more general correction formula

$$R_j = I_A \times R_{SA} - I_B \times R_{SB} + (d_{EB} - dE_A)/[(dE_A/R_{mA}) - I_A \times (1 + R_{SA}/R_{mA})]$$

with R_{SA}, R_{SB} being the serial resistances of electrodes A and B, I_A, I_B being the currents flowing through electrodes A and B, and dE_A and dE_B the changes in potential of *electrodes* A and B.

$$dV_A = dE_A - I_A \times R_{SA}$$
$$dV_B = dE_B - I_B \times R_{SB}$$

dV being the change in voltage in the *cell*. The basic principle is to calculate the voltage drop that occurs over the serial resistance and minimizes or alters the voltage in the cell or over the gap junctions.

The Problem of Cytoplasmic Access Resistance

Another problem is the existence of cytoplasmic access resistance, which is not artificial. It has been observed by many authors that voltage dependence is more pronounced if gap junction conductance is low (see Wilders and Jongsma 1992). At the first glance one might attribute this phenomenon to the problem of series resistance, since large gap junctions conduct more current, this would result in a larger voltage drop across the serial resistance than in the case of a small gap junction. However, as elegantly shown in the paper of Wilders and Jongsma (1992), the effect of series resistance alone is not large enough to account for the complete observed effect. It was suggested that the tight packing of gap junctional channels within a gap junction results in an access resistance that causes a cytoplasmic voltage drop, thereby masking the voltage sensitivity (Rook et al. 1988, 1990). Using a computer simulation, Wilders and Jongsma (1992) showed that even in the case of complete compensation for series resistance, the number of channels might be underestimated.

Thus, the overestimation of the normalized steady-state conductance may mask transjunctional voltage sensitivity. This is, at least in part, caused both by the fact that at high transjunctional potentials the number of open channels is reduced, which may cause a decrease in cytoplasmic access resistance, and by a reduction in the potential drop across the pipettes due to reduced gap junctional current (Wilders and Jongsma 1992).

Under physiological conditions, i.e. in the beating heart, the cytoplasmic access resistance should attenuate the voltage differences between two neighbouring cells, resulting in less transjunctional current than could be expected from the number of channels, their open probability and their conductance.

The Problem of Membrane Resistance

In the ideal case the membrane resistance is infinitely high for both cells, so that there is no voltage drop (or current loss) across the cell membrane. However, this ideal case does not often correspond to the reality. As long as membrane resistance has a finite value there will be some voltage drop across the membrane that overshadows the voltage drop across the gap junction. If R_m is lower than 1 GΩ, F_j is significantly decreased (Van Rijen et al. 2001). The errors induced by R_m become smaller if $g_{j,t}$ is decreased, but are still present. Thus, a correction for both R_s and R_m may be recommended as proposed by Van Rijen et al. (2001).

Run down

A common problem with gap junction measurements is a rundown of g_j in these preparations, for example in neonatal rat heart cells Schmilinsky-Fluri et al. (1990, 1997) found a decrease in g_j of 16.4% in 6 minutes, which could be antagonized by addition of a phospolipase inhibitor, 20 µmol/l bromophenacylbromide, to 1.8% within 6 minutes. They suggested endogenous arachidonic acid to be involved in spontaneous uncoupling. Others favoured a washout of ATP and cyclic nucleotides as a possible cause and prevented their preparations from spontaneous uncoupling by addition of ATP, GTP or cAMP to the pipette solution (Müller et al. 1997). Thus, it is known that there is considerable run-down of gap junctional coupling if no ATP is present in the pipettes, which can be overcome by addition of ATP to the pipette solution. Since this can also be achieved using an ATP analogue which supports protein phosphorylation but not active transport processes (ATPγS), it has been suggested that the ATP effect is due to protein phosphorylation rather than to changes in intracellular calcium homeostasis (Verecchia et al. 1999). Thus, inhibition of protein kinases by a rather non-specific inhibitor such as H7 reversibly reduced intercellular coupling. Similarly, addition of a phosphatase such as alkaline phosphatase mimicked the effect of ATP deprivation (Verrecchia et al. 1999).

References

Banach K, Weingart R (1996) Connexin43 gap junctions exhibit asymmetrical gating properties.Pflügers Arch Eur J Physiol 431: 775–785

Bennett MVL, Zheng X, Sogin ML (1995) The connexin family tree. In: Kanno Y, Kataoka K, Shiba Y, Shibata Y, Shimazu T (eds) Intercellular communication through gap junctions. Elsevier Science Publishers, Amsterdam, pp 3–8

Brink PR (1998) Gap junctions in vascular smooth muscle. Acta Physiol Scand 164: 349–356

Bruzzone R (2001) Learning the language of cell-cell communication through connexin channels. Genome Biol 2: Reports 4027

Christ GJ, Brink PR (1999) Analysis of the presence and physiological relevance of subconducting states of connxin43-derived gap junction channels in cultured human corporal vascular smooth muscle cells. Circ Res 85: 797–803

Dhein S (1998) Gap junction channels in the cardiovascular system: pharmacological and physiological modulation. Trends Pharmacol Sci 19: 229–241

Dhein S (1998a) Cardiac Gap Junctions. Karger Verlag, Basel

Fallon RF, Goodenough DA (1981) Five hour half-life of mouse liver gap junction protein. J Cell Biol 127: 343–355

Giaume C (1991) Application of the patch clamp technique to the study of junctional conductance. In: Peracchia C (ed) Biophysics of gap junction channels. CRC Press, Boca Raton, pp 175–190

Grinstein S, Romanek R, Rotstein OD (1994) Method for manipulation of cytosolic pH in cells clamped in the whole cell or perforated patch configurations. Am J Physiol 267: C1152–C1159

Laird DW (1996) The life cycle of a connexin: gap junction formation removal and degradation. J Bioenerg Biomembr 28: 311–317

Müller A, Gottwald M, Tudyka T, Linke W, Klaus W, Dhein S (1997) Increase in gap junction conductance by an antiarrhythmic peptide. Eur J Physiol 327: 65–72

Müller A, Lauven M, Berkels R, Dhein S, Polder HR, Klaus W (1999) Switched single-electrode voltage clamp amplifiers allow precise measurement of gap junction conductance. Am J Physiol 276: C980–C987

Musil LS, Goodenough DA (1993) Multisubunit assembly of an integral plasma membrane channel protein, gap junction connexin43, occurs after exit from the ER. Cell 74: 1065–1077

Polontchouk L, Haefliger J-A, Ebelt B, Schaefer T, Stuhlmann D, Mehlhorn U, Kuhn-Reignier F, DeVivie ER, Dhein S (2001) Effects of chronic atrial fibrillation on gap junction distribution in human and rat atria. J Am Coll Cardiol 38: 883–891

Polontchouk LO, Valiunas V, Haefliger J-A, Eppenberger HM, Weingart R (2002) Expression and regulation of connexins in cultured ventricular myocytes isolated from adult rat hearts. Pflügers Arch Eur J Physiol 443: 676–689

Rook MB, Jongsma HJ, Van Ginneken ACG (1988) Properties of single gap junctional channels between isolated neonatal rat heart cells. Am J Physiol 255: H770–H782

Rook MB, De Jonge B, Jongsma HJ, Masson-Pévet MA (1990) Gap junction formation and functional interaction between neonatal rat cardiocytes in culture: a correlative physiological and ultrastructural study. J Membr Biol 118: 179–192

Schimilsky Fluri G, Rüdisüli A, Willi M, Rohr S, Weingart R (1990) Effects of arachidonic acid on the gap junctions of neonatal rat heart cells. Pflüger's Arch 417: 149–156

Schmilinsky-Fluri G, Valiunas V, Willi M, Weingart R (1997) Modulation of cardiac gap junctions: the mode of action of arachidonic acid. J Mol Cell Cardiol 29: 1703–1713

Spray DC, Harris AL, Bennett MVL (1981) Equilibrium properties of a voltage dependent junctional conductance. J Gen Physiol 77: 77–93

Valiunas V, Vogel R, Weingart R (2000) The kinetics of gap junction currents are sensitive to the ionic composition of the pipette solution. Pflügers Arch Eur J Physiol 440: 835–842

Spray DC, White RL, Mazet F, Bennett MVL (1985) Regulation of gap junction conductance. Am J Physiol 248: H753–H764

Van Rijen HVM, Wilders R, Rook MB, Jongsma HJ (2001) Dual Patch Clamp. Methods Mol Biol 154: 269–192

Van Rijen HVM, Wilders R, Van Ginneken ACG, Jongsma HJ (1998) Quantitative analysis of dual whole-cell voltage-clamp determination of gap junctional conductance. Pflügers Arch Eur J Physiol 436: 141–151

Veenstra RD, Berg K, Wang HZ, Westphale EM, Beyer EC (1993) Molecular and biophysical properties of the connexins from developing chick heart. In: Hall JE, Zampighi GA, Davis RM (eds) Progress in cell research, vol 3, Elsevier Science Publishers, Amsterdam, pp 89–95

Verheule S, van Kempen MJA, te Welscher PHJA, Kwak BR, Jongsma HJ (1997) Characterization of gap junction channels in adult rabbit atrial and ventricular myocardium. Circ Res 80: 673–681

Verrecchia F, Duthe F, Duval D, Duchatelle I, Sarrouilhe D, Hervé JC (1999) ATP counteracts the rundown of gap junctional channels of rat ventricular myocytes by promoting protein phosphorylation. J Physiol (London) 516: 447–459

Weingart R (1986) Electrical properties of the nexal membrane studied in rat ventricular cell pairs. J Physiol (London) 370: 267–284

Wilders R, Jongsma HJ (1992) Limitations of the dual voltage clamp method in assaying conductance and kinetics of gap junction channels. Biophys J 63: 942–953

Recording Monophasic Action Potentials

Paulus Kirchhof, Larissa Fabritz and Michael R. Franz

Introduction

Monophasic action potentials (MAP) reflect the time course of the myocardial action potential and can be used in the intact heart and *in vivo*. They represent a unique tool to study repolarization-related arrhythmia mechanisms both in experimental models and in patients. Their parallel use in experimental and clinical studies allows verification of experimental hypotheses in the clinical setting and the performance of electrophysiological studies integrated from bench to bedside. The identification of repolarization-related arrhythmia mechanisms in primary arrhythmogenic diseases (e.g. acquired and congenital Long QT syndromes) and in more common conditions such as ventricular hypertrophy and heart failure are more recent areas in which MAP recordings are proving to be useful in both experimental and clinical research.

Description of Methods and Practical Approach

Historical Aspects

MAP recordings have been measured in myocardium for over 100 years (Burdon-Sanderson and Page 1882; Schütz 1931). The first recordings were obtained using injury by cutting (Burdon-Sanderson and Page 1882; Schütz 1931) or by suction electrodes (Taggart et al. 1996; Olsson and Harper 1978; Brorson and Olsson 1976). Although suction electrodes have been used clinically and are still occasionally used experimentally (Babuty and Lab 2000), this technique has largely been replaced by the Franz contact electrode technique developed more than 20 years ago (Franz et al. 1980; Franz 1983). The MAP contact electrode can be mounted on standard electrophysiology catheters, is easy to use and does not damage the myocardium during the recording process. A "combination catheter" (see below) allows electrical stimulation at the MAP recording site (Franz et al. 1990). The contact electrode takes advantage of a closely sited reference electrode to minimize far-field potentials, thereby rendering the MAP a truly local potential (Franz 1999).

Combination MAP Catheter or Probe for Measuring APD and Refractoriness Simultaneously

A specific design of the MAP contact electrode catheter allows one to measure the effective refractory period (ERP) at a site almost identical to the MAP recording site (Franz et al. 1983). The design of this combination catheter tip is shown in Fig. 1. With the tip and reference MAP electrode spaced 5 mm apart for applications in humans and large animals (and less for smaller animals), two pacing electrodes are placed halfway between the MAP tip and reference electrode, in an orthogonal position. This design provides for an extremely low pacing threshold (approximately 10× less than standard pacing techniques) and minimizes the stimulus artefact further, due to the fact that the electrical vector of the pacing stimulus is horizontal while the recorded MAP vector is mainly vertical to the tip electrode.

Furthermore, the distance between the stimulation electrodes is small, and their surface area is low. This situation creates relatively high gradients at the catheter-tissue interface and contributes to effective stimulation with low stimulus strengths.

This technique has been used successfully in humans (Costard Jäckle et al. 1989a), dogs (Meissner et al. 2001; Eckardt et al. 2001), rabbits (Kirchhof et al. 1998a, 2003a Zabel et al. 1997) and mice (Fabritz et al. 2002, 2003a; Knollmann et al. 2001) (Fig. 2),

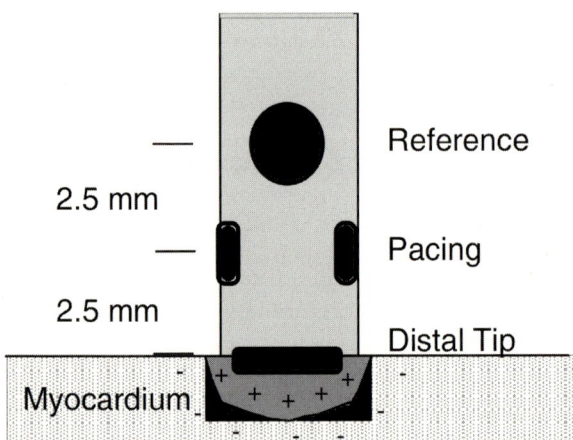

Figure 1
Schematic drawing of a monophasic action potential (MAP) contact combination catheter tip designed to record a MAP and to pace from the same site simultaneously, placed on to the myocardium in the desired, perpendicular po-sition. The *shaded area* with the (+) signs indi-cates the assumed depolarized myocardium subjacent to the catheter tip, the *greyish area* normal myocardium. On the interface between these two areas, a sink current will be created that is directly dependent on voltage changes in the normal myocardium (Knollmannn et al. 2002). The distal tip electrode is round shaped to create a constant pressure on to the myocardium. Underlying the catheter tip. 2.5 mm proximal to the distal tip electrode, 2 platinum electrodes for pacing are located opposing each other on the catheter shaft. The closely spaced reference electrode is located 5 mm proximal to the distal tip electrode. See text for details

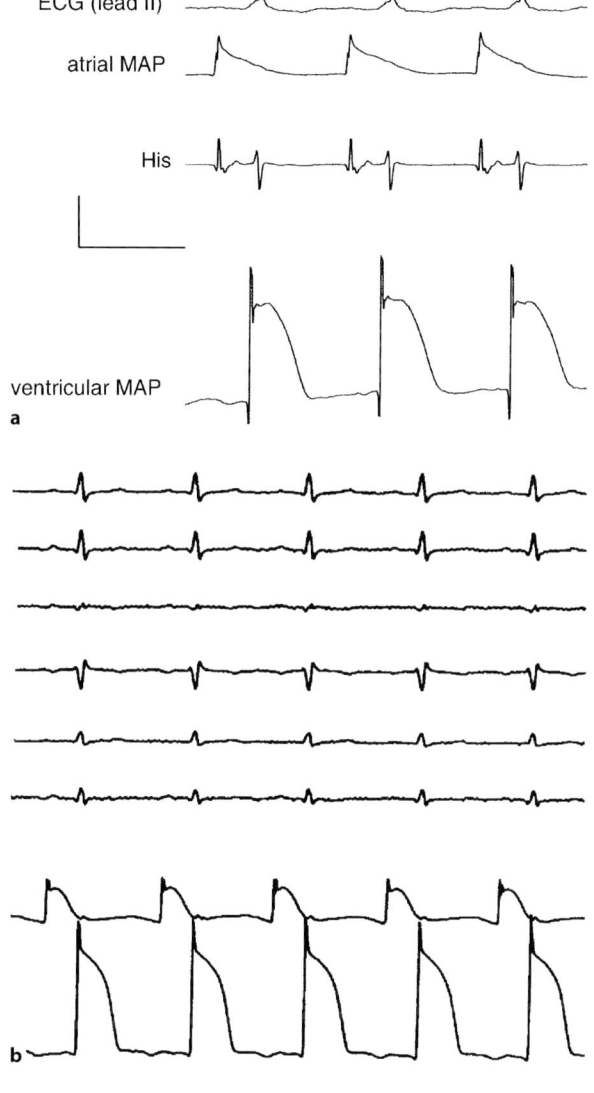

Figure 2a–e
Typical ventricular MAP recordings obtained *in vivo* from a patient (**a**), from a conscious dog (**b**), from the isolated rabbit heart (**c**) and from the isolated heart of a mouse with a LQT III mutation after AV nodal block (**d**) and during an episode of spontaneous torsade de pointes (**e**). Published with permission from Kirchhof and Franz 2001 (**a**), Eckardt et al. 2001 (**b**), Kirchhof et al. 1996 (**c**), and Fabritz et al. 2003b (**d,e**)

and in every species demonstrated a close correlation between APD and ERP. ERP ended and re-excitability occurred at between 75 and 85% of cellular repolarization at the sites examined (Fig. 3). This close relationship between APD and ERP was found to be independent of cycle length, signifying that in normal myocardium, ERP is always closely matched to APD and that post-repolarization refractoriness does not occur except in ischemic myocardium or hearts treated with ion channel-blocking drugs (Fig. 3b).

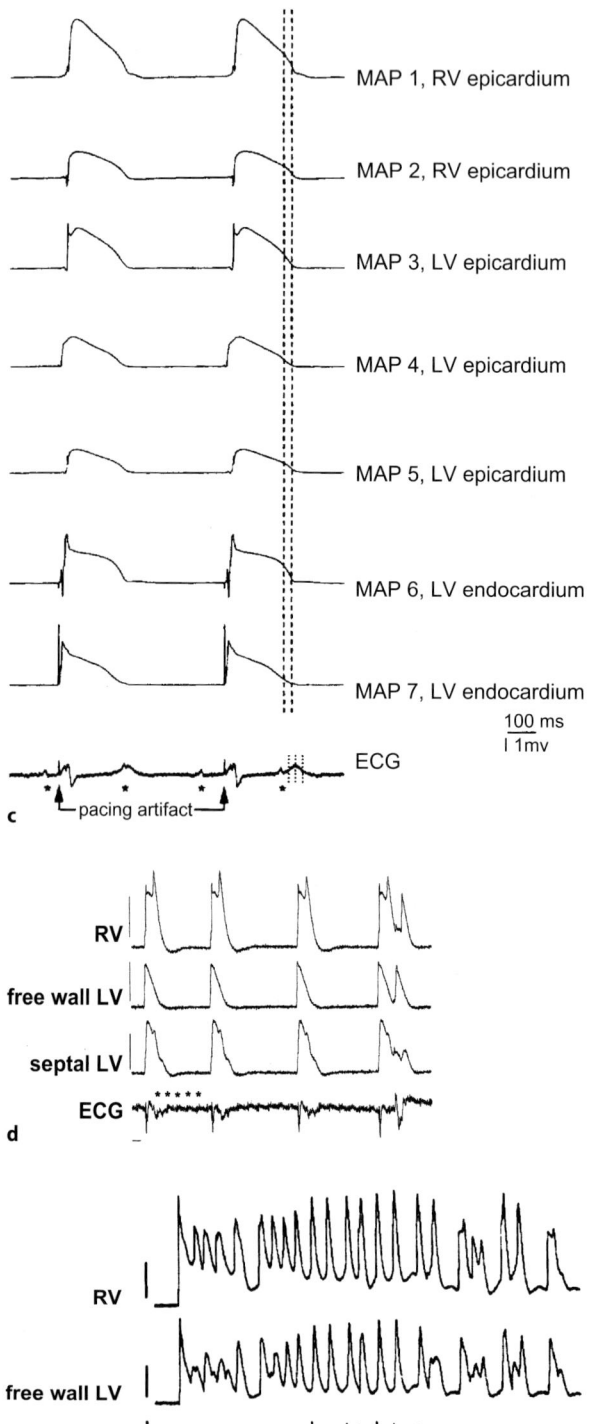

Figure 2c–e
Details see previous page

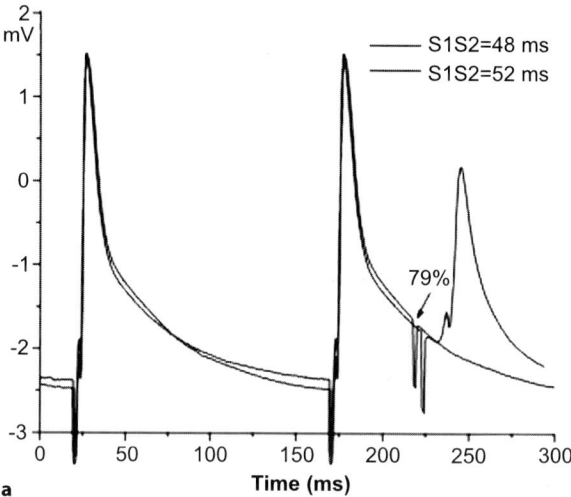

Figure 3a
Details see next page

Nature and Genesis of the MAP

It has long been recognized that the MAP signal reflects the repolarisation time course of the transmembrane action potential (Franz et al. 1986), but the genesis of the MAP signal has remained partially unexplained. The contact MAP electrode also reflects the transmembrane action potential during ventricular arrhythmias including ventricular fibrillation (Fabritz et al. 1999), suggesting that the signal is generated in only a few cardiac cells close to the catheter tip. Furthermore, recent experimental study has shown that the signal is derived from a small body of myocardial cells, probably just a few layers thick, lying underneath the MAP tip electrode (Knollmann et al. 2002). The cells just underneath the catheter tip are partially depolarized (Knollmann et al. 2002). As the depolarized tissue is electrically inactive, a "sink current" is generated during diastole and a "source current" during systole by the gradient between the depolarized cells and the action potential of surrounding active cells (Franz 1991). The driving voltage gradient is proportional to the membrane potential changes of the myocardium in this interface area. This current is most likely the source of the MAP signal that is recorded as a voltage difference between the tip electrode and a closely spaced reference electrode. (For a detailed review, see Fig. 1 and Franz 1999.)

Examples

Experimental Applications of MAP Recordings

The contact electrode has been widely used to study cardiac repolarization abnormalities in experimental models including swine and dogs as well as isolated, Langendorff-perfused hearts of rabbits or guinea pigs (see Fig. 2b,c; Kirchhof and Franz

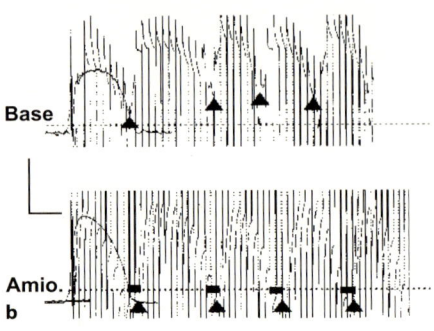

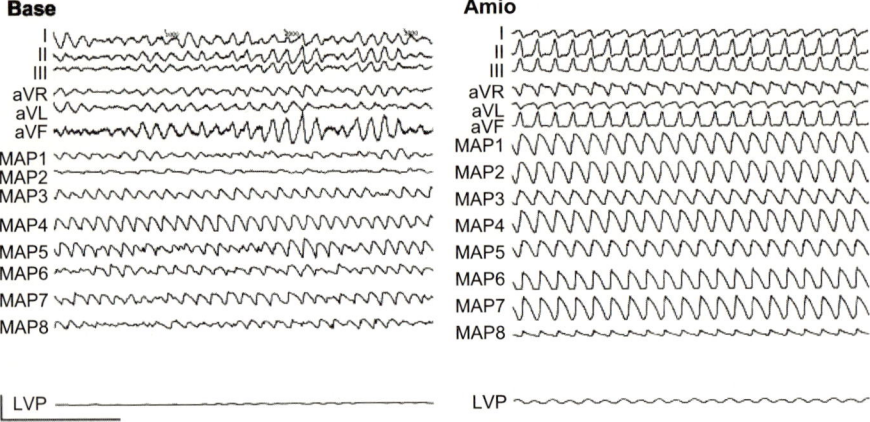

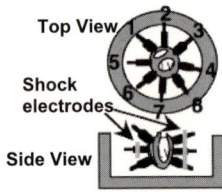

Figure 3a–c
Determination of the relationship between repolarisation and refractoriness in the intact heart. **a** Physiological relationship between action potential duration and refractoriness in the intact mouse heart. Shown are two superimposed MAPs recorded during premature stimulation with an S2 coupled at 52 ms and 48 ms. The S2 coupled at 48 ms, delivered at a repolarisation of 79% repolarisation, does not induce a new action potential. **b,c** Amiodarone-induced post-repolarisation refractoriness in the isolated rabbit heart. The MAP shown was recorded from an isolated rabbit heart during 50 Hz burst stimulation at baseline (**b**) and after oral treatment with amiodarone for 6 weeks (**c**). Amiodarone-induced post-repolarisation refractoriness, i.e. prolongation of refractoriness beyond APD90, prevents induction of ventricular fibrillation. (Published with permission from Knollmann et al. 2001 and Kirchhof et al. 2003a)

2001). Specifically, the isolated rabbit or guinea pig heart instrumented with multiple MAP contact electrodes has proved useful for studying the effects of cardiac and non-cardiac drugs on cardiac repolarization and repolarization-related arrhythmias

(Kirchhof et al. 1996, 1998a, 2003a; Zabel et al. 1994, 1997; Costard Jäckle et al. 1989b; Pinney et al. 1995; Milberg et al. 2002; Eckardt et al. 1998). The close inter-electrode spacing combined with non-depolarisable electrodes allows recording of action potentials during and after defibrillation shocks with a shock-related blanking period of only a few milliseconds (Kirchhof et al. 1996; Daubert et al. 1991; Fabritz et al. 1996; Behrens et al. 1996). The isolated heart also allows recording of MAP signals during periods of arrhythmias including ventricular fibrillation (Kirchhof et al. 1998a,b, 2003; Behrens et al. 1997; Fabritz et al. 2003b; Tovar and Jones 1997, 2000).

Human MAP Recordings *in Vivo*

MAP catheters designed for *in vivo* electrophysiological studies in humans permit comparison of experimental and clinical electrophysiological findings using the same technique, thereby bridging bench and bedside (see Fig. 2a). Many of the exciting experimental findings regarding repolarisation-related arrhythmias and antiarrhythmic drugs actions could be confirmed in humans. These include direct evidence for the genesis of the T wave (Franz et al. 1991), the relation between post-repolarisation refractoriness and protection against arrhythmia induction (Koller et al. 1995a), the physiological rate adaptation of the ventricular action potential duration (Franz et al. 1983, 1988) and, more recently, atrial action potentials and their alternation in atrial fibrillation and flutter (Franz et al. 1997; Bode et al. 2001), synchronization of repolarisation after successful defibrillation shocks (Moubarak et al. 2000), regional inhomogeneities of repolarisation in Brugada syndrome (Eckardt et al. 1999), or the occurrence of atrial afterdepolarisations and "torsade de pointes" in patients with long QT syndrome (Fig. 4, Kirchhof et al. 2000; 2003b).

Study of Mouse Hearts

The advent of transgenic technologies has shifted the focus of experimental electrophysiological studies towards transgenic mouse models, and hence towards the mouse as an experimental model of cardiac electrophysiology (Schaper and Winkler 1998; Gehrmann and Berul 2000). The MAP recording technique has been successfully transferred to isolated mouse heart preparations (Fabritz et al. 2003b; Knollmann et al. 2003; Kirchhof et al. 2003c). Preparations of intact beating hearts perfused by the Langendorff technique allow recording of multiple simultaneous MAPs from the mouse ventricles (Fig. 5; Fabritz et al. 2003a; Knollmann et al. 2001; Kirchhof et al. 1996; Franz et al. 1992).
To study transgenic mouse models with repolarization abnormalities and a suspected susceptibility to arrhythmias, a protocol for provocation of ventricular ar-rhythmias has been established in the mouse heart (Fabritz et al. 2003a). These experimental setups have been instrumental in identifying arrhythmia mechanisms in transgenic models of the long QT syndrome (see Fig. 2d,e; Fabritz et al. 2003b) and of familial hypertrophic cardiomyopathy (Knollmann et al. 2003) and of hypertensive cardiac

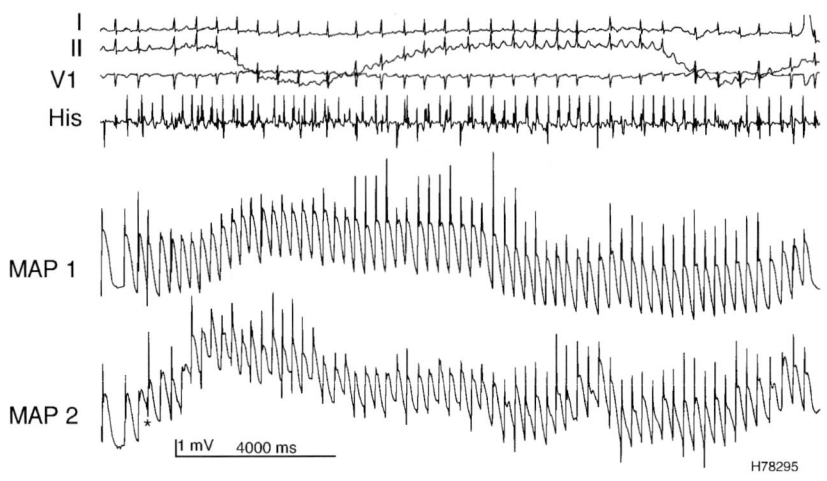

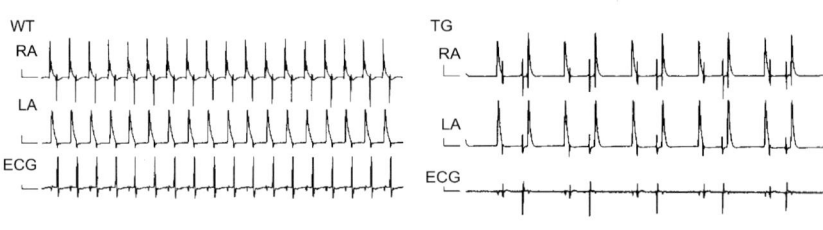

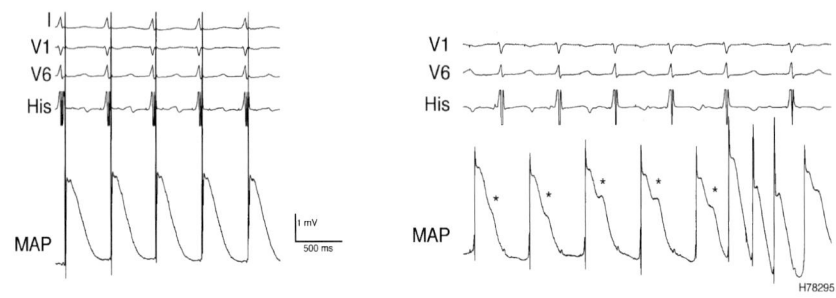

Figure 4a–d
a Recording of an atrial monophasic action potential in a patient with long QT syndrome during an episode of polymorphic atrial tachycardia. b Recording of atrial monophasic action potentials from isolated mouse hearts. *Left panel:* Recording from a wild type mouse heart (WT). *Right panel:* Recording from a transgenic mouse heart with enhanced heart-directed expression of A_1 adenosine receptors (TG). RA indicates right atrium, LA indicates left atrium. c Recording of atrial afterdepolarizations in a monophasic action potential that occur during high-rate pacing in a patient with long QT syndrome just prior to initiation of an arrhythmia episode. His indicates the His recording

hypertrophy (Kirchhof et al. 2004). Using specially designed miniaturized catheters, MAPs have also been recorded from the atrium of the isolated mouse heart (Kirchhof et al. 2003c).

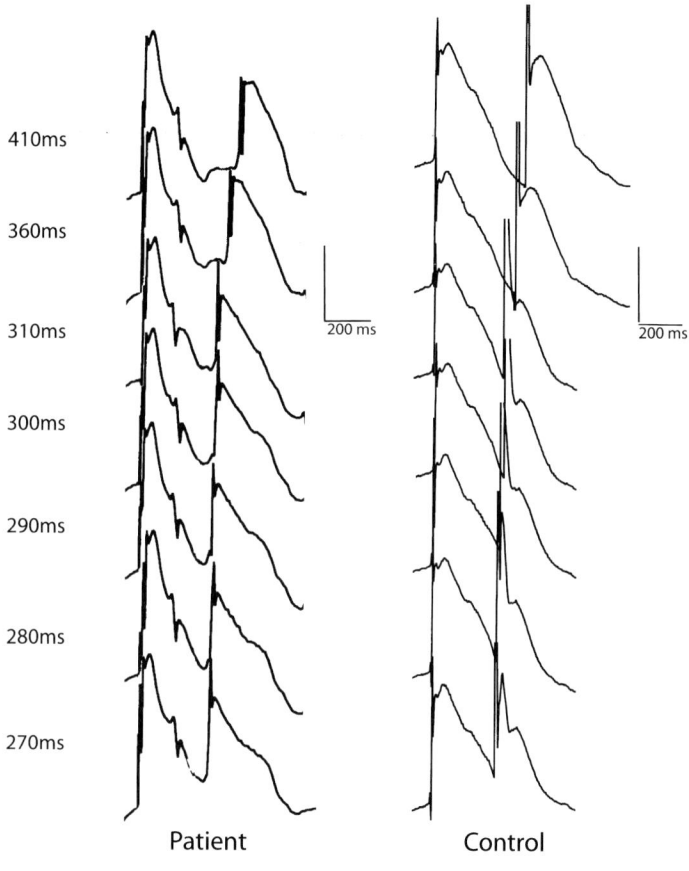

Figure 4d
Afterdepolarizations of increasing magnitude that occur during atrial stimulation in the atrium of a patient with long QT syndrome (patient, *left panel*) and in a control subject without cardiac disease (control, *right panel*). Intervals at the left of each line indicate the coupling interval of the extra stimulus, S2. In the long QT syndrome patient, paradoxical prolongation of the atrial action potential is seen, accompanied by afterdepolarizations of increasing magnitude. Published with permission from Kirchhof et al. JCE 2003b (*panels A, C*), from Kirchhof et al. 2000 (*panel D*), and from Kirchhof et al. AJP 2003c (*panel B*)

Computer-aided Analysis of MAP Signals

Using computerized semi-automated analysis programs (Franz et al. 1995), MAPs can be used to monitor the time course of action potential changes over many beats, e.g. to assess drug effects (Franz et al. 1995) or to quantify action potential alternans (Pastore and Rosenbaum 2000). The use of combination catheters allows determination of the relation between refractoriness and repolarisation in human hearts *in vivo* (Koller et al. 1995a) and in experimental settings (Kirchhof et al. 1998a, 1999, 2003a; Daubert et al. 1991). This relation is altered by antiarrhythmic agents that protect against poly-

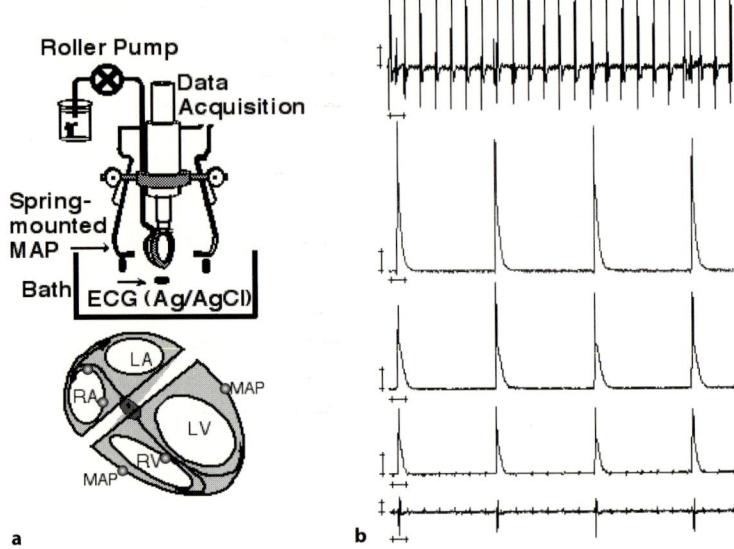

Figure 5a,b
Setup to record multiple monophasic action potentials and a volume-conducted "surface" ECG in the intact mouse heart. Shown are the perfusion system of the isolated heart, the mounting system for the MAP catheters, and the ECG electrodes (**a**). **b** Typical ventricular MAP recordings are shown after mechanical induction of AV nodal block. (Published with permission from Fabritz et al. 2003a)

morphic ventricular tachycardias and ventricular fibrillation (Kirchhof et al. 1999). Using MAP recordings, post-repolarisation refractoriness can be determined both in the ventricle (Kirchhof et al. 1998a; 1999; 2003a; Koller et al. 1995a) and in the atrium (Koller et al. 1995b; Kirchhof et al. 2002a).

On-line control of MAP signals by an experienced investigator is necessary for correct differentiation between true MAP signals and artefacts. Several parameters can be used to confirm the signal quality of MAP signals. Signal stability over long periods of time (minutes to hours) is an important criterion for a "good" MAP signal. Changing action potential morphologies over time usually suggest an unstable electrode contact, unless the changes can be explained by interventions, e.g. ischemia, drugs, cooling, or pacing, among others.

Another important quality criterion is signal amplitude. Using standard catheter tip electrodes (0.5–2 mm diameter, 5 mm inter-electrode spacing), MAP amplitude should exceed 10 mV in the adult human ventricle and 3 mV in the adult human atrium (Franz 1991). This amplitude usually develops to its full magnitude over a few beats after placement of the catheter in a stable position. As myocardial thickness influences MAP amplitude, smaller amplitudes are acceptable in small hearts, e.g. 3.5 mV for rabbit ventricle (Kirchhof et al. 1996). In the mouse, round shaped MAP catheters designed for long term recordings yield acceptable MAPs at signal amplitudes of 1.5–3 mV (Fabritz et al. 2003a,b; Kirchhof et al. 2003c, 2004). Custom-designed miniaturized electrodes with a higher contact pressure allow for higher amplitude signals, albeit with shorter recording durations (Knollmann et al. 2001,

2002, 2003). Both methods return similar action potential durations, suggesting that both techniques can be equally used. Signal amplitudes <1 mV, in contrast, are usually not sufficient to exclude relevant far-field signal recordings.

In Vivo Mapping of Repolarization using MAPs

Like most other *in vivo* techniques to record intracardiac electrograms, the MAP is recorded from a single site at a time. Placing of multiple MAP catheters in different places in the same heart is one way to record multiple action potentials simultaneously (Kirchhof et al. 1996, 2000; Behrens et al. 1996; Moubarak et al. 2000; Verduyn et al. 1997; de Groot et al. 1995). This technique, though limited to a few recording sites at a time by the maximal number of catheters that can be put into a single heart, can be useful when spatial transients in repolarisation are studied, i. e. those immediately preceding an arrhythmia like torsade de pointes, or during arrhythmia termination, e.g. by electrical defibrillation. The catheter-based MAP recording technique has also been used in non-sedated, trained dogs (see Fig. 3b; Eckardt et al. 2001; 2003).

Whenever action potential duration can be kept constant for several minutes, e.g. by pacing with a constant cycle length before and after administration of a drug, sequential mapping of MAP durations can be performed. This has so far been done using fluoroscopic verification of catheter positions, or in the open-chest heart (Eckardt et al. 1999; Franz et al. 1987; Zabel et al. 1998). The advent of non-fluoroscopic systems to assess intracardiac catheter positions, e.g. the CARTO or the LocaLisa system (Wittkampf et al. 1999; Gepstein and Evans 1998; Kirchhof et al. 2002b), is likely to improve sequential mapping of repolarisation by quantifying distances between different catheter positions, and may be used to confirm correct repositioning of catheters to a given place in the heart (Gepstein et al. 1997).

Troubleshooting

Signal Fidelity

The fidelity of the MAP signal in reflecting the transmembrane action potential relies on several factors, ranging from electrode composition and design and catheter mounting devices to assure constant electrode contact, to use of amplifiers with high bandwidth (0–5000 Hz are optimal but 0.05–1000 Hz suffice for most applications). Due to their extracellular origin, MAP signal amplitude is lower than that of transmembrane action potentials, and the signal amplitude also depends on the type of myocardial preparation and species. Signal amplitude also decreases over time, even with adequate electrode position. Therefore, the absolute voltage of MAP recordings and by inference amplitude of dV/dt is usually not used for data analysis.

Morphological characteristics of the MAP are paramount to distinguish high quality recordings from those with artefacts due to unstable contact or excessive motion. These criteria can only be applied when the investigator has ample experience with the normal action potential shape of the tissue from which the MAP is recorded. Several almost universal characteristics can, however, be defined:

The upstroke should be fast and usually monophasic. While sharp "intrinsic deflections" during phase 0 of the action potential are acceptable (reflecting extracellular activation wave fronts passing by the electrode or contamination by nearby myocardial activity), these should not exceed 5 ms duration in human and large animal ventricular myocardium, and 2 ms in small hearts, e.g. mouse hearts. When conduction velocity in the recording area is slow, this period may increase. The upstroke usually shows a small overshoot. This is an acceptable remnant of the intrinsic deflection but its amplitude should not exceed 1/2 of the MAP plateau amplitude. The overshoot is difficult to assess in mice because the murine action potential has a very rapid early repolarization phase that is followed by a slower repolarization phase at about 50% of total amplitude (Knollmann 2002).

In most species, including dog, pig, guinea pig, and humans, the plateau phase of the ventricular MAP should be horizontal, convex, or only slightly down-sloping. A triangular shaped MAP may be a sign of local ischemia, potentially induced by too much pressure (Franz et al. 1984). Due to the short action potential durations and the physiologically triangular shape of the murine action potential, these criteria are more difficult to apply to mouse and rat action potentials.

During the diastolic interval, voltage variations should not exceed 5% of MAP amplitude. This issue is especially important when the MAP is used to detect afterdepolarisations, as catheter movements during the end of systole and the beginning of diastole may create artefacts that closely resemble early afterdepolarisations (e.g. Fig. 9 in Sager 1999).

Programmed stimulation changes the timing between electrical and mechanical systole and may be a good way to discriminate between movement artefact and real potentials, especially in situations where movement artefacts are difficult to overcome as in some parts of the human atrium. Most of these morphological considerations can best be evaluated during the study or the experiment, when it is still possible to slightly reposition the catheter, or to change the amount of pressure exerted onto the catheter tip.

Intramural MAP Recordings: Possible?

Transmural differences in action potential duration have been identified as a potential arrhythmogenic factor in torsade de pointes arrhythmias, both in acquired long QT syndrome and in congenital primary electrical diseases (Sicouri et al. 1994; Shimizu and Antzelevitch 1997; Weissenburger et al. 2000; Antzelevitch et al. 1999). To record transmural action potential differences in the intact heart, several groups have tried to establish intramural MAP recordings (Weissenburger et al. 2000; Zhou et al. 2002).

So far, these attempts have been hampered by lack of a closely spaced electrically inactive reference electrode. As discussed above, a larger distance between the recording electrode and the reference electrode will include more pseudo-unipolar far-field potentials in the MAP signal, thereby trading intramural information for lack of spatial precision of the signal.

In summary, MAP recordings reliably record the local time course of myocardial depolarisation and repolarisation from a small number of cells *in vivo* and in heart tissue preparations. They can be used both in atrial and ventricular myocardium. When multiple MAPs are recorded simultaneously in the intact heart, repolarisation abnormalities preceding cardiac arrhythmias can be studied directly, and action potential characteristics during cardiac arrhythmias can be monitored. In addition to their use in the intact heart, MAP recordings can be obtained *in vivo* during invasive electrophysiological studies. MAP recordings are therefore an excellent tool to study cardiac repolarization from bench to bedside.

References

Antzelevitch C, Shimizu W, Yan GX, Sicouri S, Weissenburger J, Nesterenko VV, Burashnikov A, Di Diego J, Saffitz J, Thomas GP (1999) The M cell: its contribution to the ECG and to normal and abnormal electrical function of the heart. J Cardiovasc Electrophysiol 10: 1124–1152

Babuty D, Lab M (2000) Heterogeneous changes of monophasic action potential induced by sustained stretch in atrium. J Cardiovasc Electrophysiol 12: 323–329

Behrens S, Li C, Fabritz CL, Kirchhof PF, Franz MR (1997) Shock-induced dispersion of ventricular repolarization: implications for the induction of ventricular fibrillation and the upper limit of vulnerability. J Cardiovasc Electrophysiol 8: 998–1008

Behrens S, Li C, Kirchhof PF, Fabritz CL, Franz MR (1996) Reduced arrhythmogeneity of biphasic versus monophasic T wave shocks: Implications for defibrillation efficacy. Circulation 94: 1674–1680

Bode F, Kilborn M, Karasik P, Franz MR (2001) The repolarization-excitability relationship in the human right atrium is unaffected by cycle length, recording site and prior arrhythmias. J Am Coll Cardiol 37: 920–925

Brorson L, Olsson SB (1976) Right atrial monophasic action potential in healthy males. Studies during spontaneous sinus rhythm and atrial pacing. Acta Med Scand 199: 433–446

Burdon-Sanderson J, Page FJM (1882) On the time-relations of the excitatory process in the ventricle of the heart of the frog. J Physiol 2: 385–412

Costard Jäckle A, Goetsch B, Antz M, Franz MR (1989b) Slow and long-lasting modulation of myocardial repolarization produced by ectopic activation in isolated rabbit hearts. Evidence for cardiac „memory". Circulation 80: 1412–1420

Costard Jäckle A, Liem LB, Franz MR (1989b) Frequency-dependent effect of quinidine, mexiletine, and their combination on postrepolarization refractoriness *in vivo*. J Cardiovasc Pharmacol 14: 810–817

Daubert JP, Frazier DW, Wolf PD, Franz MR, Smith WM, Ideker RE (1991) Response of relatively refractory canine myocardium to monophasic and biphasic shocks. Circulation 84: 2522–2538

de Groot SH, Vos MA, Gorgels AP, Leunissen JD, van der Steld BJ, Wellens HJ (1995) Combining monophasic action potential recordings with pacing to demonstrate delayed afterdepolarizations and triggered arrhythmias in the intact heart. Value of diastolic slope. Circulation 92: 2697–2704

Eckardt L, Haverkamp W, Borggrefe M, Breithardt G (1998) Experimental models of torsade de pointes. Cardiovasc Res 39: 178–193

Eckardt L, Kirchhof P, Johna R, Breithardt G, Borggrefe M, Haverkamp W (1999) Transient local changes in right ventricular monophasic action potentials due to ajmaline in a patient with Brugada Syndrome. J Cardiovasc Electrophysiol 10: 1010–1015

Eckardt L, Meißner A, Kirchhof P, Weber T, Borggrefe M, Breithardt G, vanAken H, Haverkamp W (2001) *In vivo* recording of monophasic action potentials in awake dogs – new applications for experimental electrophysiology. Bas Res Cardiol 96: 169–174

Eckardt L, Meissner A, Kirchhof P, Weber T, Milberg P, Breithardt G, Haverkamp W (2003) *In vivo* recording of monophasic action potentials in awake dogs. Methods 30: 109–114

Fabritz CL, Kirchhof PF, Behrens S, Zabel M, Franz MR (1996) Myocardial vulnerability to T wave shocks: relation to shock strength, shock coupling interval, and dispersion of ventricular repolarization. J Cardiovasc Electrophysiol 7: 231–242

Fabritz CL, Kirchhof PF, Coronel R, Opthof T, Franz MR, Janse M (1999) Monophasic action potential recordings during ventricular fibrillation compared to intracellular recordings. In: Franz MR (ed) Monophasic action potentials: Bridging cell and bedside. Futura Publishing, Armonk, NY, pp 733–745

Fabritz L, Kirchhof P, Franz MR, Eckardt L, Mönnig G, Milberg P, Breithardt G, Haverkamp W (2003a) Prolonged action potential durations, increased dispersion of repolarization, and polymorphic ventricular tachycardia in a mouse model of proarrhythmia. Basic Res Cardiol 98: 25–32

Fabritz L, Kirchhof P, Franz MR, Nuyens D, Haverkamp W, Breithardt G, Carmeliet E, Carmeliet P (2002) Effect of esmolol and mexiletine on action potential duration, dispersion of repolarisation, and torsade de pointes in a transgenic mutant SCN5A (LQT3) mouse (abstract). Symposium Sodium and the Heart

Fabritz L, Kirchhof P, Franz MR, Nuyens D, Rossenbacker T, Ottenhof A, Haverkamp W, Breithardt G, Carmeliet E, Carmeliet P (2003b) Effect of pacing and mexiletine on dispersion of repolarisation and arrhythmias in hearts of SCN5A d-KPQ (LQT3) mice. Cardiovasc Res 57: 1085–1093

Franz M, Schottler M, Schaefer J, Seed WA (1980) Simultaneous recording of monophasic action potentials and contractile force from the human heart. Klin Wochenschr 58: 1357–1359

Franz MR (1983) Long-term recording of monophasic action potentials from human endocardium. Am J Cardiol 51: 1629–1634

Franz MR (1991) Method and theory of monophasic action potential recording. Prog Cardiovasc Dis 33: 347–368

Franz MR (1999) Current status of monophasic action potential recording: theories, measurements and interpretations. Cardiovasc Res 41: 25–40

Franz MR, Bargheer K, Costard-Jackle A, Miller DC, Lichtlen PR (1991) Human ventricular repolarization and T wave genesis. Prog Cardiovasc Dis 33: 369–384

Franz MR, Bargheer K, Raffelenbeul W, Haverich A, Lichtlen PR (1987) Monophasic action potential mapping in human subjects with normal electrocardiograms: direct evidence for the genesis of the T wave. Circulation 75: 379–386

Franz MR, Burkhoff D, Spurgeon H, Weisfeldt ML, Lakatta EG (1986) *In vitro* validation of a new cardiac catheter technique for recording monophasic action potentials. Eur Heart J 7: 34–41

Franz MR, Chin MC, Sharkey HR, Griffin JC, Scheinman MM (1990) A new single catheter technique for simultaneous measurement of action potential duration and refractory period *in vivo*. J Am Coll Cardiol 16: 878–886

Franz MR, Cima R, Wang D, Profitt D, Kurz R (1992) Electrophysiological effects of myocardial stretch and mechanical determinants of stretch-activated arrhythmias. Circulation 86: 968–978

Franz MR, Flaherty JT, Platia EV, Bulkley BH, Weisfeldt ML (1984) Localization of regional myocardial ischemia by recording of monophasic action potentials. Circulation 69: 593–604

Franz MR, Karasik PL, Li C, Moubarak J, Chavez M (1997) Electrical remodeling of the human atrium: similar effects in patients with chronic atrial fibrillation and atrial flutter. J Am Coll Cardiol 30: 1785–1792

Franz MR, Kirchhof PF, Fabritz CL, Koller B, Zabel M (1995) Computer analysis of monophasic action potential recordings: manual validation and clinically pertinent applications. PACE 18: 1666–1678

Franz MR, Schaefer J, Schottler M, Seed WA, Noble MI (1983) Electrical and mechanical restitution of the human heart at different rates of stimulation. Circ Res 53: 815–822

Franz MR, Swerdlow CD, Liem LB, Schaefer J (1988) Cycle length dependence of human action potential duration *in vivo*. Effects of single extrastimuli, sudden sustained rate acceleration and deceleration, and different steady-state frequencies. J Clin Invest 82: 972–979

Gehrmann J, Berul CI (2000) Cardiac electrophysiology in genetically engineered mice. J Cardiovasc Electrophysiol 11: 354–368

Gepstein L, Evans S (1998) Electroanatomical mapping of the heart: basic concepts and implications for the treatment of cardiac arrhythmias. PACE 21: 1268–1278

Gepstein L, Hayam G, BenHaim SA (1997) Activation-repolarization coupling in the normal swine endocardium. Circulation 96: 4036–4043

Kirchhof P, Degen H, Franz M, Eckardt L, Fabritz L, Milberg P, Laer S, Neumann J, Breithardt G, Haverkamp W (2003a) Amiodarone-induced post-repolarization refractoriness suppresses induction of ventricular fibrillation. J Pharmacol Exp Ther 305: 257–263

Kirchhof P, Eckardt L, Franz MR, Mönnig G, Loh P, Wedekind H, Schulze-Bahr E, Breithardt G, Haverkamp W (2003b) Prolonged atrial action potential durations and polymorphic atrial tachyarrhythmias in patients with long QT syndrome. J Cardiovasc Electrophysiol 214: 1027–1033

Kirchhof P, Eckardt L, Monnig G, Johna R, Loh P, Schulze-Bahr E, Breithardt G, Borggrefe M, Haverkamp W (2000) A patient with "atrial torsades de pointes". J Cardiovasc Electrophysiol 11: 806–811

Kirchhof P, Fabritz L, Fortmüller L, Lankford AR, Matherne G, Baba HA, Schmitz W, Breithardt G, Neumann J, Boknik P (2003c) Decreased chronotropic response to exercise and atrio-ventricular nodal conduction delay in mice overexpressing the A1-adenosine receptor. Am J Physiol 285: H145–153

Kirchhof P, Loh P, Eckardt L, Ribbing M, Rolf S, Eick O, Wittkampf F, Borggrefe M, Breithardt GG, Haverkamp W (2002b) A novel nonfluoroscopic catheter visualization system (LocaLisa) to reduce radiation exposure during catheter ablation of supraventricular tachycardias. Am J Cardiol 90: 340–343

Kirchhof PF, Fabritz CL, Franz MR (1998a) Post-repolarization refractoriness versus conduction slowing caused by class I antiarrhythmic drugs – antiarrhythmic and proarrhythmic effects. Circulation 97: 2567–2574

Kirchhof PF, Fabritz CL, Franz MR (1998b) Phase angle convergence of multiple monophasic action potential recordings precedes spontaneous termination of ventricular fibrillation. Basic Res Cardiol 93: 412–421

Kirchhof PF, Fabritz CL, Franz MR (1999) Postrepolarization refractoriness: Could it be the answer why antiarrhythmic drugs work? In: Franz MR, editor. Monophasic action potentials: Bridging cell and bedside. Futura, Armonk, NY, pp 493–509

Kirchhof PF, Fabritz CL, Zabel M, Franz MR (1996) The vulnerable period for low and high energy T wave shocks: role of dispersion of repolarisation and effect of d-sotalol. Cardiovasc Res 31: 953–962

Kirchhof PF, Franz MR (2001) Repolarization mapping using monophasic action potentials. In: Oto A, Breithardt G, editors. Myocardial repolarization: from gene to bedside. Futura, Armonk, NY, pp 139–149

Knollmann BC, Katchmann AN, Franz MR (2001) Monophasic action potential recordings from intact mouse heart: validation, regional heterogeneity, and relation to refractoriness. J Cardiovasc Electrophysiol 12: 1286–1294

Knollmann BC, Kirchhof P, Sirenko SG et al. (2003) Familial hypertrophic cardiomyopathy-linked mutant troponin T causes stress-induced ventricular tachycardia and Ca^{2+}-dependent action potential remodeling. Circ Res 92: 428–436

Knollmann BC, Tranquillo J, Sirenko SG, Henriquez C, Franz MR (2002) Microelectrode study of the genesis of the monophasic action potential by contact electrode technique. J Cardiovasc Electrophysiol 13: 1246–1252

Koller BS, Karasik PE, Solomon AJ, Franz MR (1995a) Relation between repolarization and refractoriness during programmed electrical stimulation in the human right ventricle. Implications for ventricular tachycardia induction. Circulation 91: 2378–2384

Koller BS, Karasik PE, Solomon AJ, Franz MR (1995b) Prolongation of conduction time during premature stimulation in the human atrium is primarily caused by local stimulus response latency. Eur Heart J 16: 1920–1924

Meissner A, Eckardt L, Kirchhof P, Weber T, Rolf N, Breithardt G, Van Aken H, Haverkamp W (2001) Effects of thoracic epidural anesthesia with and without autonomic nervous system blockade on cardiac monophasic action potentials and effective refractoriness in awake dogs. Anesthesiology 95: 132–138; discussion 6A

Milberg P, Eckardt L, Bruns HJ, Biertz J, Ramtin S, Reinsch N, Fleischer D, Kirchhof P, Fabritz L, Breithardt G, Haverkamp W (2002) Divergent proarrhythmic potential of macrolide antibiotics despite similar QT prolongation: fast phase 3 repolarization prevents early afterdepolarizations and torsade de pointes. J Pharmacol Exp Ther 303: 218–225

Moubarak J, Karasik P, Fletcher R, Franz MR (2000) High dispersion of ventricular repolarization after an implantable defibrillator shocks predicts induction of ventricular fibrillation as well as unsuccessful defibrillation. J Am Coll Cardiol 35: 422–427

Olsson SB, Harper RW (1978) Mexiletine effect on monophasic action potential (MAP) of right ventricle in man. Acta Med Scand [Suppl]

Pastore JM, Rosenbaum DS (2000) Role of structural barriers in the mechanism of alternans-induced reentry. Circ Res 87: 1157–1163

Pinney SP, Koller BS, Franz MR, Woosley RL (1995) Terfenadine increases the QT interval in isolated guinea pig hearts. J Cardiovasc Pharmacol 25: 30–34

Sager PT (1999) How to record high-quality monophasic action potential tracings. In: Franz MR (ed) Monophasic action potentials: Bridging cell and bedside. Futura, Armonk, NY, pp 121–134

Schaper W, Winkler B (1998) Of mice and men – the future of cardiovascular research in the molecular era. Cardiovasc Res 39: 3–7

Shimizu W, Antzelevitch C (1997) Sodium channel block with mexiletine is effective in reducing dispersion of repolarization and preventing torsade des pointes in LQT2 and LQT3 models of the long-QT syndrome. Circulation 96: 2038–2047

Sicouri S, Fish J, Antzelevitch C (1994) Distribution of M cells in the canine ventricle. J Cardiovasc Electrophysiol 5: 824–837

Taggart P, Sutton PM, Boyett MR, Lab M, Swanton H (1996) Human ventricular action potential duration during short and long cycles. Rapid modulation by ischemia. Circulation 94: 2526–2534

Tovar OH, Jones JL (1997) Epinephrine facilitates cardiac fibrillation by shortening action potential refractoriness. J Mol Cell Cardiol 29: 1447–1455

Tovar OH, Jones JL (2000) Electrophysiologic deterioration after one-minute fibrillation increases relative biphasic defibrillation efficacy. J Cardiovasc Electrophysiol 11: 645–651

Verduyn SC, Vos MA, van der Zande J, van der Hulst FF, Wellens HJ (1997) Role of interventricular dispersion of repolarization in acquired torsade-de-pointes arrhythmias: reversal by magnesium. Cardiovasc Res 34: 453–463

Weissenburger J, Nesterenko VV, Antzelevitch C (2000) Transmural heterogeneity of ventricular repolarization under baseline and long QT conditions in the canine heart in vivo: torsades de pointes develops with halothane but not pentobarbital anesthesia. J Cardiovasc Electrophysiol 11: 290–304

Wittkampf F, Wever E, Derksen R, Wilde A, Ramanna H, Hauer R, Robles de Medina E (1999) LocaLisa: new technique for real-time 3-dimensional localization of regular intracardiac electrodes. Circulation 99: 1312–1317

Zabel M, Hohnloser SH, Behrens S, Woosley RL, Franz MR (1997) Differential effects of D-sotalol, quinidine, and amiodarone on dispersion of ventricular repolarization in the isolated rabbit heart. J Cardiovasc Electrophysiol 8: 1239–1245

Zabel M, Lichtlen PR, Haverich A, Franz MR (1998) Comparison of ECG variables of dispersion of ventricular repolarization with direct myocardial repolarization measurements in the human heart. J Cardiovasc Electrophysiol 9: 1279–1284

Zabel M, Portnoy S, Franz MR (1994) Prediction of dispersion of repolarization by electrocardiographic parameters – studies in an intact rabbit heart model. PACE 17: 789 (Abstract)

Zhou X, Huang J, Ideker RE (2002) Transmural recording of monophasic action potentials. Am J Physiol Heart Circ Physiol 282: H855–861

Schütz E (1931) Monophasische Actionsströme vom in situ durchbluteten Säugetierherzen. Klin Wochenschr. 10: 1454–1456

Heart on a Chip – Extracellular Multielectrode Recordings from Cardiac Myocytes *in Vitro*

Ulrich Egert and Thomas Meyer

Introduction

Analyses of cardiac electrical potentials *in vivo*, such as in the electrocardiogram, are well known to reveal information about system properties of the heart, arrhythmia, indications of conduction failures etc., as has been described in Section I of this book. While such recordings are absolutely indispensable, the spatial resolution and the opportunities for manipulation with this approach are limited. *In vitro* investigations of isolated organs (see Section II), e.g. Purkinje fibers, papillary muscle, the Langendorff heart or patches of cardiac muscle (Yamamoto et al. 1998), have long been used to study the mechanisms of the generation and propagation of cardiac potentials at higher spatial resolution with either intra- or extra-cellular recording, or optical recording (Hirota et al. 1987). Cultures of cardiac myocytes, e.g. harvested after enzymatic digestion from cardiac tissue, on the other hand, offer the possibility of single cell or aggregate analyses, e.g. for developmental (Banach et al. 2003), pharmacological and biophysical studies (see also Section 5). Although these cultures do not maintain the structure of cardiac tissue, the functional properties of action potential generation and propagation, contractility and, depending to some extent on the culture system, the ion channel composition of the original cells are conserved or reestablished. The ease of production and the simple structure of these cell and tissue culture systems thus allow the researcher to address questions not easily accessible in organs or animal preparations. The motion of the cells in most of these preparations, however, hinders studies with conventional electrodes, in particular intracellular or patch-clamp recording, and in optical recordings with voltage sensitive dyes.

Although the motility can in principle be reduced by chemical decoupling of the contractile apparatus, this may have side effects and is thus generally not desirable. Extracellular recording of field potentials (FP) from contracting myocyte cultures is, however, facilitated considerably when the cells are grown in culture dishes with integrated microelectrode arrays (MEA, Fig. 1a,b; Halbach et al. 2003; Igelmund et al. 1999; Israel et al. 1984; Kehat et al. 2001; Meiry et al. 2001; Rohr 1990; Thomas et al. 1972). Cells grown on MEAs will adhere tightly to the substrate and contract isometrically, avoiding the motion artifacts that usually cause deterioration in the signal-to-noise ratio (SNR). These devices enable non-invasive simultaneous, multi-site, extracellular recordings from myocytes, whilst avoiding the mechanical stimulation of the cell that can hardly be avoided with conventional recording techniques. The

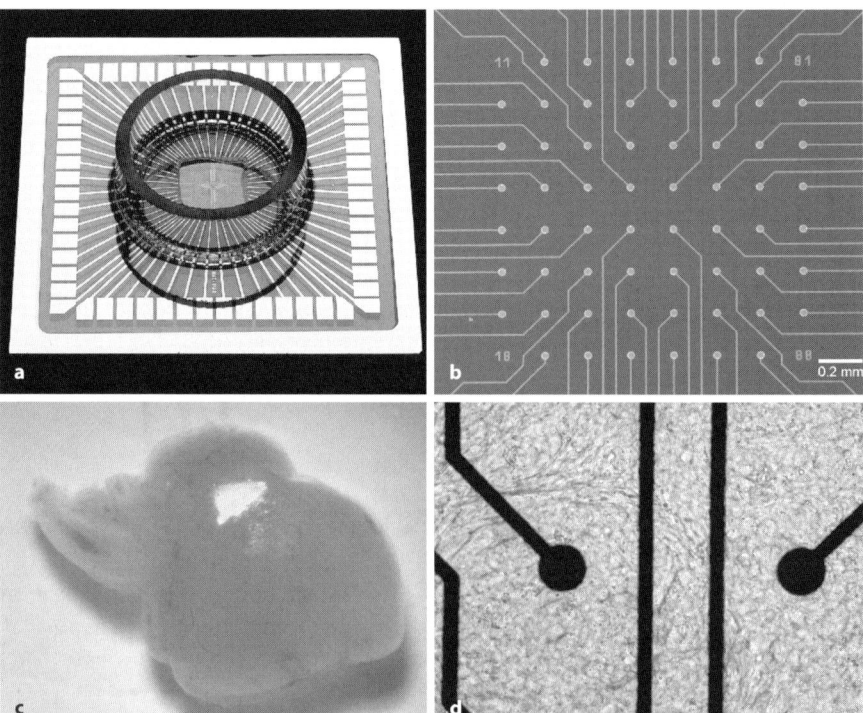

Figure 1a–d
Microelectrode arrays are produced photolithographically from thin layers of conducting and insulating materials, shaping the leads connecting the electrodes and amplifiers, in this case in gold (**a**), and the actual recording electrode surface. The latter is usually modified by galvanic deposition of platinum or microstructured titanium nitride to reduce the impedance of the electrode. The final electrode grid is shown in **b**. Whole hearts taken from chicken embryos (**c**) were dissociated and cultured to form multilayer or aggregate networks of cardiac myocytes (**d**) on the MEAs

multiplicity of recording sites also compensates for the slow structural displacements of excitable tissue, which occur when the tissue expands or when propagation pathways shift during differentiation of the cellular network or during pharmacological manipulation of the intercellular coupling. The combination of these properties enables studies that were hitherto not possible because they required long-term monitoring of activity patterns, rapid repositioning of the recording sites or were confounded by mechanical or (photo-) chemical stress. In addition, the spatio-temporal structure of activity and of the properties of the FP can be accessed even under conditions of irregular activity with changing pacemaker dominance or propagation pathways.

In this chapter we will introduce the recording of cell cultures prepared from cardiac tissue on MEAs, and the basis for the visualization and interpretation of the data obtained in such extracellular recordings. The idea is, to give the novice user a general starting point without concentrating too much on a particular application, but giving a few examples of what can be gained from such data.

MEAs with 60–70 electrodes are produced with thin-film photolithographic techniques and have become commercially available. Full recording systems are available currently as the MEA1060 system from Multi Channel Systems (MCS, Reutlingen, Germany, www.multichannelsystems.com) and as MED64 from Alpha MED Sciences (Tokyo, Japan, www.med64.com). Other groups have made their own setups or use similar MEAs produced elsewhere. To keep the details in our protocols explicit and consistent, we decided to describe the procedures as used with the MEAs and recordings systems (MEA1060) in our laboratories, knowing that this will introduce a certain bias. The techniques can be used with minor adaptations and generalizations with any other devices of this type, given that comparable properties of critical aspects are established. Where necessary, we have pointed out the goal of a particular step in the protocol, so that it can be modified in its details to suit your equipment.

System Description

The MEAs we use have 60 microelectrodes, with a diameter of 30 μm, positioned on an 8×8 grid with 200 μm spacing (Fig. 1). The recording area thus covers 1.4×1.4 mm^2. The electrodes themselves are flat, with a rough surface of TiN, 80–200 MΩ impedance (at 1 kHz) and recessed into the substrate by max. 1 μm. The culture chamber is formed by a 2 cm diameter glass ring with 6 mm height glued to the MEA base plate, resulting in a chamber volume of ca. 1.8 ml.

In addition to these standard layouts, there are modifications in the electrode material (like gold or indium-tin oxide ITO) and sizes to optimize the MEA layout for specific applications.

The recording system has amplifiers with fixed bandwidth (we used 0.1, 1 or 10 to 3.2 kHz) and amplification (we use 1000× or 1200×). It allows the continuous or triggered-window recording of all or selected channels simultaneously with sampling rates up to 50 kHz/channel (12 bit analog-to-digital conversion, mapping the input voltage range to 4096 steps).

Various analysis and display functions are provided for on line monitoring of an experiment. Further analyses are carried out off line, using tools written for Matlab (The Mathworks, Natick, USA).

Description of Methods and Practical Approach

Preparing MEAs for Cell Culture

The surface properties of the culture substrate are well known to have a decisive effect on the attachment, proliferation and differentiation of the cells. They can provide adhesion, growth-promoting, migration or differentiation cues. Pretreatment of the MEA surface is therefore important to achieve reproducible results. The insulator separating the electrode leads from the incubation medium forms most of the MEA surface, and therefore the culture substrate. In our case, this layer is formed by silicon nitride or silicon oxide; other arrays use silicon rubber, polymethylmethacrylate (PMMA), polyimide, or cured photosensitive resin (e.g. SU8, Dow Corning) used to structure the electrodes.

Pretreatment of Hydrophobic Surfaces

All of these materials tend to become hydrophobic during storage, which prevents attachment of the cells and pretreatment of the culture surface with permissive molecules. The first step in preparing the MEAs is therefore to ensure that the surfaces are hydrophilic for coating and cell adhesion. To test this without contaminating the surface, place a small drop of water on the MEA surface outside the culture chamber. If the drop does not wet the surface you probably need to perform one of the following steps, especially with new arrays:

- Laboratories with access to electron microscopy facilities probably have a sputter device or a plasma-cleaning chamber (e.g. Harrick Scientific, Ossining, NY). MEAs can be treated in these chambers with a low-vacuum plasma (2 min). This will crack surface molecules rendering them polar and thus make the surface hydrophilic. Note that the effect wears off after some days. The treatment gives a very clean (unless there is thick contamination) and sterile surface that can be coated readily with water-soluble molecules.
- If protein coating is acceptable in the experiments planned, there is a quick and simple way to render the surface hydrophilic in many cases. Sterilize the MEAs as described below. Then place approx. 1 ml of a concentrated, sterile protein solution (e.g. albumin, fetal calf serum or similar) onto the culture region for about 30 min. Wash the culture chamber thoroughly with sterile water afterwards. The MEA can then be used for cell culture directly.

Sterilization

Silicon nitride MEAs can be sterilized as usual for cell culture materials using either a 70% ethanol/H_2O mixture, UV-light, dry-heat sterilization or vapor autoclaving.

Adding Cell Culture Coating

MEA surfaces pretreated this way may then be coated with suitable surface molecules. In the following we will describe some procedures we have tested and found useful. Each coating can be used only once and needs to be removed after use with proteolytic detergent or methanol in the case of cellulose nitrate.

PEI Coating

Polyethylenimine (PEI, Sigma, Deisenhofen) is a coating agent commonly cited in the literature for cell culture (Lelong et al. 1992).

PEI works by changing the charge on the glass surface from negative to positive. It is necessary to rinse off unbound PEI thoroughly from the plates before using them to prevent the high pH (~9.5) of the solution from adversely affecting cells or tissues.

Steps

1. Prepare a 0.1% PEI solution in borate buffer (1.24 g boric acid (Riedel de Haen), 1.9 g borax (sodium tetraborate, Fluka) add 400 ml aq. dest).
2. Add 500 µl per MEA, which should cover the bottom of the culture chamber.
3. Incubate at: RT for 2 h or at 4°C overnight.
4. Remove PEI.
5. Wash three times with 1000 µl Water/MEA.
6. Dry the MEA and add cell suspension.
7. Sterilize under UV for at least 1 h after coating.

Cellulose Nitrate Coating

An alternative and fast procedure that works with several cell types and tissues and that is also successful with slightly hydrophobic MEAs is a coating with cellulose nitrate (CN). CN to our knowledge does not directly induce a cellular response.

1. For the stock solution, dissolve approx. 25 mg (5 cm^2) of blank CN blotting paper (Schleicher and Schuell, Dassel, Germany) in 2 ml of 100% methanol. Stock solution maybe stored at room temperature in polystyrene centrifuge tubes. For the final concentration add methanol in a ratio of 10:1.
2. Of the final solution we use 4 µl/cm^2, spread out carefully but quickly across the culture area with a disposable plastic pipette tip. Take care not to scratch across the central electrode field, as this may damage the electrode coating or insulator.
3. Let the coating dry completely in air. MEAs coated with CN may be stored for a few days.

Fibronectin Coating

Fibronectin (Becton Dickinson, Heidelberg, Germany) is a more biological coating alternative. Cultures tend to be more stable with respect to adhesion, which allows longer cultivation times.

1. Prepare a stock solution of 1 mg/ml fibronectin in distilled water, store it at 4 °C.
2. This solution is diluted with water to a final concentration of 10 µg/ml.
3. Cover the MEA surface with 300 µl of this solution and incubate for at least 60 min at 37 °C.
4. Wash MEAs twice with PBS, plate the cells on the MEA immediately thereafter.

Preparation of the Cell Culture

Cardiac tissue was taken from embryonic chicken ventricles (protocols for the preparation from other species are given in section 5 of this book). The hearts of 3–4 chicken embryos were removed after embryonic days 10–12 (E10-E12, see Fig. 1c).

The ventricle was isolated, minced and digested with 0.05% trypsin (original activity 10,400 U/mg) in Dulbecco's modified Eagle medium at 37 °C(DMEM, all chemicals: Sigma, Deisenhofen, Germany, unless stated otherwise). After 8 min of digestion the first supernatant was discarded and 3.5 ml of fresh, prewarmed trypsin solution were added. From now on, every 8 min the supernatant was collected in ice-cold DMEM with 10% fetal bovine serum (Gibco) and replaced by fresh trypsin solution. After 4–5 digestion cycles the heart was completely dissociated. The cells were pelleted (10 min, 800 g) and the supernatant was discarded. The pellet was washed (resuspended and centrifuged again) with 1 ml medium, then resuspended in 100–200 µl DMEM with 20% FCS, which resulted in approximately 10^7 cells/ml. 10 µl of this suspension were placed on to the electrode field of a MEA, 1 ml medium was added 1–2 min thereafter. To prevent evaporation and therefore changes in the osmolarity with medium exchange or drug application, 5 ml of sterile distilled water were added to a 12 cm Petri dish and the MEA placed into this dish when in the incubator.

The cell culture medium was exchanged every other day. After a MEA recording, the culture medium was replaced completely before returning the culture to the incubator. The ideal cultures form a homogeneous sheet of cells (see Fig. 1d). Cultures with spontaneous activity were recorded 2–5 days after preparation.

An interesting alternative is the use of 'lids' with a plastic membrane that is impermeable to water vapor but permeable to CO_2 and O_2. S. Potter has described such a technique for the use of MEAs with neuronal cell cultures (Potter 2001; DeMarse 2001) (the components are available through ALA, Westbury, NY).

Most arrays can be reused several times after cleaning with neutral, non-coating laboratory detergents; details for a particular type of MEA are indicated by the supplier. Never use cotton swabs to clean the electrode region; this will destroy the delicate surface finish of the electrodes and may damage the insulator. The durability of MEAs depends on various factors such as the insulation and electrode materials, the biological erosion of the insulator and whether they are used for electrical stimulation as well.

Recording Setup

Compared to conventional electrophysiological recording setups and given the number of electrodes, an MEA recording setup is compact and mechanically robust. Due to the compact build with integrated filters, amplifiers and computer-controlled recording interface, establishing a basic recording setup is quite simple. The standard MEA1060 system consists of a base plate with an MEA stage that is available with integrated heating, the amplifier housing with contact pins to the MEAs, the data acquisition card in the PC, and the MS-Windows based recording and analysis program MCRack.

We strongly recommend using a regulated, heated base plate since myocytes are highly sensitive to temperature changes and will often stop contracting spontaneously at room temperature. Fluctuations of 1 °C will often lead to noticeable changes in the contraction rate. In the following we therefore assume that the system has been assembled as described in the manual and that a heated base plate is available. Obviously, heating will increase evaporation and quite rapidly increase the osmolarity of the buffer in the small recording chamber. While the cells will tolerate slow changes for some time, they mostly detach if the osmolarity changes rapidly, e.g. when buffer or drug solutions are added. To reduce evaporation, cut a small notch into a plastic cover slip of 2 cm diameter and cover the chamber with it.

We generally place an Ag/AgCl pellet into the culture chamber as a reference electrode, with the connecting wire threaded through the notch. Alternatively, MEAs with substrate integrated reference electrodes are available. Components for closed systems with continuous perfusion are commercially available, e.g. from ALA (ALA Science, Westbury, NY).

Although not essential for the MEA recording itself, we work with inverted microscopes to visually monitor the cells' contraction occasionally.

Grounding the System

Although the MEA amplifier plate and the base plate already provide very good shielding, additional grounding or shielding might become necessary if line-frequency interference should be a problem. With careful grounding, however, it will almost never be necessary to use a large Faraday cage around the system. In fact, the amplifier housing and base plate already form a Faraday cage, the open top can be closed completely with a piece of wire netting or aluminum foil connected to the ground posts on the amplifier housing.

To avoid delays after mounting the MEA to the setup, the following steps should be performed in advance:
- place a dummy MEA (e.g. a worn out MEA) into the base plate,
- switch on the base plate heating and set it to 2 °C above incubator temperature,
- start MCRack and build a "Rack". For a quick start, sample racks are described in the appendix A. We suggest using a simple rack (CMC_simple_rack.rck) for the initial tests, and switch to more complex arrangements with online-analysis capabilities for the recording (CMC_adv_rack.rck).
- Assign a file name and folder to store the data to.
- Although cardiac action potentials are wider than their neuronal counterparts, they often have high-frequency components, in particular in the initial slopes at positions along the path of propagation of the excitation wave. When a detailed analysis of the waveform, and especially of this slope, is of interest, the sampling period should be set to 20 kHz. Otherwise 10 kHz are sufficient. Lower sampling frequencies may result in missing the peak amplitudes. Consequently, low-pass filters should be used with care and should be set accordingly.

Recording

For recording, mount the MEAs into the amplifier housing as described in the manual, place the Ag/AgCl pellet into the buffer and cover the recording chamber. After starting the program you should see sharp peaks for each contraction. The settings for on-line visualization should give a good overview of the SNR, the number of electrodes with spikes and changes of the beat rate. After deciding which electrodes bear useful signals and deselecting those that don't for storage, start recording to disc. Note that the saliency of the contraction bears little relation to the SNR.

Changes to Monitor during the Experiments

Critical parameters that may unexpectedly change during the experiment and influence the electrical activity are temperature, pH and osmolarity. Temperature changes, even by airflow across the MEA, will quickly change the beat rate. Since the chamber volume is small, the heating may not compensate such a change fast enough. If this is a critical issue, you may want to add a digital thermometer with an analog readout connected to an extra channel of the ADC-input (e.g. Greisinger GMH 3210 connected to an external analog-input channel of the MEA1060 system). Lacquer-insulated Ni-Cr-Ni type-K thermo-sensors are very small and can be placed inside the chamber. This allows continuous monitoring of the temperature.

During short experiments the cover slip should suffice to prevent changes in the pH. In long-term experiments the pH can be stabilized by using HEPES buffered media or by continuous perfusion with CO_2 equilibrated culture medium (low rates are sufficient, e.g. 0.1 ml/min), which would also solve any osmolarity problems.

Examples
Data Analysis and Interpretation

One major advantage of recording from cardiac tissue with MEAs is the extraordinary mechanical stability of the recording situation with isometric contractions. The extracellular signal is thus free of motion artifacts. This allows recordings over many hours or even days, facilitating, for example, developmental studies and investigations of long-term drug effects.

Comparable to conventional recording techniques, these extracellular field potentials (FP) correlate in time with the contraction cycle (FP spike rate) and can therefore be analyzed for contraction rate and spatio-temporal patterns of arrhythmia. Several aspects need to be considered in these analyses. In particular during early phases of the incubation period, the isolated or weakly coupled islets of contracting cells or cell aggregates will each have their individual pacemakers (Fig. 2). As the cells proliferate and the islets merge into a continuous sheet, the contraction will be increasingly dominated by one site, which will enslave the others depending on the intercellular resistance across the gap junctions (see Fig. 4). In the transition period, however, the current produced by that pacemaker and other excitable cells might not be large enough to depolarize the cell membrane across larger distances, allowing additional pacemakers to interfere.

The effect of this interference is often phase dependent, i.e. irregular beating because of the interacting pacemaker activity may or may not be optically visible, even when detected in the recording.

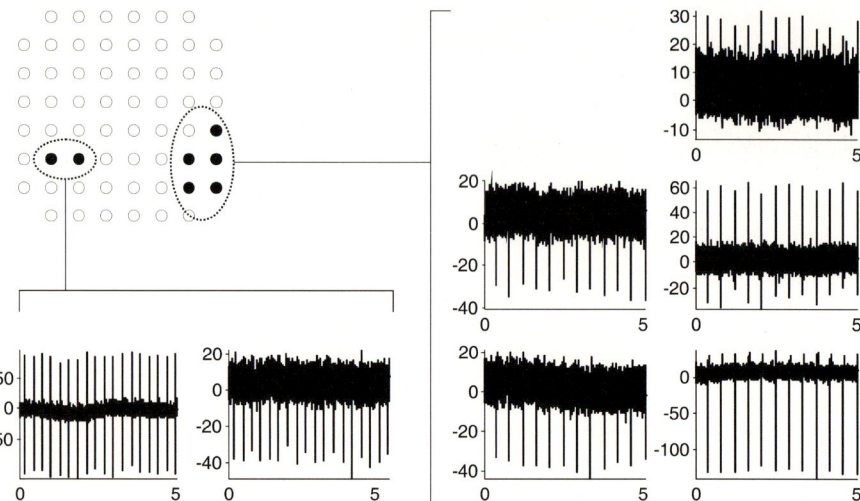

Figure 2
Within a few days, field potentials (FP) in various shapes can be recorded from CMC cultures. Initially, regions with independent pacemakers are common, identified by different rates of negative spikes (FP_{MIN}) at clusters of electrodes. In this example, these regions did not overlap. Each section had electrodes detecting FP_{MIN} only, indicating that electrical activity arose close to these electrodes. Neighboring electrodes had both FP_{MIN} and positive peaks (FP_{pre}), which we interpret as sites along the path of propagation. A third type of recording (top right trace) had FP_{pre} only, suggesting minimal early depolarizing Na^+ and Ca^{2+} currents at this location, and passive, capacitive outward currents compensating inward currents simultaneously flowing at neighboring locations. The FP initiated independently in such regions may overlap in recordings from later stages, resulting in complex mixed waveforms

Although these arrhythmias are an interesting subject in themselves, analyses of delay times between electrodes and arrhythmia patterns need to identify such artifacts, which is often possible based on the different waveforms of FPs generated by the two pacemakers at a particular electrode.

Beyond this, analyses of the FP shape are possible (Sprössler et al. 1999) (Fig. 3), which can be extended to map the spatial distribution of features of the FP (Fig. 4). The basis of this interpretation is the correlation between changes in some transmembrane currents and those of certain components of the FP. This allows an interpretation of the recording with respect to changes in the shape of the underlying action potentials and in the contribution of sodium and calcium currents (see Fig. 6b). The spike rate and the timing of spikes at different recording sites, and thus the propagation, can easily be monitored online with MCRack.

An example of how to construct a virtual setup for this purpose in MCRack and how to extract peak amplitudes, times and spike rates is described in the Appendix. While these parameters can be stored and are accessible for further processing with spreadsheet programs (e.g. Microsoft Excel), analyzing the raw data from all electrodes and creating feature maps, such as in Fig. 4, by far exceeds the capacity of such programs. In our laboratories we use Matlab (The Mathworks, Natick, MA, USA), a program with powerful analysis and visualization capabilities for more detailed

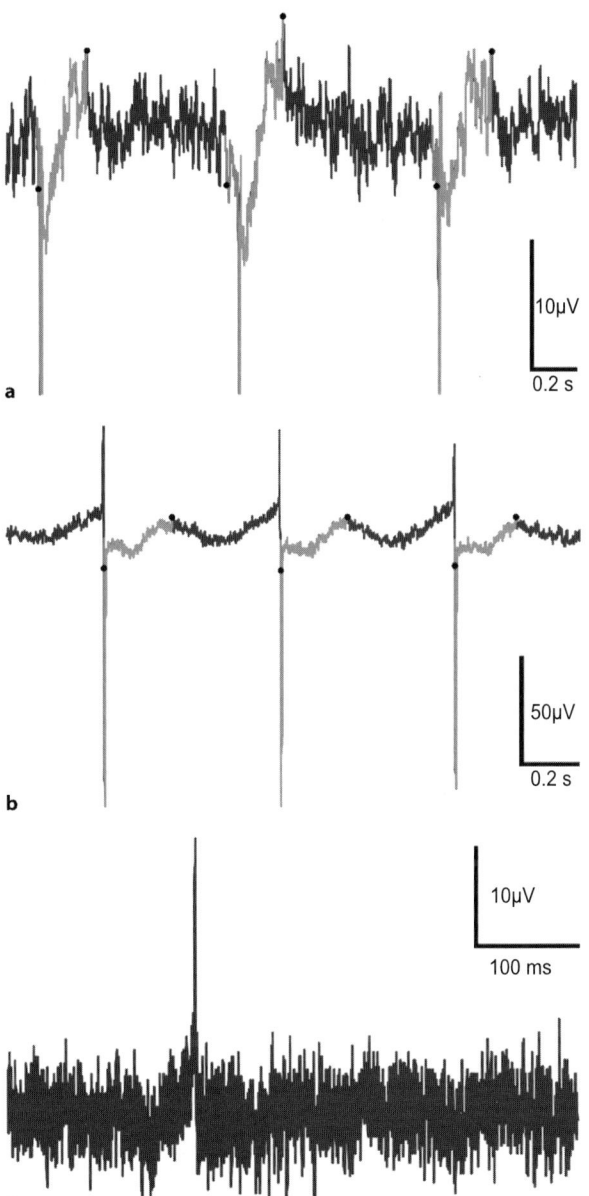

Figure 3a–c
The three standard FP types introduced in Fig. 3.10-2 in more detail. The colored sections in **a** and **b** are elements identified by the analysis program as down slope (*magenta*, **a**), FP$_{pre}$ (*magenta*, **b**), and upslope (*green*) of the FP up to FP$_{MAX}$ (*black dot*). The durations of the magenta and green sections correlate (but are not identical) with the durations of the upslope and duration of the action potentials recorded intracellularly. Even though active inward currents are not detectable in **c**, the cell layer may be moving in this region. The distribution of the electrical potentials and the types of waveforms cannot be predicted from visual inspection. *For coloured version see appendix*

offline analysis. For users of MCRack, a toolbox is available[1] to interface Matlab with MCRack data files and also various tools to specifically analyze myocyte recordings[2].

---
[1] http://www.brainworks.uni-freiburg.de/projects/mea/meatools/overview.htm
[2] The myocyte tool-box (CMC-Tools) is available as freeware to educational organizations. Please inquire to U.E.

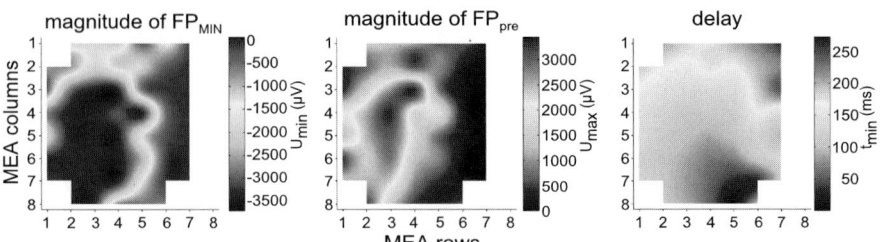

Figure 4
Pseudocolor plots of features of FP. The magnitudes of FP_{MIN}, FP_{pre} and the relative peak time of FP_{MIN}, in this example, can be used to identify the dynamics and functional status of the various regions of the culture, as well as to identify inhomogeneities. *For coloured version see appendix*

The analyses discussed thus far are largely independent of the simultaneity of the recording at different electrodes. This aspect becomes important, however, in investigations of the dynamics of excitation spreading in cardiac tissue. In particular in arrhythmic tissue, it is obvious that the beat-to-beat variation of the peak timing prohibits the reconstruction of the path of propagation based on successive recordings at different locations.

MEA recording enables the detailed assessment of event times, their variability across beats and the correlation of timing and variability between locations, and thus of the variability of dynamic processes in the tissue. The most apparent aspect of these dynamics is the propagation of the action potential across the tissue. This depends on a number of variables, predominantly the intercellular resistance across gap junctions and the magnitude of the depolarizing sodium current (Spach et al. 1979; Spach 1983; Spach and Heidlage 1995). While the spatial resolution of MEAs is not as good as in video-enhanced microscopy, we can easily identify the sharp peak associated with the Na^+ current, and thus determine the temporal succession of the depolarization across the tissue with high temporal resolution and hence the propagation of excitation (Fig. 5) (Kleber et al. 1996; Rohr et al. 1997a,b; Rohr and Kucera 1997).

When the propagation velocity is of interest, it becomes necessary to determine the pathway of excitation propagation from the succession of the peak times at the electrodes. With large electrode spacing, this may not be unequivocally feasible, as the real propagation pathway may be tortuous, masked by delays caused by high-resistance sections, bifurcation, etc.

Furthermore, it must be ensured that peak times are determined for corresponding waveform elements, i.e. the first clear negative peaks with step descending slopes in each cycle. Because of these sources of ambiguity, a general "propagation velocity" is frequently difficult to calculate and verify sufficiently.

In most cases, however, an interpretation of experimental findings can equally well be based on inter-electrode delays directly, avoiding the need to determine the length and homogeneity of the propagation pathway.

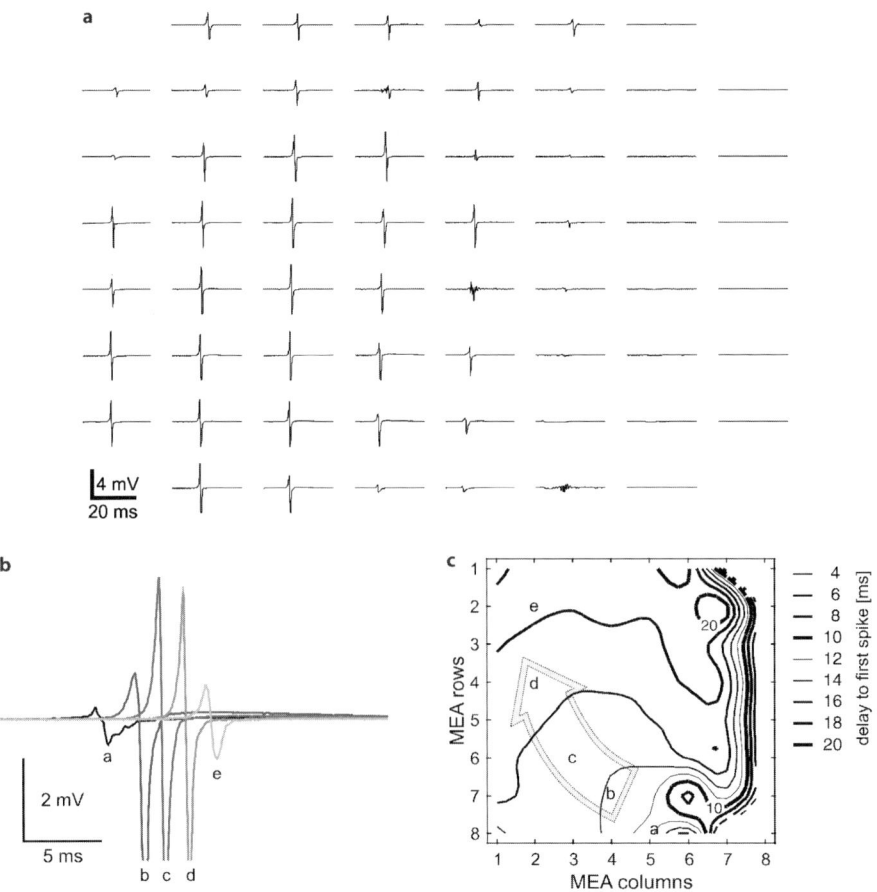

Figure 5a–c
a Based on the analysis of the distribution of FPs recorded in a confluent layer of cells (a) we identified the succession of activation across the recording area. b Overlay of FPs from a subset of electrodes along the path of propagation (marked in c). c Distribution of the delays of FP_{MIN}. The dense contours on the right of the MEA field stem from border artifacts. The slope of this FP_{MIN}-time landscape is minimal along the track marked by the large arrow, identifying the propagation pathway (Egert and Haemmerle 2002). The data were taken from the same culture as in Fig. 4. The delay contour plot is an alternative visualization for the pseudocolor plot in Fig. 4

Evaluation of Cardioactive Drugs

The interpretation of the FP shape given above suggests that these changes might be useful to predict *in vivo* responses to these compounds. Even though the mechanisms involved are certainly more complex and species dependent, we have analyzed the changes of the FP duration in response to the application of several drugs with known QT-prolonging effects (Fig. 6a,c). This change of the QT interval is highly relevant to the safety pharmacology of new drugs. We observed a concentration dependent pro-

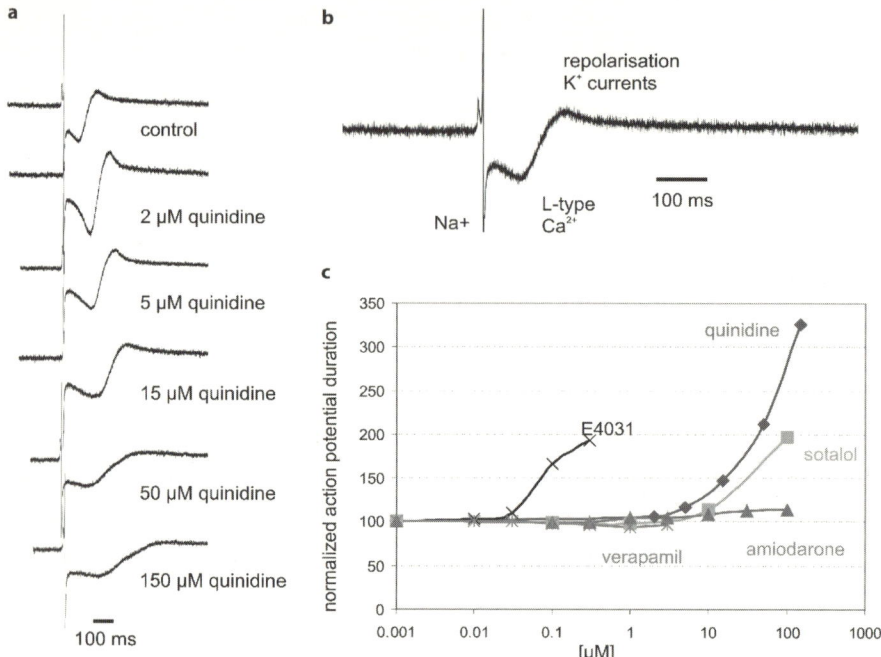

Figure 6a–c
Based on the interpretation of the FP waveform and its correlation with action potential properties, cardioactive drugs can be tested in CMC cultures. Changes of the FP in response to their application should correlate with known changes for APs measured intracellularly. Quinidine for example, is known to lengthen the QT interval, which correlates with the length of the plateau phase of the AP. This lengthening is observed in our CMC recordings (**a**). Investigations with specific ion channel blockers showed that FP_{MIN} depends on Na^+-currents, FP_{MAX} on K^+-currents and a second, negative peak, which is not always visible, is Ca^{2+}-dependent. Dose dependent changes of the FP duration correlated well with observations in *in vivo* studies on QT interval prolongation (**c**). *For coloured version see appendix*

longation of the field potential duration, which is closely related to the QT interval, with E4031 a specific blocker of the HERG channel, and the antiarrhythmics quinidine, and sotalol. Verapamil, a calcium ion influx inhibitor, and amiodarone, both with antiarrhythmic properties, did not change the QT interval. These effects, and the concentration ranges in which they occur, are comparable to those reported in the literature (Redfern et al. 2003).

Other Approaches to Spatio-Temporal Cardiac Excitation Patterns

Besides the approaches mentioned here, other techniques have been developed to investigate the structure of cardiac excitation patterns in different preparations and on various time scales. Cultures of dissociated cardiomyocytes from neonatal rats have been used with similar recording devices, e.g. to investigate structure-dependent impulse conduction and beat rate variability (Kucera et al. 2000; Rohr et al. 1997b). Lu et al. (2003) explanted whole mouse hearts, and even whole mouse embryos on MEAs to study the differentiation of cardiac activity. Myocyte cultures have also been recorded with transistor based electrode arrays (Sprössler et al. 1999).

Summary

Extracellular recordings from cardiac myocyte cultures with substrate integrated electrode arrays open a new range of experimental approaches to investigate the dynamics of electrical activity and their pharmacological modulation. The mechanical stability and fixed electrode-to-cell configuration allow long-term studies and an advanced analysis and interpretation of the field potentials recorded, extending from developmental investigations to the assessment of drug effects on the time course of the membrane potential in cardiac cells. New approaches using whole-heart explants and cultures may in the future further improve the predictive value of such studies, enabling systems analyses that are not possible with single electrode techniques alone.[3]

Appendix

The general principles in setting up recording software are necessarily the same for all systems, the means of adjusting the necessary parameters of the software are, however, very different. Below, we give instructions on how to start with the most basic arrangement and for more advanced online analyses. For recording systems other than MCRack, the basic parameters suggested are likewise valid but need to be entered into a different user interface. MCRack runs under Microsoft Windows and imposes no limit on the file size other than that which Microsoft Windows does. A Linux interface to the recording hardware is available from D. Wagenaar (www.its.caltech.edu/~wagenaar/meabench). Most systems allow the user to store the settings optimized for an experiment, so it is useful to define a setup (called virtual "Rack", in analogy with classical workplaces for electrophysiological studies) for initial tests on a culture and others for the actual experiments to be done. These Racks can be downloaded from the MCS website (www.multichannelsystems.com).

Sample Racks for MCRack version 3.1

The simplest version will allow you to record the raw, unconditioned data on all electrodes at the same time and store them to a file. It is meant to be a failsafe start requiring little computing power and is also useful to check which electrodes have activity and acceptable SNR. Note that at 20 kHz sampling rate you will record approx. 2.4 MB per s using all 60 electrodes. Except for the recording to file, this Rack during is also useful for debugging during the initial setup of the system.

---

[3]Acknowledgements: Parts of this work were funded by the BMBF grants no. 0310965, 0310968, and 0310964D.

Simple Rack (CMC_simple_rack.rck)

- Setting the input range and the sampling frequency.
  MCRack will come up with a "Recorder" in the Rack window only. Add a data source (MEA electrode field button). Select "Hardware" of the "Data Source" settings and adjust the input voltage range. For an amplification of 1200× setting this value to −2048 mV to +2047 mV is a good start. The peak voltage of the spikes multiplied by the amplification factor should fit into this window. The voltage resolution will be this range divided by the sampling resolution of the AD converter, in this setup 12 bit, which gives 4096 mV/(1200×4096) = 0.83 µV. Set the sampling frequency to 20 kHz.
- With the "MC_Card" tab selected, add a "Display". The display should give you a geometrically correct overview of the activity on all electrodes across a time span of several inter-beat intervals. By default, a window will open with small panels arranged as the electrodes on the MEA. In the 'Data' tab, activate "Electrode Raw Data". "Display Type" should be "Window". In the "Window" tab select "Continuous" mode and set both "Window Distance" and "Window Extent" to 1000 ms. In the display window itself you will find a "Peak detection" checkbox. Activating this ensures that you will see the minimum and maximum values that occurred in the time window represented by one pixel on the screen, which may span several data samples. It is not necessary to record all data you may want to visualize online. Often, an offline analysis gives the opportunity to preprocess and select relevant data with optimized tools while an online analysis gives a quick overview.
- To record exactly what you see in the display select the "Recorder" and activate "Electrode Raw Data" in the "Channels" tab.
- In the "Recorder" tab indicate path and the root name of the file in which you want to store the data. Note that MCRack will add a counter to this name and increment this number for each time a recording with storage is requested. Selecting "Auto Stop" and indicating a file size or duration target can used to limit the recording time.
- In the "Window" tab of the recorder select "Continuous" (this mode is sometimes called "gap-free" recording).
- Now you are ready to go. The data will be displayed when you press the "Start" button, but will be recorded to the file only when both the "Record" and the "Start" button are pressed.

Advanced Rack (CMC_adv_rack.rck)

During the experiment, it is generally useful to achieve a quick impression of slow changes in the spike rate and the FP peak values, e.g. when adding test substances, i.e. an online extraction of suitable parameters is desirable. These options and more will be available with the following rack. As described above, the conspicuous sodium-driven spikes mark only the early part of the corresponding action potential. To exploit the information in the FP fully it is therefore necessary to record continuously. If only the beat rate is needed, the amount of data produced can be reduced drastically by storing short cutouts and the corresponding time stamps only. In this Rack we will do both, detect spikes for online analysis and visualization, and store gap-free records.

- Start with the first Rack (the display window will be deleted later on).
- "Spikes" can be detected with individual thresholds on each electrode. These spike times can be used to determine the spike rate and delays between the electrodes. With the "Data Source" selected, add a "Spike Sorter". Select its "Channels" tab and activate "Electrode Raw Data". In the display window of the spike sorter activate "Peak Detection". We will set the detection thresholds later on when the MEA with the myocytes is in place.
- We will use one electrode as a trigger source to align the spikes on all electrodes. With the "Spike Sorter" selected, add a "Trigger Detector". In its "Trigger" tab, activate the pull down menu. You will see a list of electrodes from which you can pick one with myocyte spikes later on. This configuration will give you a trigger signal for every spike detected on that electrode.
- Configure the spike rate analysis
  Based on the time stamps generated thus far we can set up the online analysis. The number and type of analyses that can be done online ultimately depends on the computing power, the number of electrodes to be analyzed and the SNR.
  With the "Trigger Detector" selected, add an "Analyzer" window. In its "Channels" tab activate "Spikes 1". The "Analyzer" tab offers a number of parameters that can be extracted. Here we will use "rate" to calculate the beat rate from the spikes detected. The same analyzer can extract other properties of the cardiac activity simultaneously. Depending on the axes required, these can be combined in one display or need separate displays.
- An additional display in which all windows are shown triggered to one electrode is often useful to observe changes of the spatio-temporal pattern. Repeat the previous step, but set the mode in the "Window" tab to "Start on Trigger" and select "Trigger 1". Set the "Start Time" to –50 ms, "Window Extent" to 800 ms.
- With the "Analyzer" selected, add a "Parameter Display", selecting "Parameter 1" in the "Data" tab. "Plot Type" should be "Trace". This will open a second display window, which will later show the spike rate. In the "Ranges" tab set X-Axis Min to 0, Max to 600 s, set "Y-Axis Min" to 0, "Max" to 5 Hz.
- Displaying the raw signal
  With the "Analyzer" selected, add a "Display". This display will be used to display the raw signal recorded at each electrode. In the "Data" tab, activate "Electrode Raw Data", "Display Type" should be "Trace". In the "Window" tab select "Continuous" mode and set "Window Distance" and "Window Extent" to 1000 ms each. Now select the "Layout" tab and open the 8×8 mea.cmp channel map. A window will open with small panels arranged like the electrodes on the MEA. In the "Display 1" window activate "Peak Detection".
- Adjust the Recorder as described above for the first Rack, selecting "Electrode Raw Data" and "Parameter 1" in the "Channels" tab.
- Delete the display window remaining from the first rack.

Reducing CPU Load and File Size

After mounting the MEA into the amplifier we need to return to the 'Spike Sorter' to select the electrodes that actually do show activity and set suitable thresholds for spike detection (an automatic threshold finder is part of the tool). Deselected electrodes will be automatically removed from all subsequent processing stages. One of the selected electrodes then needs to be defined as the trigger in the "Trigger Detector".

In a recording, you may not detect myocyte spikes on every electrode and the SNR on some may be insufficient for certain analyses. Each tool therefore allows you to select on which electrode its function should be applied. Reducing the number of electrodes stored, analyzed or displayed will, most importantly, reduce the file size and the load on the computers CPU. Since CPU load limits the number of tools that can be used in a Rack, and therefore the number of analyses that can be performed online, using fewer electrodes gives you more flexibility.

An additional aspect to consider in the selection of the electrodes to observe is the type of FP detected. As described above, some electrodes may show positive peaks only, indicating that there is no active current sink at these sites, even though the cells at these positions may visibly move during contractions. These electrodes will not give useful information for further analysis and do not need to be stored.

Troubleshooting

The possible "troubles" we address in this section are based on, of course, our own experience, but also on the basis of questions frequently asked by other users. We did not include problems that exclusively address this particular configuration of the setup but those that are in one way or another issues common to all builds. Where we refer to particular parts of the system, these should be considered as examples and can be transferred to comparable components of other devices.

Critical Steps and Procedures during Preparation

- Blood should be removed from the hearts by a short washing to achieve clean cultures.
- It is critical to mince the ventricle into as small pieces as possible to shorten digestion time.
- Avoid too vigorous pipetting of cell suspension to minimize shear stress.
- These measures and washing of the pellet to remove trypsin enhance viability of cells.

Coating and Cell Culture

If cells do not attach:
- Check if the surface of the MEA is sufficiently hydrophilic. If not, check plasma-cleaner function or prolong treatment in the plasma-cleaner.
- If the surface is hydrophilic but cells do not attach, try new coating solution, or a different coating protocol.
- If cellulose nitrate coating does not yield sufficient cell attachment, note that the CN solutions cannot be stored indefinitely. CN forms a visible gelatinous precipitate after extended storage of at least half a year. These solutions will not produce satisfactory adhesive coatings anymore. Prepare new solutions if the precipitate shows.

If the cells do not visibly contract or contract insufficiently:
- Check the Ca^{2+}-concentration in your medium; it should be approx. 2 mM.
- Check the temperature of the medium, view only one dish at a time, and leave the others in the incubator.
- Check if potassium concentration has increased due to evaporation effects, measure osmolarity.
- Are there any single pacemaker islets, but no overall activity? – Check the culture again after one or two days. Carefully change only 50% of the medium at a time.
- If cells become too dense before contracting: reduce FCS concentration.
- Try using younger animals.

If cells aggregate/do not aggregate (depending on the experimental design):
- If cells aggregate, the coating might be bad or missing.
- The MEA surface might be hydrophobic.
- If you want to grow aggregates: use a bacteriological hydrophobic Petri dish to incubate the cells. They will not attach and will form aggregates in suspension that can be harvested after 1–2 days, depending on the size required. Aggregates can be plated carefully on MEAs pretreated as described above for monolayer cultures.

If cells detach again:
- Check all points mentioned above for non-attaching cells.
- You might want to reduce cell density or reduce FCS concentration in the proliferation phase.
- Check for increasing osmolarity in the MEA chamber, in particular if the cells detach after exchanging the culture medium.

If the osmolarity becomes too high between medium exchanges:
- Add more water to the surrounding Petri dish (prewarmed to incubator temperature).
- Place an additional small lid on the MEA chamber, e.g. the bottom of a small 3 cm Petri dish.
- Use a hygrometer, e.g. with a xy-plotter, to determine how fast the nominal humidity is reached after closing the door of the incubator.

Too Many Pacemakers

Multiple pacemaker centers prevail during the initial incubation of the cells but the culture should be dominated by one pacemaker later on. This process can be accelerated by increasing the initial cell density and by reducing the number of large aggregates. To reduce the number of aggregates, allow the suspension to settle for 10 min in a 15 ml centrifuge tube and only seed the supernatant. Alternatively, pass the suspension through a sterile nylon sieve (mesh width 50–100 μm) to skim off large aggregates. In cultures of fully dissociated cells contractions may start later than in those containing aggregates.

Low Signal-to-Noise Ratio

Low SNRs can be the result of several causes. Generally, the SNR should be judged based on the magnitude of FP_{MIN}, not of the initial positive peak. Within the recording horizon of the electrode, this depends on (i) the total inward current, mostly driven by Na^+, and thus the membrane area that depolarizes at that time. This, in turn, depends on (ii) the 3D-density of cardiac cells and (iii) the density of Na^+ channels. In consequence, the SNR can often be improved by optimizing the preparation and culture conditions to yield well-differentiated cardiomyocytes.

If the cells visibly contract in the electrode field but no FP peaks are visible:

- Dedifferentiation, a cell type mix, and low cell density will decrease the SNR. This might be prevented by reducing the digestion stress (shorter times or lower trypsin activity), increasing the seeding density, and increasing the culture period before recording.
- Sometimes the islets of active cells are so small that they come to lie between the electrodes. In this case you might detect only passive, outward currents on neighboring electrodes.
- Check if the "Peak Detection" is active in the "Display" window. The number of pixels available for each electrode is not enough to display each data sample if the temporal width of each window is larger than a few milliseconds. So the display, but not the recording, will miss data points. "Peak Detection" will ensure that the largest and the smallest values sampled in the period represented by one pixel on the screen are actually visible. The same effect will show an apparently smaller noise band when 'Peak Detection' is off.
- In some cases a worn electrode or high resistance contact to the amplifiers may lead to increased, high frequency baseline noise. Clean the outer contact pads of the MEA and the contact pins with acetone for high-frequency oscillations (see below).
- Make sure that the "Window" mode of the display is set to continuous.

Troubleshooting the Signal

If you see high frequency noise on some display panels: When the contact resistance between electrode and amplifier is high, the amplifier's input floats and may start to oscillate between the maximum and minimum voltage of the input range (e.g. −2048 mV to +2047 mV divided by the amplification factor).

- In most cases, this is due to grease or dirt on either the outer MEA contact pads or the contact pins of the amplifier. Wipe the pads with soft tissue soaked with acetone and wipe the tips of the contact pins with dry filter paper. Ask your supplier for suitable ways to clean other contacting mechanisms.
- Worn contact pads: do the contact pads on the outside of the MEA appear to have holes? Move the MEA slightly in the holding frame.
- Worn contact pins: this is the most common cause, in various ways. Spring driven pins are made from steel, coated with gold. Leakage of saline into the pins will cause corrosion, destroying the springs and finally the pin shaft itself. Initially rust may increase the contact resistances within the pins. Test if they are easily compressible and expand again, if not you may use a tiny drop of common contact spray on the pins. Inspect the very tip of the contact pins under a stereomicroscope. Dark spots or flaky appearance points to corroded gold coatings. Such contacts need to be replaced.
- If nothing helps, the electrode of the MEA itself may be damaged. On MEA1060 systems, the amplifiers can be connected to ground individually, disconnecting the damaged electrode.

50/60 Hz Components (Line Hum) and Harmonics Thereof

Because of the compact build and the housing of the amplifiers, essentially all MEA type amplifiers on the market are well shielded and grounded by their design, already. Maximal shielding will be achieved by connecting a piece of aluminum foil or wire netting to the grounding points of the amplifiers and covering the MEA with it. In most cases, the source of the line hum interference is a part of the microscope or other equipment that is not connected to the grounding point. Some microscopes need to be grounded in several places because the individual components may not be connected electrically. If used, a second source of line hum is the perfusion system. Although ground loops need to be avoided, the perfusion tubing sometimes needs to be grounded separately, e.g. by inserting a piece of steel tube cut from a syringe canula, into the tubing and connecting it to ground. Because of the frequency composition of the FP, additional high-pass filtering will lead to unacceptable distortions and therefore needs to be avoided. Additional thermo-sensors will act as antennas, in particular with power-supplies. Use a battery driven model.

Troubleshooting the Rack

If the data are not recorded to file:
- Check if the target directory is accessible for writing.
- Check if the desired data stream is checked in the "Channels" tab of the recorder.

Data Analysis

Problems during data analysis are mostly due to insufficient SNR or multiple pacemakers. Both hamper the identification of beat cycles, FP components and correlations between electrodes. While it is often possible to identify the peaks visually, an automated analysis will usually be necessary because of the large amount of data, in particular with drug testing. Depending on the frequency composition of the noise, digitally filtering the data may be suitable, especially for rate analyses, but it also may distort the FP (see above). We found a "Savitzky-Golay" filter to be very useful (Press et al. 1992; Savitzky and Golay 1964).

References

Additional illustrations and the MEA-Tools for Matlab are available from http://www.brainworks.uni-freiburg.de/projects/mea/meatools/overview.htm

Banach K, Halbach M, Hu P, Hescheler J, Egert U (2003) Development of electrical activity in cardiac myocyte aggregates derived from mouse embryonic stem cells. Am J Physiol Heart Circ Physiol 284: H2114–2123

Egert U, Haemmerle H (2002) Application of the microelectrode-array (MEA) technology in pharmaceutical drug research. In: Baselt JP, Gerlach G (eds) Sensoren im Fokus neuer Anwendungen. w.e.b. Universitätsverlag, Dresden, pp 51–54

Halbach MD, Egert U, Hescheler J, Banach K (2003) Estimation of action potential changes from field potential recordings in multicellular mouse cardiac myocyte cultures. Cell Physiol Biochem 13: 271–284

Hirota A, Kamino K, Komuro H, Sakai T (1987) Mapping of early development of electrical activity in the embryonic chick heart using multiple-site optical recording. J Physiol (London) 383: 711–728

Igelmund P, Fleischmann BK, Fischer IV, Soest J, Gryshchenko O, Sauer H, Liu Q, Hescheler J (1999) Action potential propagation failures in long-term recordings from embryonic stem cell-derived cardiomyocytes in tissue-culture. Pflügers Arch Eur J Physiol 437: 669–679

Israel DA, Barry WH, Edell DJ, Mark RG (1984) An array of microelectrodes to stimulate and record from cardiac cells in culture. Am J Physiol 247: H669–H674

Kehat I, Karsenti D, Amit M, Druckmann M, Feld Y, Itskovitz-Eldor J, Gepstein L (2001) Long term, high-resolution, electrophysiological assessment of human embryonic stem cell derived cardiomyocytes: a novel *in vitro* model for the human heart. Circ Res 18: 659–661

Kleber AG, Fast VG, Kucera J, Rohr S (1996) Physiology and pathophysiology of cardiac impulse conduction. Z Kardiol 85: 25–33

Kucera JP, Heuschkel MO, Renaud P, Rohr S (2000) Power-law behavior of beat-rate variability in monolayer cultures of neonatal rat ventricular myocytes. Circ Res 86: 1140–1145

Lelong IH, Petegnief V, Rebel G (1992) Neuronal cells mature faster on polyethyleneimine coated plates than on polylysine coated plates. J Neurosci Res 32: 562–568

Meiry G, Reisner Y, Feld Y, Goldberg S, Rosen M, Ziv N, Binah O (2001) Evolution of action potential propagation and repolarization in cultured neonatal rat ventricular myocytes. J Cardiovasc Electrophysiol 12: 1269–1277

Potter SM, DeMarse TB (2001) A new approach to neural cell culture for long-term studies. J Neurosci Methods 110: 17–24

Press H, Teukolsky SA, Vetterling WT, Flannery BP (1992) Savitzky-Golay smoothing filters. In: Numerial recipes in C. Cambridge University Press, Cambridge, pp 650–655

Redfern WS, Carlsson L, Davis AS, Lynch WG, MacKenzie I, Palethorpe S, Siegl PK, Strang I, Sullivan AT, Wallis R, Camm AJ, Hammond TG (2003) Relationships between preclinical cardiac electrophysiology, clinical QT interval prolongation and torsade de pointes for a broad range of drugs: evidence for a provisional safety margin in drug development. Cardiovasc Res 58: 32–45

Rohr S (1990) A computerized device for long-term measurements of the contraction frequency of cultured rat heart cells under stable incubating conditions. Pflügers Arch Eur J Physiol 416: 201–206

Rohr S, Kucera JP (1997) Involvement of the calcium inward current in cardiac impulse propagation: Induction of unidirectional conduction block by nifedipine and reversal by Bay K 8644. Biophys J 72: 754–766

Rohr S, Kucera JP, Fast VG, Kleber AG (1997a) Paradoxical improvement of impulse conduction in cardiac tissue by partial cellular uncoupling. Science 275: 841–844

Rohr S, Kucera JP, Kleber AG (1997b) Form and function: Impulse propagation in designer cultures of cardiomyocytes. News in Physiological Sciences 12: 171–177

Savitzky A, Golay MJE (1964) Smoothing and differentiation of data by simplified least squares procedures. Analytical Chemistry 36: 1627–1639

Spach MS (1983) The role of cell-to-cell coupling in cardiac conduction disturbances. Adv Exp Med Biol 161: 61–77

Spach MS, Heidlage JF (1995) The stochastic nature of cardiac propagation at a microscopic level: Electrical description of myocardial architecture and its application to conduction. Circ Res 76: 366–380

Spach MS, Miller WT, Miller-Jones E, Warren RB, Barr RC (1979) Extracellular potentials related to intracellular action potentials during impulse conduction in anisotropic canine cardiac muscle. Circ Res 45: 188–204

Sprössler C, Denyer M, Britland S, Knoll W, Offenhäusser A (1999) Electrical recordings from rat cardiac muscle cells using field-effect transistors. Phys Rev E 60: 2171–2176

Thomas CA, Springer PA, Loeb GW, Berwald-Netter Y, Okun LM (1972) A miniature microelectrode array to monitor the bioelectric activity of cultured cells. Exp Cell Res 74: 61–66

Yamamoto M, Honjo H, Niwa R, Kodama I (1998) Low-frequency extracellular potentials recorded from the sinoatrial node. Cardiovasc Res 39: 360–372

4 Histological Techniques

4.1 Immunohistochemistry for Structural
and Functional Analysis
in Cardiovascular Research — 457
Wilhelm Bloch, Yüksel Korkmaz and Dirk Steinritz

4.2 Classical Histological Staining Procedures
in Cardiovascular Research — 485
Wilhelm Bloch and Yüksel Korkmaz

4.3 Practical Use of in situ Hybridisation and RT
in situ PCR in Cardiovascular Research — 500
Yüksel Korkmaz, Dirk Steinritz and Wilhelm Bloch

4.4 Practical Use of Transmission Electron Microscopy
for Analysis of Structures and Molecules
in Cardiovascular Research — 525
*Wilhelm Bloch, Christian Hoffmann, Eveline Janssen
and Yüksel Korkmaz*

4.5 DAF Technique for Real-Time NO Imaging
in the Human Myocardium — 546
Dirk Steinritz and Wilhelm Bloch

4.1

Immunohistochemistry for Structural and Functional Analysis in Cardiovascular Research

Wilhelm Bloch, Yüksel Korkmaz and Dirk Steinritz

Introduction

Immunohistochemistry is one of the main methods for specific detection and recognition of molecules in cells and tissue and has a long tradition. The principle of the immunohistochemical method is localization and identification of a specific antigen in a cell or a tissue specimen. Immunohistochemical detection has been done for more then 60 years, starting with the detection of bacteria (Coons et al. 1941). The progression in development of antibodies and a series of technical developments have led to an increased sensitivity in immunohistochemical methods and made immunohistochemistry one of the most essential methods in analytical morphology. In cardiovascular research as in other fields, a large increase in the use of immunohistochemistry can be observed in the last 10 years. Because of the improved methods for immunohistochemistry, its employment has also been expanded. While in the past immunohistochemistry was mainly used for the cellular localization of molecules in the tissue, now detection of subcellular localization, colocalization with other molecules and time-dependent alterations in expression and subcellular localization are the foci of interest. Besides these aspects, a further application becomes more and more the focus of interest, the detection of molecules in the activated and/or phosphorylated form. The rapid development in the immunohistochemical field and the expanded and altered use of immunohistochemistry makes it necessary to choose the immunohistochemical method for the individual application critically. Especially the choices of fixation, primary and secondary antibody and visualization method depend upon the underlying question for an optimal result. An improvement in immunohistochemical results can also be elicited by the use of new methods that allow one to increase the sensitivity and specificity of the immunohistochemistry.

The purpose of this chapter is to summarize immunohistochemical methods and to give guidance for the use of the optimal method depending on the underlying question. Special regard will by given to the use of immunohistochemistry for the detection and time-dependent alteration of activated and/or phosphorylated molecules in cardiovascular tissues. Furthermore the possibilities of semi-quantitative analyses of immunostaining will be discussed and some rules necessary for semi-quantitative analysis will be given. Given the complexity of the subject, the technical aspects cannot be described in all detail.

Description of Methods and Practical Approach

Fixation Methods and the Appropriate Choice of Fixation

Preservation of the integrity of tissue and cellular structure is necessary for morphological investigation. Therefore tissue preservation techniques are used which allow adequate preservation of cellular components, including soluble and particular proteins, prevention of autolysis and displacement of cell constituents, including antigens and enzymes, stabilization of cellular materials against the deleterious effects of subsequent treatments and facilitation of conventional staining and immunostaining (Hayat 2002). Different preservation methods such as heating, freezing and chemical fixation are used, but only chemical fixation can claim all of these advantages. None of these preservation methods leaves the specimen in the original condition. The most widely used preservation for immunohistochemistry is chemical fixation, therefore we will mainly focus on chemical fixation.

An understanding of the effects of fixation on antigens and cell morphology is prerequisite to judging the validity of immunohistochemistry. Therefore it is necessary to know the extent and kind of antigen preservation or destruction due to fixation and dehydration/embedding. Remembering that there is no optimal universal fixative for all types of antigens, the choice of a fixative depends on the type of epitope, the tissue under study and the antibody used. Furthermore preservation of antigenicity and maintenance of cell morphology are two aspects which must be balanced for successful immunohistochemistry.

Chemical Fixation for Tissue Preservation

Chemical fixation should primarily preserve tissue structure and cellular components for a long time, therefore all fixatives lead to a denaturation of the molecules inside the cells and tissue. Depending on the way they do this, one can differentiate between fixatives which lead to coagulation of molecules and fixatives which crosslink the surrounding molecules to the antigen of interest or degenerate the molecules by direct crosslinking. The first group includes fixatives such as ethanol, methanol or acetone and the second fixatives containing aldehyde groups. Since coagulating fixatives produce poor preservation of tissue and cell structure, they should only be used if aldehyde-fixed tissue or cells are not useable for immunohistochemistry, which is seldom the case if adequate antigen retrieval techniques are used. It should be noted that antigen retrieval is not possible in tissue fixed by coagulating fixatives. The reason for the lack of the antigen retrieval option for coagulating fixatives is the stronger denaturation of the molecules, including destruction of the tertiary and quaternary structure of the proteins.

In the case of protein antigens, the structure of an epitope may involve elements of the primary, secondary, tertiary, and even quaternary structure of the protein. In the case of polysaccharide antigens, extensive side-chain branching *via* glycosidic bonds affects the overall three-dimensional conformation of individual epitopes (Hayat 2002). Therefore coagulating fixatives cannot be used if the antibody recognizes more complex molecular structures such as the tertiary or quaternary structures of proteins. Aldehyde fixatives allow, with the help of specific pre-treatment, the presentation of epitopes depending on more or less preserved molecular structure. Considering their wide use and their advantages compared to other chemical fixatives, we will take most space for aldehyde-based fixatives.

The aldehyde-based fixatives, such as the monoaldehyde formaldehyde or the dialdehyde glutaraldehyde are the most used. Formaldehyde is the preferential fixative because of its rapid penetration into the tissue and the reversible cross linking of the molecules, while glutaraldehyde penetrates slowly and introduces mostly irreversible protein crosslinks, masking the epitopes. A mixture of higher formaldehyde concentration and lower glutaraldehyde concentration can be tried, to combine preservation of antigenicity and tissue structure.

Although there is no optimal fixative for all cases of immunohistochemistry, formaldehyde fixation is usually the best choice. Formaldehyde fixation is based on the reaction of formaldehyde with amino acids that have an available hydrogen site, if hydrogen site and formaldehyde react a reactive hydroxyl group is produced. Subsequently, a second hydrogen site can react with the hydroxymethyl group produced, yielding a methylene bridge between two amino acids in the protein. Therefore formaldehyde leads to a crosslinking of proteins by production of methylene bridges. The crosslinking by methylene bridges leads mainly to a change in the tertiary and quaternary structures of proteins, whereas the primary and secondary structures are little affected.

To ensure that formaldehyde fixation leads to good preservation and maintenance of structure of cells and tissue, it is important to choose optimal fixation conditions. Too short fixation only produces a partial fixation and too long fixation results in intensive and partially irreversible cross-linking. Therefore the time of fixation and, in the case of tissue fixation, the size of specimens must be suitable. To choose the optimal fixation time it is necessary to consider several factors, including the fixative concentration, pH and temperature. Therefore, if possible, the tissue should be subdivided into small pieces, less than 2–3 mm thick, if this is not possible an increase in fixation time must be allowed from 4–6 h up to 24–48 h. In animal experiments, the optimal method is a combination of perfusion fixation for 10–20 min followed by post-fixation of subdivided tissue pieces for 4–6 h. Fixation of cells only needs 20–30 min.

It should be remembered that for cell fixation the choice of fixation conditions has increased significance for preservation of cell structure and is strongly dependent on the kind of cells fixed.

If it is not possible to choose the right fixation conditions and fixation time, which is often the case if material is used which is taken by routine surgery and stored for a prolonged time in fixative until transfer to the analytical laboratory, an intensive washing in water or aqueous buffer should be performed. Over-fixation with protein crosslinking aldehydes can be partially reversed by washing in water or aqueous solutions. Furthermore whether the material is homogenous in structure and staining should be carefully checked. Over-fixation of specimens is recognized by difficulty in sectioning because of the increased hardness of the tissue. If prolonged fixation has occurred, immunostaining can be increased by robust antigen retrieval, higher antibody concentrations, longer duration of incubations in the reagents and signal amplification. A major problem in an intensive enhancement of detected immunosignal is the risk of getting an increase in background noise. Under-fixation can be improved by post-fixation methods, which are also possible for embedded specimens. But the result of such post-fixation methods is only suboptimal; therefore they should only be performed if there is no other possibility.

Although formaldehyde fixation works under "normal conditions" at neutral pH and room temperature, an increase of formaldehyde binding occurs if the temperature is increased and the pH is set between 7.5 and 8.0, which allows shortening of the incubation time. Considering that extensive heating and pH alteration themselves cause alteration of the morphological preservation by extensive denaturation of the molecules, the influence of altered pH and temperature should be carefully tested before use.

Considering the time-dependent denaturing character of all fixatives it seems advantageous to lower fixation time by choosing adjunct methods. A powerful technique to shorten fixation time, leading to improved preservation of the tissue, is microwave heating. Besides the improvement in structural preservation, the enzymatic activity can also be preserved for enzyme cytochemistry.

Non-crosslinking fixatives such as ethanol, methanol and acetone as well as some commercially available formalin substitutes, show, beside their often coagulating nature, a further problem which abolishes an exact subcellular localization of immunodetected molecules: The non-crosslinking molecules cannot hold the free cytosolic antigens in their original location. Leakage of molecules to the extracellular space or into the nucleus from the cytoplasm occurs because of fixative-induced permeabilization of cell and nuclear membranes. This is usually not the case for aldehydes because of their crosslinking effect, which binds free cytosolic molecules to particular molecules. Aldehyde can also bind small molecules such as cGMP by crosslinking the molecule to the cell's protein matrix (De Vente and Steinbusch 1992; Bloch et al. 2001) if the fixation is performed directly after sampling.

Special attention should be given to the combined use of vital reporter molecules such as GFP and immunohistochemistry. Vital reporters such as GFP are often free in the cytosol and are lost after permeabilization of the cell membrane. Aldehydes can hold the molecules in the cell and do not denature the molecule in a way that quenches the fluorescence. An intracellular shift of the molecules cannot be prevented by aldehyde, leading in the case of GFP to an increased nuclear staining (Kazemi et al. 2002).

It should be pointed out that the best fixation method cannot work if the time between removal of the specimen and fixation is too long, so any delay in the exposure of the specimen to the fixative should be avoided to decrease proteolytic degradation of antigenicity. Tissue specimens should ideally be placed in the fixative immediately after their removal from the body and cells directly after being taken out of the incubator. If immediate fixation is not possible, the tissue or cells must be kept cool in sterile, cold saline for not more than 20–30 min. During this time the specimens should not be dried. If the tissue is not cooled and remains nearly at body temperature, at which the activity of digestive enzymes continues, the cellular structures get damaged (Grizzle et al. 1998).

Advantages and Disadvantages of Different Embedding Methods

Different methods with and without pre-fixation of the tissue can be performed for storage, preparation of specimens for cutting and subsequent immunohistochemistry. Freezing and storage of tissue at low temperature is the main method used for unfixed tissue. The advantage of this method is the option to use parts of the material for biochemical and molecular biological analyses. This kind of tissue preservation and storage is suboptimal owing to the limited preservation of the morphological structure of the tissue. The reason for the limited structural preservation of the tissue is the formation of extra- and intra-cellular ice crystals, which destroy the tissue structure. Therefore, this method should only be used if other methods are not useable. If freezing must be used, then the freezing process should be optimised by reduction of specimen size, temperature-controlled freezing and cryoprotection solutions. Recently it was also shown that the use of microwave heating can improve the cryoprotection of the tissue structure (Hanyu et al. 1992; Jackson et al. 1997).

Preferentially embedding after fixation should be used. The standard method for embedding in histology is paraffin embedding, besides this plastic embedding will often be used. Although plastic embedding gives preferable preservation of the tissue structure and allows the use of the specimens for ultrastructural investigation as well, the stronger reduction of antigenicity compared to paraffin embedding limits the use of plastic embedded material for light microscopical immunohistochemistry. It should be noted that paraffin embedding also alters specimens by additional fixation occurring during dehydration, accompanied by antigen masking and lipid dissolution. Therefore it is necessary to achieve optimal conditions of dehydration, infiltration, and embedding in paraffin to minimize chemical and physical changes that occur in specimens during these treatments, affecting the sectioning and immunostaining. The time of dehydration, infiltration and embedding in paraffin should not be too long. Longer than optimal durations of these steps is a common habit, resulting in hard and brittle tissues that are difficult to section and impaired in antigenicity.

Another method for embedding is freezing of fixed and cryoprotected tissue, which mostly works very well in our hands, especially when used for myocardial tissue (Bloch et al. 2001; Mehlhorn et al. 2003). The advantages of this embedding method in comparison to paraffin embedding are no further alterations in antigenicity, fast processing and the possibility of using it for tissue or cells that are labelled by a vital reporter.

Especially for green fluorescent protein (GFP) labelled tissue and cells, where paraffin embedding procedures destroy the GFP-fluorescence, cryoprotection of paraformaldehyde-fixed tissue and subsequent freezing can be used to preserve GFP-fluorescence (Fleischmann et al. 1998; Kazemi et al. 2002). Besides other cryoprotection substances, sucrose at concentrations around 20% is useful. We routinely incubate the specimens in 18% sucrose solution overnight and then freeze them at −80 °C, alternatively small pieces of tissue can placed in Tissue-Tek before freezing. The preservation of structure and antigenicity not only allows the performance of light microscopical immunohistochemistry on the tissue with good results, but preparation of the tissue for electron microscopy is also possible, with surprisingly good preservation of subcellular structure (Roell et al. 2002). Thick slices (30–50 μm) of this cryoprotected and frozen material are useable for pre-embedding ultrastructural immunohistochemistry.

Improvement of Antigen Presentation

The usual fixation and embedding techniques produce a masking of antigen, which makes a lot of antigens undetectable by immunohistochemical techniques. Therefore the failure of antibodies to immunostain tissues or cells does not necessarily reflect the absence of epitopes. This partially explains the different results described in the literature for the expression of an antigen, as for example the controversial findings for eNOS expression in different tissues. eNOS detection is especially strongly dependent on the antibodies and pre-treatment methods used (Bloch et al. 2001). Lack of an adequate pre-treatment method can lead to wrong negative results, as we have described for the eNOS in the heart (Addicks et al. 1994). The epitope is the part of the antigen to which the antibody is directed. Therefore the epitopes are the structures that are undetectable by the antibody, if wrong negative results are obtained. Multiple factors during tissue preparation can lead to lack of immunostaining such as kind of fixation, dehydration, kind of embedding procedure, deparaffinization, rehydration, and incubation. Examples are the building of compact protein complexes as a result of crosslinking by formaldehyde or the folding of the antigen molecule during preparation.

This raises the question of pre-treatment methods that allow unmasking of the epitopes primarily masked by fixation and/or embedding. Different enzyme digestion and antigen retrieval techniques were developed in the last 30 years to make primarily masked antigen detectable (Taylor et al. 1974; Shi et al. 1991, 1992). One major problem with antigen or epitope retrieval is the fact that different epitopes need different methods for epitope retrieval. The main reason is the enormous heterogeneity of chemical structure of not only antigens but also epitopes of any one antigen. Therefore the optimal treatment for a given epitope may not be effective for another type of epitope. This is particularly true when considering the pH of the epitope retrieval solution and the duration of pre-treatment. Especially when double-labelling immunohistochemistry is performed this could give a problem.

The choice of an adequate retrieval method is an individual process influenced by many factors such as kind of fixation, heating, retrieval fluid and the antibodies used. So one cannot give a standard method for antigen retrieval.

The antigen retrieval techniques can principally be divided into heating and non-heating methods. Both types of antigen retrieval may be based on the heat- or chemical-induced modification of the three-dimensional structure of protein, reversing the condition from a formalin-modified protein structure back towards its original structure. In other words proteins will be reversed from the fixed state to the unfixed state. Heat can be supplied by different kinds of treatment such as microwave heating, conventional heating and autoclave heating. Furthermore, the solutions in which heating is performed can strongly influence antigen retrieval. Factors influencing antigen retrieval besides the temperature chosen are the pH, the molarity and the chemical composition of the antigen retrieval solution. The non-heating antigen retrieval technique includes strong alkali or acid hydrolysis or protease treatment as well as ultrasound.

A further specific application of antigen retrieval is its use in plastic-embedded tissue, which allows detection of antigen in thin tissue sections. This can improve the morphological resolution and give the opportunity to perform ultrastructural immunohistochemistry.

Considering that an individual antigen retrieval method must be established for every tissue and antibody it is necessary to find the right conditions by variation of the main important factors. Therefore a standardized method for retrieving a given epitope in a particular tissue can be developed by using the test battery approach (Shi et al. 1996). This is a convenient and rapid means to optimise three important factors (pH, temperature, and duration of heating) responsible for the immunostaining of a given epitope-antibody combination. Besides optimising the antigen retrieval, all steps in tissue treatment should be held constant to avoid false negative and positive results. Furthermore appropriate positive and negative controls are required to rule out false-negative or false-positive staining and the reproducibility of the immunohistochemical result should be tested by duplicate immunostaining. For more detailed information about antigen retrieval procedures the reader can be referred to two excellent overviews of the technique and a long list of examples of antigen retrieval (Shi et al. 1997; Taylor and Shi, 2001). In general the selection of the individual best method for antigen retrieval must be found experimentally for each antibody and each tissue, if no description of an antigen retrieval method for the chosen antibody and/or tissue can be found in the literature. As a practical approach it seems appropriate if no information about antigen retrieval methods exists, to start without antigen retrieval and, if this does not work, to use a test approach as described by Shi et al. (1996). Thereafter further modification should be performed. Considering the long list of possible modifications of the antigen retrieval technique, the selection of the optimal method can be extremely time consuming, especially if it is remembered that intensive treatment of the tissue can also influence the morphological preservation of the specimens. Therefore a compromise between optimal antigen-antibody reaction, morphological quality and experimental expense must be found.

Avoidance and Elimination of Background Staining

For immunohistochemistry, non-specific background staining is one of the most common problems in the practical use of staining. Background staining is defined as non-specific labelling of tissue and cells by antibodies that interfere with specific immunostaining results. Background staining leads to false positive results and masking of specific staining, which makes the interpretation of the specific immunoreaction difficult or impossible. Together with false-negative staining, it presents major obstacles to successful immunohistochemistry. Although the non-specific background staining can be identified with stringent controls, it often seems impossible to interpret the specific results in the presence of the non-specific labelling. Therefore immunohistochemical protocols should be used which allow or at least reduce background staining. The strategy to avoid background staining is dependent on the kind of background staining. Each kind of background staining requires different treatment for correction. Generally, the occurrence of background staining can be divided into technical, conditional or inherited. The technically derived background staining is easy to correct. Technical mistakes can be easily abolished if they are recognized. The most common technical reasons for background staining are that the antibody solution or any of the solutions are dried or semi-dried on the preparation, the incubation duration is too long, the incubation temperature is too high, the compositions of the buffer or of any of the solutions are not correct or the washing is not long or vigorous enough.

Although the technically derived background staining causes mostly a general colouring, which can be easily recognized, sometimes only specific structures are stained. This occurs for example if endogenous peroxidase is incompletely blocked by hydrogen peroxide, in this case cells with high endogenous peroxidase activity are mainly stained, while others are nearly negative. Another example is the use of alkaline phosphatase, which, without levamisole pre-treatment, binds non-specifically to tissue structures, notably the perivascular extracellular matrix.

The last two examples can also be placed in the category of conditional or inherited background staining. These reasons for background staining are not easy to solve and often need systemic experimentation to identify the factor or factors that cause the problem. Here we will try to list some of the reasons for conditional or inherited background staining. Protein hydrophobicity, which can occur in different protein molecules and which is increased by fixation-dependent crosslinking between reactive amino acids can lead to significantly increased background staining. An effective approach to reduce background staining due to hydrophobic interaction is to use blocking protein before and/or during the application of the primary antibody. The blocking protein must compete effectively with IgG for hydrophobic binding sites in the tissue. For example bovine serum albumin can be used or other serum albumins from the host of the secondary antibody.

Cross-reactivity of an antibody can also cause background staining. Especially if polyclonal antibodies are used, a non-specific cross-reactivity with similar or dissimilar epitopes on different antigens can occur. These may occur when the epitopes share extensive sequence or structural similarities. If available, the use of a second primary antibody directed against another epitope of the antigen is the best test to identify this kind of background staining. If this is not available, Western blot analyses can help to identify non-specific binding by identification of additional bands, although additional bands in a Western blot cannot be directly interpreted as a sign for non-specific binding in the immunohistochemistry. Altogether the cross-reactivity of antibodies seems to be a major problem in immunohistochemistry.

Problems can be caused by the presence of small amounts of natural antibodies in the serum or a contamination with antibodies produced by the host's immune system as it reacts to antigens used for immunization (Boenisch 2001). An elimination of these antibodies by affinity absorption is one way to abolish this problem. But most times it can be reduced under the critical threshold by sufficiently high dilutions of the antiserum. In general it seems appropriated to increase the antibody concentration as much as possible without loss of staining intensity. The antibody at higher dilution can still achieve reasonable labelling by prolonging the incubating time or slightly raising the incubating temperature or use of amplifying detection methods.

Antigen diffusion can also lead to background staining, which must be called specific background staining because of a specific antigen-antibody reaction. The problem in this case is the diffusion of the antigen in the tissue. Fixation problems are mostly the reason for such a background staining, especially if very small molecules are being detected, as for example cGMP, which diffuse rapidly out of the cells and can often be found in the surrounding extracellular matrix (De Vente and Steinbusch 1992; Bloch et al. 2001). Fast fixation and small tissue pieces can avoid this problem best.

The content of endogenous molecules such as peroxidase, alkaline phosphatase or biotin can cause background if exogenous detection complex is bound or developed. Endogenous peroxidase can be blocked by treating the tissue sections with hydrogen peroxide and in the case of alkaline phosphatase; levamisole pre-treatment as mentioned above can avoid the problem. The biotin problem can be reduced by sequential treatment of sections (prior to staining) with up to 0.1% avidin followed by up to 0.01% biotin for 10–20 min.

Finally, some reports indicate that antigen retrieval at very high temperatures may result in non-specific staining. Considering that extreme heating can also destroy the tissue structure, such conditions should not be applied.

The best method to identify background staining is the performance of appropriated controls. The best controls include using unrelated antibodies (or non-immune serum) and the preabsorption test, as well as comparison of results with tissue with known positive and negative staining. A further test approach is the incubation of the primary antibody with its specific antigen in a test tube before applying this mixture to the tissue sample. A negative result will establish the specificity of the immunostaining when performed without a quenching step (Gu and Agrawal 1997).

Choice of the Appropriate Detection Methods

The visualization of the antigen-antibody reaction is the end point of the immunohistochemical procedure. Different detection systems are available for light and electron microscopical investigation of the immunoreaction. In general the light microscopical detection methods can be divided in two classes, the fluorescence-based methods and the enzyme-reaction based methods. More recently a third light microscopical method, the immunogold-silver staining is increasingly applied and is described as a sensitive, rapid and cheap detection method (Springall et al. 1984). All of these methods have specific advantages and disadvantages depending on the individual underlying question and the situation of use. Therefore the choice of the detection system must be made considering these individual questions and the target.

In this chapter we will give some information about the adequate selection of detection methods depending on the underlying individual need in cardiovascular research.

Detection of Antigen-Antibody Reaction by Different Labellings

The use of an adequate detection method is one of the keys for an optimal immunohistochemical analysis. It seems therefore necessary to give an overview of the mainly used detection methods in immunohistochemistry, the enzyme-based detection, the fluorescence-based detection and the detection by gold-silver staining. All of these detection methods can be performed in a direct or an indirect way. The direct method is a one step staining method, and involves a labelled antibody reacting directly with the antigen in tissue sections. This technique utilizes only one antibody and the procedure is short and fast. However, it is insensitive, due to little signal amplification and is rarely used since the introduction of indirect method. The indirect method involves an unlabelled primary antibody that reacts with tissue antigen and a labelled secondary antibody against the IgG of the species in which the primary has been raised, reacting with the primary antibody. This method is more sensitive due to signal amplification through several secondary antibody reactions with different antigenic sites on the primary antibody. In addition, it is also economical since one labelled second layer antibody can be used with many first layer antibodies to different antigens. Some advantages and disadvantages of the methods should be discussed with regard to specific applications.

Enzyme-based Visualization of Antibody Binding

The main enzymes used for visualization of the immunohistochemical reaction are peroxidase and alkaline phosphatase. A serial of technical developments in enzyme-based immunohistochemistry have created increasingly sensitive detection systems. For example, the immunoperoxidase technique can be performed as peroxidase antiperoxidase (PAP), avidin-biotin-peroxidase complex (ABC) and biotin-streptavidin (BSA) methods (Taylor and Cote 1994). All of these techniques are used in different fields of cardiovascular research.

In addition to commonly used immunohistochemical staining methods such as ABC, PAP, APAAP and LSAB, a highly sensitive detecting method, the tyramide signal amplification (TSA) method, which is 5–100× more sensitive than the ABC method is also available for detection of bound antibody.

The avidin-biotin complex method (ABC) is a sensitive and widely used technique for immunohistochemical staining. Avidin, streptavidin or extravidin can be labelled with peroxidase and have a very high affinity for biotin. Biotin, a low molecular weight vitamin, can be conjugated to a variety of biological molecules such as antibodies. The technique involves three layers. The first layer is unlabeled primary antibody. The second layer is biotinylated secondary antibody. The third layer is a complex of avidin-biotin peroxidase. The peroxidase is then developed by DAB or other substrate to produce different coloured end products. The peroxidase anti-peroxidase method (PAP) method is a further development of the indirect technique and it involves a third layer which is a rabbit or mouse antibody to peroxidase, coupled with peroxidase to make a very stable peroxidase anti-peroxidase complex. The complex, composed of rabbit or mouse gamma globulin and peroxidase, acts as a third layer antigen and becomes bound to the unconjugated goat anti-rabbit or goat anti-mouse gamma globulin of the second layer. The sensitivity is about 100 to 1000× higher since the peroxidase molecule is not chemically conjugated to the anti IgG but immunologically bound, and loses none of its enzyme activity. It also allows for much higher dilution of the primary antibody, thus eliminating many of the unwanted antibodies and reducing non-specific background staining. APAAP immunohistochemistry is related to the PAP method using alkaline phosphatase as enzyme. A further highly sensitive detection method is the labelled streptavidin-biotin system. The technique also involves three layers. The first layer is the unlabeled primary antibody. The second layer is a biotinylated secondary antibody. The third layer is, in this case, an enzyme-conjugated avidin, streptavidin or extravidin. The conjugation of more than one enzyme to the linker increases the sensitivity of this method. Tyramide signal amplification (TSA) sometimes called CARD, for Catalyzed Reporter Deposition is an enzyme-mediated detection method that utilizes the catalytic activity of horseradish peroxidase (HRP) to generate high-density labelling of a target protein. The TSA method has been reported to increase the sensitivity by up to 1000-fold compared to conventional avidin–biotinylated enzyme complex (ABC) procedures (Adams 1992; Merz et al. 1995).

A further important factor in enzyme-based immunohistochemistry is the selection of a chromogen for visualization. Peroxidase systems routinely use 3,3'-diaminobenzidine (DAB) (brown) or 3-amino-9-ethylcarbazole (AEC) (red) as chromogens. The DAB development can be modified by use of glucose oxidase or nickel sulphate (black). For alkaline phosphatase systems, 5-bromo-4-chloro-purple or fast red/nitroblue tetrazolium (BCIP/NBT) may be used to yield a blue-purple product or fast red/naphthol AS-TR phosphate to produce a red/pink product (Roche and His 2001). The choice of the chromogen can be influenced by personal preference, degree of contrast with the counterstain, incubation time and sensitivity as well as other technical issues.

The advantages of the enzyme-based methods are the possibility of strong amplification of the signal leading to high sensitivity. Furthermore, the recognisability of the unstained or counterstained tissue structures and the mostly high stability of the preparation as well as the easy detection by conventional light microscopes are advantageous.

Limitations of enzyme-based cytochemistry are the need for several amplification mechanisms to increase sensitivity resulting in several incubation steps which are time consuming, the often high background staining interfering with the quality of the results and the diffusion of the enzyme-substrate reaction products in the tissue as well as the high electron opacity of reaction products which can hinder identification of the labelled structures and give low resolution.

Visualization of Detected Antigens by Fluorescent Markers

The development of new fluorochromes and new fluorescence microscopical techniques such as confocal laser microscopy and deconvolution microscopy allows the detection of molecules with high sensitivity and local resolution. Two main advantages of the use of fluorochromes compared to enzyme based detection methods can be pointed out. The first is the possibility to make multiple staining relatively easy by use of different fluorochromes in combination with first antibodies derived from different species and/or by use of specific immunohistochemical protocols, which allow detection of different antigens in the same slice or cells with first antibodies from the same host. The second advantage is the possibility of performing high-resolution light microscopy by using confocal laser microscopy and deconvolution microscopy.

Different fluorescent dyes are available which can be selectively detected by use of adequate filters or by use of confocal laser microscopy allowing detection of single fluorescence dyes in multiply labelled specimens. Only some examples of such fluorescence dyes can be given here. Depending on the emission wavelength different colours can be seen. The following fluorescence dyes can be recognized as blue light (Amca, Alexa 350 and 405), as green light (FITC, Alexa 488, Rhodamine Green Dye, Oregon Green 488, Cy2) and as red light (TRITC, Texas red, Alexa 568, Cy3). The fluorescence dyes show great differences in fading stability, which is also dependent on the mounting medium used. In our hands Cy2 and Cy3 work very well. Cy2 and Cy3 have the advantage that the specimens can be dehydrated and covered with Entellan. If these fluorescence dyes are mounted in this way they show a high fading stability.

The advantage of the use of fluorescent dyes is that multiple antigens can easily be detected in one specimen with high resolution when the dyes are combined with high-resolution microscopy such as confocal laser and deconvolution microscopy.

Limitations of immunofluorescence are the specific and more expensive equipment, the rapid fading of fluorescence on visualization of tissue especially under UV light, the inability to visualize non-fluorescent tissue, the often high non-specific background signals due to inherent fluorescence and the partial limitations for detection of specific signals depending on tissue, microscope objectives, optical filters and fixatives used. Therefore immunofluorescence should be only preferred over enzyme-based methods if high resolution or multiple labelling of one specimen is necessary.

Immunogold-Silver Staining for Detection of Immunohistochemical Reactions

In the early eighties, a novel immunohistochemical procedure, the immunogold-silver staining technique was described (Holgate et al. 1983, Springall et al. 1984). The method is a combination of immunogold staining, originally devised for use at the electron microscopic level (Faulk and Taylor 1971), but subsequently adapted for light microscopy (Geoghegan et al. 1978), and the method of Danscher (1981). Immunogold staining for light microscopy needs relatively high concentrations of immunogold reagent for visualization (Gu et al. 1981). The immunogold-silver method requires much less of this reagent to be bound, since the gold is revealed by a silver development step, and so higher dilutions of immunogold may be used and it can be shown that the immunogold-silver technique achieves a higher sensitivity than the earlier published peroxidase anti-peroxidase method (Sternberger et al. 1979; Holgate et al. 1983; Springall et al. 1984). In the following papers it was shown, that the immunogold-silver staining resulted in greatly increased sensitivity and detection efficiency compared with other immunohistochemical techniques. The method was also useable for sections of paraffin- and resin-embedded tissues and was shown to detect antigen in very small quantities, where other methods fail to get a staining in light microscopy and electron microscopy (for review Hacker et al. 1997). Further improvements in accuracy, quality and sensitivity are made in the following papers by use of nanogold instead of colloidal gold and a new approach using an anti-horseradish peroxidase antibody-gold complex (Hainfeld and Furuya 1992; Roth et al. 1992). Detailed information about the use of immunogold-silver staining is given in Hacker et al. (1997) including a protocol for the use of this technique on paraffin sections and on semi-thin resin sections, which must be pre-treated with saturated sodium ethoxide in contrast to the paraffin section, which can be routinely handled.

Recently we tested the immunogold-silver staining on paraformaldehyde-fixed and sucrose embedded frozen myocardium with good results, showing a high sensitivity and specificity. Especially if light- and electron microscopical investigation is combined, this staining technique together with this embedding technique seems useable.

Now Streptavidin FluoroNanogold by Nanoprobes is available, which allows the combination of immunofluorescence techniques with ultrastructural immunogold techniques or with immunogold-silver staining. These new techniques open new interesting possibilities in immunohistochemistry.

Qualitative and Semi-Quantitative Recording

Immunohistochemistry was long considered as only a qualitative method and therefore held inferior to biochemical methods since they can be quantified. Quantification was restricted to counting of immunostained structures and analysis of immunostained areas, as for example the counting of proliferative cells after recognition by specific proliferation markers (Gerdes et al. 1984; Bloch et al. 1997). With the growing application and improvement of personal computer technology and image analysis systems, the possibilities of performing quantitative immunohistochemistry increase greatly. The possibility of measuring the optical density of immunostained areas is especially strongly increased. While the counting of cells and the measurement of immunostained areas are possible without computerized measurement, either by photometrical or TV-densitometrical methods, the measurement of optical density is only possible with such methods. The counting of immunostained cells or structures and the measurement of immunostained areas can also be improved and standardized by these methods.

An important prerequisite for quantitative immunohistochemistry is clear evidence of a correlation between antigen concentration and the amount of final reaction product produced by the marker enzyme (Fritz et al. 1995). For an accurate quantification of antigens using immunohistochemistry the relationship between amount of antigen and the amount of final reaction product should be nearly linear. Therefore it is necessary to find optimal concentrations of the marker enzyme and an optimal development time, which give a linear relationship between antigen content and amount of reaction product.

Even more importantly than the relationship between the marker reaction and the antigen content, the immunohistochemical staining must be reproducible. The achievement of quantitative, reproducible results requires standardized immunohistochemical procedures. The development of such a universal procedure is difficult because antigens are not equally affected by a specific processing protocol, including sampling of the specimens, fixation and embedding as well as immunohistochemical treatment. These problems of standardization can be almost avoided if the comparison of immunostained specimens is restricted to probes that are handled in the same experimental approach. If this is not the case, then it is necessary to use a standard probe. The Quicgel method described by Riera et al. (1999) is such a method. To rectify the lack of intra- and inter-laboratory reproducibility in immunostaining they processed a cultured plate of cells containing a known amount of the antigen, which yielded consistent positive staining detected by image analysis, simultaneously with the specimens. A related approach is the use of sections from embedded and sectioned cells e.g. fibroblasts (Ranefall et al. 1998) or slices of tissue with a known content of antigen.

In addition, careful choices will have to be made of the commercially available optical and recording systems as well as the application software in order to optimise quantitative immunohistochemical analyses. It appears to be of equal importance to reach consensus on which histological areas are to be analysed and which underlying question should be answered. Also using of reference cells or slices it is very difficult or nearly impossible to get absolute values, therefore the results should be handled as relative values. This makes the use of the immunohistochemical quantification methods more reliable and practicable.

If double- and triple-labelling is being performed, the use of end products that are non-spectral, such as brown or purple should be avoided. This is because these end products cannot be easily discriminated using red, green, or blue thresholding, which can make selection more problematic. In the case of single labelling, which is preferred in our hands, such non-spectral end products can be used. In addition, counterstaining may also need to be avoided, because it can interfere with the immunostaining of interest (Newman and Nelson 2000).

A detailed description of the critical technical points for the use of quantification in immunohistochemistry can be found in a review of Fritz et al. (1995). They describe the terms for qualitative control of quantitative immunohistochemistry as test of efficiency, test of specificity and precision. The efficiency is defined as intensity of specific signal against background, the specificity can be defined either as method or antibody specificity and the precision as either intra- or inter-day variability or as inter- or intra-observer variability. Furthermore methodological errors in quantitative immunohistochemistry are listed, including microscopical and camera problems as well as tissue or cell preparation problems and variation in the immunohistochemical method.

Here we will introduce quantitative immunohistochemistry a little more practically by describing an approach that does not overstress the method and allows the acquisition of detailed information on cell-type specific changes of antigens in the tissue.

Detection of Changes in Enzyme Activity or in Occurrence of Reaction Products

The rapid development of antibodies that recognize molecules depending on their phosphorylation state, their molecular configuration or as cleavage products as well as reaction products opens new approaches not only for biochemical analyses but also for immunohistochemistry. Considering the dependency of enzyme activity on phosphorylation state and molecular configuration, it is possible to get information about the activation stage of a molecule by immunohistochemistry. Especially if a cell type specific analysis of activation/phosphorylation is needed in a complex tissue containing more than one cell type, the immunohistochemical quantification method has definite advantages compared to biochemical assays and can used alone or in combination with biochemical analyses. The new possibilities of functional immunohistochemistry increase the demand for an adequate methodical approach.

An initial important step in functional immunohistochemistry is a fast fixation after sampling of the tissue, which does not make the antigen undetectable. Formaldehyde usually seems the optimal choice because of the rapid penetration into the tissue, the good preservation of the morphology and the reversible crosslinking of the molecules, which opens the possibility of antigen retrieval. Furthermore this fixation inhibits enzyme activity of most phosphatases and kinases as well as endogenous chemical reactions that can lead to an alteration of the phosphorylation state of the molecules of interest. The tissue embedding must be chosen for the preservation of antigen-antibody reaction. The cryoprotection method for paraformaldehyde-fixed tissue described above works in our hands in nearly all cases. Thereafter it must be ensured that the thickness of the sections remains in a very small range. The specimens that are to be directly compared must be handled in the same immunohistochemical procedure and the quantitative immunohistochemical analyses should be done together. We used this method for analyses of differences in activation stage of eNOS, different kinases and apoptosis signal molecules mediated by receptor stimulation or ischemia in isolated perfused heart, in organ bath experiments on myocardium and during cardiac surgery (Bloch et al. 2001; Fischer et al. 2003; Pott et al. 2003; Mehlhorn et al. 2003). The relative alterations in antigen content could easily be detected if pre- and post-stimulation conditions were directly compared. We prefer a semi-automatic approach for the measurement of the optical density in cardiomyocytes, where the individual researcher selects and surrounds the cardiomyocytes on the screen; thereafter the selected area will be measured automatically by the computer program. Additional measurement of the surrounding cell-free areas allows correction of the measured optical density in the cells of interest for the optical density of the background. This approach has the advantage that problems of inhomogeneities in the tissue and problems with the tissue preservation can be considered. If the selection of the cardiomyocytes is strongly randomised, there is a very high inter- and intra-individual reliability.

If adequate approaches are chosen and the interpretation of the data is not overstressed, quantitative immunohistochemistry is a powerful tool in addition to but not as a replacement for biochemical techniques.

Examples

The following three examples of immunohistochemistry in cardiovascular research show specific thematic and technical aspects. In the first example detection of eNOS is performed by an eNOS antibody, which is recognized as activation dependent in a study on human and rat myocardium. The second example deals with detection of molecules with relatively fast turnover and alteration e.g. free radical reaction products in human left ventricular myocardium during cardiac surgery. The third example shows the use of immunofluorescence for high-resolution light microscopical investigation of subcellular molecular distribution in cardiomyocytes.

Buffers and Fixative Used

The following solutions are common to all three described examples.
1. Sodium phosphate buffer (0.1 M PB, pH 7.4)
   [(14.40 g/l $Na_2HPO_4 \times 2H_2O$ + 2.6 g/l $NaH_2PO_4 \times H_2O$) in 1 l aqua dest]
2. Sodium phosphate-buffered saline (0.1 M PBS)
   [(14.4 g/l $Na_2HPO_4 \times 2H_2O$ + 2.60 g/l $NaH_2PO_4 \times H_2O$ + 8.76 g NaCl) in 1 l aqua dest]
3. Tris buffer (0.5 M TB, pH 7.6)
   [dissolve 60.57 g Tris in 800 ml distilled water, adjust pH to 7.6 with HCl and bring to 1 l with distilled water]
4. Tris-buffered saline (0.05 M TBS, pH 7.6)
   [dissolve 8.76 g NaCl in 900 ml distilled water and add 100 ml of 0.5 M TB pH 7.6 and adjust pH to 7.6]
5. Fixative 4% paraformaldehyde in 0.1 M PB
   20 g paraformaldehyde are dissolved in 225 ml aqua dest. by stirring and heating at 60 °C. The solution is cleared by adding 25 ml 1 N NaOH. 250 ml 0.2 M sodium phosphate buffer are added to the paraformaldehyde solution

Detection of eNOS in Rat and Human Myocardium

The following example shows the strong dependence of antibody/antigen binding on the activation stage of the eNOS. In isolated perfused rat heart, we found a direct link between ischemia time during heart preparation and the immunohistochemically detectable eNOS if we used antibodies against either amino acids of a central eNOS domain or a N-terminal domain. No alteration in eNOS immunostaining could be observed if we used an antibody against a C-terminal domain of the eNOS (Bloch et al. 2001). Further experiments, which led to receptor-mediated stimulation of the eNOS, show the same alteration of immunohistochemical signal directly after agonist treatment in rat and human myocardium (Bloch et al. 2001; Pott et al. 2003). An intensive microwave pre-treatment of the slices strongly increased the immunohistochemical signal (Bloch et al. 2001). This example gives evidence for activation/stimulation, as well as pre-treatment-dependent alteration of the antibody-antigen reaction. It must be questioned if such alterations are often not identified, which could explain controversial results in the literature. In the case of eNOS detection, we used the demonstrated dependency of eNOS immunostaining on the activation stage as a powerful tool for detection of non-phosphorylation-dependent eNOS activation. In combination with TV-densitometry, we are now able to analyse eNOS activation by immunohistochemistry (Bloch et al. 2000, 2001; Pott et al. 2003). If such relationships are not recognized, the immuno-staining results cannot be interpreted. Therefore different results with antibodies should be carefully checked for such dependency before they are held to be only technical problems.

Preparation of Tissue

The human left ventricular biopsies were fixed in 4% paraformaldehyde for 4 h and rinsed in 0.1 M PBS for 24 h. Hearts of rats were perfusion-fixed at a pressure of 60 cm H_2O with 0.1 M PBS buffered 4% paraformaldehyde for 10 min followed by 4 h immersion fixation in the same fixative. Hearts were rinsed with 0.1 M PBS pH 7.4 buffer and stored in the same buffer at 4 °C (Bloch et al. 2001).

Tissue Embedding

Frozen-embedding: The best method for antigen preservation in immunohistochemistry is freezing of cryoprotected fixed tissue. Hearts of rats and human biopsies are stored for 12 h in 0.1 M PBS containing 15% sucrose for cryoprotection. The sucrose concentration may range from 10% for soft tissues and thinner sections to 30% for hard tissues. The probes should be embedded in Tissue-Tek, frozen in liquid nitrogen and stored at –80 °C.

Tissue Sectioning

1. Cut 7 µm sections of the frozen embedded tissue on a cryostat at –24 °C;
2. Mount the section on poly (L-lysine)-coated (0.1%) slides;
3. Dry slides at room temperature for 20 min;
4. Store the sections at –80 °C.

Immunohistochemistry

1. The frozen sections are sectioned with a cryostat at 7 µm and mounted on poly (L-lysine)-coated (0.1%) slides.
2. Rinse the sections with 0.05 M TBS, 3×10 min at RT.
3. Inhibit endogenous peroxidase activity in the tissue section:
   Incubate the sections in 200 ml methanol containing 50 ml 3% H_2O_2 for 30 min at RT or in 0.05 M TBS containing 3% H_2O_2 for 20 min at RT.
4. Rinse the sections with 0.05 M TBS, 2×10 min at RT.
5. Incubate sections in 0.5 M ammonium chloride + 0.25% Triton-X100 in 0.05 M TBS at RT.
6. Wash the sections 2×10 min in 0.05 M TBS at RT.
7. Incubate the sections in 1% bovine serum albumin (BSA) solution containing 10% pre-immune serum (NGS) of the species in which the secondary antibody has been raised (diluted in 0.05 M TBS), 30 min at RT.
8. Incubate the sections with the primary antiserum diluted in 1% NGS + 20 mM sodium azide in 0.05 M TBS [1:1500, eNOS Biomol; 1:250, eNOS Santa Cruz; 1:100, monoclonal anti-mouse eNOS, Transduction], overnight at 4 °C.

9. Rinse the sections with 0.05 M TBS, 4×10 min at RT.
10. Incubate the sections with the biotinylated second antibody under the optimal conditions (biotinylated goat-anti rabbit IgG diluted in 0.05 M TBS + 1% NGS) for 1 h at RT.
11. Wash 4×10 min in 0.05 M TBS.
12. Incubate the sections in horseradish-peroxidase-complex diluted in 0.05 M TBS (1:100) for 1 h at RT.
13. Rinse the sections with 0.05 M TBS, 4×10 min at RT.
14. Incubate the sections in a solution containing 0.05% 3,3'-diaminobenzidine tetrahydrochloride (DAB), 0.01% nickel ammonium sulphate and 0.05% H_2O_2 in 0.05 M Tris-HCl buffer, pH 7.6 for 5–15 min at RT.
15. Rinse the sections with 0.05 M TBS 4×10 min at RT.
16. Dehydrate the sections in increasing concentrations of ethanol:
    – 3 min   ethanol 50%
    – 3 min   ethanol 70%
    – 3 min   ethanol 96%
    – 2×3 min   ethanol 100%
17. The sections are cleared in xylene:
    – 3 min   xylene I
    – 3 min   xylene II
18. Mount the slides with Entellan (Merck).

The Immunohistochemical Controls

1. Incubate the section in the absence of the primary antibody.
2. Incubate the sections in the absence of the secondary antibody.
3. Incubate the sections in normal non-immune rabbit IgG.
4. Pre-absorption:
    – In a microfuge tube place 2% antibody, 20% 0.05 M TBS or 0.1 M PBS and 4-, 10- and 20-fold excesses of the biologically active appropriate control peptide for the antibody.
    – Incubate at 4 °C for 24 h.
    – Spin in a microfuge at maximum speed for 15 min to pellet aggregates.
    – Remove the supernatant avoiding disturbing any pellet.
    – Make final dilutions of the supernatant as appropriate and use for immunohistochemical incubations as described above.

Interpretation of the Immunohistochemical Controls

No immunolabelling should be observed when the primary antibodies were omitted or replaced with an equivalent concentration of non-immune normal serum. In the preabsorption procedure, immunostaining should be abolished. Preabsorption of the antiserum with the appropriate active peptide should block specific labelling by the adsorbed antiserum. However, preabsorption of the antiserum with a non-specific peptide should not block a specific labelling.

Analyses of the Immunohistochemical Results

The light microscopically immunostained slices can be analysed for long time if the slices are dehydrated and covered with Entellan. If they are not dehydrated and covered with, for example, Kaiser's gelatine, fast reduction of reaction products occurs.

Besides a "classical" qualitative structural analysis, TV-densitometry is a powerful tool to detect quantitative changes also, as we have done for cardiac surgery-mediated increase of eNOS activation in human left ventricular biopsies. The advantage of such an analysis compared to biochemical assays is the small amount of tissue necessary and the cell type specific resolution.

The major problem for the use of such quantitative or semi-quantitative analyses is the standardization of the procedure. Therefore we only compare immunostained samples that were sampled from the same patient or experiment and were stained in the same batch.

Investigation of Free Radical Formation, Apoptosis Induction and Enzyme Activation During Cardiac Surgery

The following example gives evidence of the effective use of immunohistochemistry for detection of free radical reaction products, activated apoptosis signal molecules and activated kinases. During cardiac surgery, induction of cellular damage is suggested in the left ventricular myocardium.

A major problem is the limited availability of tissue for ethical and technical reasons; therefore an optimal use of the tissue that can be sampled by left ventricular biopsy is appropriate.

Furthermore, it is necessary to distinguish the cellular components damaged by the cardiac surgery. Biochemical assays are limited by the amount of tissue that is necessary for the measurement of a parameter and by the lack of cell type-specific resolution. The direct comparison of intra-individual sampled specimens, an optimal prerequisite for quantitative immunohistochemistry, gives an opportunity to compare pre- and post-surgery sampled specimens from a patient.

If the specimens are then handled together from fixation up to the densitometrical measurement, a direct comparison between the pre- and post-surgery status of the myocardium with a cell type-specific resolution is possible. We were able to detect on one biopsy more than 10 different antigens, so we can show complex interactions of free radicals, apoptosis signal pathways and activation of kinases (Bloch et al. 2001; Mehlhorn et al. 2003; Fischer et al. 2003, Tossios 2003).

Preparation of Tissue

The human left ventricular biopsies were fixed in 4% paraformaldehyde for 4 h and soaked in 0.1 M PBS for 24 h. Specimens were rinsed with 0.1 M PBS pH 7.4 buffer and stored in the same buffer at 4 °C (Bloch et al. 2001).

Tissue Embedding

Frozen-embedding: The best method for antigen preservation in immunohistochemistry is freezing of cryoprotected fixed tissue. Human biopsies are stored for 12–24 h in 0.1 M PBS containing 18% sucrose for cryoprotection. The sucrose concentration may range from 10% for soft tissues and thinner sections to 30% for hard tissues. The probes should be embedded in Tissue-Tek, frozen and stored at –80 °C.

Tissue Sectioning

1. Cut 7 µm sections of the frozen embedded tissue on a cryostat at –24 °C.
2. Mount the section on poly (L-lysine)-coated (0.05%) slides.
3. Store the sections at –80 °C.

Immunohistochemistry

1. The frozen sections are dried at RT for at least 30 min.
2. Rinse the sections with 0.05 M TBS, 3×10 min at RT.
3. Inhibit endogenous peroxidase activity in the tissue section by incubating the sections in methanol containing 3% H_2O_2 for 20 min at RT.
4. Rinse the sections with 0.05 M TBS, 3×10 min at RT.
5. Incubate the sections in 0.5 M ammonium chloride + 0.25% Triton-X100 in 0.05 M TBS at RT.
6. Wash the sections 3×10 min in 0.05 M TBS at RT.
7. Incubate the sections in 5% bovine serum albumin (BSA) solution for 60 min at RT.
8. Incubate the sections with the primary antibody in 0.05 M TBS containing 0.8% BSA [1:1500 8-Isoprostan Oxford Biochemicals; 1:500 Nitrotyrosine, Upstate], overnight at 4 °C.
9. Rinse the sections with 0.05 M TBS, 4×10 min at RT.
10. Incubate the sections with the biotinylated second antibody (anti-goat IgG for 8-Isoprostan, anti-rabbit IgG for nitrotyrosine) diluted 1:400 in 0.05 M TBS for 1 h at RT.
11. Wash 4×10 min in 0.05 M TBS.
12. Incubate the sections in horseradish-peroxidase-complex diluted in 0.05 M TBS (1:150) for 1 h at RT.
13. Rinse the sections with 0.05 M TBS, 4×10 min at RT.
14. Incubate the sections in 15 ml 0.1 M PB containing 7.5 mg 3,3'-diaminobenzidine tetrahydrochloride (DAB), 6.0 mg ammonium chloride, 3.9 mg nickel sulphate, 30 mg glucose and 0.06 mg glucose oxidase. Develop the sections for up to 30 min.
15. Rinse the sections with 0.05 M TBS 4×10 min at RT.
16. Dehydrate the sections in increasing concentrations of ethanol:
    - 3 min   ethanol 50%
    - 3 min   ethanol 70%
    - 3 min   ethanol 96%
    - 2×3 min   ethanol 100%

17. Clear the sections in xylene:
    — 3 min   xylene I
    — 3 min   xylene II
18. Mount the slides with Entellan (Merck).

The Immunohistochemical Controls and Analyses

The controls and analyses were performed as described above.

Immunohistological Detection of the Subcellular Distribution and Colocalization of Signal Molecules in Cardiomyocytes

In the last decades the significance of the subcellular distribution and interaction of structural and signal molecules for cellular function was recognized. Besides biochemical analyses of molecular interaction, high resolution morphology is needed to get information about the subcellular molecular distribution. This gives an increasing impact to the high-resolution fluorescence techniques, which allow the detection of molecules with a maximal resolution of around 100–200 nm. Immunofluorescence techniques for the labelling of structural and signal molecules in the cell are widely used and combined with high-resolution fluorescence microscopic techniques such as confocal laser microscopy or deconvolution microscopy. The following examples deal with the subcellular distribution of molecules involved in cellular calcium regulation in embryonic and adult cardiomyocytes (Bloch et al. 2001; Böhle et al. 2001). Double immunofluorescence staining and deconvolution analyses of the colocalization of inhibitory G-proteins and cytoskeletal components allowed us to show the close relationship between the cytoskeleton and the Gi-protein-dependent regulation of the L-Typ calcium channels in cardiomyocytes (Bloch et al. 2001). This combination of immunofluorescence and deconvolution microscopy also allows recognition of the cell compartments containing calcium-handling proteins (Böhle et al. 2001).

ES Cell Preparation

Studies used embryonic stem (ES) cells of the D3 line (wt) (Wobus et al. 1991), the heterozygous $\beta 1$ integrin$^{-/-}$ ES cell line, the $\beta 1$ integrin$^{-/-}$ ES cell line generated on a D3 background (Fassler et al. 1995), and the $\beta 1$ integrin rescue ES cell line. ES cells were cultured for 3 d in hanging drops and 3 d in suspension before plating on gelatine-coated coverslips without feeder cells in medium supplemented with 5 ng/ml recombinant human leukaemia inhibitory factor.

Single cardiomyocytes were isolated from clusters of spontaneously beating areas of the EBs as previously described (Bloch et al. 2001). Murine embryonic (E11.5, E17.5) ventricular cardiomyocytes were harvested from superovulated mice (Fleischmann et al. 1998). The heart was removed from the embryo, and the cardiomyocytes were isolated by collagenase digestion. The steps of the multiple immunofluorescence staining procedure of embryonic stem cell cultures follow those described by Bloch et al. (2001), and this protocol can be adapted in general to other antibodies.

Buffer and Fixation

1. 0.2 M PBS
   - 28.8 g Di-sodium hydrogen phosphate dihydrate ($HNa_2PO_4 \times 2H_2O$)
   - 5.2 g Na-di-hydrogen phosphate monohydrate ($NaH_2PO_4 \times H_2O$)
   - 17.53 g NaCl
   - add 1000 ml distilled water
2. 0.05 M TBS
   - 6.057 g Tris in about 250 ml aqua dest
   - 8.766 g NaCl
   - adjust pH to 7.6 with 1 N HCl
   - add aqua dest to 1000 ml
3. 4% PFA in 0.1 M PBS
   - 4 g paraformaldehyde in 50 ml aqua dest
   - heat to 50 °C, and add 2 drops of 1 N NaOH
   - add 50 ml 0.2 M PBS
   - filter with filter paper
   - adjust pH to 7.35–7.4

The Multiple Immunofluorescence Protocol for the ES Cell Cultures

1. The cells should be prepared from embryonic stem cells (ES) or murine embryo heart tissues.
2. Wash the EBs in 0.1 M PBS (1×10 min).
3. Fix the EBs with 4% paraformaldehyde in 0.1 M PBS for 30 min at room temperature (RT).
4. Wash in 0.1 M PBS at pH 7.4 (4×10 min).
5. Wash in 0.05 M TBS at pH 7.4 (2×10 min).
6. Put the cells into 0.05 M TBS solution containing 0.5 M ammonium chloride (NH_4Cl) and 0.25% Triton X100 for 10 min.
7. Wash the cells 2× with 0.05 M TBS at pH 7.6.
8. Incubate the cells in 0.05 M TBS containing 5% bovine serum albumin for 1 h at RT.
9. Wash the cells in 0.05 M TBS at pH 7.6 (1×10 min).
10. Incubate the cells with one or two kinds of first antibodies, which should be diluted in 0.05 M TBS containing 0.8% BSA, at 4 °C for 24 h.
    - The antibodies that should be used include monoclonal and polyclonal antibodies.
    - The monoclonal antisera
    - Anti-actinin (1:800; Sigma), a mouse anti-rabbit monoclonal antibody specific for cardiac or skeletal myocytes.
    - Anti-vinculin or anti-talin, mouse monoclonal antibodies, (1:100; Sigma, Saint Louis, Missouri, USA), two of the major linkage proteins between integrin and the actin cytoskeleton.
    - Anti-β1 integrin, a rat anti-mouse monoclonal antibody, (1:100; Chemicon International Inc.).

- The polyclonal antisera
- The polyclonal antibodies for G proteins (i.e., anti-$G_{\alpha i-3}$ which reacts with anti-$G_{\alpha i-1}$, anti-$G_{\alpha i-2}$ and anti-$G_{\alpha i-3}$, anti-$G_{\alpha 1/o/t/z}$, anti $G_{\alpha s}$ and anti-$G_{\alpha o}$) (1:500, Santa Cruz Biotechnology, Inc. Santa Cruz, USA).
- Anti-Girk1 (1:200, alomone Labs., Jerusalem, Israel),
- Anti-αIC (anti-cardiac type αIC, 1:200, alomone Labs.)
- Anti-M_2 receptor (1:2000, Research & Diagnostic Antibodies, Berkeley, CA).

11. Wash the cells with 0.05 M TBS at pH 7.6 (4×10 min). All subsequent incubations should be carried out in the dark.
12. Incubate the cells with Cy3 (or Cy2) conjugated goat anti-rabbit (or goat anti-mouse) secondary antibodies (1:800, Sigma) for 1 h at room temperature.
13. Wash the cardiac cells with 0.05 M TBS (4×10 min).
14. Incubate the cells with a biotinylated secondary goat anti-rabbit (or goat anti-mouse) IgG (1:400; Dako, Glostrup, Denmark) for 1 h at RT.
15. Wash the cells with 0.05 M TBS (4×10 min).
16. Incubate the cells with
    a) Streptavidin-conjugated Cy2 (1:100; Amersham, Braunschweig, Germany).
    b) Streptavidin-conjugated Cy3 (1:600; Amersham)
    c) Alexa FluorTM488 (1:200; Mo Bi Tec, Göttingen).
    d) FITC (1:200, Sigma Immuno Chemical, St. Louis).
17. Wash the cells with 0.05 M TBS (4×10 min).
18. The cells are dehydrated with 50%, 70%, 90% ethanol, (each step for 1 min) and 100% ethanol (2×2 min) successively. The cells labelled by FITC should not be dehydrated in ethanol.
19. The coverslips are taken from the dishes and cleared with xylene for 4 min.
20. Mounting
    a) Entellan (Merck KGaA, Darmstadt, Germany), a rapid mounting media for microscopy, should be put on each slide and the coverslips with cells placed on the Entellan at RT.
    b) For the cells which were stained with FITC, Supermount, a mounting medium, is used without ethanol dehydration.

The Double-Immunofluorescence Controls (Cross-Specificity Controls)

1. Slides incubated with rabbit polyclonal antibody should be incubated with (Cy2)-conjugated goat anti-mouse IgG.
2. Slides incubated with mouse monoclonal antibody should be incubated with Cy3-conjugated goat anti-rabbit IgG.
3. Primary antibodies should be substituted with non-immune mouse- and rabbit-IgG.

Interpretation of the Immunohistochemical Controls

In all the control experiments no immunoreactivity should be observed.

Troubleshooting

The best way is to avoid the necessity of troubleshooting, thus a detailed guideline for the experiments should be made, which is appropriate to answer the underlying question and considers the individual characteristics of antibodies and specimens. In Fig. 1 a check list for selection of the optimal experimental design is given.

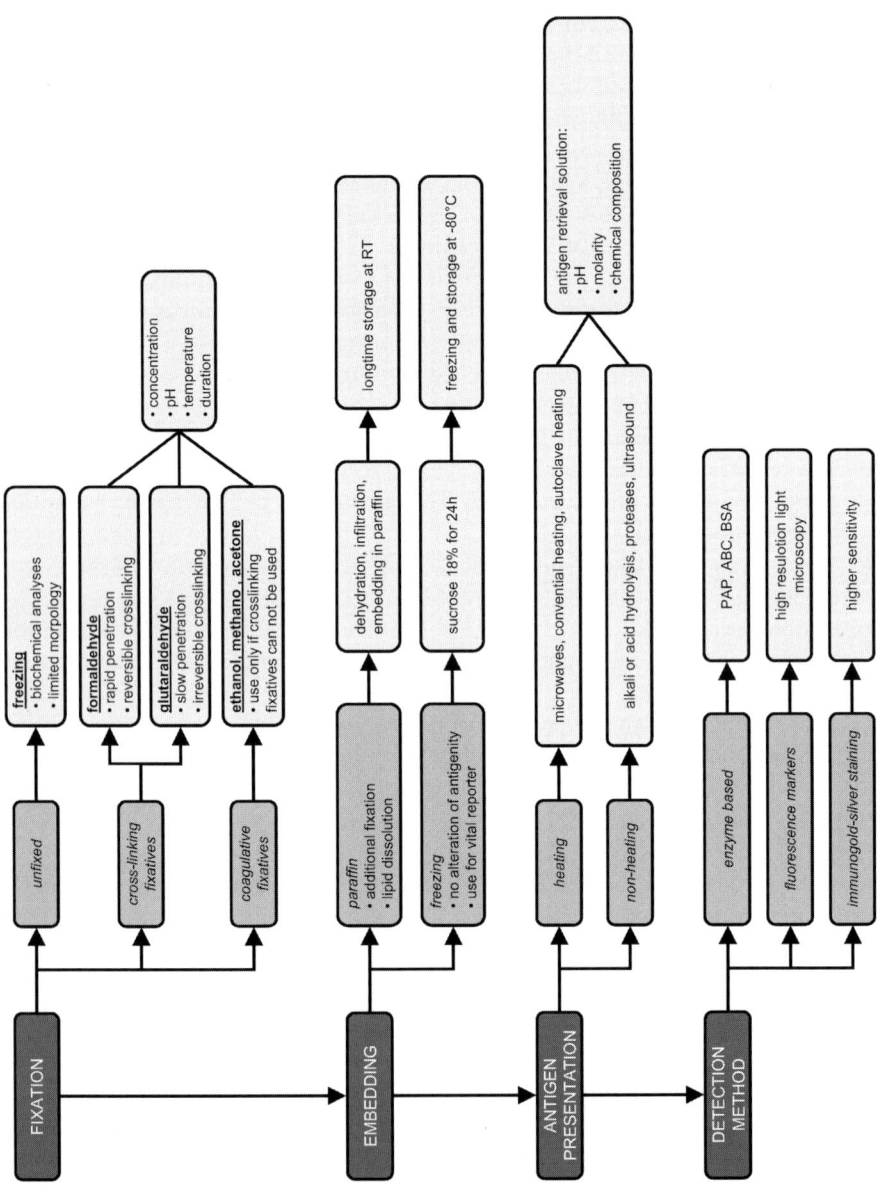

Figure 1
Checklist for development of an immunohistochemical protocol

If problems occur with the immunohistochemistry, the mistakes should be in general in two categories, lack of staining or unspecific over-staining.

At three general stages, problems can occur during immunohistochemistry: The first is sampling of the tissue and fixation, the second embedding and preparation of slices and the third the immunohistochemical procedures themselves.

In the case of a lack of immunostaining, it is appropriate to use a "positive control", tissue slices or cells with a known specific immunoreaction with the selected antibody, so that it is possible to differentiate between a general problem with the immunohistochemical procedure and problems with tissue sampling, fixation and embedding. If the failure can be classified as a tissue problem, then it is best to repeat the complete sampling, fixation and embedding procedure in a way that is comparable to the handling of the positive control. If this works, it is possible to repeat only partial steps of the procedure to localize the failure in detail and possibly allow work with the originally sampled and fixed tissue, if the reason for the lack of immunostaining was the embedding procedure. If the immunohistochemistry does not work for the positive control, a check should be made as to which steps of the immunohistochemical protocol have been changed. This is only possible if the protocol is detailed. In the case of lack of an adequate positive control, because there is no information about the suitability of the antibody for immunohistochemistry, the antibody should first be used in an experimental approach, for example a Western blot on the tissue of interest, to check if the antigen is actually present. Thereafter experiments should be performed with different fixation and embedding conditions and antibody solutions. If this does not work, works weakly or only works for preservation methods such as freezing, which show suboptimal tissue preservation, the use of an antigen retrieval test approach (Shi et al. 1996) should be tried. Alternatively the use, if available, of another antibody against the antigen of interest or an alternative method such as *in situ* hybridisation or RT *in situ* PCR should be tried.

More serious problems arise if over-staining or non-specific staining occurs, because of the risk of wrong interpretation of the immunohistochemical results, i.e. the non-specific labelling will not be recognized as such. The best way to avoid this problem is to perform a complete immunohistochemical control programme as described in the above protocols. The different control methods allow one to focus on the reason for the non-specific or over-staining. If developing solution causes a staining without primary and secondary antibody, endogenous enzyme activity, e.g. peroxidase, is eliciting the labelling. Additional pre-treatment to block the endogenous enzyme activity should help, if not another staining system can be used. A problem with the secondary antibody can recognized if there is a reaction without primary antibody. Additional blocking steps with adequate serum can help in this case or use of another secondary antibody that binds only to specific antibody fragments. A further elegant method is the *in vitro* pre-incubation of primary and secondary antibody. This should avoid incubation with free unbound secondary antibody. Problems with the specificity of the first antibody directly recognizing the antigen are the most problematic. None of the above described control methods can 100% guaranteed that there is no cross-reactivity with other antigens. Especially if polyclonal antibodies are used, but also with monoclonal antibodies this scenario cannot be excluded. Therefore the best way to check this is to use a further first antibody against another epitope of the antigen or, if this is not available, to use methods for detection of the relevant mRNA. This problem occurs mainly if new antibodies are used whose specificity has not been checked previously; if antibodies are used which have been tested the risk is relatively low.

Further problems with immunohistochemistry are inhomogeneity of the staining or increased staining of the border areas of the slices. In the first case the fixation or embedding was usually not homogenous. Such tissue should not be used because of the problems of interpretation. A limited use of such tissues is possible in the hand of a very experienced morphologist. At this point it should be mentioned that troubleshooting can be greatly reduced if an experienced morphologist is consulted. The problem with the slices' borders is derived from quenching of first and/or secondary antibodies in this region, which cannot be avoided by washing. Therefore such regions should not be investigated.

A specific problem of immunofluorescence is the occurrence of tissue autofluorescence. Especially in the heart, such autofluorescence can be found in the red and green channels. The use of band pass filters very specific for the fluorescent dyes used and the use of different fluorescent dyes as detection markers can help to recognize autofluorescence.

A successful and not too time-consuming troubleshooting can be carried out if a detailed protocol was written.

References

Adams JC (1992) Biotin amplification of biotin and horseradish peroxidase signals in histochemical stains. J Histochem Cytochem 40: 1457–1463

Addicks K, Bloch W, Feelisch M (1994) Nitric oxide modulates sympathetic neurotransmission at the prejunctional level. Microscopy Research and Technique 29: 161–168

Bloch W, Forsberg E, Lentini S, Brakebusch C, Martin K, Krell HW, Weidle UH, Addicks K, Fässler R (1997) Beta 1 integrin is essential for teratoma growth and angiogenesis. J Cell Biol 139: 265–278

Bloch W, Mehlhorn U, Krahwinkel A, Reiner M, Dittrich M, Schmidt A, Addicks K (2001) Ischemia increases detectable endothelial nitric oxide synthase in rat and human myocardium. Nitric Oxide 5: 317–333

Bloch W, Fan Y, Han J, Xue S, Schöneberg T, Ji GJ, Zu ZJ, Walther M, Fässler R, Hescheler J, Addicks K, Fleischmann BK (2001) Disruption of cytoskeletal integrity impairs G_i-mediated signaling due to displacement of G_i-proteins. J Cell Biol 154: 753–761

Boenisch T (2001) Formalin-fixed and heat-retrieved tissue antigens: a comparison of their immunoreactivity in experimental antibody diluents. Appl Immunohistochem Mol Morphol 9: 176–179

Böhle T, Brandt MC, Henn N, Schmidt A, Bloch W, Beuckelmann DJ (2001) Identification and in-situ registration of the cardiac ryanodine-receptor channel in membrane blebs of sarcoplasmic reticulum. FEBS Lett 505: 419–425

Coons AH, Creech HJ, Jones RN (1941) Immunological properties of an antibody containing a fluorescent group. Proc Soc Exp Biol Med 47: 200–202

Danscher G (1981) Localisation of gold in biological tissue: A photochemical method for light and electronmicroscopy. Histochemistry 71: 81–88

De Vente J, Steinbusch HWM (1992) On the stimulation of soluble and particulate guanylate cyclase in the rat brain and the involvement of nitric oxide as studied by cGMP immunocytochemistry. Acta Histochemistry 92: 13–38

Fassler R, Pfaff M, Murphy J, Noegel AA, Johansson S, Timpl R, and Albrecht R (1995) Lack of β1 integrin gene in embryonic stem cells affects morphology, adhesion, and migration but not integration into the inner cell mass of blastocysts. J Cell Biol 128: 979–988

Faulk WP, Taylor GM (1971) An immunogold method for the electron microscope. Immunohistochemistry 8: 1081–1083

Fischer UW, Klass O, Stock U, Easo J, Geissler HJ, Fischer JH, Bloch W, Mehlhorn U (2003) Cardioplegic arrest induces apoptosis signal-pathway in myocardial endothelial cells and cardiac myocytes. Eur J Cardiothorac Surg 23: 984–990

Fleischmann M, Bloch W, Kolossov E, Andressen C, Müller M, Brem G, Hescheler J, Addicks K, Fleischmann BK (1998) Cardiac specific expression of the green fluorescent protein during early murine embryonic development. FEBS Lett 440: 370–376

Fritz P, Tuczek H, Mulhaupt H, Schwarzmann P (1995) Quantitation in immunhistochemistry. A research method or a diagnostic toll in surgical pathology. Pathologica 87: 300–309

Geoghegan WD, Scillian JJ, Ackerman GA (1978) The detection of human B-lymphocytes by both light and electron microscopy utilizing colloidal gold-labelled anti-immuno-globulin. Immunol Commun 7: 1–12

Gerdes J, Dallenbach F, Lennert K, Lemke H, Stein H (1984) Growth fraction in malignant non-Hodgkins lymphoma (NHL) as determined *in situ* with monoclonal antibody to Ki67. Hematol Oncol 2: 365–371

Gu J, Agrawal N (1997) Elimination of background staining in immunocytochemistry. In: Gu J (ed) Analytical morphology: theory, applications and protocols. Birkhäuser Boston, Cambridge, pp 55–68

Grizzle WE, Aamodt R, Clausen K, Li Volsi V, Pretlow TG, Qualman S (1998) Providing human tissues for research: how to establish a program. Arch Pathol Lab Med 122: 1065–1076

Hacker GW, Danscher G, Hauser-Kronberger C (1997) Immunogold-silver staining – autometallography: recent developments and protocols. In: Gu J (ed) Analytical morphology: theory, applications and protocols. Birkhäuser, Boston Cambridge, pp 41–54

Hainfeld JF, Furuya FR (1992) A 1.4-nm gold cluster covalently attached to antibodies improves immunolabelling. J Histochem Cytochem 40: 177–184

Hanyu Y, Ichikawa M, Matsumoto G (1992) An improved cryofixation method: cryoquenching of small tissue blocks during microwave irradiation. J Microsc 165: 255–271

Hayat MA (2002) Microscopy, immunohistochemistry, and antigen retrieval methods. Kluwer Academic/Plenium Publishers, New York

Holgate CS, Jackson P, Cowen PN, Bird CC (1983) Immunogold-solver staining: new method of immunpstaining with enhanced sensitivity. J Histochem Cytochem 31: 938–944

Jackson TH, Ungan A, Critser JK, Gao D (1997) Novel microwave technology for cryopreservation of biomaterials by suppression of apparent ice formation. Cryobiology 34: 363–372

Kazemi S, Wenzel D, Kolossov E, Lenka N, Raible A, Sasse P, Hescheler J, Addicks K, Fleischmann BK, Bloch W (2002) Differential role of bFGF and VEGF for vasculogenesis. Cell Physiol Biochem 12: 55–62

Mehlhorn U, Bloch W, Krahwinkel A, LaRose K, Geissler HJ, Hekmat K, Addicks K, de Vivie ER (2000) Activation of myocardial constitutive nitric oxide synthase during coronary artery surgery. Eur J Cardiothorac Surg 17: 305–311

Mehlhorn U, Krahwinkel A, Geissler H, LaRose K, Suedkamp M, Fischer UM, Klass O, Hekmat K, Bloch W (2003) Nitrotyrosine and 8-isoprostane formation indicate free radical-mediated injury in hearts of patients subjected to cardioplegia. J Thorac Cardiovasc Surg 125: 178–18

Merz H, Malisius R, Mannweiler S, Zhou R, Hartmann W, Orscheschek K, Moubayed P, Feller AC (1995) Immunomax. A maximized immunohistochemical method for the retrieval and enhancement of hidden antigens. Lab Invest 73: 149–156

Newman SJ, Nelson P (2000) Image analysis and Statistics. In: Beesley (ed) Immunocytochemistry and *in situ* hybridisation in the biomedical sciences, Birkhäuser, Boston, pp 175–199

Pott C, Brixius K, Bundkirchen A, Bölck B, Bloch W, Steinritz D, Mehlhorn U, Schwinger RHG (2003) The preferential β_3-adrenoceptor agonist BRL 37344 increases force via β_1-/β_2-adrenoceptors and induces endothelial nitric oxide synthase via β_3-adrenoceptors in human atrial myocardium. Br J Pharmacol 138: 521–529

Ranefall P, Wester K, Andersson AC, Busch C, Bengtsson E (1998) Automatic quantification of immunohistochemically stained cell nuclei based on standard reference cells. Anal Cell Pathol 17: 111–123

Riera J, Simpson JF, Tamayo R, Battifora H (1999) Use of cultured cells as a control for quantitative immunocytochemical analysis of estrogen receptor in breast cancer. The Quicgel method. Am J Clin Pathol 111: 329–335

Roche PC, His ED (2001) Immunohistochemistry: theory and practice. In: Lloyd RV (ed) Morphology methods: cell and molecular biology techniques. Humana Press, Totowa, pp 229–237

Roell W, Lu ZJ, Bloch W et al. (2002) Cellular cardiomyoplasty improves survival after myocardial injury. Circulation 105: 2433–2439

Roth J, Saremaslani P, Zuber C (1992) Versatility of anti-horseradish peroxidase antibody-gold coplexes for cytochemistry and *in situ* hybridisation: preparation and application of soluble complexes with streptavidin-peroxidase conjugates and biotinylated antibodies. Histochemistry 98: 229–236

Shi SR, Key ME, Kalra KL (1991) Antigen retrieval in formalin-fixed, paraffin-embedded tissues: An enhancement method for immunohistochemical staining on microwave oven heating of tissue sections. J Histochem Cytochem 39: 741–748

Shi SR, Cote C, Kalra KL, Taylor CR, Tandon AK (1992) A technique for retrieving antigens in formalin-fixed, routinely acid-decalcified, celloidin-embedded human temporal bone sections for immunohistochemistry. J Histochem Cytochem 40: 787–792

Shi SR, Cote RJ, Yang C, Chen C, Xu HJ, Bendict WF, Taylor CR (1992) Development of an optimal for antigen retrieval: a "test battery" approach exemplified with reference to the staining of retinoblastoma protein (pRB) in formalin-fixed paraffin sections. J Pathol 179: 347–352

Springall DR, Hacker GW, Grimelius, Polak JM (1984) The potential of the immunogold-silver method for paraffin sections. Histochemistry 81: 603–608

Sternberger LA (1979) The unlabelled antibody peroxidase-anti-peroxidase (PAP) method. In: Sternberger LA, Immunocytochemistry, 2nd edn. John Wiley and Sons, New York, pp 104–169

Taylor CR, Burns J (1974) The demonstration of plasma cells and other immunoglobulin containing cells in formalin-fixed, paraffin-embedded tissues using peroxidase labelled antibody. J Clin Pathol 27: 14–20

Taylor CR, Tandon A (1994) Theoretical and practical aspects of the different immunoperoxidase techniques. In: Taylor CR, Cote RJ (eds) Immunomicroscopy: A diagnostic tool for the surgical pathologist, WB Saunders, Philadelphia, pp 21–41

Taylor CR, Shi S (2001) Antigen retrieval technique for immunohistochemistry. In: Lloyd RV (ed) Morphology methods: cell and molecular biology techniques, Humana Press, Totowa, pp 229–237

Tossios P, Bloch W, Huebner A, Dodos F, Suedkamp M, Kasper S, Hellmich M, Mehlhorn U (2003) N-acetylcysteine prevents reactive oxygen species-mediated myocardial injury in cardiac surgery patients: results of a randomized double-blinded placebo-controlled clinical trial. J Thorac Cardiovasc Surg 126: 1513–1520

Wobus AM, Wallukat G, Hescheler J (1991) Pluripotent mouse embryonic stem cells are able to differentiate into cardiomyocytes expressing chronotropic responses to adrenergic and cholinergic agents and Ca^{2+} channel blockers. Differentiation 48: 173–182

Classical Histological Staining Procedures in Cardiovascular Research

Wilhelm Bloch and Yüksel Korkmaz

Introduction

The development of new methods for qualitative and quantitative morphological investigations has been growing exponentially. In particular, methods allowing the detection of proteins and mRNA such as immunohistochemistry and in situ hybridisation have been widely expanded in their use. Although these methods are more and more important in morphology, the classical staining procedures can bring further advantages compared to these methods and can be used to get basic and supplementary information in cardiovascular research, so it is no wonder that they remain standard methods in cardiovascular research. The classical stains cannot be replaced if various components of tissues are to be distinguished. Hematoxylin-eosin (HE) for paraffin-embedded tissue and methylene blue or toluidine blue for resin-embedded tissue are probably the most widely used. The object of histological staining is to demonstrate tissue and cell components in their native localization by using chemically well-defined methods. The two main tissue units are the cell and the extracellular matrix, therefore the targets for histological staining are the molecular and structural components of the cells and the extracellular matrix. Histological staining often permits initial recognition of the molecular and structural components of the tissue. The heterogeneous chemical composition of the tissue, which leads to the molecular and subsequently to the structural composition, is a prerequisite for the histological staining. The chemical components of the cell and the extracellular matrix are the direct targets for the dyes, which can be defined as chromogens of aromatic or heteroaromatic nature, soluble in water or polar solvents and capable of binding to other substances (Anderson et al. 1992). The chemical components are of inorganic (water and salts) and organic (proteins, nucleic acids, carbohydrates and lipids) nature. Proteins, nucleic acids, carbohydrates, and lipids can occur as pure substances in the tissue, but they are more frequently found as molecular complexes or mixed compounds. The different affinities of the dyes for these tissue components allow the specific labelling of cell and extracellular matrix structures and molecules. Unfortunately the staining result is not only dependent on the chemical composition of the tissue. It is also dependent on environmental factors. Fixation and embedding are clearly important factors. Differences in the preparation of tissue will produce differences in the staining. Therefore standardization of a staining method for cytological and histological specimens requires consideration of all steps in the procedure; the subsequent interpretation of the staining results can only be performed with consideration of the conditions.

Considering that basically all morphological investigation should start with histological staining of the tissue, it seems necessary to get an overview about preservation of the tissue and the alterations that occur. It is not surprising that standard stainings such as HE and methylene blue or toluidine blue are so often used in cardiovascular research. Besides the simple detection of structural integrity or alteration of the integrity, histological stainings can also help to detect specific molecules or groups of molecules in cardiovascular tissue. For example, alteration of calcium content in infarcted myocardium can be detected by alizarin red (Chatelain and Kapanci 1984) or oil red O staining revealing deposition of fine lipid droplets in the ischemic cardiac muscle cells bordering on the necrotic areas (Lindal et al. 1986). But mostly, light microscopic histological staining is used to visualize alterations in the extracellular matrix (Rösen et al. 1995; Tagarakis et al. 2000; Röll et al. 2002) and to identify deposition of calcium in the extracellular space by specific staining methods (for review Puchtler and Meloan, 1978) as well as for detection of both (Rajamannan et al. 2003).

This chapter can give only a small insight into classical staining procedures. Therefore the chapter is focused on the most frequently used basic staining methods and those which can be used to find alterations in the extracellular spaces of vessels and myocardium.

Description of Methods and Practical Approach

Histological staining is based on physical and chemical reactions. The following mechanisms involved in the staining process can be described. A dye, which is dissolved in a staining solution, may be absorbed on the surface of a structure, or dyes may be precipitated within the structure, simply because environmental factors (such as pH, ionic strength, temperature) favour absorption or precipitation. Most staining reactions involve a chemical reaction between dye and stained substance through salt linkages, hydrogen bonds, van der Waals forces, coulombic attractions or covalent bonding.

Staining with such dyes results in a predictable colour pattern based in part on the acid-base characteristic of the tissue. In general, the staining of tissues is also affected by the number and distribution of binding sites for dyes in the tissues. However, colour and colour distribution are not absolutely reliable for discrimination between tissue components. Colour will vary with the specific stain used and also with the conditions that exist during preparation of the slide. These include everything from the initial fixing solution to the ionic strength of the staining solution and the differentiating solvents utilized after staining.

The dyes most used for histological staining can be subdivided into acidic and basic dyes. An acid dye exists as an anion in solution, while a basic dye exists as a cation. Often the staining solutions are composed of basic dyes and acidic dyes, as for example the widely used hematoxylin-eosin staining, where the hematoxylin-metal complex acts as a basic dye and the eosin as an acidic dye. This allows detection of different structures in a specimen dependent on their charge. A further commonly used staining mechanism, called trichrome staining, is a dye competition technique, which allows tissue component-specific staining with dyes of different molecular weight. In the following, staining methods, such as HE, methylene blue, trichrome stainings, Sirius red, silver impregnation and von Kossa, often used in cardiovascular research are described in more detail.

Hematoxylin and Eosin Staining (HE)

H.E. is a good general stain and is therefore the most used. It is a staining method which uses a basic and an acidic dye. A hematoxylin-metal complex acts as a basic dye, staining nucleic acids in the nucleus and the cytoplasm blue, brown, or black. Eosin, an acid aniline, stains the more basic proteins within cells (cytoplasm) and the extra-

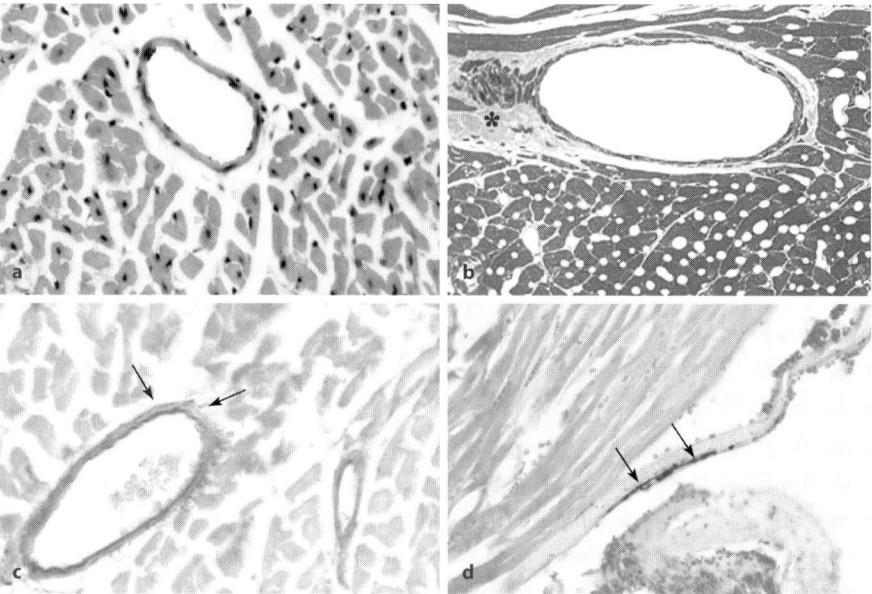

Fig. 1a–d
Histological staining of paraffin (**a, c, d**) and araldite-embedded murine heart tissue (**b**). **a** Micrograph section stained with hematoxylin-eosin. Note the dark blue to purple staining of nuclei and the pink staining of the cytoplasm. **b** Methylene blue stained semi-thin sections reveal a blue staining of cytoplasm and nuclei, which are only distinguished by colour intensity. Metachromatic colouring of the extracellular matrix leads to a blue to lilac staining of the extracellular matrix (*asterisk*). **c** Sirius red staining produces a yellow colouring of the cells and a red staining of the extracellular matrix including the thin basement membrane of the cardiomyocytes and thin collageneous fibres (*arrows*). **d** A relatively homogeneous red staining of the sections is produced by von Kossa staining, while calcium deposits in a heart valve are black (*arrows*)

cellular matrix pink to red (Fig. 1a). In myocardium, the nuclei are blue-black, while the muscle fibres are pink to red. The staining is strongly dependent on the acidic or alkaline conditions. Under acidic conditions, proteins have a net cationic charge and have an affinity for the basic dyes. Under alkaline conditions, basic dyes will stain all the tissue and selectivity will be lost. Rates of dye binding and loss may vary between different structures in a tissue, thus aiding differentiation.

HE staining can be used for frozen and chemically fixed tissues by appropriate changes in the staining procedure. A detailed staining procedure is only given for formaldehyde-fixed and paraffin-embedded tissue, which show good structural preservation. HE staining is a basic method usable for nearly all morphological investigations in cardiovascular research to get information about the structure of the tissue.

Solutions

- Mayer's haemalum
    - Dissolve the following, in the order given, in 750 ml of water
    - 50 g Alumminium potassium sulphate [$KA(SO_4)_2\ 12H_2O$]
    - 11.0 g Haematoxylin
    - 0.1 g Sodium iodate ($NaIO_3$)
    - 1.0 g Citric acid (monohydrate)
    - 50 g Chloral hydrate
- Eosin
    - 2.5 g eosin
    - 0.5 ml glacial acetic acid
    - 495 ml water
- Acid-alcohol
    - 500 ml 95% alcohol
    - 5 ml concentrated hydrochloric acid

Method

1. De-wax and hydrate paraffin sections. Frozen sections should be dried on to slides.
2. Immerse the sections in Mayer's haemalum for 1–15 min (usually 2–5 min, but this should be tested before staining a large batch of slides).
3. Wash in running tap water for 2–3 min or until the sections turn blue.
4. Immerse the sections in eosin for 30 s with agitation.
5. Wash and differentiate the sections in running tap water for about 30 s.
6. Dehydrate the sections in 70, 95% and two changes of 100% ethanol (2–3 min in each change).
7. Clear the sections in xylene and cover, using a resinous medium.

Interpretation of results

1. Nuclear chromatin should be stained blue to purple.
2. Cytoplasm, collagen, keratin and erythrocytes should be stained pink.

Methylene Blue and Toluidine Blue Staining

Toluidine blue as well as methylene blue are basic dyes, which stain nucleic acids blue (the orthochromatic colour), but polyanions such as sulphated polysaccharides purple (the metachromatic colour). When dye molecules bound to sulphate groups are stacked closely together, the dye results are colour-shifted from blue to purple. Thus, a metachromatic reaction often indicates the presence of numerous closely packed sulphate groups. Therefore extracellular matrix deposits containing a large amount of proteoglycans, which contain a sulphated glycosaminoglycan side chain such as heparan, chondroitin or dermatan sulphate, can be visualized by use of metachromatic colouring (see Fig. 1b).

Both stainings are simple staining methods for resin-embedded tissue.
- Toluidine stock solution
    - 1 g toluidine blue
    - 5 g borax
    - 100 ml distilled water
    - Mix and stand overnight then filter before use.
- Methylene blue stock solution
    - 1 g methylene blue
    - 1 g borax
    - 100 ml distilled water

Method

1. Flood a section, on a hot plate, with toluidine blue or methylene blue solution for up to 30 s (do not allow the section to dry).
2. Wash in running tap water for a few seconds.
3. Remove excess water from around the section then dry on a hot plate.
4. The section can be examined uncovered or mounted if a permanent preparation is required.

Interpretation of results

1. The end result is an intense blue staining of the section.
2. Purple stained areas give evidence of metachromatic colouring.

Trichrome Staining

In the trichrome stains, which commonly employ more than one acid dye, use is made of dye competition. Consider preparations stained with a mixture of dyes of the same charge but of markedly different sizes, and so probably of different staining rates. In the early stages of staining at least, it would be expected that whilst the fast-staining tissue substrates would take up both the large and the small dyes, slow-staining substrates would be predominantly coloured by the small fast-staining dye. Taking these

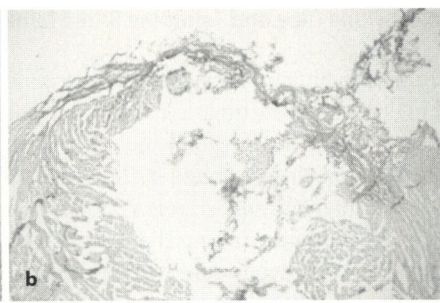
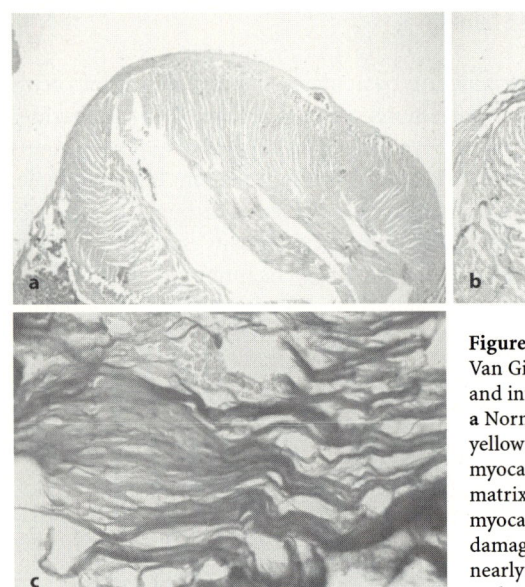

Figure 2a–c
Van Gieson staining is performed on normal (**a**) and infarcted murine myocardium (**b**).
a Normal myocardium shows a homogeneous yellow colour in all cellular components of the myocardium, while the sparse extracellular matrix is red. **b** The fibrotic replacement of the myocardium can be seen as red staining of the damaged area. **c** At higher magnification the nearly complete loss of cardiomyocytes and the replacement by collagen fibres are recognizable

facts into account one might expect that fast-staining components such as collagen fibres would be coloured by the larger dye of the pair whereas slow-staining substrates such as cardiomyocytes will be coloured predominantly by the smaller dye.

For example, acid fuchsin and picric acid are used in Van Gieson's trichrome stain (Fig. 2). In the picric acid-fuchsin mixture, the small picric acid molecule reaches and stains the available sites in muscle before the larger fuchsin molecules can enter. Used by itself, acid fuchsin has no difficulty in staining muscle. The van Gieson methods give the most selective staining of collagen fibres. The 25- to 50-fold excess of picric acid relative to the collagen dye in a van Gieson solution renders the cytoplasmic background yellow. For collagen staining, different red dyes can be used such as Sirius red or acid fuchsin. If besides larger collagen fibres, reticulin fibres and basal membranes should be demonstrated, long planar molecules such as Sirius red can be used. Sirius red stains the thinnest collagen fibres, so reticulin fibres and basal membranes can also be stained (Lyon et al. 1992).

Another trichrome staining method is the Goldner staining, a variant of the Masson staining. As the name implies, three dyes are employed, selectively staining muscle, collagen fibres, fibrin, and erythrocytes. The general rule in trichrome staining is that the less porous tissues are coloured by the smallest dye molecule; whenever a dye of large molecular size is able to penetrate, it will always do so at the expense of the smaller molecule. Trichrome staining is requested if alterations in the collagen content of heart, valves and vessel wall are to be investigated (Rösen et al. 1995; Röll et al. 2002, 2002b; Ray et al. 2002; Rajamannan et al. 2003) or if structural alterations in the myocardium, as occur during early myocardial infarction, are to be investigated (Vargas et al. 1999).

Van Gieson's Staining

Solutions

- Weigert's iron-hematoxylin
- Stock solutions
- Solution A
  - 5 g hematoxylin
  - 500 ml 95% ethanol
- Solution B
  - 5.8 g ferric chloride ($FeCl_3.6H_2O$)
  - 495 ml water
  - 5 ml concentrated hydrochloric acid
- Working solution
  - Mix equal volumes of A and B. The mixture should be made just before using. It may be re-used many times and can be kept for 2 days at room temperature or for 10–14 days at 4 °C. Older solutions stain nuclei brown or bluish-grey rather than black (Kiernan 1999).
- van Gieson's solution
  - 0.5 g acid fuchsin
  - 500 ml saturated aqueous picric acid
  - Optionally, add 2.5 ml of concentrated hydrochloric acid
  - This mixture can be reused many times, and it retains its staining power for more than 5 years (Kiernan 1999).
- Acidified water
  - Add 5 ml acetic acid (glacial) to 1 l of water (tap or distilled).

Method

1. De-wax and hydrate paraffin sections.
2. Stain in working solution of Weigert's hematoxylin for 5 min (may need 10 min if the solution is more than 4–5 days old).
3. Wash in running tap water. Check the wet section with a microscope to ensure that nuclei are selectively stained.
4. Stain in van Gieson's solution, 2–5 min. The time is not critical.
5. Wash in two changes of acidified water.
6. Dehydrate rapidly in three changes of 100% ethanol. This step also differentiates the picric acid.
7. Clear in xylene and mount in a resinous medium.

Interpretation of results

1. Nuclei should be stained black.
2. Collagen should be stained red.
3. Cytoplasm (especially smooth and striated muscle), keratin and erythrocytes should be stained yellow.

Goldner's Trichrome Staining

Solutions

- Acid fuchsin, 0.5%
  - 1.0 g acid fuchsin
  - 200 ml water
- Phosophomolybdic acid-orange solution
  - 5 g phosphomolybdic acid (molybdophosphoric acid)
  - 5 g phosphotungstic acid
  - 200 ml water
  - 4 mg orange G
- 2.5% fast green FCF
  - 5 g fast green FCF
  - 195 ml water
  - 5 ml glacial acetic acid
- For "Weigert's iron-hematoxylin" see van Gieson's Method.
- Acidified water with 1% acetic acid
  - 5 ml acetic acid
  - 1000 ml water

Method

1. De-wax the sections and bring to water.
2. Stain nuclei in a working hematoxylin for 3 min.
3. Wash in running tap water for 10 min.
4. Immerse in 0.5% acid fuchsin for 5 min.
5. Wash in acidified water.
6. Immerse in the phosphomolybdic acid-orange solution for 1 min.
   One minute may not be enough. Therefore, check a slide under a microscope to ensure that the red dye has been removed from collagen.
   Return to the phosphomolybdic acid-orange solution if necessary.
7. Wash in acidified water.
8. Stain for 5 min in 2.5% fast green FCF.
9. Wash for 5 min in acidified water.
10. Dehydrate in three changes of 100% ethanol.
11. Clear in xylene.
12. Apply coverslips using a resinous mounting medium.

Interpretation of Results

1. Nuclei should be stained red.
2. Collagen should be stained blue.
3. Cytoplasm should be in various shades of red, pink and orange.
4. Cartilage matrix should be stained blue.

Picro-Sirius Red Staining

Collagen forms the ground substance of connective tissue. It is composed of three amino- acids and stains strongly with acid red dyes due to the affinity of the cationic groups of the proteins for the anionic reactive groups of the acid dyes. Sirius red has the advantage of being a long, planar molecule, which becomes oriented parallel to the collagen fibre structure and increases birefringence. Red staining with picro-Sirius accompanied by a pronounced increase in birefringence is an unequivocal indication of the presence of collagen and reticulin fibres (Junqueira et al. 1979). Therefore this staining is useful if thin collagen fibres (see Fig. 1c) need to be detected in cardiovascular tissue (Van Kerckhoven et al. 2000; Ammarguellat et al. 2001)
- Picro-Sirius red
    - 0.5 g Sirius red
    - 500 ml saturated aqueous solution of picric acid
    - Add a little solid picric acid to ensure saturation
- Acidified water
    - Add 5 ml glacial acetic acid to 1 l of water (tap or distilled).

Method

1. De-wax and hydrate paraffin sections.
2. Stain nuclei with Weigert's hematoxylin (see under the van Gieson method), then wash the slides for 10 min in running tap water.
3. Stain in picro-Sirius red for 1 h.
4. Wash in two changes of acidified water.
5. Dehydrate in three changes of 100% ethanol.
6. Clear in xylene and mount in a resinous medium.

Interpretation of Results

1. In ordinary bright-field microscopy collagen is red on a yellow background (see Fig. 1c).
2. Nuclei, if stained, are black.

The intensity of the red colour can be measured by microdensitometry to provide estimates of collagen content in different parts of a tissue (Kratky et al. 1996). Under examination through crossed polars the larger collagen fibres are bright yellow or orange, and the thinner ones, including reticular fibres, are green.

Silver Staining for Visualisation of Basal Membrane

Silver staining, or more precisely silver impregnation, leads to an impregnation of reticular fibres with silver salt; the fibres then appear sharply black. Collagenous fibres usually stain purple. This stain can be used with a counterstain or without, if the silver stain turns out to be very dark. Beside of the staining of reticular fibres, silver impregnation is widely used in neurohistology to stain neurons and their processes. The sections are processed in solutions containing silver, which attach to specific components in tissues. The silver is then further processed and developed into dark deposits.

This staining can be used to detect alterations in the extracellular matrix, including the basal membrane, in the myocardium and vessels (Chiu et al. 1999).

Solutions

1. 0.5% periodic acid in water
2. 0.2% gold chloride in water
3. 3% sodium thiosulphate ($Na_2S_2O_3.5H_2O$) in water
4. Hexamethylentetramine-silversolution
   100 ml 3% hexamethylentetramine
   5 ml 5% silver nitrate

Dissolve 3 g hexamethylenetetramine in 100 ml water.
Dissolve 250 mg silver nitrate in 5 ml of water or use 5 ml of a 5% aqueous silver nitrate stock solution.
Combine the two solutions in a very clean glass bottle and mix thoroughly. A precipitate forms and redissolves. This solution should be stored at 4 °C as a stock solution.
— 50 ml hexamethylentetramine-silver stock solution
— 6 ml 5% sodium tetraborate ($Na_2B_4O_7.10H_2O$; borax)

This is made immediately before beginning to stain the sections.

Method

1. De-wax and hydrate paraffin sections.
2. Wash the sections in distilled water.
3. Immerse the sections in 0.5% periodic acid for 15 min.
4. Wash the sections in distilled water.
5. Place the slides in the hexamine-silver working solution for 1.5 –3 h at 50 °C in dark.
6. Wash the sections in distilled water.
7. Immerse in the gold toning solution for 2 min.
8. Wash the sections in distilled water.
9. Immerse in 3% sodium thiosulphate for 2 min.
10. Wash in running tap water for 5 min.
11. Apply hematoxylin and eosin as a counterstain if desired.
12. Dehydrate, clear and apply coverslips using a resinous mounting medium.

Interpretation of Result

Basal membrane should be stained in grey-black.

Von Kossa's Silver Staining

Tissue sections are treated with silver nitrate solution, the calcium is reduced by strong light and replaced with silver deposits, which are visualized as metallic silver. The replacement is based on inorganic precipitation, and the range of possibilities for satisfactory histochemical procedures using inorganic reactions is limited. For counterstaining fast red is used.

This staining leads to a black colouring of calcium-deposits (see Fig. 1d), while the cytoplasm is pink and the nuclei are red coloured. The staining can be performed on sections of formalin-fixed and paraffin-embedded tissue. The staining can be used to detect calcification in tissue, such as occurs in atherosclerosis and in cell cultures (Wada et al. 1999; Ray et al. 2002; Rajamannan et al. 2003).

Solutions

1. 1% aqueous silver nitrate ($AgNO_3$). Solution A must be made up in the purest available water.
2. 5% aqueous sodium thiosulphate ($Na_2S_2O_3 \cdot 5H_2O$).
3. Counterstain.

0.5% safranine or neutral red is suitable. All these solutions can be used repeatedly until precipitates form in them.

Method

1. De-wax and hydrate paraffin sections. Wash in water.
2. Immerse in silver nitrate in bright sunlight or directly underneath a 100 W electric light bulb for 15 min.
3. Rinse in two changes of water.
4. Immerse in sodium thiosulphate for 2 min.
5. Wash in three changes of water.
6. Counterstain nuclei, about 1 min.
7. Rinse briefly in water.
8. Dehydrate (and differentiate the counterstain) in 95% and two changes of absolute alcohol.
9. Clear in xylene and mount in a resinous medium.

Interpretation of Results

1. Sites of insoluble phosphates and carbonates should be stained as black, brown or yellow.
2. Nuclei should be stained pink or red.

Examples

Trichrome Staining for Detection of Myocardial and Perivascular Fibroses

Alterations in extracellular matrix amount and composition are found in several cardiovascular diseases such as myocardial infarction and diabetic cardiomyopathy (Rösen et al. 1995, 1998; Röll et al. 2002, 2002b). To evaluate the role of oxidative stress in the increased fibrosis in diabetic hearts, we analysed the myocardial and perivascular amounts of extracellular matrix and the composition of the extracellular matrix by Goldener trichrome staining and by immunohistochemistry against collagens I and III. Subsequent computerized morphometrical analyses of the perivascular connective tissue of coronary vessels were performed with a Leitz CBA 8000 image analysing system for detection of real colour. The area of connective tissue was given by the trichrome-stained area related to the circumference of the vessel. A good correlation was found between alterations in the sizes of immunohistochemically (for collagens I and III) stained areas and the changes in Goldner trichrome stained areas in the investigated groups.

Considering the quality and reproducibility of trichrome staining results in cardiac tissue, the method is well suited to simple detection of connective tissue, especially if no differentiation between extracellular matrix components is requested. If a more detailed analysis of extracellular matrix composition is required, Goldner trichrome staining is an excellent control and back-up method. In the study described the trichrome result allowed us to document the beneficial role of anti-oxidants in diabetes.

More severe alterations in the myocardium, as they occur after infarction of the heart, can be effectively shown by trichrome staining. Cellular replacement therapy represents a novel strategy for the treatment of heart failure. Before cellular replacement therapy can be used in clinical applications, a lot of questions must be answered. Therefore animal studies are required which allow further development of and prove the efficacy of this strategy.

A major problem of the experimental myocardial injury models is the great variation in lesion size. A relatively good reproducible lesion is induced in mouse hearts by cryoinjury. This approach instead of coronary artery ligation was chosen since the latter is known to result in large variations in infarct size in rodent hearts due to marked differences in collateralization. But variations of lesion sizes occur with the cryoinjury also. Therefore it is important to control the size of the lesion for every single experiment. Remembering that the lost myocardium will be replaced by fibrotic tissue after more than 6 days (Roell et al. 2002b), detection of fibrotic tissue by van Gieson trichrome staining is an excellent method for demonstrating the infarcted area (see Fig. 2).

The subsequent use of computerized morphometric analyses allows measurement of the infarct size on cross-sections of the heart. Recently van Gieson staining was also discussed as a suitable method for detection of infarcted areas at early time points (Vargas et al. 1999). Using the van Gieson tri-chrome staining at early time points after infarction seems to be appropriate.

Methylene Blue Staining of Semi-thin Sections of Araldite Embedded Tissue for Qualitative and Quantitative Morphological Analyses

Resin embedding allows the cutting of slices of less than 100 nm for electron microscopy, but also for light microscopical observation. Thin slices in combination with adequate staining procedures elicit a high structural resolution, which cannot be attained by other methods. Especially if microvascular vessels are to be investigated, resin-embedded and methylene blue- or toluidine blue-stained tissue has advantages as compared with paraffin-embedded material. Therefore we have chosen araldite embedding and methylene blue staining for investigation of myocardial capillaries. Semi-thin sections (0.5 mm) of perfusion-fixed myocardium allow recognition of the capillary density and the lumen width of the capillaries (Bloch et al. 1995; Tagarakis et al. 2000), if adequately stained by methylene blue. Other embedding methods do not give the good preservation of the tissue structure, which allows the high-resolution morphological investigation necessary for quantitative analysis of the capillary density and capillary lumen width. We used this method to detect maladaptation of the cardiac capillary network in a mouse exercise model evoked by anabolic steroids (Tagarakis et al. 2000). For this analysis, animals were perfusion-fixed and embedded in araldite. Methylene blue staining of 0.5 mm slices of the myocardium allowed recognition of all the myocardial capillaries, which is a prerequisite for the measurement of capillary density.

Another application for araldite embedding and subsequent staining of semi-thin sections by methylene blue was the investigation of the alteration in capillary diameter in isolated perfused hearts which depends on the nitric oxide pathway. Using automated detection of capillary diameter on methylene blue stained semi-thin section of perfusion-fixed myocardium after modulation of the nitric oxide pathways in isolated perfused hearts, fast changes of capillary diameter could be investigated. It could be shown, that NO influences the dilation of the capillary microvasculature independently of flow regulation (Bloch et al. 1995)

Troubleshooting

Different artefacts can arise from tissue selection up to the mounting of the stained sections, which make the interpretation of the histological staining difficult. A common reason for artefacts is late or poor fixation of the tissue. Late fixation allows the accumulation of acid metabolites in the tissue. Therefore the time up to the fixation of the tissue should be shortened. Another problem is that changes in volumes of cells and tissue are often observed, especially during dehydration. This may be accentuated by pathological changes. To overcome the change in volume, the osmolarity of the buffer should be optimised. Also the fixation process can lead to a shrinkage of the tissue, especially if strong cross-linking fixatives such as glutaraldehyde are used. If quantitative analyses of the amount of tissue components are required, the concentration and composition of the fixative may need to be optimised.

A further problem is the loss of material from the tissues. This may be various small molecules such as peptides or ions or large molecules such as glycogen. Lipids are lost by being dissolved in the organic solvents used in processing. This can cause problems, if the content of specific molecules is being analysed. The loss of material can occur before and during fixation as well as, depending on the fixation, also at later stages of the staining procedure. False positive localization may also occur. This is found especially with soluble intercellular proteins. The use of cross-linking fixatives can reduce this problem.

But problems can also be derived from the staining procedures themselves. This is mainly detected by unusual colouring of tissue structures and inhomogeneous colouring of the specimen. The protocol should then be carefully checked for the concentrations of the dyes and the composition of the dye solution and the pH of the solution should be tested. Furthermore the differentiation times and conditions of the staining must be controlled. If all of these parameters are as described in the protocol, a control tissue, which is optimally handled, can be stained to recognize tissue-specific problems. Such tissue-specific problems can be derived from late fixation, wrong fixation conditions or inhomogeneous fixation. Detailed descriptions of troubles, which can occur in the different stainings, are found elsewhere (for example Horobin and Bancroft 1998).

References

Ammarguellat F, Larouche I, Schiffrin EL (2001) Myocardial fibrosis in DOCA-salt hypertensive rats. Circulation 103: 319–324

Andersen AP, Prento P, Lyon H (1992) General theory for tissue staining. In: Lyon H (ed) Theory and strategy in histochemistry. Springer, Berlin, pp 283–291

Bloch W, Hoever D, Reitze D, Kopalek L, Addicks K (1995) Exogenously supplied nitric oxide influences the dilation of the capillary microvasculature in vivo. Agents and Actions [Suppl] 45: 151–156

Chatelain P, Kapanci Y (1984) Histological diagnosis of myocardial infarction: the role of calcium. Appl Pathol 2: 233–239

Chiu YT, Liu SK, Liu M, Chen SP, Lin YH, Mao SJ, Chu R (1999) Characterization and quantitation of extracellular collagen matrix in myocardium of pigs with spontaneously occurring hypertrophic cardiomyopathy. Cardiovasc Pathol 8: 169–175

Horobin RW, Bancroft JD (1998) Troubleshooting Histology Stains. Churchill Livingstone, Edinburgh

Junqueira LCU, Bignolas G, Brentani RR (1979) Picrosirius staining plus polarization microscopy, a specific method for collagen detection in tissue sections. Histochem J 11: 447–455

Kiernan JA (19999 Methods for connective tissue. In: Kiernan JA (ed) Histological and histochemical methods, theory and practice. Butterworth-Heinemann, Oxford, pp 144–164

Kratky RG, Ivey J and Roach MR (1996) Collagen quantitation by video-microdensitometry in rabbit atherosclerosis. Matrix Biology 15: 141–144

Lindal S, Smiseth OA, Mjos OD, Myklebust R, Jorgensen L (1986) Reversible and irreversible changes in the dog heart during acute left ventricular failure due to experimental multifocal ischaemia. Acta Pathol Microbiol Immunol Scand [A] 94: 177–186

Lyon H, Hoyer PE, Prento P (1992) Proteins. In: Lyon H (ed) Theory and strategy in histochemistry. Springer, Berlin, pp 283–291

Puchtler H, Meloan SN (1978) Demonstration of phosphates in calcium deposits: a modification of von Kossa's reaction. Histochemistry 56: 177–185

Rajamannan NM, Subramaniam M, Rickard D, Stock SR, Donovan J, Springett M, Orszulak T, Fullerton DA, Tajik AJ, Bonow RO, Spelsberg T (2003) Human aortic valve calcification is associated with an osteoblast phenotype. Circulation 107: 2181–2184

Ray R, Choudhary SK, Kumar AS (2002) Pathological aspects of explanted homograft mitral valve. Cardiovasc Pathol 11: 177–180

Roell W, Fan Y, Stoecker E et al. (2002) Cellular cardiomyoplasty in a transgenic mouse model. Transplantion 73: 462–465

Roell W, Lu ZJ, Bloch W et al. (2002b) Cellular cardiomyoplasty imporves survival after myocardial injury. Circulation 105: 2433–2439

Rösen P, Ballhausen T, Bloch W, Addicks K (1995) Endothelial relaxation is disturbed by oxidative stress in the diabetic rat heart: influence of tocopherol as antioxidant. Diabetologia 38: 1157–1168

Rösen P, Hönack C, Müssig K, Bloch W, Addicks K. (1998) Influence of AT_1 receptor inhibition on cardiac function and structure of diabetic rats. In: Dhalla NS, Zahradka P, Dixon I, Beamish R (eds) Angiotensin II receptor blockade: physiological and clinical implications. Kluwer Academic Publishers, Boston, pp 245–260

Tagarakis C, Bloch W, Hartmann G, Hollmann W, Addicks K (2000) Testosterone-propionate leads to maladaptation of the cardiac capillary bed to muscular exercise. Med Sci Sports Exerc 32: 946–953

Van Kerckhoven R, Kalkman EA, Saxena PR, Schoemaker RG (2000) Altered cardiac collagen and associated changes in diastolic function of infarcted rat hearts. Cardiovasc Res 46: 316–323

Vargas SO, Sampson BA, Schoen FJ (1999 Pathologic detection of early myocardial infarction: a critical review of the evaluation and usefulness of modern techniques. Mod Pathol 12: 635–645

Wada T, McKee MD, Steitz S, Giachelli CM (1999) Calcification of vascular smooth muscle cell cultures: inhibition by osteopontin. Circulation 84: 166–178

Practical Use of *in situ* Hybridisation and RT *in situ* PCR in Cardiovascular Research

Yüksel Korkmaz, Dirk Steinritz and Wilhelm Bloch

Introduction

The past twenty years brought progress in the incorporation of molecular techniques into life sciences. This development in molecular biology also affects the morphological field. The questions for techniques which allow the detection of DNA and RNA at the cellular level increase greatly. The technique of *in situ* hybridisation, in its various forms, has been developed as the standard technique for detection of DNA and RNA at cellular level. Besides this technique, RT *in situ* PCR is a further method for detection of DNA and RNA. In contrast to *in situ* hybridisation, only a relatively small number of applications of this technique have been described until now.

In situ hybridisation is defined as the reaction between two complementary single-stranded nucleic acid molecules. These molecules bind by means of hydrogen bonding of complementary base pairs. Hybridisation performed *in situ* includes techniques that detect these hybrids in a cell or tissue section by radioactive labelling, cytochemistry, heavy metal labelling or fluorescence labelling (for review Childs 2000). While early groups of investigators used radiolabelled probes, in the last twenty years more efficient non-radioactive detection systems have been developed. They may involve the attachment of a signalling hapten molecule such as biotin or digoxigenin to the cDNA, mRNA or oligonucleotide probe for indirect detection or fluorescent dyes for direct detection. The haptens can then be indirectly visualized by streptavidin-bound enzymes, fluorescent dyes or heavy metals or by anti-digoxigenin coupled to such detection molecules.

Furthermore amplification by sandwich techniques, as for example layers of biotin and streptavidin-peroxidase increase the sensitivity of these methods (MyQuaid and Allan 1992). Although the technical improvement of *in situ* hybridisation increases the sensitivity of the method, small numbers of DNA and RNA copies are often under the detection threshold of non-radioactive methods. Recently, polymerase chain reaction (PCR) *in situ* methods have been described, allowing the amplification and analysis of small numbers of DNA or RNA copies in cells and tissue sections (Hasse et al. 1990; Zehbe et al. 1992; Nuovo et al. 1994; Nuovo 1996; Doneda et al. 1997).

As in other fields of biological science, an increasing interest in cellular and subcellular resolution of alterations in gene expression in cells and tissue can be found in cardiovascular research. Therefore techniques are required which allow detection of mRNA in cells and tissue sections with high sensitivity and specificity. Besides mRNA detection, DNA detection by use of the FISH technique has shown high impact in recent years of cardiovascular research, especially for stem cell research. In the following chapter we will show an overview of the different methodical approaches in *in situ* hybridisation and RT *in situ* PCR and we will give some examples for practical use as well as deal with troubleshooting.

Description of Methods and Practical Approach

Principles of *in situ* Hybridisation

Since the late 1970s techniques have been developed which allow the localization of mRNAs and DNA in cells and tissue in several areas of biological research including the cardiovascular field. Besides other very sensitive methods, *in situ* hybridisation can be used to detect mRNA or DNA in tissue and, in contrast to most other techniques, *in situ* hybridisation has the ability to reveal patterns of gene content and expression with cellular resolution. Although *in situ* hybridisation has retained a reputation as one of the more difficult molecular biological techniques, the principles of the technique are very straightforward and over recent years protocols have evolved that make its practice equally simple. The objective is to fix the tissue so that all the mRNA being transcribed at the time or the DNA is retained within the cells. The mRNA or DNA is then detected *in situ* by hybridisation with a probe labelled so that it can be detected by autoradiography, chromogenic stains, heavy metals, or fluorescence.

The procedure of *in situ* hybridisation can be divided into the following component steps (Jowett 1997):
1. Fixation and storage of tissue.
2. Synthesis of labelled DNA or anti-sense RNA probes.
3. Pretreatment to permeabilize the tissue and block non-specific binding of the probe.
4. Hybridisation of the probe.
5. Washing to remove unbound probe.
6. Incubation in blocking solution to prevent non-specific binding of the detection antibodies.
7. Incubation in antibody against the probe-hapten.
8. Washing to remove unbound antibody.
9. Visualization of the bound antibody either with chromogenic stain, heavy metal stain or by epifluorescent microscopy.

In the following, the reader is introduced to non-radioactive *in situ* hybridisation methods in general and suggestions for the application of the different techniques in cardiovascular research will be given. The key steps in *in situ* hybridisation are fixation, the choice of the probes, the pre-treatment and hybridisation conditions, the

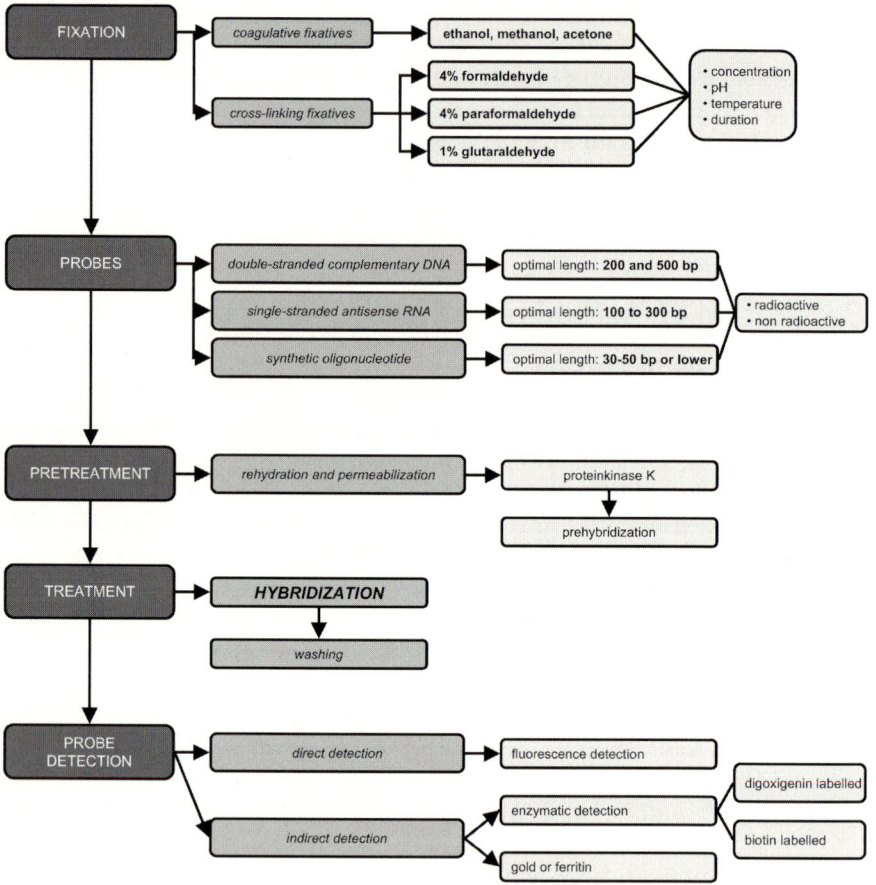

Figure 1
Flow chart for selection of an adequate *in situ* hybridisation protocol

immunolocalization of the transcript and the visualization of the signal. Therefore we will describe and discuss the principles of these steps and give suggestions for the selection of an individual protocol (Fig. 1).

Choice of Adequate Fixation

A fast and sufficient fixation is the absolute prerequisite for a successful *in situ* hybridisation; it is comparable to chemical fixation in immunohistochemistry. The chemical fixation methods can be divided into crosslinking fixatives and coagulating agents (such as ethanol/acetic acid). The crosslinking aldehyde fixatives are the most commonly used fixatives for tissue and cells as well as for whole-mounts. They crosslink the material retaining the RNA and DNA, but still allow penetration of the probe and detection of antibodies. Three commonly used fixatives in order of increasing crosslinking ability are 4% paraformaldehyde, 4% formaldehyde and 1% glutaraldehyde, each in phosphate buffered saline (PBS). Tissue must be incubated in fixative for different times dependent on the size of the tissue pieces, in principal the size of the tissue piece should be as small as possible to guarantee an optimal tissue and RNA, as well as DNA, preservation.

Selection of Probes for *in situ* Hybridisation

The requirement for successful *in situ* hybridisation starts, besides the optimal preservation of mRNA or DNA, with the selection of appropriate DNA or RNA probes. Three principal types of probes can be used for *in situ* hybridisation, namely double-stranded complementary DNA probes, single-stranded anti-sense RNA probes, and synthetic oligonucleotide probes (Jin et al. 2001). The advances in molecular biology open the possibility of generating DNA or RNA probes in different ways. DNA probes can be produced from cloned DNA in a number of ways, such as nick translation, random priming, or polymerase chain reaction (PCR) amplification, while RNA probes can be prepared by in vitro transcription of cloned DNA using the bacteriophage SP6, T3 or T7 polymerases; promoters for these polymerises are incorporated into a number of commonly used and highly versatile cloning vectors such as BluescriptTM (Jowett 1997). Oligonucleotide probes can be generated with an automated DNA synthesizer. RNA probes especially prove to be highly sensitive and reliable. This can be explained by the higher sensitivity of anti-sense probes compared to single-stranded DNA probes because the anti-sense probes form double-stranded RNA with the target transcripts, which are considerably more stable than DNA/RNA hybrids. This allows the use of more stringent conditions, which reduces problems with non-specific background signals. In general the strength of non-specific background stainings decreases in the order RNA-RNA, DNA-RNA, DNA-DNA (Wetmur et al. 1981). A further criterion for successful and specific *in situ* hybridisation is the choice of an optimal probe size. The size of the double-stranded DNA, which can be generated by reverse transcription of mRNA and by amplification of specific sequences of DNA or from cDNA using cloning vectors, should be between 200 and 500 bp. For optimal hybridisation the sizes of anti-sense RNA, which are generated by in vitro transcription from a linearized DNA template by incorporation of labelled nucleotides, range between 100-800 bp. Optimal signals are obtained with probe lengths of 100 to 300 bp, owing to very good penetration of the specimen and strong hybridisation to the target sequences (Baumgart et al. 2000). Probes shorter than 80 bp show a poorer binding to the target nucleic acid at high temperatures, leading to lower sensitivity or higher background, a principal problem of oligonucleotide probes consisting of 30–50 bases.

The disadvantage of the lower sensitivity of oligonucleotides can be overcome by using multiple oligonucleotide probes that are complementary to different regions of the target molecules (Lloyd and Jin 1995). The lower sensitivity makes the oligonucleotide probes useful especially for detection of more abundant gene expression (Jin et al. 2001).

The probes can be radioactively or non-radioactively labelled. DNA probes can be labelled by nick translation or random primer methods; RNA probes are usually labelled by the in vitro transcription method. For these methods labelled nucleotides are incorporated, while 3' or 5' end labelling methods are mainly used for oligonucleotide probes.

Besides radioactive labelling by incorporation of isotopically-labelled nucleotides, in the last 20 years non-radioactive labelling using non-isotopically labelled nucleotides and probes has replaced the radioactive method more and more. The development of non-isotopic labelling methods for nucleic acid probes has facilitated the diffusion of *in situ* hybridisation techniques to the research as well as to the cardiovascular laboratory. Digoxigenin or fluorescein labellings were mostly used besides biotin labelling. Non-radioactive probes have several advantages over the radiolabelled ones, including cost, shelf life, safety and, last but not least, resolution of the signal.

Pre-treatment and Hybridisation Conditions

Before the hybridisation procedure can start, the tissue must be rehydrated and permeabilized to allow easy penetration of the probe and detection antibodies. This is usually performed by incubation with proteinase K that punctures the cell membranes. It is also important for paraffin-embedded specimens, as the wax appears to mask the material of the transcript reducing the efficiency of hybridisation. Considering that this treatment may be detrimental to the morphology, it should be not performed more intensively and longer than necessary. Furthermore considering that protease digestion causes the specimens to become fragile, special care must be taken not to damage the tissue when changing the solutions. The incubation time in proteinase K may also depend on the particular batch of enzyme, every proteinase batch must be individually tested. Treatment with proteinase K can be followed by a second fixation step to stabilize the material and prevent over-digestion by the protease, which otherwise causes some RNA loss.

The tissue is then prehybridised in the hybridisation solution using the same conditions as for hybridisation but without probe. This step is performed to block non-specific binding sites for the probe. It should be initially as long as possible. This step can possibly be omitted, if it is seen that no increase of unspecific labelling occurs without pre-hybridisation, but it is always advisable to include it in initial experiments. After prehybridisation, the tissue can be incubated in hybridisation solution containing probe overnight.

Probe Detection and Visualization of the Signal

Direct and indirect systems of probe detection are available for non-radioactive *in situ* hybridisation and can be employed as labelling strategy. Directly labelled probes with appropriate fluorescent dyes are sufficient to visualize the site of hybridisation directly using a fluorescence microscope. Indirect methods that are similar to indirect immunohistochemical procedures are widely used. In this method, appropriate antibodies raised against the corresponding hapten, generally digoxigenin or biotin, are employed, yielding signals with a higher quality of resolution. An improvement of signal-to-noise ratio can be obtained by incubating specimens in blocking reagents to prevent non-specific staining. For visualization of biotin or digoxigenin-labelled DNA, RNA or oligos, fluorescent dyes can be used. This method is also compatible with non-fluorescent detection systems such as horseradish peroxidase or alkaline phosphatase based systems. These enzymes convert substrates from a colourless, water-soluble compound to a coloured precipitate. Several different enzyme substrates such as nitroblue tetrazolium or DAB are available. They are of varying sensitivity and produce differently coloured precipitates. Besides enzyme-based and fluorescent dye-based detection systems, colloidal gold or ferritin can also be used, which has also expanded the approach of *in situ* hybridisation to electron microscopy.

The detection and visualization steps after the hybridisation with the biotin and digoxigenin labelled probes are comparable to the detection steps in immunohistochemistry. In general, digoxigenin labelling, whatever technique used (nick translation or random priming) is held to be superior to biotin labelling. The main reason is the higher specificity of digoxigenin, which is a steroid from Digitalis, found only in plants, while biotin is also to be found in different organs as well as the heart. A further reason is the observed 50× higher sensitivity of digoxigenin compared to biotin in Western blots (Brunet et al. 1994).

Digoxigenin as well as biotin can be detected by immunohistochemistry with labelled antibodies. This is also the case for fluorescent dye-labelled probes, which can be detected by antibodies against the fluorescent dye. In contrast to digoxigenin, biotin can also be detected by avidin, streptavidin or extravidin, which are available in conjugation with horseradish peroxidase, alkaline phosphatases, fluorescent dyes, colloidal gold, ferritin and further markers. In principal all of the detection systems that are used for immunohistochemistry can also be used for detection of the bound probes in tissue and cells. The multiple amplification methods known for immunohistochemistry can therefore also be used for *in situ* hybridisation, which allows a significant increase in the sensitivity of the method.

The possibility of labelling probes with different haptens, such as fluorescent dyes, digoxigenin and biotin allows a detection of multiple transcripts in one specimen. To perform multiple labelling, the probes must be differentially labelled to allow alternative methods of detection. Thereafter the probes can be mixed and hybridised with the tissue simultaneously, followed by individual visualizing steps for the different haptens.

Principles of RT *in situ* PCR

RT *in situ* PCR allows for the routine and rapid detection of low copy RNAs with cellular resolution in complex tissue, consisting of more than one cell type. The use of formalin or paraformaldehyde-fixed and paraffin-embedded or cryo-protected tissue allows the widespread use of this technique. It is therefore surprising that the technique is not very often used. In the cardiovascular field only a very limited number of studies which use RT *in situ* PCR have been published. It seems appropriate to introduce this technique a little more to motivate more cardiovascular groups to apply it. Contrarily the RT PCR itself is performed in many laboratories as a routine method. Therefore it seems appropriate to give at the beginning of this part of the chapter a short description of the differences between RT *in situ* PCR and RT PCR (done in solution). One difference is the marked difference in the surface to volume ratio. In a 0.5 ml tube, the ratio of the surface to volume is about 1:2, while with RT *in situ* PCR on a 10 mm coverslip and in a volume of 10 μl, the surface to volume ratio is over 20× greater. This difference will alter the cycling parameters one uses for RT *in situ* PCR, especially the time and temperature of denaturation (Nuova 1996). A further difference is that the amplifying solution in RT PCR (done in solution) is mostly water, and the test sample provides relatively scanty amounts of DNA and even smaller amounts of proteins.

The amplifying specimen in RT *in situ* PCR consists of a relatively dense matrix of DNA, RNA and proteins (in the nucleus) and RNA and proteins (in the cytoplasm), if fixed in formalin, it will be extensively crosslinked to form a complex, 3-dimensional labyrinth. The relatively concentrated collection of proteins and nucleic acids in a fixed cell are the basis of some fundamental differences in the various DNA synthesis pathways that can be operative during *in situ* PCR versus solution phase PCR (Nuovo 1996). There are four potential synthesis pathways that may be operative inside the cell during *in situ* PCR. The first is the requested target-specific amplification, while the other three synthesis pathways are pitfalls for a successful RT *in situ* PCR. These unlikely DNA synthesis pathways are non-target primer-dependent amplification (mis-priming), primer oligomerization and DNA repair (a primer-independent pathway). Therefore great efforts must be made to eliminate the three non-specific synthesis pathways.

DNA repair can be avoided by optimal DNAse digestion, after sufficient protease digestion, which leads to a complete degradation of the DNA or by prevention of DNA nicks. The second is not possible with paraffin-embedded tissue. The paraffin-embedding process leads every time to a cleavage of the DNA. An alternative for avoiding a false positive result is selective labelling of the primers without use of labelled nucleotides, which lead to the labelling of the repaired DNA. The low sensitivity of only directly labelling the primers limits the availability of this method to highly expressed RNAs.

The mis-priming of DNA by non-target primer-dependent amplification can also be avoided by DNAse digestion. A second way to eliminate the mis-priming is optimal design of the primers used. Primer pairs should be used which flank spliced sequences of mRNA, as these particular sequences will be found only in RNA and will be split into sections in the DNA (Bagasra et al. 2001). A third way is the use of a hot start technique, which does not allow priming if homology between primer and the target sequence is lower, which is typical for mis-priming (Nuovo 1997).

False positive results evoked by primer oligomerization can also be avoided by hot start techniques and stringent washing steps to eliminate the short labelled DNA from primer oligomerization. In contrast to staining derived from DNA repair or mis-priming, the staining is not primarily found in the nucleus, but in the cytoplasm, on the cell membrane and surrounding the cells in the extracellular matrix.

False positive results can also be derived from specific amplification if the amplified DNA migrates to cells that do not have the target RNA.

An adequate protocol and the performance of appropriate controls can help to make RT *in situ* PCR, a specific detection method for RNA in laboratory use in spite of the problems described above. Therefore we will describe some key points for optimising the RT *in situ* PCR protocol, although most steps in the protocol must be optimised for each type of tissue or cells and for different targets.

Fixation and Embedding

In principle, precipitating as well as crosslinking fixatives can be used. The precipitating fixatives such as ethanol, methanol and acetone preserved the integrity of the nucleic acid, but most of the PCR products get lost in the supernatant. Furthermore the structural preservation is bad, leading to interpretation problems in the result. The crosslinking fixatives such as formalin and paraformaldehyde have the advantage of better structural preservation and keep the nucleic acid in the tissue. Furthermore they create a "charge" or ionic" barrier by rigidly fixing the positively and negatively charged side chains of amino acids in space inside the cell (Nuovo 1996). Therefore crosslinking fixatives are preferable, especially if they are combined with protease digestion.

The embedding can be done in paraffin or alternatively fixed cryo-protected tissue can be frozen. It must be remarked that paraffin embedding shows a problem with the occurrence of DNA nicks, which make a pre-treatment with DNAse necessary, as described above.

Protease Digestion and DNAse Treatment

The formation of meshwork by crosslinking fixatives can prevent adequate penetration of the enzymes and other reagents needed for amplification and detection. A partial digestion of proteins usually helps in restoring the permeability of the tissue. Considering that tissue structure will be greatly altered by protease digestion, an equilibrium between fixation and protease digestion must be found. The optimal conditions for protease treatment must be experimentally tested. DNAse treatment must be performed if DNA nicks are formed. If this digestion of the DNA is complete, it eliminates a source of competition during the PCR. But if the digestion is incomplete, the problems with DNA repair increase.

While some authors describe DNAse treatment as a necessary key step of a successful RT *in situ* PCR (Nuovo 1996, 1997; Baasgara et al. 2001), other authors found that the best way to avoid the problem is to omit the digestion altogether and reduce genomic amplification by other methods, such as good primer design, a short time at the extension temperature during the cycle and few cycles (Martinez et al. 2000).

PCR Reaction Solution

In principle the design of the PCR reaction solution for RT *in situ* PCR is comparable to that for PCR in solution. It consists of a mixture of nucleotides, primers, DNA polymerase, and the proper bivalent cation (either Mg^{2+} or Mn^{2+}, depending on the enzyme) in a suitable buffer. Several factors can influence the generation of a specific amplicon such as the pH of the solution, salt concentration, annealing temperature and number of cycles.

All these parameters must be optimised to get a specific amplicon. For more detailed description several excellent reviews can be recommended (Nuovo 1996, 1997; Martinez 2000; Basgara et al. 2001).

Controls

Although RT *in situ* PCR is a powerful technique that combines high sensitivity with exact localization of the signal in the tissue structure or in cell cultures, it also produces some artefacts. Therefore very special care is required to ensure the efficiency and specificity of the results. Negative and positive controls should be performed to increase confidence in the results. As negative controls, the DNA polymerase should be removed from the PCR mixture or the primers should be substituted with water in the PCR mixture. The slides can be incubated with RNAses before performing reverse transcription of RNA, the amplification should be done without reverse transcriptase and RT *in situ* PCR can be done with an irrelevant primer.

As positive controls Martinez et al. (1995) propose running a gel with the results of the *in situ* experiment. The DNA in the supernatant and the DNA trapped in the tissue section or in the cells should run separately in the gel. A further positive control can be performed by scraping the tissue or cells off the slide, digesting with DNAse-free proteases, and recovering DNA by phenol-chloroform extraction. The presence of a band of the expected size in the lane containing the tissue extract and its absence from the supernatant lane is a clear sign of a perfect RT *in situ* PCR. A further control, which deals with successful protease treatment allowing the optimal amplification of the DNA inside the tissue, can be performed if the DNAse step is omitted and labelled nucleotides are present. Variation of control experiments can be necessary depending on the use of direct or indirect methods and on the use of labelled nucleotides or labelled primers.

Examples

Detection of Endostatin in Skin Wound Healing by Use of a cDNA Probe

In this *in situ* hybridisation method a labelled "anti-sense" RNA or DNA strand is hybridised to a "sense" RNA strand present in cells in thin tissue sections. This method enables precise localization through base paired nucleotide interactions between a labelled probe (anti-sense) strand and the endogenous mRNA (sense strand).

In situ hybridisation methods are sensitive, specific and can provide important information about the sites of mRNA synthesis. In principle, types of probes for *in situ* hybridisation studies are complementary DNA probes, anti-sense RNA probes and synthetic oligonucleotides. For detection of the mRNA of endostatin and its precursor collagen XVIII, we have chosen a cDNA probe. Endostatin was originally reported as an anti-angiogenic and tumour inhibitory protein (O'Reilly et al. 1997) and was also shown to be an angiomodulatory molecule in wound healing (Bloch et al. 2000). *In situ* hybridisation with a cDNA probe against the mRNA of endostatin/collagen XVIII gave evidence for increased expression during wound healing (Bloch et al. 2000).

The sensitivity of *in situ* hybridisation depends on the preservation of mRNA integrity in the tissue or cell preparations.

Throughout the procedure, all steps should be taken in RNAse-free equipment and reagents. Solutions can be treated with an RNAse-inhibitor, 0.1% diethylpyrocarbonate (DEPC). This step is not necessary if all reagents are autoclaved.

Preparation of Tissue and Fixation

The murine skin wounds were fixed in 4% paraformaldehyde for 4–6 h then rinsed in 0.1 M PBS for 24 h. Skin wounds were rinsed with 0.1 M PBS pH 7.4 buffer and stored in the same buffer at 4 °C.

Tissue Embedding

Skin wounds are stored for 12 h in 0.1 M PBS solution with 18% sucrose for cryoprotection, embedded in Tissue-Tec, frozen in liquid nitrogen and stored at –82 °C.

For paraffin embedding, skin wounds are dehydrated in a graded series of ethanol dilutions (50%, 70%, 90%, 100%), then treated with two changes of 100% chloroform and embedded in paraffin.

Tissue Sectioning

Frozen-embedded tissue sectioning:
- Cut 7 µm sections of the frozen embedded tissue on a cryostat at –24 °C.
- Mount the section on poly (L-lysine)-coated (0.1%), RNAse-free slides.
- Dry slides at room temperature for 20 min.
- Store the sections at –82 °C.

Paraffin-embedded tissue sectioning:
- Prepare a distilled water bath at 42 °C.
- Cut 5 µm sections of the paraffin embedded tissue on a microtome.
- Place the sections into the distilled water bath. The sections should flatten.
- Mount the sections on poly (L-lysine)-coated (0.1%), RNAse-free slides and allow the sections to dry overnight at 42 °C.

Post-Fixation of Sections

For the preservation of mRNA, the sections were immediately fixed in freshly prepared 4% paraformaldehyde in 0.1 M PBS at 4 °C for 20 min. It has been found that prolonged thawing of unfixed sections or fixation at room temperature reduced signal intensity (Yang et al. 1999).

Buffer and Solutions for *in situ* Hybridisation

- 0.1 M PBS pH 7.2–7.4
  [10.8 g Na_2HPO_4, 2.0 g NaH_2PO_4, 6.6 g NaCl, 750 ml A.D.]
- 1 M $MgCl_2$
  [16.3 g $MgCl_2$, 80 ml A.D.]

- 0.1 M Triethanolamine pH 8.0
  [50 ml 0.1 M Triethanolamine pH 8.0, 125 µl acetic anhydride]
- Proteinase K-Buffer
  [200 ml Tris-HCl 1 M pH 7.5, 200 ml EDTA 0.2 M, 8 ml NaCl 5 M]
- 0.1–0.2 M, Glycine-Tris, pH 7.4
  [120 ml Tris-HCl 1 M pH 7.5, 4.5 g glycine, 600 ml A.D.]
- 2× SSC (standard saline citrate: 0.3 M NaCl, 30 mm sodium citrate, pH 7.0)
  [123 g NaCl, 62 g tri-Na-citrate, 700 ml A.D.]
- 1 M Tris-HCl pH 7.5/9.5
  [91 g Tris, 750 ml A.D.]
- 10× PBS pH 7.2/7.4
  [60.0 g NaCl, 2.2 g KCl, 10.8 g Na_2HPO_4, 1.5 g KH_2PO_4, 750 ml A.D.]
- 5 M NaCl
  [102.3 g NaCl, 350 ml A.D.]
- 10 mm NaAc pH 5.2
  [2.3 g NaAc, 170 ml A.D.]
- 0.2 M ethylenediaminetetraacetic acid (EDTA), pH 8.0
  [26 g EDTA, 350 ml A.D.]
- Tris-EDTA
  [1.4 ml Tris-HCl 1 M pH 7.5, 0.7 ml EDTA 0.2 M, 170.0 ml A.D.]
- 0.5 M Tris-NaCl pH 7.6
  [45.4 g Tris, 750 ml A.D.]
- Tris-NaCl 50 mM
  [7.5 g NaCl, 75 ml Tris-NaCl, 750 ml A.D.]
- 1 M PIPES (piperazine-N'-N'-bis[2-ethanesulfonic acid]) pH 6.8
  [Make up 3.024 g in 10 ml 1N NaOH and store in 400 µl aliquots at –20 °C]
- 1 M dithiothreitol (DTT)
  [3,09 g DTT in 20 ml of 0.01 M Na-acetate pH 5.2 stored in 400 µl aliquots at –20 °C]
- 100× Denhardt's
  [Make up 1 g Ficoll, 1 g polyvinylpyrolidone, 1 g BSA, 50 ml A.D. and store at –20 °C in 400 µl aliquots]
- Hybridisation mix
  4 g PEG 6000, 4.8 ml NaCl 5 M, 400 µl $MgCl_2$ 1 M, 400 µl Pipes 1 M, 400 µl DTT 1 M, 200 µl EDTA 0.2 M, 400 µl salmon sperm DNA 10 mg/ml, 400 µl Denhardt's 100×, 200 µl tRNA 5 mg/ml and 1.8 ml aqua dest. Filter through a 0.2 µm sterile filter into autoclaved Eppendorf tubes and store at –20 °C in 900 µl aliquots.
- ISH-wash buffer
  [500 ml formamide, 300 ml A.D., 200 ml 20× SSC]
- Buffer I pH 7.5
  [70 ml Tris-HCl 1 M pH 7.5, 21 ml NaCl 5 M, 700 ml A.D.]
- Buffer II
  [1 g blocking-reagent, 100 ml buffer I]
- Buffer III
  [60 ml Tris-HCl 1 M pH 9.5, 12 ml NaCl 5 M, 30 ml $MgCl_2$ 1 M, 600 ml A.D.]

In situ Hybridisation Protocol

1. 7 μm thick frozen-sections are cut with a cryostat at −24 °C and mounted on poly (L-lysine)-coated (0.1%) slides. 5 μm thick paraffin sections are cut on a microtome and mounted on poly (L-lysine)-coated (0.1%) slides.
2. Fix the sections with 4% paraformaldehyde for 20 min at room temperature [RT].
3. Deparaffinize the sections in xylene 2×5 min at RT (not required for frozen sections).
4. Rehydrate the sections through a graded series of ethanols and finally in distilled H_2O (not required for frozen sections).
   - 2×5 min   ethanol 100%
   - 1×5 min   ethanol 90%
   - 1×5 min   ethanol 70%
   - 1×5 min   ethanol 50%
5. The slides are rinsed in Tris-NaCl pH 7.6 for 10 min.
6. The sections are rinsed in 0.1 M PBS (50 ml)/$MgCl_2$ (250 μl) for 10 min.
7. Treat the sections with proteinase K (10 mg/ml) for 10 min at 37 °C (not required for frozen sections).
8. Acetylate the sections by incubating in 0.1 M triethanolamine pH 8.0 containing 0.25% acetic anhydride for 10 min at RT.
9. The slides are washed in Tris-NaCl pH 7.6 for 1 min at RT.
10. Rinse the sections with 0.2 M Tris-HCl, pH 7.4 containing 0.1 M glycine for 10 min at RT.
11. Prehybridisation of sections:
    The slides are incubated for 1 h at 42 °C in a solution containing 50% formamide, 2× SSC (standard saline citrate: 0.3 M NaCl, 30 mm sodium citrate, pH 7.0) and 0.1 mg/ml salmon sperm DNA (Sigma).
12. Denaturation of probe/hybridisation solution:
    Denature the probe/hybridisation solution at 92 °C for 10 min and immediately place the solution on ice until it is applied to the sections.
13. Hybridisation of sections:
    The sections are incubated in hybridisation solution for 24 h in a humidity chamber at 42 °C. The hybridisation probes (cDNA) are diluted (100 ng/section) in 50 μl hybridisation solution which contains 50% formamide, 5% distilled water and 45% buffer consisting of PEG 6000 [polyethylene glycol], 5 M NaCl, 1 M MgCl2, 1 M piperazine-N'-N'-bis[2-ethanesulfonic acid] [PIPES], 0.2 M ethylenediaminetetraacetic acid [EDTA], 1 M dithiothreitol [DTT], 10 mg/ml salmon sperm DNA, 100× Denhardt, 5 mg/ml yeast tRNA and distilled water [10:12:1:1:0.5:1:1:1:0.5:4.5, v/v].
14. The sections are rinsed in 2× SSC and 50% formamide at 42 °C for 3×15 min at 42 °C in a humidity chamber.
15. The slides are washed in buffer I (0.1 M Tris-HCl, pH 7.5, 0.15 M NaCl) for 2 min at RT.
16. Incubate the slides in buffer II (buffer I + 1% bovine serum albumin) for 30 min at RT.

17. The sections are incubated with an alkaline phosphatase-conjugated digoxigenin-antibody (Roche Diagnostics GmbH, Mannheim, Germany) diluted 1:100 in buffer II for 30 min at RT.
18. The sections are rinsed in buffer I (0.1 M Tris/HCl, 0.15 M NaCl) for 2×15 min at RT.
19. The slides are washed in buffer III (0.1 M Tris-HCl, 0.1 M NaCl, 0.05 M $MgCl_2$; pH 9.5) for 2 min at RT.
20. Hybridisation is visualized by incubating the slides in a detection solution which consists of 175 µl 5-bromo-4-chloro-3-indolylphosphate (BCIP) (Roche) and 225 µl nitro blue tetrazolium chloride (NBT) (Roche) in 50 ml buffer III for 1 h at RT or overnight at 4 °C.
21. The sections are rinsed in Tris-EDTA for 15 min at RT.
22. The sections are then washed in A.D. for 10 min at RT.
23. The slides are mounted using glycerol-gelatine (optimal) or the sections are dehydrated through ascending series of ethanol:
    - 5 min   ethanol 50%
    - 5 min   ethanol 70%
    - 5 min   ethanol 96%
    - 2×5 min   ethanol 100%
24. The sections are cleared in xylene:
    - 5 min   xylene I
    - 5 min   xylene II
25. The slides are mounted in Entellan (Merck).

In situ Hybridization Control Protocol

The following controls should be performed for cDNA probes:
1. Incubation of the control sections without labelled anti-sense probe.
2. Competition of the labelled cDNA probe with excess unlabelled cDNA: incubations performed with unlabelled cDNA probe (concentration 10-fold higher than that of the labelled cDNA probe) prior to incubation with labelled cDNA probe.
3. The hybridisation procedure should be performed without use of the digoxigenin antibody.

Interpretation of the control incubations
1. The sections incubated without labelled cDNA probe should be negative.
2. In the sections treated competitively, the hybridisation signal should be decreased or absent.
3. No signal should be recognizable without the detection antibody.

Detection of Galanin in Vascular Endothelium by Use of Anti-Sense RNA Probes

Neuropeptides can act as neurotransmitters, neuromodulators or neurohormones. Some are produced in endocrine glands and circulate as hormones, while others are contained in cardiac myocytes, neurons, or endothelial cells in proximity to the sino-atrial node and can therefore act in a paracrine or autocrine way on the pacemaker cells to modulate heart frequency (Beaulieu and Lambert, 1998). Their endothelial localization also suggests that non-neuronal derived neuropeptides are involved in vascular regulation.

Recently we found that the neuropeptide galanin is present in the endothelium by immunohistochemistry and *in situ* hybridisation using an anti-sense RNA probe against galanin (Baumann et al. 2003).

Tissue Preparation, Embedding, and Sectioning:

See Preparation of tissue and fixation, Tissue embedding, Tissue sectioning, Post-fixation of sections above.

Buffer and Solutions for in situ Hybridisation

See buffer and solutions for *in situ* Hybridisation above.

In situ Hybridization Protocol

In situ hybridization was performed as described in detail by Wevers et al. (1994).
1. Ten micrometer thick sections should be cut with a cryostat and mounted on silane coated slides
2. Fix the sections with 4% paraformaldehyde for 20 min at room temperature (RT).
3. Wash the slides in 0.1 M TBS containing $MgCl_2$ for 10 min at RT
4. Acetylate the sections at RT for 10 min by incubating in 0.1 M triethanolamine pH 8.0 containing 0.25% acetic anhydride.
5. Wash the slides in Tris-NaCl pH 7.6, for 1 min at RT
6. Rinse the sections with 0.2 M Tris-HCl, pH 7.4 containing 0.1 M glycine for 10 min at RT
7. Prehybridisation of sections:
   Incubate the sections for 1 h at 50 °C in a prehybridisation solution containing 50% formamide, 2× SSC (0.3 M NaCl, 30 mm sodium citrate, pH 7.0) and 0.1 mg/ml salmon sperm DNA (Serva).
8. Denaturation of probe/hybridisation solution:
   Denature the probe/hybridisation solution at 92 °C for 10 min and immediately place the solution on ice until it is applied to the sections.
9. Hybridize the sections over night in a humidity chamber at 42 °C or for 1 h at 50 °C
   Probes should be diluted (50 ng/section or 100 ng/section) in 50 µl hybridization solution which contains 50% formamide, 5% distilled water and 45% buffer consisting of PEG 6000, 5 M NaCl, 1 M $MgCl_2$, 1 M Pipes, 0.2 M EDTA, 1 M DTT, 10 mg/ml salmon sperm DNA, 100× DenhardM, 5 mg/ml yeast tRNA [10:12:1:1: 0.5:1:1:0.5, v/v].
10. Rinse the sections in 2× SSC and 50% formamide at 42 °C for 3×15 min at 42 °C in a humidity chamber.
11. Wash the slides in buffer I (0.1 M Tris-HCl, pH 7.5, 0.15 M NaCl) for 2 min at RT.
12. Wash the slides in buffer II (buffer I + 1% bovine serum albumin) for 30 min at RT.

13. Incubate the sections with an alkaline phosphatase-conjugated digoxigenin-antibody (Roche Diagnostics GmbH, Mannheim, Germany) diluted 1:100 in buffer II for 30 min at RT
14. Wash the sections in buffer I for 2×15 min at RT.
15. Wash the sections in buffer III (0.1 M Tris/HCl, 0.1 M NaCl, 0.05 M $MgCl_2$) for min at RT.
16. Visualize the hybridization by incubating the sections in a detection solution which consisted of 175 µl 5-bromo-4-chloro-3-indolylphosphate (Roche Diagnostics GmbH) and 225 µl nitro blue tetrazolium chloride (Roche Diagnostics GmbH) in 50 ml buffer III for 45 min at RT or overnight at 4 °C
17. The sections are rinsed in Tris-EDTA for 15 min at RT.
18. The sections are then washed in distilled water for 10 min at RT.
19. The slides are mounted using glycerol-gelatine (optimal) or the sections are dehydrated through ascending series of ethanol (50, 70, 96 and 100%) 4 min each.
20. The sections are cleared in xylene:
    Clear the sections in xylene I and II, 4 min each
21. The slides are mounted in Entellan (Merck).

In situ Hybridization Control Protocol

The following controls should be performed:
1. Incubation of the control sections with labelled sense probe.
2. Incubation of the control sections without labelled anti-sense probe.
3. Competition of the labelled anti-sense probe with excess unlabelled anti-sense: incubations were performed with unlabelled anti-sense probe (concentration 10-fold higher than that of the labelled anti-sense probe) prior to incubation with labelled anti-sense probe.
4. The hybridisation procedure should be performed without use of the digoxigenin antibody.

Interpretation of the control incubations:
1. The sense probe controls should show either abolition of specific signal or only weak labelling.
2. The sections incubated without labelled anti-sense probe should be negative.
3. In the sections treated competitively, the hybridisation signal should be decreased or absent.
4. No signal should be recognizable without the detection antibody.

Application of the FISH Technique in Stem Cell Research

Recent studies have identified cardiomyocytes of extra-cardiac origin in transplanted human hearts, but the exact origin of these myocyte-progenitors is currently unknown. The investigation of Y chromosome-positive cardiomyocytes in patients with sex-mismatched bone marrow transplantation has been shown to be an effective method of investigating the transdifferentiation of bone marrow-derived cells to cardiomyocytes. Fluorescence *in situ* hybridisation (FISH) for the Y chromosome was performed on paraffin-embedded sections to identify cells of bone marrow origin, with concomitant immunofluorescent labelling for alpha-sarcomeric actin to identify cardiomyocytes (Deb et al. 2003). In this study the benefit of the FISH method for stem cell research was shown. Therefore you will find below a protocol for the FISH technique adapted for use in cardiovascular research. In this application chromosomes will be detected in interphase, which is possible with commercially available satellite probes, specific for tandem repeats of DNA sequences of individual chromosomes (Kontogeorges et al. 2001).

In principal fluorescence *in situ* hybridisation (FISH) is a labelling technique that is used for localization of specific DNA or RNA sequences in cells or tissue sections. The DNA probe is labelled, allowed to hybridise with complementary target sequences in the cell and visualized using specific markers (Nath and Johnson 1997). *In situ* hybridisation provides precise information about the location of specific DNA sequences. It is a sensitive technique for studying the presence or expression of cell- or tissue-specific gene sequences, and for chromosome mapping (Pinkel et al. 1986; Trask et al. 1991). The DNA probes may be produced by a variety of techniques including site-specific and random primer PCR and cloning. The detection of the probes can be accomplished by different techniques including PCR labelling and nick translation and random-primer labelling.

The FISH Protocol

The fluorescence *in situ* hybridisation (FISH) technique is described in detail as performed by See (2001). The *in situ* hybridisation should be performed after the fluorescence immunohistochemistry for detection of cardiomyocytes using cardiac specific markers such as a-actin or a-actinin have been done (Deb et al. 2003).

First day

Solutions:
200 ml 2× standard sodium citrate (SSC) (20 ml 20× SSC + 180 ml H_2O)
200 ml 2× standard sodium citrate (SSC) (20 ml 20× SSC + 180 ml H_2O)
RNAse solution (10 µl RNAse 10 mg ml^{-1} stock + 990 µl 2× SSC)
100 ml proteinase K solution (10 mL 10× proteinase K buffer + 90 ml H_2O)
1. The following reagents should be added to a 1.5 ml Eppendorf tube:
2. 28 µL (200 ng) biotinylated probe DNA 10 µL sonicated salmon sperm DNA (10 mg ml^{-1} stock) 10 µL human cot-1-DNA (10 mg ml^{-1} stock)
    3 µL E. coli DNA (10 mg ml^{-1} stock)
    5 µL 3 M ammonium acetate
    112 µL ice cold ethanol
    Mix gently and leave in either a –20 °C freezer for 1 h or a –70 °C freezer for 30 min
    Add 200 µL RNAse solution to each slide; place a 24×50 mm coverslip over it and place it in a humidity chamber. The humidity chamber should be placed at 37 °C for 1 h.
3. Rinse the slides in 2× SSC 4× in a Coplin jar.

4. Transfer the slides to a Coplin jar with 50 ml proteinase K buffer pre-warmed to 37 °C in a water bath for 10 min.
5. Incubate the slides in 50 ml proteinase K buffer with 35 µL proteinase K enzyme stock solution (50 µg ml^{-1}) pre-warmed to 37 °C for 7 min.
6. Take the tubes out of the freezer from step 1 and spin at 14,000 rpm for 5 min.
7. Drain away the supernatant and either air dry the probe or freeze-dry it using a DNA SpeedVac.
8. From step 5, wash the slides in 0.1 M phosphate buffered saline (0.1 M PBS) for 5 min.
9. Incubate the slides in the formaldehyde mixture [50 ml PBS, 0.5 g magnesium chloride, and 1.3 ml 37% formaldehyde solution] for 10 min in a fume cupboard.
10. Rinse the slides in PBS for 5 min.
11. From step 7, add 40 µL hybridization mix [50% formamide in 2× SSC, 10% dextran sulphate] to each of the tubes of dried labelled probe and mix well to aid dissolution.
12. Place the tubes in a 70 °C water bath kept in the fume cupboard for 4 min to denature the probe. Then, place the tubes on floaters in a 37 °C water bath for 15 min to allow the repetitive sequences to anneal.
13. From step 9, dehydrate the slides in an alcohol series and air dry.
14. Denature the chromosomes and cells on the slides. Plunge the slides into a Coplin jar containing 70% formamide in 2× SSC pre-warmed in a 70 °C water bath for 4 min. The timing is critical.
15. Immediately plunge the slides into ice cold (−20 °C) 70% ethanol for 3 min and dehydrate the slides in the alcohol series as per normal.
16. Take up 40 µl of denatured probe from step 11 and apply it to the denatured chromosome slide.
17. Mount the slides with long coverslips and seal the edges with cow gum or any rubber sealing glue.
18. Incubate the slides in a humidity chamber at 37 °C overnight.

Second day

Solutions:
250 ml 2× SSC (25 ml 20× SSC stock + 225 ml H$_2$O)
150 ml 50% formamide in 2× SSC (15 ml 20× SSC + 60 ml H$_2$O + 75 ml formamide)
500 ml 4× SSC (100 ml 20×SSC + 400 ml H$_2$O)

From the 500 ml 4× SSC:
To 50 ml add 2.5 g Marvel non-fat milk powder, mix well, and filter into a Coplin jar.
To the remaining 450 ml, add 1.125 ml 20% Tween solution.
To 1 ml of 4× SSC-Marvel add 5 µl FITC stock in an Eppendorf tube.
To 1 ml 4× SSC-Marvel add 10 µl biotinylated anti-avidin stock in an Eppendorf tube.

1. Take the slides out of the humidity chamber and peel away the rubber seal. If the coverslip does not slide out with the rubber seal, apply a little pressure to the coverslip and push it off the slide.

2. Rinse the slides in 50% formamide in 2× SSC at 42 °C for 5 min (2×) in a water bath kept in the fume cupboard.
3. Rinse the slides in 2× SSC at 42 °C for 2 min (4×) in the same water bath.
4. Rinse the slides in 4× SSC Tween at room temperature for 5 min.
5. Incubate the slides in 4× SSC Marvel at room temperature for 20 min.
6. Add 100 µl avidin-FITC solution to each slide, place a coverslip on each, and incubate in a humidity chamber at 37 °C for 20 min.
7. Rinse the slides in 4× SSC Tween at room temperature 3× for 5 min.
8. Add 100 µl biotinylated anti-avidin solution to each slide, place a coverslip on each, and incubate in a humidity chamber at 37 °C for 20 min.
9. Rinse the slides in 4× SSC Tween at room temperature 3× for 5 min.
10. Add 100 µl avidin-FITC solution to each slide, place a coverslip on each, and incubate in a humidity chamber at 37 °C for 20 min.
11. Rinse the slides in 4× SSC Tween at room temperature for 5 min.
12. Rinse the slides in 0.1 M PBS at room temperature for 5 min (2×).
13. Dehydrate the slides through the ethanol series (described above).
14. Add anti-fade solution with 0.5 µg ml^{-1} propidium iodide and 2.5 µg ml^{-1} DAPI and apply a coverslip to the slides.
    Allow the slides to stain for 5 min before examination with a fluorescence microscope.

Microscopic Identification of Fluorescent Signals

Different filters are required to visualize the various fluorescent dyes, and must be selected carefully to ensure that all fluorescent signals are detected. In addition more than one fluorescent dye can be detected simultaneously by utilizing dual or triple band-pass filter sets (Nath and Johnson 1997).

Use of RT *in situ* PCR for Detection of sGC Isoforms

The NO-cGMP pathway is one of the key signal pathways in cardiovascular research. The binding of NO to the soluble guanylyl cyclase causes the conversion of GTP to cGMP, which can lead to different cellular responses, including vasorelaxation and regulation of growth and differentiation of endothelial cells and cardiomyocytes. At least four subunits of NO-sensitive enzyme sGC, forming these heterodimeric enzyme complexes, have been cloned (α_1, β_1, α_2 and β_2) and only two isoforms (a_1/b_1, a_2 and b_2) have been shown to exist at the protein level (Denninger and Marletta 1999). This makes methods necessary which can detect the mRNA of sGC isoforms with cellular resolution. Detection of sGC mRNA by RT *in situ* PCR can help to identify the sGC-isoform expression pattern in cardiovascular tissue and endothelial cells.

The protocol described can be varied by omission or inclusion of the DNAse digestion. Considering the expected higher expression level of sGC we do not use labelled nucleotides, only the primers are labelled. This makes omission of the DNAse treatment possible, at least if the experiments do not show nuclear staining.

Tissue Preparation and Tissue Section

Fixed paraffin or fixed cryoprotected tissue sections can be amplified quite successfully. This method permits the evaluation of individual cells in the tissue for the presence of a specific RNA or DNA sequence. In our laboratory we routinely use cardiac tissues, urogenital tract tissues, CNS tissues, etc., which are sliced to a 5 μm thickness. Tissue sections should be cut at 5 μm, floated on a water bath, mounted on poly-L-lysine-coated slides and dried in an oven at 60 °C for 1 h. Two adjacent sections are placed on one slide. The sections should be stabilized with a heat treatment at 105 °C for 5–120 s (Bagasra et al. 1994).

RT in situ PCR Buffer and Solutions

- 0.1 M PBS pH 7.2-7.4
  [10.8 g Na_2HPO_4, 2.0 g NaH_2PO_4, 6.6 g NaCl, 750 ml A.D.]
- 1 M $MgCl_2$
  [16.3 g, $MgCl_2$, 80 ml A.D.]
- 2× SSC (standard saline citrate: 0.3 M NaCl, 30 mm sodium citrate, pH 7.0)
  [123 g NaCl, 62 g tri-Na-citrate, 700 ml A.D.]
- 1 M Tris-HCl pH 7.5/9.5
  [91 g Tris, 750 ml A.D.]
- 5 M NaCl
  [102.3 g NaCl, 350 ml A.D.]
- 10 mm NaAc pH 5.2
  [2.3 g NaAc, 170 ml A.D.]
- 0.2 M ethylenediaminetetraacetic acid (EDTA), pH 8.0:
  [26 g EDTA, 350 ml A.D.]
- 0.1 M PBS-1 M $MgCl_2$
  [0.5 ml 1 M $MgCl_2$+99.5 ml 0.1 M PBS]
- Proteinase K buffer
  [200 ml Tris-HCl 1 M pH 7.5, 200 ml EDTA 0.2 M, 8 ml NaCl 5 M]
- DNAse solution
  [35 μl of 3 M sodium acetate, 5 μl 1 M $MgSO_4$, and 60 μl water, 1 μl of RNAse-free DNAse (Boerhinger Mannheim, 10 U/μl)]
- 0.1 M glycine/0.2 M Tris-HCl buffer pH 7.4
  [100 ml 1 M Tris HCl pH 7.5 + 3.75 g Glycine + 500 ml aqua dest]
- Tris-EDTA
  [1.4 ml Tris-HCl 1 M pH 7.5, 0.7 ml EDTA 0.2 M, 170.0 ml aqua dest]
- Wash buffer
  [500 ml formamide, 300 ml aqua dest , 200 ml 20× SSC]
- Buffer I pH 7.5
  [70 ml Tris-HCl 1 M pH 7.5, 21 ml NaCl 5 M, 700 ml A.D.]
- Buffer II
  [1 g blocking-reagent, 100 ml buffer I]
- Buffer III
  [60 ml Tris-HCl 1 M pH 9.5, 12 ml NaCl 5 M, 30 ml $MgCl_2$ 1 M, 600 ml aqua dest]

RT *in situ* PCR Method

1. Deparaffinize tissue sections through xylene, ethanols and rehydrate to distilled water:
   1×5 min   xylene I
   1×5 min   xylene II
   2×4 min   ethanol 100%
   1×4 min   ethanol 90%
   1×4 min   ethanol 70%
   1×4 min   ethanol 50%
   1×5 min   distilled water
2. Heat Treatment.
   Place the slides with adherent sections on a heat-block at 105 °C for 5–120 s, 90 s for DNA target sequence and 5–10 s for RNA sequences. The shorter treatment is recommended for RNA targets, because mRNAs may be unstable at high temperature (Bagasra et al. 1994).
3. Fixation
   Place the sections in a fixation solution containing 4% paraformaldehyde in 0.1 M PBS for 2–24 h at room temperature (RT).
4. Wash the sections with 0.1 M PBS (3×10 min)
   The sections may be stored at –80 °C until use.
   Before storage, the sections should be dehydrated with 100% ethanol.
5. Wash the sections in two changes of 0.1 M PBS–1 M $MgCl_2$.
   2×5 min 0.1 M PBS–1 M $MgCl_2$
6. Preincubate with 3% hydrogen peroxide methanol solution for 30 min to block the endogenous peroxidase activity.
   20 min in [40 ml methanol +9 ml distilled water +1 ml H_2O_2]
7. Wash in two changes of 0.1 M PBS–1 M $MgCl_2$.
   2×10 min 0.1 M PBS–1 M $MgCl_2$
8. Proteinase K treatment:
   – Treat samples with 10 mg/ml for 10 min at 37 °C.
   – Wash the sections with 0.1 M PBS–1 M $MgCl_2$ for 5 min to inactive the proteinase K or equilibrate the sections in 0.1 M glycine/0.2 M Tris-HCl buffer pH 7.4, at room temperature (RT) for 5 min to inactive the proteinase K.
9. Wash the sections in distilled water for 2 min at RT
   Digest the DNA with RNAse-free DNAse solution overnight at 37 °C in a humidity chamber, in which the solution is covered with the inside of an autoclaved polypropylene bag to prevent drying
   Remove the coverslip, wash the slides for 1 min in water and ethanol and air dry
10. The sections should be subjected to amplification. Prepare an amplification cocktail containing the following:
    – Master mix I:
      0.8 µl DNTP-mix (25 mM), 2.5 µl DMSO (7%), 2.5 µl DTT-solution (5 mM), 0.5 µl RNAse inhibitor (20 U), 2.0 µl 1. primer (300 nM), 2.0 µl 2. primer (300 nM) and 14.7 µl sterile water (total volume = 25 µl).

- Master mix II:
  10 µl 5× RT PCR buffer, 2 µl c-therm. polymerase [c-therm polymerase (Roche Molecular Biochemicals, Mannheim) can be used for both reverse transcription and PCR.], 13 µl sterile water (total volume = 25 µl).
- Mix the master mix I and master mix II.
- Centrifuge the mixture briefly.
- Apply amplifying solution to the appropriate tissue section:
  Layer 10 µl of amplification solution on to each well with a micropipette so that the whole surface of the well is covered with the solution
- Coverslip:
  Sections should be covered with coverslips, and placed at RT for 10 min to allow the solution around the edges of the coverslips to dry.
- Seal each coverslip using clear nail polish:
  Each corner of the coverslip should be mounted with a drop of nail polish and the edges of the coverslips should be sealed with two layers of nail polish
- Air-dry thoroughly:
  Place the sections at RT for 10 min to allow the nail polish to dry.
- Place the sections on a heat-block and load into a thermocycler. In our laboratory, amplifications are performed for
  1 cycle at 94 °C (120 s)
  10 cycles at 94 °C (30 s)
  10 cycles at 59 °C (30 s)
  10 cycles at 72 °C (60 s)
  25 cycles at 94 °C (30 s)
  25 cycles at 59 °C (30 s)
  25 cycles at 72 °C (60 s)
  1 cycle at 72 °C (420 s)

11. Place the sections at 4 °C for 4 h or overnight.
12. Immerse the sections in 100% ethanol for 10 min, to dissolve nail polish and dissociate the coverslip.
13. Wash the sections in
    - 4×20 min with 0.1 M PBS
    - 3×10 min with 0.05% Tween-20 in 0.1 M PBS
    - 4×15 min with 0.1 M PBS
14. Incubate the section with horseradish-peroxidase-complex (1:150 dilution) for 45 min at RT.
15. Wash the sections in
    - 2×10 min with Tween-20/0.1 M PBS
    - 3×10 min with 0.1 M PBS
16. Incubate the sections in a chromogen detection solution containing 0.05% 3,3'-diaminobenzidine tetrahydrochloride (DAB), 0.01% nickel ammonium sulphate and 0.05% H_2O_2 in 0.05 M Tris-HCl buffer, pH 7.6 for 15 min at RT.
17. Wash the sections with 0.1 M PBS 3×10 min at RT.
18. Sections should be mounted in
    - Glycerine-gelatine
    - Aqua Mount

- Entellan (in our laboratory):
  dehydrate the sections in increasing concentrations of ethanol
  3 min   ethanol 50%
  3 min   ethanol 70%
  3 min   ethanol 95%
  2×3 min   ethanol 100%
  clear the sections in xylene
  3 min   xylene I
  3 min   xylene II
  mount the slides in Entellan.

The RT in situ PCR Controls

Negative controls:
- RT *in situ* PCR can be done without primers.
- The reaction can be performed without c-therm. polymerase
- Incubation of the sections with irrelevant primers.
- RNAse pre-treated sections can be used.
- Incubate sections of unrelated tissues.
- Incubation of non-treated sections with enzyme-complex and chromogen

Positive controls:
- RT *in situ* PCR should be done on a tissue with known expression of the relevant mRNA.
- Treated tissue and the supernatant run separately in a gel

Interpretation of controls:
- The sections should be unstained.
- Positive signal should be found with specific localization.
- A specific band should be found in the treated tissue. If a band is detected in the supernatant, a washout of the amplicon is responsible.

Troubleshooting

Troubleshooting for *in situ* Hybridisation

Three major problems can occur: no signal, high background staining and poor morphology.

No Signal Can Be Detected

The reasons for the lack of a signal can be different, such as no target RNA is in the specimen, the probe is not labelled, the antibody staining does not work, RNA degradation by RNases destroyed the RNA, RNA has been lost from the tissue, pre-treatment and/or hybridisation conditions are not working for the applied probe, hybridisation conditions are too stringent or the staining conditions are wrong.

The content of RNA can be checked by Northern blot or RT PCR. The probe labelling and the antibody staining can be tested on a nitrocellulose or nylon filter, to which the probe should be transferred and labelled. Antibody staining can also be checked separately on nitrocellulose and nylon filters. The possible degradation of RNA or loss of RNA from the tissue, which can occur from initial and post-prehybridisation fixation problems, can be tested by use of a well-known probe. Problems with pre-treatment and/or hybridisation conditions as well as too stringent hybridisation conditions should be tested by use of a specimen with a known content of detectable RNA. If neither a known RNA probe nor a known tissue with the specific probe works, then a problem with the staining procedure, possibly the pH of the staining buffer, is the reason for the missing signal.

High Background Staining is Found

Three different reasons for the high background staining can occur generally. The probe could be hybridising non-specifically or the antibody be binding non-specifically or it could be caused by incomplete blocking of the endogenous enzyme activity. Probe and antibody problems can be differentiated by performing a control hybridisation with no probe but normal antibody visualization. If the probe is recognized as the problem, prehybridisation, concentration of the probe, temperature and/or formamide concentration in the hybridisation mix can be changed. Furthermore an RNAse A incubation step after hybridisation can be tried. Non-specific binding of the antibody can be avoided by preabsorption of the antibody against fixed material before use in probe detection or by blocking the hybridised specimen prior to incubation with the antibody. Endogenous enzyme activity will be found by performing a staining reaction on a hybridised specimen that has been through blocking solution without antibody. In the case of detection of an endogenous enzyme activity, levamisole for alkaline phosphatase activity and H_2O_2 for peroxidase should be used.

Morphological Preservation is Too Bad

The main reason for a poor morphology is an insufficient fixation. Modification of fixation time and/or fixative can help. Furthermore it should be checked that the fixation starts directly after sampling of the specimen. Further reasons for inadequate morphology are excessive proteinase K, too high a hybridisation temperature and wrong pH. Modification of temperature and pH of the buffer should be tested.

A more detailed description of troubleshooting can be found in Jowett (1997).

Troubleshooting for RT *in situ* PCR

In principal two problems can be differentiated, the lack of a signal and the occurrence of wrong positive results. These problems can easily be detected if adequate controls as described above were performed.

If no signal is visible it must be checked that the RNA is preserved, the primer works, the procedure, including the protease digestion, is running and the detection system is working. If available, a RT *in situ* PCR can be done with a known working primer and the primer of interest in the target specimen and in a control specimen containing the target RNA. A lack of signal in the control specimen for the control primer suggests that the procedure is not running or the detection system is not working. If the control specimen and the target specimen are positive for the control primer but not for the specific primer, a problem with the primer or a loss of amplicon in the supernatant can be assumed. In the first case, alteration of the protease digestion and staining system as well as the reaction solutions should be tried, and especially it should be ensured that all steps are performed in RNAse-free solution. In the second case, the primer should be used in a solution RT PCR and the tissue and supernatant should be run in a gel after the RT *in situ* PCR is done.

The second principal problem, false positive results, can be pre-screened by an exact morphological investigation. Positive nuclei and/or a relatively homogenous staining of the tissue, especially if the extracellular matrix surrounding the cells is also stained, give clear evidence for false positive results. Besides problems with the detection system, which can be handled as described above for *in situ* hybridisation, different ways that lead to incorporation of labelled nucleotides must be checked. These are the non-target primer-dependent amplification (mispriming), primer oligomerization and DNA repair (a primer-independent pathway). If a homogenous labelling of the cells and the extracellular matrix are found, a migration of the amplicon out of the target cell or an oligomerization of the primers could be the reason. A hot start procedure can be tried to avoid the oligomerization. The migration of the amplicon can be influenced by choice of another primer pair which leads to a longer amplicon and/ or by shortening the protease digestion. An intensive staining of the nuclei can derive from DNA repair or from mispriming. This can be tested by an intensive DNAse digestion, which should reduce or abolish the nuclear staining and by omission of the reverse transcription step, which should also avoid a signal. DNA repair and mispriming can be differentiated, if labelled primers and labelled nucleotides are used. In the case of DNA repair, the staining of the nucleus should be strongly reduced or abolished if no labelled nucleotides are included in the reaction solution. If the nuclear staining is further observable under these conditions and the use of labelled primers, a mispriming is likely. A hot start technique can be tried to reduce or abolish the mispriming, while DNA repair as a reason for the signal can be avoided if DNAse digestion is optimised and/or only the primers are labelled.

References

Bagasra O, Seshamma T, Hansen J, Bobroski L, Saikumari P, Pestaner JP and Pomerantz RJ (1994) Application of *in situ* PCR methods in molecular biology: I. details of Methodology for general use. Cell Vision 1: 324–335

Bagasra O, Bobroski LE, Amjad M (2001) Detection of nucleic acids in cells and tissues by *in situ* polymerase chain reaction. In: Lloyd RV (ed) Morphology methods. Cell and Molecular biology techniques. Humana Press, Totowa, pp 209–227

Baumann MA, Korkmaz Y, Bloch W, Schmidt A, Addicks K, Schröder H (2003) Localization of the neuropeptide galanin in nerve fibers and epithelial keratinocytes of the rat molar gingiva. Eur J Oral Sci 111: 175–178

Baumgart E, Schad A, Grabenbauer M (2000) *In situ* hybridization: general principles and application of digoxigenin-labeled cRNA for the detection of mRNAs. In: Beesly JE (ed) Immuncytochemsitry and *in situ* hybridization in the biomedical sciences. Birkhäuser, Boston, pp 108–137

Beaulieu P, Lambert C (1998) Peptidic regulation of heart rate and interactions with the autonomic nervous system. Cardiovasc Res 37: 578–585

Birtsch C, Wevers A, Traber J, Maelicke A, Bloch W and Schröder H (1997) Expression of α4-1 and α5 nicotinic cholinoceptor mRNA in the aging rat cerebral cortex. Neurobiol Aging 18: 335–342

Bloch W, Huggel K, Sasaki T, Grose R, Bugnon P, Addicks K, Timpl R, Werner S (2000) The angiogenesis inhibitor endostatin impairs blood vessel maturation during wound healing. FASEB J 14: 265–278

Brunet JF, Berger F, Amalfitano G, Benabid AL (1994) Chemolabeling of frozen cerebral tissue proteins and immunopurified products with biotin and digoxigenin: physicochemical characteristics of biotinylated and digoxigeninated products. Anal Biochem 222: 76–0

Childs GV (1992) *In situ* Hybridization with nonradioactive probes. In: Darby IA (ed) Methods in Molecular Biology. Humana Press, Totowa, pp 131–141

Deb A, Wang S, Skelding KA, Miller D, Simper D, Caplice NM (2003) Bone marrow-derived cardiomyocytes are present in adult human heart: A study of gender-mismatched bone marrow transplantation patients. Circulation 107: 1247–1249

Denninger JW, Marletta MA (1999) Guanylate cyclase and the NO/cGMP signaling pathway. Biochim Biophys Acta 1411: 334–350

Doneda L, Bulfamante G, Grimoldi MG, Volpi L, Larizza L (1997) Localization of fos, jun, kit and SCF mRNA in human placenta throughout gestation using *in situ* RT-PCR. Early Pregnancy 3: 265–271

Haase AT, Retzel EF, Staskus KA (1990) Amplification and detection of lentiviral DNA inside cells. Proc Natl Acad Sci USA 87: 4971–4975

Jin L, Qian X, Lloyd RV (2001) *In situ* hybridisation: Detection of DNA and RNA. In: Lloyd RV (ed) Morphology Methods. Cell and molecular biology techniques. Humana Press, Totowa, pp 27–44

Jowett T (1997) Principle of the technique. In: Jowett T (ed) Tissue *in situ* hybridisation. Methods in animal development   John Wiley & Sons, Inc. and Spektrum Akademischer Verlag Co-Publication, New York and Heidelberg, pp 1–8

Kontogeorgos G, Kapranos N, Thodou E (1992) Practical applications of the FISH technique. In: Lloyd RV (ed) Methods in Molecular Biology. Humana Press, Totowa, pp 131–141

Lloyd RV, Jin L (1995) *In situ* hybridisation analysis of chromogranin A and B mRNAs in neuroendocrine tumors with digoxigenin-labeled oligonucleotide probe cocktails. Diagn Mol Pathol 4: 143–151

Martinez A, Miller MJ, Quinn K, Unsworth EJ, Ebina M, Cuttitta F (1995) Non-radioactive localization of nucleic acids by direct *in situ* PCR and *in situ* RT-PCR in paraffin-embedded sections. J Histochem Cytochem 43: 739–747

Martinez A, Man Y, Zullo SJ, Cuttitta F (2000) *In situ* amplification and detection of nucleic acids. In: Beesly JE (ed) Immuncytochesmitry and *in situ* hybridisation in the biomedical sciences. Birkhäuser, Boston, pp 156–174

MyQuaid S, Allan, GM (1992) Detection protocols for biotinylated probes. Optimization using multistep techniques. J Histochem Cytochem 40: 569–574

Nath J and Johnson KL (1997) Fluorescence *in situ* hybridization (FISH): DNA probe production and hybridization criteria. Biotechnic and Histochemistry 73: 6–22

Nuovo GJ, Gallery F, MacConnell P, Braun A (1994) *In situ* detection of polymerase chain reaction-amplified HIV-1 nucleic acids and tumor necrosis factor-alpha RNA in the central nervous system. Am J Pathol 144: 659–666

Nuovo GJ (1996) The foundations of successful RT *in situ* PCR, Front Biosci. 1: c4–c15

Nuovo GJ (1997) Reverse transcriptase *in situ* PCR. In: Nuovo GJ (ed) PCR *in situ* hybridization. Protocols and applications. Lippincott-Raven, Philadelphia, pp 271–333

O'Reilly KH, Boehm T, Shing Y, Fukai N, Vasios G, Lane WS, Flynn E, Birkhead JR, Olsen BR, Folkman J (1997) Endostatin: an endogenous inhibitor of angiogensis and tumor growth. Cell 88: 277–285

Pinkel D, Straume T and Gray J (1986) Cytogenetic ananlysis using quantitative hichg sensitivity fluorescence hybridization. Proc Natl Acad Sci 83: 2934–2938

See CG (2001) Fluorescence *in situ* hybridization. In: Beesley JE (ed) Immunocytochemistry and *in situ* hybridization in the biomedical sciences. Birkhäuser Boston, pp 138–156

Trask BJ, Massa H, Kenwrick S and Gitschier J (1991) Mapping of human chromosome Xq28 by two-color fluorescence *in situ* hybridization of DNA sequences in interphase cell nuclei. Am J Hum Gen 48: 1–15

Wetmur JG, Ruyechan WT, Douthart RJ (1981) Denaturation and renaturation of Penicillium chrysogenum mycophage double-stranded ribonucleic acid in tetraalkylammonium salt solutions. Biochemistry 20: 2999–3002

Wevers A, Jeske A, Lobron Ch, Birtsch Heinemann S, Maelicke A, Schröder R, Schröder H (1994) Cellular distribution of nicotinic acetylcholine receptor subunit mRNAs in the human cerebral cortex as revealed by non-isotopic *in situ* hybridization. Mol Brain Res 25: 122–128

Yang H, Wanner IB, Roper SD, and Chaudhari N (1999) An optimized method for *in situ* hybridization with signal amplification that allows the detection of rare mRNAs. J Histochem Cytochem 47: 431–445

4.4 Practical Use of Transmission Electron Microscopy for Analysis of Structures and Molecules in Cardiovascular Research

Wilhelm Bloch, Christian Hoffmann, Eveline Janssen and Yüksel Korkmaz

Introduction

This chapter is designed for unestablished and established researchers in the field of electron microscopy. It gives basic information about the handling of tissue for electron microscopy and more specialized information for use of electron microscopy to detect specific molecules by ultrastructural immunohistochemistry (Fig. 1). Electron microscopy was for a long time mainly restricted to high-resolution structural analysis. In the last 20 years an increasing application for molecule detection with the help of the immunogold technique has occurred. In cardiovascular research, electron microscopy is more and more used to detect specific molecules at high resolution with the help of the immunogold technique. Classical electron microscopy remains a helpful technique in cardiovascular research, although molecular biological and cell biological techniques take more and more part in cardiovascular research. New concepts for the use of ultrastructural analyses that allow observation of dynamic alterations at the highest resolution strongly increase the impact of electron microscopic investigation. High-resolution light microscopy cannot reach a resolution comparable to that possible with electron microscopy. Considering the time consuming preparations for electron microscopy, it seems appropriate to combine high resolution light microscopy and electron microscopy to get information about the structural relationships between molecules (Bloch et al. 2001a,b). A further area where ultrastructural analyses take place is the analysis of transgenic or knockout animals or cell systems with a cardiovascular phenotype (Bloch et al. 1997; Costell et al. 199; Kostka et al. 2001). Furthermore ultrastructural analyses can give important information in angiogenesis and stem cell research (Bloch et al. 2000; Röll et al. 2002). In this chapter we will describe conventional electron microscopic preparation and examples of pre- and post-embedding immunoelectron microscopy. Furthermore, we will give an example of the use of electron microscopy that shows the possibility of investigating the dynamic processes in experimental models with electron microscopy.

For transmission electron microscopy, ultrastructure must be preserved as close to the in vivo situation as possible. This is done by either chemical or cryofixation; the later will not be in the scope of this chapter, because of the great technical difficulty that accompanies this kind of fixation for electron microscopy. Cryofixation does not seem to be a routine method and is used mainly by specialized laboratories. The time between removal of the tissue and fixation should be kept as short as possible to avoid structural damage of the tissue before the tissue is fixed. Therefore a perfusion fixa-

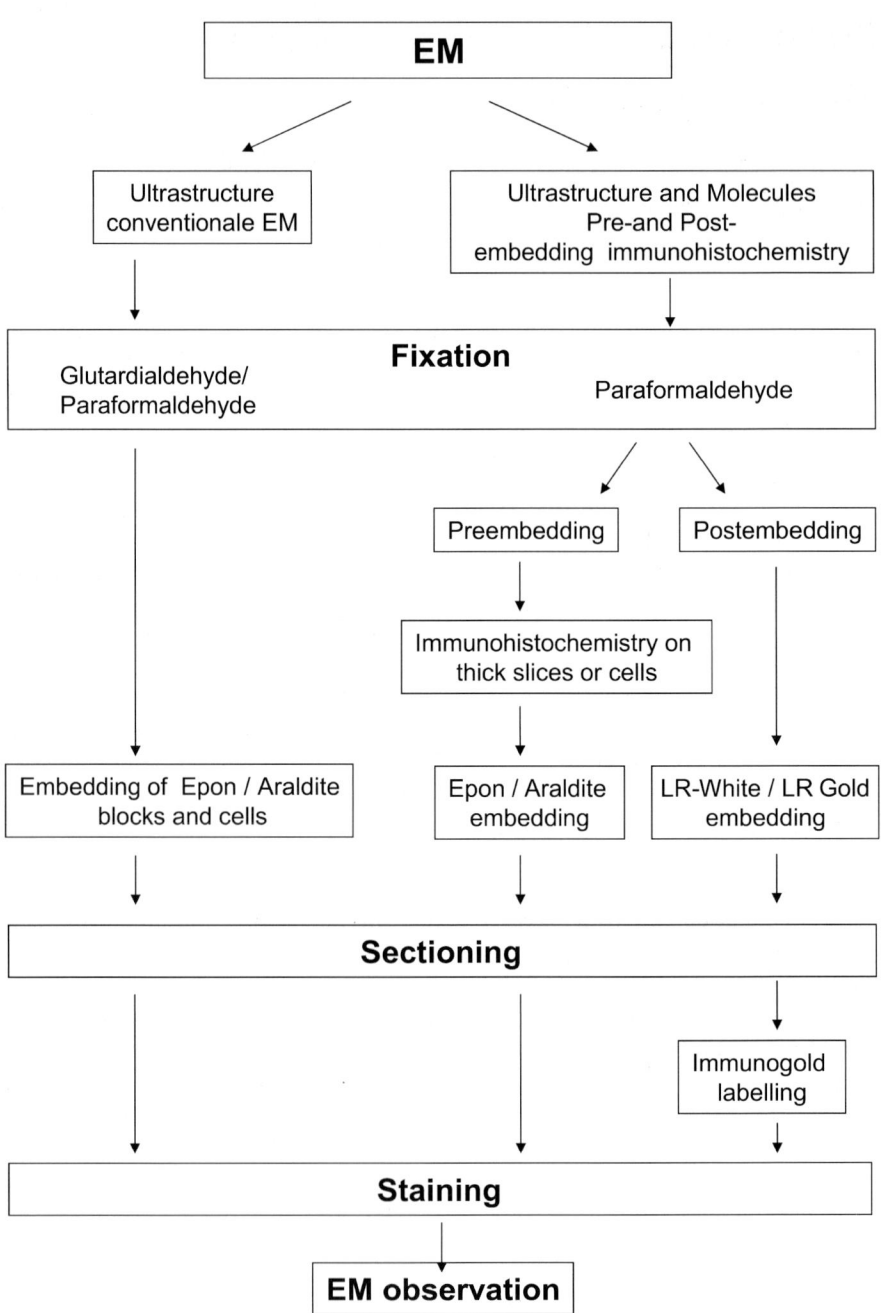

Figure 1
Flow diagram of electron microscopic techniques

tion is preferable if possible. For electron microscopic immunocytochemistry, the fixation procedure is always a compromise between good morphological preservation and retention of antigenicity.

Description of Methods and Practical Approach

Fixation

Fixation is one of the key steps in electron microscopy. If fixation is inadequate, it is impossible to get acceptable ultrastructural preservation. Therefore, a fast and sufficient fixation must be performed. There are two methods of fixation of tissue from organs, cardiovascular perfusion and immersion fixation, while cells are generally immersion fixed. The principal fixatives are paraformaldehyde and glutaraldehyde, which can be used with different buffers. Paraformaldehyde is a monoaldehyde and penetrates faster than glutaraldehyde, but results in poorer ultrastructure. An optimal solution is to use a mixture of both aldehydes in perfusion fixation. Dependent on the underlying aim of the study, it might be necessary to use varying concentrations of these two fixatives. Especially if immunogold analysis is to be performed, lower glutaraldehyde concentrations must be used, because of the strong crosslinking of the molecules by glutaraldehyde. Intensive crosslinking can decrease antigenicity of tissue.

Preparation of Fixatives for Normal and Immunoelectron Microscopy

Fixative for Standard Electron Microscopy. The standard fixative for electron microscopy is a mixture of 2% paraformaldehyde, 2% glutaraldehyde, 0.1 M cacodylate buffer, pH 7.35.

Fixative for Immunoelectron Microscopy. For higher antigenicity in immunoelectron investigations, fixative(s) should be used containing 0.1–2% concentrations of glutaraldehyde with 2–4% concentrations of paraformaldehyde. In this fixative 0.5–2% saturated acid and 0.5 mM $CaCl_2$, 0.1 M HEPES buffer pH 7.3 should be added.

Some cases use a fixative, in which 1 vol% tannic acid rather than saturated picric acid is added. If tannic acid is added, the buffer should be 0.1 M HEPES, pH 7.25.

Buffer and Solutions Necessary for Preparation of the Fixatives, Embedding and Block Staining

Tyrode Solution, a Modified Krebs-Henseleit Solution. Tyrode solution serves as a physiological, iso-osmolar buffer solution for isolated tissue perfusion. It contains NaCl (37 mmol/l), KCl (5.4 mmol/l), $MgCl_2$ (1.05 mmol/l), $CaCl_2$ (1.8 mmol/l) Na_2HPO_4 (0.5 mmol/l), Na_2CO_3 (24 mmol/l) and glucose (11 mmol/l).

Tyrode solution is used for 5–10 min to rinse the vascular circulation, before the real perfusion fixation with fixative starts.

The pH value should be adjusted to pH 7.4 with 1 N hydrochloric acid (ca. 100 ml) and the mixture diluted to 1000 ml with distilled water.

Cacodylate Buffer, 0.2 M. 42.8 g cacodylic (dimethylarsinic acid) sodium trihydrate salt; brought to 1000 ml with deionised glass-distilled water, pH adjusted to 7.4 with HCl. Either paraformaldehyde solution or osmium tetroxide solution may be used for dilution (Reiner 2002).

HEPES-Na Buffer. HEPES-Na buffer was prepared at a concentration of 0.1 M. 26.02 g HEPES-Na (2-[4-(2-Hydroxyethyl)-1-piperazinyl]-ethanesulphonic acid sodium salt) was dissolved in distilled water to give 450 ml of solution. The pH value should be adjusted to 7.2 with appr. 35 ml of 1 N hydrochloric acid and distilled water added to 1000 ml.

Osmium Tetroxide (OsO4) Solution.
Stock solution:
- 1 g OsO_4 and 25 ml deionised glass-distilled water.

Application solution:
- Stock solution should be diluted 1:1 with 0.2 M cacodylate buffer.
- The mixture should be stored at 4 °C in a dark glass container that is both capped and sealed with Parafilm.

Uranyl Acetate. Uranyl acetate solution was prepared in different ways:
- 2% in 70% ethanol for block contrast in the standard procedure
- 0.1 M maleate buffer for block contrast for immunohistochemistry
- 2% in aqueous solution for section contrast

Saturated Picric Acid. 30 g picric acid should be dissolved in 1 l hot distilled water under a well-ventilated fume hood, to get a 1.2% saturated solution.

Tannic Acid (stock solution). Heat a solution containing 25 g tannic acid (Fa. Merck, Darmstadt, Merck Nr. 773) and 25 ml distilled water with constant stirring to 70 °C, until the solution just becomes a clear dark-brown colour. Fill into a brown glass vessel and store at 6 °C.

4% Paraformaldehyde. Heat a solution containing 4 g in 45 ml distilled water with constant stirring to 60 °C under a well-ventilated fume hood. Add 1 N NaOH drop wise until the solution just clears. Cool on ice and filter through a 5 μm membrane filter under vacuum. This solution is stable for a week at 4 °C.

Before use it must be diluted with 0.2 M PBS 1:1, the pH-value adjusted to 7.35 and distilled water added to 100 ml.

25% Glutardialdehyde. 25%ige aqueous solution, Merck AG, Darmstadt. In order to preserve the ultrastructural detail, it is desirable to include glutardialdehyde in the fixative. However, some antigens are extremely sensitive to crosslinking by glutaraldehyde. Therefore, the concentration of glutardialdehyde will have to be reduced or, in the most extreme cases, omitted entirely (Oliver and Jamur 1999).

Embedding

The main interest of conventional electron microscopy is an optimal preservation of the tissue ultrastructure. To achieve this, the preparation of samples for conventional electron microscopy is harsh. The infiltration of the samples with Epon or Araldite resins after aldehyde fixation, the osmium post-fixation, and the dehydration with ethanol and propylene oxide do almost prevent antigenicity being preserved. From the beginning of the eighties the rapid development of immunohistochemistry led to the expansion of this field at the ultrastructural level. For electron microscopic immunocytochemistry, the fixation procedure is always a compromise between good morphological preservation and retention of antigenicity (Romano and Romano 1984). Besides the choice of the fixation solution and conditions, the embedding process must be altered compared to conventional electron microscopy. In general two different kinds of embedding techniques for immunoelectron microscopy can be used, the pre-embedding and the post-embedding techniques. The main advantage of the pre-embedding technique is the smaller influence of the embedding procedure on the staining result. But serious disadvantages of this method lead to the use of post-embedding techniques.

Besides the smaller influence of the embedding procedure, the pre-embedding technique possesses further advantages. Large areas of the tissue may be immunostained and examined, it is possible to flat embed the material in such a way that the same immunostained section is used for both light and electron microscopic examination and sensitivity is very high and allows the detection of low-concentration antigens. A disadvantage of the pre-embedding technique is poor penetration of antibody into the tissue leading to limited staining of the tissue. Treatments that are necessary to improve penetration of antibody have a further deleterious effect on the ultrastructure. A further disadvantage is that the electron-dense product of the peroxidase reaction often diffuses from the original side of deposition and/or masks the underlying structures, thus not allowing a reliable subcellular localization of the antigens. In addition, multiple labelling experiments are relatively difficult to perform (Merighi and Polak 1993).

The main advantages of post-embedding immunogold staining are no penetration problems, the antigens are marked more precisely by the use of gold particles as label, gold particles can be prepared in different sizes, thus allowing simultaneous visualization of more than one antigen in the same preparation by use of different primary antibodies and different sections from the same block can be labelled with different primary antibodies. However, the post-embedding technique has also a number of drawbacks, mainly related to the fact that the antigenicity of the tissue is generally reduced by the post-fixation and the embedding. Only small areas of the tissue can be immunostained compared to the pre-embedding procedure and it is more difficult to correlate light and electron microscopic findings on the same material than after pre-embedding immunostaining. The several advantages and disadvantages of both general procedures make it clear that the choice of the procedure is dependent on different factors such as lability of the antigen, distribution and relative concentration of the antigen within the tissue, subcellular localization and the necessity of quantitative immunohistochemical analysis (Merighi and Polak 1993). However, a combination of pre- and post-embedding procedures is also possible, for example the first antibody can be incubated before embedding and the second after embedding, if lability of the first antibody is too high for post-embedding.

Although virtually any embedding resin may be used for immunogold staining, for post-embedding methods, the resin can strongly affect the immunostaining. The hydrophilic resins, such as LR Gold, LR White, and Lowicryl, generally give better results than the epoxy-based hydrophobic resins, such as the Epon substitutes or Spur. Below we describe protocols for conventional resin embedding and for post-embedding using Araldite as resin and for post-embedding using LR White as resin.

Resin Embedding of Tissue Blocks and Thick Slices for Electron Microscopy

Osmification and Embedding of Tissue Blocks. Following perfusion-fixation for 10–20 min, the samples should be post-fixed in the same fixative for 12–24 h at 4 °C. After post-fixation, prepare the heart regions of interest.
- Wash the samples in buffer (pH 7.2–7.3) for 3×15 min.
- The samples should be post-fixed in 2% osmium tetroxide solution in 0.1 M buffer for 4 h.
- Wash samples in buffer for 3×15 min.

Dehydration and Resin Embedding (Araldite or Epon)

- 15 min   50% ethanol
- 15 min   70% ethanol**
- 15 min   90% ethanol
- 15 min   96% ethanol
- 3×20 min   100% ethanol

**Incubate the samples in 1% uranyl acetate in 70% ethanol, overnight in dark conditions.
Incubate the samples in propylene oxide:100% ethanol (1:1) for 15 min.
Incubate the samples in propylene oxide for 2×20 min.
Treat the tissues in Araldite:propylene oxide (1:1) for 2–12 h.
Treat the samples with Araldite:propylene oxide (3:1) for 4–24 h.
Incubate the samples in Araldite (100%).
Evaporate propylene oxide for 2 h in an incubator at 40 °C.
Flat embed the samples (Agar Aids, Essex, UK).
Cure the Araldite-blocks at 45 °C in an incubator for 12 h.
Cure the Araldite-blocks at 60 °C in an incubator for 48 h.

Dehydration and Epon Embedding of Thick Slices (also possible with Araldite)

- 5 min   50% ethanol
- 5 min   70% ethanol
- 5 min   90% ethanol
- 5 min   95% ethanol
- 2×10 min   100% ethanol
- 10 min   100% propylene oxide

Overnight in 1:1 Epon:propylene oxide mixture
2 h in 2:1 Epon:propylene oxide
2 h in 100% Epon

Flat embed using an acetate sheet, fixed with masking tape to the rack of the oven, and plastic coverslips
Cure for 24 h at 55 °C
Separate the Epon from the acetate foil and label the coverslips
Examine by light microscopy to select the areas for re-embedding
Trim the relevant areas with a knife
Re-embed on the base of plastic capsules whose tops have been cut out
Fill the capsule with Epon and cure at 60 °C for 48 h.

Modified Araldite Embedding for Post-embedding Immunohistochemistry (Brorson 1996; Brorson and Skjorten 1996; Reiner 2002). Dehydration of the sample in ethanol and treatment of tissue samples with propylene oxide.
- 20 min   50% ethanol
- 20 min   70% ethanol
- 20 min   90% ethanol
- 3×20 min   100% ethanol
- 3×20 min   100% propylene oxide

Araldite [8% DMP-30 (accelerator)]:propylene oxide 1:1, for 6 h.
Araldite (6% DMP-30):propylene oxide 3:1, for 8 h.
Absolute Araldite in 4% DMP-30 for 8–12 h.
Transfer to polyethylene- or gelatine-embedding capsules containing completely fresh absolute Araldite (6% accelerator).
Polymerize at 56 °C for 72 h.

LR-White Embedding for Post-embedding Immunohistochemistry. LR-White may be polymerised by two procedures (Reiner 2002):
- The exothermic method:
    The samples are treated with 0.75% tannin acid for 4 h at RT.
    Dehydration of samples:
    - 20 min ice-cold   50% ethanol at −18 °C.
    - 20 min ice-cold   70% ethanol at −18 °C.
    - 20 min ice-cold   90% ethanol at −18 °C.
    - 20 min ice-cold   100% ethanol at −18 °C.
    Treat the samples in ice-cold LR-White: ethanol (1:1) for 20 min at −18 °C.
    Treat the samples in fresh LR-White for 1 h at −18 °C.
    Treat the samples in fresh LR-White overnight at −18 °C.
    Treat the samples in fresh LR-White for 1 h at −18 °C.
    Transfer the samples to gelatine capsules, fill the capsules with 100% LR-White and cap. Oxygen will inhibit polymerization.
    Polymerize at 56 °C for 24 h.
- The catalyst and UV-light methods:
    The samples are treated with 0.75% tannin acid for 4 h at RT.
    Dehydration of samples:
    - 20 min ice-cold   50% ethanol at −18 °C.
    - 20 min ice-cold   70% ethanol at −18 °C.

- 20 min ice-cold 90% ethanol at −18 °C.
- 20 min ice-cold 100% ethanol at −18 °C.

Treat the samples in ice-cold LR-White:ethanol (1:1) for 20 min at −18 °C.
Treat the samples in fresh LR-White for 1 h at −18 °C.
Treat the samples in fresh LR-White overnight at −18 °C.
Treat the samples in fresh LR-White for 1 h at −18 °C.

- Polymerisation by the catalyst method:
  Transfer the samples to 1.0 ml polyethylene-embedding capsules
  Prepare a mixture of pre-cooled 100% LR-White (1.0 ml) with LR-White catalyst (15 µl).
  Fill up the capsules quickly and place in a freezing chest at −25 °C.
  Polymerize the samples at −25 °C for 24 h.
- Polymerization by the UV-light method:
  Mix pre-cooled 100% LR-White (1.0 ml) with LR-White catalyst (15 µl).
  Place the capsules in a freezing chest at −25 °C.
  Polymerize the resin with UV-light (360 nm, 6 Watt, Black Light Blue, Fa. Sylvania, Japan) placed 25–30 cm from the capsules. Expose the capsules to the UV-light at −20 °C for 5 days.

Materials for Embedding

Epon. Epon mix: Epon 20 g + DDSA 1 g + NMA 10 g + DMP30 0.8 ml (measure with a 1 ml syringe and add in the fume hood). Stir for 10 min. Bubbles in the Epon can be quickly removed under vacuum.

Araldite 502 (Oliver and Jamur 1999). 100 g Araldite 502 resin and 75 g dodecenyl succinic anhydride (DDSA); add 2.5–3.5 g 2,4,6-tri(dimethylaminomethyl)phenol (DMP-30) just prior to use. Mix components together in a glass screw-cap bottle. The resin solution may be stored at 4 °C for at least 6 months. Let it come to room temperature before opening.

LR-White (Oliver and Jamur 1999). LR White resin: Store at 4 °C; let the bottle come to room temperature before opening. The LR White resin should not be used longer than suggested on the bottle by the manufacturer.

LR Gold resin: 25 ml LR Gold resin and 25–50 mg benzoin methyl ether; mix just prior to use.

Semithin and Ultrathin Sections

Semithin and ultrathin sectioning are described according to Davies (1999).

Semithin Sections

Trimming the Block and Semithin Sectioning (Webster 1999). Start by positioning the block in front of the trimming tool and cut into the block until a flat surface is produced. Then position one corner of the trim tool at one side of the block and cut

500 nm increments into the block. Move the trimming tool to the other side of the block and repeat the trimming. Turn the block one quarter turn clockwise and repeat the side trimming process. Turn the block one quarter turn counter clockwise and examine the block. Make sure the face of the block is mirror smooth and that the sides of the block are parallel to each other and perpendicular to the knife edge. The top and bottom of the block should be parallel to the knife edge. The edges of the block should be sharp, showing no signs of chipping, and clear of debris.

The most important factor in obtaining good semithin and ultrathin sections is the quality of the knife. Until recently, glass knives were the preferred tools for production of sections. Recent improvement in diamond knife production allows them to be used routinely for the production of good semithin and ultrathin sections.

Trim the blocks and cut plane parallel sections at 500 nm (semithin sections) from the flat surface of the blocks using an ultramicrotome (Leica Ultracut UCT) equipped with a glass or diamond knife.

Mount the sections on a slide and counter-stain the sections with methylene blue-Azure II:

- Drop the methylene blue/Azure II mixture (1:1) on the sections
- Place the slides on a hotplate at 60 °C for 2 min
- Wash the sections in distilled water and dry at room temperature
- Mount the sections in Entellan
- Examine by light microscopy to select the areas of the interest

The methylene blue solution according to Richardson et al. (1960) contains:
- 0.5 g Azure II
- 2.25 g methylene blue
- 0.25 g sodium tetraborate
- made up to 100 ml with double distilled water

Ultrathin Sectioning

Select an area under light microscopy and trim the face to a trapezium shape of approx. 0.5–1 mm2 for ultrathin sectioning:
- Trim the excess resin from the block face using the glass knife.
- Cut a semithin section of 500 nm, collect on to water and use a sable paintbrush to transfer to a drop of water on a microscope slide.
- Dry on a hotplate and stain at 60 °C with a drop of methylene blue-Azure II mixture (1:1) for 20 s until a gold rim is visible around the drop of stain. Wash off with distilled water, dry on the hotplate and mount in Entellan.
- Select an area and trim the face to a trapezium shape of approx. 0.5 mm^2 for ultrathin sectioning.
- Take a diamond knife, fill the bath with water, and collect ultrathin sections, silver interference colour.

Sections should be collected carefully on to copper or nickel grids (for immunogold labelling) (150 mesh):
- Place the grid in the water beneath them and raise it at a slight angle so the first section of the ribbon sticks to the edge of the grid.

- Slowly raise the grid out of the water and the rest of the ribbon will adhere to the grid.
- Blot the edge to remove excess water. Do not blot the flat surfaces of the grid.

If the sections are in ones, twos, or threes:
- Touch the grid onto the section(s) from above. This does introduce creases into the sections but is far easier than trying to collect from beneath.
- Blot the edge to remove excess water.
- Place the grids in a filter paper lined Petri dish before staining.

The grids may be later examined in the electron microscope to evaluate the staining, therefore stain the grids with uranyl acetate and lead citrate.

Uranyl Acetate Staining

- Place drops of 2% aqueous uranyl acetate onto a clean Parafilm surface.
- Transfer the labelled grids from the final water wash with forceps and touch each on to the first two drops to wash away excess water.
- Leave each grid on the final, larger drop, for 10 min.
- Remove each grid individually from the 2% aqueous uranyl acetate solution with a wire loop.
- Place the loop on to a hardened filter paper and let excess solution drain off.

Lead Citrate Staining

Use the clean side of Parafilm, and stain inside a Petri dish. A drop of lead citrate stain is placed on to a clean surface in a Petri dish with a few NaOH pellets around and the grid placed into the drop with the section side up. Stain for 1–7 min. The grid is washed five times with fresh deionised water and then air-dried.

Staining Solutions

Uranyl Acetate. Uranyl acetate solution was prepared as two different solutions:
- 2% in 70% ethanol for section contrast in the standard procedure
- 2% in aqueous solution for section contrast in the immunoelectron microscopy procedure

Lead Citrate Solution for the Standard Procedure. Stock solution:
- Solution A 1.3 M Na citrate
- Solution B 1.0 M Pb nitrate
- Solution C 1.0 M NaOH

Preparation of the final solution:
- 800 µl .bidest
- Add 155 µl solution A to 800 µl distilled water
- Mix carefully

- Add 100 µl solution B, getting a white precipitate
- Add 200 µl solution C and shake it until the mixture is clear
- After 5 min ultrafilter the solution
- Examine the sections in the electron microscope.

Pre-embedding and Post-embedding Ultrastructural Immunohistochemistry

In general two methods can be used to perform immunohistochemistry at the ultrastructural level, pre-embedding and post-embedding immunohistochemistry. Furthermore a combination of both these methods can also be performed.

Buffer for Immunoelectron Labelling

Tris-HCl buffered saline, 0.05 M:
- 6.057 g Tris (tris(hydroxymethylaminomethane)
- 8.766 g NaCl
- made up to 200 ml with distilled water

Maleate-buffer, 0.05 M:
- 4.9 g maleic acid anhydride made up to 400 ml with distilled water
- the pH value should be adjusted to 6.5 with 90 ml of 1 N hydrochloric acid and distilled water added to 500 ml.

Pre-embedding Immunoelectron Microscopy

Thick Sections of the Tissue for Immunohistochemistry on Free-Floating Sections (Côté et al. 1993). The tissue sections were cut at 50 µm on a Leica VT 1000 E Vibratome, floated out in 0.05 M TBS pH 7.6 and stored at 4 °C. The incubations were performed in 24-well tissue culture plates, in which solutions can be easily applied and removed with a pipette (Eppendorf) or with glass or plastic transfer pipettes. In our experience, a volume of 800 µl of antisera or wash solution is sufficient to incubate six free-floating sections.

Immunohistochemistry is preferably performed on free-floating sections, as there will be two incubation surfaces instead of one when compared to sections mounted on slides.

Immunohistochemistry. The Avidin-Biotin Peroxidase Complex (ABC) immunohistochemical technique with free-floating sections (Hsu 1993):
- Wash sections in 0.05 M TBS pH 7.4 for 2×15 min
- Incubate sections in 0.3% H_2O_2 +0.05 M TBS for 20 min to eliminate the endogenous peroxidase activity
- Wash the sections for 2×15 min
- Preincubate the sections with a mixture containing 0.05 M TBS pH 7.6 + 5% bovine serum albumin + 10% normal serum (from the same animal species which provided the secondary or link antibody) for 30 min

- Incubate the sections with primary antibody which should be diluted in 0.05 M TBS pH 7.6 + 1% normal serum for 24–48 h at 4 °C
- Wash the sections in 0.05 M TBS pH 7.6 for 2×15 min
- Incubate the sections with biotin-labelled secondary antibody which should be diluted in 0.05 M TBS pH 7.6 + 1% normal serum for 1 h
- Wash in 0.05 M TBS pH 7.6 for 2×15 min
- Incubate the sections with the ABC reagent for 1 h at 1:100 dilution in 0.05 M TBS pH 7.6
- Wash in 0.05 M TBS pH 7.6 for 2×15 min
- Develop the sections in a substrate mixture containing a 0.06% solution of 3.3'-diaminobenzidine tetrahydrochloride (DAB, Sigma), 1% nickel ammonium sulphate and 0.01% H_2O_2 in 0.05 M Tris HCl-buffer pH 7.6 for 5–10 min (the different incubation times are dependent on the antibodies)
- Wash the sections in 0.05 M TBS pH 7.6 for 2×15 min.

The Immunohistochemical controls:
- Incubate the section in the absence of the primary antibody
- Incubate the sections in the absence of the secondary antibody
- Incubate the sections in normal non-immune rabbit IgG
- Pre-absorb the primary antibodies with the appropriate control peptide.

Osmification of Thick Slices (Riberio-Da-Silva et al. 1993)

- Add 1% OsO_4 solution to cover the immunolabelled sections. Stopper and seal each vial with Parafilm for 4 h
- Remove the OsO_4 solution with a pipette and pour the discard into kitchen vegetable oil. If the immunohistochemical reaction is strong enough, in-block staining in uranyl acetate should be used. If the immunohistochemical reaction is not very intense, just rinse the sections twice in 0.1 M PBS pH 7.4 and proceed to 4
- Wash the sections with distilled water for 10 min. Stain the sections for 45 min in 1.5% uranyl acetate (in water) at 4 °C. then, wash the sections with 50% ethanol and start dehydration.
- Embedding and sectioning as described above.

Post-embedding Immunogold Method

Fixation, Post-fixation and Tissue Preparation of Heart. Following isolated perfusion-fixation of the rat heart by Fixation C, the samples should be post-fixed in same fixative for 24 h at 4 °C. After post-fixation, prepare the heart tissue regions of interest [here the left ventricular papillary muscle of the heart (Reiner 2002)].
- Immerse the samples in HEPES buffer + tannic acid (1 vol.%) solution for 4 h
- Wash the samples with HEPES buffer for 3×20 min
- Treat the samples with 50 mM ammonium chloride in HEPES buffer for 1 h at 4 °C
- Wash the samples with HEPES buffer for 3×20 min
- Incubate the samples in maleate buffer for 24 h at 4 °C
- Wash the samples with maleate buffer for 3×20 min.
- Treat the samples with 2% uranyl acetate + maleate buffer for 4 h

- Wash the samples with maleate buffer for 3×20 min.
- Alternatively the incubation of the samples in maleate buffer can be omitted. In this case the samples will be incubated in 2% uranyl acetate +70% alcohol for 4 h.
- Embedding as described above.

Immunogold and Double Immunogold Staining of Ultrathin Sections

General immunolabelling method of the ultrathin sections (Webster 1999):
- Attach a long piece of Parafilm to a bench surface with a drop of water. As this will form a clean surface on which to label and wash, only expose as much of the Parafilm as needed and do not contaminate the clean Parafilm surface.
- Float the specimen grid, section side down on a drop (100 µl) of 0.05 M TBS placed on the clean Parafilm surface. It is important to always keep the section side of the grid wet and the back surface dry.
- Transfer and float the grid on a drop of 0.05 M TBS containing 3–10% bovine serum albumin (blocking solution). Use a 3.5 mm diameter loop to transfer the grid.
- Use forceps to transfer the grid to an antibody dilution drop. The antibody, diluted to a suitable concentration, is centrifuged prior to use. This will remove any aggregates formed during storage.
- Place a wet piece of filter paper close to the antibody drop (for dilution see below) and cover with a plastic dish.
- Remove the grid from the antibody drop with forceps and float on TBS. Wash by transferring the grid to five drops of TBS.
- Use forceps to transfer the grid to a 5 µl drop of protein X-gold (for dilution see below).
- Again cover with a plastic dish in a humidity chamber.
- Remove the grid with forceps and wash by transferring the grid to 5 drops of TBS.
- Wash with water, 4 changes. Although only a short wash, this step removes salts prior to incubation with uranyl acetate. Phosphates present in the sections will precipitate the uranyl salts. This step is essential for fine structure preservation as well as for producing enough contrast to visualize subcellular detail in the electron microscope (Webster 1999):
- Place drops of cold 2% aqueous uranyl acetate onto a clean Parafilm surface, on ice.
- Transfer the labelled grids from the final water wash with forceps and touch each on to the first two drops to wash away excess water.
- Leave each grid on the final, larger drop, for 10 min.
- Remove each grid individually from the cold 2% aqueous uranyl acetate solution with a wire loop.
- Place the loop on to a hardened filter paper and let excess solution drain off.
- If the grid falls out of the loop it can be rapidly transferred back to the solution on ice with forceps and the process repeated.

A Modified Method for Immunogold Labelling of the Ultrathin Sections. Immunogold labelling on grid-mounted thin sections in drops of antibody solution according to Brorson et al. (1994) and Reiner et al. (2001). This method can be performed manually but there is an automatic machine commercially available. Here, the manual method is described in detail.

- Incubate the grids in 3% defatted milk diluted in 0.05 M TBS pH. 7.6 for 30 min
- Incubate the primary antibodies (normally polyclonal rabbit antibodies are used) diluted in 0.05 M TBS pH 7.6 containing 0.3% defatted milk for 2 h at RT or at 4 °C overnight in a humidity chamber
- Wash the grids in 0.05 M TBS containing 0.05% Tween-20
- Incubate the grids with secondary antibody, i.e. an IgG against the host of the primary antibody conjugated to 10 nm gold particles (Sigma), diluted in 0.05 M TBS containing 0.05% Tween-20 for 1 h:
- Wash the grids with 3× 0.05 M TBS pH 7.6 + 0.05% Tween-20, 3× TBS and 2× double distilled water
- Transfer the grids to 2% aqueous uranyl acetate for 10 min in the dark
- Leave the grid in the loop to dry and store section-side up or immediately examined in the transmission electron microscope

A Double Immunogold Labelling of the Ultrathin Sections (Reiner et al. 2001).
- Incubate the grids in 3% defatted milk diluted in 0.05 M TBS pH 7.6 for 30 min
- Incubate the grids e.g. with polyclonal rabbit anti-eNOS (Biomol, Hamburg, Germany; 1:250) diluted in 0.05 M TBS pH 7.6 containing 0.3% defatted milk for 2 h at RT or at 4 °C overnight in a humidity chamber
- Wash the grids in 0.05 M TBS containing 0.05% Tween-20
- Incubate the grids with goat anti-rabbit IgG conjugated to 10 nm gold particles (Sigma) diluted in 0.05 M TBS containing 0.05% Tween-20 for 1 h.
- Wash the grids with 0.05 M TBS pH 7.6 and distilled water.
- Incubate the grids in 1.5% defatted milk diluted in 0.05 M TBS pH 7.6 for 30 min.
- Incubate the grids e.g. in polyclonal rabbit anti-caveolin-1 (Transduction Labs., Lexington, KY; 1:300) diluted in 0.05 M TBS pH 7.6 containing 0.3% defatted milk for 2 h at RT.
- Wash the grids in 0.05 M TBS containing 0.05% Tween-20.
- Incubate the grids with goat anti-rabbit IgG conjugated to 5 nm gold particles (Sigma) diluted in 0.05 M TBS containing 0.05% Tween-20 for 1 h.
- Wash the grids with 3× 0.05 M TBS pH 7.6 + 0.05% Tween-20, 3× TBS and 2× double distilled water
- Transfer the grids to 2% aqueous uranyl acetate for 10 min in the dark.

Example

Double Immunogold Labelling for Detection of Endothelial Nitric Oxide Synthase (eNOS) and Caveolin-1

Caveolin-1/eNOS interaction is an excellent example of the usefulness of immunogold labelling for detection of dynamic alterations in molecular interaction.

Biochemical investigation showed that eNOS interacted directly with caveolin-1 in its inactive form in the resting endothelial cell (Ju et al. 1997) and was redistributed by adequate stimuli such as bradykinin treatment (Prabhakar et al. 1998). Thus, eNOS activation and NO release are supposed to be a competitive interaction between the inactive eNOS scaffolding caveolin and the metabolically active Ca^{2+}-calmodulin-NOS complex (Michel et al. 1997). To investigate the caveolin/eNOS interaction at the subcellular level a post-embedding method adapted from the low-temperature LR-White post-embedding method of Berryman and Rodewald (1990) was performed.

To investigate the interaction of caveolin and eNOS in unstimulated and stimulated isolated perfused rat hearts the following procedure was performed (Reiner et al. 2001)

Rat hearts were harvested from male Wistar rats (350–450 g) subjected to CO_2 anaesthesia and cervical dislocation. After 25 min of retrograde perfusion via the aorta according to the Langendorff technique, further perfusion was performed for 2 min with 10^{-7} M/l bradykinin (Sigma, St Louis, MO) or with normal solution for controls.

Hearts were perfusion-fixed with 4% formaldehyde and 0.2% picric acid in 0.1 M HEPES buffer (pH 7.3 +0.5 mM $CaCl_2$). After 10 min, hearts were stored in the same fixative at 4 °C for 4 h to 8 days.

After post-fixation, samples were taken from the heart's left ventricle. The following steps were carried out at 4 °C. Without washing out the fixative, specimens were directly immersed for 4 h in 0.1 M HEPES containing 3.5% sucrose w/v and 0.75% (v/v) tannic acid (from the stock solution) followed by buffer rinsing. Remaining free aldehydes were quenched for 1 hr with 50 mM NH_4Cl in HEPES/sucrose buffer at 4 °C, followed by rinsing. Next, samples were transferred to 0.05 M maleate/sucrose buffer (pH 6.0 + 0.5 mM $CaCl_2$, 3.5% sucrose w/v). En bloc staining was done at 4 °C in the same buffer with 1% uranyl acetate for 4 h.

During graded ethanolic dehydration (20 min steps), the temperature was lowered down to –20 °C at the stage of 70% ethanol. After an infiltration step of a 1:1 mixture of 100% ethanol and LR-White, and three changes with pure resin (60 min), samples were kept at –20 °C overnight. Then, samples were transferred to microtubes placed in a steel block in a heat sink. Pre-cooled LR-White was mixed with 15 µl LR-White catalyst per ml. The activated resin was placed in the cooled microtubes which were immediately sealed. After 12 h, microtubes were left at room temperature for a further 48 h. Thin sections with silver interference colour, cut on a Leica Ultracut UCT ultramicrotome were mounted on formvar coated nickel grids.

Immunolabelling was carried out "free-floating". After 15 min equilibration in 0.05 M TBS (pH 7.6), a 30 min blocking step using 3% defatted milk was performed. Polyclonal antibodies against caveolin-1 (Transduction Labs., Lexington, USA, 1:300, Cat.No C13630) or eNOS (Biomol, Hamburg, Germany, 1:250) were applied in TBS +1% defatted milk for 2 h at room temperature. After rinsing in TBS + 0.05% Tween-20, grids were incubated with secondary goat-anti-rabbit antibodies conjugated to 10 nm gold particles (Sigma, St Louis, MO) for 1 h in TBS/Tween-20.

After repetitive rinsing with TBS and distilled water, grids were transferred to 1% aqueous uranyl acetate and stained for 20 min.

For sequential double labelling, the immunoprocedure described above was carried out for eNOS. After a further blocking step with TBS +3% defatted milk to minimize artefactual cross-labelling, sections were incubated as for caveolin-1 antibodies and then coupled with 5 nm-gold-conjugated secondary antibodies.

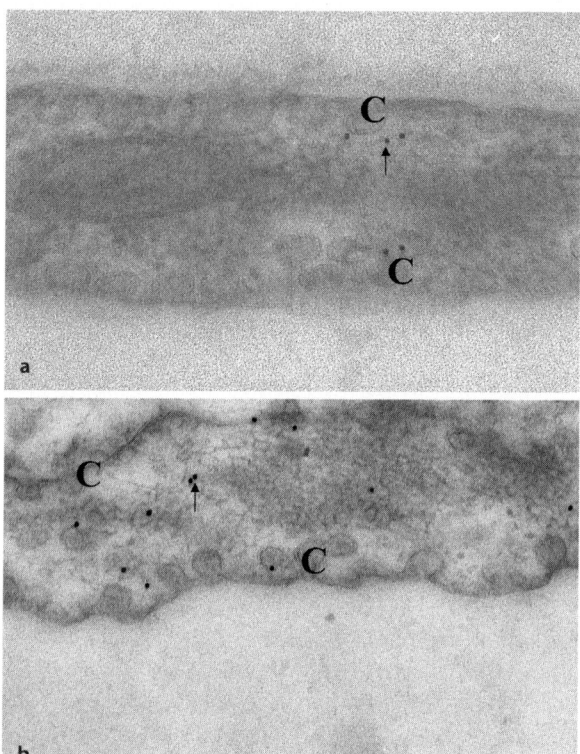

Figure 2a,b
eNOS immunogold labelling in isolated perfused rat hearts without (**a**) and with 2 min bradykinin treatment. **a** The 10 nm gold particles (*arrows*) are located adjacent to caveolae (C). **b** After 2 min bradykinin stimulation, the amount of detectable immunogold particles and their localization are greatly altered. Most gold particles are widely distributed in the cytoplasm, only some gold particles are adjacent to caveolae. Moreover the number of visible gold particles is increased (Bloch et al. 2001a; Reiner et al. 2001). Bar = 200 nm

Sections were observed with a Zeiss EM 902A electron microscope at 80 kV. Images of capillary endothelium were taken at ×85,000 magnification and analyzed with morphometric PC-software (Analysis, SIS, Münster, Germany). Endothelial cells from five randomly chosen capillaries of 2 control and 2 bradykinin-treated rat heart samples were evaluated. eNOS signals (10 nm) either co-localizing with caveolin-1 (5 nm) or isolated were counted and related to the cell area. Further, co-localized signals were investigated independently by measuring the distance between two gold particles.

The immunogold labelling procedure used allowed us to localize caveolin-1 and eNOS at caveolae and supported their tight co-localization under unstimulated conditions. Short-term bradykinin stimulation provoked a detectable dissociation of eNOS from caveolae/caveolin (Fig. 2) and its redistribution to different cell compartments, while caveolin itself remained stationary at caveolae. Morphometrical analysis revealed that more than 80% of detectable eNOS was co-localized with caveolin-1 at caveolae under control conditions. After brief stimulation for 2 min with 10^{-7} M bradykinin, only 26% of the eNOS signals were associated with caveolin-1 and were randomly distributed over the endothelial cells (see Fig. 2). After stimulation, eNOS was found at the plasmalemmal and intracellular membranes, freely in the cytoplasm and at outer mitochondrial membranes (Reiner et al. 2001).

Altogether the technique described allowed us to make observations regarding the subcellular distribution of eNOS and caveolin-1 using structural caveolae in cells of intact tissue as a reference landmark, providing an independent method of examining protein interaction besides the commonly used biochemical techniques (Reiner et al. 2001).

Troubleshooting

Problems Occurring During Conventional Electron Microscopy

Structural preservation is influenced by many aspects. Therefore problems leading to bad structural preservation can occur at different steps of the whole procedure, some of the common ones are highlighted in the following.

One of the main reasons for inadequate structural preservation is a poor fixation of the tissue. Observation of the mitochondria, nucleus and extracellular space can give information about such fixation problems. If mitochondria show dilated, misshapen cristae and there is distension of the space between the nuclear membranes and the presence of extracellular space, bad structural preservation has occurred.

Reasons for bad fixation are the time between acquisition of the material and fixation when post-mortem changes may have occurred (mostly if immersion fixation is used), wrong pH or osmolarity and quality of the fixative.

Insufficient polymerisation leading to soft blocks. Bad polymerisation can be caused by insufficient infiltration or polymerisation time as well as problems with the accelerator. Out of date accelerator is a common problem. To avoid soft blocks, the accelerator can be replaced, the infiltration time can be increased and/or the percentage of resin can be gradually increased during the infiltration.

If soft blocks are unsectionable, they must be reinfiltrated and embedded. Excess soft resin should be cut away from the tissue block and the block soaked in sodium ethoxide on a rotator for 24 h at RT. The tissue block is rinsed in four changes of ethanol, then infiltrated and embedded as usual.

The block may be unequally polymerised, especially the centre of the block may be insufficiently polymerised. This may happen in one block of a batch due to poor infiltration of that solitary block or it may happen in a complete batch of blocks. If it occurs in the whole batch of blocks, the reason could be bad dehydration. Small electron dense material found throughout the slices may be from lead citrate stain.

Check the tissue-free areas on the grid, where only support film or resin are found. If electron dense material is present, there is a staining problem, so repeat the staining procedure on unstained grids and take more care not to introduce CO_2 from breath. If absent, precipitates have been formed earlier from a contaminant in the fixative, osmium or buffer. In this case change the fixative, the osmium and the buffer.

Lastly problems can occur in the sectioning process e.g. sections will not cut, sections are lost after cutting, only a small part of the block is cut or the section is shattered or separated in small strips. In this case you can use the following checklist for solution of the problems:

- Check the knife angle
- Check the speed of the arm-drop
- Check the height of the water
- Check the glass or diamond knife for shattering
- Check if the size of the block surface is too big
- Check the position of the block
- Check the alignment of the block
- Check if the sides of the block are jagged

Main Problems Influencing a Successful Immunogold Staining

Besides the above problems in conventional electron microscopy, some specific problems can arise in ultrastructural immunolabelling, which lead either to lack of staining or unspecific and/or background staining.

A lack of labelling can occur from antigen destruction, masking or extraction. You should check the fixation and/or embedding procedures carefully and also compare with light microscopic immunostaining, and the results produced by using the pre-embedding procedure and the post-embedding technique with the antibody and tissue of choice.

A further problem could be that the primary antibody does not work. Causes of this problem may be a wrong dilution of the antibody or destroyed antibody. Therefore you can perform serial dilutions for ultrastructural immunohistochemistry and you can check the antibody used by light microscopic immunostaining. The amount of antigen available in the tissue may be too low.

You should calculate the amounts of antigen present if possible. Most often an estimation of antigen amounts can be obtained from biochemical experiments. If calculation indicates a sufficient antigen amount, increasing antigen accessibility by detergent treatment may help.

Gold particles present are not detectable. The reason could be the use of too low a magnification or too strong an image contrast. An increase in the magnification (30,000× is usual) or a reduction of specimen contrast can help.

The primary antibody leads to non-specific labelling. Suitable controls can reveal this problem. Adequate control experiments can be performed e.g. incubation in the absence of the primary antibody and incubation with antibodies from the same species as the primary antibody but which do not react with the cells or tissue under study. If background labelling is detected, treatment with additional blocking agents can be performed and/or treatment with primary amines, which quench any free aldehyde groups crosslinking antibodies, can be performed. High dilution of the antibody is also possible to reduce background.

Background can also be caused by blocking agents. You should try alternative blocking solutions.

Antigen migration could lead to the impression of background staining. This can occur if the antigen has not been properly immobilized by the fixation step, it may become redistributed throughout the cell. You should test and compare different fixation conditions (Webster 1999).

References

Berryman MA, Rodewald RD (1990) An enhanced method for post-embedding immunocytochemical staining which preserves cell membranes. J Histochem Cytochem 38:159–170

Bloch W, Forsberg E, Lentini S, Brakebusch C, Martin K, Krell HW, Weidle UH, Addicks K, Fässler R (1997) beta1 Integrin is essential for teratoma growth and angiogenesis. J Cell Biol. 139:265–278

Bloch W, Huggel K, Sasaki T, Grose R, Bugnon P, Addicks K, Timpl R, Werner S (2000) The angiogenesis inhibitor endostatin impairs blood vessel maturation during wound healing. FASEB J v10.1096/fj.00–0490fje

Bloch W, Mehlhorn U, Krahwinkel A, Reiner M, Dittrich M, Schmidt A, Addicks K (2001a) Ischemia increases detectable endothelial nitric oxide synthase in rat and human myocardium. Nitric Oxide 5:317–333

Bloch W, Fan Y, Han J, Xue S, Schöneberg T, Ji GJ, Zu ZJ, Walther M, Fässler M, Hescheler J, Addicks K, Fleischmann BK (2001) Disruption of cytoskeletal integrity impairs Gi-mediated signaling due to displacement of Gi-proteins. J Cell Biol 154:753–76

Brandtzaeg P (1982) Tissue preparation methods for immunohistochemistry. In: Bullock GR and Petrusz P (eds) Techniques in Immunhistochemistry, vol.1. Academic Press, New York, p 1–76

Brorson SH (1996) Improved immunogold labeling of epoxy sections by the use of propylene oxide as additional agent in dehdyration, infiltration and embedding. Micron 27:345–353

Brorson SH, Skjorten F (1996) Improved technique for immunoelectron microscopy. How to prepare epoxy resin to obtain approximately the same immunogold labeling for epoxy sections as for acrylic sections without any etching. Micron 27:211–217

Brorson SH, Roos N, Skjørten F (1994) Antibody penetration into LR-White sections. Micron 25:453–460

Côté SL, Riberio-Da-Silva A, and Cuello AC (1993) Current protocols for light microscopy immunohistochemistry. In: Cuello AC (ed) Immunohistochemistry II. John Wiley & Sons, New York, p 148–167

Costell M, Gustafsson E, Aszodi A, Mörgelin M, Bloch W, Hunziker E, Addicks K, Timpl R, Fässler R (1999) Perlecan maintains the integrity of cartilage and some basement membranes. J Cell Biol 147:1109–1122

Davies HA (1999) General preparation of material and staining of sections. Methods Mol Biol 117:1–11

Hsu S-M (1993) The use of the avidin-biotin interaction in immunohistochemistry. In: Cuello AC (ed) Immunohistochemistry II. John Wiley & Sons, New York, p 169–179

Ju H, Zou R, Venema VJ, Venema RC (1997) Direct interaction of endothelial nitric-oxide synthase and caveolin-1 inhibits synthase activity. J Biol Chem 272:18522–18525

Kostka G, Giltay R, Bloch W, Addicks K, Timpl R, Fässler R, Chu ML (2001) Perinatal lethality and endothelial cell abnormalities in several vessel compartments of fibulin-1 deficient mice. Mol Cell Biol 21:7025–7034

Mehlhorn U (1997) Improved myocardial protection using continuous coronary perfusion with normothermic blood and b-blockade with esmolol. Thorac Cardiovasc Surg 45:224–231

Michel JB, Feron O, Sacks D, Michel T (1997) Reciprocal regulation of endothelial nitric-oxide synthase by Ca^{2+}-calmodulin and caveolin. J Biol Chem 272:15583–15586

Oliver C, Jamur MC (1999) Fixation and embedding. Methods of Molecular Biology. 115:319–326

Prabhakar P, Thatte HS, Goetz RM, Cho MR, Golan DE, Michel T (1998) Receptor-regulated translocation of endothelial nitric-oxide synthase. J Biol Chem 273:27383–27388

Reiner M (2002) Caveolen des kontinuierlichen Kapillarendothels. Die Anwendung eines weiterentwickelten Verfahren der hochauflösenden Immunoelektronenmikroskopie. Dissertation, Medizinische Fakultät der Universität zu Köln

Reiner M, Bloch W, Addicks K (2001) Functional interaction of caveolin-1 and eNOS in myocardial capillary endothelium revealed by immunoelectron microscopy. J Histochem Cytochem 49:1605–1609

Riberio-Da-Silva A, Priestley JV, and Cuello AC (1993) Pre-embedding Ultrastructural Immunocytochemistry. In: Cuello AC (ed) Immunohistochemistry II. John Wiley & Sons, New York, p 182–222

Richardson K (1960) Studies on the structure of autonomic nerves in small intestine, correlating the silver impregnated image in light microscopy with permanganate-fixed ultrastructure in electron microscopy. J Anat 94:457–472

Roell W, Lu ZJ, Bloch W et al. (2002) Cellular cardiomyoplasty improves survival after myocardial injury. Circulation 105:2433–2439

Webster P (1999) The production of cryosections through fixed and cryoprotected biological material and their use in immunohistochemistry. Methods Mol Biol 117:49–76

Appendix

Commercial Embedding Method for Electron Microscopy

- After fixation wash the samples in buffer (pH 7.2–7.3) for 3×15 min.
- 2% osmium tetroxide solution in 0.1 M buffer for 4 h.
- Wash samples in buffer for 3×15 min.

- 15 min   50% ethanol
- 15 min   70% ethanol**
- 15 min   90% ethanol
- 15 min   96% ethanol
- 3×20 min   100% ethanol

**Incubate the samples in 1% uranyl acetate in 70% ethanol, overnight in dark conditions.
- Incubate the samples in propylene oxide:100% ethanol (1:1) for 15 min.
- Incubate the samples in propylene oxide for 2×20 min.
- Treat the tissues with Araldite:propylene oxide (1:1) for 2–12 h.
- Treat the samples with Araldite:propylene oxide (3:1) for 4–24 h.
- Incubate the samples in Araldite (100%).
- Evaporate the propylene oxide for 2 h in an incubator at 40 °C.
- Embed the samples in Beem capsules
- Cure the Araldite blocks at 45 °C in incubator for 12 h.
- Cure the Araldite blocks at 60 °C in incubator for 48 h.

LR-White Embedding for Post-Embedding Immunohistochemistry

Exothermic Method

The samples are directly bloc contrasted in 0.75% tannic acid for 4 h at RT.
- Dehydration of samples:
    - 20 min ice-cold   50% ethanol at –18 °C.
    - 20 min ice-cold   70% ethanol at –18 °C.
    - 20 min ice-cold   90% ethanol at –18 °C.
    - 20 min ice-cold   100% ethanol at –18 °C.
- Treat the samples in ice-cold LR-White: ethanol (1:1) for 20 min at –18 °C.
- Treat the samples in fresh LR-White for 1 h at –18 °C.
- Treat the samples in fresh LR-White overnight at –18 °C.
- Treat the samples in fresh LR-White for 1 h at –18 °C.
- Transfer the samples to gelatine capsules, fill the capsules with 100% LR-White and cap. Oxygen will inhibit polymerization.
- Polymerize at 56 °C for 24 h.

Modified Method for Immunogold Labelling of Ultrathin Sections

- Incubate the grids in 3% defatted milk diluted in 0.05 M TBS pH 7.6 for 30 min
- Incubate the primary antibodies (normally polyclonal rabbit antibodies are used) diluted in 0.05 M TBS pH 7.6 containing 0.3% defatted milk for 2 h at RT or at 4 °C overnight in a humidity chamber
- Wash the grids in 0.05 M TBS containing 0.05% Tween-20 four times

- Incubate the grids with secondary antibody, i.e. an IgG against the host of the primary antibody conjugated to 10 nm gold particles, diluted in 0.05 M TBS containing 0.05% Tween-20 for 1 h
- Wash the grids with 3× 0.05 M TBS pH 7.6 + 0.05% Tween-20, 3× TBS and 2× double distilled water.
- Transfer the grids to 2% aqueous uranyl acetate for 10 min in the dark.

DAF Technique for Real-Time NO Imaging in the Human Myocardium

Dirk Steinritz and Wilhelm Bloch

Introduction

Nitric oxide (NO), synthesized from L-arginine by NO-synthases (NOS), is involved in the regulation of many physiological and pathophysiological mechanisms in nearly every organ system. Many of the proposed NO mediated-functions are controversially discussed because direct evidence for the involvement of NO is missing. One reason is the difficulty of NO detection. NO is a gaseous small, hydrophobic molecule with chemical properties that allow it to act as an intra- or extra-cellular messenger. Furthermore NO has a very labile nature. It exists only for a few seconds (3–10 s) before it is converted by O_2 and H_2O into NO_2^- and NO_3^- or it reacts with oxygen radicals to form peroxynitrite. Before NO is eliminated it affects several target structures, e.g. soluble guanyl cyclase (sGC), ion channels and other intracellular proteins. Commonly NO reacts within cell signalling cascades and the NO signal gets amplified during this process. This implies that only a very small amount of NO is necessary to affect the target structures. This circumstance is a further problem of NO detection. Several methods such as chemiluminescence assays, electron paramagnetic resonance spectroscopy or NO measurement with electrochemical electrodes have been developed to detect NO. But these detection methods are limited because of their relatively low sensitivity on the one hand and their low spatial resolution on the other hand. The investigator receives little information about the actual NO-producing cell type. For the development of a fluorescence-based NO detection system, a reaction is needed in which NO is directly and specifically involved. NO has only little reactivity with organic molecules and furthermore the formation of a nitro-group leads to elimination of fluorescence. The fluorescence detection of intracellular NO by using 2,7-dichlorofluorescein has been reported. Unfortunately, this dye is not able to distinguish between NO and reactive oxygen species (ROS) and the detection limit of NO is rather high (~16 µM). In 1998, Kojima et al. (1998a) developed a new method, based on fluorescein chromophores, that specifically detects NO under physiological conditions in living cells such as vascular smooth muscle cells or endothelial cells. Different diaminofluoresceins (DAFs) have been developed for NO imaging in specific experimental setups. After NO imaging in living cells had been established, DAFs were also used to evaluate NO production in tissue slices. Kojima et al. (1998b) used DAF-2 DA to show NO production in hippocampal and cortical slices. In 1999, Brown et al. followed with imaging NO-producing neurons in slices of rat brain with imaging and in 2000 followed with imaging NO production in neuronal varicosities in hippocampal slices.

Description of the Methods and Practical Approach

Principally two sorts of DAFs can be distinguished. The first sort of DAF, DAF DA (diacetate) is able to diffuse into the living cell, where it gets hydrolyzed by nonspecific esterases and is trapped within the cell (Fig. 1). The NO formation is measured intracellularly. This setup is useful to obtain information about the actual cell type that produces NO in the tissue. The other sort of DAF (the non-esterified form) is unable to cross cell membranes. This DAF is only able to react with NO outside the cell and the NO formation is determined in the supernatant. This setup is useful if there is only one single cell type that produces NO, and the investigator has not to differentiate between different NO sources. The following instructions focus on DAF FM DA that is used for intracellular NO imaging. DAFs react specifically with NO which leads to the formation of an intensively green fluorescent triazole (DAF-T) (Fig. 1). Kojima et al. (1998a) reported no interaction with other nitrogen species such as NO_2^- NO_3^- or ROS, including the $ONOO^-$ that is built by the reaction between oxygen radicals and NO. The DAFs do not directly react with NO, but they do react with NO^+ equivalents such as N_2O_3, that is produced during auto-oxidation of NO. For this auto-oxidation, oxygen is required as a co-factor. It becomes obvious that the formation of N_2O_3 is possible only under aerobic conditions. If oxygen is available, DAFs are able to react with NO and form the strongly fluorescent triazole-fluoresceins (DAF-T) (see Fig. 1). In the absence of nitric oxide, no DAF-Ts are formed. Therefore DAF-imaging is a very potent tool for measuring nitric oxide in living tissues. Whereas the fluorescence signal of older DAF types was dependent on intracellular pH values, the improved DAF FM is independent of the pH value. We used DAF FM DA, a DAF of the newest generation, which is not dependent on cellular pH values. Normally cells have to load DAF

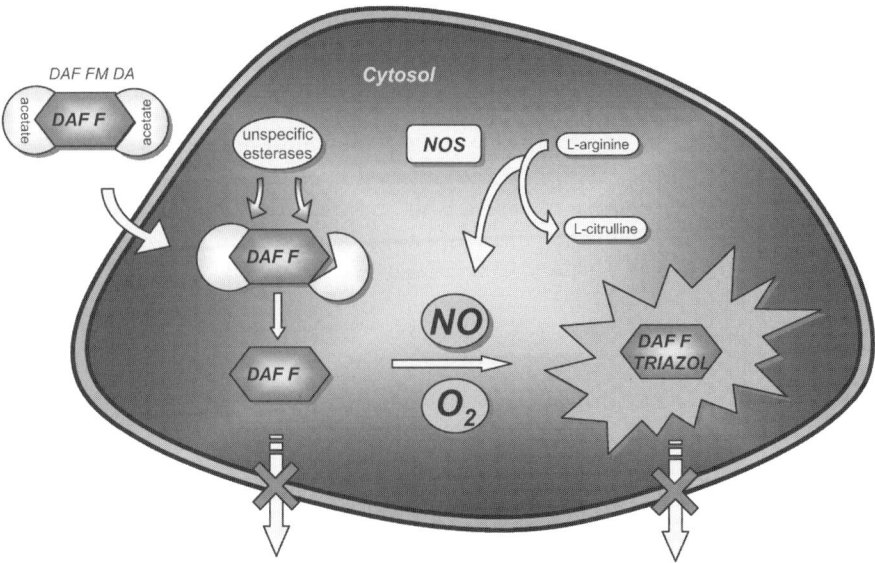

Figure 1
Reactions of DAF FM DA within intact cells. DAF and DAF-T are trapped within cell boundaries

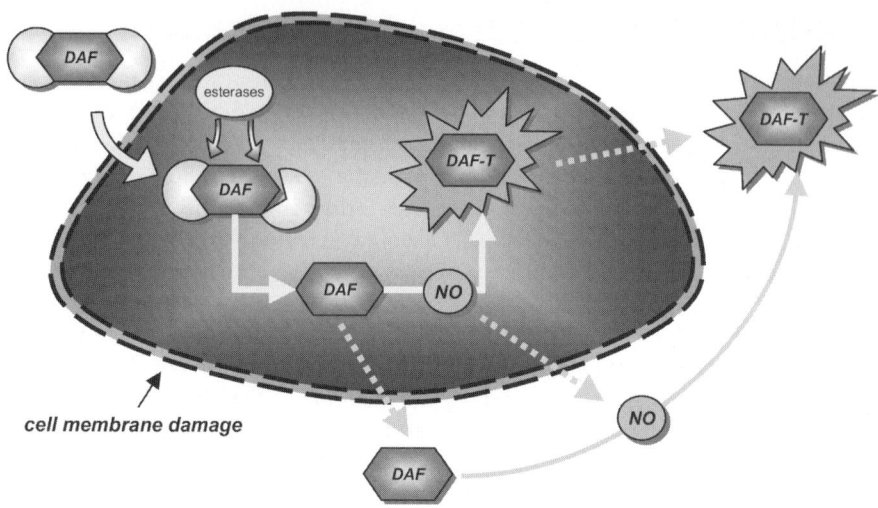

Figure 2
Reactions of DAF FM DA within cells with membrane damage. DAF, NO and DAF-T can diffuse out of the cell (yellow pointed arrows), the fluorescent signal can also be found outside the cell

DA for up to 60 min. During this loading time DAF DA is converted into a highly water-soluble DAF that is unable to cross cell membranes and is therefore trapped within the cell. After this loading process, the cells are washed and the experiment is started. This is practical for cells with intact cell membranes. If the cell membrane is damaged, the converted DAF is able to diffuse out of the cell. This implies that the converted DAF DA can also react with NO outside the cell due to the cell membrane damage and also that the formed DAF-T is able to diffuse out of the cell. The fluorescence signal does not stay within the cell boundaries (Fig. 2). During tissue freezing the cell membrane gets damaged, even if the freezing is done under cryo-protection. Furthermore during the tissue slicing process the upper and lower cell layers are cut and their cell membrane is damaged. If the cells are washed then, most of the converted DAF is washed out of the cells and the DAF concentration is too low for NO imaging. For investigating cryo-protected tissue slices it is better not to wash the tissue after DAF has been added, but to start imaging the cells with the addition of the DAF.

Tyrode Solution

The experiments are performed in a Tyrode solution containing:
- $CaCl_2 \times 2H_2O$ 1.8 mM (M=147.02 g/mol)
- $MgCl_2 \times 6H_2O$ 1.1 mM (M=203.30 g/mol)
- KCl 5.4 mM (M=74.56 g/mol)
- $NaCl$ 136.9 mM (M=58.44 g/mol)
- NaH_2PO_4 0.4 mM (M=137.99 g/mol)
- Glucose 10.1 mM (M=198.17 g/mol)

- NaHCO$_3$ 23.8 mM (M=84.01 g/mol)
- L-arginine 1.0 mM (M=174.1 g/mol)

If experiments are performed at room temperature, the solution is kept at 25 °C. If experiments are performed at 37 °C the solution should also be stored at this temperature.

Technical Equipment

For the experiments either an inverse fluorescence microscope or a normal fluorescence microscope is required. The maximum excitation wavelength is 500 nm and the maximum for emission is 515 nm. Time-lapse software for taking the images at pre-defined time-points is useful.

Analyzing software (e.g. ImageJ; website: http://rsb.info.nih.gov/ij/) is needed to evaluate the fluorescence signal.

General Tissue Preparation

The tissue must be frozen after sampling. Therefore a Wollenberger clamp is stored in liquid nitrogen. The tissue is placed within the clamp for a few seconds and then put in liquid nitrogen itself and stored at –80 °C. Other rapid freezing techniques can also be used. For experiments the tissue is allowed to equilibrate for 1 h at –20 °C. Then cryosections of 15 to 25 µm are made depending on the tissue's frangibility. In our experiments we used 20 µm sections.

Tissue Preparations for Experiments using an Inverse Microscope

The still frozen tissue slice is placed on a glass slide that is suitable for inverse microscopy, at a temperature of –20 °C. The investigator has to cover the slice with a mesh that fits into the glass slide to fix the tissue to the bottom of the slide. Be certain that the mesh does not interfere the experiments. The mesh must not have auto-fluorescence. Furthermore the mesh pores must have a diameter which allows oxygen to reach the tissue. A predefined volume of Tyrode solution is added carefully. The experiment starts by adding DAF FM DA to the slide.

Tissue Preparations for Experiments using a Normal Microscope

A 15% gelatine solution is prepared and stored at 60 °C. A slide with no auto-fluorescence is coated thinly with this 15% gelatine. The coated slide can be stored at 37 °C for up to 1 h. The still frozen cryo-section is placed on to the slide that has just been taken out of the 37 °C incubator. The tissue will attach to the surface of the slide when it touches it. Immediately a predefined volume (e.g. 1 ml) of Tyrode solution must be added so the slice cannot dry out. The tissue stays attached to the surface for at least 15 min. If experiments will take longer, the investigator has to cover the slice with a mesh to prevent movement. But the mesh pores must have a diameter which allows oxygen to reach the tissue. The experiment starts by adding DAF FM DA to the slide.

Starting the Experiment by Adding DAF FM DA

To start the NO measurement DAF FM DA is added to the slide. The final DAF concentration should be 10 µM. To reach this concentration 1 ml of undiluted DAF has to be added to 500 µl solution. After adding DAF, the solution must be carefully mixed to prevent the DAF being highly concentrated in one area ("hot spot" of DAF) of the solution. Experiments should be undertaken for 10–15 min.

Controls

Control experiments are done with a NO inhibitor, e.g. L-NAME (100 µM), and a NO donor, e.g. DETA-NONOate (10 mm). For data references a control condition is needed where only DAF is admitted to the Tyrode solution.

Densitometry

In order to evaluate the changes in fluorescence during DAF experiments computer-based densitometry is useful. There are two possibilities to evaluate the data. On the one hand the received DAF value at time point t=0 min is taken as the starting value and is set as 100%. The following values are related to the starting value. By using this way of evaluating it is possible to demonstrate endogenous NO production. On the other hand if each DAF value from each time point from the control experiment is set as 100%, the NO production under stimulation becomes more clearly visible.

Examples

We measured the real-time NO production in human atrial myocardium after stimulation of the β3-adrenoceptors (β3-AR) with the preferential β3-adrenoceptor agonist BRL 37344. Moniotte et al. showed the protein expression of β3-AR in human cardiac tissue. Gauthier et al reported a decrease in the force of contraction (FOC) in the human heart due to β3-AR stimulation and these effects could not be observed while NO antagonists were used. This has led to the suggestion that the decrease of FOC *via* stimulation of β3-AR is NO-dependent.

We used DAF-FM DA to detect changes in NO level induced by BRL. Therefore right atrial myocardial tissue was collected from patients suffering from coronary heart disease or valvular disease during sternotomy. Immediately after excision the

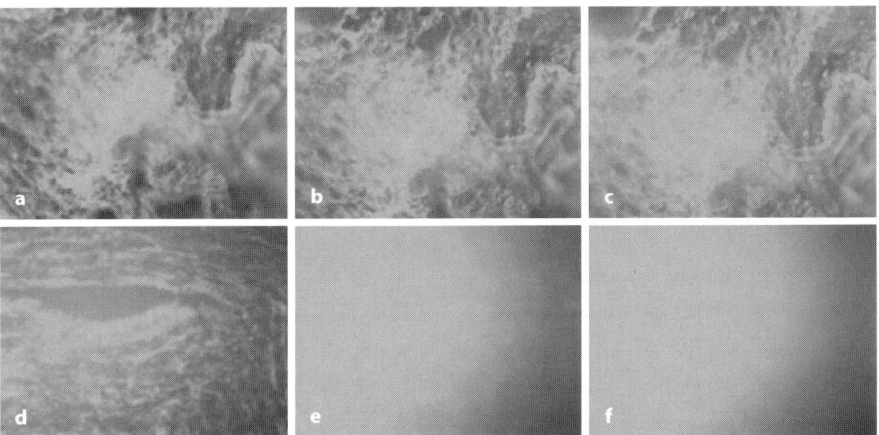

Figure 3a-f
A-C DAF control experiment with left atrial myocardium (A=0min, B=5 min, C=10 min). D-F BRL experiment (A=0 min, B=5 min, C=10 min). A distinct increase in the fluorescence signal with BRL can be observed whereas almost no increase can be detected during control conditions. *For coloured version see appendix*

tissue was placed in ice-cold cardioplegic solution. It was then shock-frozen in liquid nitrogen by using the Wollenberger clamp as described above and was stored at −80 °C. For experiments the tissue was equilibrated at −20 °C for at least 1 h and sliced to 25 mM thickness. Slices were fixed to a plastic slide (diameter 2 cm) which had been coated with 15% gelatine. 1 ml Tyrode solution was added immediately. For measurements DAF (10 µM), BRL (10 mM), NONOate (10 µM) and L-NAME (100 µM) were added for the relevant experiment The intensity of DAF-FM fluorescence was then measured every 10 s over 10 min. The intensity of DAF-FM fluorescence in the absence of the transmitters listed above was set as the 100% reference value for each time point. The effects of BRL and of BRL + L-NAME on the NO-level were then investigated in relation to the DAF-FM fluorescence intensity. For negative and positive controls we repeated experiments with L-NAME or the NO donor NONOate instead of BRL. Compared to control conditions (Fig. 3a-c) the NO detection significantly increased during 10 min in the presence of BRL (Fig. 3d-f). This increase in NO release could be blocked by the NO antagonist L-NAME. One single measurement is shown in Fig. 4. As reference point, the DAF fluorescence signal from the control condition (only with DAF and without any transmitters) at time point t=0 s has been chosen. It becomes obvious that there is an endogenous NO production (Fig. 4, green), and L-NAME is able to block this NO release (Fig. 4, red). As a positive control we used the NO donor DETA-NONOate (NOC-18) that releases NO spontaneously (t1/2=1200 min). We showed a slow, but distinct increase in DAF-T fluorescence (Fig. 4, blue). Finally BRL led to a 10-fold increase in NO production within 10 min (Fig. 4, yellow). This was partial blocked by L-NAME (Fig. 4, purple). Summarizing our results we were able to demonstrate that BRL leads to a significant increase in NO production compared to control conditions (Fig. 5). Surprisingly the starting points of control conditions and BRL conditions were not identical. By the use of trend lines

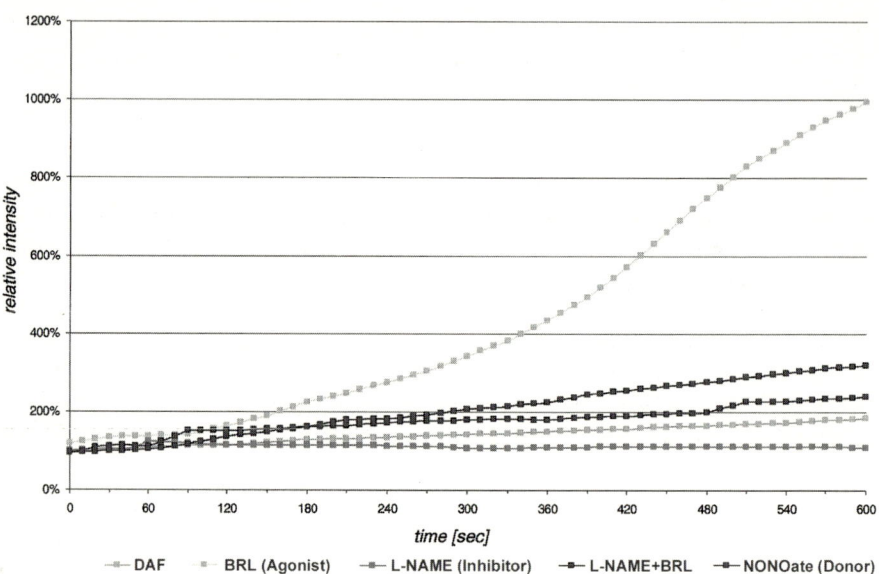

Figure 4
Results from one single experiment. The change in fluorescence intensity under different experimental conditions is shown. A 10-fold increase with BRL can be shown. *For coloured version see appendix*

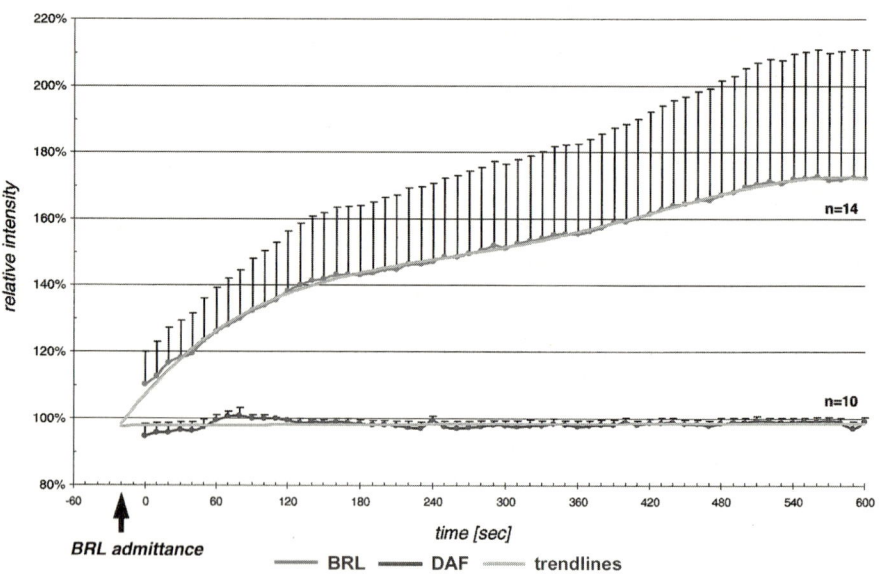

Figure 5
Results from all experiments. There is an significant increase in the fluorescence signal with BRL (BRL: *red curve*) compared to control conditions (DAF: *blue curve*). Trend lines are added (*green curves*). The probably time point of BRL addition is also shown (*black arrow*). *For coloured version see appendix*

(Fig. 5, green) we could calculate that the starting point of the BRL conditions was localized about 20 s before starting the imaging process. This can be explained by the time the investigator has to spend adding the DAF to the Tyrode solution and focussing the tissue slice. During our experiments we had to manage diverse problems. Our main problem was the fixation of our tissue slices to the glass slide. Sometimes the gelatine coating was too thick so the tissue slice was embedded into the gelatine and during observation we were not able to detect a change in the fluorescence signal. One other problem was that with raised temperatures the gelatine stayed liquid and the slice was not fixed to the plastic slide. Hard movements or vibrations were able to dislodge the slice from the surface. Sometimes the slice became loose after the observation had been started. These experiments are hard to evaluate because the slice can get out of focus during the observation and the fluorescence signal is strongly influenced if the tissue changes focus. Other problems that occurred are discussed in Troubleshooting.

Troubleshooting

Errors During Tissue Preparation

The time from taking the tissue to freezing may take too long. Avoid long-term preparation. After tissue is frozen, store it as soon as possible in liquid nitrogen. If this procedure takes too long you will possibly receive only a little fluorescent signal during the experiment, due to tissue damage at the beginning.

If the tissue is placed into liquid nitrogen directly without using the Wollenberger clamp, or if the time the Wollenberger clamp is used is too short, the tissue might suffer serious membrane damage. The fluorescent signal will not stay within the cell boundaries.

The Wollenberger clamp itself has to be stored in liquid nitrogen before the tissue can be placed in the clamp. The clamp has to reach the low temperature of liquid nitrogen. This will take some minutes. So be sure to put the clamp into the nitrogen early enough.

The tissue must equilibrate at –20 °C for at least 1 h. If the equilibration time is too short the slicing process becomes quite difficult due to the tissue's very low temperature.

After the tissue slice has been put on to the slide be sure that it cannot dry out. To avoid this, Tyrode solution has to be added immediately. If this takes too long, the slice may dry out and the investigator receives almost no fluorescence signal during the experiment.

The scale should be coated with 15% gelatine as thinly as possible. If too much volume of gelatine is used, the slice may be embedded within the gelatine. If so, no reaction can take place and the investigator will not detect a change in the fluorescence signal.

After adding the Tyrode solution the slice may not stay attached to the slide. One reason can be that the gelatine on the slide has become too cold and does not function as a glue. The tissue slice must be added immediately after taking the coated slide out of the 37 °C incubator The investigator has to take care that the slice is not embedded. If the surrounding temperature is too high, the gelatine will stay liquid and there is no glue effect at all. Try to lower the (room) temperature or use a mesh if you want to keep the temperature high.

Errors During Observation

If just after adding DAF there is a very intense diffuse green fluorescent signal over just one small area, the DAF is probably not very well dispersed in the solution. As a result the investigator focuses on an area which contains very highly concentrated DAF ("hot spot" of DAF). To avoid this, be sure that the DAF is well distributed in the Tyrode solution.

There may be no signal at all or the signal does not change even if a NO donor is used. We have some suggestions for this occurrence. One reason could be a non-optimal DAF concentration. The DAF concentration should be about 10 µM depending on the sensitivity of the detection system. Another reason could be that no oxygen is available. Do not cover the tissue slice completely (e.g. with glass) otherwise oxygen is not able to reach the cells and the reaction cannot take place.

If during observation the slice swims in the solution, try to use a mesh to prevent movement. But be certain that the mesh pores are big enough to allow oxygen to reach the tissue. The best technique is to use a ring to cover the tissue at the edges and observe the tissue through the central hole.

References

Broillet MC, Randin O, Chatton JY (2001) Photoactivation and calcium sensitivity of the fluorescent NO indicator 4,5-diaminofluorescein (DAF-2): implications for cellular NO imaging. FEBS Letters 491:227–232

Brown LA, Key BJ, Lovick TA (2000) Fluorescent imaging of nitric oxide production in neuronal varicosities associated with intraparenchymal arterioles in rat hippocampal slices. Neurosci Lett 294:9–12

Brown LA, Key BJ, Lovick TA (1999) Bio-imaging of nitric oxide-producing neurons in slices of rat brain using 4,5-diaminofluorescein. J Neurosci Meth 92:101–110

Itoh Y, Ma FH, Hoshi H et al.(2000) Determination and Bioimaging Method for Nitric Oxide in Biological Specimens by Diamnofluorescein Fluorometry. Anal. Chem. 287:203–209

Kojima H, Nakatsubo N, Kikuchi K et al. (1998a) Detection and Imaging of Nitric Oxide with Novel Fluorescent Indicators: Diaminofluorsceins. Anal. Chem. 70: 2446–2453

Kojima H, Nakatsubo N, Kikuchi K et al (1998b) Direct evidence of NO production in rat hippocampus and cortex using a new fluorescent indicator: DAF-2 DA. NeuroReport 9:3345–3348,

Leikert JF, Rathel TR, Muller C et al (2001) Reliable *in vitro* measurement of nitric oxide released from endothelial cells using low concentrations of the fluorescent probe 4,5-diaminofluorescein. FEBS Letters 506:131–134

Nagano T (1999) Practical methods for detection of nitric oxide. Luminescence 14:283–290

Pott C, Brixius K, Bundkirchen A et al (2003) The preferential b3-adrenoceptor agonist BRL 37344 increases force via b1-/b2-adrenoceptors and induces endothelial nitric oxide synthase via b3-adrenoceptors in human atrial myocardium. Brit J Pharmacol 138:521–529

Sugimoto K, Fujii S, Takemasa T et al (2000) Detection of intralcellular nitric oxide using a combination of aldehyde fixatives with 4,5-diaminofluorescein diacetate. Histochem Cell Biol 113:341–347

Suzuki N, Kojima, Urano Y et al (2002) Orthogonality of Calcium Concentration and Ability of 4,5-Diaminofluorescein to Detect NO. JBC 277(1):47–49

5 Cell Culture Techniques

5.1 Isolation and Culture of Adult Ventricular
Cardiomyocytes — 557
Klaus-Dieter Schlüter and Hans Michael Piper

5.2 Culture of Neonatal Cardiomyocytes — 568
Aida Salameh and Stefan Dhein

5.3 Culture of Embryoid Bodies — 577
*Cornelia Gissel, Dirk Nierhoff, Bernd Fleischmann,
Jürgen Hescheler and Agapios Sachinidis*

5.4 Culturing and Differentiation of Embryonic
and Adult Stem Cells for Heart Research
and Transplantation Therapy — 592
Marcel A.G. van der Heyden and Henk Rozemuller

5.5 Preparation of Endothelial Cells from Micro-
and Macrovascular Origin — 610
Saskia C. Peters, Anna Reis and Thomas Noll

5.6 In Vitro Cultivation of Vascular Smooth
Muscle Cells — 630
Daniel G. Sedding and Ruediger C. Braun-Dullaeus

5.7 Engineering Heart Tissue for In Vitro
and In Vivo Studies — 640
*Wolfram-Hubertus Zimmermann, Ivan Melnychenko,
Michael Didié, Ali El-Armouche and Thomas Eschenhagen*

Isolation and Culture of Adult Ventricular Cardiomyocytes

Klaus-Dieter Schlüter and Hans Michael Piper

Introduction

The current understanding of the physiological and pathophysiological behaviour of the heart depends on the general features of the interaction of different cell types and the knowledge of the functional behaviour of individual cells. Any analysis of the functional characteristics of ventricular cardiomyocytes with regard to size control, contractility, and biochemical or molecular properties requires the isolation of functionally and morphologically intact cells. This has been a challenge for many years due to the fact that adult ventricular cardiomyocytes are fully differentiated and do not grow by cell division. Techniques for the isolation of cardiomyocytes have been difficult to establish, because the heart muscle cells are firmly connected to each other by intercalated discs and the extracellular matrix network and these connections are difficult to cleave without injuring the cells.

The success of any experiments performed on a single cell basis with adult ventricular cardiomyocytes depends on the number of cells isolated from the heart, their purification from other cardiac cell types and the ability to maintain their main characteristics for a reasonable length of time. Normally, cells are cultured for days or weeks to perform experiments requiring long-term exposure of the cells. Although a certain set of experiments can be performed with small cell numbers, i.e. microscopic observations like the analysis of cell contraction or experiments linked to electrophysiological questions, one remaining question will always be whether the cells under investigation represent the normal behaviour of a typical cell. Thus, even in these cases it should always be an aim to isolate large cell numbers and use randomly selected cells. In general, the challenge of isolating adult ventricular cardiomyocytes can be subdivided in two problems; how can we isolate great numbers of calcium-tolerant rod-shaped physiologically intact cells and how can we keep these cells in culture allowing them to maintain their specific characters? The following chapter will give examples as to how these problems can be solved and thus make isolated ventricular cardiomyocytes a suitable model for the study of basic cardiac function.

Description of Methods and Practical Approach
Isolation of Cells from Hearts

The rat heart is still the most commonly used model for isolation of ventricular cardiomyocytes for two reasons. First, the size of the heart fits easily into commercially available perfusion systems, it is more or less easy to handle, the animal itself is not expensive and the isolation normally gives reasonable cell numbers that can be used within the next day. Second, the rat is the most commonly used animal model in cardiac biology. Therefore, any data acquired at the single cell level can be compared to a broad field of data available in the literature. Finally, myocytes from *in vivo* variations, i.e. spontaneously hypertensive rats, genetically modified rats, or rats receiving surgery before use, can also be investigated. In general, ventricular cardiomyocytes can also be isolated from the hearts of other species. However, the protocol has to be modified slightly for the mouse as explained later. For the reasons explained above, we will first describe the isolation of ventricular cardiomyocytes from rat heart.

General Features of Isolation

The isolation of ventricular cardiomyocytes from adult rat hearts is performed in several steps. In general, the heart is quickly removed from the animal, connective tissue trimmed away and the heart connected to a Langendorff perfusion system and perfused retrogradely with a buffer to remove any blood. The whole heart is then treated with collagenase for a certain length of time in the absence of exogenous calcium. This step allows firstly the disruption of connections of individual cells with the extracellular network and secondly the dissociation of Ca^{2+}-dependent desmosome structures. Thereafter, the heart is removed from the perfusion system and the ventricle cut from the rest of the heart and minced into small pieces. These are further treated with collagenase, and the isolated cells separated from the larger tissue pieces by filtration through a nylon mesh (mesh size 200 µm). The isolated cells can then be re-exposed to physiological calcium concentrations by increasing the calcium concentrations stepwise and separated from non-cardiomyocytes by centrifugation. Figure 1 summarizes these steps. The final cell pellet can be re-suspended in cell culture medium (see below) and cultured. The following description is suitable for male normotensive rats (300–400 g).

Preparation of the Heart

To remove the heart, animals must be anaesthetized. There are no specific methods known to influence the final outcome of the preparation. Thus, we do not recommend a specific method for anaesthetizing the animals. The thorax should be opened, flooded with ice-cold physiological NaCl (0.9% wt/vol) solution, and the heart removed from the thorax, beginning to cut from the back of the heart. The heart should be removed with parts of the lung and transferred into a Petri dish filled with ice-cold physiological NaCl solution. The adhering lung tissue can now be removed and the

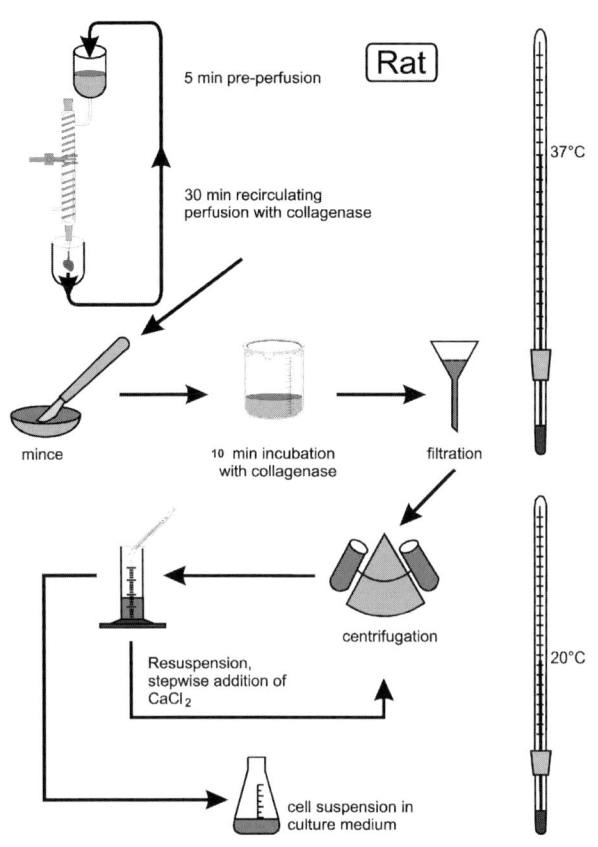

Figure 1
Schematic drawing of the isolation procedure described in the text for isolation of adult ventricular cardiomyocytes from rats. The heart is adjusted in the Langendorff perfusion system and perfused for approximately 30 min with collagenase. Then the ventricle is separated from the atrium and minced. A second collagenase treatment is performed before filtration. Finally, cardiomyocytes are separated by centrifugation from non-myocytes and the cell pellet is re-exposed to physiological calcium concentrations

aorta cut after the first aortic arch. The heart can then be connected by the aorta to a Langendorff perfusion system. It is important to perform these steps quickly. In order to avoid blood thrombosis during the time the heart is not perfused, the animals can receive heparin with the anaesthetics. People without experience of Langendorff preparations should practise these techniques before attempting the next steps.

Perfusion of the Heart

The perfusion should be started first (1 drop per second) and then the aorta should be connected to the system. With the heart immersed in saline, open the aortic lumen with two pairs of forceps, lift the heart to the cannula, slip the aorta over the cannula, and fix the aorta with crocodile clamps. Do not insert the cannula too deeply into the heart to ensure that perfusion *via* the coronary vessels is possible. Once the heart is well perfused, fix the heart to the perfusion system with thread. Continue to perfuse the heart with oxygenated perfusion buffer for 3–5 min to remove blood from the organ. Then add collagenase to the system and continue perfusion for 20 min. When necessary, readjust the perfusion to approximately 10 ml per minute.

Perfusion buffer (Powell medium):
- NaCl 110.0 mmol/l
- KCl 2.6 mmol/l
- KH_2PO_4 1.2 mmol/l
- $MgSO_4$ 1.2 mmol/l
- $NaHCO$ 25.0 mmol/l
- Glucose 5.0 mmol/l

Collagenase buffer
- Perfusion buffer
- add Collagenase 400.0 mg/l

All buffers are constantly bubbled with carbogen (95% O_2/5% CO_2).

Collagenase is not a specific term and the amount of collagenase added to the buffer as well as the time to perfuse a heart are not fixed criteria. They depend on the specific quality of the collagenase. It is impossible to give any specific recommendation for collagenase treatment. The best way to start is to test several batches from different distributors and modify the amount of collagenase and the time suggested for perfusion moderately.

Post-Perfusion Digestion

The collagenase treatment should be stopped when the hearts are smooth. Please note, that the physical behaviour of the heart itself is more important than the time you have perfused the heart. The latter depends on the activity and quality of the collagenase. Then cut the ventricle from the atrium and aorta and transfer the ventricles to a separate glass dish. Cut the heart carefully using a scalpel or, as recommended, a tissue chopper that can be used at a width of 0.7 mm to produce a cell suspension. Put this suspension into a Teflon-coated glass container and add more collagenase buffer as used before, plus 400 mg bovine serum albumin per 30 ml. Bubble with carbogen for the next 10 min. You can improve the success of the post-perfusion digestion by pipetting the solution moderately several times.

Separation of Myocytes from non-Myocytes

After 10 min take the cell suspension and filter the material through a nylon mesh (mesh size 200 µm). The cell suspension is then centrifuged for 3 min at 25 g. The cell pellet contains the myocytes, while the supernatant contains small non-myocytes. This fraction can either be used to isolate endothelial cells or fibroblasts or can be discarded. The myocyte-containing pellet is resuspended in Powell medium (see above) with added 0.2% (vol/vol) $CaCl_2$ (stock solution 100 mmol/l, final concentration 200 µmol/l)) and centrifuged again as before. The pellet is then resuspended in Powell medium containing 0.4% (vol/vol) $CaCl_2$ (stock solution 100 mmol/l, final concentration 400 µmol/l) and centrifuged again. The pellet is resuspended in Powell medium containing 1% (vol/vol) $CaCl_2$ (stock solution 100 mmol/l, final concentration 1 mmol/l) and layered over the following medium:

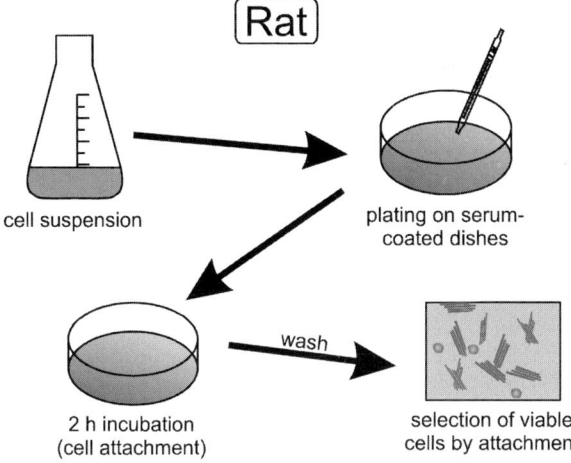

Figure 2
Plating of cardiomyocytes: The cell pellet isolated from the heart is loaded on to culture dishes pre-coated with 4% (vol/vol) foetal calf serum. After 2 h for cell attachment, the cells are washed to remove most of the round and non-viable cells

- BSA gradient
  - Powell Medium see above
  - add bovine serum albumin: 4 g/100 ml
  - $CaCl_2$ (100 mmol/l): 1 ml/100 ml

This "gradient" is centrifuged again at 15 g for 1 min. The pellet contains rod-shaped and calcium-tolerant cardiomyocytes. These can be plated on culture dishes pre-coated with 4% foetal calf serum (see Cell Attachment). Figure 2 summarizes these final steps.

Success of Isolation

Two criteria allow one to quantify the success of the isolation procedure, firstly, the total number of cardiomyocytes isolated and secondly the ratio between rod-shaped calcium-tolerant and round non-tolerant myocytes. Both criteria can only give a gross view of the quality of the cell preparation. The number of initially isolated calcium-tolerant cells might decrease during the subsequent recovery period of approximately 2–4 h. On the other hand, rounded cells will not attach to the culture dishes and thus the ratio between calcium-tolerant cells and rounded cells can be improved by washing the culture dishes after 2–4 h. In general the number of cells should be of the order of 4×10^6 cells per heart and the ratio of rod-shaped to round cells should be approximately 70:30.

We recommend suspending the final cell pellet from one ventricle in 25 ml medium and plating the cells at 1 ml per 3 cm dish (normally called "six-well dishes"). In any case, to perform reproducible experiments it is more important to work with a constant quality of the preparation than with the highest quality. In other words, a constant preparation of approximately 10^6 cells with a ratio of 50:50 may be sufficient for most experiments.

Isolation of Ventricular Cardiomyocytes from Mice

The frequent use of transgenic mice has led to an increased number of experiments using ventricular cardiomyocytes isolated from mice. In general the protocol described above for isolation of ventricular cardiomyocytes from rats can be used with slight modifications.

Firstly, the perfusion system and volumes of buffers have to be reduced because of the smaller size of the heart. Second, reconstitution of a physio-logical calcium concentration should be performed more carefully. We suggest a four-step procedure that increases the calcium concentration to 125 µmol/l, 250 µmol/l, 500 µmol/l and 1 mmol/l. The proportion of cardiomyocytes yielded by this procedure is comparable to that from rat hearts. However, due to the smaller size of the hearts, one heart will yield only 10% of the total number of cells normally got from rat hearts. This is a great limitation for biochemical experiments requiring large amounts of cells. The third and last point which differs from the procedure for rat hearts is the more difficult cultivation process. No modifications must be taken into account in regard to the medium. However, cells from mouse hearts do not attach on cell culture dishes precoated by FCS. Therefore, it is essential to use laminin precoating as described below for rat cells.

Cultivation of the Cells

As pointed out in the introduction, the second challenge in working with isolated ventricular cardiomyocytes is to cultivate the cells. In principle, two different forms of cultures should be kept in mind. First, the use of freshly isolated, attached, rod-shaped cardiomyocytes and second, the use of long-term cultures of cardiomyocytes undergoing a certain amount of differentiation during the cultivation process including morphological differentiation. Nevertheless, the common challenge in both cases is to find a way to get the cells attached to the culture dish.

Cell Attachment

There are two different types of attachment substrates found suitable. The first protocol requires pre-treatment of the culture dishes for 8–20 h prior to cell plating with cell culture medium supplemented with 4% foetal calf serum (FCS). This procedure has two main advantages over other methods: First, cell attachment *via* FCS pre-treatment allows the cells to contact *via* variable components of the serum, resulting in preferentially attachment of rod-shaped calcium-tolerant cells. Therefore, simply washing the culture dishes within the next few hours is sufficient to increase the ratio of rod-shaped to rounded cells. Second, the method is cheap and can thus be widely used even with large amounts of cultures. Culture dishes not specified for primary cells are strongly recommended.

As in cell culture procedures, use of FCS depends on batch variations. Therefore, as said before for collagenase batches, several batches of FCS should be screened for suitability prior to the start of experiments. The second method generally used to attach cardiomyocytes is to pre-treat cell dishes with laminin (1 g/ml) prior to cell plating. Compared to FCS this method cannot be used to increase the ratio of rod-shaped to round cells and is relatively expensive. However, it allows pre-treatment of dishes shortly before cell plating (10–30 min) and is suitable in cases in which FCS pre-treatment does not work properly, i.e. in case of ventricular cardiomyocytes isolated from mice.

Cell Culture Medium

Ventricular cardiomyocytes represent a finally differentiated cell type that requires complex media. The most commonly used medium is medium 199. However, even this quite complex medium should be modified by addition of creatine (5 mmol/l), carnitine (2 mmol/l) and taurine (5 mmol/l). Also, the recovery of ventricular cardiomyocytes from preparation stress can be further improved by addition of 4% (vol/vol) FCS.

As the cells are often isolated under non-sterile conditions, penicillin (100 IU/ml) and streptomycin (100 µl/ml) should be added as antibiotics.

Cell Cultures

To maintain ventricular cardiomyocytes for a certain period of time in the rod-shaped manner, the above medium should be used without addition of FCS. This allows the cells to survive without major morphological changes for approximately 36 h. During this time the amount of protein synthesis is more or less unchanged as well as the total amount of protein per cell (Pinson et al. 1993). Also, the ability of the cell to contract if it is exposed to electric stimulation is quite stable. However, cells cannot be used as confluent cultures under these conditions, because rod-shaped cells cannot attach to the culture dish without leaving spaces in between. Therefore, cell connections between individual cells, which are normal in the native tissue, are rarely present in these cultures.

To maintain ventricular cardiomyocytes for a longer period of time in culture, i.e. one or two weeks, the medium must be supplemented with 20% (vol/vol) FCS. The cells then initially undergo a period of atrophy, round up and change their morphology completely (Piper et al. 1988). After six days they reach a stable situation in which the cell spreads around the centre. These cells have obviously lost some of their *in vivo* characteristics, i.e. rod-shaped morphology. However, energy metabolism and coupling of specific receptors, i.e. that of α-adrenoceptors to the regulation of protein synthesis is still intact (Schlüter et al. 1998). The cells start to build up new cell contacts, as present in native tissue (Schwartz et al. 1985). Also one has to keep in mind that some of the alterations found under these conditions, mimic the situation found during the development of heart failure, i.e. the cells secrete growth factors like TGF-β and such factors can be activated by proteases in the FCS (Taimor et al. 1999). Thus, although some of the changes seen in these spread cells limit their use in cardiovascular experimental biology, this system represents a suitable model for many questions.

Examples

The success of any work with isolated cardiomyocytes depends on the reproducibility of cell isolation, because the cells do not divide. The morphological and biochemical characteristics of cultured adult ventricular cardiomyocytes from rat have been described previously in great detail (Piper et al. 1982, 1988, 1990). The following examples indicate the yield of cells and the quality of cell preparations based on the ratio of rod-shaped to rounded cells found with different preparations. In addition, approximately 5% of the isolated cells undergo apoptotic cell death (Taimor et al. 1999). As indicated, the number of cells and ratio of rod-shaped cells is quite stable over the next 24 h (Fig. 3). As shown elsewhere, cells maintain their protein content and rate of protein synthesis during this time period (Schlüter and Piper 1992). The preparation is therefore quite stable and suitable for biochemical or physiological analysis. However, the energy metabolism and rate of protein synthesis are the basal values for non-contracting myocytes without the energy demand of a working heart. These non-loaded and non-contracting myocytes can be used to investigate the regulation of protein synthesis by neurohumoral factors independently from mechanical influences. The example shown in Fig. 4 indicates stimulation of protein synthesis by

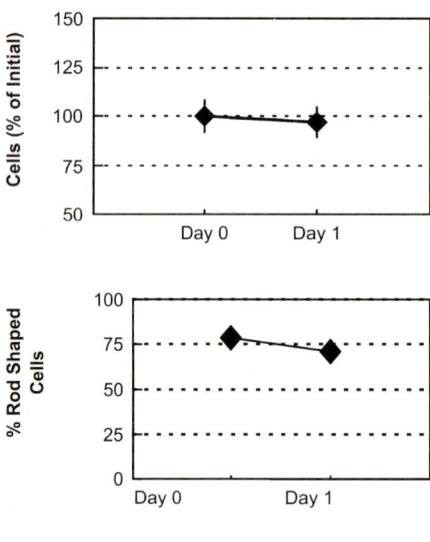

Figure 3
Change in number of cells (*right*) and percent of rod-shaped cells (*left*) during 24 h cultivation of cardiomyocytes

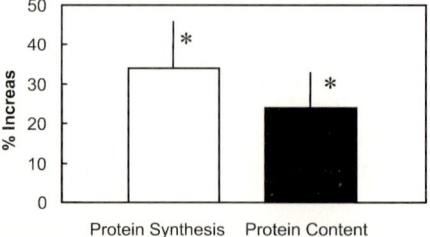

Figure 4
Influence of phenylephrine (an α-adrenoceptor agonist) on protein synthesis and protein content of cardiomyocytes cultured for 24 h in the absence (basal value) and presence of the agonist (10 µmol/l). *p <0.05 *vs.* untreated cultures

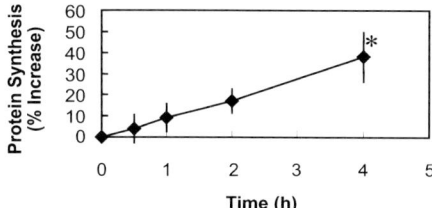

Figure 5
Effect of different times of reconstitution of mechanical activity (0.5 Hz). Cells were paced for 0.5, 1, 2, or 4 h starting 4 h after isolation. The rate of protein synthesis was determined by incorporation of ^{14}C-phenylalanine into cell protein during the next 24 h

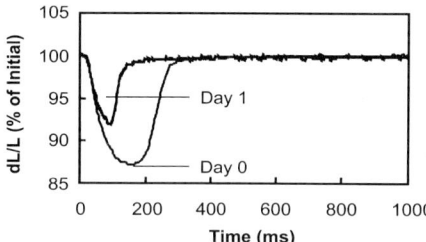

Figure 6
Cell contraction of cardiomyocytes paced at 0.5 Hz 4 h after the isolation (day 0) and 24 h later (1 day). Cell contraction is expressed as cell shortening relative to the diastolic cell length

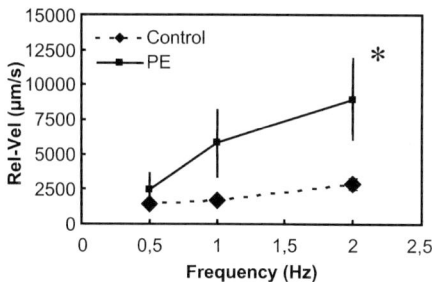

Figure 7
Influence of phenylephrine (PE), an α-adrenoceptor agonist and hypertrophic stimulus, on the relaxation velocity of isolated cardiomyocytes. Cells were cultured for 24 h in the presence of the agonist (10 μmol/l) and paced at 0.5 Hz thereafter. * $p < 0.05$ vs. control cultures, which were not treated with phenylephrine

α-adrenoceptor stimulation. As indicated, protein synthesis, determined by incorporation of ^{14}C-phenylalanine, increased by 34%, and in parallel total protein content increased by 24%. The basal value of protein synthesis can be increased by mechanical loading of the myocytes by reconstitution of mechanical activity. As shown on Fig. 5, a brief period of electrical pacing is sufficient to increase the amount of protein synthesis. In a similar way, external loading of the cells increases basal rates of protein synthesis, allowing analysis of the response of the individual cells to passive load. To perform such experiments, cells can be attached to flexible silicone materials by pre-coating with poly-L-lysine. Loading of the cells must be increased stepwise to allow the cells to adapt to the external load. The contractile activity of isolated cardiomyocytes can be analyzed by cell edge detection techniques, allowing the determination of the mechanical properties. As shown in Fig. 6, cardiomyocytes paced at between 0.5Hz and 2.0 Hz contract regularly under basal conditions when stimulated four hours after preparation. After 24 h, cell contraction is still inducible, however, the basal values are slightly reduced. The isolated cells are able to react to hypertrophic stimuli as they do in the intact heart, i.e. induction of hypertrophy by α-adrenoceptor stimulation causes a significant increase in relaxation velocity, caused by an up-regulation of SERCA2A (Fig. 7). These examples clearly indicate the usefulness of the isolated cell system in analyzing the biology of isolated cardiomyocytes.

Troubleshooting

During the isolation and cultivation of ventricular cardiomyocytes from adult animals problems may occur at various steps. At the end of the isolation procedure, the yield of cells may be quite large but nearly all of the cells are hypercontracted and round. The problem can arise at different steps. First, the heart might not be smooth at the end of the collagenase treatment period. Mostly the reason is that the blood was not fully removed from the heart initially and coagulated in some of the vessels. Thus, the heart has not been perfused adequately. You can resolve this problem either by reducing the time between the isolation of the heart from the animal and the connection to the perfusion system or alternatively by injecting heparin into the circulation of the animal shortly before starting the preparation to avoid coagulation. The second problem can be that even though the heart has been smoothly, cells are round. In this case, view the morphology of the cells after each step of the calcium gradient. If the cells are initially rod-shaped and round up during the increasing of the calcium gradient, then they are obviously not calcium tolerant. Reduce the time of collagenase treatment or re-establish a physiological calcium concentration more carefully, i.e. as suggested for mouse hearts (see above). If the cells are already round at the beginning of the calcium reconstitution, than repeat with new buffers and new collagenase batches. We found, that the system is very sensitive to the quality of water. Use the highest quality of water purification to prepare your buffers.

The next problem may occur after the initial isolation. One problem that often occurs is that the cells looked quite nice initially, but hypercontract during the next few hours. This is often the case, if the cells tend to beat spontaneously. Again, the cells are not perfectly calcium tolerant. Reduce the time of collagenase treatment. Even if you lose a small amount of rod-shaped cells by reducing the time of collagenase treatment, the resulting cells are much more calcium tolerant and survive much better. One of the most common problems is that people focus too much on the initial morphology of the cells. It is more important to have a look at the cells after 4 h, when replacing the medium and removing the round and non-attached cells, than to examine the initial morphology.

Another problem that often occurs is that the cells do not attach to the culture dishes. In general, cells should attach to culture dishes pre-treated with 4% (vol/vol) FCS. If not, test different batches of FCS. If the problem persists, then reduce the time of collagenase treatment. Never use culture dishes specially prepared for primary cultures. Falcon dishes (3001 or 3004) were found to be quite useful. If necessary, replace FCS by laminin.

When you culture cells in the presence of FCS for a couple of days, they may be overgrown by non-myocytes. This can be avoided by the addition of cytosine-β-D-arabinofuranoside (Ara-C, 10 µmol/l) for the first 5 days.

Finally, it should be noted that even in laboratories with long-standing experience of the isolation of cardiomyocytes, the quality of cell preparations declines from time to time. It is important to establish a routine procedure and to repeat experiments with several cell preparations. Some general guidelines may help to shorten the search for the cause of failure. Avoid the use of detergents in cleaning the glassware used for cell isolation. A record should be kept of the use of all materials involved in cell preparations, particularly of all chemicals. If some doubt about the purity of chemicals arises, all should be exchanged for unopened batches. A possible cause of failure is the quality of the water used to make up the solutions. In some places distillation or ion exchange systems are fed with water from a common primary ion-exchange purification system that releases volatile organic impurities. It is also important to keep the perfusion system clean. In general, the system should be flushed with water after the preparation to avoid proteins from the perfusate drying on the glass. Even if the perfusion system does not need to be sterile, it is advisable to flush the glassware after use with 70% ethanol for 30 min and subsequently dry it with a stream of clean gas (e.g. filtered compressed air).

References

Pinson A, Schlüter K-D, Zhou XJ, Schwartz P, Kessler-Icekson G, Piper HM (1993) Alpha- and beta-adrenergic stimulation of protein synthesis in cultured adult ventricular cardiomyocytes. J Mol Cell Cardiol 25:477–490

Piper HM, Jacobsen SL, Schwartz P (1988) Determinants of cardiomyocyte development in long-term primary culture. J Mol Cell Cardiol 20:825–835

Piper HM, Probst I, Schwartz P, Hütter JF, Spieckermann PG (1982) Culturing of calcium stable adult cardiac myocytes. J Mol Cell Cardiol 14:397–412

Piper HM, Spahr R, Schweickhardt C, Hunnemann D (1988) Importance of endogenous substrates for cultured adult cardiac myocytes. Biochem Biophys Acta 883:531–541

Piper HM, Volz A, Schwartz P (1990) Adult ventricular rat heart muscle cells. In: Piper HM (ed) Cell culture techniques in heart and vessel research. Springer Verlag, Berlin, p 36–60

Schlüter K-D, Goldberg Y, Taimor G, Schäfer M, Piper HM (1998) Role of phosphatidyl 3-kinase activation in the hypertrophic growth of adult ventricular cardiomyocytes. Cardiovasc Res 40:174–181

Schlüter K-D, Piper HM (1992) Trophic effects of catecholamines and parathyroid hormone on adult ventricular cardiomyocytes. Am J Physiol Heart Circ Physiol 263:H1739–H1746

Schwartz P, Piper HM, Spahr R, Hütter JF, Spiekermann PG(1985) Development of new intracellular contacts between adult cardiac myocytes in culture. Basic Res Cardiol 80 [Suppl. 1]:75–78

Taimor G, Lorenz H, Hofstaetter B, Schlüter K-D, Piper HM (1999) Induction of necrosis but not apoptosis after anoxia and reoxygenation in isolated adult cardiomyocytes of rat: Cardiovasc Res 41:147–156

Taimor G, Schlüter K-D, Frischkopf K, Flesch M, Rosenkranz S, Piper HM (1999) Autocrine regulation of TGFβ expression in adult cardiomyocytes. J Mol Cell Cardiol 31:2127–2136

Culture of Neonatal Cardiomyocytes

Aida Salameh and Stefan Dhein

Introduction

In many experimental approaches in cardiovascular research it is necessary to study processes in cultured cells. There are two options at present, either adult cardiomyocytes (preferably rat) are studied (see chapter on culture of adult cardiomyocytes by K-D. Schlüter and H.M. Piper) or neonatal rat cardiomyocytes are investigated. The latter method has the advantage that the cells grow and divide (at least several times) provided the neonatal rat was not older than 48 h. These cells form spontaneously beating clusters within about 2–3 days.

The technique of isolating and culturing spontaneously beating cells from embryonic, foetal or newborn heart tissue started in 1912 using embryonic chick hearts (Burrows 1912). At the same time the first reports on sub-cultivation of cells appeared (Carrel and Burrows 1910) and the technique of tryptic digestion of tissue was described (Rous and Jones 1916). Despite these early successful attempts, it was the 1950ies before these techniques were used by a broader scientific community. It started with the description of embryonic chick heart cell cultures by Moscona in 1952 and Cavanough (1955). The first neonatal rat heart cell culture was then established by Harary and Farley (1960). It was shown in the early studies that these cells started to beat spontaneously and synchronized when they came into contact, forming synchronously beating clusters. Moreover, it was observed that these cells generated typical cardiac action potentials and might therefore form an interesting model for electrophysiologists (Fange et al. 1956). Furthermore, it was shown in the 1960s and 1970s that these cells responded to pharmacological and physiological stimuli similarly to the adult heart (using e.g. isoprenaline) so that they seemed to be suitable as a model system for pharmacologists. For a more complete review of species and culture techniques for heart cells see Pinson et al. (1987).

However, when comparing results obtained from these cultures caution is necessary and the methods of isolation, cultivation and coating and the age of the cells have to be taken into account. These cells change with time and may up- or down-regulate the expression of certain proteins depending on the status of the culture, e.g. depending as to whether the cells are more or less isolated or are in close contact.

While adult cells are post-mitotic and do not divide, embryonic heart cells may divide. Cells obtained from newborn rats are somewhat in between and can divide several times until they become post-mitotic, which resembles the normal behaviour in the intact animal with the heart cells becoming post-mitotic on day 21 after birth (Pinson 1990). However, the cardiomyocytes' mitotic cycle seems to be 2.5-fold longer than that of non-cardiomyocytes (Kasten 1972). The cardiomyoblast can synthesize myosin and divide, thus representing a cell between an embryonic cell and a post-mitotic adult cardiomyocyte. In the neonatal rat heart, cardiomyocytes or cardiomyoblasts of various stages of development are present. On day 1 after birth it has been estimated that about 55% of the cells are dividing cardiomyoblasts whereas on day 4 this number drops down to 40% (Masse and Harary 1981). This is important to notice, since it shows that the type of culture depends critically on the age of the newborn rats and should be exactly documented. In order to obtain comparable cultures, one should use animals of the same post-birth day for all cultures. This may also affect the yield of certain cell types and the resistivity of the cells to the proteolytic treatment.

Cultures of neonatal rat cardiomyocytes are widely used today for patch clamp experiments, for experiments on propagation of action potentials using optical dyes (Rohr 1995) (and see chapter 3.1) and for investigation of regulation of protein synthesis using Western blots (see chapter on Western blots by A. Salameh) or PCR. Moreover, these cultures may be used for histological or immunohistological experiments.

Description of Methods and Practical Approach

For cultivation of neonatal rat cardiomyocytes neonatal rats of 12–48 h are used. If the rats are older than 48 h, in our experience the cells do not grow. In most protocols, the rats are killed by decapitation and the heart is removed and transferred to a phosphate buffer on ice. Thereafter, the associated tissue and the atria are removed (optionally the atria may be used to cultivate atrial cardiomyocytes), and the hearts are minced with scissors into small pieces of about 1 mm length. Next, the tissue has to be digested using collagenase and protease as digesting enzymes. This step is carried out at 37 °C to allow the enzyme to be active. After 5–10 min of digestion the supernatant is collected and the digestion is stopped with FCS/medium. The remnant pellet is again subjected to the digesting enzyme solution for another 5–10 min period. These steps are repeated several times, until all the material is digested and finally stopped with FCS/medium.

Subsequently, the cell-containing solution is centrifuged and the pellet resuspended. Next, it is necessary to remove non-cardiomyocytes, which can be achieved using a differential attachment technique, i.e. cells are incubated for 1 h at 37 °C in a cell culture flask so that the non-cardiomyocytes such as fibroblasts or endothelial cells, which attach more easily to plastic surfaces than cardiomyocytes, can attach to the surface. After 1 h the supernatant is collected and plated in Petri dishes coated with either gelatin or laminin (which is however rather expensive) for cultivation. For the first day we use a medium containing 5% foetal calf serum (FCS). On the second day and for the further cultivation FCS is reduced to 1%. Cell culture medium should be changed every day or at least every second day. In order to avoid excessive growth of fibroblasts, 10% horse serum should be added. Using this technique, clusters of spontaneously beating cardiomyocytes are obtained and can be observed after the second day. If the cells are used for patch clamp experiments they are best at days 3 to 5. Thereafter, the cells become flat and are difficult to patch. Moreover, in our experience older cells are rather fragile and do not tolerate a patch pipette well. Within 4 to 7 days the cultures become more or less confluent (depending on the number of cells which were initially seeded) and may be used for investigation of protein synthesis or biochemical experiments.

Many variations of this protocol are possible using other enzymes or mixtures, times, and temperatures. Below, we give an example as it is routinely used with good success in our laboratory. The optimal enzyme depends on the age and species of the animal. Often crude enzyme preparations are found to be more efficient than purified enzymes. On the other hand, the enzyme mixture may alter the cardiomyocytes or cardiomyoblasts as well. Thus, it is recorded that trypsin can damage myocardial cells. If purified collagenase is applied, this has to be combined with trypsin or another protease, since collagenase alone is a poor digesting enzyme. Enzymes often used are pronase and elastase (e.g. for embryonic chick heart cell cultures) or crude trypsin preparations, which also contain chymotrypsin and elastase. When using crude trypsin, one should document the activities of chymotrypsin and elastase (which may vary from batch to batch, the manufacturers can normally provide information on the other enzyme activities), in order to allow the finding of comparable batches of the enzyme if the old batch is running out. An alternative may be the use of Viokase (Viobin Corp.), a mixture of proteolytic enzymes, which is more consistent in its composition than crude preparations. It is also possible to purify an enzyme mixture from a crude preparation. Thus, Speicher and McCarl (1978, 1978a) described a procedure for purifying a mixture of chymotrypsin, elastase and trypsin from a crude trypsin preparation, resulting in a preparation which was highly efficient but less toxic to the cells than the crude preparation.

Although some experimenters argued that trypsin may lead to damage of the cardiomyocytes, trypsin is widely and successfully used in cell isolation protocols, mostly in concentrations of 0.05 to 0.1%. To keep cell damage to a minimum trypsinization cycles should be kept short, i.e. 10 to 20 min. Moreover, one may add glucose during the dissociation, which has been shown to result in better cell yield. Another factor which has to be controlled is the purity of water used. In our experience the quality of water used is very important.

Since growth and differentiation of cells is normally controlled by cell contacts, the cell types involved (i.e. the non-myocardial cells), humoral factors, the extracellular matrix and hormones, the extracellular milieu of the cells in culture, the medium, and the frequency of changes of the medium are highly important. Media used in neonatal rat heart cell culture are Ham's F10, M199 (which can both be obtained from most manufacturers) and CMRL 1415ATM (Connaught Medical Research Laboratories). In our lab we normally use M199. Since most of these media contain $NaHCO_3$, they require constant CO_2 presence (around 5%) in the incubator, to maintain a pH of 7.4. The exact concentration of CO_2 has to be determined. Most manufacturers give information on their media.

In most protocols, sera are added, such as foetal calf serum (FCS), foetal rat serum, horse serum or embryo extracts. These sera have detoxifying properties, help the cells to attach and promote cell growth by the presence of a number of hormones and growth factors. The composition of a serum may change from batch to batch, which makes it necessary to test a batch of serum first and, if it works well, buy a lot of it. Unfortunately, the use of serum promotes the growth of non-myocardial cells, which will, due to their shorter cell cycle, overgrow the cardiomyocytes. Thus, the amount of serum may also be critical. Most groups use FCS in concentrations of 1 to 10% as an additive to their media. A compromise, with which we have had good experiences, may be to use a higher FCS concentration (5%) on the first day after isolation, and to reduce the serum content to 1% on the second day. Horse serum (about 10%) often is added since it is said to reduce fibroblast growth.

Alternatively, serum-free cultures may be used. This will reduce the number of non-myocyte cells (Kessler-Icekson 1987; Claycomb 1980). In that case it is important to coat the Petri dishes with fibronectin or collagen to allow cell adhesion. Some authors coat their dishes with FCS first, then wash the dish and afterwards use it for serum-free culture. The FCS serves as an attachment factor in these protocols. In serum-free cultures, nutrients, hormones and fatty acids may be supplemented. In such protocols, the serum glucoprotein fetuin has been shown to be an essential factor to be added (Claycomb 1980; Mohamed et al. 1983).

Glucocorticoids, which have been shown to maintain the beating capacity of the cardiomyocytes and to lead to growth retardation of non-cardiomyocytes, may be added Ascorbic acid and selenium are often used as antioxidants in serum-free cultures. Transferrin may be used for detoxification of toxic metals and as a carrier for iron. Albumin may be used in order to carry fatty acids. Other hormones such as insulin, adrenaline or noradrenaline may be used depending on the requirements of the experiment. Hormonally defined media may also be used (Kessler-Icekson et al. 1983). The use of growth factors in serum-free cultures is questionable since this will enhance non-cardiomyocyte growth (which should be avoided by using the serum-free protocol). However, serum-free protocols may also be useful for the investigation of hormone or drug/cardiomyocyte interactions in order to exclude interference with serum factors.

For cell culture either glass Petri dishes, plastic Petri dishes or plastic culture flasks may be used. They should be coated with either gelatin, FCS, fibronectin, laminin or collagen. Gelatin is an easy to use, mostly collagen-containing coating factor which is used in many labs. If glass is used, the quality of glass is important, since the polarity of the glass surface may be different between various glass qualities. If cells are to be seeded in the culture dishes, it is necessary to determine the cell number/ml using e.g. a Neubauer counting chamber. If cells are used for patch clamp experiments the cell number should be low. Otherwise, if cells are used for biochemical experiments, it is often desired to have a more or less pure cardiomyocyte culture with a minimum of non-myocardial cells. This is achieved by seeding higher cell numbers such as 10^6 cells/ml which will lead to confluence within 24–48 h. Reaching confluence means contact inhibition to non-cardiomyocytes and thus prevents overgrowth of the culture with these cells.

While the heart contains about 50% non-cardiomyocytes, mostly fibroblasts/fibrocytes and endothelial cells, a mixture somewhat enriched in cardiomyocytes is obtained after the cell isolation protocol with about 80% cardiomyocytes and 20% non-cardiomyocytes. It has been assumed that a minimum of non-cardiomyocytes is necessary *in vivo* and *in vitro* for proper functioning of the cardiomyocytes. On the other hand these non-cardiomyocytes sometimes complicate the interpretation of the results.

Within the finally obtained cell culture the cardiomyocytes can be identified by their beating capacity, by their action potentials or visually by their dense cytoplasm, well-developed mitochondria and Golgi system, myofibrils, intercalated disks and cross-striated contractile proteins. Moreover, they express cardiotypic proteins such as α-actinin and troponin I.

From our point of view the most important rule in cell culture to obtain comparable results is a high standardization of protocols, solutions, enzyme preparations, water, media and sera.

Example

The following equipment will be needed: a sterile hood, best equipped with a UV-sterilized area, an inverted-phase microscope, an incubator (37 °C, 5% CO_2), an autoclave, a thermocontrolled water bath, a centrifuge, plastic Petri dishes, forceps, scissors, scalpel, 10 ml pipettes, 8 Falcon tubes (50 ml), 10 ml syringes. Scissors and forceps need to be sterile.

The following protocol is our daily use protocol. It should be stated that this is one possible example. Other protocols or modifications may also work. The interested reader may adapt this protocol to his needs according to the outlines given in the paragraphs above.

Prepare ice in a styropor container and the following solutions:
1. stop-solution
   - M199 (Hanks salts, HEPES): 474.5 ml
   - 5% FCS: 25 ml
   - PenStrep: 0.5 ml
2. collagenase solution
   - PBS-glucose: 50 ml
   - Bovine serum albumin (BSA): 0.5 g
   - Collagenase Type II: 50 mg (204 U/mg) (total about 10.000 U)
3. day 1 medium (500 ml)
   - M199 (Hanks salts, HEPES): 424,5 ml
   - 5% FCS: 25 ml
   - 10% horse serum: 50 ml
   - PenStrep: 0.5 ml
4. phosphate buffered saline (PBS) with glucose (50 ml)
   - NaCl 137 mM: 401 mg
   - KCl 2.7 mM: 0.01 g
   - Na_2HPO_4 8.3 mM: 0.073 g
   - KH_2PO_4 1.5 mM: 10.2 mg
   - Glucose 20 mM: 0.198 g
   - pH 7.4

5. penicillin/streptomycin solution (PenStrep)
   - 100 mg/ml penicillin
   - 100 mg/ml streptomycin
6. gelatin 1% (for coating of Petri dishes)
   - 1.5 g gelatin in 150 ml H_2O; then autoclave
7. Dulbecco's wash solution
   - NaCl 137 mM
   - KCl 2.68 mM
   - Na_2HPO_4 6.48 mM
   - KH_2PO_4 1.47 mM
   - $MgCl_2$ 0.49 mM
   - $MgSO_4$ 0.81 mM
   - $CaCl_2$ 0.9 mM
   - pH 7.2
8. day 2 medium (500 ml)
   - M199 (Hanks salts, HEPES): 444.5 ml
   - 1% FCS: 5 ml
   - 10% horse serum: 50 ml
   - PenStrep: 0.5 ml

All solutions must be sterile either by sterile filtration or autoclaving.

Place the following items under the sterile hood: PBS-glucose in a large Petri dish, a glass with 70 % ethanol, a sterile filter and a syringe, collagenase solution, stop solution, several sterile 50 ml Falcon tubes. First decapitate the neonatal rats (10 for 1 cultivation) using large scissors, open the thorax, and remove the hearts with small scissors and forceps. The hearts have to be transferred immediately to a Petri dish with 10 ml ice-cold PBS-glucose to avoid ischemia. Remove the blood by gently shaking. Transfer the dish under the sterile hood. Warm the stop solution and the medium (day 1) in a water bath at 37 °C. Fill a second Petri dish with ice-cold PBS-glucose solution.

Now remove the supernatant solution but leave about 1 third of the solution to avoid drying of the tissue. Next, the atria and the associated tissue have to be removed using small scissors and forceps (instead, it might be interesting to use only the atria). The ventricles are transferred to the second dish with 10 ml ice-cold PBS-glucose. The ventricles are now minced into small pieces of about 1 mm length and then the total 10 ml containing the hearts are transferred into a sterile Falcon tube (50 ml). 7 ml of the collagenase solution are added and the Falcon tube is closed. Then, *gently* shake the solution in a 37 °C water bath for 5–6 min. Thereafter, the supernatant, which contains the first isolated cells, is transferred into another sterile 50 ml Falcon tube (FT-II) and 7 ml stop solution are added. With the remaining tissue the same procedure is repeated, i.e. 7 ml collagenase solution are added again, the tube is shaken for another 5–6 minutes at 37 °C. Then, the supernatant is transferred into the Falcon tube (FT-II) and 7 ml stop solution are added. This procedure is repeated until the 50 ml of collagenase solution are completely used up.

Next, the solution in the Falcon tubes containing the cardiomyocytes is centrifuged at 700 rpm/min for 5 min. The supernatant is removed and the resulting cell pellet is resuspended in 13 ml day 1 medium. Thereafter, the solution has to be trans-

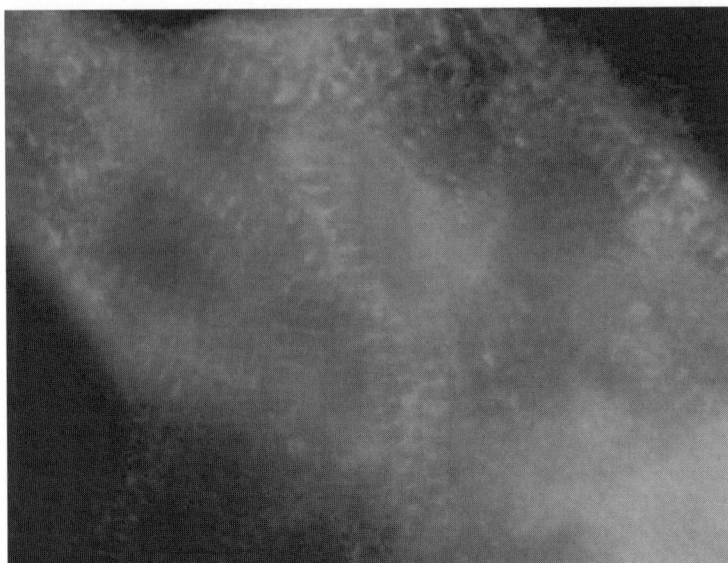

Figure 1
Fluorescence microscopy of ventricular neonatal rat cardiomycytes with anti-α-actinin staining. *For coloured version see appendix*

ferred to a 75 cm^2 culture flask and incubated in the incubator at 37 °C (5% CO_2) for 1 hour. During that time, mainly non-cardiomyocytes attach to the plastic surface. During this hour the Petri dishes for the cardiomyocyte culture are coated with 1% gelatin solution. After 1 h the supernatant of the culture flask is removed and transferred to a Falcon tube for cell counting. Thereafter, the cell suspension is diluted with day 1 medium to the correct cell number (e.g. 1 million/ml) transferred to the Petri dishes and incubated for 24 h.

Next day, the Petri dishes are washed twice with Dulbecco's wash solution. Then the cells are fed with the day 2 medium Subsequently, the medium should be changed every 24–48 h until the cells are used for the experiments. Normally, you should observe the first spontaneously beating cells or cell clusters on day 2.

The culture should be monitored by histological /immunohistological methods. The cells should be stained for α-actinin, actin, troponin I and connexin 43. The contractile proteins should exhibit a cross-striated pattern. Cx43 should be localized at the cell borders and at the cell-cell contact zones. Figure 1 shows neonatal rat cardiomyocytes.

Troubleshooting

The most common problems with this type of primary cell culture are infections. In case of an infection, the infected culture dishes have to be removed. To avoid infections, sterility of all solutions has to be controlled very strictly. Thus, the gelatin solution may be infected, especially if it is used for a long time, or the FCS solution by using a pipette several times. In order to find the source of infection, it is sometimes helpful to incubate the suspected solutions for 24 h in an incubator at 37 °C. The use of additional antibiotics/antimycotics etc. should be strictly avoided since you may select multiresistant bacteria this way. To keep infections at a minimum, you may wash the neonatal rats with isopropanol prior to opening the thorax.

Another common problem is a small cell yield after the isolation steps. This may be related to ischemia during the isolation procedure. It is essential to perform the first steps on ice and to avoid all unnecessary delays. Another factor, which might compromise the result, is the shaking of the collagenase/cell solution. It seems necessary to shake this solution *gently* and not to stir it. It may be suspected that during this step the cells are more susceptible to mechanical stress.

Sometimes, after a good cell yield at the first day, the cell number is markedly reduced after the second day. A typical problem is the washing step to remove the day 1 medium. It is essential to use the Dulbecco's wash solution as stated in this chapter, i.e. containing Ca^{++} and Mg^{++}. Some Dulbecco's wash solutions which can be obtained commercially do not contain calcium. If these, i.e. Ca^{++}-free solutions, are used for washing, the cardiomyocytes will lose their contact to the surface, since many of the contacts are calcium-dependent.

Another problem often encountered with neonatal rat heart cell culture is contamination with non-cardiomyocytes. There are several strategies discussed in the first part of this chapter to keep the number of contaminating cells at a minimum. However, it should be noted that a number of authors have argued that a minimum number of non-cardiomyocytes (10–20%) may be necessary to maintain a proper functioning cardiomyocyte culture, as in the heart there are also non-cardiomyocytes, which may influence the cardiac cells by humoral and non-humoral factors such as direct contact. In order to minimize the percentage of non-cardiomyocytes, differential attachment as described above may be used. It might be useful to adapt the times to special requirements and to monitor the two fractions (that in the culture flask and that in the supernatant). In addition, the use of 5–10% horse serum is recommended to retard fibroblast growth. Since non-cardiomyocytes are stimulated with FCS, we recommend the reduction of FCS at the second day to 1% (day 1 medium 5%; day 2 medium 1%). This might be adapted. Another possibility is the use of a serum-free culture method (see above); Moreover, several investigators recommend the addition of 7-β-OH cholesterol. Finally, since the non-cardiomyocytes exhibit a faster cell cycle with higher DNA synthesis, DNA synthesis may be inhibited by BrdU incubation and subsequent UV irradiation or by other chemical inhibitors of DNA synthesis. However, it is questionable whether this may not also alter the physiology of the cell culture and might compromise the results. If such treatments are used, very careful controls have to be performed to exclude effects of the treatment.

References

Burrows MT (1912) Rhythmical activity of isolated heart muscle cells in vitro. Science 3:90-92
Carrel A, Burrows MT (1910) Culture de tissus adultes en dehors de l'organisme. CR Soc Biol (Paris) 69: 293-294
Cavanough MW: Pulsation migration and division in dissociated chick heart cells. J Exp Zool 128:573-589, 1955
Claycomb WC (1980) Culture of cardiac muscle cells in serum-free medium. Exp Cell Res 131:231-236
Fange R, Persson H, Hesleff T (1956) Electrophysiologic and pharmacologic observations on trypsin disintegrated embryonic chick hearts cultured in vitro. Acta Physiol Scand 38:173-183

Harary I, Farley B (1960) In vitro studies of isolated beating heart cells. Science 131:1674-1675
Kasten FH (1972) Rat myocardial cells in vitro: mitosis and differentiated properties. In Vitro 8:128-150
Kessler-Icekson G, Wassermann L, Yoles E, Aampson SR (1983) Characterization of cardiomyocytes cultured in serum-free medium. In: Fischer G, Weiser RJ (eds) Hormonally defined media. A tool in cell biology. Springer Verlag, Berlin, p. 383
Kessler-Icekson G (1987) Cardiomyocytes grown in serum-free medium. In: Pinson A (ed) The heart cell in culture. CRC, Boca Raton, p 23-28
Masse MJO, Harary I (1981) The use of fluorescent antimyosin and DNA labelling in the estimation of the myoblast and myocyte population of primary rat heart cell cultures. J Cell Physiol 106:165-172
Mohamed SNW, Holmes R, Hartzell CR (1983) A serum-free chemically defined medium for function and growth of primary neonatal rat heart cell cultures. In Vitro 19:471-478
Pinson A, Padieu P, Harary I (1987) Techniques for culturing heart cells. In: Pinson A (ed.) The heart cell in culture, vol 1. CRC, Boca Raton, p 7-22
Pinson A (1990) Neonatal rat heart muscle cells. In: Piper HM (ed.) Cell culture techniques in heart and vessel research. Springer Verlag, Berlin, p 20-35
Rohr S (1995) Determination of impulse conduction characteristics at a microscopic scale in patterned growth heart cell cultures using multiple site optical recording of transmembrane voltage. J Cardiovasc Electrophysiol 6: 551-568
Rous P, Jones FS (1916) A method for obtaining suspensions of living cells from fixed tissues and for plating individual cells. J Exp Med 23:549-555
Speicher DW, McCarl RL (1978) Isolation and characterization of the proteolytic enzyme component from commercially available crude trypsin. Anal Biochem 84:205-217
Speicher DW, McCarl RL (1978) Evaluation of a proteolytic enzyme mixture isolated from crude trypsins in tissue disaggregation. In Vitro 14:849-853

Culture of Embryoid Bodies

Cornelia Gissel, Dirk Nierhoff, Bernd Fleischmann, Jürgen Hescheler and Agapios Sachinidis

Introduction

Regenerative medicine offers a novel therapeutic approach to a wide variety of human diseases. It is based on stem cells and their capability to self-renew indefinitely and to differentiate into several tissue-specific cell types. In the past, embryonic stem (ES) cells were shown to maintain their proliferative and undifferentiated state *in vitro* using special cell culture conditions. ES cells are fully pluripotent and can be differentiated into all cell types of the three embryonic germ layers. ES cells are isolated from the inner cell mass (ICM) of the early mammalian blastocyst-stage embryo (Fig. 1) and are purified using special cell-sorting facilities (Bradley et al. 1984). Due

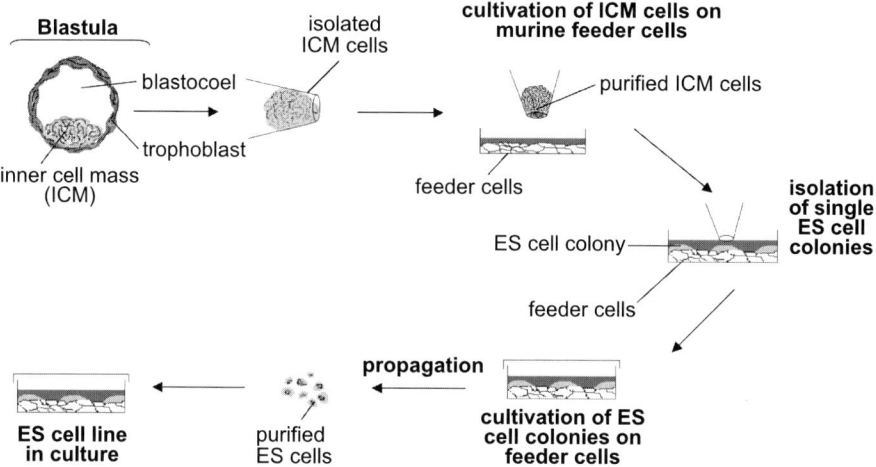

Figure 1
Generation of embryonic stem (ES) cell lines. Cells of the inner cell mass (ICM) of the blastula-stage are isolated and separated. These purified ICM cells are cultured on murine mitotically inactivated fibroblasts called feeder cells. Feeder cells produce, apart from other factors, the leukemia inhibitory factor (LIF), which inhibits a further differentiation of ES cells. Within a short period, ES cells growing on the feeder cell layer form colonies. These colonies are isolated by a pipette and propagated once more on feeder cells to increase the purity of the ES cell population. These purified ES cells are used for the generation of ES cell lines

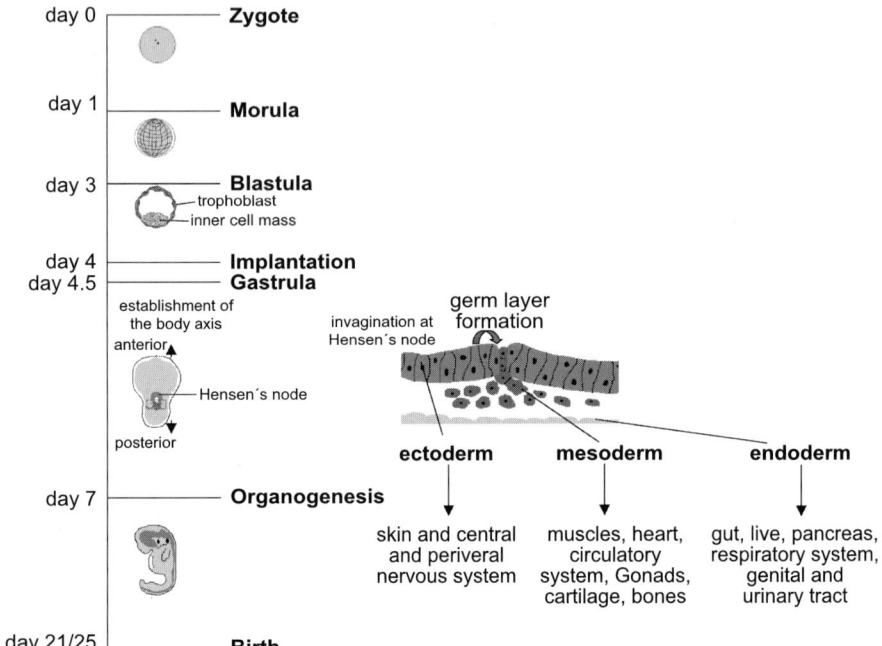

Figure 2
Developmental process *in vivo*. The developmental process is initiated by the fusion of egg and sperm and the subsequent migration of the zygote from the ovary to the uterus. Within the first day, the zygote develops into the morula stage by rapid cell divisions. The inner cells loosen their intercellular adhesion and generate a cavity called a blastocoel. The outer cells build up stronger intercellular adhesion contacts. This is called the blastula stage. The inner cells differentiate into the inner cell mass (ICM) cells, while the outer cells differentiate into the trophoblast. At day 4 after fertilization, the embryo is embedded into the uterus. From now on, the embryo receives all nutrients from the maternal organism, leading to an increase in size and further differentiation. The following gastrulation is a cell migration process with the formation of the three embryonic germ layers (ectoderm, mesoderm and endoderm) and is also decisive for the establishment of the body axis (anterior/posterior, the ventral/dorsal axis and left-right asymmetry). While the ectoderm develops by the diffentiation of the outer cells of the ICM cells, endoderm and mesoderm emerge from cells having passed during the cellular migration process. Each of these three embryonic germ layers differentiates into specialized organs. The date of birth varies between different mouse strains (Gilbert 1991)

to ethical restrictions, the use of human ES cells has begun only recently and protocols are not yet established. In 1998, Thomson succeeded for the first time in isolating and cultivating human ES cells (Thomson et al. 1998). Murine ES cells have already been demonstrated to be an ideal tool to study developmental processes. They can be used in cell culture and for *in vitro* differentiation as well as for the generation of transgenic mice.

A crucial step at the beginning of *in vitro* differentiation is the formation of spheroidal aggregates, also referred to as embryoid bodies (EBs). With regard to the spatial and temporary gene expression pattern, EBs reveal physiological processes similar to the native development of ICM cells (Rathjen et al. 1999; Sachinidis et al. 2003). These EBs resemble early post-implantation embryos and the first structures generated by EBs are quite like the first embryonic structures. At the time of gastrulation, these structures are the three embryonic germ layers and the embryonic body axes. After the formation of the three embryonic germ layers, cells will continue to differentiate into tissue-specific cell types (Fig. 2). Therefore, the formation of EBs represents an optimal *in vitro* model to study the basic cellular and molecular mechanisms of differentiation. Moreover, EBs are derived from pluripotent ES cells and they do not have the potential to develop into a mature organism. For this reason, they are not classified as living organisms with all the resulting ethical and technical limitations.

The transplantation of differentiated tissue-specific cells derived from ES cells may restore the lost function in damaged organs. Therefore, ES cells offer a stem cell-based therapy for several human diseases including diabetes mellitus, Parkinson's disease and severe heart failure (Odorico et al. 2001). Using special protocols, ES cells are able to differentiate *in vitro* into cardiomyocytes (Sachinidis et al. 2003), hematopoietic progenitors, yolk sac, skeletal myocytes, smooth muscle cells, adipocytes, chondrocytes, endothelial cells, melanocytes, neurons, glia and pancreatic islet cells (Doetschman et al. 1985; Lowell 2000; Odorico et al. 2001). Our working group has concentrated on the generation of functionally mature cardiomyocytes from ES cells for the treatment of cardiovascular diseases (Sachinidis et al. 2003). Heart failure is one of the most common cardiovascular diseases in the world. It develops due to a loss of functional cardiomyocytes, a condition also known as cardiomyopathy. This defect is irreversible because of the inability of adult cardiomyocytes to regenerate. Therefore, heart transplantation is the only effective treatment for patients suffering from end-stage heart failure. In recent years, transplantation of isolated precursor cardiomyocytes has been tested in several animal studies as an alternative approach for the treatment of severe heart failure. This technique is known as cardiomyoplasty and the successful grafting of the transplanted cells into the adult heart has been clearly demonstrated (Delcarpio and Claycomb 1995; Roell et al. 2002). As the precursor cardiomyocytes must be isolated from embryonic hearts from aborted fetuses, cardiomyoplasty is not applicable for the treatment of heart failure in humans. The differentiation of ES cells into functionally mature cardiomyocytes might offer an alternative source of transplantable cells. In our recent work, we have focused on the development of strategies for the specific differentiation of ES cells into early cardiomyocytes and for lineage-selection (Hescheler et al. 1997; Rathjen et al. 2001; Sachinidis et al. 2003).

In this chapter, the basic methods used for the generation of EBs from murine *D3* ES cells are described. The generation of EBs is the crucial step in the differentiation of ES cells into any type of tissue-specific cells.

Description of Methods and Practical Approach

Description of Methods

The preparation of EBs is described using ES cells derived from the *D3* cell line. This cell line is distributed by the American Type Culture Collection (ATCC). The cell line was established from the mouse strain *129/Sv+C/+P* (Threadgill et al. 1997).

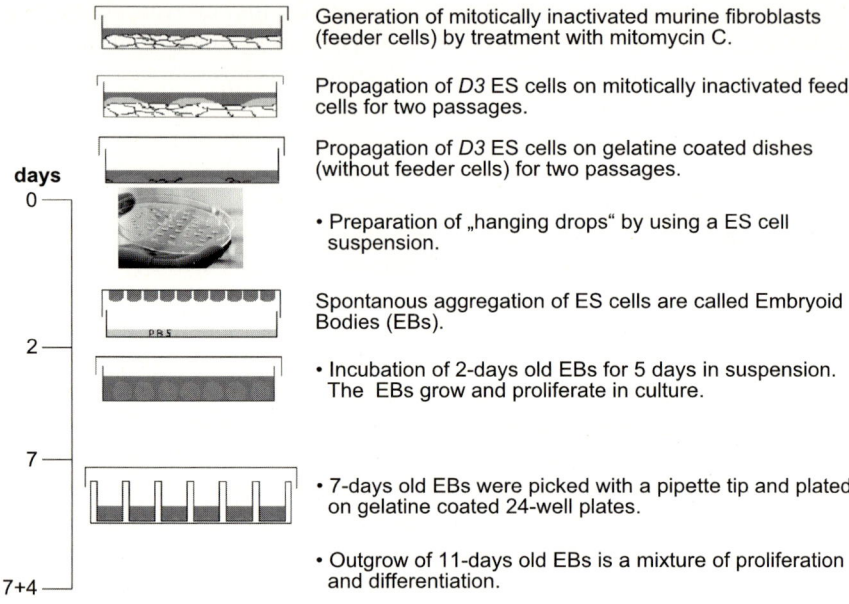

Figure 3
Generation of EBs

In general, ES cells are cultured on mitotically inactivated fibroblasts, also referred to as feeder cells. In the presence of leukemia inhibitory factor (LIF), ES cells remain undifferentiated (see Fig. 1) and they form cell colonies consisting of small and tightly packed single cells. In the absence of LIF, ES cells differentiate spontaneously into different cell types (Ling and Neben, 1997). The basic principle of EB generation and differentiation is schematically illustrated in Fig. 3.

Cell culture of *D3* ES cells requires feeder cells for propagation after thawing. Afterwards, ES cells have to be cultured on gelatine-coated dishes to minimize the number of fibroblasts. In our laboratory, EBs are generated by the "hanging drops" method. In brief, a defined volume of an ES cell suspension is cultivated in the form of a "hanging drop" in the lid of a Petri dish for two days. In order to allow further proliferation and to increase their size, EBs are transferred into bacteriological dishes and are cultivated in renewed medium for a further period of 5 days. Finally, the EBs are plated on multi-well culture plates for their definitive differentiation.

Practical Approach

It is important to maintain sterile conditions and to avoid contamination during cell culture. Apart from a sterile working place, it is important to use sterile cell culture dishes, autoclaved solutions and single-use plastic material. Clean all materials (bottles, plastic packs and surfaces) with 70% ethanol (EtOH). The incubator and water bath should be sterilized with 10% $CuSO_4$ solution overnight. Rinse the incubator and water bath with distilled autoclaved water and clean afterwards with 70% EtOH the day before use. In addition, 50–100 units per millilitre (units/ml) of penicillin/streptomycin can be added to the respective culture media. However, penicillin/streptomycin as well as L-glutamine remain stable only for a couple of days and media should be renewed after two or three days. Warm up all solutions and media 30 min before use in a 37 °C warm water bath. Standard conditions for the incubation of mammalian cells require 37 °C in a humid atmosphere with 5% carbon dioxide (CO_2).

Solutions, Tissue Culture Media and Materials

Materials, commercially available:
- 10 cm Petri dishes (bacteriological) (Greiner 664102)
- 10 cm cell culture dishes (Falcon 35-3003)
- 15 ml tubes (Falcon 35-2097)
- 50 ml tubes (Falcon 35-2098)
- 6-well cell culture plates (Merck 35-3046)
- 24-well cell culture plates (Merck 35-3047)
- 5 ml pipettes (Merck 356543)
- 10 ml pipettes (Merck 356551)
- cryotubes (Nunc 375418)
- 0.2 mm sterile filter (Merck 2004-10)
- Neubauer cell counting chamber (Merck)
- Pasteur pipette (Merck 61271722)
- 10–100 µl Multipipette (Eppendorf)
- 1000 µl micromolecular-pipette Gilson (Amersham)
- Blue tips (Biolabs 70762)

Solutions, commercially available:
- Phosphate-buffered saline (PBS) (v/o Ca^{2+}/Mg^{2+}) (Invitrogen 14190-094)
- Dulbecco's modified Eagle medium (DMEM), supplemented with L-glutamine and 4500 mg/l glucose, but free from sodium pyruvate (Invitrogen 41965-039)
- Iscove's modified Dulbecco's medium (IMDM) (supplemented with L-glutamine and 25 mM HEPES) (Invitrogen 21980-065)
- Fetal calf serum (FCS, heat-inactivated) (Invitrogen 40F4498K/0602015K). (Note: FCS and fetal bovine serum (FBS) are the same sera)
- Trypsin/EDTA solution (Ca^{2+}/Mg^{2+}-free), stored at -20 °C (Invitrogen 25300-054)
- Crystalline trypsin type XII (Sigma Aldrich C6645)
- Gelatine type II (Sigma, G2500)
- Non-essential amino acids (MEM) (100×concentrated) (Invitrogen 11140-035)
- L-glutamine (100× concentrated, 200 mM), stored at -20 °C (Invitrogen 25030-024)
- β-Mercaptoethanol (14.3 M) (Sigma M7522)
- LIF (aliquots stored at 4°C) (Chemicon ES61107)
- Penicillin/streptomycin (100× concentrated), stored at −20 °C (Invitrogen 15070-063)
- Mitomycin C (Serva, 29805)
- Dimethylsulfoxide (DMSO) (Merck)

Materials, self-prepared. Preparation of gelatine-coated dishes:
- Dilute the stock solution 1:10 with PBS to prepare a 0.1% gelatine solution under sterile conditions.
- Use naked cell culture dishes or 6-well plates and fill with 7 ml or 4 ml respectively of this 0.1% gelatine solution.
- Incubate gelatine-coated dishes or plates for at least 3 h (or overnight).
- Aspirate the gelatine solution shortly before use (*Note:* prevent drying of gelatine-coated dishes or plates).

Solutions, self-prepared
- *Punks balanced salt saline* (BSS) (self-prepared, using 8 g NaCl, 0.3 g KCL, 0.073 g Na_2HPO_4, 2 g D(+) glucose, 0.2 g EDTA and 0.02 g phenol-red, dissolved in one litre double-distilled (dd) H_2O and sterilized by autoclaving for 15 min).
- *Trypsin-diluted* (TD) *medium* (self-prepared, using 100 mg crystalline trypsin type XII, dissolved in 5 ml Punks BSS). As crystalline trypsin is volatile, we recommend that the flask delivered by the manufacturer is used to avoid contamination. Afterwards prepare 5 ml aliquots and store at –20 °C.
- 14.3 M β-*mercaptoethanol* is diluted in PBS to obtain a final concentration of 0.1 mM.
- Dissolve 5 g type II gelatine in 500 ml PBS and incubate it for 30 min at 37 °C. Autoclave this 1% gelatine stock solution twice for 30 min.

ES cell culture medium (see Table 1):
- DMEM supplemented with 15%FCS
- 1000 units/ml LIF
- 0.1 mM β-mercaptoethanol
- L-glutamine (200 mM solution), finally 1×- concentrated (2 mM)
- Non-essential aminoacids (MEM), finally 1× concentrated
- 50 units/ml penicillin/streptomycin.

Table 1

	ES cell culture	EB culture	Feeder cell culture
Medium	DMEM	IMDM	DMEM
LIF	1000 units/ml	–	–
β-mercaptoethanol	0.1 mM	0.1 mM	0.1 mM
L-glutamine	2 mM	2 mM	2 mM
MEM	1-fold	1-fold	1-fold
FCS	15%	20%	10%
Penicillin/Streptomycin	50 units/ml	50 units/ml	50 units/ml

EB cell culture medium (see Table 1):
- IMDM supplemented with 20%FCS
- 0.1 mM β-mercaptoethanol
- L-glutamine (200 mM solution), finally 1× concentrated (2 mM)
- Non-essential amino acids (MEM), finally 1× concentrated
- 50 units/ml penicillin/streptomycin.

Feeder cell culture medium (see Table 1):
- DMEM supplemented with 10% FCS
- 0.1 mM β-mercaptoethanol
- L-glutamine (200 mM solution), finally 1× concentrated (2 mM)
- Non-essential amino acids (MEM), finally 1× concentrated
- 50 units/ml penicillin/streptomycin.

ES cell wash medium
- DMEM supplemented with 5% FCS

Cryoconversation medium
- 10% DMSO and 90% FCS – ice cold!

Cell Culture of Murine Fibroblast (Feeder) Cells

Preparation of murine fibroblast (feeder) cells:
1. Decapitate a pregnant mouse (at day 13–14 of pregnancy).
2. Clean the abdomen with 70% EtOH and carefully remove the complete uterus. Bath the uterus in a 50 ml tube with 20 ml 70% EtOH.
3. From now on work should be carried out in a sterile atmosphere. Remove all uterine and embryonic walls step by step. After removing one wall, the embryos are transferred into a new Petri dish filled with ice cold PBS.
4. Remove head, legs, tail and all inner organs and transfer the embryos after each step into a new dish with ice cold PBS.
5. Use two scalpels to cut the embryo into small pieces (place it for this purpose in an empty Petri dish on ice).
6. Transfer the tissue pieces into a 15 ml tube and wash them with ice cold PBS. (*Note:* Do not spin down, let the pieces settle down slowly by gravitation!).
7. Dissolve the tissue pieces in 5 ml TD medium. Incubate the suspension for 3 min at 37°C and pipette it up and down.
8. Stop the digest by adding 3 ml FCS and homogenize the solution with pipettes.
9. Spin down the cells for 15 min at 1000 revolutions per minute (rpm).
10. Remove the supernatant and resuspend the cells in 10 ml feeder cell culture medium. (*Note:* Resuspend the cells carefully, first using a pipette with a larger diameter (10 ml pipettes), then a smaller one (5 ml pipettes) and finally a Pasteur pipette. Pipette the suspension up and down each time!).
11. Spin down as before and remove the supernatant and resuspend the cells in 10 ml feeder cell culture medium.

12. Plate 1 ml of this cell suspension into a 10 cm cell culture dish filled with 14 ml feeder cell culture medium.
13. Incubate the cells overnight at 37 °C with 5% CO_2 and humidity and renew the medium the next day.
14. When cells are 70–90% confluent, passage cells of these dishes in the ratio 1:4 (see next section). Up to 4 passages with each dish are possible.
15. The process of feeder cell inactivation is described below.

Passaging murine fibroblast (feeder) cells:
1. Aspirate the medium from a confluent dish and wash the cells twice with warm PBS (37 °C).
2. Aspirate the supernatant and add 3 ml trysin/EDTA solution.
3. Incubate at 37 °C for about 3 min until the cells have lost their contact with the dish or with each other.
4. Add 3 ml feeder cell culture medium and transfer the cell suspension into a 15 ml tube.
5. Spin down for 15 min at 1000 rpm and remove the supernatant.
6. Resuspend the cells in 10 ml feeder cell culture medium.
7. Spin down again, remove the supernatant and resuspend in 4 ml feeder cell culture medium.
8. Plate 1 ml of this suspension into a 10 cm cell culture dish and add 12 ml feeder cell culture medium. Incubate the cells at 37 °C with 5% CO_2 and humidity until they are confluent.

Preparation of murine mitotically-inactivated fibroblast (feeder) cell dishes
1. Prepare murine feeder cells as described above.
2. Dissolve 1 g mitomycin C in 1 ml PBS to get a 0.001% concentrated solution and sterilize this solution by passing it through a 0.2 µm sterile filter.
3. Aspirate the medium from a confluent feeder cell culture and wash twice with 37 °C warm PBS.
4. Pour 6 ml of feeder cell culture medium into each cell culture dish and add 60 µl of the freshly prepared mitomycin C solution.
5. Incubate the cells for 2.5 h at 37 °C with 5% CO_2 and humidity. Remove the supernatant and wash the cells three times with 37 °C warm PBS.
6. Passage the cells using the trypsin/EDTA solution.
7. Re-plate the cells from the 10 cm cell culture dish in one 6-well cell culture plate. Mitotically inactivated fibroblast (feeder) cells can be used for ES cell culture or can be stored frozen in liquid nitrogen (see below).

    After thawing cells as described in the following section, cells from one vial (analogous to one 10 cm cell culture dish) can be plated into a one 6-well cell culture plate using feeder cell cul-ture medium.

Cell Culture of D3 ES Cells

See Figs. 3 and 4.

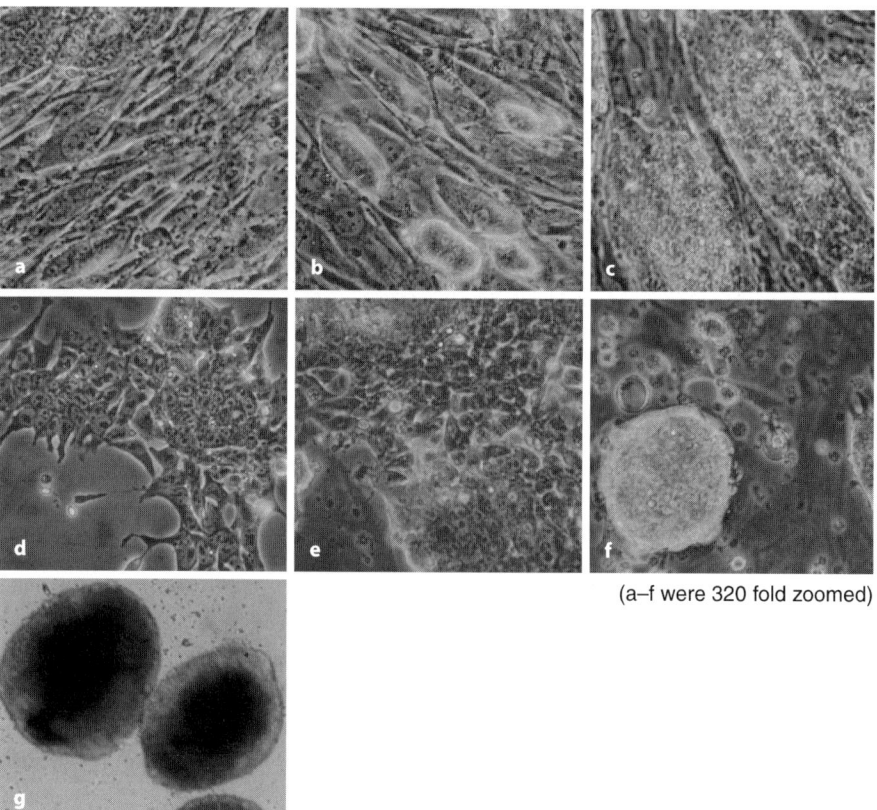

(a–f were 320 fold zoomed)

Figure 4a–g
Morphology of *D3* ES cells and EBs. **a** Mitotically inactivated murine fibroblasts plated on cell culture dishes and cultured for several days. The cellular monolayer appears homogeneous and all cells show similar morphology. Co-cultured ES cells generate colonies (bright spots) on the feeder cell layer. **b** 24 h after thawing and plating, ES cells start to form small colonies (*bright spots*). **c** 48 h after plating, colonies are bigger in size and their morphology looks homogeneous (even in colour and contour), indicating an undifferentiated state. **d** *D3* ES cells cultured on gelatine-coated dishes for 18 h. This culture does not show any colonies, but single cells, which are small in size and tightly packed. Cells at the edge show offshoots and spikes. These had disappeared within the following 6 h (see **e**). **f** ES cell culture two days after the 4th passage on gelatine-coated dishes. ES cells have generated multi-cellular colonies (*bright spots*). This culture has been used for the generation of EBs. **g** The ES cell aggregates proliferate in suspension. These are 4 day old EBs with a diameter of 1.2–1.4 mm. All cell culture pictures were taken with a 320× zoom

Thawing of cells
1. Fill a 50 ml tube with 30 ml 37 °C warm wash medium.
2. Take out a frozen vial from liquid nitrogen (wear protective clothes) and place it immediately for 2 min into a 37 °C warm water bath.
3. Slowly add some wash medium to the vial and transfer the suspension into the 50 ml tube containing the prepared wash medium.

4. Spin down for 5 min at 1000 rpm.
5. Aspirate the medium and resuspend the pellet in 4 ml ES cell culture medium, pipetting up and down to get a homogenized solution.
6. Aspirate the medium from a dish prepared with mitotically inactivated feeder cells as described in the previous section.
7. Transfer all of the cell suspension from 50 ml tube into the prepared feeder cell dish.
8. Place the dish into the incubator at 37 °C with 5% CO_2 and humidity and incubate overnight.
9. Monitor the cellular morphology and check for contamination each day. Change the medium after 24 h.

Passaging of ES cell cultures:
1. Aspirate the medium and wash the ES cell culture twice with 37 °C warm PBS.
2. Aspirate the PBS and add 2–3 ml cold (room temperature (RT)) trypsin/EDTA solution. Incubate at 37 °C for 3–5 min until the cells have lost their adhesion to the surface and with each other. Monitor the reaction under the microscope.
3. Rock the dish, add 5–7 ml wash medium. Transfer the suspension into a 15 ml tube.
4. Pipette the suspension up and down several times to generate a single cell suspension. Monitor under the microscope to be sure that there are no more clumps left.
5. Spin down for 15 min at 1000 rpm and RT.
6. Aspirate the supernatant and resuspend the cells in 5 ml wash medium.
7. Spin down for 15 min at 1000 rpm and RT.
8. Estimate the cell titer in your suspension using a cell counting chamber. Prepare the cell counting chamber as described by the manufacturer. Add the appropriate volume of the cell suspension. Count the cells under a microscope and calculate the total cell number in your cell suspension as described below.
   - Cell titre (cells/ml) = number of counted cells × chamber factor (Neubauer chamber = chamber factor 10^4)
   - Total number of cells = cell titre × volume of available cell suspension
   - Number of ES cells = total number of cells – 10^6 cells.
     Note: 10^6 cells represents the estimated number of 10^6 feeder cells left in your cell suspension. This is not required for ES cells obtained from gelatine-coated dishes.
   - Volume to resuspend the pellet = number of ES cells/1×10^6
     Note: To evaluate the vitality of your cells, Trypan blue can be added to the aliquot reserved for cell counting. White cells surrounded by Trypan blue are vital, dead cells are coloured blue.
9. Aspirate the supernatant and resuspend the cells in the calculated volume of ES cell culture medium to obtain a cell suspension with 1×10^6 cells/ml.
10. Depending on the number of passages after thawing, the ES cells have to be plated once more on mitotically inactivated feeder cell dishes or on gelatine-coated dishes. Aspirate the medium or solution from the dishes and fill them with 3.7 or 3.5 ml ES cell culture medium, respectively.
11. Inoculate the dish with 0.3 ml (feeder cell dish) or 0.5 ml (gelatine-coated dish) of the 1×10^6 cells/ml ES cell suspension, corresponding to 3×10^5 or 5×10^5 ES cells, respectively.
12. Check that the cells are adherent within 12 h after replating.

13. Change the medium after 24 h or passage the cells after two days if they are confluent. (*Note:* Do not passage ES cells 24 h after plating/replating)

Preparation of EBs:
1. Choose 65–70% confluent ES cells 4 passages after thawing (2 passages on feeder cell dishes and 2 passages on gelatine-coated dishes).
2. Trypsinize ES cells and follow the instructions for thawing of cells, as described above, until step 8. Afterwards, dissolve the pellet in EB culture medium in order to obtain a 1×10^6 cells/ml cell suspension.
3. Dilute this suspension with EB culture medium to obtain 2×10^4 cells/ml.
4. Fill 30 Petri dishes with 7 ml PBS each.
5. Pipette the cell suspension up and down a couple of times to get a homogenized cell suspension.
6. Use the multi-pipette to drop 20 µl/drops of this cell suspension into the lid of the Petri dish, placing about 60–70 drops/lid (see Fig. 3) (*Note:* keep 0.5 cm distance between the drops and 1 cm distance from the edge).
7. Close the Petri dish carefully and incubate the drops as hanging drops for 2 days.
8. Open the dish after two days in a sterile atmosphere.
9. Use a 5 ml pipette and 3 ml EB culture medium to remove the drops from the lid.
10. Collect the EBs from 3 lids in one new Petri dish in a total volume of 12 ml EB culture medium.
11. Incubate the 2-day old EBs for another 5 days at 37 °C with 5% CO_2 and humidity.

Freezing cells:
1. Prepare the cryoconservation medium and keep it on ice for 30 min
2. Label a cryotube with all the important data (date, passage, cell line) and place it on ice as well.
3. Aspirate the medium from a confluent ES cell culture dish and continue to passage the cells following the protocol for cell thawing until step 5.
4. Remove the supernatant.
5. Rock the tube to loosen the pellet and add a defined volume of ice cold cryoconservation medium to obtain a suspension with 1×10^6 cells/ml.
6. Fill 1–1.8 ml of this cell suspension into each cryotube and close it.
7. Store the cryotube for the next 48 h in a freezer at –80°C.
8. Place it into liquid nitrogen and store it until use.

Examples

EB Differentiation Protocol: Generation of Beating Cells in Plated EBs.

This protocol requires 7-day old EBs. Beating cells can be detected more easily in plated EBs (gelatine-coated multi-well plates) than in unplated EBs. Therefore, EBs were plated as 7-day old EBs in EB culture medium. Beating cells can be found in 11-day old EBs very easily (beating cells are visible in 9-day old EBs up to 7-day old EBs. An example of a plated EB is shown in Fig. 5.

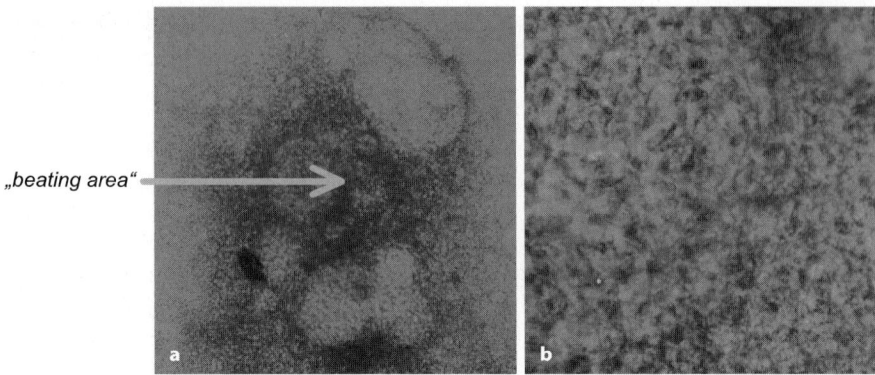

Figure 5
"Beating area" in plated EB. This EB was generated as described in our example in the section above. EBs collapse within the first day after plating and the spheroidal structure of the EBs has disappeared. **a** EB 4 days after plating (100-fold zoomed). The area with beating cells is indicated by the arrow. It is characteristic that cells at the border of the collapsed center start the beating activity. **b** Area with beating cells (320-fold zoomed).

1. Prepare *D3* EBs as described in the section Preparation of EBs above.
2. Aspirate the gelatine solution from a 24-well plate and fill 0.5 ml EB culture medium into each well.
3. Use a blue tip and a micromolecular pipette to pick up the EBs from the suspension and transfer 20 EBs into each well. Count the number of EBs per well under the microscope. (*Note:* Counting the plated EBs is necessary to ensure comparable experimental conditions in each well)
4. Incubate the plates at 37 °C with 5% CO_2 and humidity and check daily under the microscope for beating areas and changes in their cellular morphology.
5. Change the medium every second day.
6. Beating cells can be monitored and documented by photography or by video film.

Troubleshooting

Finding Only Cellular Debris After Thawing

- Freezing and thawing is difficult in cells, because DMSO is a toxic agent. Cool the cryoconservation medium on ice before use and do the same with the cryotubes. Reduce the time of incubation and handling in DMSO to a minimum.
- Prepare the cell culture dishes thoroughly for thawing (do not use dried dishes or dishes with inhomogeneous feeder cell layers).
- Place the cryotubes in a protective Styrofoam box in a –80 °C freezer for 24 h before freezing. Keep the cryotubes for another 24 h in a –80 °C freezer without a box and transfer them finally into liquid nitrogen.

ES Cells Become Confluent Overnight

The titre of the plated cells was probably higher than calculated. You cannot continue the protocol with these cells, as they will start to differentiate due to a high number of intercellular interactions.

ES Cells Start to Differentiate in the Presence of LIF

- LIF might have been inactivated. Notice that LIF should be stored at 4 °C.
- ES cells that were passaged more than 12× often start to differentiate. To prevent this, freeze and thaw cells during propagation. For the generation of EBs, you should use only ES cells which have been passaged no more than 4×.
- Cells were not optimally homogenized after passaging, so that the solution contains clumps (aggregates). These clumps should be removed by passing the suspension through 100 µm and 50 µm meshes.
- Use a newly stored vial of frozen cells and freshly prepared feeder cell dishes and start again.

No EBs Obtained from "Hanging Drops"

There are a number of possible explanations for this observation, only a small selection of which are presented here.

- Use a higher cell titre for the cell suspension than was used for the generation of "hanging drops" and try again (titre should be from 2×10^4 cells/ml up to 3×10^4 cells/ml corresponding to 200–400 cells/"hanging drop").
- The ES cell culture used in the experiment might be contaminated by mycoplasm or fungi.
- The presence of differentiated cells can lead to important changes in EB formation.
- MEM and L-glutamine might have been degraded.
- Different batches of FCS vary significantly in their potency to generate EBs.

EBs are Small

- The cell number in the cell suspension was less than 2×10^4 cells/ml.
- Contaminations prevent normal cellular proliferation.
- The cellular density was higher than defined. Therefore, the cells produce more CO_2, which increases the acidity of the medium. This difference in pH value can reduce cellular proliferation.
  Moreover, L-glutamine, MEM and glucose concentrations are reduced by increased metabolism.

EBs are Sticky

Use only bacteriological Petri dishes, because the surface of cell culture dishes is treated with special agents, which makes the ES cells adhere to the surface.

Media from Plated EBs is Yellow

- The number of plated EBs/well was higher than defined (20 EBs/24-well) leading to an increased metabolism in this well.
- Bacterial contamination might have occurred. Use a higher concentration of penicillin/streptomycin and work very carefully.

Self-Prepared Feeder Cells Do Not Grow After Plating

- Self-prepared feeder cells might contain mycoplasms. Occasionally, this kind of contamination leads to a reduced proliferation rate. Different companies, like ATCC, offer STO feeder cells or CF1 feeder cells. These cells are mitotically inactivated by gamma irradiation and tested for mycoplasm contaminations.
- In order to improve the quality of the feeder cell cultures, you have to be sure to remove all differentiated cells from the embryos.

Mitotically Inactivated Feeder Cells Differentiate And Proliferate After Inactivation

The mitomycin C solution must be prepared freshly before use because mitomycin C might degrade in solution. Do not use frozen solutions.

How to Evaluate the Quality of Feeder Cells

Criteria for good quality feeder cells include the formation of a homogeneous cellular layer and a homogeneous cellular morphology. Ideally, feeder cells have the same colour, similar size and smooth cellular borders. The quality of feeder cells is critical for ES cell culture.

Getting no Reproducable Data

- Check all culture conditions and the quality of your cells and document your data by photography or video film to compare with earlier observations.
- Check your cultures for contamination (mycoplasm, bacteria or fungi) using commercial kits.

References

Bradley A, Evans M, Kaufman MH, Robertson E (1984) Formation of germ-line chimaeras from embryo-derived teratocarcinoma cell lines. Nature 309:255–6

Delcarpio JB, Claycomb WC (1995) Cardiomyocyte transfer into the mammalian heart. Cell-to-cell interactions *in vivo* and *in vitro*. Annals of the New York Academy of Sciences 752:267-85

Doetschman TC, Eistetter H, Katz M, Schmidt W, Kemler R (1985) The *in vitro* development of blastocyst-derived embryonic stem cell lines: formation of visceral yolk sac, blood islands and myocardium. J Embryol Exp Morphol 87:27–45

Gilbert S.F (1991) Developmental Biology. Edition 3, Sinauer Associates

Hescheler J, Fleischmann BK, Lentini S, Maltsev VA, Rohwedel J, Wobus AM, Addicks K (1997) Embryonic stem cells: a model to study structural and functional properties in cardiomyogenesis. Cardiovasc Res 36:149–62

Ling V, Neben S (1997) *In vitro* differentiation of embryonic stem cells: immunophenotypic analysis of cultured embryoid bodies. J Cell Physiol 171:104–15

Lowell S(2000) Stem cells show their potential. Trends Cell Biol 10:210–1

Odorico JS, Kaufman DS, Thomson JA (2001) Multilineage differentiation from human embryonic stem cell lines. Stem Cells 19:193–204

Rathjen J, Dunn S, Bettess MD, Rathjen PD (2001) Lineage specific differentiation of pluripotent cells *in vitro*: a role for extraembryonic cell types. Reprod Fertil Dev 13:15–22

Rathjen J, Lake JA, Bettess MD, Washington JM, Chapman G, Rathjen PD (1999) Formation of a primitive ectoderm like cell population, EPL cells, from ES cells in response to biologically derived factors. J Cell Sci 112 (Pt 5): 601–12

Roell W, Lu ZJ, Bloch W et al. (2002) Cellular cardiomyoplasty improves survival after myocardial injury. Circulation 105:2435–41

Sachinidis A, Fleischmann BK, Kolossov E, Wartenberg M, Sauer H, Hescheler J (2003) Cardiac specific differentiation of mouse embryonic stem cells. Cardiovasc Res 58:278–91

Thomson JA, Itskovitz-Eldor J, Shapiro SS, Waknitz MA, Swiergiel JJ, Marshall VS, and Jones JM (1998) Embryonic stem cell lines derived from human blastocysts. Science. 282:11457 Erratum in Science 282:1827

Threadgill DW, Matin YD, Nadeau JH and Magnuson T (1997) Genealogy of the strain 129 inbred strains: 129/SvJ is a contaminated inbred strain. Mammalian Genome 8:390–393

Culturing and Differentiation of Embryonic and Adult Stem Cells for Heart Research and Transplantation Therapy

Marcel A.G. van der Heyden and Henk Rozemuller

Introduction

Stem cells are unspecialised cells capable of self-renewal, which give rise to multiple differentiated cell types in the body. Embryonic stem (ES) cells are totipotent. They are the founder cells for all the tissues of the three different germ layers of the developing organism. Adult stem cells in contrast are pluripotent, reside within differentiated tissues and are primarily involved in the self-renewal of that specific tissue.

Once brought into culture, ES cells are, in principle, still able to differentiate into all cell types, including cardiac myocytes and endothelial cells. The plasticity of adult stem cells appears to be surprisingly great. Whole bone marrow samples and different small populations of bone marrow-derived haematopoietic stem cells show a potential to transdifferentiate into heart cells *in vitro* and *in vivo*. Currently, stem cell derived cardiomyocytes are considered to be a potential donor source for cell replacement therapy in diseased hearts, but also represent a good *in vitro* cardiomyocyte cell model for basic heart cell research at the molecular and physiological level, a fact appreciated for many years.

Embryonic Stem Cells

The mammalian blastocyst stage embryo contains a confined population of stem cells, the inner cell mass that gives rise to all the tissues of the developing organism. Following microsurgery, this type of cell was brought into culture and clonal cell lines were established (Evans and Kaufman 1981). Since then, murine ES cells have represented an invaluable model for studying embryonic development, including cardiac differentiation.

The electrophysiological differentiation has been studied extensively (Hescheler et al. 1997), and it was concluded that the ES cell derived cardiomyocytes display a late embryonic/neonatal phenotype. In an animal model for heart dystrophy, transplantation of purified mES derived cardiomyocytes led to the formation of stable cardiac grafts (Klug et al. 1996), emphasizing the potential of stem cells for cell transplantation technology.

Recently, embryonic stem cell lines have been isolated from human blastocysts (Thomson et al. 1998). Initial studies also demonstrated the potency of these stem cells in differentiation into cardiomyocytes (Kehat et al. 2001; Mummery et al. 2003), which holds promise for cell based transplantation therapy in diseased human hearts.

Embryonal Carcinoma Cells

Teratocarcinomas are spontaneous tumours found in the testes of mice and humans. They have a remarkable phenotype, in that they consist of numbers of differentiated tissues as diverse as hair, muscle, bone and even complete teeth. Besides fully differentiated cells, these tumours contain small numbers of rapidly dividing undifferentiated stem cell-like cells, named embryonal carcinoma (EC) cells. Once brought into culture, it was established that these stem cells could be differentiated into more specialised cell types. In 1982, pluripotent murine P19 EC cells (reviewed by Van der Heyden and Defize 2003) were derived from an experimental teratoma formed after ectopic transplantation of a 7.5 dpc mouse embryo. These cells can be easily differentiated into either neurons or cardiomyocytes following embryoid body formation in combination with retinoic acid or DMSO. The resulting cardiomyocytes have been reasonably phenotyped with respect to contractile proteins, electrophysiological properties and cardiac specific transcription factors. Furthermore, these cells have provided a good tool for studying cardiac differentiation factors and gene products, since the cells are easy to transfect and select for stably expressing cell lines. Subsequent differentiation efficiency assays determine the ability of any given factor to induce, enhance or inhibit cardiomyocyte differentiation.

Bone Marrow Derived Haematopoietic Stem Cells

Evidence was shown that circulating stem cells engraft the adult heart and differentiate into mature cardiac myocytes. Several research groups observed this plasticity of bone marrow derived cells in animal models (Hirschi and Goodell 2002; Krause 2002; Jackson et al. 2002). Bone marrow (BM) contains different subsets of stem cells; e.g. the mesenchymal stem cells (MSC), the haematopoietic stem cells (HSC), and endothelial progenitor cells (EPC). The phenotype and origin of stem cells, responsible for the regeneration of cardiomyocytes and coronary vessels, is still not known. Data were published in which differentiation into cardiomyocytes was observed from different types of bone marrow cells, e.g. unpurified whole bone marrow (Bittner et al. 1999), cultured human and rat stromal cells (Makino et al. 1999; Toma et al. 2002; Jiang et al. 2002a) and subpopulations of highly purified haematopoietic stem cells (HSC) (Orlic et al. 2001a; Goodell et al. 2001). The purified stem cell populations are very homogeneous, well characterised cells and can be reproducibly isolated from bone marrow but also from non-haematopoietic tissues. There is no evidence that one of the approaches is superior.

Description of the Method and Practical Approach
Embryonic Stem Cells

mES Cells

mES cells can be obtained from various sources, e.g. the American Type Culture Collection (ATCC). mES D3 line (ATCC #CRL-1934) cells have proved to differentiate efficiently into cardiac myocytes. Murine embryonic cell lines depend on either feeder layers (most often irradiated- (12,000 rads) or mitomycin C (0.01 mg/ml; for 90 min) treated-mouse embryonic fibroblast (MEF) or STO cells) or addition of leukaemia inhibitory factor (LIF) to the culture medium (Glasgow MEM/20% FCS) to retain an undifferentiated, pluripotent state. Often, researchers use a combination of feeder cells and LIF addition. Undifferentiated mES cells express the marker protein Oct4, which can be easily stained in cell cultures thus confirming the undifferentiated state of the cells.

Differentiation is initiated by spontaneous aggregation in hanging drops of Glasgow MEM/10% FCS without LIF, from the lid of a PBS-filled Petri dish (~40 hanging drops on a lid of a 10 cm diameter bacterial Petri dish). Each 20 µl drop contains 400 cells. After five days of hanging drop culture, the resulting embryoid bodies are transferred to culture dishes and are allowed to attach and grow out. From day 8 onwards, spontaneously beating cardiomyocytes appear.

Dissociation and replating of the cardiac cells can be essential for certain subsequent procedures, such as immunohistochemistry or patch clamp electrophysiology. Therefore, clusters of beating cells are excised under microscopical inspection in a laminar flow cabinet. Clusters are collected in low Ca^{2+} medium (120 mM NaCl, 5.4 mM KCl, 5 mM $MgSO_4$, 5 mM Na pyruvate, 20 mM glucose, 20 mM taurine, 10 mM HEPES pH7.4) and cells are dissociated in the above medium containing 30 µM $CaCl_2$ and 1 mg/ml collagenase B for approximately 45 min at 37 °C under repetitive up-and-down trituration. Dissociated cells are centrifuged, resuspended in differentiation medium and replated on 1% gelatine coated coverslips or 3.5 cm culture dishes for immunofluorescence and electrophysiology respectively.

mES Differentiation and Dissociation Protocol

Materials:
- MEF medium (Glasgow MEM, 10% FCS, L-glutamine, sodium pyruvate, non-essential amino acids, penicillin/streptomycin)
- ES medium (Glasgow MEM, 20% FCS, LIF)
- EB medium (Glasgow MEM, 10% FCS)
- TVP (0.025% trypsin, 1% chicken serum, 1 mM EDTA, in PBS)
- Low Ca^{2+}-medium (120 mM NaCl, 5.4 mM KCl, 5 mM $MgSO_4$, 5 mM Na pyruvate, 20 mM glucose, 20 mM taurine, 10 mM HEPES, pH7.4)
- Dissociation medium, low Ca^{2+}-medium supplemented with 30 µM Ca^{2+} and 1 mg/ml collagenase B
- Bacterial dish 10 cm diameter
- Tissue culture dish

- Cell counter
- Inverted phase contrast microscope
- Microscalpel

Protocol
- Day 1
  - Irradiated or mitomycin treated MEFs can be frozen in liquid nitrogen. They are available from commercial sources or can be produced and frozen in house. These cells are cold-sensitive and media should be prewarmed to 37 °C
  - Thaw MEF and suspend in 12 ml medium
  - Plate MEFs in 24 well plates, 0.5 ml per well
  - Incubate overnight in a CO_2 incubator
- Day 2
  - Thaw mES cells from liquid nitrogen, or trypsinise from another culture
  - Count cells
  - Remove medium from MEFs and plate mES at various concentrations (2.10^3 to 1.10^4) on MEF feeders in mES medium
- Day 5, 6 or 7
  - Choose wells in which mES forms nice round colonies to trypsinise
  - Remove medium and wash cells twice with PBS
  - Add 0.1 ml of TVP and incubate at 37 °C for 5 to 10 min
  - Add 1 ml of mES medium
  - Transfer to a tube and centrifuge for 5 min at 800×g
  - Remove excess supernatant
  - Resuspend cells in remaining medium and count cells
  - Make a dilution of 20 cells/µl in EB medium
  - Fill the base of a 10 cm diameter bacterial dish with PBS
  - Make 20 µl drops of mES cells (= equivalent of 400 cells) on the lid of the bacterial dish, about 40 drops per lid
  - Invert lid and place on the PBS filled base
  - Incubate in CO_2 incubator for 5 days, embryoid bodies will form in the hanging drops
- Day 10
  - Transfer embryoid bodies to tissue culture plates containing EB medium, 10 embryoid bodies per dish of 3 cm diameter.
- Day 14 and onwards
  - Beating cells can be observed
  - Refresh differentiation medium every two days until further processing of the cardiomyocytes
  - Excise clusters of beating muscle under microscopical examination in the laminar flow cabinet, using a sterile microscalpel
  - Collect excised beating clusters with blue pipette tip and put in low Ca^{2+}-medium
  - After a maximum of 30 min, remove excess medium and add low Ca^{2+}-medium supplemented with 30 µM Ca^{2+} and 1 mg/ml collagenase B
  - Incubate at 37 °C for 45 min under repetitive up-and-down trituration
  - Collect dissociated cells at the bottom of the tube by 5 min centrifugation at 800×g

- Remove as much dissociation solution as possible
- Carefully resuspend cells in EB medium using a wide mouthed pipette
- Transfer cells to tissue culture dishes or 0.1% gelatin coated coverslips

P19 EC Cells

P19 cells can be obtained from ATCC (#CRL-1825), and are regularly grown on α-MEM supplemented with 10% FCS, without the need for feeder cells or LIF. P19 cells grow very rapidly and cultures should be split every 2 days, using standard trypsin solutions.

Cardiac differentiation is initiated by embryoid body formation in the presence of 1% DMSO for four days. Cells can be aggregated using the hanging drop method (see mES cells), or embryoid bodies can be produced in bulk by putting 1×10^6 cells/ml in a bacterial dish, or on a 2–3 mm layer of 0.5% agar dissolved in culture medium containing 1% DMSO.

As a result, cells will spontaneously aggregate. Add DMSO-containing medium at day 1, and replace 40% of the medium on day 2. Embryoid bodies can be plated to culture tissue dishes on day four, and areas of beating cardiomyocytes occur between days 8 and 10 after the start of aggregation. Medium should be refreshed regularly.

To obtain single cells, beating clusters are excised under microscopical inspection in a laminar flow cabinet and collected in Hanks solution without Ca^{2+} and Mg^{2+}. Cells are dissociated in the same buffer supplemented with 0.13% trypsin and 20 µg/ml DNAse I at 37 °C. The tube should be swirled every 3 min. After 25 min, dissociated cells are collected by centrifugation ($800\times g$), suspended in normal medium using a pipette with a wide mouth opening, and replated on, for instance, 0.1% gelatin coated coverslips or 3.5 cm dishes.

P19 Differentiation and Dissociation Protocol

Materials:
- α-MEM medium containing 10% differentiation tested FCS
- DMSO (tissue culture grade)
- 5% agar in PBS (sterilized)
- Hanks solution without Ca^{2+} and Mg^{2+}
- Bacterial dishes, 10 cm diameter
- Tissue culture dishes
- Cell counter
- Inverted phase contrast microscope
- Microscalpel
- Trypsin
- DNAse I

Protocol
- Day 0
    - Prewarm 13.5 ml medium with optimal FCS for differentiation and 1% DMSO (differentiation medium) at 37 °C.

- Melt sterile 5% agar in PBS in a microwave
- Quickly add 1.5 ml 5% agar solution to prewarmed differentiation medium, and transfer 7 ml to a 10 cm diameter bacterial dish, swirl till the complete surface is covered
- Cool at room temperature for at least 1 h
- Trypsinise P19 EC cells as usual and count cells
- Dilute P19 cells to 1×10^6/ml in differentiation medium
- Tilt the agar plate and slowly add 9 ml of P19 cells (1×10^6 cell/ml) at the edge of the plate.
- Allow cells to aggregate for 24 h in a CO_2 incubator
- Day 1
  - Add 4 ml of differentiation medium
- Day 2
  - Carefully remove 4 ml of medium without embryoid bodies
  - Add 4 ml of differentiation medium
- Day 4
  - Fill dishes with differentiation medium (i.e. 8 ml in a 10 cm diameter tissue culture dish)
  - Carefully remove embryoid bodies with a blue tip and add to prefilled tissue culture plate (i.e. 5–10 embryoid bodies per dish)
  - Allow aggregates to attach for 24 h
- Day 6 and further
  - Refresh differentiation medium every two days until further processing of the cardiomyocytes
  - Excise clusters of beating muscle under microscopical examination in the laminar flow cabinet, using a sterile microscalpel
  - Collect each excised beating cluster with a blue pipette tip and put it in 7 ml of Hanks solution
  - After collecting the last beating cluster (within 1 h from the first) carefully remove Hanks solution from the excised clusters
  - Add 7 ml fresh Hanks solution containing 0.13% trypsin and 20 µg/ml DNase I
  - Incubate for 25 min in 37 °C water bath and swirl the tube every 3 min
  - Collect dissociated cells at the bottom of the tube by 5 min centrifugation at $800\times g$
  - Remove as much Hanks solution as possible
  - Carefully resuspend the cells in normal differentiation medium using a wide mouthed pipette
  - Transfer the cells to tissue culture dishes or 0.1% gelatin coated coverslips

Adult Stem Cells

MSC (Makino et al. 1999; Toma et al. 2002; Tomita et al. 1999)

Human, goat, mouse and rat MSC's are isolated by loading the BM cells over Percoll solution. Mononucleated cells (MNC) are collected from the upper and interphase layers and washed in PBS. The cells are cultured in DMEM/low glucose containing

10% FCS. After a series of passages, attached marrow stromal cells become homogeneous and are devoid of haematopoietic cells. This population of pure MSCs can be used at different passages for *in vivo* differentiation into cardiomyocytes. To induce cell differentiation *in vitro*, cells are treated with 3 µM of 5-azacytidine for 24 h followed by washing with PBS and continued culturing in medium.

MAPC (Jiang et al. 2002a,b)

Multipotent adult progenitor cells (MAPCs) can be isolated from mice, rats, or humans and from various organs such as BM, brain and muscle. The MNC are obtained by Ficol-hypaque density gradient centrifugation. MNC's from the interphase are incubated for at least 20 min at 4 °C with anti CD45 and anti GpA for human cells, or anti murine CD45 and anti TER119 for mouse and rat cells, conjugated to micromagnetic beads. The $CD45^+$ and GpA^+ cells are depleted using magnetic activated cell sorting (MACS) technology. $CD45^-$ GpA^- cells are cultured in 60% low glucose DMEM and 40% MCDB-201 (Sigma), supplemented with 1× insulin/transferrin/selenium (working concentrations of 10, 5.5 and 5 mg/L, respectively), 1× linoleic acid-BSA (working concentration of 1 mg/ml), 10^{-8} M dexamethasone, 10^{-4} M ascorbic acid 2-phosphate, 2% FCS, 10 ng/ml epidermal growth factor (EGF) and 10 ng/ml platelet derived growth factor (PDGF). This stem cell population (0.01% of MNC) is enriched for the MAPC, but mesenchymal stem cells are co-purified and have to be eliminated by exhaustion through prolonged culturing. MAPC are purified by prolonged culturing (~3 months) in basic MAPC medium. The frequency of MAPC has been determined as 10^{-7} of MNC. MAPC can be cultured and expanded indefinitely while maintaining their plasticity. The cells are characterised by their potential to differentiate into endothelial, hepatocytic and neural cells.

MAPC Isolation and Growth Protocol

Materials:
- Basic MAPC medium: DMEM medium low glucose containing, MCDB201, ITS, ascorbic acid, dexamethasone, 2% differentiation tested FCS (Hyclone), EGF/PDGF-BB both 10 ng/ml
- Differentiation medium: basic MAPC medium without FCS, EGF and PDGF
- PBS/2 mM EDTA (sterilized)
- Ficol-hypaque
- Fibronectin (5 ng/ml)
- Trypsin (0.25%)
- Tissue culture 96, 48, 24, 12 and 6 wells plate (Falcon)
- Tissue culture flasks T25, T75 and T175
- CD45 beads, GpA beads (Miltenyi)
- Variomacs and depletion CS-columns
- Cell counter
- Inverted phase contrast microscope

Protocol for isolation MAPC cells:
- Dilute bone marrow sample with PBS/2 mM EDTA (1:1)
- Add 20 ml of BM sample slowly to 15 ml of Ficol-hypaque
- Centrifuge 15 min, 1400×g, RT no brake
- Use cells from the interphase
- Wash the cells twice in excess PBS/2 mM EDTA
- Count the cells
- Incubate the cells with CD45-beads and GpA beads (Miltenyi) according to the manufacturers' manual (20 µl beads per 10^7 MNC)
- Sort the CD45⁻ and GpA⁻ cells using the CS column of Miltenyi
- After depletion, plate the cells at a density of 2,000 cells/well in a fibronectin (5 ng/ml) coated 96-well plate in basic MAPC medium
- Change the medium every 3–4 days and check for clones
- The first clones will appear 10 days after the purification
- At 50% confluency, passage cells to a FN-coated 48 well plate, using 0.25% trypsin/2 mM EDTA
- Passage cells at 80% confluency from 48 to 24 to 12 and finally to a 6 well plate (all FN coated)
- Count cells and transfer to a T25 culture flask
- Plate the cells at a density of 2000 cells/cm^2 and passage the cells at 80% confluency (8000 cell/cm^2)
- Start differentiation studies after 25–30 population doublings

SP Cells (Goodell et al., 1996)

Murine bone marrow is isolated from the femurs and tibias and resuspended in a concentration of 10^6 cells/ml in prewarmed DMEM containing 2% FCS, penicillin, streptomycin, and 5 µg per ml Hoechst 33342. The cells are incubated for 90 min at 37 °C. After the Hoechst staining, the cells are incubated with a cocktail of lineage specific antibodies, e.g. T-lymphocytes (CD4 and CD8), B-lymphocytes (B-220), macrophages (Mac-1), granulocytes (GR-1) and erythrocytes (TER-119). After incubation, the cells are washed in an excess of buffer and the cell pellet resuspended in media containing goat anti-rat antibody conjugated to phycoerythrin (PE). The cells are then stained with biotinylated anti Sca1, followed by avidin conjugated to FITC. The cells are isolated by using the fluorescence activated cell sorter (FACS) with a dual-laser flow cytometer. The Hoechst dye is excited at 350 nm and the fluorescence is measured at two wavelengths, e.g. the blue fluorescence using a 450 BP optical filter and the red fluorescence through a 610 long pass edge optical filter. A 610 nm short pass dichroic mirror is used to separate the emission wavelengths. The side population (SP) is defined using the Hoechst red and blue fluorescence on a linear scale. The population has a low fluorescence due to the actively extruded Hoechst dye. The cells falling into the SP-region, negative for the lineage markers and positive for the Sca1 are sorted into FCS coated glass tubes. An aliquot is reanalysed to establish the purity of the cells. This highly purified population of stem cells contains ~0.1% of the total MNC.

Lin-c-kit^{POS} Cells (Orlic et al. 2001a, c)

Bone marrow is harvested from femurs and tibia and suspended in PBS containing 5% FCS. To isolate lin-c-kit^{POS} cells, the cells are incubated for 30 min on ice with lineage specific anti-mouse antibodies as described above (CD4, CD8, CD5, B220, Mac-1 and GR-1). After the labelling, the cells are rinsed in an excess of PBS and incubated with magnetic beads coated with a goat anti-rat immunoglobulin secondary antibody. The lineage positive cells are removed by MACS. The 10% remaining lineage negative cells are stained with a biotinylated anti c-kit monoclonal antibody. After rinsing the cells in PBS, the cells are labelled with streptavidin-conjugated PE and sorted by FACS. The Lin-c-kit^{POS} cells are sorted into FCS coated plastic and suspended at a concentration of 3×10^4 to 2×10^5 cells per 5 µl PBS. This population of stem cells comprises ~1–0.5% of total MNC.

Examples

In vitro/in vivo Versatility of mES Cells

To create a method to identify stem cell derived cardiomyocytes by fluorescence detection methods, stem cells were stably transfected with a construct in which the gene encoding enhanced cyan fluorescent protein was put under the control of a fragment of the ventricular myosin light chain 2 (MLC2v) promoter (Meyer et al. 2000). Following cardiac differentiation, the ECFP gene switched on in ventricular-like cardiomyocytes only. After dissociation, the cardiomyocytes could be purified using FACS, and subsequently used for *in vitro* or *in vivo* studies. When the non-differentiated cells were placed into an adult mouse heart, a portion of the cells differentiated into cardiac myocytes as identified by the presence of blue fluorescence and other cardiac markers (Behfar et al. 2002).

The efficiency of this *in vivo* differentiation was dependent on intact TGF-β/BMP signalling as measured by the appearance of blue cells in transgenic mice affected in this signalling pathway.

Similarly engineered mES cells, in this case EGFP driven by the α-cardiac myosin heavy chain, were used to screen 880 different drugs from a complete compound library, for their capability to induce cardiac differentiation (Takahashi et al. 2003).

P19 EC Cell Differentiation and Characterization

Cell Morphology

When observed by phase contrast microscopy, undifferentiated P19 cells are relatively small with a high nucleus to cytoplasm ratio (Fig. 1a), which in fact is a common feature of embryonic stem cells. Aggregation of cells leads to the formation of embryoid bodies (Fig. 1b) in which the first differentiation occurs, i.e. the outer layer of the embryoid body differentiates towards primitive or visceral endoderm. Following

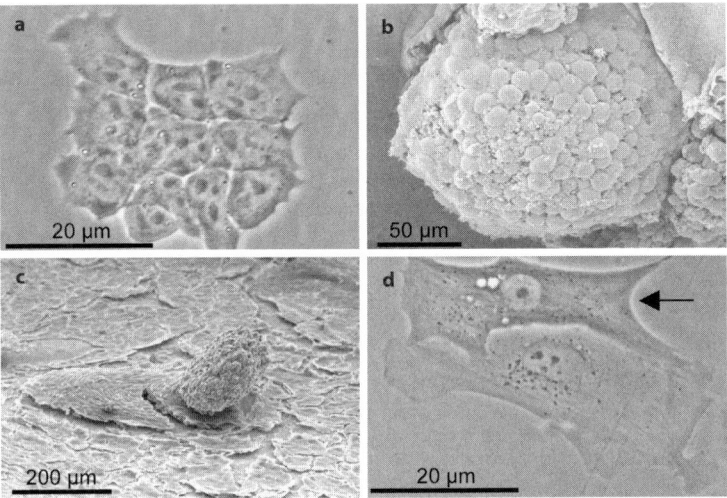

Figure 1a–d
P19 EC cell morphology during cardiac differentiation. **a** Phase contrast image of a small cluster of undifferentiated P19 EC cells. **b** Scanning electron microscopy image of a 4 day old P19 embryoid body. **c** Scanning electron microscopy image of an aggregate outgrowth area, 12 days after plating of the embryoid body (not visible). **d** Phase contrast image of a dissociated day 18 beating cardiomyocyte (*arrow*) and an attached non-cardiomyocyte

plating of the embryoid body, many differentiated cell types can be found in the aggregate outgrowth (Fig. 1c). Often, the outgrowths still contain undifferentiated cells, which can overgrow the slower growing, differentiated cells. Dissociated and replated beating myocytes display a denser cytoplasmic appearance combined with a bright halo around the cell (Fig. 1d, arrow), in contrast to non-myocytes.

Regulation of Ion Channels

The ability of P19 cells for large-scale differentiation, offers the opportunity to combine biochemical approaches with single cell electrophysiology. During the differentiation phase, samples can be taken at every stage. As depicted in Fig. 2a, RNA can be isolated and subsequently used for RT-PCR approaches. In this example, cells are harvested at days 0, 14 and 24 of differentiation and compared to adult mouse heart material. β-tubulin serves as an input control, and from the cardiomyocyte marker MLC2v it can be seen that cardiac differentiation is already obvious at day 14. Regulation of ion channels at the mRNA level can be studied, for example the L-type calcium channel α1c or the transient outward channel I_{TO} (Fig. 2a). Following cell dissociation, action potentials and single cell currents can also be measured. Most early (day 16–18) spontaneously active cells display action potentials with a clear diastolic depolarization and a nodal-like phenotype (Fig. 2b). Application of specific stimulation protocols elucidates the presence of several different inward and outward ion currents (Figs. 2c–e). Data shown suggest the presence of cardiac sodium and slow inward (I_{CaL}) channels.

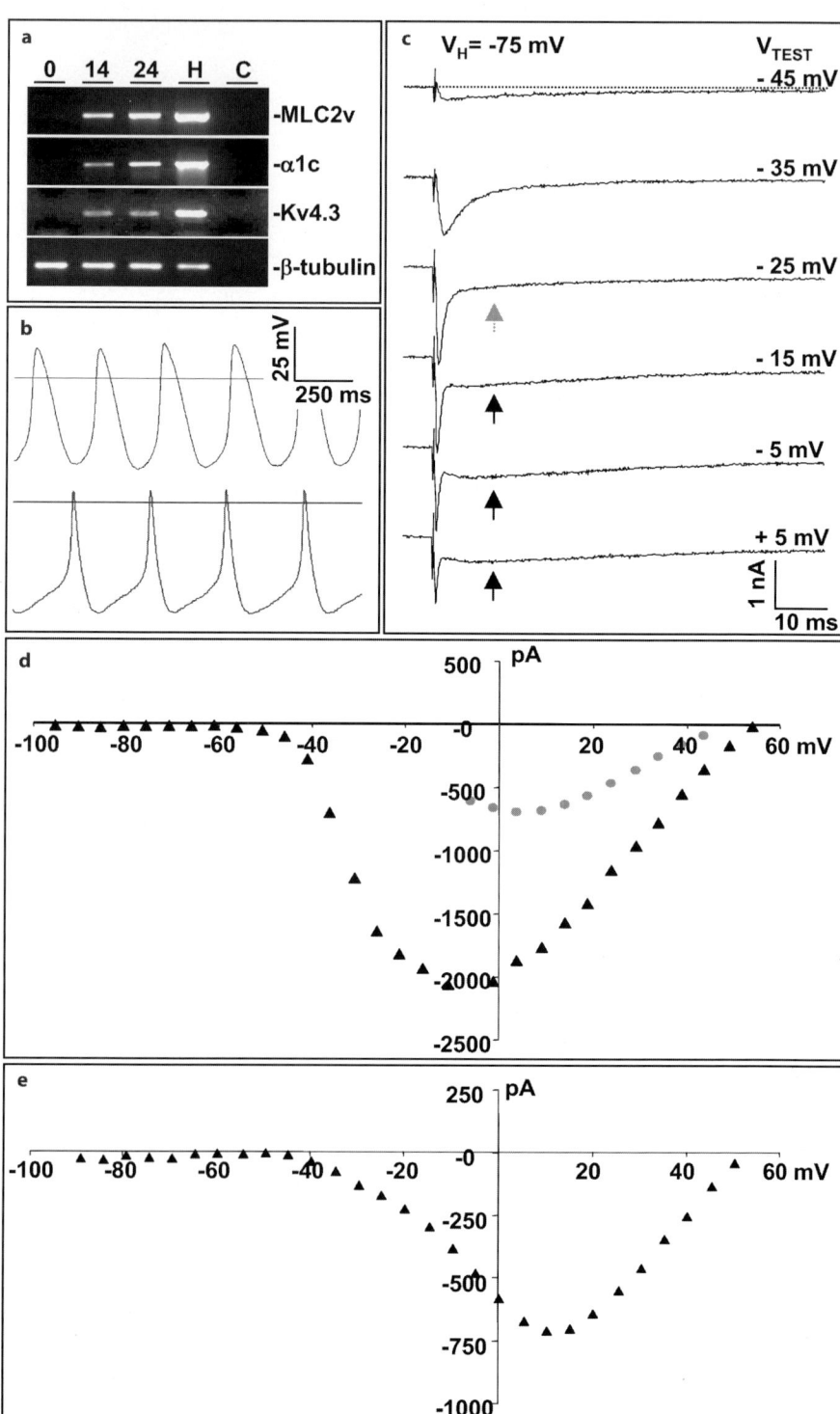

Role of Cardiac Specific Transcription Factors in Cardiomyocyte Differentiation

Because of their ability to generate clonal cell lines efficiently in combination with their high susceptibility to ectopic gene incorporation and expression, P19 cells offer an attractive system to study genetic pathways involved in cardiac differentiation, as illustrated in the following examples.

The cardiac specific transcription factor GATA-4 is exclusively expressed in the cardiac lineages of differentiating P19 cells. Expression was found near maximal levels after 3 days of DMSO treatment. This expression precedes the up-regulation of putative GATA-4 target genes such as the cardiac muscle markers BNP, cTpC and αMHC. To investigate the necessity of GATA-4 for cardiac differentiation, antisense RNA was stably expressed in P19 cells (Grépin et al. 1995). This had no effect on undifferentiated growth or RA-induced neuronal differentiation. However, DMSO-induced P19 aggregates spread poorly after aggregation, cultures contained many undifferentiated cells and apoptosis was observed by day 5 of differentiation. Most importantly, neither beating muscle nor cardiac marker expression was found, in contrast to control cells. Endoderm and early mesoderm are formed normally as detected by the specific markers, indicating no requirement for GATA-4 in very early differentiation processes. After analysis of early cardiac marker expression, it was concluded that antisense GATA-4 P19 clones are unable to differentiate beyond the precardiac, or cardioblast stage (Grépin et al. 1997). GATA-4 over-expression (P19[GATA-4]) on the other hand, increased cardiac differentiation even without DMSO treatment, although it was still dependent on aggregation. The combination of GATA-4 and DMSO potentiated differentiation in time and extent.

◀ **Figure 2a–e**
a Cardiac differentiation of P19 embryonal carcinoma as revealed by semi-quantitative RT-PCR. Undifferentiated cells (0) were allowed to aggregate for 4 days and subsequently plated. On days 14 and 24 samples were taken from whole cultures and excised beating clusters respectively. After RNA was isolated, DNAse-treated and transcribed to cDNA, samples were amplified with primers for ventricular myosin light chain 2 (MLC2v), cardiac L-type calcium channels (α1c) and transient outward channels (Kv4.3). β-tubulin served as input control. Adult mouse heart was used as positive control (H). C indicates the water control. Undifferentiated P19 EC cells express no MLC2v or the cardiac ion channels α1c and Kv4.3. During cardiac differentiation, the mRNAs from these genes increase, but expression levels remain lower than in adult murine heart. **b** Action potentials recorded from spontaneously beating P19 derived cardiomyocytes (day 21–22) display different morphologies with a predominant nodal-like character, slow upstroke velocities and relatively long AP duration. Action potential 2 displays a clear diastolic depolarization. Horizontal line, 0 mV. **c–e** P19 derived cardiomyocytes show a mix of fast (TTX sensitive) and slow inward voltage dependent currents that activate and inactivate at different potentials. **c** Example of voltage clamp recordings of inward currents at test potentials of -45 mV to +5 mV, the holding potential was -75 mV. Within the first 5 ms of the test pulse, inward currents activated and inactivated increasingly faster with increasing depolarization test pulses. At -25 mV and more positive, the fast current component is followed by a slow activating and inactivating current component (arrows). **d** IV-relationship of peak inward current measured between -95 mV and +55 mV. Triangles: amplitude of fast activating and inactivating component, dots: amplitude of the slow component (as far it could be discriminated from the fast component). I_{max} of the fast component is approximately at -15 mV, that of the slow component at +5 mV. **e** IV curve of inward currents recorded in the presence of 50 μM TTX (another cell). These currents were slow activating and inactivating (not shown) and peak amplitude was reached at +15 mV

Like GATA-4, the transcription factors Nkx2.5 and MEF2c, whose up-regulation follows that of GATA-4 in time, are able to induce beating muscle independently of DMSO when stably transfected in P19 cells, following aggregation (Skerjanc et al. 1998). Up-regulation of MEF2c and GATA-4 is observed in differentiating P19 [Nkx2.5] cell cultures and *vice versa* Nkx2.5 and GATA-4 are enhanced in differentiating P19[MEF2c] cells. Like GATA-4, Nkx2.5 turns out to be essential for cardiac differentiation of P19 cells as demonstrated by the introduction of a dominant negative version of Nkx2.5 (P19[Nkx/EnR]) (Jamali et al. 2001). Cells remain arrested in the precardiac stage as no up-regulation of GATA-4 and MEF2c was observed, while mesoderm marker expression remained unaffected. Specificity for the cardiac pathway was demonstrated by the observation that skeletal muscle differentiation occurred normally in P19[Nkx/EnR] cells. So, with the use of P19 cells, it can be concluded that GATA-4, Nkx2.5 and MEF2c most probably form a self-amplifying genetic system leading to cardiac commitment and differentiation.

Adult Stem Cells

Unpurified Bone Marrow

In the majority of experiments on the direct introduction of the BM-derived cells into the cardiac environment, an injury to the tissue was essential for differentiation. The first publication of differentiation of bone marrow cells into cardiomyocytes was published by Bittner (Bittner et al. 1999). His group performed a study of BM transplantation in dystrophic mdx mice. He used whole bone marrow from male donors and performed a sex-mismatched BM transplantation. In sections of cardiac muscles from different atrial and ventricular regions of the mdx mice, single cardiomyocytes containing bone marrow-derived Y chromosomes were found. This was direct evidence that cardiac muscle is capable of undergoing regeneration by recruiting circulating BM derived progenitors.

Mesenchymal Stem Cells

More defined populations of the bone marrow were used by others. Cultured MSC's were able to differentiate into cardiomyocytes *in vitro* by treatment with the cytosine analog 5-azacytidine. 1×10^6 cells were injected into the centre of scar tissue and after 5 weeks the heart function was analysed, and confirmed by immunohistochemistry (Makino et al. 1999; Toma et al. 2002; Tomita et al. 1999). It was also shown that the cultured cells were able to differentiate into ventricular scar tissue and improve myocardial function.

Verfaillie and coworkers reported a new population of adult MSCs, the so-called multipotent adult progenitor cells (MAPC) (Jiang et al. 2002a). After introducing a single MAPC into an early blastocyst, the MAPC contributed to most, if not all, somatic cell types including cardiomyocytes, indicative of the potency of these cultured cells. The MAPCs were marked with the reporter gene LacZ, and differentiation into cardiomyocytes was analysed by co-localization with cardiac troponin-I. However, in experiments in which high numbers of MAPC were injected into irradiated NOD/SCID mice, no contribution was seen to skeletal or cardiac muscle. An explanation would be the absence of tissue injury.

Haematopoietic Stem Cells

Not only stromal cells but also the population of haematopoietic stem cells were able to differentiate into cardiomyocytes. Goodell and coworkers examined the contribution of SP cells to newly formed cardiomyocytes by employing BM transplantation of LacZ transgenic SP cells in lethally irradiated mice (Goodell et al. 2001). Ten weeks after transplantation, the left anterior descending coronary artery was occluded for 1 h and subsequently reperfused. The mice were sacrificed 2–4 weeks after the induced infarct and analysed for SP cell contribution. They observed incorporation of LacZ-positive cells, which were co-stained with antibodies against α-actinin. They also reported that LacZ positive cells participated in neovascularization in regenerating heart functions.

Orlic (Orlic et al. 2001a, c) describes an experiment in which they injected male $GFP^+Lin^-c-kit^{POS}$ cells into the border zone of acute infarcts in female non-transgenic mice. These BM cells were able to differentiate into myocytes and vascular structure, ameliorating the function of the infarcted heart. The origin was confirmed by detection of enhanced GFP and the Y-chromosome. As a negative control he used Lin^-c-kit^{NEG} cells, which did not result in new myocytes, indicating that a specific population of stem cells were responsible for the regeneration of heart muscle. The BM derived cardiomyocytes expressed MHC as well as cardiac transcription factors (myocyte enhancer factor 2, GATA-4 and Csx/Nkx2.5).

In a later publication, this group showed that in the presence of an acute myocardial infarct, mobilized BMC were involved in a significant degree of tissue regeneration (Orlic et al. 2001b). Obviously, cytokine mobilization brings the same population of Lin^-c-kit^{POS} stem cells into circulation.

A publication of the group of Kocher reported the results of experiments with a comparable population of cells. They injected G-CSF-mobilized human $CD34^+$ cells into rats with acute infarction and observed improved myocardial function due to neovascularization of the ischemic myocardium (Kocher et al. 2001). However, they did not report any regeneration of cardiomyocytes.

The mobilization of adult stem cells offers a less invasive therapeutic strategy for restoration of heart function by vascularization of injured tissue and differentiation into cardiomyoblasts.

Clinical Studies

So far 3 papers have been published with nonrandomized clinical trials (Assmus et al. 2003; Strauer et al. 2002; Stamm et al. 2003). In these studies, the cells were injected along the circumference of the infarct border. Although the stem cell populations differ in cell subfractions (whole bone marrow versus the purified $AC133^+$ stem cell population), they all demonstrated that the heart function was improved. But all these stem cell transplantations for myocardial regeneration have been done in association with surgical or inventional revascularisation, so that the effect of transplantation cannot be assessed. The hypothesis is, however, that both processes, e.g. myocardial regeneration and neovascularization benefit from the stem cell transplantation.

Troubleshooting

Mouse ES Cells

Care has to be taken to keep the stem cells undifferentiated, since this influences the efficiency of subsequent differentiation into cardiomyocytes. The use of a combination of feeder cells and LIF is recommended. Also, the percentage of undifferentiated stem cells can be regularly checked by determining the expression of the stem cell marker Oct4 using immunofluorescence microscopy.

The efficiency of differentiation into cardiomyocytes is variable. Important factors are the number of cells per hanging drop and the FCS batch. It is advisable to test different batches of FCS for differentiation efficiency and choose the batch that performs best for all subsequent differentiation assays.

The efficiency of dissociation of the beating clusters into individual cardiomyocytes is dependent on the batch of collagenase B used. Again, it is advisable to test different batches simultaneously.

Compared to P19 cells, mouse ES cells have a normal karyotype and differentiate into cardiomyocytes independently of DMSO. Once genetically manipulated, mouse ES cells can be easily used to generate transgenic animals. This offers an opportunity to combine *in vitro* and *in vivo* experiments using the same cells. However, undifferentiated mouse ES cells depend on feeder cells and LIF addition in culture, which makes them less attractive for bulk biochemical approaches or well-defined culture conditions.

Finally, many studies demonstrate that mES derived cardiomyocytes have an embryonic-like phenotype.

P19 EC Cells

Like mES cells, differentiation of P19 EC cells also depends on the serum batch used, and an initial test of several batches should be performed to select the one best suited for induction of cardiac differentiation.

Though P19 cells form a good model system for several kinds of studies, the system also has its limitations. The dependence on 1% DMSO for cardiac specific differentiation might influence several responses. Furthermore, P19 cells have an abnormal, euploidic, karyotype (40:XY).

Based on the studies performed thus far on expression of contractile markers, the functional properties of the ion channels and the resulting action potentials, P19 derived cardiomyocytes appear to have an embryonic phenotype. During heart development, cardiomyocytes alter their transcriptional activity, morphology and electrical properties, resulting in stage dependent characteristics. In P19 derived cardiomyocytes, the contractile apparatus consists of a mixture of atrial and ventricular light and heavy chains and, in addition to cardiac actin, the skeletal form of actin is expressed, another characteristic of embryonic cardiomyocytes. The contractile proteins are organized in sarcomeres, not however of the robust type found in adult, working myocytes. P19 derived cardiomyocytes beat spontaneously, they express calcium channels and limited amounts of functional sodium channels. The maximal diastolic potential is rather low (–40 to –60 mV). The action potential shape and characteristics resemble primary isolated embryonic cardiomyocytes, in that they have a relatively long action potential duration with a slow upstroke velocity (Van der Heyden et al. 2003).

Notwithstanding the limitations, no doubt within the next few years much more information will be obtained using this model system, in which bulk biochemical approaches as well as single cell studies can be carried out.

Bone Marrow Derived Stem Cells

So far, the preliminary experiments with unfractionated bone marrow cells and purified haematopoietic stem cells are promising but still require an extensive research effort. In animal models, regeneration of a large area with new mature cardiomyocytes has not been found. A small group of immature cells scattered in the area of injured tissue was observed without any or only a few cardiomyocyte properties. None of the investigations showed normal functional and electrophysiological properties in the *novo* cardiomyocytes. Also the long-term engraftment of the *novo* cardiomyocytes is still unknown.

Wagers et al. (2002) showed that differentiation of adult stem cells into other tissues is an extremely rare event. Using a slightly different source of murine haematopoietic stem cells (c-kit$^+$Thy1.1^{lo}Lin-Sca-1$^+$), plasticity of the HSC was tested by transplanting GFP marked cells into lethally irradiated nontransgenic recipients. They did not find any transdifferentiation in the cardiac muscle. However the data cannot rule out the potential of HSCs to be recruited into atypical functions in the face of severe injury and/or selective pressure.

We must be very cautious in interpreting plasticity results. Terada and coworkers demonstrated an alternative hypothesis, i.e. that transplanted bone marrow cells might turn into all lineages by fusion of the donor cells to the cells of the new origin (Terada et al. 2002). In this study, adult cells from mouse BM tagged with GFP were cocultured with ES cells that did not carry the marker. They soon detected GFP$^+$ ES cells, but these cells had twice as many chromosomes. Furthermore, using an *in vivo* mouse model, Wang and coworkers demonstrated that bone marrow-derived hepatocytes are mainly the result of cell fusion (Wang et al. 2003). Although the rate of cell fusion may differ between tissues, it might partly explain the plasticity of stem cells. In the experiments of Orlic, the number of newly formed cardiomyocytes was far greater than the spontaneous fusion of cells.

Although in some studies the haematopoietic stem cell populations are highly purified, it is still possible that contaminating non-haematopoietic cells are responsible for the generation of cardiomyocytes. Data from retroviral marking studies to demonstrate the plasticity of individual HSCs are missing. Only in the case of the MAPC is there clear evidence that bone marrow-derived adult stem cells are able to generate cardiomyocytes. In mice it was shown that one single MAPC could form cardiomyocytes by direct transplantation into the blastocyst. Regarding the origin of the MAPC, it is still unknown whether the MAPC have this multipotential activity as a natural phenomenon or whether it is an alteration due to long-term culture.

All these studies showed that different subsets of adult stem cells participate in regenerating cardiomyocytes. Further studies are needed to select the most successful population of bone marrow derived stem cells. Expanding this population would be probably essential for employment of stem cell technology in the treatment of cardiac diseases.

Acknowledgements. We thank Wally Müller (Utrecht University), Nancy Mutsaers and Ingrid de Grijs (UMC Utrecht) for Fig. 1b,c, and Martin Rook for Fig. 2b–e. This work is in part financed by STW grant #MKG.5942 (MvdH).

References

Assmus B, Schächinger V, Teupe C, Britten M, Lehman R, Döbert N, Grünwald F, Aicher A, Urbich C, Martin H, Hoelzer D, Dimmeler S, Zeiher AM (2002) Transplantation of progenitor cells and regeneration enhancement in acute myocardial infarction (TOPCARE-AMI). Circulation 106:3009–3017

Behfar A, Zingman LV, Hodgson DM, Rauzier JM, Kane GC, Terzie M, Pucéat M (2002) Stem cell differentiation requires a paracrine pathway in the heart. FASEB J 16:1558–1566

Bittner RE, Schofer C, Weipoltshammer K, Ivanova S, Streubel B, Hauser E, Freilinger M, Hoger H, Elbe-Burger A, Wachtler F (1999) Recruitment of bone-marrow-derived cells by skeletal and cardiac muscle in adult dystrophic mdx mice. Anat Embryol (Berl) 199:391–396

Evans MJ, Kaufman MH (1981) Establishment in culture of pluripotential cells from mouse embryos. Nature 292:154–156

Goodell MA, Brose K, Paradis G, Conner AS, Mulligan RC (1996) Isolation and functional properties of murine hematopoietic stem cells that are replicating in vivo. J Exp Med 183:1797–1806

Goodell MA, Jackson KA, Majka WM, Mi T, Wang H, Pocius J, Hartley CJ, Majesky MW, Entman ML, Michael LH, Hirschi KK (2001) Stem cell plasticity in muscle and bone marrow. Ann N Y Acad Sci 938:208–18; discussion 218–220

Grépin C, Robitaille L, Antakly T, Nemer M (1995) Inhibition of transcription factor GATA-4 expression blocks in vitro cardiac muscle differentiation. Mol Cell Biol 15:4095–4102

Grépin C, Nemer G, Nemer M (1997) Enhanced cardiogenesis in embryonic stem cells overexpressing the GATA-4 transcription factor. Development 124:2387–2395

Hescheler J, Fleischmann BK, Lentini S, Maltsev VA, Rohwedel J, Wobus AM, Addicks K (1997) Embryonic stem cells: a model to study structural and functional properties in cardiomyogenesis. Cardiovasc Res 36:149–162

Hirschi KK, Goodell MA (2002) Hematopoietic, vascular and cardiac fates of bone marrow-derived stem cells. Gene Ther 9:648–652

Jackson KA, Majka SM, Wulf GG, Goodell MA (2002) Stem cells: a minireview. J Cell Biochem Suppl 38:1–6

Jamali M, Rogerson PJ, Wilton S, Skerjanc IS (2001) Nkx2-5 activity is essential for cardiomyogenesis. J Biol Chem 276:42252–42258

Jiang Y, Jahagirdar BN, Reinhardt RL et al. (2002a) Pluripotency of mesenchymal stem cells derived from adult marrow. Nature 418:41–49

Jiang Y, Vaessen B, Lenvik T, Blackstad M, Reyes M, Verfaillie CM (2002b) Multipotent progenitor cells can be isolated from postnatal murine bone marrow, muscle, and brain. Exp Hematol 30:896–904

Kehat I, Kenyagin-Karsenti D, Snir M, Segev H, Amit M, Gepstein A, Livne E, Binah Ol, Itskovitz-Eldor J, Gepstein L (2001) Human embryonic stem cells can differentiate into myocytes with structural and functional properties of cardiomyocytes. J Clin Invest 108:407–414

Klug MG, Soonpaa MH, Koh GY, Field LJ (1996) Genetically selected cardiomyocytes from differentiating embryonic stem cells form stable intracardiac grafts. J Clin Invest 98:216–224

Kocher AA, Schuster MD, Szabolcs MJ, Takuma S, Burkhoff D, Wang J, Homma S, Edwards NM, Itescu S (2001) Neovascularization of ischemic myocardium by human bone-marrow-derived angioblasts prevents cardiomyocyte apoptosis, reduces remodeling and improves cardiac function. Nat Med 7:430–436

Krause DS (2002) Plasticity of marrow-derived stem cells. Gene Ther 9:754–758

Makino S, Fukuda K, Miyoshi S, Konishi F, Kodama H, Pan J, Sano M, Takahashi T, Hori S, Abe H, Hata J, Umezawa A, Ogawa S (1999) Cardiomyocytes can be generated from marrow stromal cells *in vitro*. J Clin Invest 103:697–705

Meyer N, Jaconi M, Landopoulou A, Fort P, Pucéat M (2000) A fluorescent reporter gene as a marker for ventricular specification in ES-derived cardiac cells. FEBS Lett 478:151–158

Mummery CL, Ward-van Oostwaard D, Doevendans P, Spijker R, Van den Brink, Hassink R, Van der Heyden MAG, Opthof T, Pera M, Brutel de la Riviere A, Passier R, Tertoolen L (2003) Differentiation of human embryonic stem cells to cardiomyocytes, role of coculture with visceral endoderm-like cells. Circulation 107:2733–2740

Orlic D, Kajstura J, Chimenti S, Jakoniuk I, Anderson SM, Li B, Pickel J, McKay R, Nadal-Ginard B, Bodine DM, Leri A, Anversa P (2001a) Bone marrow cells regenerate infarcted myocardium. Nature 410:701–705

Orlic D, Kajstura J, Chimenti S, Limana F, Jakoniuk I, Quaini F, Nadal-Ginard B, Bodine DM, Leri A, Anversa P (2001b) Mobilized bone marrow cells repair the infarcted heart, improving function and survival. Proc Natl Acad Sci USA 98:10344–10349

Orlic D, Kajstura J, Chimenti S, Bodine DM, Leri A, Anversa P (2001c) Transplanted adult bone marrow cells repair myocardial infarcts in mice. Ann N Y Acad Sci. 938:221–229; discussion 229–230

Skerjanc IS, Petropoulos H, Ridgeway AG, Wilton S (1998) Myocyte enhancer 2C and Nkx2-5 up-regulate each other's expression and initiate cardiomyogenesis in P19 cells. J Biol Chem 52:34904–34910

Stamm C, Westphal B, Kleine H, Petzsch M, Kittner R, Klinge H, Schümichen C, Nienaber CA, Freund M, Steinhoff G (2003) Autologous bone-marrow stem-cell transplantation for myocardial regeration. The Lancet 361: 45–46

Strauer BE, Brehm M, Zeus T, Köstering M, Hernandez A, Sorg R, Kögler G, Wernet P (2002) Repair of infarcted myocardium by autologous intracoronary mononuclear bone marrow cell transplantation in humans. Circulation 106:1913–1918

Takahashi T, Lord B, Schulze C, Fryer RM, Sarang SS, Gullans SR, Lee RT (2003) Ascorbic acid enhances differentiation of embryonic stem cells into cardiac myocytes. Circulation 107:r61–r65

Terada N, Hamazaki T, Oka M, Hoki M, Mastalerz DM, Nakano Y, Meyer EM, Morel L, Petersen BE, Scott EW (2002) Bone marrow cells adopt the phenotype of other cells by spontaneous cell fusion. Nature 416:542–545

Thomson JA, Itskovitz-Eldor J, Shapiro SS, Waknitz MA, Swiergiel JJ, Marshall VS, Jones JM (1998) Embryonic stem cell lines derived from human blastocysts. Science 282:1145–1147

Toma C, Pittenger MF, Cahill KS, Byrne BJ, Kessler PD (2002) Human mesenchymal stem cells differentiate to a cardiomyocyte phenotype in the adult murine heart. Circulation 105:93–98

Tomita S, Li RK, Weisel RD, Mickle DA, Kim EJ, Sakai T, Jia ZQ (1999)Autologous transplantation of bone marrow cells improves damaged heart function. Circulation 100(19 Suppl):II247–256

Van der Heyden MAG, Defize LHK (2003) Twenty one years of P19 cells: what an embryonal carcinoma cell line taught us about cardiomyocyte differentiation. Cardiovasc Res 58:292–302

Van der Heyden MAG, Van Kempen MJA, Tsuji Y, Rook MB, Jongsma HJ, Opthof T (2003) P19 embryonal carcinoma cells: a suitable model system for cardiac electrophysiological differentiation at the molecular and functional level. Cardiovasc Res 58:410–422

Wagers AJ, Sherwood RI, Christensen JL, Weissman IL (2002) Little evidence for developmental plasticity of adult hematopoietic stem cells. Science 297:2256–2259

Wang X, Willenbring H, Akkari Y, Torimaru Y, Foster M, Al-Dhalimy M, Lagasse E, Finegold M, Olson S, Grompe M (2003) Cell fusion is the principal source of bone-marrow-derived hepatocytes. Nature 24:897–901

Preparation of Endothelial Cells from Micro- and Macrovascular Origin

Saskia C. Peters, Anna Reis and Thomas Noll

Introduction

Endothelial cells (EC) compose a flat cell monolayer lining the inner surface of the entire vascular system. In many vascular regions they function as the principle barrier between the vessel lumen and the interstitial space. Due to their strategic position, EC control the passage of water, solutes, macromolecules, and leukocytes through the vascular wall.

EC are continuously exposed to haemodynamic forces and signalling molecules arriving via the blood stream or the surrounding tissue. In response to these diverse stimuli, EC express cell adhesion molecules (e.g. ICAM or VCAM) and release a multitude of mediators (e.g. nitric oxide, prostaglandins, cytokines, growth factors, or von Willebrand factor). They can also dynamically change their barrier function. Due to thes multiple functions, EC may be considered as a signal transduction surface, that integrates various signals to adapt vascular functions to the needs of the surrounding tissue. Accordingly, EC are involved in the control of vascular tone and haemostasis and play a crucial role in angiogenesis and vascular repair mechanisms, e.g. re-endothelialization of an injured intima.

In order to analyse the diverse physiological functions independently of the surrounding tissue, ambitious efforts have been made to isolate and culture EC. During the past three decades, the development of isolation and culture techniques of EC from numerous vascular regions and species has revolutionized our understanding of EC function (for a comprehensive survey of isolation techniques of EC from diverse origins ref. to Piper 1990). Today, several techniques have been established to prepare EC either from macrovascular origins such as aorta (Booyse et al. 1975; Watanabe et al. 1991, 1992), vena cava, vena saphena (Watkins et al. 1984), and umbilical vein (Jaffe et al. 1973), or from microvascular origins such as heart (Cirillo et al. 1999; Gräfe et al. 1994; Nees et al. 1981; Oxhorn et al. 2002; Watanabe et al. 1991), brain (Bowman et al. 1981; Mischeck et al. 1989), liver (Rauen et al. 1993), lung (Hewett and Murray 1993; Magee et al. 1994), and eye (Bowman et al. 1982). Depending on the availability of organs and the preparatory access to the vascular region, EC have been isolated from diverse species such as pig (Mischeck et al. 1989; Slater and Sloan 1975; Watanabe et al. 1991), cattle (Booyse et al. 1975, Bowman et al. 1982), rabbit (Cirillo et al. 1999), guinea pig (Nees et al. 1981), and rat (Bowman et al. 1981; Magee et al. 1994; Rauen et al. 1993; Watanabe et al. 1991, 1992). The increasing availability of 'knockout' mice has raised great interest in isolating endothelial cells from this rodent (Dong et al. 1997). Due to its clinical importance, great effort has been focused on the development of isolation techniques for human EC. Most commonly, human EC are isolated from macrovasculature, e.g. umbilical veins (Jaffe et al. 1973), aorta (Draijer et al. 1995), large veins (Watkins et al. 1984), and coronary vessels (Gräfe et al. 1994), or microvasculature, e.g. myocardium (Gräfe et al. 1994), lung (Hewett and Murray 1993), foreskin (Davison et al. 1980), adipose tissue (Hewett et al. 1993), and placenta (Ugele and Lange 2001). Apart from the use of freshly isolated, primary endothelial cell cultures, there are also a variety of endothelial cell preparations commercially available. In addition, a number of endothelial cell lines have been generated from endothelial cells of micro- and macrovascular origin (Adamson et al. 2002; Fitzgerald et al. 2000). However, one great disadvantage of cell lines is that cell morphology and function may change during long-term culture. Therefore, isolation of primary EC is preferable.

Within this article, basic protocols are described for the isolation of EC from microvascular and macrovascular beds of rodents, swine, and humans. With some modifications, these procedures can be adapted to prepare EC from other vascular regions and species. Descriptions of basic staining techniques are given to characterise EC and to discriminate them from cells most commonly responsible for the contamination of endothelial cell preparations.

Description of Methods and Practical Approach

Material

General Equipment and Cell Culture

- Laminar flow hood with a High Efficiency Particulate Air filter (HEPA-filter) equipped with pipette aid and a Bunsen burner
- CO_2 incubator with controlled temperature (37 °C) and humidity (95%)
- Phase contrast microscope (objectives 10× and 20×)
- Autoclave
- Centrifuge
- pH meter
- Adjustable pipettes (5 µl–1 ml) with sterile tips (e.g. Eppendorf)

Cell Culture Utilities

- Culture medium bottles (0.5–1 l)
- Disposable 50 ml polypropylene conical tube (e.g. Falcon)
- Disposable sterile plastic pipettes (10 ml, e.g. Falcon)
- Disposable 100 mm tissue culture dishes (e.g. surface-modified polystyrene dishes PRIMARIA™, Falcon)
- Disposable sterile filter (0.22 µm pore diameter)

Isolation of Microvascular Coronary EC from Mouse

The availability of 'knock-out' mice enables us to characterise vascular function under physiological and pathophysiological conditions. A broad variety of 'knock-outs' evoke a strong demand for isolating murine EC to identify the impact of endothelial key factors on a cellular level.

A method is provided to obtain coronary EC from isolated mouse hearts perfused with a collagenase solution. EC are harvested from the cell suspension of the digested tissue. This method makes use of the fact that EC attach faster on culture dishes than any other myocardial cells. For perfusion of mouse hearts, a special system adapted to small organs is essential. Technical training is required to mount the heart onto the system and re-establish the circulation of the dissected organ quickly. Mouse EC sometimes require special additives to their basal medium, e.g. amino acids and growth supplements.

Preparation Apparatus and Instruments

- Langendorff perfusions system (Fig. 1)
- Y-branch with male Luer lock at both ends for mounting a 20 Gauche 1½" needle
- Temperature-controlled water circulator
- Roller pump
- Teflon beaker (50 ml)
- Tissue chopper equipped with a razor blade (Bachofer, Reutlingen, Germany)
- Scissors, small curved forceps, scalpels and a watch glass
- Disposable sterile 5 ml pipette
- Carbogen (95% O_2, 5% CO_2)

Culture Media and Substances

- Dulbecco's Modified Eagle's Medium (DMEM; e.g. Sigma-Aldrich)
- Foetal Calf Serum (FCS)
  alternatively for higher cell yield Horse Serum (e.g. Invitrogen, Sigma-Aldrich, PAA Laboratories)
- Penicillin and Streptomycin (10,000 IU/ml)
- Collagenase from Clostridium histolyticum (Worthington class II; e.g. Biochrom, PAA Laboratories, Serva)
- Trypsin (e.g., Invitrogen)
- 1 N NaOH
- $NaHCO_3$
- Aqua bidest.
- Non-essential amino acids (e.g. Invitrogen)
- Endothelial growth supplement (e.g. Sigma)
- Heparin (e.g. Roche)

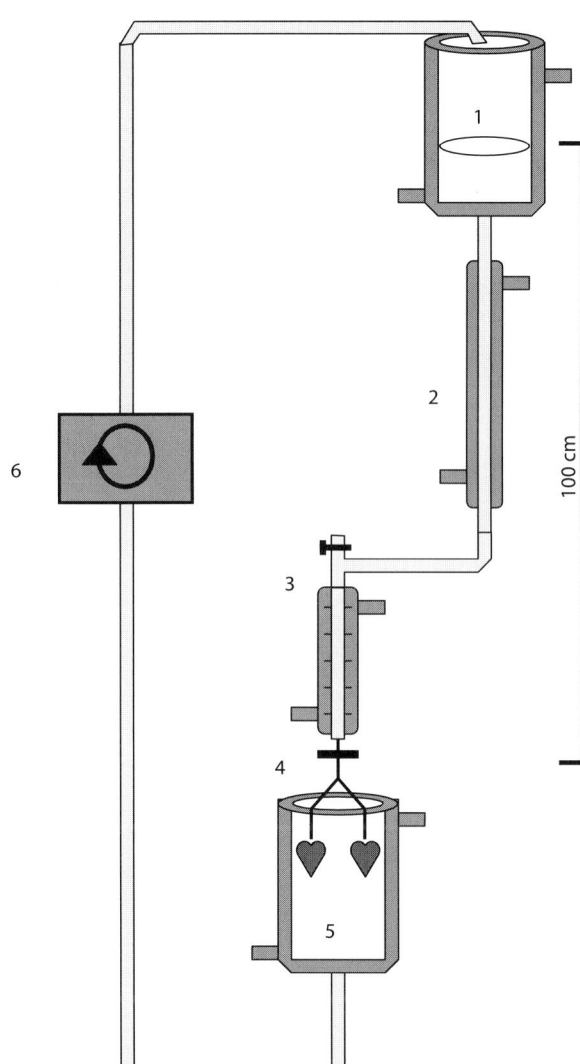

Figure 1
Heart perfusion system.
1. Reservoir (100 ml), containing basic perfusion medium with a temperature of 37 °C, aerated with carbogen (95% O_2, 5% CO_2), 2. Connector for constant height (1 m), 3. Heat exchanger for final temperature equilibration of the perfusate (37 °C), 4. Inverted Y-connector for simultaneous perfusion of two hearts, 5. Funnel as a temperature-controlled chamber, 6. Roller pump, 7. Flow reducer. No. 1–3, and 5 are double-walled and temperature-controlled

Preparing Culture Media and Tissue Solutions

- Dulbecco's Modified Eagle's Medium (DMEM)
  - DMEM dry powder, for 1 l
  - 2.1 g $NaHCO_3$
  Adjusted to pH 7.3 at room temperature with NaOH
  Sterile filtered and stored at 4°C
- DMEM complete; high antibiotics

- 20% FCS
- 1% non-essential amino acids
- 50 U/ml heparin
- 180 µg/ml endothelial growth supplement
- 250 U/ml penicillin; 250 µg/ml streptomycin
- DMEM complete; low antibiotics
  - 20% FCS
  - 1% non-essential amino acids
  - 50 µg/ml endothelial growth supplement
  - 100 U/ml penicillin; 100 µg/ml streptomycin
- Basic perfusion medium
  - NaCl: 110.0 mM
  - KCl: 2.6 mM
  - KH_2PO_4:   1.2 mM
  - $MgSO_4$:   1.2 mM
  - $NaHCO_3$:   25.0 mM
  - HEPES: 25.0 mM
  - Glucose: 11.0 mM

  Aerated with carbogen (pH 7.4)
- $CaCl_2$ stock solution (100 mM)
  - 110 mg $CaCl_2$/10 ml basic perfusion medium
- HEPES-Solution
  - NaCl: 125.0 mM
  - KCl: 2.6 mM
  - KH_2PO_4:   1.2 mM
  - $MgCl_2 \times 6\ H_2O$: 1.2 mM
  - HEPES: 25.0 mM

  Adjust to pH 7.4 with NaOH
- Isotonic sodium chlorid solution: 9 g NaCl/1l distilled water

Procedure

- Euthanasia and Dissection

  One commonly used is cervical dislocation. The thumb and index finger are placed on either side of the neck at the base of the skull. Alternatively, a rod is pressed to the base of the skull. Shortly after that, the base of the tail is quickly pulled (45° angle), causing the dislocation of the cervical vertebrae. Although cervical dislocation in mice does not require anaesthesia, it is preferable for persons only using this method sporadically.

  For sedation and euthanasia, ether has been used extensively in cardiovascular research due to its low effects on blood flow parameter even after long-term exposure. However, it is no longer acceptable for euthanasia and is dangerous to the operator. Carbon dioxide (>70%) is used for quick loss of consciousness (15–30 s) without hypoxia. To prevent cardiovascular effects (e.g. contracted heart), the length of time of exposure to CO_2 should only be as long as it is necessary to reach unconsciousness.

After killing, the thorax is opened very quickly on both sides using small scissors. The thoracic organs are completely removed by cutting the oesophagus, trachea, aorta and caudal part near the diaphragm. The pluck is immediately placed in cold 0.9% NaCl solution for final dissection.

- Mounting on the perfusion system
    1. Heat the perfusion system and fill it with approximately 100 ml bubble-free basic perfusion medium.
    2. Kill two mice, dissect the hearts, and transfer them into cold 0.9% NaCl solution.
    3. Remove connective tissue to prepare the arch of the aorta, and cut the aorta caudally at the branch of the brachiocephalic trunk. Use a dissection microscope to identify the arch of the aorta and the branching brachiocephalic trunk, the left common carotid artery, and left subclavian artery.
    4. Adjust the flow rate to 3 ml/min.
    5. In order to connect the heart to the perfusion system, fix the aorta with two thin curved forceps and pull it over the cannula. Use gauche 20 cannulas, where the sharp tip is cut off.
    6. Place the cannula's end between the first aortic branch and the aortic valve, to ensure that the myocardium is retrogradely perfused via the coronary arteries. Fix the aorta with a crocodile clamp. The epicard turns pale within a few minutes, if coronary perfusion is sufficient. Fix the aorta with a ligature. Mount the second heart using the same procedure.
    7. Place the funnel underneath and adjust the perfusion speed to 1–2 drops per s.
- Tissue dissociation and digestion
    1. Adjust the perfusion medium to 40 ml and add 30 mg collagenase (750 mg/l final concentration) and 12.5 μl $CaCl_2$ stock solution into the basic perfusion medium of the upper reservoir (see Fig. 1).
    2. Continue perfusion under recirculating conditions for 40 min. This step is critical for the cell yield of the preparation. The perfusion time depends on the effective activity of the collagenase. Thus, the appropriate collagenase concentration and perfusion time must be determined for each individual batch of collagenase used. A measure for optimal conditions is the yield of attached and dividing EC after 1 and 12 h of plating on culture dishes, respectively.
    3. Cut the hearts from the cannula and remove residual non-myocardial tissue including atria.
    4. Open both ventricles and chop the tissue with a razor blade to a size of 0.3×0.3 mm pieces. For this step, use of a chopper (see above) equipped with a razor blade is recommended.
    5. Transfer chopped tissue into 30 ml of collagenase-containing basic perfusion medium and allow further 10 min of incubation at 37 °C. During that period aerate buffer with carbogen and gently disperse the cells by aspiration of the suspension with a disposable pipette.
    6. Centrifuge the suspension at 30×g for 3 min, transfer the supernatant into a Teflon beaker, and adjust the volume to 40 ml with basic perfusion medium. Add 10 mg trypsin (250 mg/l final concentration) and 30 μl $CaCl_2$ stock solution. Continue incubation for 5 min at 37°C and aerate the suspension with carbogen.

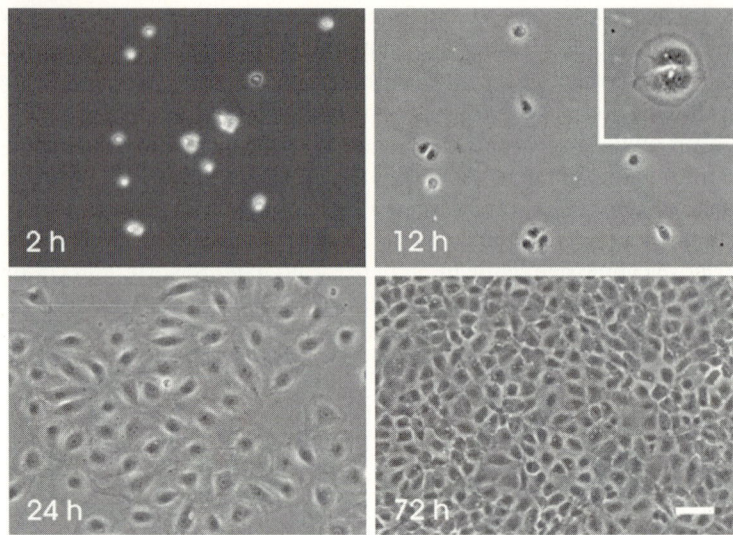

Figure 2
Phase contrast microphotographs of EC after various times in culture. EC harvested from porcine aortas 2 h, 12 h, 24 h, and 72 h after seeding. 2 h: EC attach on the bottom of the culture dish. 12 h: EC are spreading and start to divide (insert). 24 h: EC form a pre-confluent monolayer. 72 h: EC have reached confluency and display cobblestone pattern typical for static EC cultures. Bar = 100 µm

- Culturing of EC (Fig. 2)
    1. Transfer equal volumes of the suspension into two tubes and add 20 ml DMEM (complete high antibiotics) into each tube.
    2. Centrifuge for 8 min at 260×g and discard supernatant.
    3. Under sterile conditions (laminar flow), add 2 ml of sterile DMEM (complete; high antibiotics) to the pellet. Resuspend the pellet by gentle aspiration of the suspension with an Eppendorf pipette, the total volume on a 100 mm Petri dish (PRIMARIA™) containing 8 ml of DMEM (complete; high antibiotics).
    4. Leave the dishes in the CO_2 incubator for 1 h. Afterwards, shake the dishes vigorously several times, aspirate medium containing debris and unattached cells and add 15 ml of DMEM (complete; high antibiotics).
    5. After 24 h change the medium and add 15 ml of DMEM (complete; low antibiotics). Change the medium every second day.
    6. After 5–6 days, EC should have formed confluent monolayers.
    7. Flush the perfusion system immediately after use with a minimum of 1 l distilled water or 70% ethanol for 30 min. to prevent contamination. Alternatively, low-dose antibiotic solution (e.g. 0.1% gentamycin) can be used.

Isolation of Microvascular Coronary EC from Rat

If higher amounts of coronary EC from rodents are needed, perfusion of rat hearts can be an appropriate alternative to mouse hearts. Coronary EC from rat hearts are isolated by almost the same protocol as described for mouse hearts, with slight modifications. Due to its larger aortic diameter, mounting of rat hearts is less technically ambitious, but interruption of organ perfusion must be reduced to an absolute limit.

Preparation Apparatus and Instruments

See above (Isolation of Microvascular Coronary EC From Mouse).

Culture Media and Substances

- Medium 199 (M199, e.g. Biochrom AG)
- Mixed serum: 10% foetal calf serum (FCS) plus 10% newborn calf serum (NCS)
- For other components, see above (Culture Media and Substances)

Preparing Culture Media and Tissue Solutions

- Medium 199
  - M199 dry powder, for 10 l
  - 36 g HEPES
  - 15 g $NaHCO_3$
  Adjusted to pH 7.3 at room temperature with NaOH
  Sterile filtered and stored at 4°C
- Medium 199 complete; high antibiotics
  - 20% mixed serum
  - 250 U/ml penicillin; 250 µg/ml streptomycin
- Medium 199 complete; low antibiotics
  - 20% mixed serum
  - 100 U/ml penicillin; 100 µg/ml streptomycin
- Basic perfusion medium: For composition, see page 614
- $CaCl_2$ Stock Solution (100 mM): For composition, see page 614
Isotonic sodiumchlorid solution: 9 g NaCl/1 l distilled water

Procedure

- Euthanasia and dissection:
  - To receive adequate cell amounts, hearts from rats with a minimum age of 3 months (250–300 g) should be used.
  - For euthanasia, rats should be sedated with CO_2 (see above) or stunned, prior to dislocation. Thoracic organs are removed completely and finally dissected in isotonic sodium chlorid solution.
- Mounting on the Perfusion System
  - Step 1–7: are almost the same as described above for mouse hearts
  - Step 2: For dissection of the rat heart, a dissection microscope is not needed.
  - Step 5: Use cannulas with a tip diameter of ≥1.5 mm
- Tissue dissociation and digestion
  - Step 1–7: are almost the same as described above for mouse hearts, with the following exception:

— Step 1: 20 mg collagenase (500 mg/l final concentration) is added to the basic perfusion medium.

- Culturing of EC
   1. Transfer equal volumes of the suspension into two tubes and add 20 ml M199 into each tube.
   2. Centrifuge for 8 min at 260×g and discard supernatant.
   3. Under sterile conditions (laminar flow), add 20 ml of sterile M199 (complete; high antibiotics) to the pellet. Resuspend the pellet by gentle aspiration of the suspension with an Eppendorf pipette, and transfer 8 ml of suspension to one 100 mm Petri dish (PRIMARIA™) containing 20 ml of M199 (complete; high antibiotics).
   4. After 1 h, shake the dishes vigorously several times, aspirate medium containing debris and unattached cells, and add 20 ml of M199 (complete; high antibiotics).
   5. Change the medium (M 199 complete; low antibiotics) after 24 h and then every second day.
   6. After 5–6 days, EC should have formed confluent monolayers.
   7. Flush the perfusion system immediately after use with a minimum of 1 l distilled water or 70% ethanol for 30 min to prevent contamination. Alternatively, low-dose antibiotic solution (e.g. 0.1% gentamycin) can be used.

Isolation of Macrovascular EC from Pig Aorta

If high amounts of cells are needed, EC isolation from pig aortas is an inexpensive and simple procedure. EC are harvested from vessel segments by gently scratching the cells from the intimal surface using a scalpel. For the isolation procedure no complicated perfusion system is needed. EC from swine and cattle are undemanding and easy to maintain in culture. With some minor changes, this technique is easily adapted to harvest EC from other macrovascular provinces.

General Equipment and Cell Culture

- Pin board (tinfoil covered Styrofoam™ plate 40×40 cm)
- Pins (hypodermic needles)
- Scissors
- Forceps
- Disposable scalpel with a curved blade
- 50 ml polypropylene conical tube (e.g. Falcon)
- 100 mm culture dishes (Falcon 3003 or 3800 PRIMARIA™)
- Glass pipette
- Centrifuge

Culture Media, Substances and Solutions

- Isotonic sodium chloride solution: 9 g NaCl/1 l distilled water
- Medium 199 (Composition, see page 617)

- Medium 199 (complete; high antibiotics)
  - 20% NCS
  - 250 U/ml penicillin; 250 µg/ml streptomycin
- Medium 199 (complete; low antibiotics)
  - 20% NCS
  - 100 U/ml penicillin; 100 µg/ml streptomycin

Procedure

- Getting Aortic Material

  The source of pig aortas are slaughterhouses or local butchers. To prevent contaminations, only pluck with intact aorta and without severely affected lungs should be chosen.

  Dissect 20 segments of porcine thoracic aortas beginning from arcus aortae 15–30 cm out of pluck. Touching and pressing of the aorta should be kept to a minimum.

  Transfer the segments immediately into a bucket containing isotonic sodium chloride solution.

  Make sure that the time between dissection, transport to the laboratory and preparation does not exceed 3 h, but is not less than 1 h.

- Harvesting of EC
  1. Remove the adventitial tissue with scissors (without cutting into the media of the vessel), and transfer the segments into fresh isotonic sodium chloride solution.
  2. Cut the segments between the branches of posterior intercostal arteries in a longitudinal direction. Fix the segment, intima surface up, with pins onto the Styrofoam™ plate. Reposition the pins to stretch the segments slightly to flat sheets.
  3. Scrape off the EC by gently sliding the blade over the intimal surface. Incline the blade to an angel of nearly 45°, and move your hand with constant velocity and pressure while sliding over the intimal surface in a longitudinal direction. Avoid scratching at the cutting edges of the aortic segments. Transfer the smear material accumulating at the blade's edge after each scratch into a 50 ml Falcon tube filled with 30 ml M199 (medium without serum).
  4. Centrifuge the tube at 250×g for 10 min, decant the supernatant, and resuspend the pellet in 30 ml of M199 (complete; high antibiotics) by gently dispersing the sediment using a glass pipette.

- Culturing of the cells
  1. Add 15 ml of M199 (complete; high antibiotics) into six 100 mm dishes, and add 5 ml of the cell suspension.
  2. Incubate the dishes for not more than 4 h at 37 °C in a CO_2 incubator. Afterwards, shake the dishes vigorously several times, aspirate medium containing debris and non-attached cells, and add 20 ml of M199 (complete; high antibiotics).
  3. Change the medium and add 20 ml of M 199 (complete; low antibiotics) after 24 h, and then every second day.
  4. After 3–4 days, EC should have formed confluent monolayers.

Isolation of Macrovascular EC from Human Umbilical Vein

It is of particular interest to use EC of human origin because species-specific differences sometimes make it difficult to extrapolate findings from animals to humans. Differences in metabolic rate, pharmacological profile or applicability of monoclonal antibodies and human specific mediators are reasons why human EC are frequently preferable. To avoid infections, special care has to be taken in handling human material. Cells derived from human tissue are often difficult to obtain. It is mainly limited to post mortem material, leftover specimen or intentionally removed material.

Human umbilical cords are commonly used because they are easily accessible. EC are obtained by collagenase digestion of the interior vein and flushing out the detached cells. In contrast to scratching aortas, this procedure is more complicated. Furthermore, one has to screen for an appropriate collagenase to get high cell yield. Generally, human EC are critically affected even by low contaminations of endotoxin and demand special growth factor additives. The technique described below can also be applied to large vessels from other provinces.

General Equipment and Cell Culture

- Sterile tissues
- 2 feeding needles
- 2 crocodile clamps
- 2 three-way stopcocks
- Cable fixer
- 50 ml syringes
- Incubator at 37 °C

Culture Media, Substances and Solutions

- Hanks' balanced salt solution (HBSS; e.g. Invitrogen)
- Foetal Calf Serum, FCS
- Collagenase type II
- PromoCell™ Endothelial Growth Medium Kit Cat.-No.: C-22110 containing
  - 10% FCS
  - 0.4% Endothelial Cell Growth Supplement with Heparin
  - 0.1 ng/ml human EGF
  - 1.0 µg/ml Hydrocortison
  - 1.0 ng/ml human bFGF
  - 50.0 µg/ml Gentamicin
- 50 ml HBSS with 0.025% collagenase type II
- 30 ml HBSS + 1 ml FCS

Procedure

- Tissue dissociation and digestion
    1. Umbilical veins should not be older than 24 h (stored at 4 °C).
    2. Clean the umbilical vein with a sterile tissue.

3. Cut both ends with a sterile scalpel.
4. Insert sterile feeding needle into the vein at each end and fix it first with a crocodile clamp.
5. Be sure that the feeding needle is placed correctly, then fix it with a cable fixer.
6. Connect both feeding needles with three-way stopcocks and perfuse vein 2× with 50 ml HBSS.
7. Be sure that there is no leakage.
   Then fill the vein with 50 ml collagenase solution until vein is stretched very well.
8. Transfer the vein into a CO_2-free incubator for 30 min at 37 °C.
9. After incubation, massage vein softly to detach EC from their layer.

- Culturing of EC
  1. Open the stopcocks and flush the collagenase solution, including EC, out of the vein with 30 ml HBSS/FCS.
  2. Centrifuge 180×g for 5 min.
  3. Disccard supernatant and resuspend pellet with 15 ml PromoCell™ Medium per 100 mm dish.
  4. Wash the dishes after 3–4 h 3× with HBSS by roughly shaking the dishes several times to remove debris and unattached cells.
  5. Change medium every third day.

Characterization and Identification of Culture Purity

Fixation of EC

For fixation of EC, three methods are commonly used and are listed below. The method finally chosen is dependent on the antibody used.

Para-formaldehyde (PFA)-Fixation

- Materials
  - Phosphate buffer (0.1 M, pH 7.44), store at +4 °C
    Aqua bidest.:   800 ml
    $NaH_2PO_4 \times H_2O$:   3.0 g
    $Na_2HPO_4 \times 2\ H_2O$: 21.7 g
    Adjust pH 7.44 with 1 M NaOH or 1 M H_3PO_4
    Aqua bidest.:   fill up to 1 l
  - 3–4% (wt/vol) para-formaldehyde in phosphate buffer
  - Phosphate-buffered saline (PBS, pH 7.44), store at +4 °C
    NaCl: 8.8 g
    Aqua bidest: 800 ml
    Phosphate buffer (pH 7.44): 116 ml
    Aqua bidest: fill up to 1 l
  - HEPES-solution (see page 614)
- Procedure
  - Wash EC twice with HEPES-solution (37 °C).

- Remove solution and fix confluent cells with PFA for 15 min at 37 °C.
- Remove PFA and wash 3× with PBS.
- For long-term storage, use PBS with 0.1% NaN$_3$.

Methanol or Acetone Fixation

- Procedure
    - Place methanol or acetone into a freezer for about 30 min.
    - Use glass dishes for acetone.
    - Wash EC twice with HEPES-solution (37 °C).
    - Remove solution and fixate EC immediately with ice-cold methanol or acetone.
    - Incubate in a freezer for 10 min.
    - Remove methanol or acetone and wash 3× with PBS at room temperature.
    - For long-term storage, use PBS with 0.1% NaN$_3$.

Passaging of the Cells

- Materials
    - HEPES-solution (see page 614)
    - Trypsin-EDTA (e.g. Invitrogen)
    - Neubauer chamber for cell counting
    - Sterile 25 mm glass coverslips (e.g. Type # 1, Menzel)
    - EC-specific medium (complete; low antibiotics)
    - 30 mm plastic culture dishes (e.g. Falcon 3001)
    - 50 ml Falcon tube
- Procedure
    - Wash confluent cell layer 3× with HEPES-solution (37 °C).
    - Add 5 ml pre-warmed Trypsin-EDTA per 100 mm dish.
    - Incubate without CO_2 at 37 °C for 2–3 min.
    - Detach EC with a 1 ml pipette and resuspend them by triturating gently.
    - Add cell suspension to 5 ml pre-warmed medium containing 20% serum.
    - Take off an aliquot and count cells in counting chamber.
    - Add desired volume of cell suspension to the dishes (with/without coverslips).
    - Fill up with medium (complete; low antibiotics) and shake carefully to spread cells over the dishes.

DiI-Ac-LDL-Uptake (Fig. 3)

- Materials and Solutions
    - Culture medium (complete; low antibiotics)
    - DiI-Ac-LDL solution (concentration 200 µg/ml; e.g. Paesel and Lorei)
    - Fixative solution: 4% PFA
    - Embedding solution: 65% glycerol in $NaHCO_3/Na_2CO_3$ (0.5 M, pH 8.6)
    - Staining solution for nuclei: 1 µg Hoechst 33 258 (e.g. Riedel-de Haen)/1 ml PBS
    - 30 mm plastic culture dishes (e.g. Falcon 3001)
    - 25 mm glass coverslips (e.g. Type # 1, Menzel)

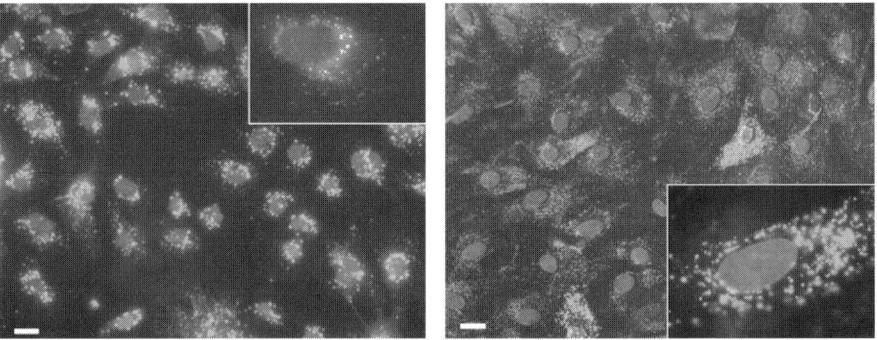

Figure 3
Fluorescence microphotographs of DiL-Ac-LDL uptake by HUVEC and microvascular coronary EC. EC were incubated for 4 h in presence of 10 μg DiI-Ac-LDL in the incubator. *Left:* DiI-Ac-LDL is predominantly localised around the cell nuclei in HUVEC. *Right:* In microvascular coronary EC DiI-Ac-LDL is accumulated in small vesicles distributed in the whole cytosol. Bar = 50 μm. *For coloured version see appendix*

- Procedure
    - Place sterile 25 mm glass coverslips into 30 mm culture dishes.
    - Trypsinize EC and seed them on glass coverslips (approximately 2×10^4 cells/cm^2).
    - Use monolayers after 2 days, when they have reached 70–80% of confluency.
    - Remove the culture medium, wash the monolayers 3× with the respective culture medium (37 °C), add 1 ml of culture medium containing 10 μg DiI-Ac-LDL.
    - Leave the cell in the incubator for 4 h, wash 3× with culture medium (37 °C) and 2× with PBS to remove residual DiI-AC-LDL.
    - Aspirate the PBS and add 2 ml fixative solution (15 min at 37 °C).
    - Aspirate the fixative solution and rinse the dish thoroughly 3× with PBS.
    - Add 1 ml of Hoechst solution and incubate the specimens for 15 min at room temperature.
    - Aspirate the Hoechst solution and wash with PBS 3× for 10 min.
    - Carefully take the coverslips out of the culture dish using fine forceps.
    - Place a drop of embedding solution onto a slide. Turn the coverslip cell side down, and place it slowly onto the drop. Avoid the inclusion of air bubbles. Remove surplus embedding medium with an absorbing paper tissue.
    - For examination under a fluorescence microscope for DiI-Ac-LDL use an excitation filter of 530–560 nm and an emission filter of above 570 nm, and for Hoechst 33258 an excitation filter of 340–380 nm and an emission filter of 460–490 nm staining.

F-Actin Staining

Phalloidin is a toxin from the toadstool *Amanita phalloides*, which specifically binds to filamentous actin (F-actin) but not to actin monomers (G-actin) (Faulstich et al. 1993; Low and Wieland 1974). To visualize overall F-actin in EC staining with fluorophore-coupled phalloidin is an easy and convenient technique (Fig. 4, 5b).

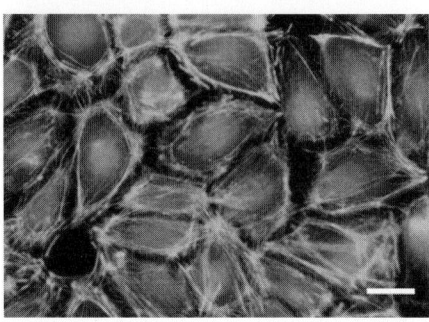

Figure 4
Fluorescence microphotograph of F-actin. In confluent endothelial monolayers, cultured under static conditions, F-actin fibres are typically arranged in fibre strands adjacent to cell boarders (dense peripheral band). HUVEC are stained with TRITC-phalloidin. Bar = 25 µm.
For coloured version see appendix

- Materials
  - 4% PFA
  - Phalloidin Fluorophor-coupled 1:200 (e.g. Alexa Fluor 350 phalloidin, Molecular Probes)
  - PBS with 0.1% Triton-X 100
  - PBS
  - PBS with 0.1% NaN_3
- Procedure
  - Fix confluent cells with PFA for 15 min at 37 °C (see page 621).
  - Permeabilise cells for 10 min with PBS plus 0.1% Triton-X 100.
  - Aspirate the supernatant and wash 2× with PBS.
  - Incubate with phalloidin for 24 h in humidified CO_2-free incubator.
  - Remove supernatant and wash 3× for 10 min with PBS at room temperature.
  - Embed coverslip with Citifluor™ AF 1 (Canterburry, UK).
  - For examination of Alexa Fluor 350 phalloidin under a fluorescence microscope, use an excitation filter of 340–380 nm and an emission filter of 460–490 nm.

α-Smooth Muscle Actin

Actin is one of the most conserved proteins and is expressed as six isoforms. Two of them are found in almost all cells, whereas four are expressed tissue-specifically in muscle. One of these is α-smooth muscle actin (Fig. 5a), which is expressed in smooth muscle cells and can be identified by the use of specific antibodies (Skalli et al. 1986).

- Materials
  - 4% PFA
  - Primary antibody: mouse monoclonal anti-α-smooth muscle actin (e.g. Clone 1A4, Sigma A2547), diluted 1:100 in PBS/NaN_3
  - Secondary antibody: anti-mouse Cy3 (e.g. Dianova), diluted 1:500 in PBS/NaN_3
  - PBS with 0.1% Triton-X 100
  - PBS
  - PBS with 0.1% NaN_3
- Procedure
  - Fix cells with PFA (see page 621).
  - Permeabilise cells for 10 min with PBS with 0.1% Triton X100, and wash 3× for 10 min with OBS

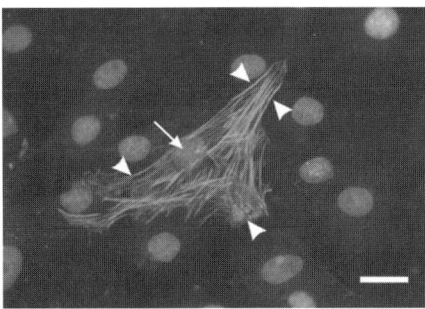
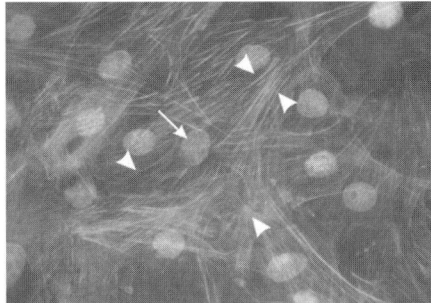

Figure 5
Fluorescence microphotographs of α-smooth muscle actin, F-actin and cell nuclei of a pre-confluent HUVEC culture. *Left:* EC culture stained with an anti-α-smooth muscle actin antibody. Cell nuclei are visualized with Hoe 33258. One cell expressing α-smooth muscle actin is identified, indicating contamination with non-EC. *Right:* Same section as *left*, stained for F-actin with phalloidin-coupled Alexa Fluor 350. All cells show a characteristic F-actin positive staining. In pre-confluent endothelial monolayers actin is assembled in stress fibres. Arrow heads point to identical α-smooth muscle actin stress fibres in both figures. The *arrow* points to the same nucleus in either figure. Bar = 25 µm. *For coloured version see appendix*

- Incubate with primary antibody for 24 h in humidified incubator.
- Remove supernatant, and wash 3× for 10 min with PBS at room temperature in order to remove the remaining antibody completely.
- Incubate with secondary antibody for 4 h in a humidified incubator.
- Remove supernatant and wash 3× for 10 min with PBS at room temperature.
- Embed coverslip with Citifluor™ AF 1 (Canterburry, UK).
- For examination under a fluorescence microscope, use an excitation filter of 530–560 nm and an emission filter of above 570 nm.

Von Willebrand Factor

Von Willebrand factor (vWF) is expressed by EC and also by megakaryocytes (Bahnak et al. 1989). vWF staining is often more pronounced in EC from macrovasculature than from microvascular origin due to regional variations in vWF expression within the vascular tree. It is stored in Weible-Pallade bodies and is secreted into the plasma and the vascular extracellular matrix. It initiates platelet adhesion to extracellular matrix of injured intima, and is also involved in anchorage of EC to the extracellular matrix. Due to its exclusive expression in EC, it is widely used as an EC marker (Fig. 6).
- Materials
  - 4% PFA
  - Primary antibody: Anti-vWF rabbit polyclonal (H-300 Santa Cruz Biotechnology), dilute 1:500 in PBS/ NaN_3
  - Secondary antibody: anti-rabbit Cy2 (e.g. Dianova), 1:500 diluted in PBS/ NaN_3
  - PBS with 0.1% Triton-X 100
  - PBS
  - PBS with 0.1% NaN_3

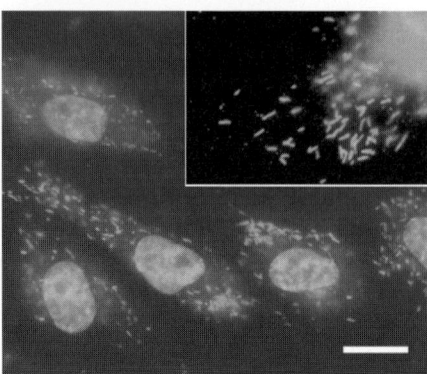

Figure 6
Fluorescence Microphotograph of von Willebrand Factor and Cell Nuclei of HUVEC. Von Willebrand factor is visualised with an anti-vWF antibody. It is characteristically localised in cytoplasma in rod-shaped granules (Weibel-Pallade bodies), which can be seen at higher magnification in the insert. Bar = 50 μm. *For coloured version see appendix*

- Procedure
    - Fix confluent cells with PFA (see page 621).
    - Permeabilise cells for 10 min with PBS with 0.1% Triton-X 100.
    - Aspirate the supernatant and wash 2× with PBS.
    - Incubate with primary antibody for 24 h in a humidified incubator.
    - Remove supernatant, and wash 3× for 10 min with PBS at room temperature in order to remove the remaining antibody completely.
    - Incubate with secondary antibody for 4 h in a humidified incubator.
    - Remove supernatant and wash 3× for 10 min with PBS at room temperature.
    - Embed coverslip with 80% glycerol/20% PBS (pH 7.0).
    - For examination under a fluorescence microscope, use an excitation filter of 470–490 nm, a dichotic mirror of 505 and an emission filter of 510–530 nm.

Troubleshooting

General Aspects

EC Do Not Attach

- Prevent detergent contamination in all materials used for cell isolation culturing.
- Choice of disposable culture dishes.
  EC typically grow only when attached to specially coated surfaces. In general, EC are no more demanding than other cells in culture. However, selection of specifically modified surfaces (e.g. surface-modified polystyrene dishes PRIMARIA™, Falcon) can enhance EC attachment and proliferation and thus increase cell yield.
- Test every new charge of serum, collagenase or trypsin, because change in composition or enzyme activity can substantially affect cell attachment and proliferation.

- EC may need special attachment aids like gelatin (0.2–2.0%), laminin (30–60 µg/ml), fibronectin (10–20 µg/ml), vitronectin (1–10 µg/ml), or poly-L-lysine (0.01%). Dilute the substances in PBS, and preincubate dishes for more than 2 h. Aspirate the solution and start with EC seeding.
  Sometimes, preincubation of culture dishes with culture medium supplemented with 20% serum (for 1–12 h) is sufficient to facilitate cell attachment.
- The presence of too many non-EC, especially erythrocytes or cell debris, may hinder EC attachment.
  Improve organ perfusion to flush out erythrocytes, and shorten preparation time between dissecting and mounting of the organ to avoid blood coagulation.
- Control the pH of your medium.
- Check your incubator, to see whether CO_2 level and temperature are constant.
- Think of detergent contamination

EC Do Not Grow

- Primary rather than passaged cultures do not grow on glass or untreated plastic
- Some endothelial cell preparations are more sensitive to antibiotic/antimycotics e.g. gentamycin (>50 µg/ml) or amphotericin B (5–12.5 µg) than others. Try to restrict use of those antibiotics/antimycotics to a minimum. In general, penicillin (100 U/ml) or streptomycin (100 µg/ml) is sufficient to prevent bacterial growth.
- Add special additives to medium, e.g. essential amino acids, growth supplements (e.g. Invitrogen, Sigma).
- Change your serum batch or try serum from other species (e.g. from adult horse).

Organ Perfusion of Rodent Hearts

Only a Few EC can be Isolated

- Removal of the heart and onset of Langendorff perfusion takes too long. The total cell amount will decrease because blood coagulates and occludes the vascular system. Therefore, the digestion of the heart would be incomplete.
- Control your aerating system during perfusion and dissociation. Reduced aeration of perfusion medium will reduce cell yield.

Primary Cultures are Contaminated

- Clean and autoclave the components of your perfusion system and your instruments
- Disinfect your perfusion system every time with 70% ethanol.
  Attention! Do not use detergents for cleaning or disinfecting. Use diluted NaOH or acetic acid solutions.

Cannulation of Single Vessels

Only a Few EC Can Be Isolated or Cell Amount is Suddenly Reduced

- Never use glassware while working with HUVEC. These cells adhere to glass surfaces.
- The umbilical cord is probably too old (> 24 h).

EC Culture Contains Non-EC

- Shorten the digestion period or reduce the amount of collagenase.
- In the case of HUVEC, reduce the pressure while you knead the vein.

Scratching

Primary Cultures are Contaminated

- Take no vessels from lung-infected animals from the slaughterhouse.

EC Culture Contains Non-EC

- Reduce the pressure while scratching.
- Reduce the time between dissection of aortas and EC preparation.

References

Adamson RH, Curry FE, Adamson G, Liu B, Jiang Y, Aktories K, Barth H, Daigeler A, Golenhofen N, Ness W and Drenckhahn D (2002): Rho and Rho Kinase Modulation of Barrier Properties: Cultured Endothelial Cells and Intact Microvessels of Rats and Mice. J Physiol 539: 295–308

Bahnak BR, Wu QY, Coulombel L, Assouline Z, Kerbiriou-Nabias D, Pietu G, Drouet L, Caen JP and Meyer D (1989): Expression of von Willebrand Factor in Porcine Vessels: Heterogeneity at the Level of von Willebrand Factor mRNA. J Cell Physiol 138: 305–310

Booyse FM, Sedlak BJ and Rafelson ME, Jr (1975): Culture of Arterial Endothelial Cells: Characterization and Growth of Bovine Aortic Cells. Thromb Diath Haemorrh 34: 825–839

Bowman PD, Betz AL, Ar D, Wolinsky JS, Penney JB, Shivers RR and Goldstein GW (1981): Primary Culture of Capillary Endothelium from Rat Brain. In Vitro 17: 353–362

Bowman PD, Betz AL and Goldstein GW (1982): Primary Culture of Microvascular Endothelial Cells from Bovine Retina: Selective Growth using Fibronectin Coated Substrate and Plasma Derived Serum. In Vitro 18: 626–632

Cirillo P, Golino P, Ragni M, Guarino A, Calabro P and Chiarriello M (1999): A Simple Method for the Isolation, Cultivation, and Characterization of Endothelial Cells from Rabbit Coronary Circulation. Thromb Res 96: 329–333

Davison PM, Bensch K and Karasek MA (1980): Isolation and Growth of Endothelial Cells from the Microvessels of the Newborn Human Foreskin in Cell Culture. J Invest Dermatol 75: 316–321

Dong QG, Bernasconi S, Lostaglio S, De Calmanovici RW, Martin-Padura I, Breviario F, Garlanda C, Ramponi S, Mantovani A and Vecchi A (1997): A General Strategy for Isolation of Endothelial Cells from Murine Tissues: Characterization of Two Endothelial Cell Lines from the Murine Lung and Subcutaneous Sponge Implants. Arterioscler Thromb Vasc Biol 17: 1599–1604

Draijer R, Vaandrager AB, Nolte C, de Jonge HR, Walter U and van Hinsbergh VW (1995): Expression of cGMP-Dependent Protein Kinase I and Phosphorylation of its Substrate, Vasodilator-Stimulated Phosphoprotein, in Human Endothelial Cells of Different Origin. Circ Res 77: 897–905

Faulstich H, Zobeley S, Heintz D and Drewes G (1993): Probing the Phalloidin Binding Site of Actin. FEBS Lett 318: 218–222

Fitzgerald U, Hettle S, MacDonald C and McLean JS (2000): Umbilical Cord Endothelial Cells Expressing Large T Antigen: Comparison with Primary Cultures and Effect of Cell Age. In Vitro Cell Dev Biol Anim 36: 222–227

Gräfe M, Auch-Schwelk W, Graf K, Terbeek D, Hertel H, Unkelbach M, Hildebrandt A and Fleck E (1994): Isolation and Characterization of Macrovascular and Microvascular Endothelial Cells from Human Hearts. Am J Physiol 267: H2138–H2148

Hewett PW and Murray JC (1993): Human Lung Microvessel Endothelial Cells: Isolation, Culture, and Characterization. Microvasc Res 46: 89–102

Hewett PW, Murray JC, Price EA, Watts ME and Woodcock M (1993): Isolation and Characterization of Microvessel Endothelial Cells from Human Mammary Adipose Tissue. In Vitro Cell Dev Biol Anim 29A: 325–331

Jaffe EA, Nachman RL, Becker CG and Minick CR (1973): Culture of Human Endothelial Cells Derived from Umbilical Veins: Identification by Morphologic and Immunologic Criteria. J Clin Invest 52: 2745–2756

Low I, and Wieland T (1974): The Interaction of Phalloidin: Some of its Derivatives, and of other Cyclic Peptides with Muscle Actin as Studied by Viscosimetry. FEBS Lett 44: 340–343

Magee JC, Stone AE, Oldham KT and Guice KS (1994): Isolation, Culture, and Characterization of Rat Lung Microvascular Endothelial Cells. Am J Physiol 267: L433–L441

Mischeck U, Meyer J and Galla HJ (1989): Characterization of Gamma-Glutamyl Transpeptidase Activity of Cultured Endothelial Cells from Porcine Brain Capillaries. Cell Tissue Res 256: 221–226

Nees S, Gerbes AL, Gerlach E and Staubesand J (1981): Isolation, Identification, and Continuous Culture of Coronary Endothelial Cells from Guinea Pig Hearts. Eur J Cell Biol 24: 287–297

Oxhorn BC, Hirzel DJ and Buxton IL (2002): Isolation and Characterization of Large Numbers of Endothelial Cells for Studies of Cell Signalling. Microvasc Res 64: 302–315

Piper HM: Cell Culture Technique in Heart and Vessel Research. Berlin (1990): Springer-Verlag

Rauen U, Hanssen M, Lauchart W, Becker HD and de Groot H (1993): Energy-Dependent Injury to Cultured Sinusoidal Endothelial Cells of the Rat Liver in UW Solution. Transplantation 55: 469–473

Skalli O, Ropraz P, Trzeciak A, Benzonana G, Gillessen D and Gabbiani G (1986): A Monoclonal Antibody Against Alpha-Smooth Muscle Actin: A New Probe for Smooth Muscle Differentiation. J Cell Biol 103: 2787–2796

Slater DN and Sloan JM (1975): The Porcine Endothelial cell in Tissue Culture. Atherosclerosis 21: 259–272

Ugele B and Lange F (2001): Isolation of Endothelial Cells from Human Placental Microvessels: Effect of Different Proteolytic Enzymes on Releasing Endothelial Cells from Villous Tissue. In Vitro Cell Dev Biol Anim 37: 408–413

Watanabe H, Kuhne W, Schwartz P and Piper HM (1992): A2-Adenosine Receptor Stimulation Increases Macromolecule Permeability of Coronary Endothelial Cells. Am J Physiol 262: H1174–H1181

Watanabe H, Kuhne W, Spahr R, Schwartz P and Piper HM (1991): Macromolecule Permeability of Coronary and Aortic Endothelial Monolayers Under Energy Depletion. Am J Physiol 260: H1344–H1352

Watkins MT, Sharefkin JB, Zajtchuk R, Maciag TM, D'Amore PA, Ryan US, Van Wart H and Rich NM (1984): Adult Human Saphenous Vein Endothelial Cells: Assessment of Their Reproductive Capacity for use in Endothelial Seeding of Vascular Prostheses. J Surg Res 36: 588–596

In Vitro Cultivation of Vascular Smooth Muscle Cells

Daniel G. Sedding and Ruediger C. Braun-Dullaeus

Introduction

Vascular smooth muscle cell dysfunction is a major factor contributing to the development of vascular proliferative diseases, which are still major of mortality in the Western World (Tunstall-Pedoe et al. 1999). Current therapeutic strategies are directed towards enhancing blood flow by angioplasty or surgical revascularization. However, patients undergoing percutaneous interventions will often experience restenosis within the first few months (Nobuyoshi et al. 1988; Serruys et al. 1988), even the placement of stents is accompanied with a high rate of restenosis. Patients with severe and diffuse restenosis will finally require additional interventions such as bypass surgery, a procedure that is itself limited by graft failure, due to luminal obstruction caused by excessive cell proliferation. Occlusive vascular disease involves cellular growth, programmed cell death (apoptosis), cell migration, matrix modulation, and vascular remodeling. Neointimal hyperplasia, which is mainly due to vascular smooth muscle cell (SMC) proliferation, contributes significantly to vessel narrowing after angioplasty, in bypass vein grafts, during transplant vasculopathy, and in atherosclerotic plaque formation and progression (Dzau et al. 2002).

Therefore, beside describing the mechanisms of vascular proliferative disease *in vivo*, there is the obvious need for *in vitro* systems, which allow us to further investigate the molecular mechanisms involved in physiological and pathophysiological regulation of vascular smooth muscle cell function.

Since rabbits were used most often in the earlier years of atherosclerosis research, today researchers tend to establish cell-isolation techniques in smaller animals i.e. rats or mice. The use of genetically 'engineered' mice especially, offers exciting new possibilities to elicit the role of specific genes during the development of cardiovascular diseases. Facing the requirement of isolating cells from genetically modified mice for further *in vitro* studies, we describe isolation techniques that are suitable for isolation of SMC from both rat and mouse tissues.

In this article we have provided a short description and discussion of cell culture techniques for vascular smooth muscle cells currently used in cardiovascular research.

Methods and Practical Approach
Material

General equipment and cell culture

- Lamina Flow equipped with pipette aid and fire boy
- CO_2-air incubator with controlled temperature (37 °C) and humidity (95%)
- Phase contrast microscope (objectives 10× und 20×)
- Autoclave
- Centrifuge
- pH-meter
- Eppendorff pipettes (5 µl–1 ml) with sterile filter tips

Instruments for Cell Preparation and Isolation

- Small forceps
- Surgical scalpel
- Small scissors

Cell Culture Utilities

- Culture medium bottles (500 ml)
- Polypropylene conical tubes (50 ml and 15 ml)
- Disposable sterile plastic pipettes (5, 10, 25 ml)
- Disposable tissue culture dishes (Petri dishes, 75 mm^2 and 25 mm^2 cell culture dishes)

Cell Culture Media and Substances

- Dulbecco's Modified Medium (DMEM-F12), low glucose content
- Fetal Calf Serum (FCS)
- Penicillin and streptomycin (each 100 IU/ml)
- Trypsin/EDTA
- Carbogen (95%O_2, 5%CO_2)

Preparing Culture Media and Tissue Solutions

To 500 ml DMEM-F12 add
- 250 U/ml penicillin
- 250 µg/ml streptomycin
- 50 ml FCS
- Glutamine

Methods

Isolation of Rat Aortic Smooth Muscle Cells

Preparation of the aorta:
- Euthanize a Wistar rat ~200–250 g (Charles River) by CO_2 inhalation
- Under sterile conditions, perform thoracotomy and dissect the thoracal aorta using sterile forceps and scissors
- Place aorta into a Petri dish, add preparation medium (1× PBS + Pen/Strep) and clean gently of remaining blood
- Remove adhering connective and fatty tissue by blunt dissection
- Transfer aorta into a new Petri dish with fresh media several times to avoid contamination with suspended cells. The vessel should always be covered with medium to avoid drying
- Cut the aorta longitudinally and open it
- Gently remove the intimal layer (consisting of endothelial cells and a few intimal smooth muscle cells normally present in the intima) by scraping gently with bent forceps
- Intensely rinse vessel surface with preparation medium to remove adherent intimal cells, and place the vessel into a new Petri dish containing preparation medium.

Primary Explant Technique

The thoracic aorta is used preferentially to obtain media explants, because it is easier to strip the media off the adventitia of this part of the aorta than of the abdominal part of the aorta. The size of media explants should be ~0.1–0.25 mm^2. Exceeding this size results in an increased risk of explant detachment during further cultivation.
- The differences in the texture between media and adventitia allow easy separation of the medial and adventitial layer
- Grasp the vessel at the lateral margin with straight forceps, and carefully strip off the medial layer in small pieces using bent forceps
- Place the media pieces into a new Petri dish
- If necessary cut media explants into ~1 mm^2 pieces
- To prevent detachment of explants, do NOT add culture medium to the cells
- Place the Petri dish upside down in an incubator at 37 °C and allow explants to attach for 12–18 h
- Now add 7 ml of culture medium containing 20% FCS to the cells
- Change medium every 48 h
- After approximately 5–7 days, single cells will spread out of the tissue samples
- As soon as they reach confluency within their local environment, remove tissue samples with a sterile needle and trypsinize cells as described
- Plate cells into a small dish (max. 25 cm^2). If seeded too sparsely, cells will not proliferate further

Enzymatic Disaggregation

- Isolate media pieces as described above
- If necessary, cut explants into smaller pieces (~1 mm^2) using a scalpel
- Place explants into a 15 ml tube (Falcon)
- Add enzyme solution (approx 1 ml solution/mg medial tissue) containing collagenase (1 mg/ml), elastase (0.25–0.5 mg/ml) and soy bean trypsin inhibitor (1 mg/ml), and rinse explants to the bottom (either enzyme solution had been 0.2 µm filter sterilized prior to use)
- Close tube with a cap and place it into a water bath (constantly shaking, 37 °C)
- Allow cells to disaggregate for ~120 min
- Do not exceed a digestion time >150 min
- If the solution appears turbid, obtain a small aliquot to microscopically determine the sufficient digestion of the explants
- If single cells are visible, stop the digestion and gently pipette (1 ml pipette) the suspension up and down to completely disperse the tissue
- To remove undispersed tissue, filter the suspension through a 100 µm mesh
- Centrifuge cell suspension at 800 g for 5 min and remove supernatant
- Resuspend cells in DMEM-F12 + 20%FCS
- Count cells
- Plate cells at a seeding density of ~10000 cells/cm^2
- Change medium every 48 h

Modified Protocol for Enzymatic Disaggregation of Vascular Smooth Muscle Cells

The following protocol resulted in a higher purity of SMC:
- Take aorta and dissect loose adventitia as described above – do not cut aorta open longitudinally or pin to dish
- Pre-digest in 5 ml enzyme solution for 5–15 min until adventitia becomes loose – like "cotton candy"
- After pre-digestion, separate adventitia from media, which will come off in about 1 mm^2 sections
- Keep immersed in medium and minimize time
- Transfer media pieces to centrifuge tube and cut into tiny fragments
- Add enzyme solution to media fragments, digest at 37 °C, shaking for 60–90 min
- Titrate with 5 ml plastic pipette every 15–20 min and check for free cells
- Filter with sterile 100 µm mesh
- Spin down cells, resuspend in 2–3 ml culture medium supplemented with 20% FCS
- Change medium every 48 h

Sub-Cultivating SMC

After enzymatic disaggregation, ~25–75% of cells attach to the cell culture dish. Dead cells and debris will not attach and should be removed by changing the medium to avoid any toxic effects. Following isolation, the cells will not start proliferating or migrating for ~6 days (lag phase). After this lag phase, cells will start to proliferate and cell numbers increase logarithmically (log phase). When cells become confluent they stop to proliferate, due to contact inhibition and enter a post-confluent, quiescent state (plateau phase).

During further sub-cultivation, cells should always be kept in the log phase. When reaching ~80–90% confluency, cells should be 'split' to allow further proliferation:
- Remove cell culture medium
- Rinse cells twice with PBS
- Add 1 ml trypsin-EDTA/50 cm^2 cell dish
- Incubate for ~1 min at 37 °C
- Microscopically control cell detachment (~80% of cells should be detached)
- Mechanically detach remaining cells by rapping the flask against the palm of your hand ~5×.
- Immediately add cell culture medium containing 10% FCS.
- (At least an equal amount of cell culture medium containing 10% FCS is required to neutralize the Trypsin-EDTA).
- Resuspend cells by gently pipetting
- Count cells in a haemocytometer
- (A confluent SMC culture in a 25 cm^2 culture dish consists of ~1.5×10^6 cells)
- Seed cells at a density of 10,000 cells/cm^2

Characterization of SMC

After isolation and sub-cultivation of SMC, contamination with endothelial cells or fibroblasts has to be excluded. As a first step, SMC can be identified by their specific morphology and growth pattern using a light microscope. However, further characterization is essential, and immunocytohistochemical staining has become the standard method for the characterization of primary SMC cultures.

Morphology

Primary SMC have a spindle-shaped appearance. However, after further sub-cultivation, SMC may increase in size and cell volume and may appear as polygonal cells. As SMC become confluent, they form multilayers with isles of monolayered cells, and show the characteristic 'hill and valley' pattern (Fig. 1). With a higher *in vitro* age, the monolayered areas become more dominant. When SMC are allowed to grow further without splitting after being 'post confluent', the formation of 'nodules' can be observed in areas of highest cellular density. These nodules consist of cell debris surrounded by viable SMC.

Immunofluorescence Staining for SMC-Marker Proteins

Contaminated endothelial cells in a SMC culture can be easily detected by their typical polygonal cell form, and the formation of a 'cobblestone' pattern when reaching confluency. However, after several passages, SMC as well as endothelial cells dediffer-

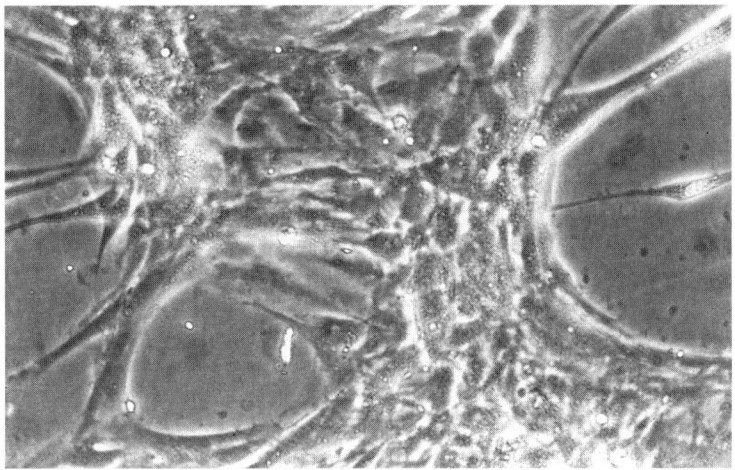

Figure 1
Freshly isolated primary rat aortic smooth muscle cells grown to confluence show a characteristics 'hill and valley' pattern

entiate and change morphology, so that it is almost impossible to distinguish between these cells using light microscopy. Furthermore, contaminated fibroblasts will not be detected by light microscopy. Therefore, there is a need to clearly characterize the primary cell culture using specific markers of SMC.

Alpha Smooth Muscle Actin

Actin is the dominant protein in cells and exists as at least six different isotypes. Ultrastructurally, actin forms diffusely distributed cytoplasmic 6 nm microfilaments. The distribution of the α-isoform, α-smooth muscle actin is restricted to vascular smooth muscle cells, and α-SMA is not expressed in endothelial cells or fibroblasts, allowing a good characterization of cultured SMC.

Smooth Muscle Myosin Heavy Chain

Smooth muscle myosin heavy chain (SM-MHC) is a cytoplasmatic structural protein that is a major component of the contractile apparatus in smooth muscle cells. Expression of smooth muscle myosin is developmentally regulated, appearing early in smooth muscle development (Glukhova et al. 1990; Frid et al. 1992).

H-Caldesmon

Caldesmon is a developmentally regulated protein involved in smooth muscle and nonmuscle contraction (Glukhova et al. 1990; Sobue and Sellers 1991). Two closely related variants of caldesmon have been identified, which differ in their electro-

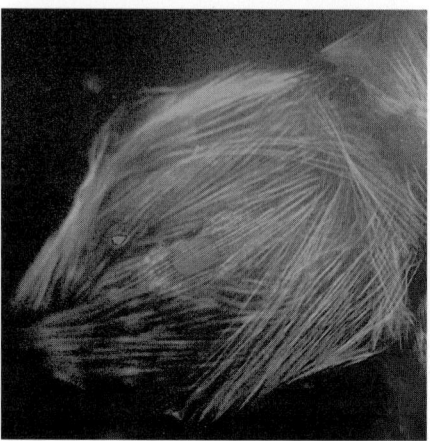 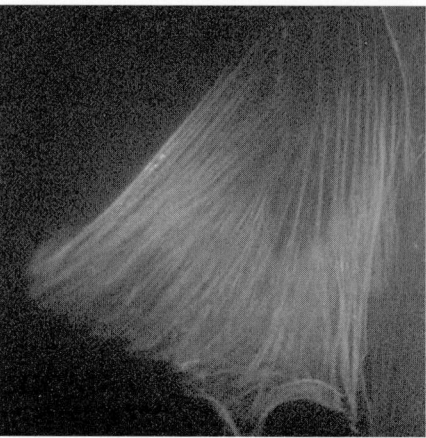

Figure 2a,b
Primary rat aortic smooth muscle cells were serum starved for 48 h to achieve quiescence. Cells were fixed and stained as described. Representative pictures of cells stained for α (*left*) and calponin (*right*) are shown. *For coloured version see appendix*

phoretic mobility and cellular distribution. Since the *l*-caldesmon is found in non-muscle tissue, *h*-caldesmon is predominantly expressed in smooth muscle cells and not in endothelial cells or fibroblasts (Frid et al. 1992).

Calponin

Calponin has been identified to be a calmodulin, F-actin and tropomyosin binding protein that is thought to be involved in the regulation of smooth muscle contraction (Takahashi et al. 1986). Calponin expression is restricted to smooth muscle cells, and has been shown to be a marker of the differentiated (contractile) phenotype of developing smooth muscle (Takahashi et al. 1986; Gimona et al. 1990).

Staining of Cryosections (Fig. 2)

- Fix slides 10 min in 2% paraformaldehyde
- Rehydrate sections for 15 min
- Block sections for 10 min at room temperature using 10% goat serum.
- Dilute primary antibodies to appropriate concentration in freshly prepared antibody dilution buffer (PBS + 2.5% FCS + 0.2% Triton X)
- Incubate for 60 min with primary antibody.
- Wash 2×5 min in antibody dilution buffer.
- Dilute a fluorescein-isothiocyanate- (FITC-) labeled secondary antibody to appropriate concentration.
- Incubate for 40 min at room temperature, in the dark!
- Wash 2×5 min in antibody dilution buffer.
- Add 2 μl DAPI (nuclear counter stain) to 1 ml 'Vectashield' mounting medium and vortex well.

- Add a small amount of mounting medium and cover with a cover slide.
- Evaluate cells by fluorescence microscopy.

Cryopreservation

Primary cells can be kept in a seed stock in frozen nitrogen for nearly unlimited time.
- Rinse cells twice with PBS
- Add 1 ml Trypsin-EDTA/50 cm^2 cell dish
- Incubate for ~1 min at 37 °C
- Microscopically control cell detachment (~80% of cells should be detached)
- Mechanically detach remaining cells by rapping the cell culture vessel against your palm ~5×
- Immediately add cell culture medium containing 10% FCS to neutralize trypsin-EDTA
- Centrifuge cells at 300 g for 5 min and remove supernatant
- Resuspend ~1×10^6 cells in 1 ml ice cold (0 °C) freezing medium [DMEM-F12 + 20% FCS + 10% dimethylsulfoxide (DMSO)]
- Immediately transfer cells to precooled cryoconservation caps
- Transfer cells to a Styrofoam box
- Store cells at –80 °C overnight
- Transfer cells to liquid nitrogen (–196 °C)

Recovery of SMC from Cryopreservation

Cryoconserved cells should be kept at –196 °C. Short or long-term storage at –70 °C after freezing or before thawing will result in severe decrease in cell culture viability.

Caution: Cryopreserved cells are very delicate. Cells should be thawed and returned to culture as quickly as possible with minimal handling. Eye protection is recommended when handling frozen cells, because rapid temperature changes may cause splattering of liquid nitrogen.
- Add 1 ml DMEM-F12 + 10% FCS/5 cm^2 surface area to a cell culture flask (e.g. 5 ml growth medium/25 cm^2 (T25) flask)
- Allow the culture vessel to warm and equilibrate in a 37 °C, 5% CO_2/95% air humidified incubator for at least 30 min
- Remove the cryopreservation vial from –196 °C storage
- Twist the cap partially open to relieve the internal pressure, then retighten it
- Place cryovial in a 37 °C water bath and swirl for 1–2 min until contents are thawed
- Wipe the cryovial with 70% Ethanol before opening in a sterile field
- Resuspend cells by gently up and down pipetting with a 1000 µl pipette ~5×
- Dispense cells in the prewarmed cell culture vessel
- Gently rock the vessel to evenly distribute cells
- Return the vessel to 37 °C, 5% CO_2 incubator
- Change the growth medium the day after seeding to remove DMSO and unattached cells

Troubleshooting

Cells Do Not Recover From Cryopreservation

1. Washing cells immediately after thawing to remove DMSO is not recommended, since it will be more damaging to the cells than further cultivation in medium containing DMSO for 24 h. However, if cells do not recover adequately, removal of DMSO before seeding by a wash/spin step is worthwhile trying.
2. Cells may not consequently have been held at −196 °C: isolate new cells.

Cells Do Not Grow After Trypsinization

1. Try to use less trypsin and closely follow their detachment under the microscope. Cells detach better by banging against the palm of the hand than waiting for the cells to detach by themselves
2. Although removal of trypsin after neutralization with FCS-containing media is not usually necessary, it should now be considered. For this, cells are spun down in 15 ml Falkon tube after neutralization (3 min at 300 g), and resuspended in medium containing 10% FCS.

Cells Do Not Reach the Log Phase of Proliferation But Rather Grow Slowly

As stated earlier, freshly isolated cells do not grow if seeded too sparsely. During the first two passages, do not split with a ratio >1:2, and during passage 3 to 4 >1:4. Later on, cells can even be passaged up to 1:10.

Growth Characteristics Change, Some Cells Enlarge Covering Other Cells

Between passage 12 and 14 smooth muscle cells usually become senescent characterized by retarded growth, enlargement, and lost of spindle shape. Therefore, smooth muscle isolates should not be used beyond passage 12.

Recurrent Problems With Infections (Bacterial Or Fungal)

Do not forget to remove everything used during cultivation (remaining media, trypsin solution). Sometimes, even the entire cryopreserved isolate has been contaminated. Also, check cell culture bench for flow characteristics.

References

Dzau VJ, Braun-Dullaeus RC, Sedding DG (2002) Vascular Proliferation and Atherosclerosis: New Perspectives and Therapeutic Strategies. Nat Med. 8:1249–56

Frid MG, Shekhonin BV, Koteliansky VE, Glukhova MA (1992): Phenotypic Changes of Human Smooth Muscle Cells During Development: Late Expression of Heavy Caldesmon and Calponin. Dev Biol. 153:185-934

Gimona M, Herzog M, Vandekerckhove J, Small JV (1990): Smooth Muscle Specific Expression of Calponin. FEBS Lett. 274:159–62

Glukhova MA, Frid MG, Koteliansky VE (1990): Developmental Changes in Expression of Contractile and Cytoskeletal Proteins in Human Aortic Smooth Muscle. J Biol Chem. 265:13042–6

Nobuyoshi M, Kimura T, Nosaka H, Mioka S, Ueno K, Yokoi H, Hamasaki N, Horiuchi H, Ohishi H (1988): Restenosis After Successful Percutaneous Transluminal Coronary Angioplasty: Serial Angiographic Follow-Up of 229 Patients. J Am Coll Cardiol. 12:616-23

Serruys PW, Luijten HE, Beatt KJ, Geuskens R, de Feyter PJ, van den Brand M, Reiber JH, ten Katen HJ, van Es GA, Hugenholtz PG (1988): Incidence of Restenosis After Successful Coronary Angioplasty: A Time-Related Phenomenon - A Quantitative Angiographic Study in 342 Consecutive Patients at 1, 2, 3, and 4 months. Circulation. 77: 361-71

Sobue K, Sellers JR (1991): Caldesmon, a Novel Regulatory Protein in Smooth Muscle and Nonmuscle Actomyosin Systems. J Biol Chem. 266:12115-8

Tunstall-Pedoe H, Kuulasmaa K, Mahonen M, Tolonen H, Ruokokoski E, Amouyel P (1999): Contribution of Trends in Survival and Coronary-Event Rates to Changes in Coronary Heart Disease Mortality: 10-Year Results from 37 WHO MONICA Project Populations. Monitoring Trends and Determinants in Cardiovascular Disease. Lancet. 353:1547-57

Takahashi K, Hiwada K, Kokubu T, (1986): Isolation and Characterization of a 34,000-Dalton Calmodulin- and F-Actin-Binding Protein from Chicken Gizzard Smooth Muscle. Biochem Biophys Res Commun. 141:20-6

Engineering Heart Tissue for *In Vitro* and *In Vivo* Studies

Wolfram-Hubertus Zimmermann, Ivan Melnychenko, Michael Didié, Ali El-Armouche and Thomas Eschenhagen

Introduction

Cardiac tissue engineering is an emerging field. Possible applications are *in vitro* heart modelling and cardiac replacement therapy *in vivo*. Cardiac muscle constructs should display structural and functional properties of native myocardium for either application. These are mainly an electrical syncytium, synchronous contractile function, and a high degree of differentiation. The general principle of tissue engineering and seeding of scaffold material with cells, was proposed by Langer and Vacanti in the early 90's (Langer and Vacanti 1993). Accordingly, most approaches in cardiac tissue engineering focus on scaffold fabrication and identification of cell sources for scaffold seeding (Carrier et al. 1999; Li et al. 1999; Leor et al. 2000; Kofidis et al. 2002; van Luyn et al. 2002).

Our group has developed an alternative approach in cardiac tissue engineering over the past 8 years (Eschenhagen et al. 1997; Fink et al. 2000; Zimmermann et al. 2000, 2002b). In contrast to seeding of prefabricated matrices, we utilize liquid cell-collagen mixtures with casting moulds and culture under mechanical strain, to construct Engineered Heart Tissue (EHT) with functional and morphological properties of native myocardium.

Our idea to construct EHT emanated from *in vitro* studies with standard monolayer cardiac myocyte cultures when highly efficient genetic manipulations became available by adenovirus mediated gene transfer technologies. Despite having good tools for cardiac target validation, the standard 2-dimensional culture system is limited by relatively poor functional read out with respect to cardiac myocyte contractility. Most importantly, isometric force measurement of cultured cardiac myocytes is not possible. Thus, we aimed to construct 3D heart muscle constructs *in vitro* that would allow gene transfer similar to monolayer cultures which also behave like a papillary muscle with respect to contractile function.

Our first steps in cardiac tissue engineering were prompted by studies that had been performed by Kolodney and Elson (Kolodney and Elson 1993) with embryonic chick fibroblasts in a 3D collagen I matrix. This culture format allowed measurement of (tonic) contractile forces of fibroblasts in standard organ baths. By adapting the method to embryonic chick cardiac myocytes, we generated synchronously and regularly beating cardiac tissue-like structures (Eschenhagen et al. 1997). Further modifications yielded cardiac constructs from neonatal rat heart cells and opened the way

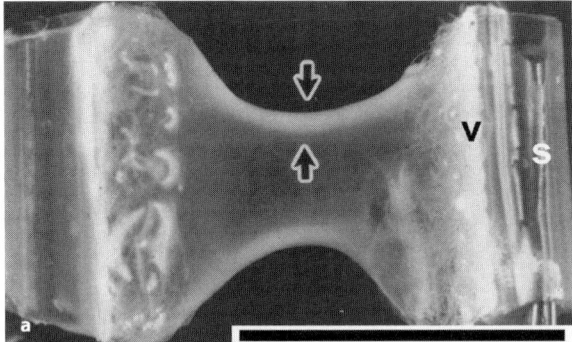
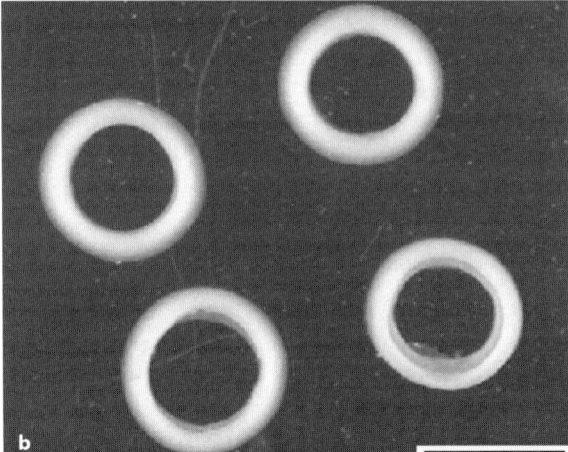

Figure 1a,b
Construction of EHT Lattices or Circular EHTs. a Construction of EHT lattices requires holding devices made from silicone tubing (s) and Velcro (v). EHTs span the gap in between the holding devices. Note the less translucent concave edges (arrows) that contain well organized and differentiated cardiac myocytes (see Fig. 2a). In contrast, the EHT center contains fewer and less organized heart cells (see Fig. 2b). (b) Circular EHTs can be constructed without artificial holding devices in a highly reproducible shape and size. Cells within circular EHTs show no spatial preference and spontaneously organize to form a dense network of interconnected muscle strands (see Fig. 5). Bars: 10 mm

for a broader utilization of this technology in target validation, due to the availability of more comprehensive gene sequence information in rats and the smaller phylogenetic distance between rats and men (Zimmermann et al. 2000). At that time, we termed our newly developed heart muscle constructs Cardiac Myocyte Populated Matrix (CMPM) but changed the terminology later to Engineered Heart Tissue (EHT) to address the tissue engineering aspect of our approach.

Initially, neonatal rat heart cardiac myocytes did not yield beating muscle constructs when cultured according to the chick embryonic myocyte protocol. This was in line with earlier reports showing that cardiac myocytes from neonatal rats do not grow inside a collagen I matrix, but can only be cultured on top of a preformed collagen I matrix (Souren et al. 1992). By systematically varying reconstitution conditions we defined matrigel supplementation as an essential component for rat EHT (Zimmermann et al. 2000). Matrigel is collected from ascites of mice with Engelbreth-Holm-Swarm tumours and is rich in extra-cellular matrix components including laminin, collagen IV, entactin, and various growth factors (IGF-1, TGFβ, EGF a.o.). Matrigel did not improve chick EHTs. Thus, our findings indicate species' specific requirements for construction of EHT.

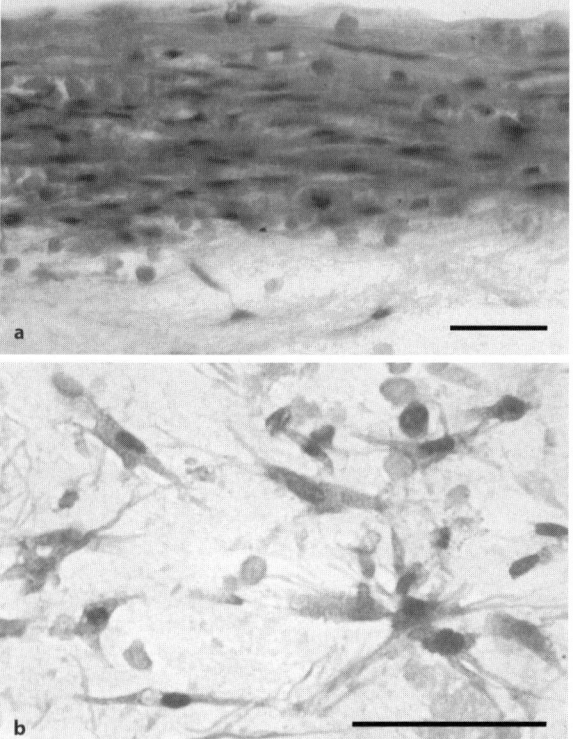

Figure 2
Spatial preference of cells within EHT lattices. Longitudinally oriented cardiac muscle strands form at the concave edges of EHT lattices. In contrast, EHT lattices contain fewer none oriented cardiac cells in the construct's center. Formalin fixed EHTs were embedded in paraffin, sectioned, and stained with hematoxylin and eosin. Bars: 50 μm

In our initial experiments, EHTs were constructed as lattices according to the fibroblast 3D culture technique developed by Kolodney and Elson (Kolodney and Elson 1993). This 3D tissue culture technology utilizes two Velcro covered glass tubes held at a defined distance by a metal spacer and a liquid mixture from freshly isolated cardiac myocytes and neutralized liquid collagen I in chicken EHTs and collagen I/matrigel in rat EHTs (Eschenhagen et al. 1997; Zimmermann et al. 2000). Casting of the cell-matrix, in-between the Velcro covered tubes, resulted in consolidation and adhesion of the EHTs to the Velcro fabric. During culture, biconcave lattices formed that spanned the gap between the glass tubes. EHTs can easily be attached to a fixed holder and a force transducer to measure isometric force of contraction in standard organ baths (Fig. 1a).

Another important aspect for optimization of EHT, is culture under mechanical strain. At the free concave edges of EHT lattices, the region of increased strain, cells formed a dense network of muscle bundles that were oriented in parallel to the edges, i.e. in the direction of the strain (Fig. 2a). In contrast, cells formed only a loose randomly oriented network in the central parts of the lattices (Fig. 2b). Thus, it appeared as if the orientation of cells reflected the biomechanical strain throughout the lattice, which is in accordance with current concepts (Tomasek et al. 2002). The importance of strain was substantiated by detailed stretch experiments. EHTs were subjected to a 5-day cyclic stretch regimen in a motorized device (Fink et al. 2000). This resulted in a 3–5-fold increase in contractile force development, hypertrophy of cardiac myocytes, and an improvement of tissue formation at the free edges. A systematic analysis of the relation between the degree of stretch and force development, showed that strain had a threshold effect and that approximately 5–7% stretch was necessary to optimize tissue properties in EHTs (Fink et al. 2000). A larger degree of stretch did not further improve force and at more than 20%, EHTs tended to disrupt under chronic phasic strain.

Despite the improvement in lattice EHT morphology and function by culture under mechanical strain, inhomogeneity of cell orientation and tissue formation and the need to produce slightly variable holding devices (Velcro-covered glass tubes) led us to think about an easier set-up. The solution was a ring-shaped casting mould in which the cell-collagen-matrigel mixture was pipetted. These casting moulds are made from silicone, are easily produced in large quantities at reproducible size, and can be used indefinitely (Zimmermann et al. 2000). In addition to these practical advantages, ring-shaped EHT (Fig. 1b) turned out to develop much better tissue homogeneity, likely due to more homogeneous distribution of biomechanical strain in a circular geometry. Hence, all our present studies are carried out with the improved circular EHT system.

EHTs proved to be a valuable *in vitro* system to measure pharmacological responses to β-adrenergic and muscarinic agonists and extracellular calcium (Fink et al. 2000; Zimmermann et al. 2000; Eschenhagen et al. 2002), gene transfer of cardiac genes (Most et al. 2001; El-Armouche et al. 2003), and the investigation of effects of chronic growth factor stimulation (Zimmermann et al. 2002b). Having a contractile heart muscle-like construct and given the increasing interest in cell based cardiac regeneration, it was obvious to test the applicability of EHT grafting for cardiac repair (Eschenhagen et al. 2002; Zimmermann et al. 2002a). First EHT implantation studies have demonstrated that EHTs survive for at least 8 weeks *in vivo*, become vascularized and innervated, and regain a high degree of differentiation. Presently, large longitudinal animal studies are underway in infarcted rats to address whether or not EHTs can be utilized to repair infarcted hearts.

Description of Methods and Practical Approach

The principle of EHT preparation is simple. Freshly isolated neonatal rat heart cardiac myocytes are mixed with freshly neutralized rat tail collagen type I, Matrigel (BD Biosciences; alternatively Harbor Extracellular Matrix [ECM], Tebu can be utilized), and a medium-concentrate calculated to yield a concentration of 1× DMEM, 10% horse serum and 2% chick embryo extract in the final reconstitution mixture. This reconstitution mixture is prepared on ice, well mixed by gentle trituration, and then pipetted into ring-shaped casting moulds at room temperature. After transfer to a CO_2 incubator at 37 °C the reconstitution mixture quickly (30 min) consolidates, yet remains soft, and thus traps the cells in a defined viscose 3D environment. During the first 2–3 days, cultured cells start to spread out to develop cell-cell contacts, and to form spontaneously contracting aggregates. In parallel, the collagen matrix is condensed considerably. Condensation induces biomechanical strain, and over time the cell aggregates organize to longitudinally oriented strands (diameter up to 200 µm but mostly thinner) that become highly interconnected throughout the matrix and thus form a dense muscular 3D network. During the consolidation process, EHTs undergo extensive matrix modelling and change from an initially slack gel that fills the entire circular well (outer/inner diameter: 16/8 mm, height: 5 mm) to a dense and mechanically stable ring (outer/inner diameter: 10/8 mm; thickness: 1 mm). We routinely transfer EHTs on culture day 7 into a motorized stretch device to continue culture under chronic mechanical strain (10%, 2 Hz) for 5–7 days. Under these conditions, improved maturation of EHTs has been observed. Longer periods of stretching often resulted in EHT disruption. Alternatively, EHTs can be cultured without phasic but static stretch, on simple stainless steel holders. This allows for prolonged *in vitro* culture for at least 4 weeks.

Isolation of Neonatal Rat Cardiac Myocytes

Cardiomyocytes are isolated from 1–3 day old neonatal rat hearts by a modification of the technique described by Webster and Bishopric (Webster and Bishopric 1992). After decapitation, hearts are excised, freed of atria and great vessels, and kept in 20 ml CBFHH (calcium and bicarbonate-free HEPES-buffered Hanks solution; mmol/l: 136.9 NaCl, 5.36 KCl, 0.81 $MgSO_4$ $(H_2O)_7$, 5.55 Dextrose, 0.44 KH_2PO_4, 0.34 Na_2HPO_4 $(H_2O)_7$, 20 HEPES; pH adjusted to 7.5 with NaOH) in a 15 cm culture dish, at room temperature until all hearts are prepared. For our routine cell isolations, we utilize 30–60 neonatal rat hearts. Hearts are cut in half, washed 3 times with CBFHH, and then extensively minced in 5 ml of CBFHH with scissors to a size of approximately 1 mm^3. Tissue fragments are washed again in CBFHH and then transferred to a 50 ml plastic tube for a serial trypsin/DNase digestion. After sedimentation by gravity, the supernatant is discarded and 10 ml trypsin solution (2.6 mg/ml trypsin, 24 µg/ml DNase II; 100 U/ml penicillin, 100 µg/ml streptomycin) is added. Digestion is performed at room temperature for 10 min. under gentle agitation. Subsequently, the supernatant of this pre-digestion is discarded and 10 ml of trypsin solution are added for an additional 10 min. digestion under gentle agitation. From this point, the supernatant is collected in 50 ml Falcon tubes filled with 2.5 ml foetal calf serum (FCS) to inactivate trypsin. Collection tubes are kept on ice for the duration of the cell isolation. Subsequently, 9 ml DNase solution (24 µg/ml DNase II; 3.4% FCS; 100 U penicillin; 100 µg/ml streptomycin) is added to digest traces of DNA that may interfere with sedimentation and release of isolated cells. DNase digestion is facilitated by extensive trituration with a wide-bore pipette. The turbid supernatant is then collected as described above. Cycles of trypsin/DNase digestions are repeated until near complete break-up of the heart tissue fragments. Trypsin digestion times are adjusted to the cell release, judged by an increase in turbidity of the supernatant, and kept for less than 5 min. for all subsequent digestion cycles. According to the amount of remaining tissue fragments, we gradually reduce the volumes of trypsin and DNase to 7.5 ml and 6.5 ml, respectively. After approximately 4 h, most tissue fragments are resolved. This procedure will yield approximately 5–6 collection tubes (50 ml each). Isolated cells are sedimented out by centrifugation at 60×g for 15 min at 4 °C, supernatants are discarded and cell pellets are re-suspended in 2 ml complete culture medium (DMEM, 10% horse serum, 2% chick embryo extract, 100 U penicillin, 100 µg/ml streptomycin) and pooled. 1/100 volume of DNAse II stock solution (2 mg/ml DNAse II) is added, the solution is triturated 25× and centrifuged as above. The supernatant is discarded and the cell pellet re-suspended in 32 ml complete medium. The cell suspension is filtered through a stainless steel cell strainer with a pore size of 100 µm^2 into four 10 cm culture dishes (Falcon series 3003) and incubated for 1 h in a CO_2 incubator. During this time, fibroblasts and other non-cardiac myocytes adhere. Non-adherent cells, mostly cardiomyocytes, are transferred to a 50 ml tube, sedimented by centrifugation, re-suspended in fresh complete medium and counted. The cell concentration is adjusted to 5.04×10^6 cells/ml. Cell yield per animal is generally 2×10^6 viable cells/heart as judged by trypan blue exclusion.

Engineered Heart Tissue Reconstitution Mixture

A typical reconstitution mixture for 4 EHTs is shown in Table 1 and is prepared in 10 ml tubes on ice. The optimal reconstitution mix has been the result of extensive testing of the effect of different original cell numbers ($1-10 \times 10^6$ cells per EHT) as well as the concentrations of collagen type I (0.4–1 mg/EHT = 0.44–1.1 mg/ml), ECM (0, 5, 10, 15%) and serum supplements (chick embryo extract, horse serum, fetal calf serum) on EHT formation and contractile function.

Part of these culture conditions were studied in the original lattice model (Zimmermann et al. 2000), part in the ring model (Zimmermann et al. 2002b). An increase in cell number between 1×10^6 and 2.5×10^6 cells per EHT enhanced contractile force, further increases did not improve function, but led to faster condensation of the cell/matrix mix. Whereas we could observe a narrow threshold for increasing the cell number in lattices (Zimmermann et al. 2000), it was noted that circular EHTs remained contractile despite a massive increase in original cell number (tested up to 10×10^6 cells/EHT). However, this maneuver did also result in EHTs with inferior contractile function when compared to EHTs constructed from 2.5×10^6 cells (unpublished data).

Table 1 Typical reconstitution mixture for 4 EHTs

	Mastermix (4 × EHT)
Collagen type I (5.5 mg/ml)	40 µl
2 × DMEM, 20% HS, 4% CEE, P/S	640 µl
NaOH (0.1 N)	140 µl
ECM	400 µl
Cells (5.04×10^6/ml)	2180 µl
Volume	**4000 µl**

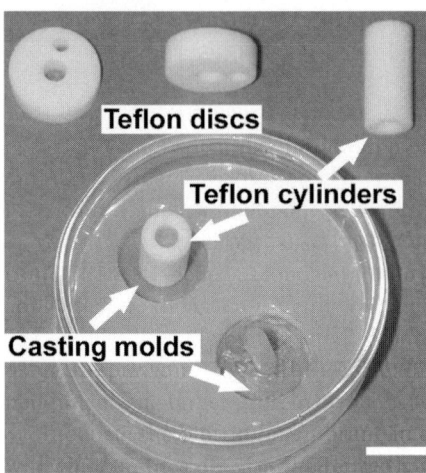

Figure 3
Casting mould assembly for circular EHTs. Circular casting moulds (diameter: 16 mm, depth: 5 mm) were prepared in glass culture dishes (diameter: 50 mm). First, 2 silicone tubes were glued to the surface of culture dishes to hold reversible Teflon discs (diameter: 16 mm, depth: 5 mm) that act as spacers while liquid silicone glue is poured into the culture dish. After hardening of the silicone glue, the Teflon spacers are removed (bottom casting mould). For EHT casting, removable Teflon cylinders (diameter: 8 mm) are placed over each silicone tube to yield ring-shaped wells (~750 mm^3, top casting mould). The size of a casting mould was sufficient to hold the viscous reconstitution mixture (900 µl) in place. Casting moulds could be re-used indefinitely after sterilization. Bar: 10 mm

Collagen type I was found to be optimal at 0.5–0.8 mg/EHT. A lower collagen content resulted in unstable and only weakly contracting EHTs, whereas a higher collagen content yielded EHTs that were rigid and developed less active force. A collagen content of 0.8 mg/EHT was chosen as a compromise between mechanical stability and optimal contractile function. ECM was essential for development of contractile rat EHTs and improved force when the construction mixture was supplemented with 5 to 15% ECM. We chose 10% (v/v) in our standard EHT construction mixture as a compromise between function and costs. Extensive testing was necessary to identify collagen (CVS, Germany) and ECM (Tebu, Germany) suppliers and batches that were suitable for EHT construction. Chick embryo extract could be omitted on day 7 without significant effect on force development, but was found to be important at the initial reconstitution phase (Zimmermann et al. 2004). In contrast, even small reductions in horse serum concentration starting on day 7, 8 or 9 of culture impaired condensation of the cell/matrix mix and led to a loss of contractility (Eschenhagen et al. 2002).

Preparation of Casting Moulds

Circular casting moulds (Fig. 3; diameter: 16 mm, depth: 5 mm) are prepared in glass culture dishes (diameter: 50 mm). Silicone tubes (height: 10 mm; diameter: 2 mm) are glued to the surface of a culture dish to hold reversible Teflon discs (height: 5 mm; diameter: 16 mm) with a central bore hole (diameter: 2 mm) that act as spacers while liquid silicone glue (Dow Corning 734) is poured into the culture dish. After hardening of the silicone glue, Teflon spacers can be removed. Instead of the Teflon discs, removable Teflon cylinders (height: 15 mm; diameter: 8 mm) with central bore holes (diameter: 2 mm) are placed over each silicone tube to yield ring-shaped wells (depth: 5 mm; outer/inner diameter: 16/8 mm). Casting moulds can be autoclaved and re-used indefinitely.

Casting of Engineered Heart Tissue

The ice cold, freshly prepared, EHT reconstitution mixture is cast into the circular moulds at room temperature. The volume of the casting moulds (750 mm^3) is sufficient to hold the viscous reconstitution mixture (900 µl) in place. Cast EHTs are transferred into a CO_2 (10%) incubator for 30–60 min to allow consolidation of the construct. Thereafter, complete culture medium has to be added with care not to disrupt the initially fragile EHT.

Culture of Engineered Heart Tissue

EHTs are cultured in the casting moulds for 7 days. Culture medium (6 ml) is changed after initial overnight culture and then every other day. Thereafter, EHTs are transferred into a stretch device consisting of motor driven bars that allow adjustment of initial EHT strain, the range of deviation during phasic stretch, and the frequency of stretch. EHTs are mounted on the stretch device in an initially relaxed state 10% below zero strain (–10% strain; internal circumference at zero and –10% strain: 25.1 and 22.6 mm, respectively), a stroke of +10% (from –10% to zero strain), and a frequency of 1 Hz. Within 24 h EHTs retract to the adjusted minimal strain (internal circumference: 22.6 mm) and are stretched by 10% to original zero strain. Stretch frequency is adjusted to 2 Hz, which resembles the frequency of spontaneous EHT contraction.

This stretch protocol minimizes EHT rupture during mounting and continuous phasic stretch for 5–7 days. Two EHTs are placed on each stretch unit and suspended in 6 ml complete culture medium. While being stretched, culture medium is changed every day.

Force Measurement in EHT

EHTs are mounted individually at slack length in thermostatically controlled (37 °C) organ baths containing modified Tyrode's solution (mmol/l: NaCl 119.8, KCl 5.4, $MgCl_2$ 1.05, $CaCl_2$ 0.4 , NaH_2PO_4 0.42 , $NaHCO_3$ 22.6 , glucose 5.05 , Na_2EDTA 0.05 , ascorbic acid 0.28, pH is maintained at 7.4 by bubbling with 95% O_2/5% CO_2) between a lower fixed pole and a stainless steel wire connected to a force transducer (Ingenieurbüro Jäckel, Hanau, Germany). After 30 min equilibration without pacing, EHTs are electrically stimulated with rectangular pulses (2 Hz, 5 ms, 80–100 mA) and stretched to L_{max}, i.e. the length where EHTs develop maximal active force (twitch tension). Resting tension at L_{max} normally amounts to 0.2–0.3 mN. All together, equilibration and pre-load adjustment takes on average 60 min. Thereafter, EHTs can be subjected to various stimuli to study inotropic and lusitropic responses of EHTs. Data is acquired by Bmon software (Ingenieurbüro Jäckel, Hanau, Germany) for later off-line analysis of twitch tension (TT), resting tension (RT), contraction duration (T1: time from 10% to peak force development), and relaxation duration (T2: time from peak contraction to 90% relaxation).

Gene Transfer in EHT

The most efficient way to transfect cardiac myocytes (and other cell types in EHT) is adenoviral gene transfer. We generally purify adenovirus by cesium chloride gradient centrifugation and dialysis and store virus stocks in virus storage buffers (VSB: 10 mM Tris, 100 mM NaCl, 0.1% BSA, 30% glycerol) at –20°C. Virus titration is performed in neonatal rat cardiac myocytes by serial dilutions. The amount of virus that gives 100% transfection efficiency in 2 million cells, is considered to contain 2 million biologically active virus (bav). This titer is used to calculate the multiplicity of infection (MOI). An MOI of 1 is, by our definition, sufficient to yield 100% transfection of cultured neonatal rat cardiac myocytes. We use an MOI of 50 to get similarly high transfection rates in EHTs. The necessity to utilize higher virus titers than in 2D culture of neonatal rat cardiac myocytes could result from the advanced maturation of cardiac myocytes in EHTs. Accordingly, high titers (MOI of 100–10.000) are employed to reach comparable transfection rates in adult cardiac myocytes (El-Armouche et al. 2003). This phenomenon might be attributed to the down-regulation of the common coxsackievirus and adenovirus receptor (CAR) during cardiac myocyte differentiation and aging (Communal et al. 2003; Fechner et al. 2003). Generally, we perform adenovirus infections in EHTs at culture day 10 under serum free conditions. Therefore, complete culture medium is replaced and EHTs are washed twice in DMEM before being re-suspended in serum free culture medium (5 ml; DMEM, 100 U/ml penicillin, 100 µg/ml streptomycin). Transfection is performed by directly pipetting adenovirus concentrate into the medium. After 1 h, serum-free medium is supplemented with 10% horse serum and 2% chick embryo extract to continue culture under standard medium conditions. Functional consequences of adenovirus mediated gene transfer are evaluated 48 h after infection by isometric contraction experiments. Adenovirus mediated transduction of β-galactosidase (β-Gal) or green fluorescence protein (GFP) serve as controls. Transgenes with bicistronic expression cassettes that include GFP allow for live imaging of transfection efficiency in EHT.

Histological Procedures in EHTs

We generally perform paraffin, vibratome, cryo, and ultra-thin sections for light, confocal, and electron microscopy. For light microscopy EHTs are fixed in 4% formaldehyde/1% methanol in phosphate buffered saline (PBS), pH 7.4, containing 1 mmol/l $CaCl_2$ and 30 mmol/l 2,3-butanedione monoxime (BDM) for 24 h at 4 °C or for 15 min at room temperature. Subsequently, fixed samples are washed overnight in PBS and embedded in 2% agar blocks for better handling. Dehydration in graded concentrations of isopropanol, paraffin infiltration, and paraffin embedding are performed according to standard protocols. We usually stain horizontal and cross sections (4 µm) of EHTs with hematoxylin & eosin (H&E), Masson Goldner trichrome, or Sirius red to evaluate cell-matrix composition of EHTs.

For confocal laser scanning microscopy and immunofluoresence studies, EHTs are fixed and embedded in agar as described above for later vibratome sectioning (100 µm slices) or used as whole mount samples after fixation. Whole mount and thick section staining is an attractive method to see the 3-dimensional organization of cells within EHTs. However, this technique brings about the requirement for extended antibody incubation time to allow sufficient diffusion in thick samples and extensive washing to minimize background due to high antibody binding capacities of collagen and other extracellular matrix components. The experimental procedures explained below have been adapted accordingly. Sections (100 µm) of agar embedded EHTs are prepared with a vibratome slicer (Campden Instruments, UK). Whole mount samples are used without prior embedding. Vibratome and whole mount samples are blocked and permeabilized at 4 °C overnight in tris-buffered saline (TBS), pH 7.4 containing 10% FCS, 1% bovine serum albumine (BSA), 0.5% Triton-X 100, and 0.05% thimerosal. After two washes in TBS, sections/whole mounts are incubated with primary antibodies at 4 °C for 48 h with gentle agitation. Sections/whole mounts are washed repeatedly (4×) in TBS and left in TBS over night at 4 °C with gentle agitation. After the overnight wash sections/whole mounts are incubated with secondary antibodies at room temperature for 3 h. Again, extended washing as described above, is performed before EHTs are mounted in Mowiol 4-88 with additional anti-fade protection by 2.5% diazabicyclo[2.2.2]octane (DABCO). Alternatively, EHTs are fixed, as described above, suspended in 10% sucrose overnight at 4°C for cryo protection, subsequently snap frozen in pre-cooled (–80°C) isopentane, and mounted in Tissue Tek. Generally, we perform 10 µm cryo sections. Staining is performed according to the protocol outlined above with shorter washing stages. Fluorescent imaging is performed by confocal laser scanning microscopy (CLSM) with a Zeiss LSM 5 Pascal system using a Zeiss Axiovert microscope. Especially in thick sections, this includes cryosections, it is in our view mandatory to perform CLSM if high spatial resolution is aimed for.

For transmission electron microscopy (TEM) EHTs are fixed in 2.5% glutaraldehyde in PBS, pH 7.4 containing 1 mmol/l $CaCl_2$ and 30 mmol/l BDM overnight at 4 °C. Subsequently, fixed EHTs are washed in PBS overnight and post fixed in osmiumtetroxyd/PBS (1:1) for 2 h at room temperature. Following an overnight wash in PBS at 4 °C, samples are dehydrated in graded concentrations of ethanol and acetone, epon infiltrated, and epon embedded according to standard protocols. Semi-thin sections (1 µm) are stained with toluidin blue for gross orientation. For TEM, ultra-thin sections (50 nm) are cut (Ultracut UCT, Leica) and contrasted with uranyl acetate and lead citrate. We examine sections with a Zeiss Leo 906 EM system.

EHT Grafting

We have performed initial EHT grafting studies in the peritoneum and on the heart of syngeneic Fischer 344 and outbred Wistar rats (Eschenhagen et al. 2002; Zimmermann et al. 2002a). Implantation studies were performed either after intraperitoneal injection of ketamine (20–50 mg/kg) and xylazine (3–10 mg/kg) or in volatile isoflurane (2–4% in 400 ml/min 95% oxygen and 5% CO_2) anesthesia. The latter protocol is by far superior since it allows adjustment of narcosis according to vital signs, echocardiography, and breath rate. In contrast ketamine/xylazine anesthesia can be variable with respect to cardiac parameters and most importantly exhibits negative inotropic effects. Effects on cardiac contractility become of great importance especially when animals with experimentally impaired myocardial function are operated on. Isoflurane anesthesia is performed via a mask or after intubation for studies on peritoneal and cardiac implantation, respectively. Intubation is performed in light isoflurane anesthesia and after injection of atropin (0.5 mg/kg).

Peritoneal implantation was performed in our initial experiments to study EHT survival *in vivo* and was chosen because of easy access to the peritoneal cavity, with no need for intubation, and low rate of complications (Eschenhagen et al. 2002). Briefly, after midline laparotomy EHTs were sutured to the peritoneal wall or in artificially prepared pockets underneath the peritoneum parietale. The fate of grafted EHTs was followed for up to 8 weeks.

We could demonstrate that EHTs survive, retain a high degree of differentiation, and become vascularized in this heterotopic position. All our present grafting studies are performed in an orthotopic position on the heart after left lateral thoracotomy. Briefly, rats are intubated and ventilated with positive endexpiratory pressure (PEEP) to avoid collapse of the lungs. The thoracic cavity is accessed after blunt dissection of the latissimus dorsi and pectoralis muscles through the 4th intercostal space. The intercostal space is held open by a retractor. After removal of the pericardium, EHTs are fixed onto the myocardium with 5/0 prolene sutures. Thereafter, the thoracic cavity is closed by layered sutures and the rats are weaned from anesthesia. Presently, all grafting studies are performed in outbred Wistar rats under triple immunosuppression with azathioprin (2 mg/kg/d), ciclosporin A (5 mg/kg/d), and methylprednisolon (2 mg/kg/d).

Examples

We have utilized EHTs for *in vitro* and *in vivo* studies. In this paragraph we will briefly describe some studies that have been performed in our lab to give a more detailed overview on experimental applications of EHT.

Study of Isometric Force Development

To define contractile properties of EHTs we performed a series of isometric contraction experiments (Zimmermann et al., 2002b). EHTs (n=12–15) were mounted as described above and equilibrated. Preload was adjusted stepwise from slack length to L_{max}. At L_{max}, twitch tension (TT) amounted to 0.36±0.06 mN at a resting tension (RT) of 0.27±0.03 mN. Contraction and relaxation time (T1 and T2) were 83±2 ms and 154±9 ms, respectively. An increase in extracellular calcium enhanced TT from 0.34± 0.06 to 0.75±0.11 mN with a maximal inotropic response at 1.6 mmol/l, RT and twitch kinetics remained unchanged. β-adrenergic stimulation with isoprenaline induced a maximal increase of TT from 0.28±0.06 to 0.69±0.09 mN at 1 µmol/l isoprenaline.

Additionally, isoprenaline shortened T1 from 86±4 to 56±2 ms and T2 from 144±8 to 83±3 ms, respectively, and reduced RT from 0.15±0.02 to 0.05±0.02 mN. The decrease in RT may be mediated by smooth muscle cells that line the surface of EHTs

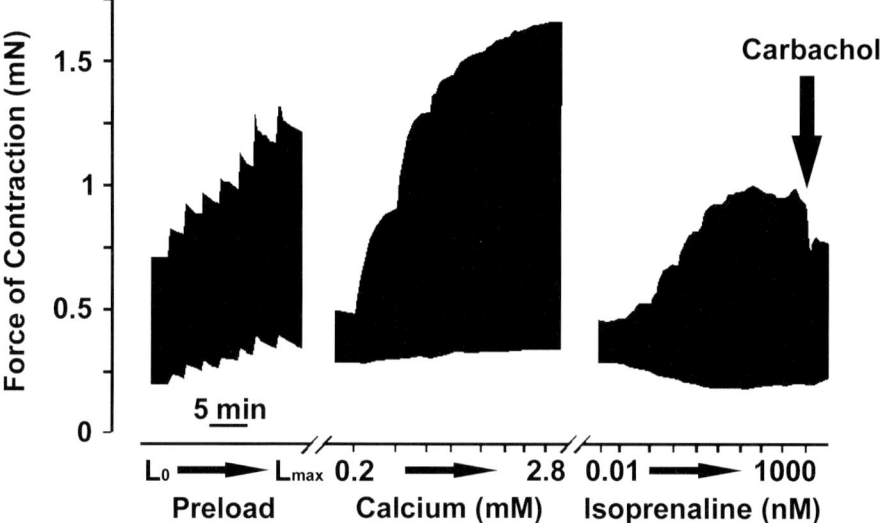

Figure 4
Contractile Function of Circular EHTs. Contractile properties of EHTs can be assessed in standard organ baths by isometric contraction experiments. A representative tracing of a contraction experiment demonstrates an increase in force of contraction after adjustment of preload to L_{max} (Frank-Starling mechanism), a positive inotropic response to an increase in extracellular calcium, and increasing concentrations of isoprenaline. Addition of carbachol (1 μM) at maximal isoprenaline stimulation leads to a drop in force of contraction (indirect negative inotropic effect of carbachol)

and respond to β-adrenergic stimulation via $β_2$-adrenoceptors by relaxation. Addition of the muscarinergic agonist carbachol to isoprenaline stimulated EHTs results in a decrease in contractile function (indirect negative inotropic effect of carbachol) and complete reversal of the isoprenaline-induced positive lusitropic effect. Carbachol effects were completely abolished by overnight incubation with pertussis toxin (100 ng/ml) (Zimmermann 2000). Thus, our findings indicate that EHTs elicit contractile properties of native heart muscle including effective coupling of stimulatory and inhibitory G-proteins with the adenylyl cyclase, albeit, that EHTs demonstrate a high calcium-sensitivity (apparent EC_{50}: 0.2–0.5 mmol/l calcium). A representative tracing of a contraction experiment with a circular EHT is included in Fig. 4.

Study of EHT Differentiation

The degree of cardiac differentiation in EHTs was compared with native heart muscle from neonatal and adult rats (Zimmermann et al. 2002b). Paraffin sections of EHTs (n=7) were prepared 14 days after casting as described above and stained with hematoxylin and eosin. Tissue sections from native myocardium were performed accordingly. In contrast to planar EHTs where cardiac myocytes were mainly concentrated at the lateral free edges [see above and (Zimmermann et al. 2000)] serial sections of paraffin-embedded circular EHTs revealed no spatial preference of cell distribution. Moreover, complexes of multicellular aggregates and longitudinally oriented cell

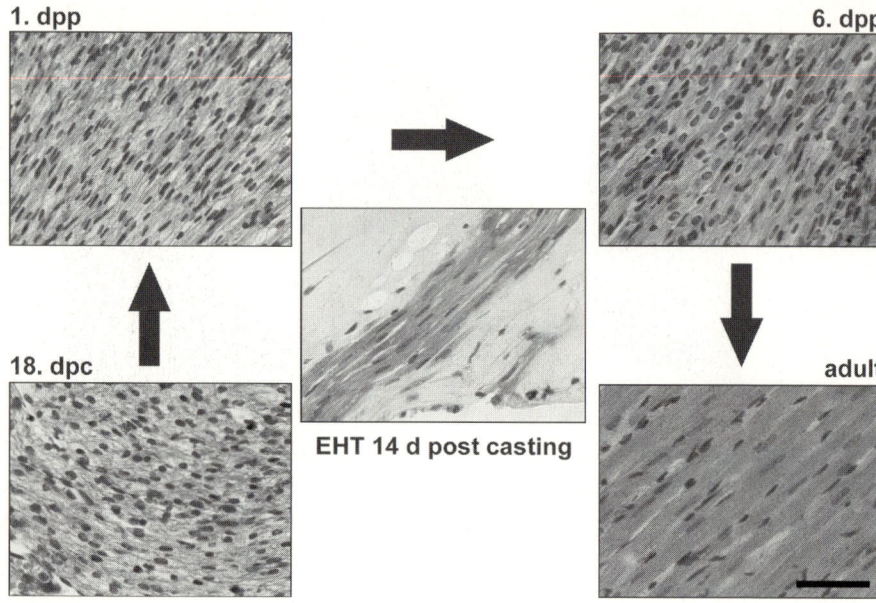

Figure 5
Morphology of EHTs and Native Myocardium. Hematoxylin and eosin staining of paraffin sections from native myocardium foetal (day 18 post conception), neonatal (days 1 and 6 post-partum), and adult Wistar rats (300 g) and EHTs (day 14 post casting). All sections were prepared, fixed, and stained in parallel to allow direct comparison of eosin staining. Note that EHTs are constructed from heart cells that were derived from neonatal rats (days 1–3 post-partum) and contain muscle strands that resemble cardiac morphology in the adult heart more closely than in neonatal myocardium

bundles mainly consisting of cardiac myocytes (Fig. 5) were found throughout circular EHT and formed an extensive 3-dimensional network. The width of these muscle bundles ranged from 30–100 µm. Whereas, native myocardial tissue was by far more compact (Fig. 5), we found that on the single cell level cardiac myocytes within EHTs (derived from neonatal rat hearts, Fig. 5) developed an intense eosin stain and clear cross striation, indicating a high amount of sarcomeric proteins and a high degree of sarcomeric organization. Additionally, nuclei were elongated and centrally localized. Despite being clearly distinguishable from adult myocardium (Fig. 5) our data indicates that cardiac myocytes within EHTs surpass the degree of differentiation of the original (Fig. 5; 1. dpp) and even further developed (Fig. 5; 6. dpp) tissue.

Target Validation

Our group has been interested over the past years in validation of potential targets for new treatment strategies in heart failure. To study the impact of gene products on cardiac myocyte function, we have extensively utilized EHT (Eschenhagen et al. 2000; Zolk et al. 2002; El-Armouche et al. 2003) and adenovirus mediated gene transfer. The principle technology has been described above and is exemplified by the following

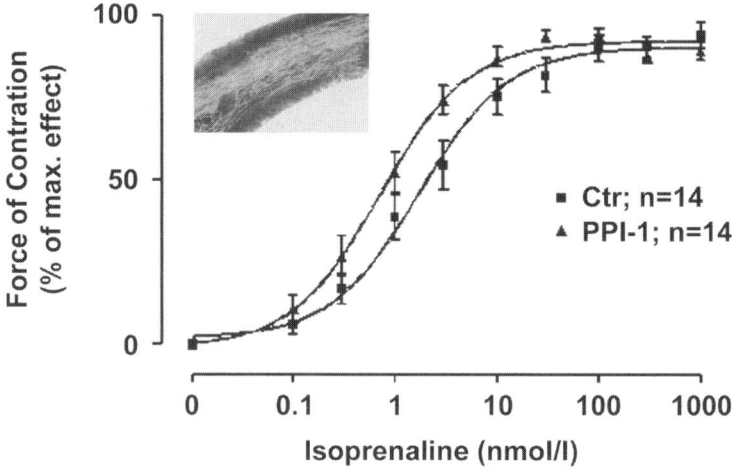

Figure 6
Utilization of EHTs for Target Validation. EHTs were transfected with adenovirus encoding for protein phosphatase inhibitor-1 (PPI-1) and green fluorescent protein (GFP). Highly efficient transfection is evidenced by GFP expression (inset). A left shift of the isoprenaline concentration response curve in PPI-1 over-expressing EHTs is in line with our hypothesis of PPI-1 regulated sensitization of cardiac myocytes to β-adrenergic stimulation. Significance of left shift was analyzed by Mann-Whitney-Test (P<0.05).

study on protein phosphatase inhibitor-1 [PPI-1; (El-Armouche et al. 2003)]. PPI-1 is a target of protein kinase A and has been reported to be a positive regulator of myocyte contractility, when phosphorylated, by preventing dephosphorylation of other protein kinase A phosphorylated proteins including phospholamban (PLB). In a phosphorylated state, PLB loses its inhibitory action on the sarcoplasmic reticulum calcium transporter (SERCA2a) and thus facilitates calcium loading of the sarcoplasmic reticulum (SR). By increasing the calcium influx in the SR relaxation is hastened (positive lusitropic effect), due to a faster calcium decay in end systole, and SR calcium stores are increased, making more calcium available for calcium release via the ryanodin receptor at the beginning of systole (positive inotropic effect). Naturally, PLB phosphorylation is controlled by catecholamine stimulation via β-adrenoceptors in the heart. In heart failure, decreased PPI-1 expression might account for decreased catecholamine responsiveness, aside from β-adrenoceptor down-regulation, and diminished cardiac contractility (El-Armouche et al. 2003). Thus, we hypothesized that PPI-1 over-expression might restore catecholamine responsiveness, increase contractility, and eventually might serve as a target for heart failure therapy. To test this hypothesis, EHTs were generated and transfected with adenovirus encoding for full-length rat PPI-1. Utilization of a bicistronic vector, encoding also for GFP, allowed us to follow transgene expression *in vitro* (Fig. 6 inset). In line with our hypothesis PPI-1 over-expression resulted in increased catecholamine (isoprenaline) sensitivity in EHTs (Fig. 6) and future studies will have to determine if manipulation of expression or pharmacological targeting of PPI-1 *in vivo* will indeed serve as a treatment strategy in heart failure.

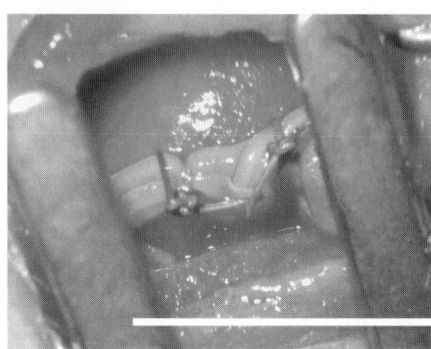

Figure 7
EHT Grafting. Different implantation techniques were employed to fix EHTs onto the recipients' hearts. Here EHTs were sutured onto the heart in apical-valvular direction

EHT Grafting

Cardiac regeneration by means of cell implantation has been emerging over the past years (Reinlib and Field 2000). In this context, grafting of EHTs might be applicable to replace diseased myocardium after myocardial infarction or to reconstruct congenital cardiac malformations. In initial experiments, EHTs were grafted into the abdomen of rats in a syngeneic implantation model (Eschenhagen et al. 2002) to study the fate of EHTs *in vivo*. After having observed that EHTs survive for up to 8 weeks *in vivo*, we have shifted our focus to implant EHTs directly onto the heart of healthy rats. Suturing of EHTs to the epicardial surface of the heart is relatively easy to perform and does not result in significant impairment of ventricular function and survival (Zimmermann et al. 2002a; Fig. 7). After 2 weeks we observed that EHTs are firmly affixed to the host heart, yet they remained contractile. Histological analysis revealed that cardiac myocytes gained a highly differentiated phenotype making them indistinguishable from native myocardium. Additionally, vascularization and innervation of EHT-grafts was observed. Presently, grafting studies in rats after induction of a myocardial infarction are performed in our laboratory to study the applicability of EHT grafting in disease, including functional coupling and consequences on contractile function in the long run. Whether or not EHT grafting will serve to refurnish infarcted hearts remains open at present. In order to have a realistic perspective for a clinical application, present stem cell based technologies will have to be improved dramatically to yield ideally autologous cardiac myocytes in large quantities. To allow reconstruction of large cardiac defects, like a myocardial infarction, approximately 109 cells will be needed (Gepstein 2002).

Troubleshooting

Construction of EHTs is highly reproducible but critically depends on the utilization of suitable collagen, culture medium supplements, matrigel in rat EHTs, cell number, geometry, and mechanical strain during culture. In studies of target validation with adenovirus mediated gene transfer, transfection efficiency can be variable and virus toxicity has to be taken into consideration. Grafting studies require highly trained individuals to perform surgeries and are compromised by immune rejection even in a syngeneic animal model. In this paragraph, critical aspects in EHT construction, adenovirus mediated gene transfer in EHTs, and EHT grafting will be addressed.

EHT Construction

Extensive collagen type I batch testing was found to be essential for EHT construction. Additionally, we found that a narrow window exists for the optimal collagen I content. The optimal concentration in terms of contractile force was between 0.5 and 0.7 mg/EHT, lower and higher concentrations yielded less contractile force. Additionally, EHTs are more prone to disruption at lower collagen concentrations and tend to become rather rigid at higher concentrations (Eschenhagen et al. 2002; Zimmermann and Eschenhagen 2003). We chose 0.8 mg/EHT as a standard concentration as a compromise between mechanical stability and function. ECM supplementation was found to be critical in rat but not in chick EHTs. Currently, we have not succeeded in isolating essential factors for rat EHT construction from ECM. It is likely that soluble growth factors are more essential than extra-cellular matrix components (Zimmermann 2000; Zimmermann et al. 2000).

Serum supplementation of culture medium is also essential for EHT construction. Whereas only slight reduction of horse serum (to 3%) for as short as 3 days leads to deterioration of EHT formation, we found that chick embryo extract can be omitted after 7 days in culture. However, complete withdrawal of CEE similarly leads to deterioration of EHT formation. We chose horse serum instead of calf serum due to its higher content in triiodothyronin (T3). T3 has been described as an essential factor for myofilament development. CEE has been chosen for its high content in growth and differentiation promoting growth factors (Coon and Cahn 1966).

The effect of cell density on EHT construction was tested in lattice and ring shaped EHTs. We could observe a marked biphasic effect on force development in EHT lattices with an increase in force of between 0.5 and 2.5 Mio cells/EHT. Above this, formation of contractile EHTs was not possible as contractions ceased and the amount of rounded cells within the EHT matrix increased. This steep threshold effect on contractile function is likely to be explained by increasing metabolic problems within the matrix. In contrast, we did not observe complete deterioration in circular EHTs at higher cell numbers. However, force of contraction was diminished at cell concentrations above 2.5×10^6/EHT.

Geometry and Strain

EHT geometry was apparently important for improved EHT structure. Whereas in lattices, cells were preferentially located along the free concave EHT edges, we could not observe a similar pattern in circular EHTs. In contrast, cardiac myocyte strands formed throughout the matrix with no apparent spatial preference. We attributed this finding to more homogeneously distributed biomechanical strain in circular EHTs.

The importance of strain was further exemplified when EHTs were subjected to phasic stretch. Whereas lattice shaped EHTs can be markedly improved in function and morphology by actively stretching, this was not observed in circular EHTs. This difference is most likely explained by the more homogeneous distribution of biomechanical strain in circular EHTs, which is likely to be induced by non-myocyte supported matrix retraction. The latter is also expected to occur in lattice EHTs. However, in our lattice geometry homogeneous matrix retraction is inhibited by the peripherally attached holding devices. Regardless of the need for phasic strain in lattice shaped EHTs, it also remains essential in circular EHTs, to continue the culture under at least static strain. Freely floating circular EHTs retract quickly and loose contractile function completely. Thus, mechanical strain remains an important issue in either culture geometry.

Adenovirus Mediated Gene Transfer

Successful application of EHTs for target validation depends on efficient gene transfer. To achieve this goal, extensive testing of virus titers and transfection efficiency has to be performed in EHTs. As described above, differentiation in EHTs seems to go along with a reduced susceptibility of EHTs to transfection by adenoviruses. We routinely employed MOIs of 50 to yield transfection efficiencies of 100%. Utilization of bicistronic adenovirus encoding for a gene of interest and GFP facilitates MOI finding. However, toxicity of the virus itself and of the transgene, including GFP marker genes has to be taken into consideration. Important control experiments include GFP-only adenovirus and eventually mutated non-functional genes of interest to rule out non-specific confounding effects by the virus itself, the transgene of interest and GFP. In contrast to monolayer cell cultures, EHTs appear to be extremely sensitive to virus infections, which may be due to the fact that force measurements in EHTs integrate the influence of "tissue development" as well as cardiac myocyte function. The possibility exists that adenovirus toxicity also occurs in monolayer cultures but cannot be detected.

Grafting of EHTs

Our initial studies on EHT grafting were performed in syngeneic Fischer 344 rats. Care was taken to utilize neonates and collagen I from Fischer 344 rats. Additionally, prolonged washing prior to implantation was performed in Tyrode's solution to get rid of soluble xenogenic medium and matrix components. Despite these precautions, we observed significant immunorejection that was most prevalent in our cardiac grafting experiments. Immunosuppression, as described above, prevented rejection. The reasons of rejection in the syngeneic Fischer rat model are not entirely clear, but likely involve impregnation of cardiac myocytes with xenogenic proteins (from matrigel or chick embryo extract) or self-antigen expression. All our present studies are performed in outbred Wistar rats under triple immunosuppression. A practical advantage of the Wistar rat is a higher rate of reproduction and eventually lower costs.

We have not tested the utilization of nude rats so far. This might be a good alternative in short term experiments (weeks) but will most likely be complicated by high morbid-ity of nude rats and a partial recurrence of immune competence in long term studies (6–12 months). Presently, we are looking at the possibility of reducing immunosuppressants in long-term experiments (6 months). However, our initial study with a complete withdrawal of azathioprine after 3 months and a gradual weaning from prednisolone leaving ciclosporine A as the only immunosuppressant failed. Whether or not other immunosupressants or tolerance induction strategies will prevent rejection in the long run remains unclear.

Acknowledgements. This study was supported by the German Research Foundation (Deutsche Forschungsgemeinschaft) to T.E. (Es 88/8-2) and W.H.Z. (GRK 750, A1) and the German Ministry for Education and Research to T.E. and W.H.Z. (BMBF FKZ 01GN 0124).

References

Carrier RL, Papadaki M, Rupnick M, Schoen FJ, Bursac N, Langer R, Freed LE, and Vunjak-Novakovic G: Cardiac tissue engineering: cell seeding, cultivation parameters, and tissue construct characterization. Biotechnol Bioeng 64:580–589, 1999

Communal C, Huq F, Lebeche D, Mestel C, Gwathmey JK, and Hajjar RJ: Decreased efficiency of adenovirus-mediated gene transfer in aging cardiomyocytes. Circulation 107:1170–1175, 2003

Coon HG and Cahn RD: Differentiation *in vitro*: effects of Sephadex fractions of chick embryo extract. Science 153:1116–1119, 1966

El-Armouche A, Rau T, Zolk O, Ditz D, Pamminger T, Zimmermann WH, Jackel E, Harding SE, Boknik P, Neumann J, and Eschenhagen T: Evidence for protein phosphatase inhibitor-1 playing an amplifier role in beta-adrenergic signaling in cardiac myocytes. Faseb J, 2003

Eschenhagen T, Fink C, Remmers U, Scholz H, Wattchow J, Weil J, Zimmermann W, Dohmen HH, Schafer H, Bishopric M, Wakatsuki T, and Elson EL: Three-dimensional reconstitution of embryonic cardiomyocytes in a collagen matrix: a new heart muscle model system. Faseb J 11:683–694, 1997

Eschenhagen T, Fink C, Rau T, Remmers U, Weil J, Zimmermann WH, Aigner S, Eppenberger HM, Wakatsuki T, and Elson EL: Transfection studies using a new cardiac 3D gel system. In: Molecular Approaches to Heart Failure Therapy; Ed: Hasenfuss G, Marbán E; Springer Verlag; Darmstadt, 2000

Eschenhagen T, Didie M, Munzel F, Schubert P, Schneiderbanger K, and Zimmermann WH: 3D engineered heart tissue for replacement therapy. Basic Res Cardiol 97 Suppl 1:I146–152, 2002

Fechner H, Noutsias M, Tschoepe C, Hinze K, Wang X, Escher F, Pauschinger M, Dekkers D, Vetter R, Paul M, Lamers J, Schultheiss HP, and Poller W: Induction of coxsackievirus-adenovirus-receptor expression during myocardial tissue formation and remodeling: identification of a cell-to-cell contact-dependent regulatory mechanism. Circulation 107:876–882, 2003

Fink C, Ergun S, Kralisch D, Remmers U, Weil J, and Eschenhagen T: Chronic stretch of engineered heart tissue induces hypertrophy and functional improvement. Faseb J 14:669–679, 2000

Gepstein L: Derivation and potential applications of human embryonic stem cells. Circ Res 91:866–876, 2002

Kofidis T, Akhyari P, Boublik J, Theodorou P, Martin U, Ruhparwar A, Fischer S, Eschenhagen T, Kubis HP, Kraft T, Leyh R, and Haverich A: *in vitro* engineering of heart muscle: artificial myocardial tissue. J Thorac Cardiovasc Surg 124:63–69, 2002

Kolodney MS and Elson EL: Correlation of myosin light chain phosphorylation with isometric contraction of fibroblasts. J Biol Chem 268:23850–23855, 1993

Langer R and Vacanti JP: Tissue engineering. Science 260:920–926, 1993

Leor J, Aboulafia-Etzion S, Dar A, Shapiro L, Barbash IM, Battler A, Granot Y, and Cohen S: Bio-engineered cardiac grafts: A new approach to repair the infarcted myocardium? Circulation 102:III56–61, 2000

Li RK, Jia ZQ, Weisel RD, Mickle DA, Choi A, and Yau TM: Survival and function of bio-engineered cardiac grafts. Circulation 100:II63–69, 1999

Most P, Bernotat J, Ehlermann P, Pleger ST, Reppel M, Borries M, Niroomand F, Pieske B, Janssen PM, Eschenhagen T, Karczewski P, Smith GL, Koch WJ, Katus HA, and Remppis A: S100A1: a regulator of myocardial contractility. Proc Natl Acad Sci U S A 98:13889–13894, 2001

Reinlib L and Field L: Cell transplantation as future therapy for cardiovascular disease? A workshop of the National Heart, Lung, and Blood Institute. Circulation 101:E182–187, 2000

Souren JE, Schneijdenberg C, Verkleij AJ, and Van Wijk R: Factors controlling the rhythmic contraction of collagen gels by neonatal heart cells. In Vitro Cell Dev Biol 28A:199–204, 1992

Tomasek JJ, Gabbiani G, Hinz B, Chaponnier C, and Brown RA: Myofibroblasts and mechano-regulation of connective tissue remodelling. Nat Rev Mol Cell Biol 3:349–363, 2002

van Luyn MJ, Tio RA, Gallego y van Seijen XJ, Plantinga JA, de Leij LF, DeJongste MJ, and van Wachem PB: Cardiac tissue engineering: characteristics of in unison contracting two- and three-dimensional neonatal rat ventricle cell (co)-cultures. Biomaterials 23:4793–4801, 2002

Webster KA and Bishopric NH: Molecular regulation of cardiac myocyte adaptations to chronic hypoxia. J Mol Cell Cardiol 24:741–751, 1992

Zimmermann WH: Entwicklung und Charakterisierung einer neuen Methode zur Herstellung von künstlichem Herzgewebe aus Herzmuskelzellen neonataler Ratten. Dissertation at the University of Hamburg, Germany, 2000

Zimmermann WH, Fink C, Kralisch D, Remmers U, Weil J, and Eschenhagen T: Three-dimensional engineered heart tissue from neonatal rat cardiac myocytes. Biotechnol Bioeng 68:106–114, 2000

Zimmermann WH, Didie M, Wasmeier GH, Nixdorff U, Hess A, Melnychenko I, Boy O, Neuhuber WL, Weyand M, and Eschenhagen T: Cardiac grafting of engineered heart tissue in syngenic rats. Circulation 106:I151–157, 2002a

Zimmermann WH, Schneiderbanger K, Schubert P, Didie M, Munzel F, Heubach JF, Kostin S, Neuhuber WL, and Eschenhagen T: Tissue engineering of a differentiated cardiac muscle construct. Circ Res 90:223–230, 2002b

Zimmermann WH and Eschenhagen T: Cardiac tissue engineering for replacement therapy. Heart Fail Rev 8:259–269, 2003

Zimmermann WH, Melnychenko I, Eschenhagen T: Engineered heart tissue for regeneration od diseased hearts. Biomaterials 25: 1639–1647, 2004

Zolk O, Frohme M, Maurer A, Kluxen FW, Hentsch B, Zubakov D, Hoheisel JD, Zucker IH, Pepe S, and Eschenhagen T: Cardiac ankyrin repeat protein, a negative regulator of cardiac gene expression, is augmented in human heart failure. Biochem Biophys Res Commun 293:1377–1382, 2002

6 Biochemical and Analytical Techniques

6.1 High-Performance Liquid Chromatography (HPLC) — 661
Veronika R. Meyer

6.2 Protein Biochemistry — 686
Aida Salameh, Stefan Lehr, Jürgen Weiss and Peter Rösen

6.3 Receptor and Binding Studies — 723
*Peter Hein, Martin C. Michel, Kirsten Leineweber,
Thomas Wieland, Nina Wettschureck and Stefan Offermanns*

6.4 Recording and Analysing Concentration-Response Curves — 784
Stefan Dhein

6.5 Measurement of NO and Endothelial Function
in Cardiovascular Research — 799
*Renate Roesen, Anke Rosenkranz, Dirk Taubert
and Reinhard Berkels*

6.6 Biomechanical Stimulation
of Vascular Cells In Vitro — 813
Henning Morawietz and Andreas Schubert

6.7 Measurement of Function and Regulation
of Adrenergic Receptors — 829
Marc Brede, Melanie Philipp and Lutz Hein

6.8 Measurement of Function and Regulation
of Muscarinic Acetylcholine Receptors — 848
Björn Kaiser and Chris J. van Koppen

6.9 Cytometry in Cardiovascular Research — 863
Attila Tárnok

High-Performance Liquid Chromatography (HPLC)

Veronika R. Meyer

Introduction

The potential of high-performance liquid chromatography (HPLC) becomes obvious when looking at the chromatogram presented in Fig. 1. It shows the separation of the calcium channel antagonist verapamil and its seven metabolites. Although all eight compounds are chemically similar (some of them differ only in the structural detail that a methoxy group has been replaced by a hydroxyl group), they appear as distinct peaks. Their position in the chromatogram is a characteristic of their chemical nature and can be used for qualitative identification. The size of the peaks, their height as well as their area, is proportional to the concentration of the particular analyte in the sample solution; therefore quantitative analysis is possible when pure compounds are available for calibration.

Together with electrophoresis, HPLC is one of the powerful techniques that allow the isolation, identification and quantitative determination of minor and major compounds present in body fluids, whether of endogenous or exogenous origin. As with all laboratory techniques, HPLC also needs good knowledge and practical experience, but the method is mature and the necessary instruments and columns are commercially available from a large number of companies. A wealth of books, technical descriptions and method protocols has been published and the literature is still growing.

Simple HPLC instruments are available for 20000 Euro but a system with higher versatility costs 50000 Euro and even more. The price is markedly higher if coupling with mass spectroscopy is necessary but this combination is a most powerful tool for the structural elucidation of analytes to be detected in complex mixtures (Ermer and Vogel 2000).

What must not be forgotten is that in many cases the sample preparation prior to the HPLC separation is an important and sometimes difficult part of the whole laboratory protocol.

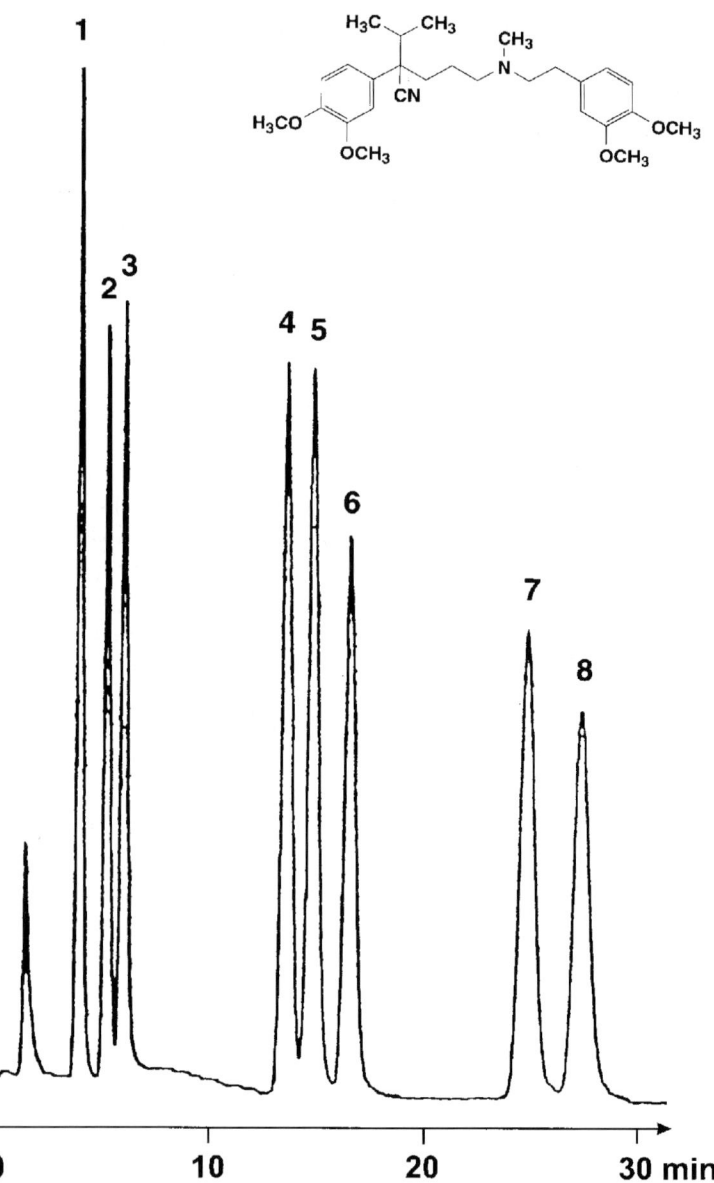

Figure 1
HPLC separation of verapamil and metabolites. Column: 3.9 mm×15 cm; stationary phase: NovaPak C_{18}; mobile phase: water/acetonitrile 65:35 with 0.03% triethylamine and phosphoric acid to obtain pH 3.8; flow rate: 0.9 ml/min; detection: fluorescence 276/310 nm; temperature: ambient. Peaks 1–7 are metabolites, peak 8 is verapamil. (After Brandsteterova and Wainer, J. Chromatogr. B 732:395–404, 1999)

Description of Methods and Practical Approach

General Remarks

Chromatography is a technique for the separation of chemical compounds. Their molecules are distributed between two phases of which they prefer one to a certain degree, in accordance with their physico-chemical properties. Since one of the phases is moving whereas the other stays in place, the different compounds of a mixture are travelling at different velocities. If the phase system has been chosen carefully, the compounds will be separated after some travelling distance and time. The chromatogram obtained yields information that can be used for both qualitative and quantitative analysis.

The moving (or mobile) phase can be a gas, and then the process is called gas chromatography GC. If it is a liquid, the stationary phase is usually solid (although in rare cases it is a immiscible liquid). A liquid chromatographic separation can take place on a plate (and is then called thin-layer chromatography TLC) or in a tube, the so-called column, which is packed with the porous stationary phase material. If this packing has a particle diameter of 10 µm or less it is possible to separate even complex mixtures of chemically similar compounds on a column of 10–30 cm in length, requiring 5–60 min of time. This method is called high-performance liquid chromatography HPLC (formerly also high-pressure liquid chromatography).

HPLC stationary phases can be chosen from an extremely large selection of commercially available materials. The mobile phase can be an organic solvent of any polarity or a mixture of water with salts, buffers, acids, bases, other additives and organic solvents. Due to this broad variety of phase systems, HPLC can be used for the separation of any mixture of chemical compounds soluble in a solvent. Theoretically it is possible to find a phase system for any two (and hopefully more) compounds even if they are very similar, such as homologues or isomers, including the extreme case of enantiomers. On the other hand, this versatility of HPLC can make it difficult to find the appropriate phase pair for a given separation problem.

Another drawback of all chromatographic methods is the fact that the separation process needs some time. This is in contrast to most spectroscopic analytical techniques where the actual measurement requires virtually no time.

HPLC columns are expensive (100–1000 Euro), therefore a single column will be used for hundreds of analyses. Only in rare cases it is possible to inject a sample of a body fluid directly into the HPLC system. It is usually necessary to clean the material by tedious and time-consuming sample preparation steps. It can even be more demanding to set up an effective cleaning protocol than to find the appropriate HPLC system for the final analysis.

The Chromatogram

A chromatogram such as the one shown in Fig. 1 can be characterized by a number of terms.

Dead Time t_0

Time elapsed between injection and the elution of a non-retained compound (a compound which was not adsorbed at all by the stationary phase). In many but not all cases, the first disturbance of the baseline or the first peak represents t_0. The dead time signal in Fig. 1 at 1.1 min is not caused by analyte but perhaps by the sample solvent.

Retention Time t_R

Time elapsed between injection and peak maximum. t_R is a characteristic of an eluted compound as long as the phase system (mobile and stationary phase), column dimensions, eluent flow rate, and perhaps the temperature are constant. Many other compounds may have the same retention time. In Fig. 1 verapamil has a retention time of 27.5 min.

Retention Factor k (Formerly Capacity Factor k')

$$k = \frac{t_R - t_0}{t_0}$$

k is dimensionless and is a characteristic of an eluted compound for a certain phase system and perhaps temperature. It is independent of other factors. The retention factor of verapamil is (27.5-1.1) min/1.1 min = 24.0. Again, many compounds can have identical retention factors in a given separation system.

Resolution R

R is a measure of how well two adjacent peaks are separated from each other. An ideal peak has the shape of a Gaussian curve with base width $w = 4\sigma$ (σ = standard deviation), and R is expressed as a function of w. Two peaks with resolution R = 1.0 are not completely separated but have some overlap. Both peak pairs 2 and 3 as well as 4 and 5 of Fig. 1 are resolved with a resolution of slightly better than 1.0. The pair 7 and 8 has a resolution of approx. 2.

The peaks should be of symmetrical shape but in many cases they show some asymmetry, usually tailing. The front half of a tailed peak is narrower than the trailing side. (In rare cases the opposite behaviour is observed and the front side of the peak is broader than the back half, a shape called fronting.) Tailing is unfavourable because it reduces the resolution between adjacent peaks, it impairs the peak area determination by the integrator, and it always occurs at the expense of peak height.

The HPLC Instrument

The HPLC instrument or chromatograph consists of several parts that can be bought as individual instruments or packed into a housing. Neither set-up is superior. The latter may need less bench space whereas the former may offer easier access to the

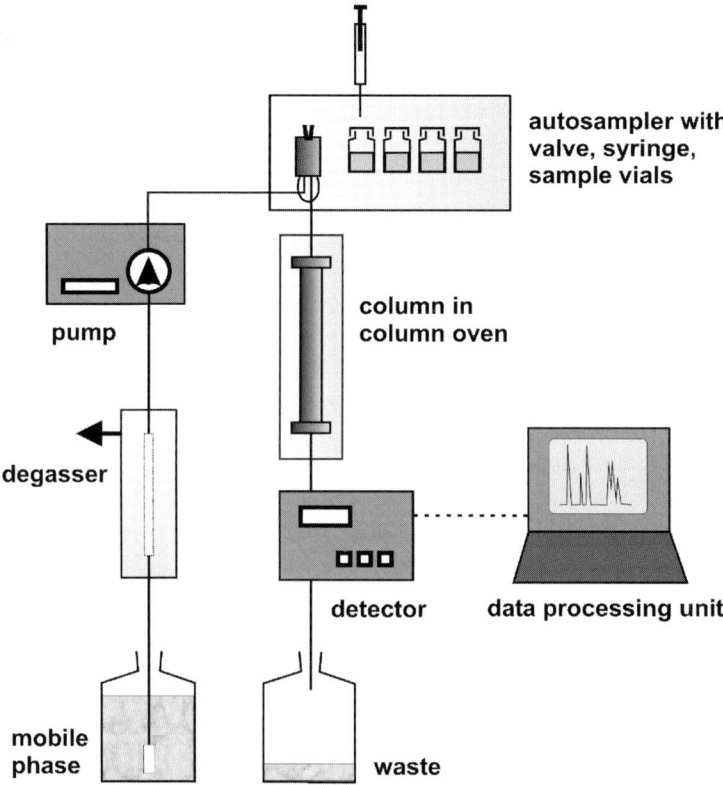

Figure 2
The HPLC instrument

failed part if a repair is needed. The set-up of the HPLC instrument is shown in Fig. 2. The parts are:

Mobile Phase

The mobile phase or eluent is a solvent of high purity or a mixture of solvents. Additives such as salts, acids, bases, reagents, etc. can be dissolved in the mobile phase. They should be easily soluble. The eluent must be particle-free; therefore it is necessary to filter any self-prepared solution through a membrane that retains fines larger than 0.5 µm. It should not interfere with the detection method; e.g., if a UV detector is used the mobile phase needs to be optically transparent at the chosen wavelength. It is advisable to buy solvents of "HPLC quality". Even water, a common constituent of eluents, should be of HPLC grade if the laboratory is not equipped with a water purification system that produces ultrapure water. Additives must be detector compatible as well.

Degasser

Air-free eluents are recommended; therefore a degasser is part of the HPLC instrument. Degassing allows the proper functioning of the pump and detector. In addition, it decreases the noise of the baseline of the chromatogram, therefore degassing is mandatory in trace analysis. It can be performed using a flow-through vacuum system with a gas-permeable membrane or by purging the solvent reservoir with helium.

Pump

HPLC separations are performed at pressures of 50–300 bar (0.5–3×10^7 Pa). The flow-rate chosen by the analyst is usually between 0.5 and 2 ml/min (or in the range of 0.1 ml/min if a narrow-bore column is used). The pump must deliver an accurate flow of mobile phase at any flow-rate without pulsations, irrespective of the viscosity of the solvent and of the backpressure of the column.

Injector, Autosampler

Usual sample sizes for HPLC analyses are between 10 and 100 µl of liquid. The sample can be injected manually into an injection valve although an autosampler is a common part of most HPLC instruments. The samples to be analyzed are filled into small vials (with a volume of e.g. 2 ml), capped and put into the sample rack. Cooled racks are commercially available for the investigation of thermally labile samples. The minimum amount of sample that is needed by an autosampler is between 10 µl (under optimum circumstances and if the injected sample volume is not higher than 1–3 µl) and 50 µl, depending on construction and vial details. No autosampler can inject the full amount of liquid that is present in a vial; part of it will be left. Manual injection is an option if not enough sample is available. Instead of vials it is also possible to inject directly from well plates if an appropriate rack is used.

Column and Column Oven

The column is the heart of the chromatograph because the separation takes place here. It is a stainless steel tube of 2–4.6 mm inner diameter and 5–30 cm length. Microcolumns with less than 1 mm inner diameter are also available; they should only be used with specially designed micro HPLC instruments. The column is installed between the injector valve and the detector. Most columns come without a preordained direction of flow but once a column has been used the flow should not be reversed. A short precolumn can be mounted between injector and column in order to protect the column from dirt or clogging substances. The precolumn is rather cheap and is replaced when necessary. For many separations it is advisable or necessary to control the column temperature or to work at elevated temperatures. Therefore column ovens are a standard part of many HPLC instruments, but they can also be installed subsequently.

Detector

In HPLC, the sample is injected at one end of the column and the separated peaks are eluted at the other. Concentrations are low and the eluted bands are narrow, therefore a highly sophisticated instrument is needed for their detection. A broad variety of measuring principles are in use. Some detectors measure a bulk property of the eluate such as the refractive index or the electrical conductivity. Most detectors, however, are built to register compounds with certain properties. Commercially available instruments are, amongst others, ultraviolet (UV)/visible, fluorescence, refractive index, conductivity, electrochemical, evaporative light scattering (for non-volatile compounds), or polarimetric detectors. In addition, the on-line coupling of HPLC with mass spectroscopy MS or nuclear magnetic resonance spectroscopy NMR is possible. The detector transforms the observed phenomenon into an electric signal, usually a voltage.

Integrator, Data Processing Unit

The signals of the detector are presented on screen or paper as graphs of intensity versus time. These chromatograms give qualitative information (are there eluted peaks, at which time did they appear?) and a quantitative one as well (what is the size of the peaks?). The necessary peak size determinations and calculations are usually done by a personal computer that is also used for the control of the whole HPLC instrument.

Waste

It is a drawback of HPLC that expensive and in some cases toxic and/or environmentally harmful solvents must be used. The best way to keep the volume of fresh eluent, and of waste as well, low is to use columns with small inner diameters, e.g. 3, 2 or 1 mm instead of the frequently used 4.6 mm columns.

Connections

The various parts of the chromatograph are connected with capillaries of 0.25 or 0.18 mm inner diameter and the appropriate fittings. They are made from stainless steel or chemically resistant plastics. Not all materials are compatible with all possible mobile phases, and plastics have a certain upper pressure limit depending on their chemical composition, wall thickness and the mobile phase used.

Gradient Designs

Figure 2 shows one single solvent reservoir; therefore it is an apparatus for so-called isocratic separations. In this mode, the composition of the mobile phase is constant over the whole duration of the chromatogram. The later a peak is eluted the broader and less high is its shape. The separation of Fig. 1 was performed using an isocratic

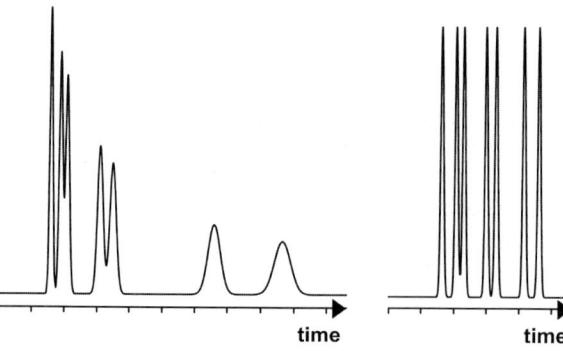

Figure 3
Schematic comparison of isocratic (*left*) and gradient (*right*) separations. For better clarity, the areas of all peaks are identical

approach. The number of compounds that can be separated is limited. For complex mixtures it is necessary to work in the so-called gradient mode where the composition of the eluent is altered during the separation. This can be done by using two (or more) pumps, one for every solvent used, and a mixing unit; this is the high-pressure gradient design. A cheaper alternative is to use one single pump and to deliver the necessary proportions of the various solvents by a computer-controlled switching valve; this is the low-pressure gradient design. With gradients, the duration of a separation can be as long as one hour and very complex mixtures can be analyzed. The compounds can have similar properties or strongly differing ones. There is no noticeable peak broadening with time. Figure 3 is a comparison of what idealized isocratic and gradient separations look like. The drawback of gradient separations is that some time is needed for back-conditioning, i.e. for bringing the separation system to its starting condition.

Post-Column Reactor

What can also be added to any HPLC instrument is a post-column reaction system. A tee junction is placed between the column outlet and the detector and a reagent solution is fed to the mobile phase by a low-pressure pump. The reagent converts the analytes of interest to products with properties suitable for specific and/or highly sensitive detection.

One of the important derivatisations is, e.g., the reaction of primary amines with o-phthaldialdehyde which gives fluorescent products. Some derivatisation reactions are fast, others need reaction times up to 10 min or longer and/or elevated temperature. For the slow reactions suitable instrumental provisions are necessary to prevent excessive broadening of the separated peaks.

Electrochemical Detection

Every HPLC detection principle has its own features and possibilities of pitfalls. In the context of this essay the UV, fluorescence, and electrochemical detectors are the most important ones. The former two are easy to understand and simple to use but the latter need some deeper knowledge for successful usage.

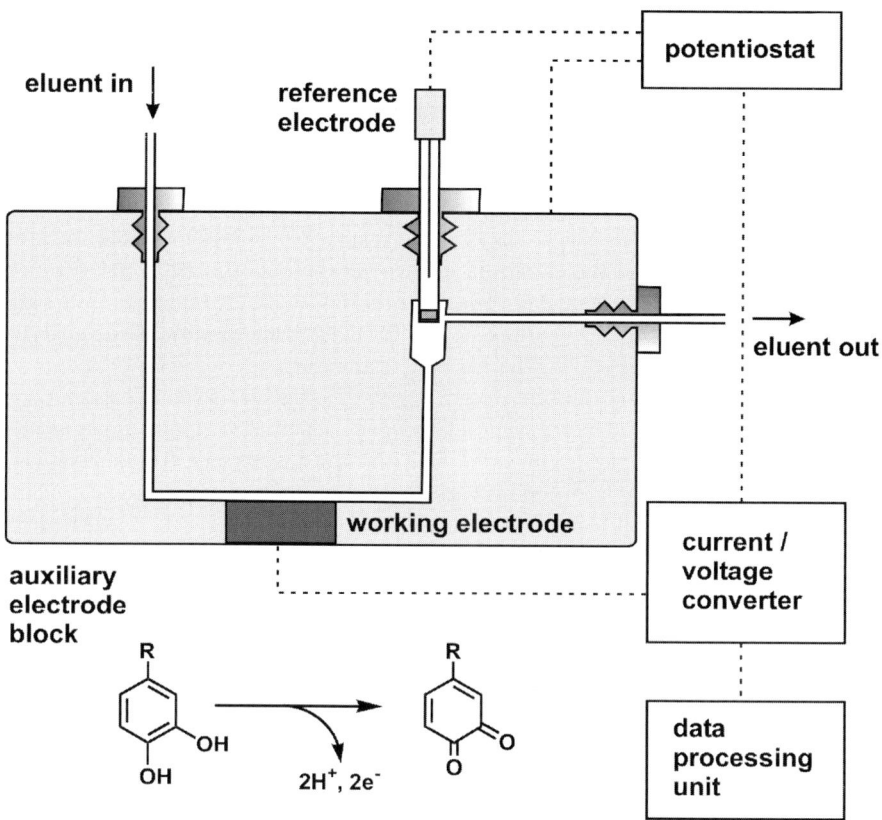

Figure 4
Electrochemical detector. As an example, an aromatic o-dihydroxide is oxidized to the o-quinone at the working electrode

An electrochemical detector oxidizes analytes that carry suitable functional groups such as aromatic hydroxy compounds, aromatic amines, indoles, phenothiazines or mercaptans by the withdrawal of electrons. (Reductive detection is also possible but less convenient.) A common set-up is shown in Fig. 4. Usually 3 electrodes are built together into the detector cell: a working electrode, e.g. from glassy carbon, a reference electrode, typically of the silver/silver chloride type, and an auxiliary electrode which can be the stainless steel block from which the cell is made. The potential between working and reference electrodes can be chosen; it determines whether a certain functional group will be oxidized or not. The auxiliary electrode draws the current that arises from the electrochemical reaction, thereby keeping the potential in the cell constant. The principle of measuring the current at a given potential is referred to as amperometric detection.

Working and reference electrodes are prone to contamination, and their lifetime is limited. Whereas the reference electrode needs to be replaced regularly (every 3–12 months), the working electrode must be polished with a slurry of alumina from time to time in order to reconstitute a clean surface.

A set-up as shown in Fig. 4 converts only approx. 5% of the electroactive analyte molecules flowing through the cell. Other detectors use porous flow-through working electrodes with a conversion rate of almost 100%; this is the coulometric detection principle. The detection limits of both approaches are similar because detector noise increases with increasing current; therefore the signal-to-noise ratio remains constant.

A special technique is pulsed amperometric detection for the detection of carbohydrates (Cataldi et al. 2000). They can be oxidized by a silver or gold working electrode at high pH but the electrode surface is rapidly poisoned by the reaction products. Therefore the potential of the cell is not constant but varied in definite steps over approx. half a second. One of the steps is for the actual detection of the analytes whereas others are necessary for the cleaning of the electrode surface.

Since the mobile phase must be electrically conductive, electrochemical detection is well suited for reversed-phase and ion exchange separations where aqueous eluents are used (see next paragraph). Chloride ions must be absent. Gradient separations are possible but not favoured because they can give rise to considerable baseline drift.

Phase Systems

The versatility of HPLC is based on the fact that a number of totally different phase systems can be used. Only the most important ones are described here.

Normal-Phase Systems

The stationary phase is polar, e.g. silica or alumina, whereas the mobile phase is less polar or non-polar. The eluents are organic solvents, ranging in polarity from pentane to tetrahydrofuran. The more polar an analyte is, the later it will be eluted. Normal-phase systems are less suitable for gradient separations. They are not suitable for aqueous samples. For the investigation of body fluids or tissues it is necessary to extract the analytes into an organic solvent prior to injection.

Reversed-Phase Systems

The stationary phase is non-polar, in most cases silica covered with chemically bonded n-alkane chains or other groups such as $C_{18}H_{37}$ ("octadecyl phase"), C_8H_{17} ("octyl phase") or C_6H_5 ("phenyl phase"). The mobile phase is very polar, i.e. aqueous, usually a mixture of water with methanol, acetonitrile, tetrahydrofuran or isopropanol. Buffer salts and other additives can be present. Polar analytes are eluted earlier than less polar ones. The separation in Fig. 1 was performed on a C_{18} reversed-phase column. Usually metabolites are more polar than their parent compound; therefore they have shorter retention times than verapamil. Reversed-phase systems are well suited for gradient separations because back-conditioning is fast. Due to the aqueous nature of the mobile phase they are the first choice for the investigation of biological samples. The analytes should be in a well-defined neutral or fully ionized state; therefore the suppression of ions by the choice of an appropriate pH for the mobile phase (e.g., acidic analytes are uncharged in acidic solution) is often necessary.

Ion-Exchange Systems

The stationary phase is an ion exchanger, either of the acidic type with carbonic acid or sulphonic acid groups (cation exchanger) or of the basic type with amine groups (anion exchanger). The mobile phase is an aqueous buffer. Its pH determines whether the stationary phase is charged or neutral. As long as the ion exchanger is in the charged state it can bind analytes of opposite charge; it releases them when the pH is altered towards a value where it is uncharged. Ion exchange is an important alternative to reversed-phase systems if the analytes in an aqueous sample are ionized or ionisable.

Ion-Pair Systems

The stationary phase is of the reversed-phase type but the aqueous mobile phase contains a charged reagent of partially hydrophobic character. A typical ion-pair reagent is tetrabutylammonium phosphate. If it is dissolved in a buffer of pH 7.5 the cation $N(C_4H_9)_4^+$ will form an ion-pair with acidic analytes which are dissociated at this pH. On the contrary, heptanesulphonate $SO_3C_7H_{15}^-$ at pH 3.5 makes ion-pairs with basic analytes. This approach is useful for the chromatography of amphoteric analytes (compounds with acidic and basic groups in the same molecule). The dissociation of one of their functional groups is suppressed by the appropriate pH of the mobile phase whereas the other one is masked by the ion-pair reagent. As a whole, the analytes appear as neutral compounds and can be separated on a versatile reversed-phase system. Ion-pair chromatography is not only useful for the separation of amphoteric compounds but also if both acidic and basic analytes are present in a sample.

Stationary phases of different brands that may look identical at first sight, such as the octadecyl reversed phases, can have very different properties. In many cases it is only possible to reproduce a published separation by using exactly the same type of column. In publications, all details concerning the phase system must be disclosed.

Analytical HPLC

Qualitative Analysis

A chromatographic peak marks the presence of an eluted compound whose identity is unknown in principle. To make things worse, even a peak of excellent, narrow shape can represent more than one co-eluting compound. For the identification of totally unknown analytes it is necessary to use spectroscopic techniques, mainly mass spectrometry. The on-line coupling of HPLC with UV, MS, and NMR spectroscopy, although demanding, allows immediate structural elucidation (Wolfender et al. 2003). In many cases the nature of the analytes is known and they can be identified by the injection of standards. Identity is only proven if the standard and the unknown compound show identical retention times in more than one separation system, preferably of different characters such as normal and reversed phase or reversed phase and ion exchange.

Quantitative Analysis

Either peak area or peak height can be used for quantification. The relationship between the injected amount of an analyte and the peak size can only be described by an empirical response factor; therefore it is necessary to perform calibration separations with known amounts or concentrations of analyte if quantification is required. If the analyte peak is well resolved from adjacent peaks it is possible to use the pure reference compound. Otherwise it is better to use a mixed reference material with a known amount of analyte or to dissolve the reference compound in an artificial mixture. This approach allows a calibration under realistic conditions. A sound calibration has 5–8 reference points of different concentration; the expected analyte concentration of the sample should lie in the middle of the calibration range.

Internal Standard

For many quantitative analyses it is advisable to work with an internal standard. This is a compound with high chemical similarity to the analytes of interest, e.g. an isomer. It will therefore behave similarly during sample preparation and chromatography. As one of the first steps in the analysis, it is added to both the sample and the reference in identical amounts. From the known mass or concentration ratio of internal standard and analyte in the reference it is possible to calculate the "true" amount of analyte in the sample by comparison of the peak size ratios. Losses of analyte during sample preparation or injection problems can be compensated to a high degree with this approach.

Sample Preparation

Many drug preparations contain the analytes in rather high concentration and in a relatively simple mixture. With samples of biological origin the situation is totally different. Blood, urine or tissues represent a motley of compounds, many of them in very low concentrations. To find and even quantitate a certain analyte is not simple at all, and elaborate sample preparation steps are necessary for isolation and concentration. Moreover, most HPLC protocols do not allow the direct injection of untreated body fluids due to the possible rapid contamination or clogging of the column. As a general rule, at the end of the sample preparation the analytes of interest should be dissolved in the mobile phase that is used for the HPLC separation; exceptions are possible but as a minimum requirement it is necessary that the sample solution is readily soluble in the mobile phase.

Of the many possible techniques and strategies for sample preparation, the most important ones in our context are liquid-liquid and liquid-solid extraction. The latter can be performed as a separate working step called solid-phase extraction or on-line with the chromatographic separation using the technique of column switching. Other approaches are pre-column derivatisation or physico-chemical methods such as filtration, centrifugation, dialysis or precipitation. In most cases a combination of several techniques is necessary. With all possible procedures the recovery, i.e. the percentage of analyte originally present that will be found in the final solution, can be rather low and the use of an internal standard is often necessary.

Liquid-Liquid Extraction

Two immiscible liquids are necessary and the sample is partitioned between them by shaking. The extraction can be performed on the 100 ml scale with a separating funnel or with less than 1 ml by using conical vials and centrifugation for the necessary phase separation. The pH of the aqueous phase is usually the driving force for the analytes. As an example, acidic compounds can be selectively brought into an organic solvent by working at a pH below 6. Later they can be re-extracted into an aqueous phase (necessary for reversed-phase and ion-exchange chromatography) by shaking with a basic buffer. A different approach is to evaporate the organic solvent (if necessary under nitrogen to prevent oxidation of the analytes) and to dissolve the residue in the mobile phase.

Solid-Phase Extraction

The sample, e.g. urine or diluted serum, is cleaned by passing it through a small column or cartridge that is packed with a solid, porous material. This can be an adsorbent (silica, alumina), a non-polar phase (octylsilica, polystyrene), an ion exchanger, a highly specific affinity phase or something else. The cartridge is operated by gravity or by the application of a slight vacuum at the exit. The working steps with solid-phase extraction are shown in Fig. 5. The packing material usually needs some con-

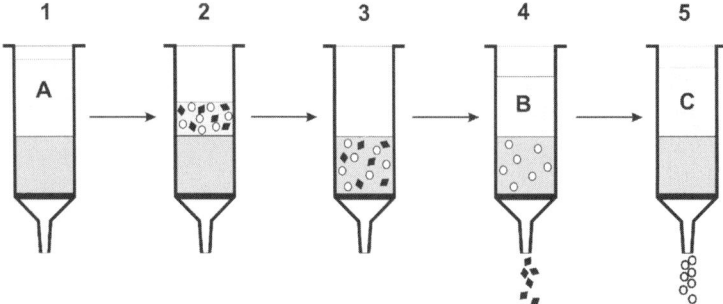

Figure 5
Solid-phase extraction. Step 1: cartridge with stationary phase is conditioned with solvent A. Step 2: sample is loaded. Step 3: sample is adsorbed. Step 4: interfering compounds are eluted with solvent B. Step 5: analytes are eluted with solvent C

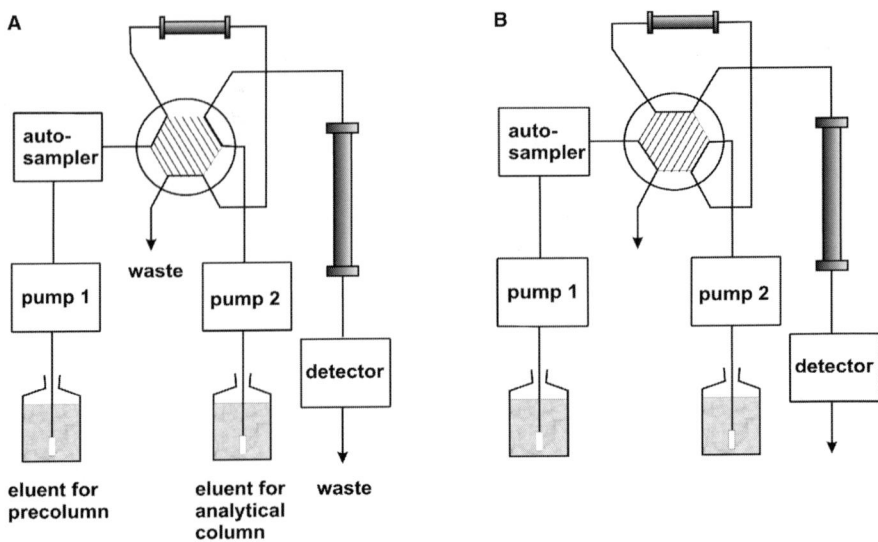

Figure 6
Column switching. Step A: Injection of a sample onto the small precolumn and separation of the previous sample on the analytical column. Interfering compounds are eluted from the precolumn, analytes of interest are retained. Step B: The six-port valve is turned by 60°. Transfer of the analytes to the analytical column and separation

ditioning with an appropriate solvent, which is sucked through. Then the cartridge is loaded with sample. In most cases the phase system is chosen in such a way that the analytes of interest are adsorbed. The other compounds are removed by washing the cartridge with a suitable solvent or buffer. Finally the analyte molecules are eluted with a third solvent or a buffer with different pH.

Column Switching

Instead of the off-line sample treatment it is possible in many cases to use an on-line procedure. The above-mentioned cartridge is replaced by a short HPLC column that is packed with any suitable stationary phase. The sample is injected on to this column, washed, and transferred to the separation column with a different phase by switching a six-port valve, as shown in Fig. 6. Two solvents and therefore also two high-pressure pumps are necessary. The procedure can be automated.

Examples

HPLC of Catecholamines

The chemical structures of epinephrine (E) (adrenaline), norepinephrine (NE) (noradrenaline) and dopamine (DA) are shown in Fig. 7. 3,4-dihydroxybenzylamine (DHBA) is used as internal standard, if necessary; its structure is also presented in

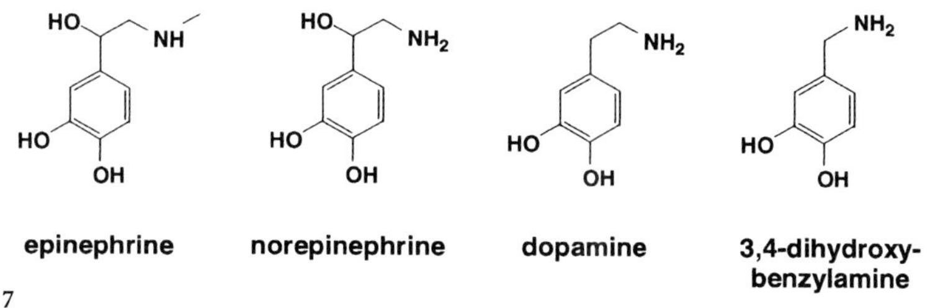

Figure 7
The structures of the catecholamines and a possible internal standard

Fig. 7. Since the elution order in reversed-phase systems goes with decreasing polarity of the analytes, the retention times increase in the order NE, E, DHBA and DA.

The common analytical technique for these compounds is ion-pair chromatography on a C_{18} or C_8 reversed phase with electrochemical detection. An interesting property of the catecholamines is the fact that their electrochemical oxidation is reversible at negative potential. Therefore a design with three working electrodes in series is frequently used. The first one, at approx. +0.5 V oxidizes the analytes but also some other compounds present in the sample. Many of them can be reduced at approx. +0.1 V and will therefore not influence the current of the third electrode that is run at approx. –0.2 V. Only the output of this last electrode is used for the detection of the catecholamines. Catecholamine analyzers, especially designed for this class of compounds and based on HPLC with electrochemical detection, as well as so-called catecholamine columns, are commercially available.

Fluorescence detection is also possible because the catecholamines show native fluorescence; for even lower detection limits they can be derivatised with reagents that enhance the fluorescence.

In all biological samples, the catecholamines are only found in low concentrations. Because they are susceptible to oxidation and are unstable in basic solution, special precautions such as the addition of antioxidants (e.g. sodium bisulphite, ascorbic acid, EDTA), the acidification of samples, and working at low temperatures are necessary. If samples need to be stored it should be done at –80 °C. Urine samples are stabilized by the addition of hydrochloric acid. For blood samples, tubes with EDTA or heparin are used. They are stored on ice immediately after collection until centrifugation can be performed.

Sample Preparation

Urine samples are worked up by extraction with phenylboronic acid, cation exchanger or alumina, either with solid-phase cartridges or with column switching (although other procedures such as the manual addition of alumina powder have also been published). These materials bind the catecholamines and related molecules more or less selectively whereas other compounds are not retained and can be washed out. All cleaning steps can be fully automated and coupled on-line to the HPLC separation. Plasma samples are treated with similar procedures. Tissue samples are sonicated in cold 0.2 M perchloric acid with 0.1% sodium bisulphite and centrifuged. The supernatant can be injected directly into the HPLC system.

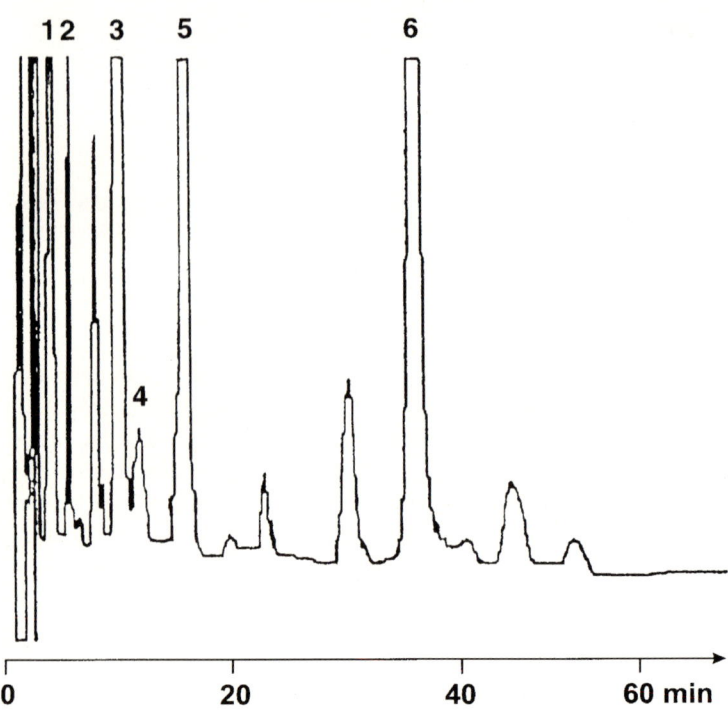

Figure 8
HPLC separation of catecholamines and related compounds in human plasma. For sample preparation and separation conditions see text. Peak 1: dihydroxyphenylglycol; 2: norepinephrine; 3: dihydroxyphenylalanine; 4: epinephrine; 5: dihydroxybenzylamine (internal standard); 6: dihydroxyphenylacetic acid. For the better presentation of the small peaks the large ones are not shown in full size. (After Holmes et al. 1994)

Example for HPLC with Alumina Sample Preparation and Electrochemical Detection (Holmes et al. 1994) – A Protocol for Catecholamines and Other Endogenous Catechols in Plasma

To 1 ml freshly thawed plasma in a plastic 1.5 ml sample tube add 5 mg acid-washed alumina, 0.5 ml TRIS/EDTA buffer pH 8.6, and 20 µl DHBA internal standard solution. Shake vigorously for 30 min, centrifuge for 1 min and discard the supernatant. Add HPLC grade water, shake for 15 s, centrifuge for 1 min and discard the supernatant. Perform this washing step with water once again. Add 100 µl of 0.04 M phosphoric acid/0.2 M acetic acid (20:80 v/v), shake vigorously for 5 min and centrifuge for 1 min. Transfer the supernatant to an autosampler vial and put it into a rack that is cooled to 4 °C. HPLC conditions: Column: 4.6 mm×25 cm. Stationary phase: Beckman Ultrasphere ODS 5 µm. Mobile phase: water with 13.8 g/l monobasic sodium phosphate, 40 mg/l (or less) octanesulfonic acid, 50 mg/l EDTA, 5 ml/l (or less) acetonitrile, adjusted to pH 3.2–3.3 with phosphoric acid 85%; the amounts of ion pair reagent and organic solvent need to be adapted to the batch of stationary phase used. Flow: 1 ml/min. Temperature: 15 °C, i.e. the column is cooled. Detector: amperometric with three working electrodes in series at +0.30 V, +0.16 V, and −0.35 V; the output of the last electrode is recorded. Figure 8 shows a separation of two catecholamines and related compounds together with DHBA as the internal standard. The plasma concentration of dopamine is in many cases too low for detection. It would be eluted near the peak at 30 min. The k values of the analytes depend on the temperature of the separation and thermostatting of the column decreases the variability of retention times. A good resolution of the first eluted analyte, dihydroxyphenylglycol, is only obtained at a temperature below ambient.

Example of HPLC with Column Switching, Post-Column Derivatisation and Fluorescence Detection (Boos et al. 1987; Hansen et al. 1999)

The catecholamines are converted to fluorescing trihydroxyindoles (THI) by the post-column addition of three different reagents. Urine samples are collected in bottles with 1 g citric acid per 50 ml. After filtration through a 0.45 µm filter, 100 µl are directly injected into the precolumn with nitrophenylboronic acid on Co-polymer 40–60 µm. Impurities are washed out with a buffer of 0.2 M di-ammonium hydrogen phosphate, 10 mM EDTA, and 1 mM sodium azide, adjusted to pH 8.7 with ammonia solution 25%. Then the catecholamines are transferred to the analytical column with buffer/methanol 80:10 (v/v). The buffer consists of 0.1 M sodium dihydrogen phosphate, 5 mM sodium 1-octane sulphonate, and 1 mM sodium azide, adjusted to pH 3 with phosphoric acid 20%. The buffer/methanol mixture is also the eluent for the separation on the analytical column, a LiChrospher RP C-18, 5 µm phase kept at 40 °C. The principle of column switching is shown in Fig. 6. To the eluate from the analytical column three reagents are added consecutively. Reagent A is 0.1 M sodium dihydrogen phosphate, 0.2 M disodium hydrogen phosphate, and 2 mM potassium hexacyanoferrate adjusted to pH 7; it yields the corresponding adrenoquinones after a reaction time of 45 s at 40 °C. Reagent B is 1.5 mM ascorbic acid and reduces any excess trivalent iron. Reagent C is 5 M sodium hydroxide, which allows intramolecular rearrangement to the fluorescing trihydroxyindoles within 30 s at 40 °C. Fluorescence is measured at 410/520 nm.

HPLC of Cardiac Glycosides

The most important cardiac glycosides are digitoxin and digoxin whose structures are shown in Fig. 9. A steroid structure is linked to an unsaturated lactone; this aglycone part of the molecule is bonded to three digitoxose sugar moieties. In some pharmaceutical preparations the OH groups at positions α and β are replaced by acetyl or methoxy groups. The metabolites are digitoxose (the cleaved monosaccharide), the cardiac glycoside structure minus one or two sugars (bis- and mono-digitoxoside, respectively), and the aglycone, the so-called genin (digitoxigenin or digoxigenin).

The standard procedures in clinical laboratories for the analysis of digitoxin and digoxin are based on immunoassays. Their drawback is the possible cross-reactivity with the above-mentioned metabolites and with endogenous digoxin-like compounds that may be present in the body. HPLC can be performed with detection in the low UV,

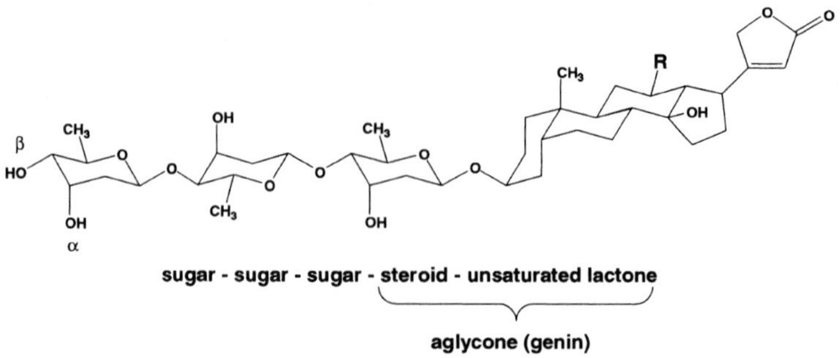

Figure 9
The structure of the cardiac glycosides. R = H: Digitoxin. R = OH: Digoxin

with fluorescence detection after derivatisation or preferably with pulsed amperometric detection. Recently interest has grown in studies with HPLC coupled to mass spectroscopy (Guan et al. 1999). Sample preparation is done with liquid-liquid or solid-phase extraction.

Example of HPLC with Pulsed Amperometric Detection (Kelly et al. 1995)

This kind of detection does not only work with carbohydrates but also with the aglycones of the cardiac glycosides. With standard reversed-phase separation systems a selective analysis method is obtained. Isocratic separation is possible for a single cardenolide series, e.g., digoxin and its metabolites, see Fig. 10, whereas a gradient is necessary if a mixture of digoxin, digitoxin and metabolites is to be analyzed. Chro-

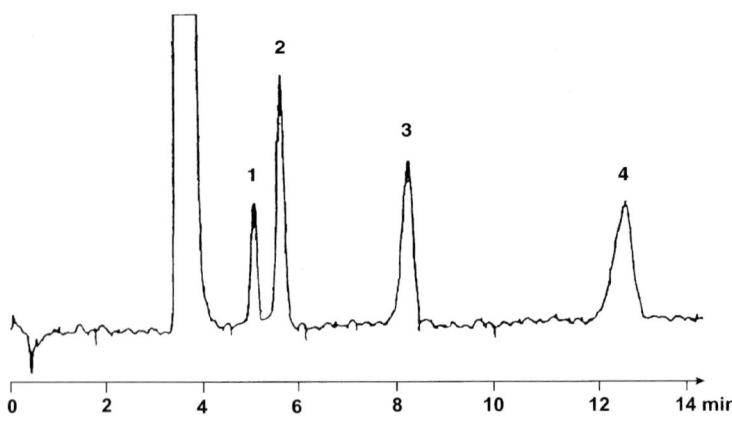

Figure 10
HPLC separation of digoxin and metabolites with pulsed amperometric detection. Mobile phase is water/acetonitrile 77:23, other conditions see text. Peak 1: digoxigenin; 2: digoxigenin monodigitoxoside; 3: digoxigenin bisdigitoxoside; 4: digoxin. The large peak at 4 min is methanol that is used as the sample solvent. (After Kelly et al. 1995)

matographic conditions: Column: 4.6 mm × 25 cm. Stationary phase: Deltabond C_{18}. Mobile phase for digoxin and metabolites: water/acetonitrile 77:23 (v/v); for digitoxin and metabolites: water/acetonitrile 67:33; for both series of compounds: linear gradient from 10% to 45% acetonitrile in water within 8 min. Flow: 1.0 ml/min for isocratic separation, 1.3 ml/min for the gradient. As with all reversed-phase systems, the mobile phase composition and gradient shape need to be adapted to the stationary phase in use. Temperature: ambient. Post-column reagent addition: 0.5 ml/min NaOH 1 M in order to shift the pH to the necessary basic conditions for the detection; uniform mixing is obtained with a 500 µl reaction coil between tee junction and detector. Electrodes: gold working electrode, stainless steel counter electrode, and Ag/AgCl reference electrode. Detection potentials: +0.07 V for 400 ms (of which 300 ms are used for the actual data collection), +0.7 V for 120 ms, −1 V for 300 ms. The working electrode needs to be re-polished after approx. 200 h of operation. Gradient separations show a distinct drift of the baseline due to the adsorption of acetonitrile on the electrode surface. Oxygenated organic solvents such as methanol or tetrahydrofuran cannot be used as a constituent of the mobile phase.

HPLC of Proteins

The most important technique in protein research and proteomics is two-dimensional gel electrophoresis. In comparison to such approaches, HPLC protocols are much faster and reproducible, they can be automated and allow simple quantification due to the linear relationship between peak size (area or height) and analyte concentration over several orders of magnitude. The on-line or off-line coupling of HPLC with mass spectroscopy is straightforward and various ionization or measurement principles can be used.

Proteins have different features from small molecules; they therefore show different behaviour in chromatography. Experiences and protocols that are valid for other classes of compounds do not necessarily work with proteins.

HPLC of proteins is possible with a number of separation modes with complementary discrimination powers.

Reversed-Phase Separations

The main difference between proteins and small molecules in a reversed-phase system is that the former show a strong dependence of their k values on the composition of the mobile phase. A small change in % B (acetonitrile or methanol) can result in a major change of the retention time. At a given concentration of the organic solvent a certain protein may have no adsorption at all to the stationary phase, i.e. no retention. Another protein will be strongly adsorbed and not eluted even with a long duration of separation. Therefore isocratic chromatography is almost never used for mixtures of proteins. However, the gradients used must be shallow and should not run to a higher amount of organic solvent than 50% acetonitrile or 65% methanol. A higher concentration, very common for small molecules, can result in long retention times or no elution at all.

If an additive such as trifluoroacetic or phosphoric acid is needed, it should be present in equal concentration in both the water and the B solvent. Stationary phases especially designed for proteins are worth their cost.

Hydrophobic Interaction Separations

This is a separation method that is almost exclusively used for proteins. The stationary phase is of the reversed-phase type but with short alkyl chains such as butyl or ethyl. The mobile phase is an aqueous salt solution. The analytes are eluted with a gradient from high to low salt concentration. A typical starting condition is 1.5 M ammonium sulphate that decreases linearly to 0 M during the separation whereas a constant concentration of 0.1 M potassium phosphate, buffered to keep the pH within a narrow range, is maintained. Without buffering, the ionic state of the proteins is ill-defined, resulting in poor reproducibility of the separation. Hydrophobic interaction chromatography is a mild procedure and the eluted proteins keep their biological activity. If necessary or advantageous, the separation can be performed at subambient temperatures.

Ion-Exchange Separations

With this mode it is possible to separate proteins with subtle differences in their amino acid composition (in some cases even two compounds which differ in a single position). The separation is based on the presence of ionized amino acids on the outer surface of the molecule. Therefore the pH of the mobile phase should be chosen 1–2 units away from the isoelectric point of the protein of interest (otherwise it will not be charged). Eluent A is e.g. a 0.05 M buffer which matches this pH, i.e. its pK_a value is not more than 0.6 units away from the necessary pH. A linear gradient with eluent B is then used which is composed of 1 M sodium acetate in the same buffer.

Size-Exclusion Separations

This is a technique that separates the analytes according to their size (which is more or less correlated to their molecular mass). Separation times are short and predictable. The stationary phase is an inorganic or organic porous material whose pore width is of such a dimension that the smaller analytes will find a larger space that is accessible to them than the larger molecules do. Therefore the large proteins will be eluted earlier than the small ones. The mobile phase must be chosen with regard to maximum solubility of the analytes in order to prevent unwanted interactions with the stationary phase. For proteins this is e.g. a 0.2 M potassium phosphate or sodium phosphate solution at pH 7. Gradients are not necessary. A drawback of size-exclusion chromatography is the limited number of peaks that can be separated in one run, often restricted to a maximum of ten compounds.

Troubleshooting

General Remarks

The most important points to keep in mind are the following:
1. A separation can only be taken for granted if it can be reproduced.
2. Usually a peak indicates that there is a compound (although there are even exceptions to this rule). No peak does not mean that there is no compound in the sample; perhaps it was absorbed on the column, the wrong detector has been used or the injection failed.
3. A peak can represent more than one compound even if it is perfectly narrow in shape and if all compounds that are eluted at the retention time in question are detector-active.

The HPLC instrument and separation system is more intricate than it may seem at first sight, and the possible pitfalls are numerous. In the case of unexpected phenomena or results it can be difficult to find the reason. Some simple rules are helpful in troubleshooting:
1. Change only one parameter at time. E.g., prepare a new batch of mobile phase and check the result. Clean the detector cell only after this first measure did not help, and so on.
2. A problem is only a problem if it can be reproduced. If something unexpected happens only once without showing up again, it is not worth wasting your time to identify the reason.
3. If it is not possible to confirm the proper functioning of a part of the instrument (check valve, fitting, lamp, detector cell, and others) it should be thrown away if a repair is not possible. Otherwise the drawers in the laboratory will soon be full of dubious gadgets.

General Hints Regarding the Mobile Phase

Many reversed phases should not be used with a lower amount of organic solvent than 10%. If the water content is close to 100% there is the risk of the collapse (or folding) of the long hydrocarbon chains of the stationary phase. As a consequence, the phase system changes its character (but it is stable and can be used in this conformation). After a change in the solvent composition it will take a long time to obtain the typical reversed-phase behaviour. Note the distinct viscosity maximum with mixtures of methanol and water that leads to much higher backpressures than with pure water or methanol. This effect is not observed with acetonitrile/water mixtures.

Buffering of the mobile phase is mandatory in many cases in order to get the analytes in a well-characterized state, either fully ionized or neutral. As a starting point, a buffer concentration of 25 mM is favourable. An increase in buffer strength decreases the retention of polar compounds whereas nonpolar ones will be eluted later. Therefore changes in selectivity or even peak order can be expected. Too high a salt concentration can give rise to solubility problems, precipitation, and clogging of an instrument part or of the column.

Buffer solutions must be filtered after preparation. The compatibility of an aqueous buffer must be checked with all proportions of the organic solvent used. Buffers should not remain in the HPLC system or in the column due to the danger of salt crystallization. If no analyses are running overnight, it is necessary to maintain a low flow rate or to rinse the whole system first with water and then with pure organic solvent.

A small amount of an additive in the mobile phase can be advantageous: 0.1% (or less) of trifluoroacetic acid for biomolecule separations or trimethylamine for basic analytes. Additives should only be used if necessary because detection problems can be the consequence. It is always best to use a stationary phase that gives good peak shapes and resolutions without the need of additives, if available.

Problem: Noisy Baseline

1. The HPLC instrument is in poor shape
   Replace the pump seals. Clean the check valves of the pump or replace them. Check all fittings for leaks. Replace a UV or fluorescence lamp after the time interval that is noted in the manual. Move the instrument to a place without disturbing electrical fields, draught, temperature fluctuations or direct sunlight.
2. The mobile phase is not thoroughly mixed
   For isocratic separations it can be helpful to prepare the eluent in a single bottle instead of mixing the components in the instrument. Even with gradient separation, lower noise can be observed if the initial mobile phase (such as 80% water with additives/20% organic solvent) is pre-mixed in reservoir A. Poor degassing increases the noise. In some cases, e.g. with electrochemical detection, a two-step degassing procedure (helium plus a membrane degasser) is necessary.
3. Solvents and reagents are detector-active
   Use a better quality. It is very possible that a reagent with perfect UV compatibility cannot be used with electrochemical detection, and vice versa. In many cases it is not possible to obtain a phase system without any detector activity that can give rise to unexpected phenomena such as extra peaks or negative peaks (e.g. if UV detection at 210 nm or lower is necessary).
4. Time constant of the detector is too low
   Select the next higher time constant (but beware of too high a time constant which can lead to tailed peaks).

Problem: Baseline Drift

Baseline drift is very common with gradient separations. Its slope depends on the mobile phase composition and the detector used. High-quality reagents and solvents may be mandatory, as mentioned above. Some detection principles such as refractive index detection are not compatible with gradients.

Drift can be observed with temperature fluctuations, with changes in the composition of pre-mixed mobile phases (evaporation, too intense helium degassing), with incomplete purging of the pump or too short a column equilibration time when the eluent is changed.

Problem: Poor Peak Shape

Poor peak shape, strong tailing or even double peaks are observed with a column that is no longer fit for its purpose and must be replaced. Tailing can also occur with too large extra-column volumes in the HPLC system such as capillaries with a large inner diameter, poor fittings or poor connections between the individual parts of the instrument or even worn rotor seals. A detector cell with too high an internal volume can also give rise to tailing. Tailing or other asymmetric peak shapes can be the result of too high a sample volume or too high a sample concentration. In this case the simple remedy is to inject a smaller volume or to dilute the sample.

In many cases the poor peak shape comes from too low a buffer concentration, from working with an unbuffered system although buffering is necessary and from the use of an unfavourable phase system. See also the discussion of additives above.

General Hints Regarding Ion-Pair Separations

Ion-pair separations can be tedious and should only be used if necessary, e.g. with analytes with acidic and basic groups in the molecule such as the catecholamines. For solubility reasons it is better to use methanol as the organic part of the eluent instead of acetonitrile. Long-chain ion-pair reagents give longer retention times than short-chain ones, thus better resolution (in theory), but the selectivity can be higher with short-chain reagents and the solubility will be better. The reagent concentration is usually between 50 and 200 mM; short-chain reagents need somewhat higher concentrations than the long-chain types. The buffer concentration must be higher than in reversed-phase separations without ion-pair reagent, namely 60 mM or higher. Since ion-pair equilibria depend on temperature, thermostatting of the column can be necessary.

It is advisable to use a column for either general reversed-phase separations or for ion-pair chromatography because the reagent will only be removed from the stationary phase after a long washing cycle. Be aware of the poor stability of most silica-based stationary phases at pH above approx. 7.5. If necessary, use a specially designed phase that is stable at high pH.

Specific problems can be: High pressure or clogged column due to the precipitation of the ion-pair reagent: Flush the column with a large volume of water, check the solubility with all possible ratios of water and organic solvent (preferably methanol) and use a composition which is not critical. Decrease the concentration of the reagent (retention times will decrease!). The reagent can also precipitate in the detector cell.

Variable retention times: Work at a pH where the analytes are fully ionized, i.e. two units away from their pK_a values (for acidic analytes at higher pH, for basic analytes at lower pH). Increase the buffer strength or the ion-pair concentration (and check solubility). Decrease the sample concentration.

Poor peak shape: Change the column if it has deteriorated, check the pH compatibility of the stationary phase used. Try the measures recommended under "variable retention times". Increase the amount of organic solvent in the eluent (retention times will decrease!). Try another ion-pair reagent.

References

Only original papers are mentioned in the text but the books and reviews should be consulted in order to get a deeper understanding.

HPLC

Cataldi TRI, Campa C, De Benedetto GE (2000) Carbohydrate analysis by high-performance anion-exchange chromatography with pulsed amperometric detection: the potential is still growing. Fresenius J. Anal. Chem. 368: 739–758
Dolan JW, Snyder LR (2000) Essential guides to method development in liquid chromatography. In: Wilson ID (ed) Encyclopedia of Separation Science. Academic Press, London, p 4626–4636
Erickson BE (2000) Electrochemical detectors for liquid chromatography. Anal. Chem. 72:353A–357A
Ermer J, Vogel M (2000) Applications of hyphenated LC-MS techniques in pharmaceutical analysis. Biomed. Chromatogr. 14:373–383
Hanai T (ed) (1991) Liquid Chromatography in Biomedical Analysis. Elsevier, Amsterdam
Meyer VR (2004) Practical High-Performance Liquid Chromatography. John Wiley & Sons, Chichester, 4th ed.
Papadoyannis IN (1990) HPLC in Clinical Chemistry. Marcel Dekker, New York
Parvez H, Bastart-Malsot M, Parvez S, Nagatsu T, Carpentier G (eds) (1987) Electrochemical Detection in Medicine and Chemistry. VNU Science Press, Utrecht
Patel D (1997) Liquid Chromatography Essential Data. John Wiley & Sons, Chichester
Snyder LR, Kirkland JJ, Glajch JL (1997) Practical HPLC Method Development. Wiley-Interscience, New York, 2nd ed.
Wolfender JL, Ndjoko K, Hostettmann K (2003) Liquid chromatography with ultraviolet absorbance – mass spectrometry: a powerful combination for the on-line strutural investigation of plant metabolites.. J. Chromatogr. A 1000: 437–455

Sample Preparation

Cortes HJ, Rothman D (1990) Multidimensional high-performance liquid chromatography. In: Cortes HJ (ed) Multidimensional Chromatography, Techniques and Applications. Marcel Dekker, New York, p 219–250
Hennion MC (1999) Solid-phase extraction: Method development, sorbents, and coupling with liquid chromatography. J. Chromatogr. A 856:3–54
Moldoveanu SC, David V (2002) Sample Preparation in Chromatography. Elsevier, Amsterdam
Moldoveanu SC (2004) Solutions and challenges in sample preparations for chromatography. J Chromatogr. Sci. 42: 1–14
Simpson NJK (ed) (2000) Solid-Phase Extraction, Principles, Techniques and Applications. Marcel Dekker, New York
Wells MJM (2000) Essential guides to method development in solid-phase extraction. In: Wilson ID (ed) Encyclopedia of Separation Science. Academic Press, London, p 4636–4643

Catecholamines

Boos KS, Wilmers B, Sauerbrey R, Schlimme E (1987) Development and performance of an automated HPLC-analyzer for catecholamines. Chromatographia 24:363–370
Hansen AM, Kristiansen J, Nielsen JL, Byrialsen K, Christensen JM (1999) Validation of a high performance liquid chromatography analysis for the determination of noradrenaline and adrenaline in human urine with an on-line sample purification. Talanta 50:367–379
Holmes C, Eisenhofer G, Goldstein DS (1994) Improved assay for plasma dihydroxyphenylacetic acid and other catechols using high-performance liquid chromatography with electrochemical detection. J. Chromatogr. B 653: 131–138
KrstuloviæAM (ed) (1986) Quantitative Analysis of Catecholamines and Related Compounds. Ellis Horwood, Chichester
Musso NR, Vergassola C, Pende A, Lotti G (1990) HPLC with electrochemical detection of catecholamines in human plasma. A mini-review. J. Liquid Chromatogr. 13:1075–1090
Nikolajsen RPH, Hansen AM (2001) Analytical methods for determining urinary catecholamines in healthy subjects. Anal. Chim. Acta 449:1–15
Raggi MA, Sabbioni C, Nicoletta G, Mandrioli R, Gerra G (2003) Analysis of plasma catecholamines by liquid cromatography with amperometric detection using a novel SPE ion-exchange procedure. J. Sep. Sci. 26: 1141–1146

References Hanai, Papadoyannis and Parvez of the HPLC section also include chapters on catecholamines.

Cardiac Glycosides

Guan F, Ishii A, Seno H, Watanabe-Suzuki K, Kumazawa T, Suzuki O (1999) Identification and quantification of cardiac glycosides in blood and urine samples by HPLC/MS/MS. Anal. Chem. 71:4034–4043

Kelly KL, Kimball BA, Johnston JJ (1995) Quantitation of digitoxin, digoxin, and their metabolites by high-performance liquid chromatography using pulsed amperometric detection. J. Chromatogr. A 711:289–295

Vetticaden SJ, Chandrasekaran A (1990) Chromatography of cardiac glycosides. J. Chromatogr. 531:215–234

Proteins

Cunico RL, Gooding KM, Wehr T (1998) Basic HPLC and CE of Biomolecules. Bay Bioanalytical Laboratory, Richmond

Jäger D, Jungblut PR, Müller-Werdan U (2002) Separation and identification of human heart proteins. J. Chromatogr. B 771:131–153

Kastner M (ed) (2000) Protein Liquid Chromatography. Elsevier, Amsterdam

Troubleshooting

Dolan JW, Snyder LR (1989) Troubleshooting LC Systems. Aster, Chester

Kromidas S (2000) Practical Problem Solving in HPLC. Wiley-VCH, Weinheim

Meyer VR (1997) Pitfalls and Errors of HPLC in Pictures. Hüthig, Heidelberg

Sadek PC (2000) Troubleshooting HPLC Systems, A Bench Manual. Wiley-Interscience, New York

Protein Biochemistry

Aida Salameh, Stefan Lehr, Jürgen Weiss and Peter Rösen

6.2.1
Western Blotting of Cytosolic and Membrane Proteins

Aida Salameh

Introduction

An important method in cardiovascular research is the extraction and detection of cytosolic and membrane proteins and proteins located in a sub-cellular organelle. The methods used for this approach are cell lysis, differential centrifugation, gel electrophoresis and western blot. Depending on the protein, which is to be detected, these protocols have to be adapted.

First, it is necessary to decide in which fraction of the cell the protein of interest occurs. It is important to select the correct lysis protocol. Next, the physical properties of the protein are important when choosing a suitable protocol for the sample preparation from the crude extract. Furthermore, the physical properties of the protein (molecular weight, solubility, charge) have to be taken into account when choosing suitable buffers and procedures for gel electrophoresis and electroblotting.

Methods and Practical Approach/Troubleshooting

Lysis Protocols

Extraction of Soluble Cytoplasmatic Proteins

Many soluble, cytoplasmatic proteins can be extracted by mechanical and/or osmotic force, since cell membranes are weak and can be easily disrupted using a homogeniser and a suitable buffer. Tissue like liver, kidney, brain, lung, heart etc. can be homogenised using a blender or mincer. For very fibrous tissue, it may be necessary to freeze the specimen before homogenisation. Small amounts of soft tissue and cultured mammalian cells may be homogenised using a Dounce homogeniser. Whole organs for example liver or heart may be minced in a chilled beaker and thereafter homogenised in a Potter-Elvejhem homogeniser or Ultraturrax. For some applications, the use of high frequency ultrasound may be effective to disrupt cellular integrity. However, an important disadvantage of this method is the considerable heat generation, which has to be taken into account. The use of ice-cold buffer solutions and special vessels with a cooling system may help to overcome this disadvantage.

Although the choice of homogenisation buffer may be dictated by the special properties of the target protein, a buffer of moderate ionic strength at neutral pH may generally be sufficient for extraction of cytoplasmatic soluble proteins (0,1 M phosphate buffer, if necessary with addition of 0,1 M NaCl to overcome protein attachment to cell debris or membrane fragments or a 50 mM HEPES (N-2-hydroxyethylpiperazine-N'-2-ethanesulfonic acid)/NaOH buffer to which one can add 0,33 M sucrose to achieve isotonic conditions. Nota bene that sucrose may interfere with some assays and is not always easy to eliminate from the sample preparation). Adherent cultured cells grown in a monolayer may be harvested using a cell scraper and cells growing in suspension should be concentrated by centrifugation and then re-suspended in the chosen lysis buffer. The buffer to tissue ratio should be 2:1 to 3:1 and cell lysis should be controlled under a microscope using 0,5% Trypan blue solution: only lysed cells include Trypan blue while intact cells are able to exclude the blue dye and thus are not stained.

Some proteins are susceptible to oxidation and the addition of dithiothreitol (1 mM) or β-mercaptoethanol (0,1 M) may be necessary. The homogenisation and cell lysis should be carried out at 4°C with pre-chilled buffers to minimise proteolysis. In addition, proteinase inhibitors may be included in the extraction buffer. Usually a cocktail of the various proteinase inhibitors is used. For most of the applications, the addition of the chelator ethylenediaminetetraacetic acid (EDTA, 0,1–1 mM, inhibits metalloproteinases) and phenylmethyl sulfonyl fluoride (PMSF, 1–10 µM, inhibits serine proteinases, like chymotrypsin or trypsin), may be sufficient to protect the target protein from unwanted proteolysis.

Please note that PMSF is quite unstable in aqueous solution, at room temperature and at alkaline pH with a half-life of about <1 h under these conditions. Normally a stock solution of 10–100 mM is prepared in ice-cold dry organic solvents, i.e. methanol or isopropanol and is added freshly to the lysis buffer. Stored at –20 °C the stock PMSF solutions are stable for several weeks.

Since cells differ in their content of proteinases, for example kidney or liver are known to express much more proteinase activity than skeletal or cardiac muscle, the addition of more proteinase inhibitors may be advisable: aprotinin at a working concentration of 5 µg/ ml in HEPES buffered solution (avoid repeatedly freezing and thawing cycles) may be used to inhibit trypsin, kallikrein, chymotrypsin and plasmin, pepstatin A (1 µg/ ml, stock solution of 1mg/ml in methanol or ethanol) inhibits proteinases like pepsin or cathepsin D while leupeptin 1–2 µg/ ml does not only inhibit plasmin and trypsin but also papain and cathepsin B. Beside these, which are most commonly used, other proteinase inhibitors exist, such as benzamidine, antithrombine III, antipain, cystatin, E64 and phosphoramidone. Due to the diverging targets of the proteinase inhibitors, it is necessary to adapt the inhibitor cocktail to the tissue, as well as, to the protein that is being investigated.

After homogenisation and cell lysis cell debris and other particulate matter can be removed by centrifugation at low speed (500–600 g) at 4 °C. The soluble cytoplasmatic protein is encountered in the supernatant but the remaining pellet may nevertheless contain a substantial amount of the wanted protein. To increase yields the pellet may be again re-suspended in lysis buffer with a second centrifuging step, though the dilution of the final extract may be disadvantageous and further steps to reduce volume have to be done.

In addition, a useful step to concentrate the samples and to denature proteinases, is the precipitation of the supernatants with trichloracetic acid (TCA) at a final concentration of 5% (w/v) at 4 °C for 10 min. followed by brief centrifugation. The remaining pellet will contain the wanted proteins and may be washed gently with acetone or diethyl ether to remove residual TCA. Thereafter, the protein pellet may be dissolved in sample buffer (i.e. buffer according to Laemmli) for SDS-PAGE.

In our laboratory, to investigate the gap junction proteins connexin 40, connexin 43, connexin 45 and connexin 37 in cultured heart muscle cells and cultured endothelial cells, we use as homogenisation buffer an ice-cold hypo-osmotic lysis buffer containing K_2HPO_4 20 mM, EDTA 1 mM, at pH=7,9, Triton-X 1%, aprotinin 10 µg/ml, leupeptin 0,5mg/ ml, pepstatin 1 µg/ ml and PMSF 1 mM. The cells are harvested from Petri dishes (100 µl lysis buffer per Petri dish of 60 mm diameter) using a cell scraper, transferred to 1,5 ml microtubes in which cell membranes are disrupted with the help of polypropylene pestles (that fit into the microtubes) and high frequency ultrasound (4 treatments of 10 s each). Thereafter, samples are kept at 4 °C in lysis buffer for another 4–6 h in order to allow complete lysis. The samples are centrifuged at 500 g and the supernatant is collected for protein quantitation and stored at –80 °C for longer storage.

Extraction of Integral or Membrane-Bound Proteins

Membrane proteins appear in different forms within the phospholipid bilayer: 1. Integral membrane proteins with a transmembrane unit. 2. Peripheral membrane proteins either connected to the phospholipid bilayer by electrostatic interactions and hydrogen bonds or membrane proteins that are connected by lipid-anchors to the membrane.

To extract and solubilise integral or peripheral membrane-bound proteins, the use of diverse detergents, buffer solutions at definite pH, chelators, denaturing agents or organic solvents are necessary. Depending on the nature of the membrane protein, several detergents and buffers have to be tested to receive optimal results.

Membrane bound proteins may usually be released by treatments with alkaline (pH 8,0–12,0) or acidic buffers (pH 3,0–5,0), by the use of metal chelators (i.e. 10 mM EDTA or EGTA (ethylene glycol-(bis[beta]-amminoethyl ether)-N,N,N',N'-tetraacetic acid)), by high ionic strength (1 M NaCl or KCl), by treatment with denaturing agents (i.e. urea) or organic solvents (i.e. butanol). The various buffers and agents may be used alone or in combination. Moreover, sonication of membrane fragments may be useful to increase protein yields. Usually, the employment of 1 M NaCl in combination with alkaline or acidic buffers and EDTA as metal chelator, will result in a relatively distinct separation between solubilised membrane-bound proteins and integral membrane proteins. However, non-specific association of soluble proteins with membrane fractions, and the entrapment of cytoplasmatic proteins in membrane vesicles, may be a problem that is not easy to overcome and which makes the interpretation of differential extraction procedures somewhat difficult.

After extraction of the proteins (10–30 min), the remaining membrane fragments can be separated by centrifugation (100 000 g, 30–60 min) and the released peripheral membrane- bound protein found in the supernatant. It may be advisable to also test the pellet for activity of the wanted protein.

Since control of pH is an important consideration when handling proteins, the selection of different buffers is important. Ideal buffer solutions should be chemically inert, non-toxic, water soluble, have no absorption at 280 nm, no complex formation with cations and the pKa value should not vary with temperature. These properties belong to the so-called Good-buffers: HEPES (N-2-hydroxyethylpiperazine-N'-2-ethanesulfonic acid; pKa 7,48), PIPES (piperazine-N,N''-bis(2-ethanesulfonic acid) pKa 6,76) and MOPS (3-(N-morpholino)propanesulfonic acid; pKa 7,2). These buffers where synthesised in by Good et al. (1966) and are widely used but quite expensive. It is noteworthy that, for example, HEPES may promote cell growth in some cell lines and interfere with some biochemical reactions.

Generally, to obtain a good buffer capacity, the pKa values of the selected buffer must be close to the desired pH of the resulting solution. Since the buffer capacity also depends on the ionic strength of the buffer usually buffer solutions of 20–50–100 mM are used. Furthermore, a variety of most commonly used buffers with different pKa values exist, like Mes (2-(N-morpholino)ethansulfonic acid; pKa 6,1), Bis-Tris ([bis(2-hydroxyethyl)imino]-tris(hydroxymethyl)methane; pKa 6,46) phosphate buffer (pKa$_2$ 7,2), Tris (tris(hydroxymethyl)aminomethane; pKa 8,06), Tricine (N-[tris(hydroxymethyl)methyl]glycine; pKa 8,05), TAPS (3-{[tris(hydroxy-methyl)methyl]-amino}-propanesulfonic acid; pKa 8,4), CAPS (3-[cyclohexylamino]-1-propanesulfonic acid; pKa 10,4), to give you a selection of possible examples.

Extraction of integral membrane proteins makes the application of various detergents necessary. Detergents are molecular "hermaphrodites" with a hydrophilic head and a hydrophobic tail. The hydrophobic part may consist of an aliphatic chain (Zwittergent 3-14, Lubrol PX, octylglucoside), may contain a phenyl group (Triton X-100) or may have a cholesterol-based structure (CHAPS, sodium cholate, Digitonin). The hydrophilic parts are represented by ionic (sodium cholate, sodium dodecyl sulphate, CHAPS) or glycoside groups (Digitonin, octylglucoside) or by polyethylene groups (Triton X-100, Lubrol PX). Therefore, detergents can be classified into three different classes: non-ionic detergents such as Triton X-100, Nonidet P-40 (NP-40), Lubrol PX, Digitonin and octylglycoside, ionic detergents such as sodium cholate and zwitterionic detergents like CHAPS and Zwittergent 3-14. Another important characteristic of these detergents is the critical micelle concentration (CMC), a specific value for each individual detergent, which describes the lowest detergent concentration that is needed to form micelles in aqueous solutions. Below the specific CMC, the detergent does not form micelles, but remains in solution as monomer.

It is important to mention that non-ionic detergents with high CMC, such as octylglucoside (CMC 25 mM) can be easily removed from samples using dialysis, in contrast to detergents with a low CMC value, such as Triton X-100 (CMC 0,24 mM), which cannot be removed by dialysis. The CMC of ionic detergents is dependent on the ionic strength of the buffer (the higher the ionic strength the lower the CMC) whereas, the CMC of non-ionic detergents does not depend on the ionic strength. The temperature of the buffer solution has hardly any influence on the CMC of ionic detergents but influences the CMC of non-ionic detergents significantly: the higher the temperature the lower the CMC. The CMC of a mixture of two detergents with different CMC values lies near the lower CMC (even if there is only a small amount of the detergent with low CMC in solution). Thus, the best detergent has to be found depending on the protein that is to be extracted, and on the experimental conditions. Before working with large-scale preparations, it may be useful to run some pilot experiments with different detergents. Usually an effective solubilisation may be achieved using a detergent concentration of 0,5–3% in a well buffered solution (HEPES, Tris or MOPS-buffer) with the addition of 0,1–0,4 M NaCl at physiological pH. For stabilisation of protein 10–20% glycerol, 1 mM dithiothreitol (DTT, anti-oxidative agent) and/or 0,1–1 mM EDTA as well as protease inhibitors may be supplemented.

After solubilisation, protein samples should refrigerated at 4°C, or at –80°C in liquid nitrogen for longer storage. Repeated freezing and thawing cycles should be avoided.

Preparation of Sub-Cellular Fractions

The first step in preparing sub-cellular fractions is to homogenise the organ or tissue in a suitable homogenisation buffer, for example, 50 mM HEPES at pH 7,4 containing 0,33 M sucrose, to obtain iso-osmotic conditions. For homogenisation of large-scale preparations a Waring blender with a capacity of 1,5 l may be used. For smaller amounts of tissue alternative homogenisers such as Ultraturrax are also applicable. For soft tissues, Potter-Elvehjem or Dounce homogenisers can be used.

The homogenisation, and the subsequent sub-cellular fractionation, should be carried out at 4°C with pre-chilled buffers to reduce unwanted proteolysis. The tissue to buffer relation should be 1:10. Since some proteins are quite susceptible to proteolytic degradation, the supplementation of protease inhibitors may be advisable (see Lysis protocols). After homogenisation, the next step is to isolate sub-cellular fraction using differential centrifugation. Using this method, a crude separation of the major organelles can be achieved.

First of all the homogenate is centrifuged at 4 °C in a refrigerated laboratory centrifuge (all centrifugation steps are at 4 °C) at a speed of 600 g for 3 min to remove cell nuclei, cell debris and whole cells. The pellet is then again re-suspended in homogenisation buffer and centrifuged again at 600 g, to reduce the contamination of the fraction by membrane components. The supernatant is collected and again centrifuged at 6000–15,000 g for 8–10 min in order to prepare a fraction rich in mitochondria, lysosomes and peroxisomes. This fraction (pellet) is then again re-suspended in homogenisation buffer and centrifuged at 6000–15,000 g for another 8–10 min to reduce contamination by other membranous components. If necessary this washing step can be repeated two or three times. The resulting pellets can be preserved for further analysis and the supernatants are pooled and again centrifuged at 40,000 g for 30 min. using an ultracentrifuge. The pellet formed by the last centrifugation step contains vesicles derived from plasma membrane, fragments of Golgi apparatus and endoplasmic reticulum. The supernatant is then centrifuged again at 100,000 g for 90 min. This procedure yields a pellet rich in ribosomal subunits and a supernatant containing the cytosolic fraction.

Since these centrifugation procedures do not guarantee absolutely pure fractions, it is recommended that the purity is tested by detection of lead enzymes such as LDH for the cytosolic fraction or histone-1 for the nuclear fraction.

Further purification of a particular fraction can be achieved by density gradient centrifugation either using sucrose, Ficoll or Percoll gradients. However, an important disadvantage of this method is the relatively small amounts of material that can be obtained. Nevertheless, this method is the method of choice if translocation of a certain protein from, e.g. the cytosol to the plasma membrane, is to be investigated.

If the nature of the target protein is unknown, it is advisable to run some pilot experiments trying single- or triple-detergent lysis buffers, before turning to more specialised lysis protocolls. Subsequently several lysis buffers are given:
- Single detergent lysis buffer
  - 50 mM Tris-HCl (pH 8,0)
  - 150 mM NaCl
  - 1% Triton X-100 (or 1% NP-40)
  - 100 µg/ml PMSF
  - 1 µg/ml aprotinin
- Triple detergent lysis buffer
  - 50 mM Tris-HCl (pH 8,0)
  - 150 mM NaCl
  - 0,1% SDS (sodium dodecyl sulfate)
  - 1% NP-40
  - 0,5% sodium deoxycholate
  - 100 µg/ml PMSF
  - 1 µg/ml aprotinin

- High-salt lysis buffer
  - 50 mM HEPES (pH 7,0)
  - 500 mM NaCl
  - 1% NP-40
  - 100 µg/ml PMSF
  - 1 µg/ml aprotinin
- No-salt lysis buffer
  - 50 mM HEPES (pH 7,0)
  - 1% NP-40
  - 100 µg/ml PMSF
  - 1 µg/ml aprotinin

Protein Quantitation

Prior to any immunodetection of proteins, it is necessary to determine the protein concentration in a given sample, in order to allow application of equal amounts of protein for Western blotting. In principal, there are three widely used methods of protein determination: the bicinchoninic acid (BCA) assay, the Lowry assay and the Bradford assay. However, the choice of the best method (or the modification which is needed) depends on the choice of detergents and buffers that have been used for cell lysis (see above) and on the sensitivity that is desired.

The bicinchoninic acid assay (BCA assay), which is similar to the Lowry assay, is based on the reduction of Cu^{2+} to Cu^{+}-ions under alkaline conditions. The Cu^{+}-ions are then detected by reaction with BCA and given an intense purple colour with a maximum absorbance at 562 nm. The production of reduced copper ions is a function of protein concentration and incubation time, thus the protein content of unknown samples can be determined spectrophotometrically by comparison with a calibration curve of known protein standards. The chemicals are stable at room temperature and may be purchased ready prepared (e.g. as a kit from Pierce). Both, a standard (0,1–1,0 mg protein/ ml) or a micro protein assay (0,5–10 µg protein/ ml) can be carried out.

Advantages: since BCA is stable under alkaline conditions this assay can be quickly carried out as a one-step investigation. This assay is sensitive, detection limit 0,5 g protein and rather unsusceptible to faults. Detergents like Triton X-100 and denaturing agents like urea or guanidine HCl do not interfere with the reaction.

Problems: high concentrations of chelating agents like EDTA, ammonium sulphate, glycine and reducing agents like DTT, sorbitol, glucose or other reducing sugars may interfere with the assay. One way to overcome this disadvantage is to dilute the sample (provided that the protein concentration remains above the detection limit).

It is noteworthy, that the BCA assay like the Lowry assay depends on the amino acid composition of the protein, and therefore, an absolute concentration of the target protein cannot be determined. The standard curve of known protein samples, usually a calibration curve using bovine serum albumin (BSA) samples, can for this reason only be used to compare relative protein concentration of similar protein solutions.

Standard Assay

Materials:
- Reagent A: mix 0,1 g sodium bicinchoninate, 2 g $Na_2CO_3 \cdot H_2O$, 0,16g sodium tartrate dihydrate, 0,4 g NaOH, 0,95 g $NaHCO_3$ with 100 ml aqua bidestillata. Adjust pH to 11,25 with NaOH.
- Reagent B: dissolve 0,4 g $CuSO_4 \cdot 5H_2O$ in 10 ml aqua bidestillata.
- Working solution: mix 100 vol. of reagent A with 2 vol. of reagent B.
  The solution is green in colour and is stable at room temperature for about one week.

Assay Protocol:
- Add 2 ml of the working solution to a 100 µl aqueous protein sample (10–100 µg protein) and heat at 60 °C for 30 min. Cool the sample to room temperature to stop the reaction and measure at 562 nm.

Microassay

- Reagent A: mix 0,8 g $Na_2CO_3 \cdot H_2O$, 1,6 g sodium tartrate, 1,6 g NaOH with 100 ml aqua bidestillata. Adjust pH to 11,25 with 10 M NaOH.
- Reagent B: dissolve 4,0 g BCA in 100 ml aqua bidestillata
- Reagent C: dissolve 0,4 g $CuSO_4 \cdot 5H_2O$ in 10 ml aqua bidestillata.
- Working solution: mix 1 vol. of reagent C with 25 vol. of reagent B then add 26 vol. of reagent A.

Assay Protocol:
- Add 1 ml of the working solution to 1 ml of an aqueous protein sample (0,5–1,0 µg protein/ml) and incubate at 60 °C for 60 min. Cool down the sample to room temperature and measure at 562 nm.

Lowry Assay

This assay is also based on the Biuret-reaction, where the protein reduces bivalent copper ions to monovalent copper ions under alkaline conditions, which then react with the Folin reagent. This Folin-Ciocalteau reaction gives an intense blue colour, partly dependent on the tyrosine and tryptophan content of the protein, which can be measured spectrophotometrically at 750 nm. Although requiring a great deal of work, this method exhibits the best accuracy with regard to protein concentration and is sensitive down to 0,01 mg/ml protein. Nota bene, that like the BCA-assay, the absolute concentration of a target protein cannot be obtained. The most accurate method of protein determination is probably acid protein hydrolysis followed by amino acid analysis. But as the sensitivity of the Lowry protein assay varies only slightly between different proteins, this assay is a good alternative (especially if protein mixtures or crude extracts are used).

Advantages: Widely used assay with best accuracy.

Problems: the Lowry assay is highly susceptible to potentially interfering substances like nucleic acids, mercaptoethanol, buffers for example HEPES or Tris, detergents like Triton-X-100, SDS or CHAPS, sugars like sucrose, EDTA and many other substances and drugs. To overcome this disadvantage, and to concentrate the protein solution, a precipitation step can be carried out prior to the Lowry assay:

- To precipitate the protein, add 0,1 ml of a 0,15% deoxycholate solution to 1,0 ml of the protein sample. Vortex the solution and let it stand for 10 min. at room temperature. Add 0,1 ml of 72% TCA, vortex again, and centrifuge at 1,000–3,000 g for 30 min. The protein pellet is now ready for the Lowry assay.
- Another way to precipitate the protein is to use a 10% TCA solution. After precipitation, TCA remnants can be removed by washing the pellet thoroughly with 80% ice-cold acetone.
- Alternatively, a precipitation step using acetone as precipitant can be performed: one part of the aqueous protein sample and four parts of ice-cold acetone are mixed and stored at −20°C for 1 h. Thereafter the precipitated proteins are centrifuged and the pellet is used for the subsequent procedure.

Gel Electrophoresis (SDS-PAGE; Sodium Dodecyl Sulphate Polyacrylamide Gel Electrophoresis)

SDS-PAGE, a most widely used technique, serves as a method to analyse protein mixtures and to determine the relative molecular mass of different proteins. This system is based on the following principle: the anionic detergent SDS (sodium dodecyl sulphate) binds to proteins, especially after reduction of the proteins with DTT or β-mercaptoethanol, which both reduce disulphide bonds, thereby disturbing the tertiary structure of the protein. This detergent denatures the proteins by impeding protein-protein-interactions and thereby destroying the quaternary structure of the protein.

The majority of proteins bind the detergent SDS to negatively charged protein-SDS-complexes with a constant charge-to-mass ratio and as a result the protein unfolds into a linear elongated negatively charged structure migrating to the positive pole (anode) of an electrical field. This movement is hindered by the sieve-like pores of the SDS-PAGE, due to large proteins migrating more slowly in contrast to small proteins. Thus, the migration of a certain protein only depends on its molecular mass and not on its native tertiary or quaternary structure. If the relative molecular mass of an unknown protein is to be determined, calibration proteins with known molecular weight are applied to the same gel as the unknown protein.

By comparing the mobility of the calibration proteins with that of the unknown protein, its relative molecular mass can be calculated. For that purpose, a calibration curve of $\log_{10}$ molecular weight (y-axis) versus relative mobility of the calibration proteins (x-axis) is plotted and on the basis of this linear curve the molecular weight of the unknown protein can be estimated. The relative mobility can be calculated from the following equation: R_f (relative mobility) = distance migrated by protein/ distance migrated by bromphenol blue dye. The bromphenol blue dye, as it is a small molecule, passes the gel without being retarded and is therefore used to monitor the electrophoretic run. It is important to mention that the linearity of the calibration curve is only given over a limited range of molecular masses and is dependent on the gel concentration: for a 15% acrylamide gel the linear relationship is approximately true for proteins between 10–60 kDa, for a 10% acrylamide gel between 30–120 kDa and for a 5% acrylamide gel between 60–200 kDa. Moreover, it is important to mention that, since proteins have to bind SDS in a constant charge-to-mass ratio, highly basic proteins such as histones, which have a high number of positively-charged amino acids, migrate more slowly during the gel run than one would expect from their molecular weight.

The polyacrylamide gels consist of two parts: the stacking gel with large pore sizes to concentrate the protein samples into sharp bands and the separating gel, where the proteins are separated according to their molecular mass. Both parts, the stacking and the separating gel, are composed of a mixture of acrylamide monomer and small amounts of *N,N´*-methylene-bis-acrylamide (=″bis-acrylamide″), as a crosslinker. The polymerisation of this mixture is initiated by addition of ammonium persulphate (APS) and by addition of *N,N,N´,N´*-tetramethylenediamine (TEMED). The working solution of acrylamide/bis-acrylamide is prepared by dissolving 30% (w/v) acrylamide and 0,8% (w/v) bis-acrylamide in aqua bidestillata, the solution is stable for

Microassay

- Reagent A: mix 0,8 g $Na_2CO_3 \cdot H_2O$, 1,6 g sodium tartrate, 1,6 g NaOH with 100 ml aqua bidestillata. Adjust pH to 11,25 with 10 M NaOH.
- Reagent B: dissolve 4,0 g BCA in 100 ml aqua bidestillata
- Reagent C: dissolve 0,4 g $CuSO_4 \cdot 5H_2O$ in 10 ml aqua bidestillata.
- Working solution: mix 1 vol. of reagent C with 25 vol. of reagent B then add 26 vol. of reagent A.

Assay Protocol:
- Add 1 ml of the working solution to 1 ml of an aqueous protein sample (0,5–1,0 µg protein/ml) and incubate at 60 °C for 60 min. Cool down the sample to room temperature and measure at 562 nm.

Lowry Assay

This assay is also based on the Biuret-reaction, where the protein reduces bivalent copper ions to monovalent copper ions under alkaline conditions, which then react with the Folin reagent. This Folin-Ciocalteau reaction gives an intense blue colour, partly dependent on the tyrosine and tryptophan content of the protein, which can be measured spectrophotometrically at 750 nm. Although requiring a great deal of work, this method exhibits the best accuracy with regard to protein concentration and is sensitive down to 0,01 mg/ml protein. Nota bene, that like the BCA-assay, the absolute concentration of a target protein cannot be obtained. The most accurate method of protein determination is probably acid protein hydrolysis followed by amino acid analysis. But as the sensitivity of the Lowry protein assay varies only slightly between different proteins, this assay is a good alternative (especially if protein mixtures or crude extracts are used).

Advantages: Widely used assay with best accuracy.

Problems: the Lowry assay is highly susceptible to potentially interfering substances like nucleic acids, mercaptoethanol, buffers for example HEPES or Tris, detergents like Triton-X-100, SDS or CHAPS, sugars like sucrose, EDTA and many other substances and drugs. To overcome this disadvantage, and to concentrate the protein solution, a precipitation step can be carried out prior to the Lowry assay:

- To precipitate the protein, add 0,1 ml of a 0,15% deoxycholate solution to 1,0 ml of the protein sample. Vortex the solution and let it stand for 10 min. at room temperature. Add 0,1 ml of 72% TCA, vortex again, and centrifuge at 1,000–3,000 g for 30 min. The protein pellet is now ready for the Lowry assay.
- Another way to precipitate the protein is to use a 10% TCA solution. After precipitation, TCA remnants can be removed by washing the pellet thoroughly with 80% ice-cold acetone.
- Alternatively, a precipitation step using acetone as precipitant can be performed: one part of the aqueous protein sample and four parts of ice-cold acetone are mixed and stored at –20°C for 1 h. Thereafter the precipitated proteins are centrifuged and the pellet is used for the subsequent procedure.

Lowry Protein Assay:
- Solution A: 2% (w/v) Na_2CO_3 in aqua bidestillata
- Solution B: 1% (w/v) $CuSO_4 \cdot 5H_2O$ in aqua bidestillata
- Solution C: 2% (w/v) sodium potassium tartrate in aqua bidestillata
- These reagents are stable at room temperature.
- Working solution (complex forming reagent): prepare freshly immediately before use by mixing 100 vol. of solution A with 1 vol. of solution B and 1 vol. of solution C
- $2N$ NaOH
- $1N$ Folin reagent (commercially available, Merck)

Assay Protocol:
To 0,1 ml of known standard protein samples, usually a calibration curve using bovine serum albumin (BSA) samples is done, or to 0,1 ml of an unknown protein sample 0,1 ml of $2N$ NaOH is added. The protein samples are hydrolysed at 100°C for 10 min, then cooled down to room temperature, and 1 ml of freshly mixed complex forming reagent is added. This solution should stand for 10 min. at room temperature. The reaction is pH dependent and care must be taken to maintain the pH in a range of between 10–10,5. This has to be taken into account when analysing samples in buffers outside this pH range. Subsequently, 0,1 ml of Folin reagent is added, and the samples mixed thoroughly using a vortex mixer. The mixture is incubated at room temperature for 30–60 min. (do not exceed 60 min, since Folin is not very stable under alkaline conditions). The protein samples are then measured at 750 nm in a spectrophotometer.

Bradford Assay

This assay is based on the binding of the dye Coomassie blue G250 to arginyl and lysyl residues of proteins which is accompanied by a shift in the absorbance maximum of 470 nm of the free cationic red dye, which predominates in the acidic assay reagent solution, to 590 nm absorbance maximum of the anionic blue dye which is bound to protein. Therefore, the increase of absorption at 590 nm is a function of protein concentration and the protein quantity in a given solution can thus be determined. Both, a standard (10–100 µg protein/ ml) or a micro protein assay (1,0–10 µg protein/ ml) can be carried out. The main disadvantage of this rapid and easy method is the fact that, because of the specificity of the Coomassie blue G250 dye to arginyl and lysyl residues of proteins, the resulting measurements at 590 nm vary in dependence on the content of arginyl or lysyl residues of the different proteins. BSA, which is commonly used as a protein standard to generate calibration curves, exhibits rather high signals in comparison to other cellular proteins. Thus, in many cases the Bradford assay used with BSA as standard will underestimate the protein content of the sample. Alternatively, bovine γ-globulin may be used as standard since its absorption curve is closer to that of cellular proteins. Since the Bradford assay is fast and easy to perform, this assay is advantageous in cases when a large number of samples have to be tested and relative protein contents are sufficient (in most cases of gel electrophoresis and Western blotting).

Advantages: The assay is easy to perform (only one stable reagent is needed), cheap and has low sensitivity to interfering substances.

Problems: This assay exhibits high blank values and, especially at high protein concentrations, is not strictly linear. Substances that do interfere with the assay are detergents like SDS, Triton-X or CHAPS.

Dissolve 100 mg Coomassie blue G250 in 50 ml of 95% ethanol, add 100 ml 85% phosphoric acid and make up to 1l with aqua bidestillata. The solution should be filtered to remove any dye precipitates. The reagent, which should be stored in a dark bottle, is stable at ambient temperature for several weeks. Since the Coomassie dye may precipitate during storage, it is advisable to filter the reagent solution prior to use. It is important to mention that for protein measurements with the Coomassie dye, no Quartz spectrophotometer cuvets should be used, as the dye binds to this material. Glassware, or plastic beakers, may be cleaned, by rinsing with methanol.

Assay Protocol:
- Standard Assay
  To 100 µl of γ-globulin protein standard (10–100 µg of total protein) or to 100 µl of an unknown protein sample add 5 ml of the Coomassie reagent, mix well and let stand for 2 min. at room temperature. Thereafter, the absorption at 595 nm is measured against reagent blank. The protein-dye complex remains stable for about 60 min. Since the standard curve is not strictly linear (see above), and since the exact absorbance varies depending on the age of the dye, it is necessary to run a calibration curve for each set of protein determination experiments. To overcome the non-linearity of the calibration curves (especially at high protein levels, when the free dye becomes depleted) the ratio of the absorbency at 595 nm and 465 nm should be calculated.
- Microassay
  To 100 µl of γ-globulin protein standard (1–10 µg of total protein) or to 100 µl of an unknown protein sample add 1 ml of the Coomassie reagent, mix well and let stand for 2 min. at room temperature. Thereafter the absorption at 595 nm is measured against reagent blank. For routine measurements of many probes it may be convenient to use a microplate reader. For that purpose, the assay can be adapted in the following way: put 10 µl of the protein sample into the well of the microtiter plate and add 200 µl of the Coomassie reagent. Ensure effective mixing to gain reproducible results.

To obtain a rough idea of the approximate protein content, one may measure the absorption of a protein solution at 280 nm in comparison to a given concentration of BSA, γ-globulin or ovalbumin (1 mg/ml BSA results in an absorption of 0,66 in a 1 cm light path, 1 mg/ml γ-globulin in an absorption of 1,35 and 1 mg/ml ovalbumin in an absorption of 0,75), provided that the sample does not contain other UV-absorbing substances. If a pure protein solution is used and the extinction coefficient of the protein is known, this method can be used as a relatively exact measurement of protein content. However, since in most cases cell extracts with a broad range of different proteins are used, only an approximation of the protein content is possible with that method.

Gel Electrophoresis (SDS-PAGE; Sodium Dodecyl Sulphate Polyacrylamide Gel Electrophoresis)

SDS-PAGE, a most widely used technique, serves as a method to analyse protein mixtures and to determine the relative molecular mass of different proteins. This system is based on the following principle: the anionic detergent SDS (sodium dodecyl sulphate) binds to proteins, especially after reduction of the proteins with DTT or β-mercaptoethanol, which both reduce disulphide bonds, thereby disturbing the tertiary structure of the protein. This detergent denatures the proteins by impeding protein-protein-interactions and thereby destroying the quaternary structure of the protein.

The majority of proteins bind the detergent SDS to negatively charged protein-SDS-complexes with a constant charge-to-mass ratio and as a result the protein unfolds into a linear elongated negatively charged structure migrating to the positive pole (anode) of an electrical field. This movement is hindered by the sieve-like pores of the SDS-PAGE, due to large proteins migrating more slowly in contrast to small proteins. Thus, the migration of a certain protein only depends on its molecular mass and not on its native tertiary or quaternary structure. If the relative molecular mass of an unknown protein is to be determined, calibration proteins with known molecular weight are applied to the same gel as the unknown protein.

By comparing the mobility of the calibration proteins with that of the unknown protein, its relative molecular mass can be calculated. For that purpose, a calibration curve of $\log_{10}$ molecular weight (y-axis) versus relative mobility of the calibration proteins (x-axis) is plotted and on the basis of this linear curve the molecular weight of the unknown protein can be estimated. The relative mobility can be calculated from the following equation: R_f (relative mobility) = distance migrated by protein/ distance migrated by bromphenol blue dye. The bromphenol blue dye, as it is a small molecule, passes the gel without being retarded and is therefore used to monitor the electrophoretic run. It is important to mention that the linearity of the calibration curve is only given over a limited range of molecular masses and is dependent on the gel concentration: for a 15% acrylamide gel the linear relationship is approximately true for proteins between 10–60 kDa, for a 10% acrylamide gel between 30–120 kDa and for a 5% acrylamide gel between 60–200 kDa. Moreover, it is important to mention that, since proteins have to bind SDS in a constant charge-to-mass ratio, highly basic proteins such as histones, which have a high number of positively-charged amino acids, migrate more slowly during the gel run than one would expect from their molecular weight.

The polyacrylamide gels consist of two parts: the stacking gel with large pore sizes to concentrate the protein samples into sharp bands and the separating gel, where the proteins are separated according to their molecular mass. Both parts, the stacking and the separating gel, are composed of a mixture of acrylamide monomer and small amounts of N,N´-methylene-bis-acrylamide (="bis-acrylamide"), as a crosslinker. The polymerisation of this mixture is initiated by addition of ammonium persulphate (APS) and by addition of N,N,N´,N´-tetramethylenediamine (TEMED). The working solution of acrylamide/bis-acrylamide is prepared by dissolving 30% (w/v) acrylamide and 0,8% (w/v) bis-acrylamide in aqua bidestillata, the solution is stable for several weeks at 4 °C. Since acrylamide is a strong neurotoxin, care has to be taken not to inhale the substance during weighing out and to wear gloves when handling the gels. Ready to use solutions of 30% acrylamide and 0,8% bis-acrylamide are also commercially available.

Formation of polyacrylamide gels: 10% separating gel: To make 10 ml of gel solution (sufficient for 2 mini gels) mix
- Aqua bidestillata: 4,1 ml
- Acrylamide/bis-acrylamide solution: 3,3 ml
- 1,5 M Tris-HCL, pH 8,8: 2,5 ml
- 20% SDS: 0,05 ml

Degas the solution under vacuum, and to initiate polymerisation add
- 10% APS: 0,05 ml
- TEMED: 0,005 ml

Pour the gel solution into the gel cassette and let the gel stack. To avoid desiccation of the surface of the gel, overlay a thin film of aqua bidestillata.
Meanwhile prepare the 4% stacking gel: To make 5 ml of gel solution (sufficient for 2 mini gels) mix:
- Aqua bidestillata: 3,07 ml
- Acrylamide/bis-acrylamide solution: 0,62 ml
- 0,5 M Tris-HCL, pH 6,8: 1,25 ml
- 20% SDS: 0,025 ml

Degas the solution under vacuum, and to initiate polymerisation add
- 10% APS: 0,025 ml
- TEMED: 0,005 ml

Pour off the overlaying water from the separating gel and add the stacking gel to the gel cassette. Place the well-forming comb into the gel solution and let the gel stack. Thereafter remove the comb and the gel is now ready to use.
For the electrophoretic run a Tris-glycine electrophoresis buffer is used. Dissolve 3 g Tris, 14,4 g glycine and 1 g SDS in 1 l aqua bidestillata. The pH value of this solution should be 8.9, but do not adjust pH with acid ore base since the Cl^- or Na^+ ions will disturb the balance of the ionic system which will result in blurred bands. Some investigators use a Tris-glycine electrophoresis buffer of double strength (6 g Tris, 28,8 g glycine and 1 g SDS ad 1 l aqua bidestillata) to gain sharper protein bands, which may be useful if phosphorylated and non-phosphorylated forms of proteins have to be separated.
Assemble the gel cassette in the electrophoresis tank according to the supplier's instruction and fill in the electrophoresis buffer. Remove all air bubbles trapped along the bottom edge of the gel to ensure even current distribution. Thereafter, rinse the gel slots with electrophoresis buffer to remove any non-polymerised acrylamide. The gel is now ready to load the protein samples. The amount of protein which can be applied to the gel slots depends on the thickness of the gel (0,5–1,5 mm) and on the width of

the gel slots (5–15 well combs): the upper limit of protein per slot is 1 mg if a 1,5 mm gel is used with 5 slots. In most cases 20–50 µg protein per slot is sufficient to retain good results.

Prior to electrophoresis, dilute the protein samples with an equal volume of double-strength Laemmli sample buffer and denature the probes at 96°C for 2–3–5 min. Since proteinases may still be active at room temperature, even in Laem mli sample buffer, the samples should be kept at 4 °C prior to heat denaturation. After cooling down the protein probes to room temperature, they can be loaded onto the gel together with protein standards of known molecular weight.

For double-strength Laem mli sample buffer mix 100 mM Tris-HCl (pH 6,8) with 20% (v/v) glycerol, 4% (w/v) SDS, 10% (v/v) β-mercaptoethanol (or 200 mM DTT) and 0,2% (w/v) bromphenol blue. The buffer is stable at 4 °C for several weeks. Alternatively, prepare a sample buffer lacking β-mercaptoethanol or DTT, which can now be stored at room temperature for a month, and just before use the appropriate amount of β-mercaptoethanol or DTT is added.

For running the gel, a constant current of 20–30 mA/gel or a constant voltage of 120–150 V is applied. The electrophoresis is continued until the bromphenol blue dye band has reached the bottom of the gel. This will usually take 1–3 h and can be controlled using pre-stained protein markers of definite molecular weights. Thereafter the gel is used for Western blotting. If one wishes to control the protein bands before blotting the gel, a staining with eosin Y can be carried out. This dye is able to stain all proteins down to 10ng protein/band, including sialoglycoproteins, which normally cannot be stained using the Coomassie brilliant blue dye. It has the advantage that the antigenicity of proteins remains unchanged, so that after Western blotting, the subsequent antibody detection steps will not be disturbed. The eosin Y staining solution consists of 1% (w/v) eosin Y soluble in aqua bidestillata, 40% methanol and 0,4–0,5% glacial acetic acid. The acetic acid has to be added last while stirring the solution otherwise precipitation of the eosinY dye might occur. The solution is then filtered and ready to use. After electrophoresis, the polyacrylamide gels are immersed in the staining solution for 15–45 min. at room temperature with gentle shaking. Thereafter the gels are immediately rinsed with aqua bidestillata and washed with aqua bidestillata 3× for 5 min. each. The protein bands will now appear as yellow-orange bands. If the protein bands are not visible at this point the washing step may be prolonged for another 5–10 min. Afterwards, Western blotting can be carried out as usual.

To obtain a better separation of protein solutions containing proteins with a broad range of different molecular masses (for example proteins with molecular weights from 8 to 200 kDa) the use of linear gradient polyacrylamide gels (5–20%) may be advantageous. Furthermore, proteins with very similar molecular weights may be resolved in a gradient gel, that otherwise in a fixed percentage acrylamide gel, cannot be separated. Therefore, a running gel with increasing acrylamide concentration, thus decreasing pore size, has to be prepared in the following manner:

To make 15 ml of each gel solution (A and B) mix:
- Solution A (5% acrylamide)
- Aqua bidestillata: 9,3 ml
- Acrylamide/bis-acrylamide solution: 2,5 ml
- 1,875 M Tris-HCL, pH 8,8: 3,0 ml

- 10% SDS: 0,15 ml
- 10% APS: 0,05 ml
- Solution B (20% acrylamide)
- Aqua bidestillata: 0,6 ml
- Acrylamide/bis-acrylamide solution: 10,0 ml
- 1,875 M Tris-HCL, pH 8,8: 3,0 ml
- 10% SDS: 0,15 ml
- 10% APS: 0,05 ml
- Sucrose: 2,2 g

Degas the solutions under vacuum, and to initiate polymerisation, add
- TEMED: 0,012 ml to each solution

Commercially available gradient mixer may be used to form the linear gradients. More easily, use a 30 ml glass pipette and draw up firstly the 5% acrylamide solution and thereafter the 20% acrylamide solution. The two solutions are then transformed into a linear gradient by means of air bubbles drawn up into the pipette. Pour the gradient solution into the gel cassette. The top half of the gel will then have a gradient of about 5–10%, while the gradient increases over the next half of the gel up to 20%. To visualise gradient forming, the dye bromphenol blue may be added to the 20% acrylamide solution. Preparation of the stacking gel, sample preparation and gel run are carried out exactly as described for the fixed percentage gel electrophoresis.

Since after electrophoresis, the polyacrylamide gels are further processed for Western blotting, there is usually no need to dry the gels because Western blot cannot be carried out after drying. But, nevertheless, if it is desired to dry the gel in order to store it as a record of the experiment, it is best done after staining the gel with a Coomassie blue solution (this will fix and stain the gel in one step, for protocol see next page) in the following manner: soak the stained gel in a solution of 20% methanol and 3% glycerol overnight, this will prevent the gel from breaking into pieces during the drying process. This step can be omitted if thin gels (0,5–0,75 mm) are to be dried. Thereafter, place the gel onto a piece of Wathman 3 MM filter paper slightly larger than the gel and cover the gel with a piece of Saran Wrap. Place the sandwich on the surface of the gel dryer with the Saran Wrap uppermost, close the lid of the apparatus, and connect the dryer to a vacuum source. Apply the vacuum until a tight seal around the gel is achieved. In addition, low heat (50–60 °C) may be used to accelerate the drying process. Usually for a 0,75 mm gel 2 h of drying are sufficient. After drying is complete, it is important to turn off the heat a few minutes before the vacuum is released, in order to avoid distortion of the gel. The dehydrated gels may then be stored indefinitely.

Western Blot (Electroblotting)

SDS-gel electrophoresis allows separation of proteins according to their molecular mass, but does not allow precise identification of a certain protein. For exact identification of a particular protein, a technique was developed similar to the Southern blot technique (which is used for DNA), called Western electroblotting. This method depends on the transfer of the negatively charged proteins to a membrane in anodic position and thus, depends on the pK_a of the protein and the pH of the buffer used. This method allows the transfer of proteins from the acrylamide gels onto the surface of an inert membrane, which may then be probed with antibodies or other ligands to further analyse the target protein.

The electrophoretic transfer of proteins from the acrylamide gel to a membrane can be performed using two different types of Western blot apparatus: in the older type, the so-called tank blot system, a membrane/gel/filter paper sandwich is placed vertically in an electrophoresis tank between two platinum electrodes, in the newer one, the so-called semi-dry blot procedure, the transfer membrane/gel/filter paper sandwich is placed in a horizontal position between two platinum/stainless steel electrodes. A special advantage of the semi-dry method is the reduced blotting time, the smaller amount of transfer buffer needed and its use at room temperature.

To obtain best results with the Western blot technique there are three issues to be considered: the transfer membrane, the transfer buffer and the blotting time.

With regard to the blotting matrix there are a wide range of membranes available, and depending on the protein that is to be analysed, the investigator has to choose the appropriate one. Nitrocellulose was the first blotting membrane used for electroblotting and is still probably the most widely used blotting matrix. It has good protein binding capacities and as non-specific protein binding sites may be easily blocked using, for example, non fat dry milk, this membrane allows immunodetection of proteins with a good signal to noise ratio. Membranes of different pore sizes (0,025–0,45 µm) are available and for standard procedures a pore size of 0,45 µm will be sufficient (for example Hybond-C or Hybond ECL from Amersham). However, for very small proteins (<20 kDa), nitrocellulose membranes of a pore size of 0,1–0,2 µm or even smaller should be used, to enhance the yield of the blotted protein.

Polyvinylidine difluoride (PVDF) blotting membrane is another widely used blotting matrix with high-protein binding capacity but is more expensive than nitrocellulose. The PVDF membrane is compatible with the most commonly used immunological detection systems (e.g. alkaline phosphatase reaction or detection using the ECL-system), and because this membrane is resistant to acidic and organic solvents, it may also be used for analysis of amino acid composition of the target protein.

Less commonly used blotting matrices are diazobenzyloxymethyl (DBM) modified cellulose paper or diazophenylthioether (DPT) membranes. The binding capacity of these blotting membranes is higher than that of nitrocellulose or PVDF and proteins are bound covalently via the azo groups. However, the resolution of the separated proteins is less, and glycine has to be washed out of the SDS gel as it interferes with these membranes. Nylon membranes are also used for electroblotting and have good protein binding capacities, but protein staining is difficult owing to the positive charge of the membrane and also blocking of unoccupied binding sites may be a problem resulting in high background values.

The next issue to address is the composition of the transfer buffer. There are several buffers in use, and depending on the nature of the protein, the appropriate buffer has to be chosen. The most commonly used buffer, the so-called "Towbin buffer" was introduced by Towbin in the year 1979 for electrophoretic transfer of proteins. It is composed of 25 mM Tris, 192 mM glycine and 20%(v/v) methanol, pH should be 8,3 (do not adjust pH, a pH between 8,2–8,4 is sufficient, if pH differs more than ±0,1 the buffer should be replaced). A modified Towbin buffer may also be prepared with the addition of 0,1% (w/v) SDS.

For electrophoretic transfer of proteins there are two critical factors to be taken into account: the elution efficacy of the protein out of the acrylamide gel and the binding capacity of the membrane. The elution capacity is mainly determined by the ionic strength, and the pH (alkaline pH enhances elution of proteins from the gel, acidic pH enhances absorption of proteins on the transfer membrane), of the transfer buffer and the addition or the omission of SDS and methanol. Methanol acts as a fixative and thus favours the absorption of proteins on the blotting membrane furthermore it facilitates dissociation of protein-SDS complexes. However, it reduces the efficiency of protein elution by fixing the proteins in the SDS-gel and by reducing the pore size of the gel. Thus, extended transfer times have to be used. For that reason, for proteins with a molecular weight >100 kDa, methanol should be omitted from the transfer buffer. In contrast, SDS enhances the elution efficiency of proteins out of the gel, but reduces the absorption of proteins on the blotting membrane.

In general, continuous buffers (same buffer on the anodic and cathodic side) or discontinuous blotting buffers may be used.

Examples of continuous buffers used in Western blotting (for semi-dry blot):
- Towbin buffer without SDS
  - 25 mM Tris
  - 192 mM glycine
  - 20% (v/v) methanol
  - pH 8,3
- Towbin buffer with 0,1% SDS
  - 25 mM Tris
  - 192 mM glycine
  - 20% (v/v) methanol
  - 0,1% (w/v) SDS
  - pH 8,3
- Dunn carbonate buffer pH 9,9 (advantage: enhances immunochemical detection, increases retention of small proteins)
  - 10 mM $NaHCO_3$
  - 3 mM Na_2CO_3
  - 20% (v/v) methanol
- Schäfer-Nielsen buffer pH 9,2 (buffers with higher pH have lower conductivity than the Towbin buffer and are recommended only for semi-dry transfer)
  - 40 mM Tris
  - 39 mM glycine
  - 20% (v/v) methanol
- Bjerrum buffer pH 9,2
  - 48 mM Tris
  - 39 mM glycine
  - 20% (v/v) methanol
  - 0,0375 % (w/v) SDS

- Matsudaira CAPS buffer adjust pH to 11 with NaOH (advantage: useful buffer to perform amino acid composition analysis)
  - 10 mM CAPS
  - 10% (v/v) methanol

Examples of discontinuous buffers used in Western blotting (for semi-dry blot): For some proteins, for example, for analysis of nitric oxide synthase, a discontinuous buffer system may be useful.
- Svoboda buffer pH 8,3
  The presence of methanol at the anodic side, facilitates binding of proteins to the blotting membrane, whereas, the presence of SDS at the cathodic side, enhances protein elution out of the gel.
- Cathodic side
  - 0,1% (w/v) SDS
  - 25 mM Tris
  - 192 mM glycine
- Anodic side
  - 20% (v/v) methanol
  - 25 mM Tris
  - 192 mM glycine
- Kyhse-Andersen buffer
  - Cathodic side pH 9,4
  - 40 mM 6-amino-n-hexanoic acid
  - 25 mM Tris
  - 20% (v/v) methanol
- Anodic side pH 10,4
  - 300 mM Tris
  - 20% (v/v) methanol
  - (in contact with anode)
  - 25 mM Tris
  - 20% (v/v) methanol
  - (in contact with blotting membrane)
- Laurière buffer
- Cathodic side pH 8,4
  - 0,4% (w/v) SDS
  - 60 mM lactic acid
  - 100 mM Tris
  - (in contact with cathode)
  - 0,1% (w/v) SDS
  - 15 mM lactic acid
  - 25 mM Tris
  - (in contact with acrylamide gel)
- Anodic side
  - 20% (v/v) methanol
  - 60 mM lactic acid
  - 20 mM Tris

- (in contact with blotting membrane, pH 3,8)
- 20% (v/v) methanol
- 100 mM Tris
- (in contact with anode, pH 10,4)

With this buffer system semi-dry blotting allows nearly quantitative transfer of proteins from acrylamide gels almost independently of their molecular weight.

Examples of continuous buffers used in Western blotting (for wet-(tank)-blot):
- Towbin buffer
  - 25 mM Tris
  - 192 mM glycine
  - 20% (v/v) methanol
  - pH 8,3
- Towbin buffer with SDS
  - 48 mM Tris
  - 386 mM glycine
  - 20% (v/v) methanol
  - 0,1% (w/v) SDS
  - pH 8,3
- Bolt buffer pH 8,8
  - 40 mM Tris
  - 20 mM sodium acetate
  - 2 mM EDTA
  - 0,05% (w/v) SDS
  - 20% (v/v) methanol
- Matsudaira buffer
  - Adjust pH to 11 with NaOH
  - 10 mM CAPS
  - 15% (v/v) methanol

For pilot experiments we suggest using a universal transfer buffer, for example, the Towbin buffer, a nitrocellulose or PVDF membrane of 0,45 µm pore size and a maximum blotting time to allow complete transfer of the proteins. In some cases, it may be helpful in a first experiment to use two blotting membranes placed on each other in order to optimise the blotting procedure. If the current applied is too high or the blotting time is too long, small proteins especially, may penetrate the first membrane and may be found in the second after membrane staining. In these cases current or blotting time have to be corrected.

Furthermore, it is important to mention that for semi-dry apparatus with graphite electrodes, pH should not exceed 8,5 to avoid damaging the electrodes.

The third issue to address is the blotting time. For tank blot, depending on the size of the blotting chamber (mini tank blot: cross-section of blotting chamber 150 cm^2, maxi tank blot: cross-section of blotting chamber 500cm^2), and depending on the molecular weight of the proteins, different current densities (mA/cm^2) and blotting times have to be used (Table 1).

Table 1
Current densities and blotting times for tank blot

	Current density (mA/m²)		Blotting time
	Mini tank blot	Maxi tank blot	
Proteins <80 kDa	0.8–1.5	0.2–0.5	2–8 h
Proteins >80 kDa	0.4–0.7	0.2–0.3	15–20 h

Table 2
Current densities and blotting times for semi-dry blot

	Current density (mA/m²)		Blotting time
	Gel size: 80–100 m2	200–250	
Graphit electrodes	1.5–3	1–1.3	1–3 h
Platinum/stainless steel electrodes	3–5	2.5–3	0.5–2

Tank blot should always be carried out in the cold to prevent overheating of the apparatus and to avoid formation of air bubbles in the blotting sandwich, which will result in a poor transfer. For semi-dry blot, depending on the size of the acrylamide gel and on the electrodes used: graphite or platinum/stainless steel electrodes, different current densities and blotting times are necessary (Table 2).

Protocol for Western Blotting Using Tank Blot

Assemble the transfer apparatus according to the supplier's instruction. Fill in the appropriate transfer buffer (see above) and if the transfer apparatus is equipped with a cooling device let the transfer buffer cool down to 4–8 °C. Otherwise, the transfer can also be carried out in a cold-storage room. Cut two or more pieces (depending on the thickness) of filter paper (for example Whatman 3 MM) and the transfer membrane to fit into the cassette clamp. Filter paper and transfer membrane should be soaked in transfer buffer prior to use. Remove the acrylamide gel from the electrophoresis apparatus and let it also equilibrate in transfer buffer (for various buffers see above) for about 10–15 min. This will remove electrophoresis buffer salts and excess detergent. Make a sandwich of filter paper/blotting membrane/acrylamide gel/filter paper with the blotting membrane placed towards the anode. Air bubbles trapped in the sandwich should be avoided. Place the sandwich in-between the two sponge pads normally supplied with the tank apparatus and clamp the whole sandwich securely in the transfer cassette. Carry out electroblotting for 2–8 h at 0,25–0,5 A (for details see above). Thereafter, remove the transfer membrane from the apparatus. It is now ready for immunodetection of proteins.

Protocol for Western Blotting Using Semi-Dry Blot

In this newer type of blotting apparatus, the filter paper/transfer membrane/gel sandwich is placed horizontally between two platinum/stainless steel (or graphite) electrodes. The Western blot transfer can be carried out at room temperature. Assemble the transfer apparatus according to the supplier's instruction. Cut two or more pieces of filter paper (for example Whatman 3 MM) and one piece of the transfer membrane to the exact size of the acrylamide gel to avoid a short circuit that will disturb the electrophoretic transfer. Filter paper, transfer membrane and acrylamide gel should be soaked in transfer buffer (for continuous or discontinuous systems see above) prior to use (10–20 min). If PVDF membranes are used these membranes have to be pre-wetted with 100% methanol prior to equilibration in transfer buffer. They have to be kept wet all times because proteins will not bind to dried PVDF membranes. If this occurs during use, the PVDF membrane can be rewetted using 100% methanol. Make a sandwich of filter paper/blotting membrane/acrylamide gel/filter paper with the blotting membrane placed towards the anode. Remove all air bubbles trapped in the sandwich using a glass pipette as a roller, because air bubbles will create areas of high resistance resulting in low transfer. Place the upper electrode, the cathode, on top of the sandwich and carry out electroblotting for 1–2 h at 0,25–0,5 A, or at a constant voltage of 13–18 V (for details see above). Take care not to exceed 25 V (for platinum/stainless steel electrodes) or 40 V (for graphite electrodes) because in that case the blotting unit may be damaged. Thereafter, remove the transfer membrane from blotting apparatus. The blotting matrix is now ready for immunodetection of proteins.

Recently, polyethyleneglycol polymers (PEG 1,000–2,000) have been introduced to improve electroblotting. With PEG, a better resolution, a reduced background and a sharpening of protein bands may be obtained. After SDS-PAGE the acrylamide gel is equilibrated in a 30% (v/v) PEG solution [12,5 mM Tris, 96 mM glycine and 15% (v/v) methanol]. Thereafter, electroblotting can be carried out as usual using the same PEG-solution as transfer buffer.

After Western blotting, staining of the polyacrylamide gel with Coomassie blue may be carried out to check for remaining protein bands that have not been transferred during semi-dry or tank blot. Usually no protein bands should be visible after complete transfer, but since proteins of high molecular weight are difficult to transfer by electroblotting, very often protein bands at the range of >100.000 Da will remain in the polyacrylamide gel, and for that reason staining of the gel may be useful to define the blotting time.

Coomassie blue staining solution: for 1 l of staining solution mix 1 g Coomassie brilliant blue R-250 with 50% (v/v) methanol and 10% (v/v) glacial acetic acid, stir until the dye is dissolved and filter the solution to remove any particulate matter.

De-staining solution: for 1 l solution mix 35% (v/v) methanol with 5–10% (v/v) glacial acetic acid.

Stain the gel for 10–30 min in an appropriate volume of the Coomassie blue staining solution (staining may be prolonged up to several hours) at room temperature while gently shaking. Thereafter, de-stain the gel in de-staining solution to visualise the protein bands. Change the de-staining solution three to four times. For a more rapid de-staining, include a piece of sponge in the de-staining solution. The sponge will absorb the Coomassie dye as it emerges from the gel.

Before immunodetection of the target protein is carried out, it may be useful to reversibly stain the proteins immobilised on the transfer membrane, in order to control the electrophoretic transfer and to locate the molecular-weight markers, which can then be marked with indelible ink. The dye used for reversible staining of proteins, must be compatible with the subsequent immunological probing, using primary and secondary enzyme-linked antibodies (such as alkaline phosphatase- or horseradish-peroxidase (HRP)-labelled secondary antibodies). Therefore, the red dye Ponceau S, is best used for transient staining of the membranes. This dye will not interfere with immunodetection and is rinsed out by washing the membranes with PBS (137 mM NaCl, 27 mM KCl, 10 mM Na_2HPO_4, 1,8 mM KH_2PO_4, pH 7,4) or blocking solution. To stain the transfer membranes use the following protocol:

Ponceau S Staining

Prepare a working solution of 0,1% (w/v) Ponceau S in 3% (v/v) trichloroacteic acid or 5% (v/v) glacial acetic acid, the solution should be a deep red colour. Incubate the blotting membrane for 3–5 min with gentle agitation. When protein bands become visible as pink-purple bands, wash the blotting membrane with aqua bidestillata or PBS at room temperature, and mark the molecular weight standard proteins with a waterproof pencil. Thereafter, wash the membrane several times with PBS or blocking solution to remove all remaining dye. The blotting membrane is then ready for immunological probing.

Immunodetection

After protein blotting, the membranes should be rinsed with PBS or aqua bidestillata to remove transfer buffer. Membranes should be kept wet at all times. If the hydrophilic nitrocellulose filters have been dried, they can easily be rewetted in aqua bidestillata, whereas if the hydrophobic PVDF membranes have become dry during use, they must be rewetted in 100% methanol first, before soaking the membranes in aqua bidestillata. This can be done even if the membranes already contain absorbed proteins. In most cases, rewetting will not interfere with the subsequent immunodetection of proteins.

Before immunodetection is carried out, it is necessary to block non-specific binding sites on the membrane. This will reduce background by preventing non-specific binding of probes (antibodies). Furthermore, it has been shown that the blocking step may ease monoclonal antibodies to recognise their antigenic site by renaturation of epitopes. There are several blocking solutions in use, of which the most widely used and also cheapest blocking solution is non-fat dried milk. It is compatible with nearly all immunological detection systems except, because of the biotin content in milk, the biotin-streptavidin-HRP system. In this case, blocking of the membrane can be done with a solution of 1–3% bovine serum albumine. The blotting membrane should be incubated in the blocking solution for 1–2 h at room temperature or at 4 °C overnight with gentle agitation. For the first experiment use a blocking solution of 5% (w/v) non-fat dried milk in PBS pH 7,4. For some antibodies, the use of Tris-buffer (20 mM

Tris, 145 mM NaCl, pH 7,4) instead of PBS may give better signals, and if background value is still too high the addition of non-ionic detergents such as Tween-20 (0,1–0,3% (w/v) might be advantageous.

The following blocking agents are used in Western blotting:
Bovine serum albumine (BSA): especially for nylon membranes, high concentrations of BSA must be used to obtain a satisfactory low background: 10% (w/v) BSA in PBS, incubation time of the membrane 12–15 h at 45–50 °C. BSA might also be used for low concentrations (0,5% (w/v)) together with non-fat dried milk, or at a concentration of 1–3% instead of non-fat dried milk, if the biotin-streptaviden-HRP system is used (see below).

Non-fat dried milk: used at a concentration of 3–6%, may contain biotin, which might interfere with immunodetection when using streptavidin-labelled horseradish-peroxidase.

Gelatin: We do not recommend the use of gelatin because it may mask epitopes and often gives high background values.

Non-ionic detergents (do not exceed 0,3–0,5%): Tween-20: minimises non-specific binding and may be added to non-fat dried milk blocking solutions or to blocking solutions containing BSA. On the other hand, it is known that Tween-20 may remove proteins and antibodies from the blotting membrane, so it should be used with care. For a pilot experiment, use a concentration of 0,05–0,1% (w/v).

Polyvinylpyrolidone-40 (PVP-40): this detergent can be used at a concentration of 1% (w/v) together with 0,05% (w/v) Tween-20. Doubling of the signal-to-noise ratio has been reported.

NP-40 or Triton-X 100: these detergents should be avoided since they remove antibodies and proteins from the blotting membrane to a higher extent than Tween-20.

Immunoprobing of membranes is carried out in two steps after blocking of unspecific binding sites. In principle: first an unlabelled primary antibody, specific to the target protein, is applied to the membrane. Thereafter, the membrane is incubated with either a secondary antibody raised against the primary antibody, and linked to marker enzymes such as alkaline phosphatase or horseradish peroxidase, or with protein A, which recognises the Fc region of immunoglobulins and which also may be labelled with either alkaline phosphatase or horseradish peroxidase. After several washing steps, the target protein is detected using either chromogenic reactions or the iodophenol/luminol system.

General remarks: a wide range of monoclonal antibodies raised in mice or rats are commercially available, thus in most cases it is not necessary to develop and purify antibodies in your own laboratory. If the target protein is not detected with the monoclonal antibody (for example if the protein has only a small epitope), the use of polyclonal antibodies (raised in rabbits, goats or sheep) might be advantageous. Monoclonal antibodies are often used at a final concentration of 1–10 μg antibody/ml blocking solution, polyclonal antibodies at a dilution of 1:500–1,000. The best working concentration has to be established empirically by the investigator.

As a secondary antibody, protein A (a cell wall-component of Staphylococcus aureus) that recognises the Fc region of IgG can be used. As little as 0,1ng protein can be detected using this ligand, however, protein A has the major disadvantage that it fails to bind to IgGs from rats, goats, or sheep. For antibodies raised in these animals, protein g (isolated from group g of Streptococcus) should be used instead as a secondary antibody. Due to the limited availability of suitable protein g conjugates, other secondary antibodies are preferable.

In most laboratories, anti-immunoglobulin secondary antibodies are used, which are developed against the specific primary antibodies (IgGs). These secondary antibodies are either linked to a marker enzyme or to biotin. The biotinylated secondary antibodies are then detected in a third step using (strept)avidin-labelled marker enzymes. The secondary antibody is normally raised in a species different from the primary antibody to avoid cross-reactions: for example, if a monoclonal mouse antibody is used, then an anti-mouse antibody raised in goat or sheep is suitable as a secondary antibody.

In the following paragraphs, different protocols for immunodetection of proteins are introduced:

Alkaline Phosphatase (AP)-Reaction Using BCIP/NBT

The enzyme alkaline phosphatase (AP), converts the soluble chromogenic substrates 5-bromo-4-chloroindolyl phosphate (BCIP) and nitro blue tetrazolium (NBT) to an insoluble indigo/purple dye. This is deposited on the blotting membrane and thus visualises the band of the target protein. The detection limit is 10–50 pg of protein. The following standard protocol may be used:

Incubate the blotting membrane in a 5% (w/v) non-fat dried milk solution using a TBS-buffer: 150 mM NaCl and 50 mM Tris pH 7,4, with or without the addition of 0,05–0,1% (w/v) Tween-20, for 2 h at room temperature or at 4 °C overnight. Do not use phosphate buffered saline when using alkaline phosphatase. Thereafter, discharge the blocking solution and incubate the membrane with the appropriate primary antibody for 1–2 h at room temperature with gentle agitation. For weak antigens, the primary antibody solution may be left on the membrane at 4 °C overnight. Wash the membrane thoroughly in TBS 4–5× with excess of buffer. Then incubate the membrane with the secondary AP-labelled antibody at a dilution recommended by the supplier, normally between 1:1000 and 1:10000 in blocking buffer for another 1h at room temperature.

Meanwhile prepare the AP-substrate mixture:
Dissolve 100mg BCIP in 1,9 ml 100% dimethylformamide (DMF) and 100mg NBT in 1,9 ml 70% DMF. These stock solutions are stable for about 1 year when stored at 4°C. Prepare the alkaline phosphatase buffer (AP-buffer) using the following composition: 100 mM NaCl, 10 mM Tris·HCl pH 9,5, 5 mM $MgCl_2$. For the working solution, mix 10 ml AP-buffer with 33 µl of the BCIP stock and 66 µl of the NBT stock solution. The working solution should be stored in the dark and used within 30–60 min.

After incubation with secondary antibody, wash the membrane again in TBS 4–5× for 10 min. each and equilibrate the membrane in the AP-buffer for about 5 min. Thereafter, the membrane is incubated in the alkaline phosphatase substrate mixture until the protein bands become visible, usually after 2–30 min.

To stop the reaction, transfer the membrane to a container containing the stop solution composed of 5 mM EDTA and 20 mM Tris·HCl, pH 8. Finally, dry the membrane and photograph or scan the membrane as a permanent record of the experiment. The indigo/purple bands can be analysed densitometrically using commercially available software.

Horseradish-Peroxidase (HRP)-Reaction Using DAB

Horseradish-peroxidase catalyses the oxidation of 3,3'-diaminobenzidine (DAB) in the presence of H_2O_2, resulting in a red-brown insoluble complex, thereby, visualising the specific protein bands. This method is less sensitive (detection limit: 100–500 pg protein) than when using AP-substrates, but sensitivity can be increased 50–100 fold using cobalt and nickel salts in combination with DAB, which then give a brown/black precipitate. The following standard protocol may be used:

Incubate the blotting membrane in a blocking solution of 5% (w/v) non-fat dried milk in 150 mM NaCl and 10 mM NaH_2PO_4 pH 7,3 with or without the addition of 0,05–0,1% (w/v) Tween-20, for 2 h at room temperature or at 4 °C overnight. It is also possible to use 4–8% (w/v) BSA, instead of milk, and some investigators use a Tris buffered saline (TBS, 150 mM NaCl and 50 mM Tris pH 7,5) instead of phosphate buffer. Thereafter, discharge the blocking solution and incubate the membrane with the appropriate primary antibody for 1–2 h at room temperature with gentle agitation. For weak antigens, the primary antibody solution may be left on the membrane at 4 °C overnight. Wash the membrane thoroughly in Tris or PBS 4–5× with excess of buffer. Then incubate the membrane with the secondary HRP-labelled antibody at a dilution recommended by the supplier, normally between 1:1,000 and 1:10,000 in blocking buffer for another 1 h at room temperature. Do not use sodium azide as a preservative when working with HRP since sodium azide strongly inhibits peroxidases.

Meanwhile, prepare the HRP-substrate mixture:
Dissolve 40 mg DAB in 940 µl aqua bidestillata. This stock solution may be frozen at 20°C in 100 µl aliquots and is stable for about 1 year. Prepare two stock solutions of 8% (w/v) $CoCl_2$ and 8% (w/v) $NiCl_2$ in aqua bidestillata. Hydrogen peroxide, which is needed as a 30% stock solution, can be purchased stabilised. However, since H_2O_2 decomposes with time (stable only for weeks) the exact concentration of H_2O_2 can be determined photometrically by measuring the absorbance at 240 nm (molar extinction coefficient 43,6 $M^{-1} \cdot cm^{-1}$). Instead of hydrogen peroxide, the more stable derivative urea peroxide might also be used: prepare a stock solution of 10% (w/v) (stable for several months), and use urea peroxide at a final concentration of 0,1%.

For the working solution, mix 10 ml of 50 mM Tris·HCl pH 7,5 with 200 µl DAB stock, 50 µl 8% (w/v) $CoCl_2$ and 50 µl 8% (w/v) $NiCl_2$. Filter the solution through a membrane to remove any particulate matter. Immediately before use, add 15 µl H_2O_2. The working solution should be stored in the dark and used within 30 min.

After incubation with secondary antibody, wash the membrane again in TBS 4–5× for 10 min each and equilibrate the membrane in the 50 mM Tris·HCl buffer for about 5 min. Thereafter, incubate the membrane with the HRP substrate mixture until the protein bands are of the desired intensity (2–5 min, longer exposure times of about 10–30 min. are possible, however, significant background staining might occur). Stop the reaction by washing the membrane extensively with aqua bidestillata. Finally, dry the membrane. For longer storage, because of the light sensitivity of the peroxidase-stained bands, photograph or scan the membrane as a permanent record of the experiment. The protein bands of brown/black colour can be analysed densitometrically using commercially available software.

To increase specificity of protein staining and to reduce background, instead of using an HRP-labelled secondary antibody, a biotinylated secondary antibody may be applied. Since the glycoprotein streptavidin (from Streptomyces avidinii) has a high affinity to biotin, the biotinylated secondary antibody can be detected in a third step using streptavidin-labelled HRP. The following standard protocol may be used. Depending on the target protein, which is to be detected, adaptations have to be made.

Incubate the blotting membrane in a blocking solution containing BSA (1–5%) instead of non-fat dried milk. If dried milk has to be used, then extensive washing of the membrane in PBS with addition of Tween-20 has to be carried out, in order to remove biotin, which is contained in milk and interferes with the biotin-streptavidin-HRP system. Thereafter, carry out incubation with a primary antibody as usual, then wash the blotting membrane and incubate with secondary biotinylated antibody (dilution 1:1,000–1:5,000). Wash the membrane again and then incubate it with the streptavidin-labelled HRP (dilution 1:500–1:5000 in PBS containing 0,1% BSA as stabiliser) for 1h at room temperature. Detection of the protein bands may be performed using either DAB or the enhanced chemiluminescence technique.

Horseradish-Peroxidase (HRP)-Reaction Using Enhanced Chemiluminescene (ECL) Detection

In this system, HRP catalyses the oxidation of the cyclic diacylhydrazide luminol in the presence of H_2O_2, thereby, emitting light which can be detected using a blue light sensitive X-ray film. During the reaction the phenol derivative 4-iodophenol saves as an enhancer of the luminescence by increasing the light output. A special advantage of this method is the high sensitivity: down to 1 pg of antigen can be detected. Moreover, after detection of a target antigen, the blotting membrane may be re-probed with different antibodies for other antigens. The following protocol may be used for the detection of proteins using the ECL-system:

Membrane blocking and incubation with primary and secondary HRP-labelled antibodies as well as the use of the biotin/streptavidin/HRP system can be carried out as described above.

Preparation of the ECL-mixture (also commercially available ECL-detection kits (Amersham, Pierce) can be used):
Dissolve 40 mg luminol in 10 ml dimethylsulfoxide (DMSO) and 10 mg 4-iodophenol in 10 ml DMSO. The stock solution should be stable for about 1 year if stored frozen at –70 °C. Thereafter, prepare a 100 mM Tris·HCl buffer pH 7,5. Immediately before use, mix 2,5 ml Tris buffer with 500 μl luminol and 500 μl 4-iodophenol stock, add 25 μl 30% H_2O_2 and 1,5 ml aqua bidestillata. The reagent mixture (5 ml) is sufficient

for a blotting membrane of 80–100 cm^2 and should be used directly since the chemiluminescence declines with time. Submerge the membrane in the ECL-mixture for 1 min. at room temperature, drain excess fluid off, and cover the blot with Saran Wrap. Place the wrapped membrane in an X-ray cassette and expose it to an appropriate X-ray film (X-ray films specialised for ECL-detection are sold for example from Amersham). Exposure times may vary between a few seconds and 5–10 min. For very weak antigens, the exposure time might be extended up to 30 min but it is noteworthy that prolonging the exposure time might result in high background values. Moreover, since the ECL-signal peaks in 5–20 min and declines with a half-life time of 60 min. longer exposure times are not useful. After detection of the target antigen, the blotting membrane can be stripped and re-probed with different antibodies.

Blot stripping can be carried out as follows (Western blot recycling kits are also commercially available for example from BioRad):
Prepare a stripping buffer of 50 mM Tris·HCl pH 6,8, 2% SDS and 10 mmM β-mercaptoethanol. Heat the stripping buffer to 50°C and incubate the blotting membrane for 10–30 min. Thereafter wash the membrane thoroughly with TBS or PBS. Membrane blocking and application of primary and secondary antibodies can now be performed as usual.

If immunodetection is not carried out immediately after Western blotting, the blotting membranes can be stored for several weeks at 4°C in PBS containing 0,005% (w/v) sodium azide. It is noteworthy to mention that sodium azide is poisonous and that it is a strong inhibitor of peroxidase activity. Thus, thorough washing of the membranes is necessary before immunodetection is performed.

After immunodetection of the target protein, the blotting membrane may be recycled and re-probed (only when using the ECL-technique, colour reactions using BCIP/NBT or DAB are irreversible) with different antibodies once again, or the membrane may be stained with Amido black and stored as a record of the experiment.

For the Amido black staining, dissolve 0,1% Amido black in 7% glacial acetic acid and 20% methanol and stain the membrane for about 5 min. at room temperature with gentle agitation. Thereafter, de-stain the membrane in order to reduce background in the de-staining solution (7% glacial acetic acid and 20% methanol) and until clear protein bands become visible.

Concluding Remarks

SDS-PAGE and Western blot are the most useful methods to analyse a broad variety of proteins, and also translocation from cytosol to membrane or to nucleus, if SDA-PAGE is combined with differential centrifugation methods. The success of Western blotting, however, depends on the choice of the correct protocol, buffers, antibodies, blocking solution and detecting system. Hints on how to select the best buffer or system, and on troubleshooting, are given in the respective section of this chapter.

For further information, the interested reader is referred to the literature listed below.

References

Celis JE: Cell Biology. A Laboratory Handbook, Academic Press, San Diego, 1994.
Doonan S: Protein Purification Protocols. Methods in Molecular Biology Vol. 59. Humana Press, Totowa New Jersey, 1996.
Gassen HG, Schrimpf G: Gentechnische Methoden. Spektrum Akademischer Verlag Heidelberg 1999.
Hames BD: Gel Electrophoresis of Proteins. A Practical Approach, Oxford University Press, Oxford 1998.
Rehm H: Der Experimentator: Proteinbiochemie/Proteomics. Spektrum Akademischer Verlag, Heidelberg 2002.
Roe S: Protein Purification Applications, Oxford University Press, Oxford 2001.
Sambrook J, Fritsch EF, Maniatis T: Molecular Cloning, Cold Spring Harbor Laboratory Press, 1989, USA.
Walker JM: The Protein Protocols Handbook, Humana Press, Totowa, New Jersey, 1996.

6.2.2 Phosphorylation of Proteins

Stefan Lehr, Jürgen Weiss and Peter Rösen

Introduction

Most proteins undergo co- and/or post-translational modifications, which have influence on the physical and chemical properties, folding, conformation, distribution, stability, activity and, consequently, function of the protein.

Protein phosphorylation represents one of the most important and well-studied post-translational modifications, providing a mechanism of acute and reversible regulation of protein function. Modulation of protein phosphorylation may initiate signal transduction pathways to induce rapid changes in response to hormones, growth factors, and neurotransmitters, enabling an adjustment of the cell to environmental changes. Therefore, phosphorylation plays critical roles in the regulation of many cellular processes including the cell-cycle, growth, apoptosis and signal transduction pathways.

Molecular mechanisms of phosphorylation and their regulation pave the way to understanding their alterations in various physiological states as well as in many disease processes. Therefore phosphorylation of proteins and the activities of protein kinases and phosphatases that define the phosphorylation state may become targets for pharmacological interventions.

Protein Kinases

In eukaryotes, phosphorylations are carried out by protein kinases, a family of evolutionarily related enzymes that transfer the terminal phosphate from ATP to a specific serine, threonine or tyrosine residue on protein substrates. However some kinases are also able to phosphorylate all three types of hydroxy-bearing amino acid residues.

Phosphorylation most often results in a change in protein conformation and thereby in alteration of activity. Alternatively, phosphorylation creates docking sites for other enzymes or adaptor molecules, a strategy that is common to cell membrane receptors to initiate a signalling event upon ligand binding.

Protein kinases represent about 2% of the proteins encoded by eukaryotic genomes (Kennelly 2003). They are roughly divided into several subtypes: protein kinases that requires calcium and/or phospholipid for activity such as the family of protein kinases C (Gutcher et al. 2003; Ping 2003; Takizawa et al. 2003), cAMP-dependent protein kinase (PKA) the activity of which is dependent on cyclic AMP (Biondi and Nebrada 2003; Huang and Sha'afi 1993; Kopperud et al. 2003), protein tyrosine kinase (PTK) that phosphorylates tyrosine residues only (Bogatcheva et al. 2003; Drews et al. 2003; Ferguson 2003; Grimes and Miettinen 2003; Sada and Yamamura 2003; Traxler 2003), and a group of protein kinases known as mitogen activated protein (MAP) kinases (Blanc et al. 2003; Lew 2003; Reddy et al. 2003; Seboldt-Leopold et al. 2003; Starniskova et al. 2002) that are characterized by their requirement for dual phosphorylation. Each protein kinase subtype also has a broad spectrum of substrate specificity.

Therefore, a short synthetic peptide with a defined sequence is commonly used as a substrate for assaying a specific type of protein kinase activity.

Protein Phosphatases

In contrast to protein kinases their counterparts are less characterised. Protein phosphatases are integrally associated with regulation of cellular signalling as counterparts to a variety of protein kinases. Once viewed as simple house-keeping enzymes, newer studies revealed that protein phosphatases are dynamic and highly regulated enzymes (Sim and Ludowyke 2002).

The mechanisms underlying the regulatory roles are likely to be specific for each cell system. Although a number of phosphatases have been identified and targeted to specific binding partners, knowledge about specific phosphatases involved in regulatory cycles and the underlying mechanisms is still scarce, if compared to that about protein kinases.

The PPP gene family is one of the largest families of phosphatases that specifically hydrolyse serine- and threonine-phosphate (Honkanen and Golden 2002).

In addition to serine/threonine phosphatases the human genome encodes approximately 100 phosphatases that belong to the protein tyrosine phosphatase superfamily (PTP). The active site of these phosphatases contains the C(X)5R sequence, known as the PTP signature motif (Zhang et al. 2002; Wang et al. 2003).

To acquire a better understanding of the molecular basis of these regulatory mechanisms, it is essential to elucidate the identity and activity of protein kinases and phosphatases involved in specific signalling pathways and the substrates, as well as the specific phosphorylation sites in the affected proteins. Therefore, identification of the phosphorylated amino acids and knowledge about their precise quantitative distribution within distinct proteins is an important task in protein analysis.

Description of Methods and Practical Approach

Analysis of Phosphoproteins

Phosphoamino acid residues can be divided into four different types: 1. *O*-phosphates (phosphomonoesters) are generated by phosphorylation of the hydroxyamino acids serine, threonine or tyrosine. 2. *N*-phosphates (phosphoamidates) are produced by phosphorylation of the amino groups in arginine, lysine or histidine. 3. Acylphosphates (phosphate anhydrides) are created by the phosphorylation of aspartic or glutamic acid, whereas 4. *S*-phosphates (phosphothioesters) are derivates of cysteine. Because sample preparation is the crucial step for successful investigations, it is important to take account of the chemical stability of the different amino acid derivates. Generally *O*-phosphates are stable under acidic conditions as well as in the presence of hydroxylamine or pyridine, whereas N-phosphates are stable under alkaline conditions, except for phosphoarginine. In contrast the reactive acylphosphates are labile in acid, alkali, hydroxylamine and pyridine. Phosphocysteine, on the other hand, is stable under all these conditions. Therefore the selected method for analysis has to match with these limitations.

Because of their importance for cellular signal transduction, this article will focus on the analysis of *O*-phosphates, i.e. phosphoserine, phosphothreonine and phosphotyrosine.

Analysis of Phosphoproteins Using Specific Antibodies

By now, a wide range of phosphorylation specific antibodies is commercially available for many known proteins, applicable for Western blot analysis, ELISA, etc. Antiphosphotyrosine, -serine and -threonine antibodies are also available enabling analysis of the phosphorylation state of unknown proteins. But in contrast to anti-phosphotyrosine antibodies, which show great specificity and sensitivity in detection of single phosphorylated tyrosine residues, anti-phospho-serine and -threonine antibodies generally fail to detect a single phosphoserine/-threonine with the required specificity and/or sufficient sensitivity. In the case of tyrosine phosphorylation, the phosphorylated tyrosine side chain alone provides a sufficient epitope for antibody detection by its structure. Therefore anti-phosphotyrosine antibodies represent a very useful tool to monitor complex tyrosine phosphorylation patterns, e.g. whole cell lysates. In contrast, phospho-serine/-threonine alone do not form sufficient epitopes for generation of specific antibodies. However, once the primary sequence around the phosphorylation site containing phospho-serine or -threonine has been determined, phosphorylation site-specific antibodies have been generated for a number of proteins. These antibodies are generated against synthetic phosphopeptides modelled on those phosphorylation motifs including additional amino acids in the surrounding of the phosphorylation site. This strategy is very efficient because many kinases, e.g. mitogen activated protein kinases, utilize specific consensus motifs for phosphorylation (Gonzales et al. 1991). Accordingly these phosphorylation specific antibodies are suitable for monitoring changes in the phosphorylation state of several corresponding target proteins.

With immunoassays, quantification of the results often arises as the main problem. Systems are recently commercially available which perform multiplex immunoassays (de Jager et al. 2003), providing the option of reliable quantification (e.g., Luminex 100Ô; Luminex Corporation, Austin, USA). In this system, also adapted for sets of phosphoproteins (e.g., BioRad, Hercules, California, USA), a microplate 96 well format enables simultaneous detection and quantification of up to 100 different analytes per well. Moreover, beside commercially available applications, this setup allows coupling of customized sets of antibodies to 00 different beads. Therefore this system enables achievement of a wide spectrum of information, e.g. of the cellular status, in a single step requiring only a small amount of sample in the μl range. These bead-based assays may help to overcome the limitations of traditional ELISA and Western blot based analyses, especially when multiple parameters need to be analysed from restricted sample amounts (e.g. human or mouse serum) and reliable quantification is required.

Identification of Phosphoamino Acids

The major problem in phosphoamino acid analysis is to discriminate samples containing the phosphorylated protein or peptides from unphosphorylated proteins. Usually only a few percent of the whole amount of a specific protein or peptide is phosphorylated *in vivo* and *in vitro*. Therefore, it is essential to be able to track phosphorylated proteins or peptides through the whole experiment. Up to now radioactive labelling of the proteins with $\gamma^{32}P$ has represented the best and easiest way to achieve reliable results. This approach allows monitoring of each step of the whole analytical process with high sensitivity and prevents an unnoticed loss of phosphorylated components during preparation. Furthermore, quantification of phosphate incorporation is enabled as well as determination of its precise distribution within a protein when more than one site is phosphorylated, by calculating the specific radioactivity

Recently, novel products are available (e.g., Phosphopeptide Isolation Kit; Pierce-Biotechnology, Inc., Rockford, USA) which allow specific enrichment of phosphopeptides and -proteins using immobilized metal ion affinity chromatography (IMAC). Phosphopeptide isolation is performed using the specific interaction of phosphate groups with metal chelating agents such as gallium (Posewitz and Tempst 1999). This may be an easy way to concentrate phosphorylated proteins or peptides and to reduce the complexity of the sample by separating them from unphosphorylated compounds. Even in this case labelling with ^{32}P is recommended to prevent unnoticed loss of phosphorylated compounds.

To get initial data on phosphorylated proteins, phosphopeptide mapping and phosphoamino acid analysis using two-dimensional separation on a thin-layer electrophoresis system (Boyle et al. 1991) is a suitable procedure. This technique allows discrimination between phosphoserine, phosphothreonine and phosphotyrosine. After partial acidic hydrolysis of phosphorylated proteins, phosphoamino acids are separated by two-dimensional thin-layer electrophoresis on cellulose plates. The detection of phosphoamino acids is performed either by staining with ninhydrin or in the case of ^{32}P-labelling by autoradiography. Figure 1 shows the analysis of a ^{32}P-radiolabelled protein phosphorylated solely on serine residues.

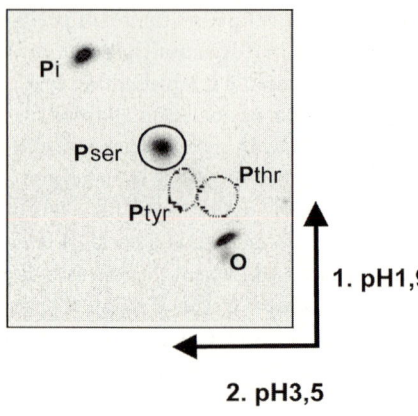

Figure 1
Separation of phosphoamino acids by two-dimensional thin-layer electrophoresis. Subsequent to partial acidic hydrolysis (6 N HCL, 1.5 h, 110 °C) radiolabelled samples (sample volume equivalent to 500 cpm) were separated by two-dimensional electrophoresis on thin-layer cellulose plates. In the first dimension (1D) formic acid (88%)/glacial acid/H_2O (5:15.6:179.4 v/v) pH 1.9 by 1.5 kV for 15 min and glacial acid/pyridine/H_2O (10:1:189 v/v) pH 3.5 by 1.3 kV for 10 min in the second dimension (2D) was used for separation. To determine the exact position of the different phosphoamino acids (Pser, phosphoserine; Pthr, phosphothreonine; Ptyr, phosphotyrosine) 1 µg each of unlabeled phosphoamino acid standard substance was added to the sample. Subsequently the phosphoamino acid standards were detected by staining with ninhydrin and ^{32}P labelled amino acids were visualized by autoradiography. The origin is indicated by (O) and position of inorganic phosphate by (Pi). *Arrows* mark directions for the 2D electrophoresis

Localisation of Phosphorylated Amino Acid Residues

Beside the detection of protein phosphorylation and identification of the different O-phosphate amino acid residues, their exact localization within the protein sequences is a very important challenge. Today mass spectrometry (MS) techniques provide a powerful tool to address this question. The phosphoprotein is digested into peptides of defined size, commonly using trypsin as proteolytic enzyme. Again primary labelling with ^{32}P is recommended, providing a marker for efficient phosphopeptide tracking. The tryptic digest of phosphoproteins may typically produce a complex mixture of up to hundreds of different peptide species resulting in signal suppression of the underrepresented phosphopeptides in MS-analysis. Therefore a high-resolution separation of the mixture, such as a two-dimensional (2D)-HPLC approach (Lehr et al. 1999, 2000; Roth et al. 2000) is essential to reduce the complexity of sample and enrich phosphorylated peptides providing a basis for their successful identification. A commonly used system separates the whole proteolytic digest by anion exchange chromatography in the first dimension with subsequent rechromatography of the radioactive phosphopeptide containing fractions in a second dimension by applying an acetonitrile/water/TFA gradient system. Since phosphopeptides may adsorb irreversibly to iron surfaces, it is recommended to use a so-called bio-inert HPLC and column system, characterized by avoiding iron components, for maximum recovery. Subsequently, separated phosphopeptides can be analysed by MS-techniques to determine their exact molecular mass. Therefore, the highly sensitive matrix-assisted-laser-desorption-ionisation (MALDI)-MS is an appropriate method. Phosphorylated peptides exhibit an increase in peptide mass of 80 D, specific for a phosphorylated amino acid side chain. Because phosphoserine, -threonine and -tyrosine show different behaviours during MS-analysis, examination procedures have to be adjusted for the different O-phosphates. In contrast to phosphotyrosine, which is more stable, phosphoserine and -threonine frequently lose their phosphate group during MS-analysis. Identification of those phosphopeptides is then possible through the detection of marker ions represented by signals at [M+H]$^+$ minus 80 Da (loss of HPO$_3^{2-}$) and [M+H]$^+$ minus 98 Da (loss of H$_3$PO$_4^-$) in the mass spectra. Determination of the primary structure of the three kinds of O-phosphopeptides can be done further through fragmentation analysis of the selected ions by MALDI-PSD (post source decay). This technique provides information about the amino acid sequence of the selected peptide including the localisation of the phosphorylation site. However, in the cases of phosphoserine and -threonine, their unstable nature during MS-analysis sometimes makes it impossible to localise the phosphorylated amino acid residue within the peptide sequence. To overcome these restrictions, classic peptide sequencing by Edman degradation provides an ideal completion, giving positive evidence for O-phosphates. Phosphorylated serine is detectable through its derivate S-ethylcysteine and threonine through methyl-S-ethyl cysteine, whereas tyrosine exhibits a gap in the sequence because it is insoluble in commonly used Edman chemicals. A combinatory strategy consisting of MS analysis and Edman degradation, furthermore gives the opportunity to validate the results. Therefore the combination of Edman degradation and MS-techniques provides the most powerful tool to identify phosphorylation sites in proteins.

As a feasible alternative, phosphopeptides in a mixture can be analysed by electrospray-ionisation (ESI) tandem mass spectrometry (MS/MS) directly coupled to a nano-HPLC system, especially when ^{32}P labelling is not practicable. Analysis of highly complex mixtures, e.g. proteolytic digests of whole cell lysates, is preferentially subjected to a multidimensional chromatography/MS approach (Wolters et al. 2001). In a first dimension the peptides are collected on a strong cation exchange (SCX) column that is positioned upstream of a reverse-phase (RP) column for the second dimension separation. Depending on their isoelectric point, successive peptide fractions are released from the SCX-column by salt steps of increasing concentration at low organic solvent concentrations and are captured by the RP-column. Subsequently, depending on their hydrophobicity, peptides are eluted from the RP-column with a gradient of increasing organic solvent concentration between each salt step, directly into a mass spectrometer. Then, to analyse the enormous quantities of acquired sequence data, dedicated software packages are used to identify potential phosphorylation sites.

Examples and Troubleshooting

Figures 2–4 show an example of an in-depth analysis of complex protein phosphorylation. The multi-docking protein Gab-1 (Grb-associated binder), being involved in signal transduction of several hormones and cytokines, exhibits 17 potential tyrosine and 47 potential serine/threonine phosphorylation sites. Therefore, the elucidation of the localisation of incorporated phosphate and its quantitative distribution corresponding to phosphorylation events by different protein kinases is essential for understanding differentially initiated signal transduction pathways. Recombinant

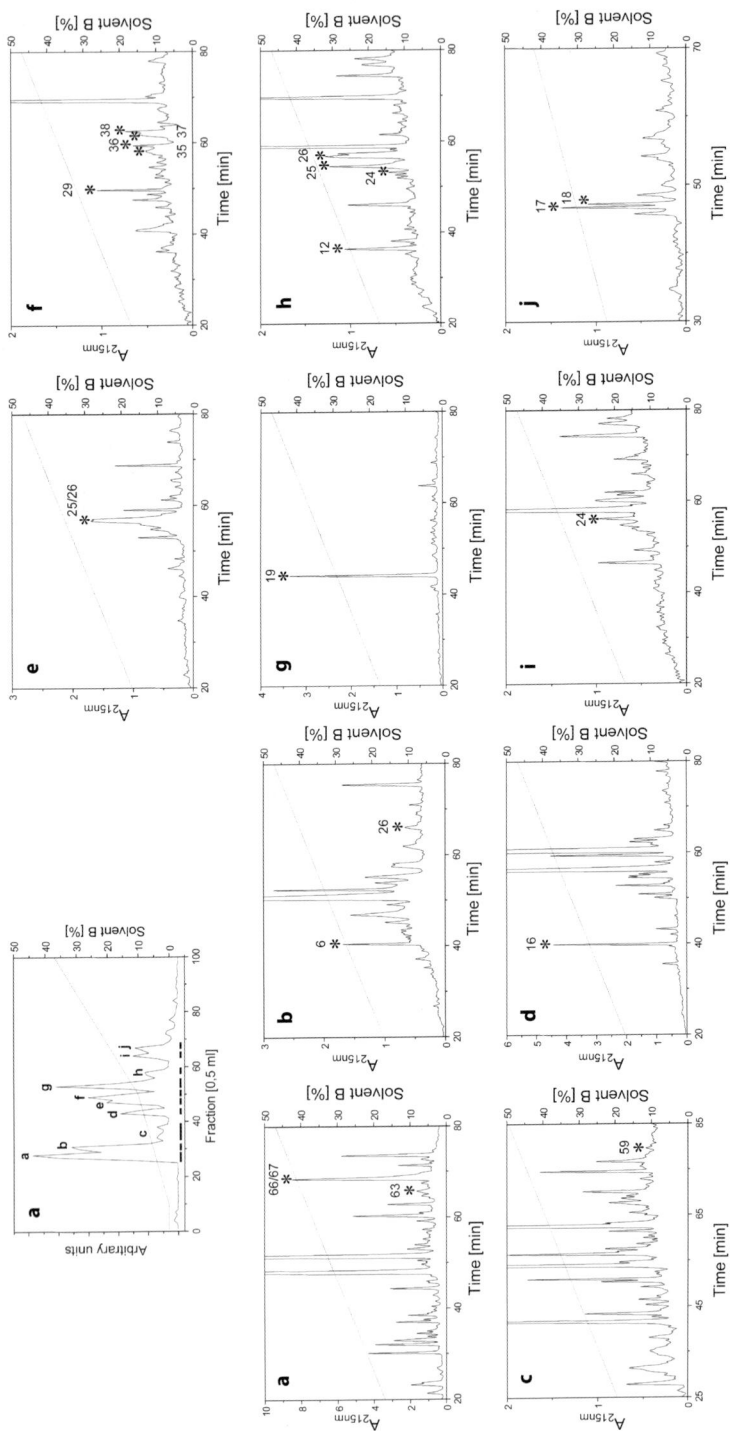

human Gab-1 protein was phosphorylated by the human insulin receptor using ^{32}P labelling, *in vitro*. For preliminary purification of Gab-1 protein SDS-PAGE separation was performed. Subsequently, the phosphorylated Gab-1 protein bands were excised from the gel and subjected to in-gel digestion with trypsin. Figure 2 shows a 2-D HPLC separation of the tryptic digest of Gab-1. In the first dimension, anion-exchange chromatography was performed (A). The fractions containing radioactivity were selected for a second dimension separation using C18 reverse phase (RP)-HPLC (a–j).

Reverse phase fractions containing radioactivity were subsequently subjected to MALDI-MS analysis. Figure 3 shows a MALDI-PSD fragment analysis of the phosphopeptide of m/z 3024.4 recovered in RP-fractions h/12, g/19 and c/59. Besides determining the exact molecular mass of the peptide, giving positive evidence of phosphorylation (shift in mass of +80 D), fragment data achieved by PSD analysis (b- and y-ion series) allowed identification of the phosphorylated amino acid residue Y_{*447} in the known primary structure [NVLTVGSVSSEELDENY$_{*447}$VPMNPNSPPR (aa 431-457)]. Overall, using this approach eight different phosphorylation sites were identified in Gab-1, specific for insulin receptor phosphorylation. Moreover, the utilisation of ^{32}P labelling allowed quantifying of the distribution of phosphate incorporation among the different phosphorylation sites of Gab-1 summarised in Fig. 4. This approach was used several times, elucidating complex phosphorylation patterns of different proteins, with great success. Nevertheless it has to be mentioned, that this strategy is only effective when sufficient sample amounts (nmoles) are available. The

◀ **Figure 2**
Two-dimensional HPLC analysis of tryptic phosphopeptides derived from human Grb-associated binder- 1 (Gab-1) phosphorylated by the human insulin receptor, *in vitro*. Initial recombinant Gab-1 (5 nmol) was phosphorylated for 30 min at 22 °C in kinase buffer (50 mM, HEPES/NaOH (pH 7.5), 5 mM MgCl$_2$, 5 mM MnCl$_2$, 1 mM DTT, 1 mM Na$_3$VO$_4$, 1 µM poly(lysine), 250 µM ATP, 0.1 mCi/ml [γ-^{32}P] ATP) using 0.3 nmol recombinant insulin receptor kinase (rIR). Subsequently phosphorylated Gab-1 was separated by SDS – PAGE and the radioactive Gab-1 protein band was excised out of the gel. Gel slices were washed in 30% acetonitrile/20 mM ammonium bicarbonate and digestion with trypsin (50 µg sequencing grade; Roche, Basel) was performed over night at 37 °C in 20 mM ammonium bicarbonate. The eluted peptides were then subjected to HPLC separation. First dimension (A): HPLC anion exchange chromatography of trypsinised Gab-1 phosphorylated by IR using ^{32}P-labelling. Peptides were separated on a Nucleogel SAX 1000-8/46, 50×4.6 mm (Macherey & Nagel, Düren, Germany) using a Beckman Gold solvent delivery system. HPLC flow rate was adjusted to 0.5 ml/min and peptides were eluted beginning with 100% solvent A (20 mM ammonium acetate, pH 7.0) and 0% solvent B (0.5 M KH$_2$PO$_4$, pH4.0). The amount of buffer B was increased to 10% over 40 min and from 10 to 50% over during the following 75 min. Fractions of 0.5 ml were collected and phosphate incorporations were determined by counting Cerenkov radiation. For second dimension analysis, radioactive fractions were pooled according to the solid bars. Second dimension (B): Reversed-phase separation (C18) of the pooled fractions (a–j) containing radioactivity. Pooled fractions a–j were subjected to rechromatography by C18 reversed phase HPLC. Peptides were separated on a C18 reversed-phase column (250×0.8 mm, 5 µM particle size, 300 Å pore size; LC Packings, The Netherlands) using an ABI 140 D solvent delivery system (Applied Biosystems, Foster City, CA, USA). HPLC flow rate was adjusted to 16 µl/min. Elution started with 95% solvent A (0.1% TFA) and 5% solvent B (0.08% TFA, 84% acetonitrile (v/v)). The content of solution B was raised to 50% within 90 min. Peptide containing fractions were measured by Cerenkov radiation. Radioactive fractions (designated by *asterisks* followed by the fraction number) were subjected to MS and Edman analysis

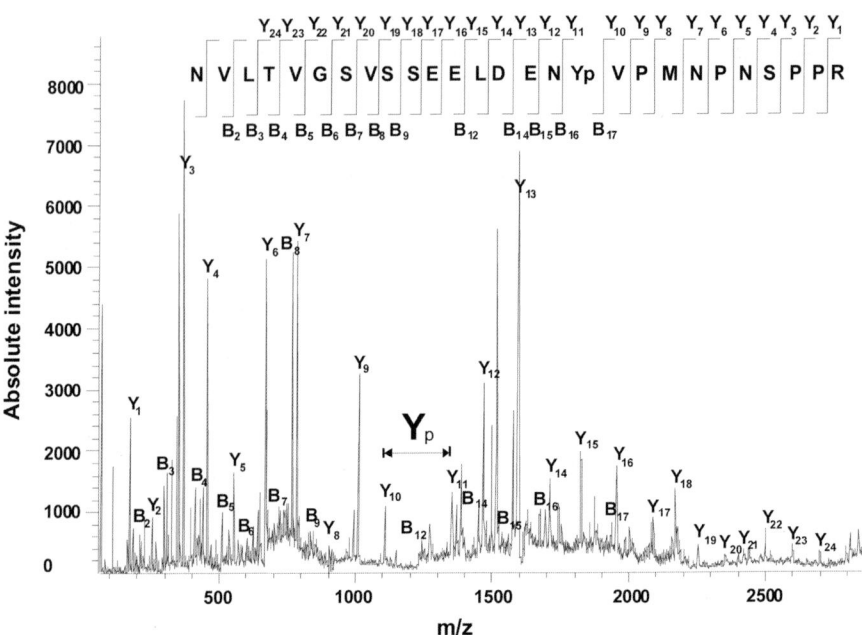

Figure 3
Fragmentation mass spectrum of a Gab-1 derived single charged phosphopeptide ion representing m/z 3024.4 (RP-fractions h/12, g/19, c/59). The phosphotyrosine peptide NVLTVGSVSSEELDENY$_{•447}$VPMNPNSPPR (aa 431-457) was identified by designated b- and y-fragment ion series. For MALDI mass spectrometry, 0.5 μl of selected fraction was directly prepared on to the MALDI target with a saturated solution of α-cyano-4-hydroxy-cinnamic acid in acetonitrile/0.1% TFA (1:1 (v/v)). Mass spectrometry was performed on a REFLEX III system (Bruker Daltonik, Bremen, Germany) equipped with a SCOUT 384 multiprobe ion source. Positive ion mass spectra were acquired in a linear and reflector mode using an acceleration voltage of 20 kV. PSD spectra were recorded in 14 windows with reflectron voltages between 21.6 kV and 0.65 kV. In addition to manual interpretation of PSD fragment ion spectra, the SEQUEST algorithm (OWL sequence database; University of Leeds) was used to identify the peptide phosphorylation sites

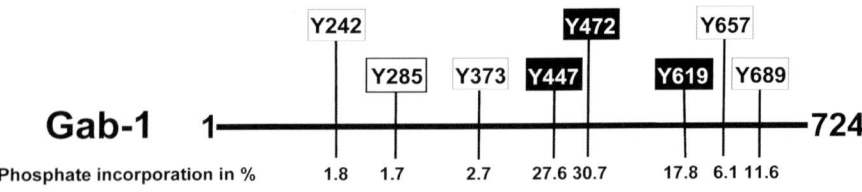

Figure 4
Identified phosphorylation sites in Gab-1 specific for the insulin receptor. Phosphorylation sites identified (MALDI-PSD-MS and Edman sequencing) are listed above the schema of Gab-1 protein. Quantitative distribution of phosphate incorporation among the different phosphorylation sites is listed below the schema of Gab-1. The specific predominant phosphorylation sites for the insulin receptor identified are displayed in black boxes

starting amount has to be so large, because usually less than 0.5–1% of the total amount of the protein to be analysed is phosphorylated. This ratio is worse for each single phosphorylation event, when several different sites are phosphorylated within a protein as shown in the example with Gab-1. Even though nmolar amounts of protein were initially used for analysis, these samples stretched the sensitivity of Edman degradation (low picomolar) and MS-analysis (subpicomolar range), because some sites were less than 0.05% phosphorylated.

The high sample amounts initially required are normally achievable with recombinant proteins. In this case, the combination of ^{32}P labelling, 2D-HPLC, MS-analysis and Edman degradation may function as a basic approach capable of analysing localisation as well as quantitative distribution of protein phosphorylation with high sensitivity and confidence.

It should be mentioned, that such combinatorial approaches to identification of phosphorylation sites are only applicable in specially equipped and trained laboratories. Because of their complex nature it is recommended to contact research groups or service units familiar with these procedures. Taking notice of this fact will prevent wasting much time and money. Preparation of the sample especially should be performed with the highest accuracy and adjusted to the following analytical steps, because it is the most critical step in the analysis.

References

Biondi RM, Nebreda AR (2003) Signalling specificity of Ser/Thr protein kinases through docking-site-mediated interactions. Biochem J. 372:1–13

Blanc A, Pandey NR, Srivastava AK (2003) Synchronous activation of ERK 1/2, p38mapk and PKB/Akt signaling by H2O2 in vascular smooth muscle cells: potential involvement in vascular disease (review). Int J Mol Med 11: 229–234

Bogatcheva NV, Garcia JG, Verin AD (2002) Role of tyrosine kinase signaling in endothelial cell barrier regulation. Vascul Pharmacol 39:201–212

Boyle WJ, van der GP, Hunter T (1991) Phosphopeptide mapping and phosphoamino acid analysis by two-dimensional separation on thin-layer cellulose plates. Methods Enzymol 201:110–49

de Jager W, te VH, Prakken BJ, Kuis W, Rijkers GT (2003) Simultaneous detection of 15 human cytokines in a single sample of stimulated peripheral blood mononuclear cells. Clin Diagn Lab Immunol 10:133–139

Drevs J, Medinger M, Schmidt-Gersbach C, Weber R, Unger C (2003) Receptor tyrosine kinases: the main targets for new anticancer therapy. Curr Drug Targets 4:113–121

Gonzalez FA, Raden DL, Davis RJ (1991) Identification of substrate recognition determinants for human ERK1 and ERK2 protein kinases. J Biol Chem 266:22159–22163

Grimes ML, Miettinen HM (2003) Receptor tyrosine kinase and G-protein coupled receptor signaling and sorting within endosomes. J Neurochem 84:905–918

Gutcher I, Webb PR, Anderson NG (2003) The isoform-specific regulation of apoptosis by protein kinase C. Cell Mol Life Sci 60:1061–1070

Honkanen RE, Golden T (2002) Regulators of serine/threonine protein phosphatases at the dawn of a clinical era? Curr Med Chem 9:2055–2075

Huang C, Sha'afi R (1993) Protein kinase in blood cell function. CRC Press, Inc., London

Kennelly PJ (2003) Archaeal protein kinases and protein phosphatases: insights from genomics and biochemistry. Biochem J 370:373–389

Kopperud R, Krakstad C, Selheim F, Doskeland SO (2003) cAMP effector mechanisms. Novel twists for an 'old' signaling system. FEBS Lett 546:121–126

Lehr S, Kotzka J, Herkner A, Klein E, Siethoff C, Knebel B, Noelle V, Bruning JC, Klein HW, Meyer HE, Krone W, Muller-Wieland D (1999) Identification of tyrosine phosphorylation sites in human Gab-1 protein by EGF receptor kinase *in vitro*. Biochemistry 38:151–159

Lehr S, Kotzka J, Herkner A, Sikmann A, Meyer HE, Krone W, Muller-Wieland D (2000) Identification of major tyrosine phosphorylation sites in the human insulin receptor substrate Gab-1 by insulin receptor kinase *in vitro*. Biochemistry 39:10898–10907

Lew J (2003) MAP kinases and CDKs: kinetic basis for catalytic activation. Biochemistry 42:849–856
Ping P (2003) A new chapter in cardiac PKC signaling studies: searching for isoform-specific molecular targets. Focus on: isoenzyme-selective regulation of SERCA2 gene expression by protein kinase C in neonatal rat ventricular myocytes". Am J Physiol Cell Physiol 285:C19–C21
Posewitz MC, Tempst P (1999) Immobilized gallium (III) affinity chromatography of phosphopeptides. Anal Chem 71:2883–2892
Reddy KB, Nabha SM, Atanaskova N (2003) Role of MAP kinase in tumor progression and invasion. Cancer Metastasis Rev 22:395–403
Roth G, Kotzka J, Kremer L, Lehr S, Lohaus C, Meyer HE, Krone W, Muller-Wieland D (2000) MAP kinases Erk1/2 phosphorylate sterol regulatory element-binding protein (SREBP)-1a at serine 117 *in vitro*. J Biol Chem 275:33302–33307
Sada K, Yamamura H (2003) Protein-tyrosine kinases and adaptor proteins in FcepsilonRI-mediated signaling in mast cells. Curr Mol Med 3:85–94
Sebolt-Leopold JS, Van Becelaere K, Hook K, Herrera R (2003) Biomarker assays for phosphorylated MAP kinase. Their utility for measurement of MEK inhibition. Methods Mol Med 85:31–38
Sim AT, Ludowyke RI (2002) The complex nature of protein phosphatases. IUBMB Life 53:283–286
Strniskova M, Barancik M, Ravingerova T (2002) Mitogen-activated protein kinases and their role in regulation of cellular processes. Gen Physiol Biophys. 21:231–255.
Takizawa T, Kato M, Suzuki M, Tachibana A, Motegi Y, Fujiu T, Kimura H, Arakawa H, Mochizuki H, Tokuyama K, Morikawa A (2003) Distinct isoforms of protein kinase C are involved in human eosinophil functions induced by platelet-activating factor. Int Arch Allergy Immunol 131 Suppl 1:15–19
Traxler P (2003) Tyrosine kinases as targets in cancer therapy–successes and failures. Expert Opin Ther Targets 7:215–234
Wang WQ, Sun JP, Zhang ZY (2003) An overview of the protein tyrosine phosphatase superfamily. Curr Top Med Chem. 3:739–748
Wolters DA, Washburn MP, Yates JR, III (2001) An automated multidimensional protein identification technology for shotgun proteomics. Anal Chem 73:5683–5690
Zhang ZY, Zhou B, Xie L (2002) Modulation of protein kinase signaling by protein phosphatases and inhibitors. Pharmacol Ther 93:307–317

Receptor and Binding Studies

Peter Hein, Martin C. Michel, Kirsten Leineweber, Thomas Wieland,
Nina Wettschureck and Stefan Offermanns

6.3.1
Radioligand Binding Studies in Cardiovascular Research (Saturation and Competition Binding Studies)

Peter Hein and Martin C. Michel

Introduction

Radioligand binding studies are an important tool to quantify and qualitatively characterize receptors and hence have become a universal tool of cardiovascular research. While radioligand binding experiments are relatively simple to perform, interpretation of the results and optimisation of the experimental settings are more complex. Several criteria must be met to consider a labelled binding site a receptor: Binding should be of high affinity, saturable, stereospecific and have a ligand recognition profile similar to that of a functional response in that tissue. A hilariously funny description of the fundamental principles of radioligand binding has been presented by Guth (1982).

Radioligand binding experiments can be divided into two major types of experiments, kinetic and equilibrium studies. Kinetic (i.e. association and dissociation) studies are required to define optimal assay conditions. On theoretical grounds they also allow the most reliable determination of the affinity of a radioligand for its cognate receptor. However, kinetic studies are cumbersome to perform and hence rarely used in routine studies. Their most frequent application is in the phase of characterization of novel radioligands. Once radioligands have been characterized and proper assay conditions have been established, the translation of such assays to cardiovascular tissues can be done in most cases without repeating the kinetic studies.

The vast majority of applications of radioligand binding studies are based on equilibrium binding studies. The key molecular principle underlying such experiments is the idea that association of a radioligand with its cognate receptor and dissociation of the resulting ligand-receptor complex are reversible processes that occur concomitantly until equilibrium has been reached. Key factors in determining the

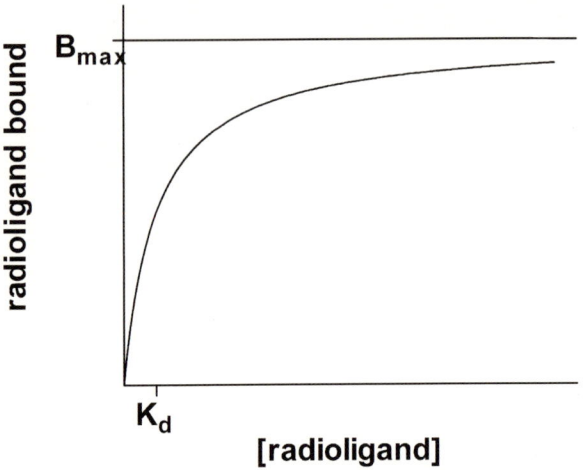

Figure 1
A saturation binding experiment allows measuring K_d and B_{max} of a ligand/receptor-pair

development of equilibrium conditions are incubation time, incubation temperature and assay volume (the latter as a measure of amount of radioligand relative to number of binding sites in the assay). Equilibrium binding studies can be divided into two main types of experiments, i.e. saturation and competition studies (with the latter often but incorrectly referred to as displacement studies). Saturation binding studies allow determination of the affinity of a receptor for a radioligand and, more importantly, receptor densities. Competition binding studies allow a pharmacological characterization of receptors and, under proper experimental conditions, identification of the receptor subtype distribution within a tissue or cell line.

Saturation binding studies are performed using several concentrations of a radioligand and allow determination of the dissociation constant (K_d) and number of binding sites in the assay (B_{max}) for the radioligand (Fig. 1). The K_d-value is a measure of the affinity of the ligand for its binding sites. Since the K_d is the concentration at which the ligand binds to half its binding sites, the ligand's affinity for the receptor is small when its K_d is large. Likewise, ligands with a high affinity have small K_ds. Sometimes the affinity is given as pK_d, i.e. the negative logarithm of K_d. K_d is a constant and, unless a new radioligand or receptor is characterized, is largely used as an internal quality control of a binding assay. The receptor density in a tissue or cell line is called B_{max}. B_{max} values are typically adjusted to account for tissue content in the assay, e.g. for protein content or tissue wet weight and expressed as fmol/mg protein or fmol/mg wet weight, respectively. Saturation binding experiments can also be used to determine whether a given drug indeed acts as a competitive antagonist at a receptor of interest. Thus, concomitant saturation binding experiments in the absence and presence of a competitor should yield identical B_{max} values but distinct apparent K_d values if the competing drug acts in a competitive manner. In this case the shift in K_d value can even be used to determine antagonist affinity in a manner analogous to that used when analyzing the shift of an agonist concentration-response curve by an antagonist in organ bath experiments with isolated tissues.

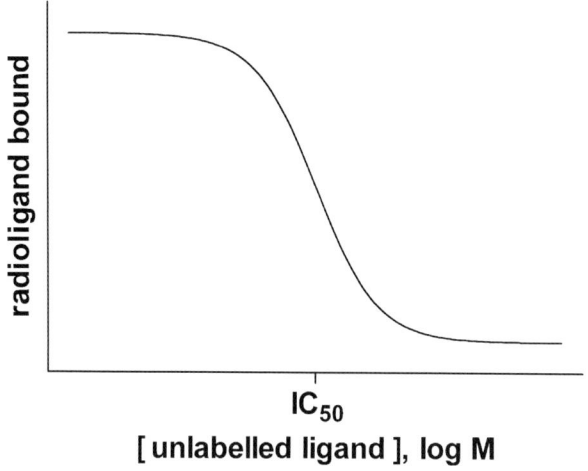

Figure 2
C_{50}, the concentration of the ligand causing 50% inhibition of radioligand binding, is determined by a competition binding experiment

Competition binding studies, sometimes also referred to as displacement studies, use a single concentration of a radioligand that is competed for by multiple concentrations of another, not radioactively labelled compound (Fig. 2). They allow the pharmacological characterization of binding sites. Competition studies primarily yield the concentration of the inhibitor causing 50% inhibition of radioligand binding (IC_{50}), which can be converted into the inhibitor constant of the inhibitor (K_i) using appropriate equations. If a tissue contains multiple binding sites for a given radioligand and the competing compound differentiates them, biphasic or even multiphasic competition curves are obtained which allow not only determination of K_i values at the various sites but also an estimate of the relative quantitative contributions of each site.

The following considerations are primarily developed for radioligand binding studies with G-protein-coupled receptors, which are the most frequent subjects of studies in cardiovascular research. While radioligand binding studies to other receptor classes such as ligand-gated ion channels, receptors with intrinsic enzyme activity or ligand-activated transcription factors (e.g. glucocorticoid receptors) follow similar principles, not all details given below apply to these other receptor classes. On the other hand, many of the approaches described hereafter can also be applied to non-receptor proteins such as uptake carriers using minor variations of the protocols given below.

Descriptions of the Methods and Practical Approach

Receptor Theory

Binding of the ligand to the receptor follows the law of mass action. The ligand and receptor associate and form a ligand-receptor-complex, or they may dissociate again.

$$\text{receptor} + \text{ligand} \leftrightarrow \text{receptor} \cdot \text{ligand} \tag{1}$$

The association rate is called K_{on}, and the amount of newly associated receptor-ligand complex depends on K_{on}, the concentration of the free ligand and the concentration of free receptors. Accordingly, the dissociation rate K_{off}, and the concentration of ligand-receptor complexes describe the number of dissociations. At equilibrium concentrations, the rate at which new receptor-ligand complexes are formed equals the rate at which they dissociate.

$$[\text{ligand}] \times [\text{receptor}] \times K_{on} = [\text{receptor} \cdot \text{ligand}] \times K_{off} \tag{2}$$

This may be rearranged to

$$\frac{[\text{ligand}] \times [\text{receptor}]}{[\text{receptor} \cdot \text{ligand}]} = \frac{K_{off}}{K_{on}} = K_d \tag{3}$$

The quotient K_{off}/K_{on} is named the equilibrium dissociation constant K_d. It has the units of a concentration and, more specifically, is the concentration at which half the receptors are occupied by the ligand or free, respectively. Note that there is a specific K_d value for each ligand/receptor-pair, and since in different tissues different receptor-subtypes (or even conformational different states of the same subtype) may be present, there may be different K_d values for the same ligand and receptor in different tissues.

K_{off} has a major effect on the time required to reach equilibrium and hence usually governs the choice of incubation time for saturation and competition equilibrium binding studies. Equilibrium is often reached after 45–60 min, but with some ligands or receptors, longer time periods may be necessary. It should also be noted that K_{off} is affected by the incubation temperature, but this has little effect on kinetic determination of K_d as long as K_{on} and K_{off} are measured at the same temperature (for criteria for choice of temperature see below).

Radioligands

Chemically, radioligands can be derived from agonists or antagonists, and it should be noted that the two classes of drugs label different receptor populations. Thus, antagonists theoretically should label all receptors while agonists typically only label a fraction thereof with high affinity. Therefore, antagonists are usually preferred as radioligand unless labelling the receptor population in a high affinity state for agonists is specifically attempted. However, for some receptor classes, e.g. for many peptide receptors, only agonist radioligands are available, which are typically radiolabelled forms of the endogenous ligand. Moreover, it should be noted that in some cases antagonist radioligands from distinct chemical classes may label different numbers of receptors, even if it is guaranteed that only one receptor subtype exists within the assay (Hein et al. 2000).

In some cases a given receptor can be labelled with either a more lipophilic or a more hydrophilic radioligand, e.g. for muscarinic acetylcholine receptors with [^{3}H]-quinuclidinyl-benzylate or [^{3}H]-N-methyl-scopolamine, respectively. While more lipophilic radioligands tend to have more non-specific binding (see below), they also tend to label greater receptor numbers. This is due to the fact that, with intact cells, some receptors are located intracellularly or, with membrane preparations, in spontaneously formed inside-out vesicles, and hence are inaccessible to hydrophilic ligands.

Different radioisotopes can be used to label ligands, with tritium ([^{3}H]) and iodine ([^{125}I]) being used most frequently. Since [^{3}H] and [^{125}I] emit distinct types of radiation, different methods for detection and hence different hardware are required. The key advantage of [^{3}H] is that it does not change the molecular structure of the ligand because a hydrogen atom is exchanged with its radioactive homologue. A practical advantage is the long half-life of [^{3}H] which allows storage of the radioligand for extended periods of time. On the other hand, tritiated radioligands have rather low specific activity (usually less than 100 Ci/mmol), which may lead to weak radioactive signals in some cases. This is mainly a problem with radioligands with very high, i.e. subnanomolar, affinity. The specific activity of the tritiated compounds slowly declines over time, as tritiated molecules become untritiated. Since this does not *per se* destroy the chemical integrity of the radioligand, the fraction of labelled molecules will become less. Because of the long half-life of tritium, this is mainly a problem when you store the radioligand for a long time (years), as long as reasonably fresh stocks are used, the decay of tritium does not have to be corrected for. In contrast, high specific radioactivity (typically 2200 Ci/mmol) is the key advantage of iodinated radioligands. This is counterbalanced by possible disadvantages. Introduction of iodine into a molecule may change its affinity for the target receptor, particularly if it is a low molecular weight compound (it seems to be less of a problem with larger ligands such as peptides). Moreover, based on the shorter half-life of [^{125}I], iodinated radioligands cannot easily be stored over extended time periods without marked loss of activity; hence, it is usually recommended to use fresh stock every month. Finally, it should be remembered that radioactive decay of [^{125}I] tends to destroy the ligand chemically. Hence, correction for radioactive decay is typically not necessary since the amount of ligand and the amount of radioactivity decline in parallel.

While the radioactivity emitted by [^{125}I] can be measured directly using appropriate hardware, the counting of [^{3}H] usually requires the use of scintillation cocktails and counters. The efficiency of counting depends on a variety of factors including hardware-specific ones and, in the case of [^{3}H] also depends on the scintillation fluid being used. The choice of scintillation fluid depends on the type of sample (e.g. relative amount of aqueous fluid contained therein) but can also involve factors such as environmental safety.

Counting efficiency must be taken into consideration when experimental results (usually obtained as counts per minute, cpm) are converted into disintegrations per minute (dpm) to ultimately allow conversion into molar units. Data-sheets for radioligands often state the specific activity in Ci/mmol. However, at the end of the experiment you are measuring dpm or cpm which can be transformed to molar concentrations, with intermediary conversion of cpm to dpm not always being necessary. By definition, 1 Ci equals 2.22×10^{12} disintegrations per minute. To convert Z Ci/mmol to Y cpm/fmol, use the following equation:

$$Y = Z \times 2.22 \times \text{counter efficiency} \tag{4}$$

If you count C cpm in a volume of V ml, you can compute the concentration according to:

$$\frac{C}{Y} \div V = \frac{C}{Y \times V} = \frac{C}{Z \times 2.22 \times e \times V} \tag{5}$$

with e being the relative counting efficiency (e.g. 0.4 for 40%) and Z the specific activity in Ci/mmol.

Buffer and Incubation Conditions

Fortunately, most radioligand binding assays are not very sensitive to changes in buffer conditions (with experiments involving receptor agonists being an exception) and buffer systems established for well-characterized radioligands can easily be picked from the literature. The choice of buffer depends on the receptor type under investigation. While radioligand binding experiments are usually carried out in cell or tissue homogenates, it is also possible to perform them with intact cells. Although it is not necessary to establish a physiological environment for binding studies with intact cells, a somewhat isotonic buffer should be used to avoid shrinkage or bloating of cells due to buffer hyper- or hypo-osmolarity, respectively. For binding studies with cell or tissue homogenates hypotonic buffers are used in most cases. Buffering is mostly achieved using Tris, HEPES or phosphate buffer. While Tris is widely used, it has the disadvantage of having a pK_A value (>10) far from physiological pH. Moreover, the pH of a Tris-buffered solution is quite temperature-dependent and hence its pH must be titrated at the desired incubation temperature.

Frequently, chelating substances such as EDTA are added to prevent endogenous enzymes from degrading membranes and/or proteins. In some cases ascorbic acid or other anti-oxidants are added to prevent oxidation of the radioligand or competing agents, but this may also be harmful since e.g. the specific binding of [^{125}I]-BE 2254 (also known as [^{125}I]-HEAT) to α_1-adrenoceptors is markedly inhibited by ascorbic acid. When an agonist is used as radioligand or competing ligand, the ionic composition of the buffer can have additional requirements such as the inclusion of magnesium. Moreover, agonist binding to some receptors is sensitive to sodium.

The choice of temperature affects the kinetics of radioligand binding to its receptor. In most cases 25 °C or 37 °C are used, with the higher temperature yielding equilibrium faster and hence requiring shorter incubation times. In some cases incubations for long times are carried out at 4 °C, e.g. in order to look at total *vs.* cell surface receptors differentially in intact cells.

Specific and Non-Specific Binding

Within the incubation mixture only a small fraction of the radioligand binds to the receptor of interest, and this fraction is designated "specific" binding. Another fraction binds to sites distinct from the receptor of interest and is called "non-specific" binding. A third fraction of the radioligand does not bind at all but remains free in solution and is referred to as "free" radioligand. The analysis of radioligand binding studies assumes that only a small fraction of the radioligand binds, and hence that the concentration of the free radioligand is approximately equal to the total concentration added. If the percentage of bound (specific and non-specific together) exceeds 10% of total radioligand, ligand depletion occurs, which prevents equilibrium conditions and hence invalidates analysis of the data. Thus, it is necessary that free radioligand is always in great excess of bound radioligand, i.e. that at least 90% of the total amount of radioligand in the assay remains unbound, with a greater percentage being even better. Ligand depletion is frequently a problem when the assay contains a very high receptor number, e.g. when transfected cells, and a tritiated radioligand with subnanomolar affinity are used. Such problems can be avoided by increasing the assay volume, thereby increasing the amount of radioligand but not that of receptors.

Non-specific binding may involve binding to receptors other than the target receptor (if the radioligand is not sufficiently specific) as well as truly non-specific binding, e.g. to cell membrane lipids or the wall of the test tube. To discriminate specific and non-specific binding, a number of samples within each assay (typically one for each radioligand concentration being tested) are incubated in the additional presence of a high concentration of an agent to define non-specific binding. Specific binding is then calculated as the difference between total binding and non-specific binding. To define non-specific binding a competing compound should be chosen that also binds to the receptor of interest with high specificity but, if possible, belongs to a different chemical class. Using the non-labelled form of the radioligand to define non-specific binding should be avoided if possible, but this may not be feasible e.g. for some peptide receptors where specific agents apart from the native agonist peptide are frequently not available. The concentration of the competing agent used to define non-specific binding should be so high that it practically occupies all receptors of interest, i.e. typically about 1000× its K_d at that receptor. Before starting a major project with a new radioligand it is useful to determine the appropriate concentration of the compound used for definition of non-specific binding experimentally in a competition-binding assay. From such a competition curve a concentration can be picked which is high enough to yield complete competition but not so high that it causes non-specific effects in its own right.

Pseudo-non-specific binding, i.e. binding to other receptors due to insufficient pharmacological specificity of the radioligand, can become a serious problem when the definition of non-specific binding involves a compound that also lacks pharmacological specificity and also binds to this additional receptor. For example, both the β-adrenoceptor radioligand [^{3}H]-dihydroalprenolol and the antagonist propranolol can also bind to certain serotonin receptors at high concentrations. Hence, attempts to label β-adrenoceptors using too high a concentration of these two compounds

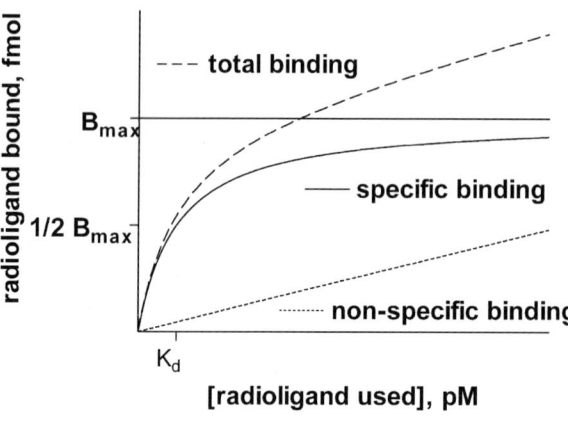

Figure 3
Specific binding is obtained by subtracting non-specific binding from total. Note that non-specific binding increases linearly with the concentration of the radioligand, while specific binding becomes saturated at B_{max}

may also label serotonin receptors, and this may masquerade as "specific" binding. Whether the "specific" binding of a given radioligand is indeed specific for the target receptor can be judged on the basis of its affinity (K_d value) as well as upon the results of competition studies with a range of chemically distinct compounds with known affinities for the receptor of interest.

When reporting results of radioligand binding experiments, the typical degree of non-specific binding should be mentioned. In this regard specific binding is by definition saturable, whereas non-specific increases linearly with the concentration of the radioligand for all practical purposes (Fig. 3). Hence, the percentage of non-specific binding within a given experiment always depends on the concentration of the radioligand. Thus, it is customary to report the percentage of non-specific binding for a radioligand concentration close to its K_d value. High levels of non-specific binding may make interpretation of the results dubious. In that case assay conditions should be carefully revised to minimize non-specific binding.

General Protocol Considerations

A radioligand binding experiment can be divided into five steps: preparing the assay, preparing the cell or membrane suspension, incubation, separating bound from free ligand, and data analysis. While the first and the last steps are somewhat different for saturation and competition binding assays, the three steps in between are typically the same for both types of experiments. Hence, we will first discuss these three steps and then the specific aspects of assay preparation and data analysis in saturation and competition binding experiments.

Preparing the Cell or Membrane Suspension

Radioligand binding experiments can be performed with cell and tissue homogenates, intact cells, tissue sections (autoradiography) or solubilised receptors. Each of these approaches has different advantages and disadvantages. Homogenates are used most frequently, and the other techniques are mainly employed for specific questions that cannot be easily answered using homogenates. Thus, we will focus on homogenates here. A detailed discussion of the pros and cons of the other techniques has been provided elsewhere (Hulme and Buckley 1992).

To avoid degradation of the receptors within a cell or tissue, it is paramount that tissues are rapidly excised and that the entire membrane preparation is performed under well cooled conditions, i.e. at 4 °C. For most applications it is possible to snap freeze tissues and to perform the homogenization later with thawed tissue or to freeze the freshly prepared membrane preparation for later use in a binding experiment. If such storage is planned, it is good to store at temperatures not exceeding -70 °C. Tissues are usually minced with scissors prior to homogenization. For the latter step, a variety of devices are commercially available. For soft tissues Potter-Elvehjem glass/glass or glass/Teflon homogenizers are most frequently used, whereas for tougher tissues Polytron-type devices are preferred (Hulme and Buckley 1992). The type and intensity of homogenization also depend on the desired outcome, i.e. whether crude homogenates or specific subcellular fractions are desired. It should be kept in mind that the homogeneity of the membrane preparation is a key determinant of data scatter in the assay.

Depending on the experimental aims, subcellular fractions are frequently prepared by centrifugation, sometimes involving density gradient centrifugations. The use of more centrifugation steps increases the purity of the preparation at the cost of yield and time. The most desirable balance between these factors depends on the cell or tissue and receptor under investigation.

For example, β-adrenoceptor binding assays have been performed on human heart biopsies weighing no more than 5 mg (Brodde et al. 1991). Since the mechanical forces of homogenization will generate heat, the vessel in which it is performed should always be cooled; a short break between homogenization bursts will potentially be helpful in keeping the temperature low.

Incubation

Incubation conditions depend on the tissue or cell line and/or radioligand under investigation. In principle, equilibrium binding has to occur during the incubation time. Since adrenoceptors and muscarinic receptors are studied most frequently in the cardiovascular system, Table 1 gives an overview of some commonly used radioligand and incubation conditions. For other receptor classes and radioligands, readers should consult recent publications for reasonable conditions.

Separating Bound from Free Radioligand

At the end of the incubation period bound and unbound radioligand must be separated. The two main methods for this are vacuum filtration and centrifugation. Since vacuum filtration is used most frequently, we will not discuss centrifugation techniques here but rather refer to an in-depth description of such techniques (Hulme 1992a). In specific instances, e.g. with solubilised receptors, other separation methods may become relevant including gel filtration (Hulme 1992b) or charcoal adsorption

Table 1
Incubation conditions for some frequently used radioligands for adrenergic and muscarinic acetylcholine receptors

Receptor	Ligand	Assay volume	Incubation time	Incubation temperature
α_1-adrenoceptors	[^{3}H]-prazosin	1000 µl	45 min	25°C
α_2-adrenoceptors	[^{3}H]-RX 821002	250 µl	60 min	25°C
β-adrenoceptors	[^{125}I]-iodocyano-pindolol	250 µl	90 min	37°C
Muscarinic receptors	[^{3}H]-quinuclidinyl-benzylate	1000 µl	60 min	37°C

(Strange 1992). For filtration assays, a variety of devices and filter types are offered. The filtration devices range from simple pots hooked up to a vacuum pump to elaborate harvesters, with the former being the cheapest and the latter being most convenient, particularly if large numbers of samples are processed on a routine basis. Glass fibre filters are used most frequently, particularly the GF/C type. Filtration plates that allow direct filtering of samples from a 96 well plate into a filter plate are being offered by some manufacturers.

After the filtration, it is helpful to rinse the filters a few times (with a total of about 10 ml incubation buffer) to minimize non-specific binding. This should be done with ice-cold buffer to minimize dissociation of bound ligand.

Saturation Binding Experiments

As stated above, saturation binding experiments are used to determine the affinity of a radioligand to a receptor (K_d), as well as the total number of receptors present in the assay (B_{max}). To obtain reliable estimates of these parameters, at least 6 different concentrations of radioligand must be tested, but particularly when a receptor is first detected in a given tissue or cell type, an even greater number of concentrations is helpful.

Preparing the Assay

To minimize experimental error all assays are performed at least in duplicate. This can be done in polypropylene vials but also in 96 well plates. The former approach is more appropriate for smaller scale experiments, whereas the latter is more economical when large numbers of samples are to be processed.

Radioligand dilutions should be prepared to cover the desired concentration range. Optimally these concentrations should cover both the high range (corresponding to 5–10×K_d and hence saturation of the receptor) and the low range (around K_d)

in order to allow reliable estimates of both K_d and B_{max}. If an assay is well established and the number of data points has to be constrained to 6 within an experiment for technical reasons, an emphasis on higher concentrations is advisable if the primary parameter of interest is B_{max} whereas it should be on the lower concentrations if the interest is primarily in precise K_d estimates. Duplicates of total binding and non-specific binding should be tested for each concentration of the radioligand.

Data Analysis

To derive K_d and B_{max} from the experimental data several steps are required. After having calculated the mean value of the duplicate, triplicate or quadruplicate measurements for total binding, non-specific binding and totals (i.e. the concentrations of the radioligand used which become the x-axis values in the subsequent analysis), it is necessary to calculate specific binding by subtracting non-specific binding from total binding at each concentration of the radioligand. It may be helpful to graph total and non-specific binding separately to get an impression of the raw data (see Fig. 3). Thereafter, two steps are required but their sequence is not relevant. In one step experimental results in cpm must be converted into molar units based on the specific activity of the radioligand as described above. In the other step, affinity and receptor number are calculated from the data. Moreover, it is customary to then correct molar units of B_{max} for tissue content in the assay. The most frequently used denominator for this is mg protein, but cell number, mg wet weight or DNA content are equally acceptable and may even be preferable e.g. when receptor number in a hypertrophied or scarred tissue is compared to a control tissue.

To obtain estimates of K_d and B_{max} from saturation binding experiments, it was customary to use the Rosenthal plot, frequently but incorrectly referred to as a Scatchard plot. This plot was very popular twenty years ago at a time when computer-assisted data analysis was not yet widely available. However, the transformations involved in the Rosenthal analysis may cause problems due to inappropriate weighing of certain data points, and the assumptions of linear regression are no longer met since x and y are no longer independent of each other. This eventually leads to inadequate results (for review see Burgisser 1984). Since saturation binding isotherms should follow rectangular hyperbolic functions based on theoretical considerations, they are best analysed by fitting such functions to the experimental data using computer-assisted non-linear iterative curve fitting programs. A variety of such programs are commercially available, with Prism (Graphpad Software, San Diego, CA, USA) and Sigmaplot (SPSS Inc., Chicago, IL, USA) being most popular.

Any of these computer programs requires that the concentration of radioligand be entered for the x-axis (the amount of radioactivity in the assay measured as explained below is more reliable than calculated theoretical concentrations). The amount of specific binding is entered for the y-axis values (if desired this can also be done for total and non-specific binding). The programs will fit a rectangular hyperbola to your data according to

$$y = \frac{B_{max} \times x}{K_d + x} \qquad (6)$$

This equation is derived as follows: When you substitute [ligand] with x and [receptor · ligand] with y in equation 2 and rearrange it, you obtain

$$y = [\text{receptor}] \times x \times \frac{K_{on}}{K_{off}} = [\text{receptor}] \times x \times \frac{1}{K_d} \quad (7)$$

[receptor] is the concentration of the free receptors and usually unknown. However, free receptors are all receptors minus the occupied ones

$$[\text{receptor}] = B_{max} - [\text{receptor} \cdot \text{ligand}] = B_{max} - y \quad (8)$$

Inserting and rearranging leads to

$$y = \frac{(B_{max} - y) \times x}{K_d} = \frac{B_{max} \times x - y \times x}{K_d} \quad (9)$$

$$y \times K_d = B_{max} \times x - y \times x \quad (10)$$

$$y \times K_d + y \times x = B_{max} \times x \quad (11)$$

$$y \times (K_d + x) = B_{max} \times x \quad (12)$$

$$y = \frac{B_{max} \times x}{K_d + x} \quad (13)$$

You will get K_d and B_{max} as results. Note that, when the concentration of the ligand (the x-value) equals K_d, you will get

$$\frac{B_{max} \times K_d}{K_d + K_d} = \frac{B_{max} \times K_d}{2 K_d} = \frac{B_{max}}{2} \quad (14)$$

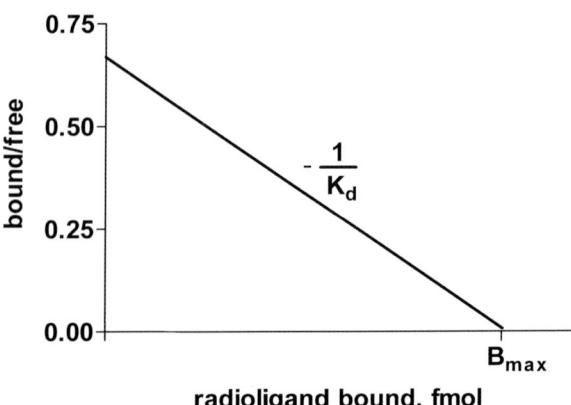

Figure 4
A Rosenthal plot was used to determine K_d and B_{max} before nonlinear regression methods were widely available. However, this analysis may yield unreliable results (see text)

In other words, when the concentration of the ligand equals K_d, half of the receptors ($B_{max}/2$) are occupied as it corresponds to the definition of K_d.

Although the Rosenthal (a.k.a Scatchard) plot is no longer considered appropriate for quantitative data analysis (Burgisser 1984), it remains helpful to gauge the experimental data visually. The principle of the Rosenthal plot is that the amount of specifically bound radioligand on the x-axis is plotted against the ratio of bound/free (unbound) ligand on the y-axis (Fig. 4). In this analysis the x-intercept corresponds to B_{max}, while the negative reciprocal of the slope corresponds to K_d. A deviation of the regression line of the data points in this representation indicates some form of lack of equilibrium in the assay.

Practical Approach (Protocol)

Note that two sets of tubes are necessary: one to perform the incubation of receptor and ligand, and one (this is actually done directly in vials) to quantify the radioactivity, and hence the concentration of radioligand, being used. Following the separation step of the experiment, the radioactivity is transferred from the incubation tubes to the vials. The vials have to be compatible with your radiation counter, too.

Not all of these steps have to be taken in the indicated order. Many of them can be done in parallel or in an intercalated way, e.g. tubes can be set up and solutions be prepared during the centrifugation steps of the membrane preparation.

1. Prepare a number of incubation tubes (or a microtitre plate) according to the planned number of data points (2 each for total and non-specific binding (in the example presented below, designated 'TB' and 'NS', respectively) for each concentration of the radioligand).
2. Prepare the same number of vials for use in your radiation counter (alternatively a corresponding filter plate which can be placed directly into the counter). Additionally, prepare 2 vials for each concentration of the radioligand to allow quantification of the amount of radioligand used in the assay (total radioactivity, 'T' in the example below) and hence its true concentration. This is necessary because the radioligand is not diluted to a certain molar concentration; rather, the concentration is calculated from the counts obtained in these vials. Place a filter in the vials to make sure that they are treated like the assay samples.
3. Prepare sufficient amounts of incubation buffer, check its pH at the desired incubation temperature, and cool it to 4 °C in an ice-bath.
4. Prepare the working solution for determining the non-specific binding.
5. Prepare the working solution of the radioligand from the stock solution provided by the radiochemical manufacturer. Dilute the working solution to obtain a separate working solution for each desired concentration of the radioligand.
6. Add the working solution for non-specific binding or corresponding amounts of incubation buffer to all incubation tubes (or wells).
7. Add the working solutions of the various concentrations of the radioligand to the respective tubes (or wells).
   Don't forget to add it to the tubes used for determination of total amount of radioligand in the assay as well (see 2).

8. Resuspend the membrane preparation (the pellet from the last centrifugation step) thoroughly in incubation buffer to ensure a homogenous suspension. Add aliquots of membrane suspension to all incubation tubes (or wells).
9. Incubate tubes (or plate) at the chosen temperature for the chosen period of time. A gently shaking water bath may be helpful to ensure constant agitation during the incubation. Since the incubation time should allow for equilibrium conditions, minor extensions of the incubation are not usually harmful to the assay.
10. Incubations are stopped by vacuum filtration of the samples either manually or with a harvester. Rinse the incubation tubes (or wells) with approximately 10 ml of ice-cold incubation buffer each and filter that as well. Apply the filtration vacuum until the filters appear dry.
11. Put the filters in the corresponding scintillation vials (not necessary in the case of filtration plates). If the radioligand is labelled with [^{3}H], dry the filters (e.g. for 1 h at 60 °C or overnight at room temperature) and then add an adequate volume of scintillation fluid to each vial.
12. Seal the vials, shake gently. Count the probes in a counter.

Competition Binding Experiments

Competition binding experiments (sometimes incorrectly referred to as displacements) can serve multiple purposes. Firstly, they characterize the ligand recognition properties of a binding site. Comparison of this pharmacological specificity with that of a given functional response allows one to determine whether the binding site indeed corresponds to a functional receptor.

Secondly, in many case a cell or tissues expresses more than one subtype of a receptor, e.g. β_1- and β_2-adrenoceptors in the heart, but measurements of each of them individually may be cumbersome or, due to the lack of proper subtype-selective radioligands, even impossible. Competition studies with suitable subtype-selective agents can reveal the relative proportions of receptor subtypes within a tissue or cell. Together with information on the total receptor density this will allow indirect determination of the individual numbers of each subtype (for an example see Brodde et al. 1991).

Thirdly, competition studies with agonist in suitable buffer conditions will also allow determination of the relative percentages of the receptor in the high and low affinity state for agonists.

Finally, competition studies can substitute for saturation binding studies in cases where true saturation curves are not feasible, e.g. for economical reasons with very expensive radioligands as is the case with some peptide receptors. This is called homologous competition binding and based on the assumption that radioligand and its unlabelled analogue have identical affinities for the receptor of interest (for details see DeBlasi et al. 1989).

The overall design of a competition binding experiment is quite similar to that of a saturation binding experiment, and hence we will focus here on its specific aspects.

Preparing the Assay

In contrast to saturation binding experiments, competition-binding assays employ only a single concentration of radioligand. The concentration of the radioligand in competition studies should be about 2–3× its K_d value as determined in saturation binding. It is also necessary to determine the total amount of radioligand in the assay and total and non-specific binding within a competition binding experiment. Additional data points are generated in which radioligand binding is quantified in the presence of various concentrations of an unlabelled compound of interest. If possible the concentrations of the competitor should be chosen so that the lowest concentration causes no inhibition (i.e. binding equals total binding) and the highest concentration causes complete inhibition of specific binding (i.e. binding equals non-specific binding).

In most cases it will be necessary to test at least 2 competitor concentrations per log unit of concentration increment. If one is attempting to look for the presence of multiple binding sites (e.g. receptor subtypes or agonist high affinity states), 4 concentrations per log unit are advisable.

Data Analysis

If a compound competes for a homogeneous class of binding sites, the competition curve should theoretically follow a sigmoidal function with a Hill-slope of unity. Thus, experiments should primarily be analyzed by fitting a sigmoidal curve to the data with a floating Hill-slope.

$$y = \text{Bottom} + \frac{\text{Top} - \text{Bottom}}{1 + 10^{\log(IC_{50}-x) \cdot \text{HillSlope}}} \quad (15)$$

If it deviates consistently from unity, the data do not support interaction with a homogeneous class of sites under equilibrium conditions. If a cell or tissue contains two subtypes of a receptor and the radioligand binds to both with similar affinity, competitors that are selective for one of them will yield shallow and biphasic competition curves, with each of the two components having a Hill-slope of unity.

To test this assumption, both a monophasic and a biphasic model may be fitted to the data. The biphasic model should only be accepted if the fit is statistically superior to a monophasic fit in an F-test. A monophasic curve is characterized by its top (corresponding to total binding), its bottom (corresponding to non-specific binding) and the position of half-maximal inhibition. The latter is referred to as the IC_{50} value. A biphasic curve is defined by top, bottom, distinct IC_{50} values for each of the two sites and the percent contribution of each site. Theoretically, it is also possible to distinguish more than two receptors but practically this is rarely feasible due to insufficiently selective competitors and/or an insufficient number of data points to reach statistical superiority over a two-site fit. While performing the curve fitting, there is no need to transform the y-values (which have the unit of cpm) to molar concentrations.

However, it may sometimes be useful to normalize them (setting top to 100% and bottom to 0%) in order to compare different experiments, or to show them on a single graph.

If radioligand and competitor interact at the receptor in a competitive manner, the IC_{50} value depends in part on the concentration of radioligand in the assay and thus gives only a very crude estimate of the competitor affinity (K_i value) at this receptor. The K_i value is computed from the IC_{50} using the Cheng-Prusoff (1973) equation

$$K_i = \frac{IC_{50}}{1 + \frac{[ligand]}{K_{d,\,ligand}}} \qquad (16)$$

This calculation requires knowledge of the concentration of the radioligand in the assay, which is determined in the same way as in a saturation binding experiment.

Practical Approach (Protocol)

The practical approach to competition binding is very similar to that used in saturation binding experiments.

1. Prepare a number of incubation tubes (or a microtitre plate) according to the planned number of data points (2 each for total and non-specific binding and for each concentration of the competitor).
2. Prepare the same number of vials for use in your radiation counter (alternatively a corresponding filter plate which can directly be placed into the counter). Additionally, prepare 2 vials for the radioligand to allow quantification of the amount of radioligand used in the assay and hence its true concentration. The latter vials should also contain a filter to make sure that they are treated like the assay samples.
3. Prepare sufficient amounts of incubation buffer, check its pH at the desired incubation temperature, and cool it to 4 °C in an ice-bath.
4. Prepare the working solution for determining the non-specific binding.
5. Prepare the working solution of the radioligand from the stock solution provided by the radiochemical manufacturer.
6. Prepare the working solutions of the competitor and its dilutions.
7. Add the working solution for non-specific binding, corresponding amounts of incubation buffer or corresponding amounts of competitor solution to all incubation tubes (or wells).
8. Add the working solution of the radioligand to all tubes (or wells). Don't forget to add it as well to the tubes used for determination of total amount of radioligand in the assay (see item 2).

All subsequent steps are identical to those for saturation binding (see above items 9–13).

Examples

Saturation Binding Experiment

A saturation binding experiment in rat heart was performed, using [^{3}H]-prazosin as the radioligand to label α_1-adrenoceptors. A rat heart (700 mg wet weight) was prepared, and 120 µg protein per assay were used.
Counts were reported as follows:

Counts for total radioactivity (T) in the assay at radioligand concentrations 1–6:

T1	T2	T3	T4	T5	T6
30300	17813	16117	7619	3417	1720
31472	17804	14251	7084	3536	1963

Remember that this is actually the amount of radioligand used at the different dilutions. These values will be used to calculate the concentration of the ligand according to equation 5.

Counts for total (TB) and non-specific (NS) binding at radioligand concentrations 1–6:

TB1	TB2	TB3	TB4	TB5	TB6	NS1	NS2	NS3	NS4	NS5	NS6
513	440	451	374	289	168	154	94	51	32	22	15
541	477	410	392	279	161	171	87	62	37	22	21

Figure 5 shows these data with the averaged total values on the x-axis and total and non-specific binding shown separately on the y-axis.

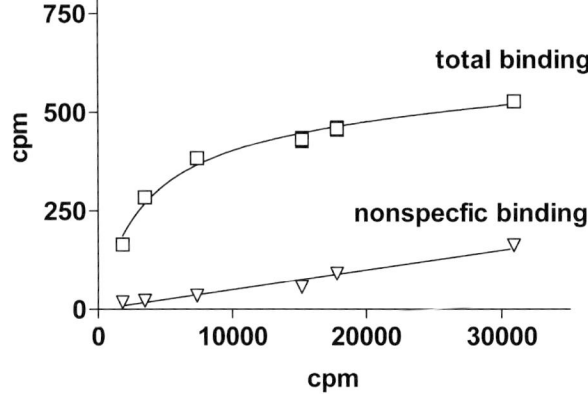

Figure 5
Total and non-specific binding, expressed in cpm

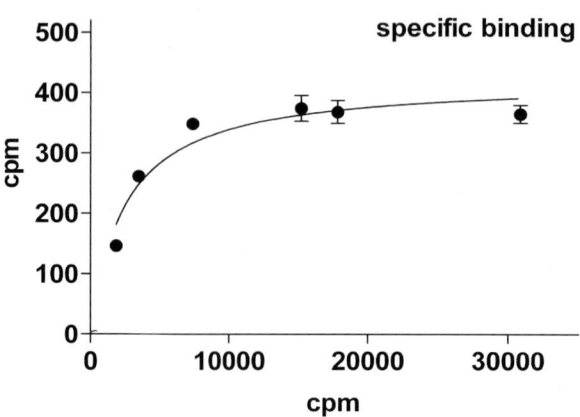

Figure 6
Specific binding, expressed in cpm

It may be helpful to look at your data this way in order to detect outliers or entry errors. However, to evaluate the experiment, total counts are averaged, and the averaged non-specific counts are subtracted from the averaged total counts:

radioligand used, cpm	30886.0	17808.0	15184.0	7351.0	3476.0	1841.0
specific binding, cpm	364.5	368.0	374.0	348.5	262.0	146.5

The resulting graph of specific saturation binding is shown in Fig. 6.

The nonlinear regression estimated a K_d of 2430 and a B_{max} of 421 cpm, which can then be converted into molar concentrations using the specific activity of the radioligand and the assay volume. Alternatively, these factors can be used to convert cpm into molar concentrations prior to curve fitting to obtain the following mean values:

radioligand used, pM	435	251	214	104	48.9	25.9
radioligand bound, fmol	5.13	5.18	5.26	4.91	3.69	2.06

When these values are used in curve fitting, Fig. 7 is obtained, which is basically identical to Fig. 6, except that the units have changed. Note that in this particular experiment two data points are close to the estimated K_d and the three points with the highest x-values define a plateau. This indicates that the experiment is indeed a saturation experiment, and that binding to the receptor is saturable (i.e. that there are a finite number of binding sites). If the smallest x-value were larger, the experiment should be repeated with less radioligand, in order to get more reliable results from the nonlinear fit.

In molar units, the K_d of prazosin for rat heart is 34.2 pM. As a last step, the receptor density is calculated relative to a denominator such as protein content. Here a B_{max} of 5.93 fmol was determined using 120 µg protein per assay, and hence receptor density was 49.4 fmol receptors/mg protein used. Note that total binding is less than 9% of the radioligand used (therefore no ligand-depletion). Non-specific binding amounts to less than 1% of total radioligand used.

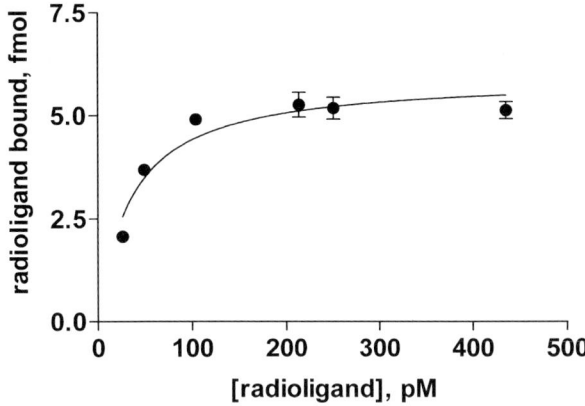

Figure 7
Specific binding, expressed in molar units. Compared with Fig. 6, only the axes have changed

Rosenthal Plot

Rosenthal plots were used before nonlinear regression by computer programs became widely available. The data was transformed in such a way that K_d and B_{max} could be calculated by linear regression. However, the step of transforming the data enhances the error, alters the relative weighting of the data and the x- and y-values will no longer be independent of each other. So, it is no longer advisable to calculate K_d and B_{max} using Rosenthal plots based on linear regression.

However, Rosenthal plots are often useful to simply display data and therefore the method of transforming the data is described briefly. X-values of Rosenthal plots are the amount of bound radioligand, and the y-values are the ratio of bound to free radioligand. So, x- and y-values have first to be interchanged, and then, the reciprocal of each y-value is multiplied by its corresponding x-value to yield Fig. 8. The linear regression line of the data will cross the x-axis at an x-value corresponding to B_{max}, and the slope of the line will be $-1/K_d$.

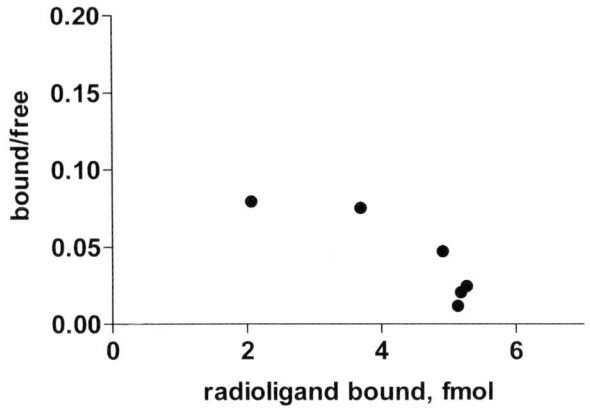

Figure 8
The same data as in Figs. 5 to 7, transformed to generate a Rosenthal plot

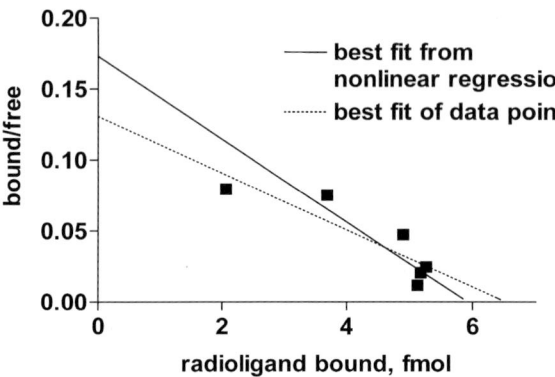

Figure 9
Linear regression (*dotted line*) of the transformed data. Note the difference from the solid line, which was generated using B_{max} and K_d obtained by non-linear regression of the same data

Figure 9 illustrates the differences in K_d and B_{max} estimates when linear regression of a Rosenthal plot and nonlinear curve fitting of untransformed data are used. The solid line was generated using the best-fit values of nonlinear regression performed on the raw data as described above. The dotted line, however, is a best-fit linear regression. In a quantitative analysis, K_d is estimated to be 34.2 pM and 50.0 pM in non-linear regression and Rosenthal plot, respectively, whereas B_{max} values of 5.93 and 6.53 fmol, respectively, are obtained. Depending on the technical quality of the data even greater differences may occur.

Competition Binding Experiment

A competition experiment was performed for rat cardiac α_1-adrenoceptors with [^{3}H]-prazosin (K_d = 34.2 pM, taken from the above example) as the radioligand and noradrenaline as the competitor (concentrations ranging from 10^{-9} to 10^{-4} M). The protein content was 1180 µg per assay. The following results were obtained (Table 2).

These counts were graphed with the logarithm of the concentrations as x- and the counts as y-values (Fig. 10). Total binding (TB) was graphed at an x-value of 10^{-12}, and non-specific binding (NS) at an x-value of 10^{-3}. Next, a sigmoidal curve with a variable Hill-slope was fitted to the data. This was characterized by a Hill-slope of -1.14 (i.e. close to unity), a -log IC$_{50}$ of 4.75, a top of 3311 and a bottom of 273. While the data nicely define a top plateau, they do not cover a bottom plateau. Hence, the calculated bottom plateau is slightly lower than the averaged non-specific binding of 289. When performing further experiments, the concentration range should be shifted to −8 to −3; however, it should be kept in mind that non-specific binding of the competitor can also increase with such high concentrations.

Since the curve fits the data nicely and the calculated bottom-plateau looks reliable, this experiment may also be evaluated further. The duplicate measurements were averaged and normalized – 3311 cpm were defined as 100% and 273 cpm as 0% (Fig. 11). Since top and bottom plateaus are defined by normalizing the data, nonlinear regression of the normalized data should fit the curve with top and bottom set constant to 100 and 0%, respectively, and the data points corresponding to total and

Table 2
Competitor concentrations given as log values

log M	Cpm		log M	Cpm	
TB	3315	3202	–6.5	3288	3126
NS	252	271	–6.3	3400	3487
–9	3077	2998	–6	3214	3355
–8.7	2906	3370	–5.7	3123	2925
–8.5	3380	3475	–5.5	3104	2960
–8.3	3270	3100	–5.3	2798	2410
–8	3336	3176	–5	2420	2219
–7.7	3408	3439	–4.7	1598	1764
–7.5	3275	3228	–4.5	1347	1223
–7.3	3527	3284	–4.3	1054	1059
–7	3572	3271	–4	670	650
–6.7	3456	3474	NS	298	337

non-specific binding should be excluded from further analysis. This normalization process is not part of the analysis of the experiment but may be helpful e.g. in order to pool results from several such experiments.

As a last step, the K_i value is calculated. The total counts, i.e. the counts of the total amount of radioligand used, were 22998 and 23050 cpm, averaging 23024 cpm. This corresponds to a concentration of the radioligand (specific activity 80 Ci/mmol)

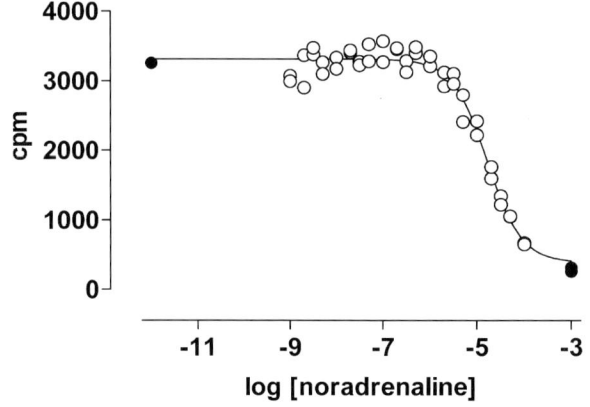

Figure 10
Total and non-specific binding (closed circles) and binding at various competitor concentrations (open circles). The IC_{50} value can already be obtained

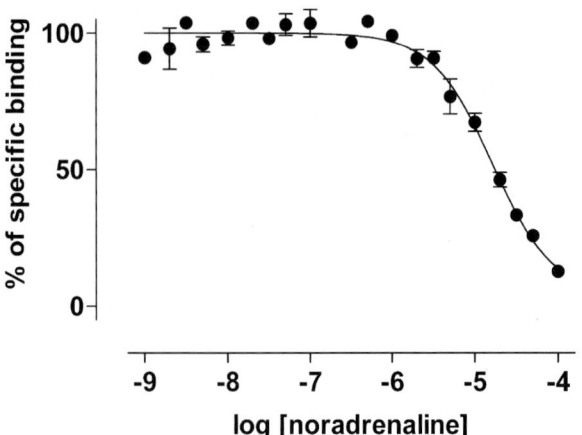

Figure 11
Data from Fig. 10 normalized (see text for details)

of 324 pM based on an assay volume of 1000 ml and a counter efficiency of 0.4. As presented in the example above, the K_d of [³H]-prazosin for rat heart is estimated to be 34.2 pM. Using the equation of Cheng-Prusoff (1973), the K_i can be calculated by

$$K_i = \frac{IC_{50}}{1 + \frac{[\text{ligand}]}{K_{d,\text{ligand}}}} = \frac{10^{-4.75} \text{ M}}{1 + \frac{324\text{pM}}{32.4\text{pM}}} = 1.70 \times 10^{-6} \text{ M} = 1.70 \text{ µM} \qquad (17)$$

This equals a pK_i for noradrenaline in rat heart of -5.77.

Troubleshooting

Problem: Duplicate values are not in good agreement with each other.

Solution: Apart from sloppy pipetting, lack of homogeneity of the membrane preparation is the most frequent reason. Try to homogenize the tissue or cell preparation more vigorously. Don't forget that the pellet from the last centrifugation step also needs to be re-homogenised. If all else fails, use triplicates or quadruplicates rather than duplicates to get more robust readings.

Problem: Non-specific binding at radioligand concentrations around K_d is high.

Solution: High non-specific relative to specific binding is a signal-noise question, and hence can result from to little signal or too much noise. Too little signal is due to too few receptors within the assay. This can sometimes be overcome by adding more membrane preparation to the assay. However, if receptor expression in the tissue of interest is very low, this will not help since non-specific binding increases as well. Too much noise can have many reasons. Some radioligands intrinsically have more non-specific binding than others (e.g. [³H]-quinuclidinyl-benzylate relative to [³H]-N-methyl-scopolamine for muscarinic acetylcholine receptors or [³H]-rauwolscine and [³H]-yohimbine relative to [³H]-RX 821002 for α_2-adrenoceptors). Some radioligands stick to certain surfaces, and attempts to use other types of vials or silicon coating of vials can be helpful. Sometimes radioligands stick to the filters. Use of alternative filter types and/or pre-treatment of the filters with polyethylimine (toxic!) can be helpful. Alternatively, a switch to other means of separation of bound and free radioligand can be considered.

Problem: Total binding (sum of specific and non-specific binding) exceeds 10% of total radio-ligand in the assay.

Solution: This situation creates ligand depletion and hence prevents a valid mathematical assessment of the data obtained. Increase the assay volume while maintaining the amount of membrane preparation in the assay. This will increase the amount of radioligand without affecting its concentration. Additionally, the amount of membrane (receptor) in the assay can be reduced to decrease binding; this can be particularly helpful when working with transfected cells expressing artificially high receptor numbers.

Problem: Confidence intervals for B_{max} estimates in saturation binding are very wide.

Solution: Use more radioligand concentrations in a range expected to cover B_{max}. This will enhance the robustness of B_{max} estimates.

Problem: Confidence intervals for K_d estimates in saturation binding are very wide.

Solution: Use more radioligand concentrations in a range around the expected K_d. This will enhance the robustness of K_d estimates.

Problem: Fitting of curves to competition data does not yield a reasonable top plateau.

Solution: Use more data points in the region where you expect the top plateau, particularly at very low competitor concentrations.

Problem: Fitting of curves to competition data does not yield a reasonable bottom plateau or even negative estimates.

Solution: A variety of possible explanations exists. Firstly, it is possible that the computer program is attempting to fit to unreasonably low values because there are insufficient data points at high competitor concentrations, i.e. the program extrapolates far beyond the data. This is best prevented by having more data points in the concentration range of competitor where the bottom plateau is expected. Secondly, it is also possible that the competitor indeed competes for more sites than the agent used for definition of non-specific binding (because the definition was chosen incorrectly in the first place or because the solution of agent used for defining non-specific binding does not contain what it is supposed to contain). Check whether the definition of non-specific binding is indeed correct, e.g. by performing a competition experiment with a range of concentrations of the agent used for definition of non-specific binding.

Problem: Confidence intervals for the estimate of IC_{50} in a competition binding experiment are very wide.

Solution: If the overall data are good, this is usually because there are an insufficient number of competitor concentrations being checked per log unit of concentration range. Increase the number of competitor concentrations per log unit.

Problem: When fitting a curve with a floating Hill-slope to competition binding data, the Hill-slope becomes considerably greater than unity (the competition curve is very steep).

Solution: If this is reproducibly so, the most likely explanation is that the mechanism of inhibition is not strictly competitive. This can be tested by performing saturation binding experiments in the absence and presence of a moderate concentration of inhibitor. A strictly competitive inhibitor should increase the apparent K_d of the radioligand but not affect its B_{max}.

Problem: When fitting a curve with a floating Hill-slope to competition binding data, the Hill-slope becomes considerably smaller than unity (the competition curve is very shallow).

Solution: This is the expected result if the radioligand labels two sites (e.g. subtypes of a receptor) that are discriminated by the competing agent. Perform a two-site fit and compare it to the results of a one-site fit (Hill-slopes must be fixed at unity for both equations) by an F-test. However, not every shallow competition curve is due to a biphasic inhibition curve. Other more complex reasons such as negative cooperativity of binding may also exist.

Problem: The fitted curve obviously does not explain the data.

Solution: This can occur due to the phenomenon of local minima in iterative curve fitting. During the iterative processes the program performs stepwise deviations from the starting parameters to test whether they improve the fit. When the starting parameters are far away from the actual data, this can lead to inaccurate parameter estimates (for a detailed discussion see Motulsky and Ransnäs 1987). Use your scientific understanding to "manually" estimate starting parameters for the curve fitting and start anew.

Problem: Curve fitting does not converge.

Solution: There are two possible explanations. The starting values of the fitting procedure may be implausible. In this case select new starting parameters using your scientific understanding. Alternatively, the mathematical model does indeed not fit the data. In this case look at the quality of your data (this problem frequently occurs if the technical quality of the data is poor and lots of scatter exists). If data quality seems good, reconsider whether the mathematical model is appropriate for these data.

Problem: I have a problem that is not resolved by any of the above hints.

Solution: Write an e-mail to the friendly authors of this chapter. Perhaps they can help.

References

Brodde O-E Khamssi M, Zerkowski H-R (1991) β-Adrenoceptors in the transplanted human heart: unaltered β-adrenoceptor density, but increased proportion of $β_2$-adrenoceptors with increasing posttransplant time. Naunyn-Schmiedeberg's Arch. Pharmacol. 344:430–436

Burgisser E (1984) Radioligand-receptor binding studies: What's wrong with the Scatchard analysis? Trends Pharmacol. Sci. 5:142–145

Cheng Y-C, Prusoff WH (1973) Relationship between the inhibition constant (K_i) and the concentration of inhibitor which causes 50 per cent inhibition (I_{50}) of an enzymatic reaction. Biochem. Pharmacol. 22:3099–3108

DeBlasi A, O'Reilly K, Motulsky H (1989) Calculating receptor number from binding experiments using the same compound as radioligand and competitor. Trends Pharmacol. Sci. 10:227–229

Guth PS (1982) The structurally specific, stereospecific, saturable binding of pepperoni to pizza. Trends Pharmacol. Sci. 3:467

Hein P, Goepel M, Cotecchia S, Michel MC (2000) Comparison of [^{3}H]tamsulosin and [^{3}H]prazosin binding to wild-type and constitutively active $α_{1B}$-adrenoceptors. Life Sci. 67:503–508

Hulme EC (1992a) Centrifugation binding assays. In: Hulme EC (ed) Receptor-Ligand Interactions. IRL Press, Oxford, p 235–246

Hulme EC (1992b) Gel-filtration assays for solubilized receptors. In: Hulme EC (ed) Receptor-Ligand Interactions. IRL Press, Oxford, p 255–264

Hulme EC, Buckley NJ (1992) Receptor preparations for binding studies. In: Hulme EC (ed) Receptor-Ligand Interactions. IRL Press, Oxford, p 177–212

Motulsky HJ, Ransnäs LA (1987) Fitting curves to data using nonlinear regression: a practical and nonmathematical review. FASEB J. 1:365–374

Strange PG (1992) Charcoal adsorption for separating bound and free radioligand in radioligand binding assays. In: Hulme EC (ed) Receptor-Ligand Interactions. IRL Press, Oxford, p 247–254

Further reading

Hulme EC (1992) (ed) Receptor-Ligand Interactions. IRL Press, Oxford, p 255–264 (An affordable, in-depth text explaining many different aspects of radioligand binding experiments)

Yamamura HI, Enna SJ, Kuhar MJ (1985) Neurotransmitter Receptor Binding. 2nd edition, Raven Press, New York (The mother of all reference books on radioligand binding)

6.3.2
Tracer Techniques for Detection of Transport

Kirsten Leineweber

Introduction

Transport can be investigated by tracer techniques. As an example for this method, in the following chapter the investigation of noradrenaline uptake will be described. Sympathetic nerve activity is altered and is a prognostic factor for many cardiovascular diseases such as hypertension, coronary syndromes, and congestive heart failure. It is now generally accepted that an increase in sympathetic nerve activity is closely associated with increased plasma noradrenaline levels and reduced myocardial catecholamine stores due to decreased cardiac neuronal noradrenaline transporter activity, which is also known as uptake$_1$, and a reduction in noradrenaline transporter density. Therefore, uptake$_1$ that removes more than 90% of the synaptically released noradrenaline into noradrenergic neurons, plays a pivotal role in the inactivation of the transmitter (for review see Esler et al. 1997).

In addition to the endogenous catecholamines, noradrenaline, dopamine and adrenaline, uptake$_1$ also transports indirectly acting amines such as tyramine and the psychostimulant amphetamine, as well as the dopaminergic neurotoxin MPP$^+$ [1-methyl-4-phenylpyridinium]. Uptake$_1$ is inhibited selectively, with nanomolar affinity, by nisoxetine and the tricyclic antidepressant desipramine and less potent by cocaine.

Accordingly, drugs acting on the noradrenaline transporter can be broadly classified as substrate analogs or as non-substrate uptake$_1$ inhibitors. The former compounds inhibit noradrenaline transport by being transported instead of noradrenaline, whereas uptake$_1$ inhibitors prevent noradrenaline uptake but are not themselves transported into the cell.

In the case of the noradrenaline transporter protein, three binding sites have been identified, one for Na$^+$, one for Cl$^-$ and one for the protonated substrate. Substrate transport as well as inhibitor binding are absolutely dependent on Na$^+$ and Cl$^-$ ions: while Cl$^-$ can be replaced by Br$^-$, and to a lesser extent by SCN$^-$ or NO$_3^-$, it is not possible to replace Na$^+$ by other cations. The Na$^+$/Cl$^-$/noradrenaline stoichiometry observed for the noradrenaline transporter protein is 1:1:1 (for review see Graefe and Bönisch 1988; Esler et al. 1997).

The noradrenaline transporter is mainly located in the axonal membranes of noradrenergic neurons and adrenal medullary cells. However, it has also been found natively expressed in some non-neuronal tissues such as glandular epithelial cells of rabbit uterine endometrium, rat phaeochromocytoma (PC12) cells, human placental brush border membrane vesicles and rat placenta trophoblasts, rabbit dental pulp fibroblasts, rabbit lingual gingiva and nasal mucosa, rat interscapular brown adipose tissue, bovine adrenal medullary cells and pulmonary endothelial cells. Evidence has accumulated that the noradrenaline transporter is also expressed in many components of the cardiovascular system since the lining of arteries (e.g. the dorsal aorta) and veins (e.g. subcardial vein), the epicardium and the cardiac trabeculae are strongly noradrenaline transporter-immunoreactive (for review see Graefe and Bönisch 1988; Esler et al. 1997).

The human noradrenaline transporter (hNAT, Gen Bank Acc No: M65105) was the first noradrenaline transporter to be cloned, followed much later by cloning of the bovine (bNAT, X79015), the rat (rNAT, Y13223), the mouse (mNAT, U76306) and the monkey (*Macaca mulatta*) noradrenaline transporter (mmNAT; AF286026). At the nucleotide level, hNAT and rNAT share 87% identity in the coding region, while hNAT and bNAT show 90% and hNAT and mmNAT show 98.9% identity. However, studies investigating these cloned transporters transfected in different cell types revealed naturally occurring variations in the properties of the various noradrenaline transporters in different species. The hNAT has higher affinities than the rNAT for substrates, such as noradrenaline and MPP+, with no differences between affinities for tricyclic and non-tricyclic antidepressants, such as nisoxetine and desipramine. On the other hand, the hNAT has a higher affinity for cocaine than the rNAT.

The gene encoding hNAT has been assigned to 16q12. It consists of 14 exons coding for a 617 amino acid protein that shows sequence similarity to the dopamine transporter, the serotonin transporter and the GABA transporter. Recently, thirteen naturally occurring single nucleotide polymorphisms within the hNAT gene have been identified: Five intron variants in flanking intron sequences that do not alter splice site acceptor/donor consensus sequences, three silent mutations (955T/C, 1287G/A, 1779G/A) and five missense variants (Val69Ile, Thr99Ile, Val245Ile, Val449Ile, Gly478Ser) located at TMDs 1, 2, 4, 9 and 10, respectively (for review see Brüss et al. 1997). Runkel et al. (2000), who investigated the functional importance of the five amino acid substitutions within the noradrenaline transporter protein *in vitro* found, however, that none of these variants affected the potency of desipramine for inhibition of uptake$_1$. Furthermore, there were no differences in the kinetic constants (K_M, V_{max}) for the hNAT Val69Ile, Thr99Ile, Val245Ile and Val449Ile variants. The hNAT Gly478Ser variant, on the other hand, exhibited a four-fold reduced substrate affinity for noradrenaline (without change in maximum rate of transport) in comparison to the wild-type hNAT. Whether these polymorphisms are of functional importance *in vivo* is still a matter of debate.

The noradrenaline transporter protein, with a molecular mass of about 80 kDa, is characterized by 12 potential transmembrane domains (TMDs) and cytoplasmic amino and carboxyl termini. A large extracellular loop, containing 2-4 potential N-glycosylation sites, is located between TMD-3 and TMD-4 and potential sites for phosphorylation by protein kinases (two for protein kinase C, and one for casein kinase II) are found at intracellular domains. Structure-function analysis using recombinant chimeras of the dopamine and noradrenaline transporter, and serotonin and noradrenaline transporter identified several functional domains within the monoamine transporter proteins where TMD-1 has been identified as being critically involved in ligand binding and substrate transport.

The process by which the noradrenaline transporter specifically binds and transfers its substrate across the membrane resembles a typical enzyme-substrate reaction and follows the saturation kinetics of the Michaelis-Menten type (Graefe and Bönisch 1988): 1. When the carrier protein is saturated (that is when all binding sites are occupied), the rate of transport is maximal (V_{max}) and 2. The noradrenaline transporter has a characteristic binding constant for its substrate (K_M, concentration of substrate when the transport rate is half its maximum value). Therefore, from the number of transporter sites estimated from inhibitor binding (B_{max}) and from the maximal transport rate of noradrenaline (V_{max}), the duration of the transport cycle for a substrate at V_{max} can be calculated (V_{max}/B_{max}). It should be noted that V_{max} for uptake$_1$ is substrate-concentration-dependent and by this is the length of the transport cycle. The transporter undergoes a conformational change in order to transfer the substrate across the membrane. This reaction includes:

1. binding of the substrate (i.e. the transported ligand) to a specific binding site
2. translocation
3. dissociation and release of the substrate to the other side of the membrane and
4. return to the unloaded state.

General characteristics of substrate transport mediated by uptake$_1$ include:
1. temperature-dependence of transport
2. requirement of Na$^+$ and Cl$^-$ ions
3. saturability of transport
4. structural substrate specificity and/or stereoselectivity (uptake$_1$ operates at low concentrations (< 3 µmol/ l) and favours the accumulation of (-)-noradrenaline that has more than twice the affinity of (–)-adrenaline)
5. sensitivity to specific competitive inhibitors (which compete for the same binding site and may or may not be transported by the carrier) or non-competitive inhibitors (which bind elsewhere and specifically alter the structure of the carrier) which differ chemically from the solute under study and
6. transport occurs via a limited number of transporter proteins.

The properties determined by the noradrenaline transporter protein permits a vectorial reaction, i.e., substrate movement from one side of the membrane to the other side. To test the characteristics of uptake$_1$ it is therefore useful to assess:
1. the time course of uptake of a labeled substrate at different temperatures (4 °C to 37 °C) to determine whether the transported substrate is accumulated and whether substrate uptake increases linearly with time (indicating a unidirectional inward transport),
2. the dependence of transport-rate or its kinetic determinants K_M and V_{max} on Na$^+$ and Cl$^-$ concentration,
3. K_M and V_{max} for a given substrate by incubating the material under investigation (vesicles, cells, tissue slices) with various concentrations (below and above the expected K_M), of the radiolabeled substrate for a short time period (initial rate) and a defined temperature,
4. whether [^{3}H]-noradrenaline uptake is inhibited by standard inhibitors to determine the IC$_{50}$-values (i.e., the concentration which causes half-maximum inhibition of either uptake or binding of a labeled ligand at a given concentration) for the unlabeled substrates,
5. whether [^{3}H]-noradrenaline uptake is inhibited by standard inhibitors of the transport system to determine the IC$_{50}$-values for the unlabeled antagonists,
6. B$_{max}$ (as mentioned above the value reflects the density (number) of carrier sites) and K$_D$ (value reflects the concentration by which half of the carriers are occupied by the radiolabeled ligand) for the transporter,
7. whether the accumulation of the substrate is dependent on the protein or tissue amount that is used.

Description of Methods and Practical Approach

The measurement of noradrenaline transporter activity and density has become routine now that many radioactively labelled ligands, substrates like [^{3}H]-noradrenaline or metaiodobenzylguanidine (MIBG) radioiodinated with ^{131}I or ^{123}I or antagonists like [^{3}H]-desipramine, [^{3}H]-mazindol and [^{3}H]-nisoxetine, are commercially available.

The use of the noradrenaline analog [^{131}I/^{123}I]-MIBG, to determine uptake$_1$ *in vivo*, was first developed and utilized clinically as an agent for scintigraphic imaging of neuroendocrine tumors, such as pheochromocytomas and neuroblastomas, but has also proven to be useful for imaging of cardiac sympathetic nerves (for review see Kiyono et al. 2001). In the myocardium, MIBG is carried like noradrenaline to the sympathetic nervous terminals by myocardial blood flow; it is taken up by cardiac sympathetic neurons via uptake$_1$ and shares noradrenaline storage in intraneuronal vesicles. Like noradrenaline, MIBG is released from synaptic vesicles into the synaptic cleft by neuronal stimulation. However, it should be noted that MIBG also shares noradrenaline extraneuronal uptake, which is not inhibited by desipramine. Therefore, a desipramine pretreatment should be considered to differentiate specific neuronal MIBG uptake by uptake$_1$ from non-specific extraneuronal uptake. Additional radiopharmaceuticals useful for PET imaging of neuroendocrine tumors or sympathetic nerves are [^{11}C]-hydroxyephedrine (Allman et al. 1993; Malizia et al. 2000) and [^{18}F]-6-fluorodopamine (FDA).

Desipramine and substrates share a common binding site and like noradrenaline the binding of desipramine is also Na$^+$ and Cl$^-$ dependent with a coupling ratio for Na$^+$/desipramine of 2 or 3 and for the Cl$^-$/desipramine ratio of 1. Both Na$^+$ and Cl$^-$ enhance the binding affinity of desipramine to the noradrenaline transporter. The radiolabeled noradrenaline transporter antagonist [^{3}H]-desipramine was reported by several investigators (for review see Lee and Snyder 1981) to bind uptake$_1$ sites for NA in rat brain. However, [^{3}H]-desipramine exhibits a high amount of non-specific binding due to its highly-lipid solubility and binds in addition to a high affinity site to a low affinity site not related to the noradrenaline transporter. If non-specific binding is properly defined so that only the high-affinity site (transporter) is measured, the percentage of specific binding is found nevertheless to be low (40% at twice the K_D concentration). Therefore, although desipramine has a high affinity for uptake$_1$ and can be used in *ex vivo* and *in vitro* experiments to locate the noradrenaline transporter, its usefulness *in vivo* is limited due to the high level of non-specific binding. Furthermore, it should be noted that the pharmacokinetics of desipramine are non-linear and related to cytochrom P450-2D6 activity, making single subject pharmacokinetics prediction (different plasma levels) difficult.

[^{3}H]-Mazindol has also been used to label uptake$_1$ sites in the rat brain or the failing human heart (for review see Böhm et al. 1995). However, [^{3}H]-mazindol binds as well to dopamine uptake sites with high affinity, necessitating the use of selective inhibitors of the dopamine uptake when measuring uptake$_1$ sites for noradrenaline. Additionally, to displace [^{3}H]-mazindol, extremely high concentrations of desipramine (30–100 mmol/l) are necessary. Thus, it is possible that desipramine also displaces [^{3}H]-mazindol from non-specific binding sites resulting in a lower than actual noradrenaline transporter density.

On the other hand, [^{3}H]-nisoxetine ([N-methyl-3-(o-methoxyphenoxy)-3-phenylpropylamine]) is a potent and selective inhibitor of uptake$_1$, being approximately 1000-fold and 400-fold more potent in blocking the uptake of NA than that of serotonin or dopamine, respectively (for review see Tejani-Butt 1992; Jayanthi et al. 1993). Furthermore, [^{3}H]-nisoxetine has little or no affinity for many neurotransmitter receptors. In contrast to [^{3}H]-desipramine, [^{3}H]-nisoxetine binds to a single class of binding sites and the percentage of specific binding is about 80% at twice its K_D concentration. It is suggested that the binding site for noradrenaline and nisoxetine are either identical or exhibit a considerable steric overlap and that [^{3}H]-nisoxetine does not bind to intracellular non-adrenergic sites as do the mentioned ligands above. Binding of [^{3}H]-nisoxetine is pH-dependent with a pK_a of 5.7, with maximal binding in the pH range of 7.0–8.5, and shows an absolute requirement for Na^+ and Cl^-. The presence of Na^+ increases the binding affinity of [^{3}H]-nisoxetine in a concentration-dependent manner.

The relationship between the binding and the Na^+ concentration is sigmoidal, suggesting a coupling ratio of Na^+/nisoxetine of 2. On the other hand, the relationship between the binding and the Cl^- concentration is hyperbolic, suggesting that the coupling ratio of Cl^-/nisoxetine is one.

Although Tris-containing buffers can be used with this radioligand, the best results with regard to total and non-specific binding can be obtained with a buffer consisting of 10 mM Na_2HPO_4, 120 mM NaCl and 5 mM KCl (pH 7.4). Binding of [^{3}H]-nisoxetine is also temperature-dependent. Maximal binding occurs within 15 min of incubation at 22 °C, whereas, a 3–4 h incubation is required to obtain maximal binding at 4 °C.

On the other hand, the dissociation at 22 °C is very rapid, the time required for 50% dissociation is less than 5 min. Although nisoxetine is an appropriate radioligand for labelling and blocking uptake$_1$ sites in *in vitro* and *ex vivo* experiments, the [^{11}C] analog of nisoxetine, created for PET imaging *in vivo* was found unsuitable.

Examples

Detection and Quantification of Uptake$_1$ Sites in Crude Cardiac Membranes

Protocol 1: Crude Membrane Preparation

1. Thaw 100–150 mg frozen tissue (after excision immediately frozen in liquid N_2 and stored at –80 °C) on ice in 5 ml ice-cold incubation buffer (10 mM Na_2HPO_4, 120 mM NaCl, 5 mM KCl; pH 7.4) containing 0.25 M sucrose.
2. Mince the tissue with scissors and gradually homogenize it with an Ultra Turrax (Ultra-Turrax T25, Jahne andKunkel IKA Labortechnik, Germany) at 24,000 rpm for 10 s. and twice at 17,500 rpm for 20 s. with 1 min intervals on ice.
3. Bring the homogenate up to 20 ml with incubation buffer (+ 0.25 M sucrose) and centrifuge it at 1,200×*g* for 10 min at 0 °C.
4. Filter the supernatant through four layers of cheese cloth and centrifuge it at 20,000×*g* for 20 min at 4 °C.
5. Re-suspend the resulting pellet in 20 ml incubation buffer (+ 0.25 M sucrose) and re-centrifuge at 20,000×*g* for 20 min at 4 °C.
6. Re-suspend the final crude membrane pellet in 1 ml ice-cold incubation buffer (without sucrose!).

7. Freeze the protein suspension immediately in liquid N_2 and store it at –80 °C (noradrenaline transporter protein in suspension is stable for up to 4 days at –80 °C).

Protocol 2: [³H]-Nisoxetine Binding

1. Thaw the protein suspension obtained in Protocol 1 on ice.
2. Determine the protein content according to Bradford (1976) using bovine γ-globulin as a standard.
3. Dilute the protein suspension with incubation buffer (without sucrose) to reach a protein concentration of 100 μg protein/400 μl incubation buffer (without sucrose) and store it on ice until further use.
4. Dilute [³H]-nisoxetine ([N-methyl-³H]-Nisoxetine; specific activity 80 Ci/mmol; NEN™ Life science Products Inc., Boston, MA, USA) with incubation buffer to reach 6 different concentrations ranging from 100 nM down to 3.125 nM.
5. Prepare a solution of 1 mM desipramine by dissolving the antagonist in distilled water and dilute it by adding 50 μl of this solution to 4.95 ml incubation buffer (without sucrose).
6. Place 12×75 mm polypropylene tubes in a tube rack standing in an ice-water bath and add 50 μl either of incubation buffer (total binding) or 50 μl desipramine (final concentration 1 μM /assay; non-specific binding) and 400 μl of the protein solution.
7. Pre-incubate the compounds for at least 15 min on ice.
8. Add to the tubes (+/– desipramine) 50 μl of the corresponding [³H]-nisoxetine dilution (final assay volume 500 μl) and incubate the compounds for 3 h at 4 °C.
9. Terminate the incubation by adding 5 ml of ice-cold incubation buffer (without sucrose) to the reaction mixture and rapidly filter them through Whatman GF/C filters using a 12-well harvester. Wash the filters twice each time with 5 ml incubation buffer (without sucrose).
10. Transfer the filters into scintillation vials and allow them to dry over night.
11. Add 4 ml scintillation cocktail (LumasafeTM Plus, Lumac, Groningen, Netherlands) to each vial and shake them for at least 10 min at room temperature.
12. Determine the radioactivity with a scintillation counter (e.g. Packard TRI-Carb 2250CA) that has a minimum efficiency of 60% for [³H]-labeled ligands.

Protocol 2 should be performed in duplicates for each [³H]-nisoxetine dilution. According to this protocol "non-specific" binding of [³H]-nisoxetine is defined as binding in the presence of 1 μM desipramine. Specific binding is defined as total binding minus non-specific binding and should amount 80% at 2.5 nM [³H]-nisoxetine.

To estimate the equilibrium dissociation constant (K_D) and the maximal number of binding sites (B_{max}) for [³H]-nisoxetine, we use the iterative curve-fitting program Prism 2 from GraphPad Software (San Diego, CA, USA), to analyze the data by non-linear regression (hyperbolic function). The non-linear regression analysis of the saturation experiment should reveal that [³H]-nisoxetine binds to a single population of binding sites.

Protocol 3: Drug Competition Experiments

1. Follow steps 1 to 3 of Protocol 2.
2. Dilute [^{3}H]-nisoxetine ([N-methyl-^{3}H]-Nisoxetine; specific activity 80 Ci/mmol; NEN™ Life science Products Inc., Boston, MA, USA) with incubation buffer to reach a concentration of 20 nM.
3. Prepare a solution of 1 mM desipramine, nisoxetine, cocaine or GBR 12909 (dopamine transporter antagonist) by dissolving each in distilled water and dilute them to get at least 8–12 different concentrations ranging from 1 mM down to 0.01 nM.
4. Place 14×12 ml polypropylene tubes in a tube rack standing in an ice-water bath and add in one tube 50 µl incubation buffer (to determine total binding), in one tube 50 µl 1 µM desipramine (final concentration 1 µM /assay; to determine non-specific binding), and in the other tubes 50 µl of the corresponding antagonist dilution. Add in each tube 400 µl of the protein solution.
5. Pre-incubate the compounds for at least 15 min on ice.
6. Add to all tubes 50 µl of the 20 nM [^{3}H]-NIS dilution (final assay volume 500 µl) and incubate the compounds for 3 h at 4 °C.
7. Follow steps 9 to 12 of Protocol 2.

Protocol 3 should be performed in duplicates for each antagonist dilution. According to this protocol "non-specific" binding of [^{3}H]-nisoxetine is defined as binding in the presence of 1 µM desipramine. Specific binding is defined as total binding minus non-specific binding. The competition binding data can be analyzed by computer-assisted non-linear regression analysis (Prism 2 from GraphPad Software) to fit a one-site competition curve to estimate the IC_{50}-value (concentration of the competitor to inhibit specific [^{3}H]-nisoxetine binding by 50%).

Determination of Uptake$_1$ Activity in Cardiac Tissue Slices

Protocol 4: [^{3}H]-Noradrenaline Uptake$_1$ Activity

1. Place the tissue immediately after excision in ice-cold oxygenated (5% CO_2/95%O_2) Krebs-Henseleit solution (118 mM NaCl, 4.7 mM KCl, 2.5 mM $CaCl_2$, 0.54 mM $MgCl_2$, 25 mM $NaHCO_3$, 1 mM NaH_2PO_4, 11 mM glucose, 0.094 mM EDTA, 1.14 mM ascorbic acid, 0.067 mM nialamide, MAO-blocker).
2. Mince about 120 mg tissue into small pieces using scissors and cut them first into 500×500 µm and then into 250×250 µm slices covered with about 500 µl ice-cold oxygenated Krebs-Henseleit solution using a tissue chopper (McIllwain; Bachhofer, Reutlingen, Germany).
3. Wash the slices twice in fresh ice-cold oxygenated Krebs-Henseleit solution.
4. Re-suspend the tissue slices in ice-cold oxygenated Krebs-Henseleit solution, containing 40 µM corticosterone (stock solution solved in 0.1% DMSO) to block extraneuronal uptake of noradrenaline), to reach a dilution of 10 mg slices per 400 µl buffer.

5. Because the K_M value is in the high nanomolar range it is necessary to dilute the labelled with unlabelled substrate to reveal high noradrenaline concentration. Therefore, prepare a solution of 250 nM noradrenaline (diluted in ice-cold oxygenated Krebs-Henseleit solution). Take 2.5 ml of the solution and add 25 µl [^{3}H]-noradrenaline (D,L-(7-^{3}H[N])-Noradrenaline hydrochloride; specific activity 13.5 Ci/mmol; NEN™ Life science Products Inc., Boston, MA, USA).
6. Dilute the 250 nM [^{3}H]-noradrenaline stock solution to get at least 5 different concentrations ranging from 250 nM down to 15.6 nM.
7. Place 10×6 ml polypropylene tubes (two tubes per noradrenaline dilution) in a tube rack standing at room temperature and 10×6 ml polypropylene tubes in a tube rack standing in an ice-water bath (to determine non-specific accumulation of radioactivity) and add in all tubes 50 µl ice-cold oxygenated Krebs-Henseleit solution. Add in each tube 400 µl (=10 mg) tissue slices.
8. Equilibrate the compounds to each temperature for at least for 15 min.
9. Add to the tubes (room temperature/4 °C) 50 µl of the corresponding [^{3}H]-noradrenaline dilution (final assay volume 500 µl) and incubate the compounds for 15 min either at 37 °C or 4 °C.
10. Terminate the incubation by adding 3 ml of ice-cold ice-cold oxygenated Krebs-Henseleit solution to the reaction mixture and rapidly filter them through Whatman GF/C filters, that had been pre-soaked for 15 min in ice-cold Krebs-Henseleit solution containing 0.05% polyethylenimine, using a 12-well harvester. Wash the filters twice each time with 5 ml incubation buffer (without sucrose).
11. Transfer the filters into scintillation vials. Add 500 µl of ice-cold 3% trichloroacetic acid (TCA) to each filter and incubate them (digestion of the slices and release of [^{3}H]-noradrenaline in the liquid phase) overnight at 4 °C.
12. Add 4 ml scintillation cocktail (LumasafeTM Plus, Lumac, Groningen, Netherlands) to each vial and shake them for at least 10 min at room temperature.
13. Determine the radioactivity with a scintillation counter as mentioned in Protocol 2, step 12.

According to this protocol, which determines the initial rate of [^{3}H]-noradrenaline uptake at low concentrations (1.56–25 nM), specific uptake$_1$ is defined as total uptake (37 °C) minus non-specific uptake (4 °C). To determine uptake$_1$ kinetic parameters the slices have to be incubated as described above with [^{3}H]-noradrenaline concentrations leading to the saturation of uptake$_1$ (final concentration about 250 nM). Again, specific uptake$_1$ must be determined by incubating the slices in parallel at 37 °C and 4 °C. Competition studies with desipramine, nisoxetine, cocaine and GBR 12909 have to be conducted as described above by incubating tissue slices with a fixed concentration of [^{3}H]-noradrenaline (25 nM) in the presence of 8–12 concentrations of each competitive drug. As described in Protocol 3 the tissue slices have also to be pre-incubated with the antagonists for at least 15 min. (the interaction between the noradrenaline transporter and inhibitors requires more time than this for substrate, implying that the binding of inhibitors might involve a significant conformational change in the transporter protein), therefore the volume of 50 µl of Krebs-Henseleit solution can just be replaced by the same volume of the antagonist dilution. Again, non-specific accumulation of radioactivity is determined by parallel incubation at

4 °C. To ensure that only uptake$_1$ is active under the experimental conditions described above, tissue slices have to be incubated with [^{3}H]-noradrenaline in the presence of 40 µM of the uptake$_2$-inhibitor corticosterone. To estimate the kinetic parameters K_M and V_{max} of the noradrenaline transporter we use the iterative curve-fitting program Prism 2 from GraphPad Software to analyze the data by non-linear regression (hyperbolic function). The competition data can be analyzed by computer-assisted non-linear regression analysis (Prism 2 from GraphPad Software) to fit a one-site competition curve to estimate the IC$_{50}$-value (concentration of the competitor to inhibit specific [^{3}H]-noradrenaline uptake by 50%).

Indirect Determination of Uptake$_1$ Activity in Isolated Trabecular Strips

Human trabecular strips can be obtained from e.g. right atrial appendages that are removed during the installation of a cardiopulmonary bypass. Each muscle preparation should be used for only one concentration-response curve to exclude β-adrenoceptor desensitization. An uptake$_1$ blocker should shift the concentration-response curve of noradrenaline to the left. As a result, an increase in the potency of noradrenaline is able to reflect a reduced inactivation of noradrenaline via uptake$_1$ and this represents indirectly the activity of the noradrenaline transporter (Leineweber et al. 2002).

To verify that the effect is clearly dependent on the uptake$_1$ activity the experiments should be repeated in the presence of isoprenaline instead of noradrenaline, since isoprenaline is not a substrate for uptake$_1$. To block a-adrenoceptors, phentolamine (1 µM) should be present throughout the experiments.

Protocol 5: Preparation and Organ-Bath Incubation of Trabecular Strips

1. Immediately after excision, transfer the cardiac tissue into carbogenated (95% O$_2$/ 5% CO$_2$) Tyrode-solution (mmol/l: NaCl 119.8; KCl 5.4; CaCl$_2$ 1.8; MgSO$_4$ 1.05; NaH$_2$PO$_4$ 0.42; NaHCO$_3$ 23.6; glucose 5.05; EDTA 0.05; ascorbic acid 0.28; at room temperature). The time that it needs to reach the laboratory where the experiment is conducted should not exceed 15–30 min.
2. Prepare the tissue in continuously aerated Tyrode-solution (see above) at room temperature to minimize inadequate oxygenation. Remove the connective tissue carefully without endocardial damage.
3. Dissect trabecular strips of uniform size (4–5 mm in length and 1 mm or less diameter) with muscle fibres running approximately parallel to the length of the strips in aerated Tyrode solution under microscopic control using scissors. (Isolated cardiac tissue should only be used if at least two functioning trabecular strips can be obtained).
4. Suspend the muscles in an organ bath maintained at 37 °C containing continuously aerated Tyrode solution (between 10 to 70 ml with respect to organ bath size).
5. Stimulate the muscles by two platinum electrodes using field stimulation from a stimulator (frequency 1 Hz, impulse duration 5 ms, intensity 10 to 20% [e.g. between 3–12 V] greater than threshold).
6. Stretch each muscle to a length at which force of contraction is maximal (the force of rest has to be kept constant throughout the experiment).

7. Measure the resultant tension isometrically with an inductive force transducer attached to a recorder.
8. To determine the functional evidence of uptake$_1$ on the potency of noradrenaline to increase force of contraction mediated by b-adrenoceptors, pre-incubate the preparations with an uptake$_1$ blocker (e.g. 1 µM desipramine) or vehicle for at least 30 min and then estimate cumulative concentration-response curves for noradrenaline within a concentration range of 10 nM to 10 µM.

Experimental data of the contraction studies can be fitted and analyzed by non-linear regression analysis (sigmoidal concentration-response curve: y = bottom + [top − bottom]/[1 + 10$^{(\log EC50-x)}$], with x = logarithm of agonist concentration and y = response), using Prism 2 from GraphPad Software.

Troubleshooting

Great Variations in IC$_{50}$ Values

The affinity of the uptake antagonists desipramine and nisoxetine (both specific uptake$_1$ blockers) as well as cocaine (monoamine-transporter blocker) and GBR12909 (dopamine uptake blocker) for the noradrenaline transporter is dependent on the cell type and species that is used. Nevertheless, for uptake$_1$ the order of potency should be in general desipramine ≥ nisoxetine >> cocaine ≥ GBR12909 independent whether noradrenaline activity or density is investigated (Leineweber et al. 2000; 2002). The concentration of desipramine that inhibits 50% of uptake$_1$ activity (IC$_{50}$ values in nM) ranges between 1.2 to 2.0 in hNAT- or mmNAT-transfected cells, 7.0 to 13 in rat cardiac slices or natively expressing rat PC12 cells and 450 nM in human placental brush border membrane vesicles. The IC$_{50}$ values (nM) of nisoxetine ranges between 1.7 to 4.2 in bNAT- or mmNAT-transfected cells, 11.8 in rat cardiac slices and 17.2 in natively expressing rat PC12 cells; that of cocaine ranges between 380 in cardiac synaptosomes, 2300 in human placental brush border membrane vesicles and 3817 in rat cardiac slices. Finally, that of GBR12909 ranges for all above 5000. Equally, the concentration of desipramine that inhibits 50% of [^{3}H]-nisoxetine binding (IC$_{50}$ values in nM) ranges between 0.73 in rat heart, 2.66 in rat palcenta, 31 in human right atria and 450 in human placenta. That of nisoxetine ranges between 3.75 in rat placenta, 10.7 in rat heart, 82 in human right atria and 600 in human placenta. For cocaine, the IC50 values (nM) are above 2000 and above 3000 for GBR 12909.

Stimulating Agents on Noradrenaline Transporter Activity and Increase In Density

In general, treatment with compounds that increase noradrenaline content (e.g. monoamine oxidase inhibitors) positively regulate mRNA expression and protein density of the noradrenaline transporter. Further modulatory/stimulating agents implicated in regulating transporter-density and -activity *in vivo* include angiotensin II, atrial natriuretic peptide, insulin, ATP, Ca^{2+} and nitric oxide. In general, protein kinase A (PKA)-dependent pathways produce an increase in V_{max} and up-regulation of the noradrenaline transporter. Furthermore, (patho-) physiological conditions, like dietary restriction or chronic hypoxia, seems to up-regulate the noradrenaline transporter-activity and density.

Inhibiting Agents on NAT Activity and Reduction in NAT Density

In general, treatment with compounds that deplete noradrenaline stores (e.g. reserpine) negatively regulate the noradrenaline transporter. Uptake$_1$ is further found to be blocked by low temperature, sodium azid and ouabain. Activation of protein kinase C (PKC) by phorbol esters results in phosphorylation of the transporter protein and decreases V_{max} of noradrenaline transport. Long-term treatment *in vitro* and *in vivo* with INF-α, nerve growth factor or desipramine leads to a down-regulation of transporter density and therefore to a decrease in uptake$_1$. On the other hand, amphetamine and metamphetamine, haloperidol, procaine, tetracaine and dibucaine, long-term treatment with propofol, thiamylal and diazepam and N-ethylmaleimide are acute inhibitors and inhibiting uptake$_1$ to a great extent (>40%). (Patho-)physiological conditions like age, cold (4 °C) exposure; long-term pressure overload, diabetic cardiomyopathy, congestive heart failure, ischemia-induced arrhythmia and orthostatic intolerance are accompanied by noradrenaline transporter malfunction.

Anesthetics

It is now commonly accepted that anesthesia depresses the activity of the sympathetic system. Enflurane and isoflurane were shown to be associated with decreases in noradrenaline spillover rates leading to results which showed lower than actual noradrenaline concentrations. Ketamine, on the other hand, has a dual effect on the noradrenaline transporter (for review see Hara et al. 2000). Whereas short-term treatment causes inhibition, long-term-treatment leads to an increase of uptake$_1$ by upregulation of transporter-density. Chloralose induces large decreases (about –38%) in the noradrenaline clearance rate, whereas diethyl ether induces a stimulation of sympathetic nerve activity with an increase in noradrenaline spillover rate and plasma concentration while the uptake$_1$ mechanism is unchanged. On the other hand, pentobarbital, a typical general anesthetic agent, does not affect the uptake of monoamines and should therefore be the first choice for anaesthesia of animals.

References

Böhm M, LaRosee K, Schwinger RHG, Erdmann E (1995) Evidence for reduction of norepinephrine uptake sites in the failing human heart. J. Am. Coll. Cardiol. 25:146–153

Bradford MM (1976) A rapid and sensitive method for the quantification of microgram quantities of protein utilizing the principle of protein-dye binding. Anal. Biochem. 72:248–254

Brüss M, Pörzgen P, Bryan-Lluka LJ, Bönisch H (1997) The rat norepinephrine transporter: molecular cloning from PC12 cells and functional expression. Mol. Brain Res. 52:257–262

Esler M, Kaye D, Lambert D, Jennings G (1997) Adrenergic nervous system in heart failure. Am. J. Cardiol. 80:7L–14L

Graefe KH and Bönisch H (1988) The transport of amines across the axonal membranes. In: Trendelenburg U, Weiner N (eds) Catecholamines I. Springer-Verlag, Berlin, p 193–245

Hara K, Yanagihara N, Min ami K, Hirano H, Sata T, Shigematsu A, Izumi F (2000) Dual effects of intraveneous anesthetics on the function of norepinephrine transporters. Anestesiol. 93:1329–35
Jayanthi LD, Prasad PD, Ramamoorthy V, Mahesh VB, Leibach FH, Ganapathy V (1993) Sodium- and chloride-dependent, cocaine-sensitive, high-affinity binding of nisoxetine to the human placental norepinephrine transporter. Biochem. 32: 12178–12185
Kiyono Y, Lida Y, Kawashima H, Tamaki N, Nishimura H, Saji H (2001) Regional alterations of myocardial norepinephrine transporter density in streptozotocin-induced diabetic-rats: implications for heterogeneous cardiac accumulation of MIBG in diabetes. Eur. J. Nucl. Med. 28:894–899
Lee CM and Snyder SH (1981) Norepinephrine neuronal uptake binding sites in rat brain membranes labeled with [^{3}H]desipramine. Proc. Natl. Acad. Sci. USA 78:5250–5254
Leineweber K, Seyfarth T, Brodde O-E (2000) Chamber-specific alterations of noradrenaline uptake (uptake$_1$) in right ventricles of monocrotaline-treated rats. Brit. J. Pharmacol. 131:1438–1444
Leineweber K, Wangemann T, Giessler Ch, Bruck H, Dhein S, Kostelka M, Mohr F-W, Silber R-E, Brodde O-E (2002) Age-dependent changes of cardiac neuronal reuptake transporter (uptake$_1$) in the human heart. J. Am. Coll. Cardiol. 40:1459–1465
Runkel F, Brüss M, Nöthen MM, Stöber G, Propping P, Bönisch h (2000) Pharmacological properties of naturally occuring variants of the human norepinephrine transporter. Pharmacogenetics 10:397–405
Tejani-Butt SM (1992) [^{3}H]-Nisoxetine: A Radioligand for quantification of norepinephrine uptake sites by autoradiography or by homogenate binding. J. Pharmacol. Exp. Therap. 260:427–436

6.3.3
Study of G proteins in Cardiovascular Research

Thomas Wieland, Nina Wettschureck and Stefan Offermanns

Introduction

Many neurotransmitters, hormones and growth factors which play important roles in the regulation of the cardiovascular system, act through seven-transmembrane-spanning G protein coupled receptors (GPCRs). Of these, adrenergic and muscarinic cholinergic receptors mediate the control of cardiovascular functions by the autonomic nervous system. Other receptors, such as those for endothelins, angiotensin II or eicosanoids are involved in the local or systemic regulation of cardiovascular functions. The cellular effects induced through these receptors depend on the type of G protein activated by the receptor (see Table 3).

There are basically four families of heterotrimeric G proteins: G_s, which couples receptors in a stimulatory fashion to adenylyl cyclase; $G_{i/o}$, which couples receptors in an inhibitory fashion to adenylyl cyclase and which mediates the activation of potassium channels as well as the inhibition of voltage-dependent Ca^{2+} channels; $G_{q/11}$, which couples receptors to the stimulation of β-isoforms of phospholipase C; and finally the $G_{12/13}$ family, which mediates the activation of the small GTPase Rho. These families of heterotrimeric G proteins play central roles in transmembrane signalling by processing and sorting of signals conveyed by GPCRs. They are also able to adjust the sensitivities of the system to certain stimuli, a function involving various mechanisms including the action of "regulators of G protein signalling" (RGS) proteins, which are able to "switch off" the active state of the G protein.

Multiple excellent reviews and book chapters have been written on the analysis of receptor G protein coupling and on the determination of G protein activity [e.g. Methods in Enzymology Vols. 237 (1994) and 344 (2002)] which can be applied to

Table 3
G protein coupled receptors (GPCRs) in the cardiovascular system.

Endogenous ligand(s)	Receptor	Coupling to G protein subclass(es)
Acetylcholine	M_2	$G_{i/o}$
Adrenaline, Noradrenaline	$\alpha_{1A}, \alpha_{1B}, \alpha_{1D}$,	$G_{q/11}, (G_{i/o}?)$
	$\alpha_{2A}, \alpha_{2B}, \alpha_{2C}$	$G_{i/o}$
	β_1	G_s
	β_2, β_3	$G_s, G_{i/o}$
Prostacyclin (PGI_2)	IP	G_s
Thromboxane A_2 (TXA_2)	TP	$G_{q/11}, G_{12/13}$
Angiotensin II	AT_1	$G_{q/11}, G_{12/13}, G_{i/o}$
	AT_2	$(G_{i/o}?)$
Bradykinin	B_1, B_2	$G_{q/11}$
Endothelin- 1, -2, -3	ET_A (ET-1, ET-2)	$G_{q/11}, G_{12/13}$
	ET_B (ET-1, -2, -3)	$G_{q/11}, G_i$
Urotensin II	UT	$G_{q/11}$
Vasopressin	V_{1a}, V_{1b}	$G_{q/11}$
	V_2	G_s
Thrombin and others	PAR-1, PAR-3, PAR-4	$G_{q/11}, G_{12/13}, G_{i/o}$
Trypsin and others	PAR-2	$G_{q/11}$

study the cellular and sub-cellular role of heterotrimeric G proteins in the cardiovascular system. To study G protein mediated signalling in the living organism, molecular biological and genetic methods are required. This chapter therefore will focus on recent progress in applying adenoviral vectors and genetic approaches to the study of heterotrimeric G protein functions in the cardiovascular system.

Adenovirus Mediated Overexpression of Negative Regulators of Heterotrimeric G Proteins to Analyze Signalling Pathways in Cardiac Myocytes

A variety of G protein coupled receptors (GPCRs) in cardiac myocytes, for example endothelin-1 receptors, angiotensin II receptors and protease activated receptors, simultaneously activate more than one subtype of heterotrimeric G proteins. They thereby regulate several effector molecules and induce a variety of cellular responses. Therefore, the contribution of a distinct G protein subtype or its subunits to the regu-

Table 4
Adenoviral constructs suitable for analyzing G protein mediated pathways in cardiac myocytes[a]

Recombinant adenovirus	Expressed protein	Function	Observed effect after overexpression
Ad5RGS2	RGS2	$G\alpha_{q/11}$- >> $G\alpha_{i/o}$-GAP	Inhibition of $G\alpha_{q/11}$-mediated effects
Ad5RGS4	RGS4	$G\alpha_{q/11}$- ≈ $G\alpha_{i/o}$-GAP	Inhibition of $G\alpha_{i/o}$ plus $G\alpha_{q/11}$-mediated effects
Ad5Lsc	Lsc-RGS domain	$G\alpha_{12/13}$-GAP	Inhibition of $G\alpha_{12/13}$-mediated effects
Ad5KIAA380	PDZRhoGEF-RGS domain	$G\alpha_{12/13}$-GAP	Inhibition of $G\alpha_{12/13}$-mediated effects
Ad5TDα	Transducin α-subunit	Gβγ scavenger	Inhibition of Gβγ-mediated effects

[a] An adenoviral construct expressing the RGS-homology domain of RGS-PX1 should theoretically be suitable to suppress $G\alpha_s$-mediated signals (Zheng et al. 2001). This concept has however not been approved in our laboratories

lation of a specific signalling pathway is often not readily evident and additionally may vary between different receptors and their subtypes. The (over)-expression of specific negative regulators of heterotrimeric G protein function, for example GTPase-activating proteins (GAPs) for Gα subunits or scavenging proteins for activated Gα subunits or free Gβγ dimers, is often used to dissect the involvement of G proteins in distinct signalling pathways in living cells. Besides the fact that isolated cardiac myocytes are difficult to culture, the transfection of cultured cardiomyocytes by standard methods such as liposomes, electroporation or calcium phosphate precipitation is known to have an extremely low efficiency. Thus, the use of these methods for the above mentioned expression of negative regulators of G protein function in cardiac myocytes is very limited.

An approach which is however widely used to express recombinant proteins in cardiac myocytes is the infection of the cells with recombinant adenoviruses. Moreover, this method can additionally be applied to express recombinant proteins in engineered heart tissue (El-Armouche et al. 2003), heart muscle strips (Janssen et al. 2002), perfused Langendorff hearts (Wiechert et al. 2003) in vitro and even in the living heart of animal models (Neyroud et al. 2002). We will describe herein the use of recombinant adenoviruses encoding the RGS homology domains of regulators of G protein signalling proteins or the α subunit of the retinal G protein transducin (Table 4) to analyze G protein coupling of several GPCRs in neonatal rat and adult rabbit cardiac myocytes. Besides the over-expression of the aforementioned negative regulators to analyze the role of endogenous G proteins, adenoviral mediated over-expression of $G\alpha_{12}$, $G\alpha_q$ and $G\alpha_s$ has been used to study the role of these G protein a subunits in cardiomyocytes, heart muscle and the hearts of living animals (Table 5).

Table 5
Adenoviral over-expression of wild type or mutant G protein α subunits in the cardiovascular system

Transgene	Tissue	Phenotype	Reference
$G\alpha_s$	Neonatal rat cardiomyocytes	Enhanced activation of adenylyl cyclase, induction of hypertrophy	Novotny et al. (1994), Biochem Mol Biol Int 34:993-1001
$G\alpha_{i2}$	Rabbit trabeculae	Impaired inotropic response to catecholamines	Janssen et al. (2002), Cardiovasc Res 55:300-308
$G\alpha_{i2}$	Catheterized porcine hearts	Reduction of heart rate during atrial fibrillation	Donahue et al. (2000), Nature Medicine 6:1395-1397
$G\alpha_{i2}$	Adult rat cardiomyocytes	Induction of the negative inotropic effect of β2-adrenoceptors	Gong et al. (2002), Circulation 105:2497-2503
$G\alpha_{i2}$	Neonatal and adult rat cardiomyocytes	Suppression of isoprenaline-stimulated adenylyl cyclase and inotropic response	Rau et al. (2003), FASEB J. 17:523-525
$G\alpha_q$ (wt)	Neonatal rat cardiomyocytes	Enhanced PGF2α- and phenylephrine-induced PLC activation and apoptosis	Adams et al. (1998) Proc Natl Acad Sci USA 95:10140-10145, Adams et al. (2000) Circulation Res 87:1180-1187
$G\alpha_q$ (Q209L) (const. active)	Neonatal rat cardiomyocytes	Activation of PLC, induction of apoptosis	Adams et al. (1998) Proc Natl Acad Sci USA 95:10140-10145, Adams et al. (2000) Circulation Res 87:1180-1187

const. active constitutively active mutant; *wt* wild type form.

Description of Methods and Practical Approach

Isolation and Culture of Neonatal Rat Cardiac Myocytes

Buffers and Media.
- CBFHH buffer, pH 7.4 (mM)
  NaCl 136, Hepes 20, glucose 5.55, KCl 5.36, $MgSO_4$ 0.81, KH_2PO_4 0.44, NaH_2PO_4

- Dnase II solution
  Dnase II (Sigma) 0.02 mg/ml, foetal calf serum (Invitrogen) 0.65% (v/v), penicillin 100 U/ml, streptomycin 0.1 mg/ml, in CBFHH buffer
- Trypsin solution
  Trypsin (Sigma) 0.3% (w/v), Dnase II (Sigma) 0.02 mg/ml, penicillin 100 U/ml, streptomycin 0.1 mg/ml, in CBFHH buffer
- MEM
  Foetal calf serum (FCS), inactivated, 10% (v/v), penicillin 100 U/ml, streptomycin 0.1 mg/ml, 5-bromo-2-desoxyuridine (BrdU, Sigma) 1 mM, in Minimum Essential Medium (Invitrogen).

Procedure. Newborn (60–80 animals) Wistar rats (1–3 d old) are decapitated and the heart is extracted from the thorax. The atria and tissues from surrounding organs are excised. The hearts are minced with scissors in CBFHH buffer and poured into a sterile 50 ml Falcon tube. After sedimentation of the tissue, the supernatant is discarded and the pellet is incubated in 10 ml freshly prepared trypsin solution for 20 min at 4 °C. Thereafter, the supernatant is discarded and the pellet is resuspended in 10 ml fresh trypsin solution. After an incubation of 10 min at room temperature with gentle shaking, the supernatant is removed and added to 2.5 ml FCS (not inactivated) and stored on ice. The pellet is resuspended in 9 ml of DNase II solution and the suspension is triturated by repeated suction through a pipette with a 3 mm wide opening 27×.

After sedimentation of the pellet, the supernatant is removed and added to the already stored supernatant. This procedure has to be repeated as long as the digest produces a detectable clouding. Thereafter, the cells in the stored supernatants are pelleted by centrifugation for 15 min at 60×g in a swingout rotor. The supernatant is discarded, the cells are resuspended in 20 ml of MEM without BrdU and 0.4 mg DNase II is added. After trituration with the pipette, the cells are again pelleted by centrifugation for 15 min at 60×g. Thereafter, the cells are resuspended in 32 ml of MEM without BrdU and plated through a 60 mm mesh filter on to four culture dishes (Ø 10 cm). The dishes are kept for about 2 h in an incubator at 37 °C. This time is sufficient to let non-myocytes adhere to the dishes whereas the cardiac myocytes are still floating. Thus, the myocytes are harvested with the supernatant and the cells are plated on new culture dishes (Ø 6 cm) in MEM, now complemented with the antimetabolite BrdU, at a density of $1-3\times10^6$ cells per dish. The cardiac myocytes adhere to the dishes and form a monolayer after 1 day of culture. Regular autonomous contractions are observed usually after 2–3 days of culture.

Isolation of Adult Rabbit Cardiac Myocytes

Buffers and Media.
- Tyrode solution, pH 7.55 (mM)
  NaCl 137, Hepes 20, glucose 15, KCl 5.4, $MgSO_4$ 1.2, NaH_2PO_4 1.2, saturated with O_2
- Enzyme Solution
  Collagenase CLS II (Biochrom) 1 mg/ml, protease fraction XIV (Sigma), 0.04 mg/ml, $CaCl_2$ 0.025 mM in Tyrode solution

- M199 (mM)
  Creatine 5.0, D,L-carnitine 5.0, taurine 5.0, L-glutamine 2, penicillin 100 U/ml, streptomycin 0.1 mg/ml, in medium 199 (Invitrogen)

Adult New Zealand White rabbits receive heparin anticoagulation (1,000 units i.v.) prior to pentobarbital (50 mg/kg i.v.). The heart is extracted and rinsed twice in ice-cold Tyrode solution. Next, the aorta is cannulated, and the heart is suspended in an insulated chamber at 35–37 °C. Langendorff perfusion is performed by retrograde flow from the cannula in the ascending aorta to the coronary arteries. The heart is perfused with Tyrode containing 1 mM Ca^{2+} at 20 ml/min until the heart beats regularly at about 130 beats per minute. Thereafter, the perfusion is switched to calcium-free Tyrode for 10 min at 20 ml/min, before perfusion with the enzyme solution for an additional 10–15 min. The digestion is stopped by perfusion with 100 ml Tyrode containing 0.05 mM Ca^{2+} and 20 mM 2,3-butanedione-monoxime (BDM). The presence of BDM is crucial as it binds reversibly to cardiac myofilaments and thereby prevents hypercontractions that might lead to sarcolemmal injury and cell death. The ventricles are excised, minced in Tyrode containing 0.05 mM Ca^{2+} and 20 mM BDM, and agitated by repeated suction through a Pasteur pipette. The resulting cell suspension is strained through a 200 mm nylon mesh filter. In general, the ventricles are uniformly digested, and the residue remaining on the filter is from the valvular and tendon structures, with only minimal myocardium. The Ca^{2+} concentration is gradually restored in several steps (0.05 mM, 0.078 mM, 0.156 mM, 0.3125 mM, 0.625 mM) before the cells are finally resuspended in M199. Viable myocytes are enriched by sedimentation through 6% (w/v) albumin fraction V (Sigma) in M199. The cells are plated at a density of 50,000 cells per dish in laminin-coated dishes (∅ 3.5 cm, 20 µg/ml laminin (Sigma) in M199 for 1 h at 37 °C) and cultured in a 37 °C incubator for a maximum of 48 h.

Construction and Amplification of Recombinant Adenoviruses

Recombinant adenoviruses are constructed using the AdEasy system developed by the group of Bert Vogelstein (He et al. 1998). As detailed information and protocols for that system are available in the World Wide Web at www.coloncancer.org/adeasy.htm, only a brief description of the system will be given here. The cDNA encoding the gene of interest is first cloned into a shuttle vector. The most commonly used pAdTrack-CMV vector additionally encodes enhanced green fluorescent protein (EGFP) under the control of an independent CMV promotor. E. Coli BJ 5183 cells are co-transformed with purified recombinant pAdTrack-CMV linearized by a PmeI digest and the adenoviral backbone vector pAdEasy-1. By homologous recombination, sequences of the pAdTrack-CMV are inserted into the pAdEasy-1. As by the homologous recombination the gene encoding resistance against ampicillin is also switched to the gene encoding resistance to kanamycin, positive recombinants can be selected on agar plates containing kanamycin. Note however that the homologous recombination has to be verified by a digest with restriction endonucleases. Thereafter, adenovirally transformed human embryonic kidney (HEK 293) cells are transfected with the positive plasmid linearized by digestion with PacI. If pAdTrack-CMV was used as shuttle vector originally, the transfected cells can be visualized 12–24 h post transfection by fluorescence microscopy. Usually the recombinant viruses are harvested 5–6 days post transfection. After several rounds of amplification to increase the numbers of infected cells, the viruses are purified from the culture medium either by centrifugation through a $CsCl_2$ gradient or using commercially available purification kits. Viral stocks can be stored in aliquots in a glycerol enriched storage buffer for several months. To determine the titres of the viral stocks an endpoint dilution assay (see below) can be recommended for EGFP encoding adenoviruses.

Endpoint Dilution Assay to Determine the Viral Titre of EGFP-encoding Adenoviruses

HEK293 cells are harvested from a culture dish (∅ 10 cm) and resuspended in 5 ml DMEM (Dulbecco's minimal essential medium (Invitrogen) supplemented with 2% (v/v) inactivated FCS, 2 mM glutamine, 100 U/ml penicillin, and 0.1 mg/ml streptomycin at a density of 20,000 cells/90 µl. 90 µl of this suspension is added into each well of a 96 well plate. For controls, the first 6 wells of the first row of the 96 well plate remain uninfected (negative control) whereas the remaining 6 wells of this row are infected with 1 µl of original virus stock (positive control). The vast majority of the cells in these six wells should become infected and can be seen by fluorescence microscopy.

Virus Dilutions

From the original virus stock a 100-fold dilution (1 µl stock + +99 µl DMEM) is prepared. This dilution is further diluted with DMEM to 10^{-4}, 10^{-5}, 10^{-6}, 10^{-7}, 10^{-8} and 10^{-9}. From these dilutions 10 µl are added to the 90 µl cell suspension (additional 1:10 dilution, see below) and mixed with the pipette. 12 wells = 1 row are used per dilution. The cells are incubated for 4 days in the 37 °C incubator. Thereafter the number of wells that contain EGFP expressing cells is determined by fluorescence microscopy. One single green cell per well scores as a positive count (infected). A well without EGFP expression is negative (uninfected). The results are noted in a result table (see under Examples).

Examples

See Table 6

Calculation of Proportional Distance PD

Use dilutions surrounding the 50% infection value: A effectivity (%) lower dilution, B effectivity (%) higher dilution
- PD = A-50/(A-B)
- Example from above (57.8-50)/(57.8-27.3) = 0.256

Table 6
Results

Final dilution	Infected	Uninfected	Total infected*	Total uninfected*	% Infected†
10^{-5}	12	0	34	0	100.0
10^{-6}	11	1	22	1	95.7
10^{-7}	5	7	11	8	57.8
10^{-8}	4	8	6	16	27.3
10^{-9}	2	10	2	26	7.1
10^{-10}	0	12	0	38	0.0
Sum	34	38			

*This calculation assumes that all wells which have been infected by the respective virus dilution would also have been infected by the higher dilutions which caused an infection. On the other hand wells, not infected at a specific dilution would also not have been infected by any lower dilution. In the example given, at a 10^{-5} dilution all 12 wells are infected. Thus, a 10^{-5} dilution would also infected the 11 positive wells at 10^{-6}, 5 at 10^{-7}, 4 at 10^{-8} and 2 at 10^{-9}, together 34 wells. On the other hand, 10 wells are not infected at a 10^{-9}. Thus a 10^{-9} dilution would also not infect the uninfected wells at 10^{-8}, 10^{-7} and 10^{-6}, in sum 26 wells. †At each dilution the percentage of total number infected is calculated, e.g. 10^{-7}. $11/(11+8) = 57.8\%$ infected.

Calculation of TCID$_{50}$ (Dilution causing 50% infection)

- Log TCID$_{50}$ = Log of lower dilution -PD
- Example: Log TCID$_{50}$ = Log 10^{-7} – 0.256 = –7 – 0.256 = –7.256 $\Rightarrow$ TCID$_{50}$ = 5.546 × 10^{-8}

Calculation of Viral Titre

Titre (pfu/µl) = 1/TCID$_{50}$ per dilution volume used × ln 2
Example: $1/(5.546 \times 10^{-8})/10(\mu l) \times 0.69 = 1.244 \times 10^{6}$ pfu/µl = 1.244 × 10^{9} pfu/ml

Infection of Cardiac Myocytes

Neonatal Rat Cardiac Myocytes. After 4 days of culture, dishes with morphologically well-shaped and contracting myocytes are selected for viral infection. The medium is removed and 1 ml fresh MEM (with 2% FCS) containing the desired amount of virus is added. For example to achieve a multiplicity of infection (MOI) of 8, 8×10^{6} pfu of the virus are given to 1×10^{6} myocytes. The dishes are placed in an incubator for 20 min at 37 °C. Thereafter 4 ml of fresh medium are added and the cells are cultured, if not otherwise required, for an additional 48 h before assay. Usually 12–24 h after infection, the efficiency of the transduction can be monitored by the expression of EGFP (see Fig. 12a).

Adult Rabbit Cardiac Myocytes. Directly after preparation of the myocytes, the required amount of adenoviral stock (e.g. 50,000 pfu for a MOI of 1) is added to 50,000 cells in the M199 medium. The cells are plated and incubated for 2 h in the incubator.

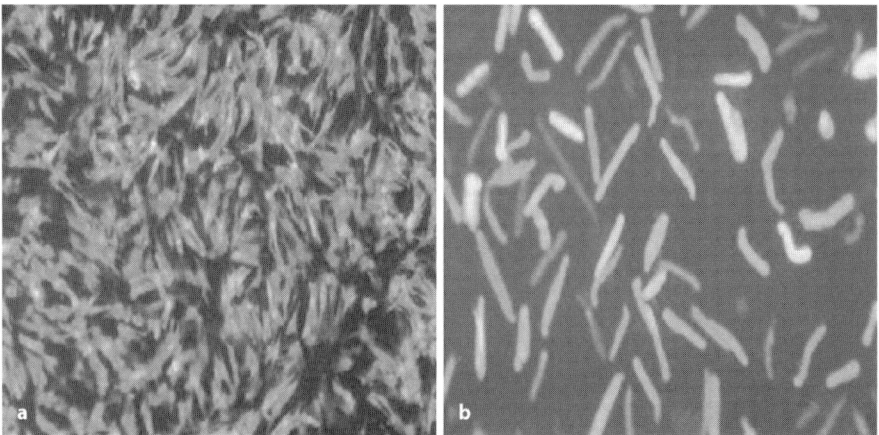

Figure 12a,b
Adenoviral expression of EGFP in neonatal rat and adult rabbit cardiac myocytes. Neonatal rat cardiomyocytes (a) and adult rabbit (b) cardiac myocytes were infected with an adenovirus encoding EGFP and RGS4 at a MOI of 10. The expression of EGFP was visualized by fluorescence microscopy 24 h (b) and 48 h (a) post infection

Thereafter, the virus-containing medium is removed and replaced by fresh M199. The efficiency of the transduction can be monitored 12–24 h after infection by fluorescence microscopy (see Fig. 12b).

Differential Activation of Neonatal Cardiac Myocyte Phospholipase D by Protease Activated Receptors, Endothelin-1 Receptors and a_1-Adrenoceptors.

Activation of the phosphatidylcholine-specific phospholipase D (PLD) in isolated cardiomyocytes has been demonstrated to occur for example by stimulation of endo-thelin-1 receptor subtype A (ET_AR), thrombin activated protease receptor type 1 (PAR1) and α_1-adrenoceptors (α_1AR). PLD and its reaction product, phosphatidic acid, are assumed to participate in cardiac hypertrophy. Therefore we analyzed the coupling of these receptors to PLD in neonatal rat cardiac myocytes. As the stimu-lation of PLD by these GPCRs is pertussis toxin insensitive in cardiac myocytes, we discriminated between the contributions of the pertussis toxin insensitive $G_{q/11}$- and $G_{12/13}$-types of heterotrimeric G proteins by adenovirus-mediated overexpression of the $G_{q/11}$-inhibiting RGS4 and the $G_{12/13}$-inhibiting LscRGS, respectively. The cultured myocytes (3×10^6 cells per culture dish, $\varnothing$ 6 cm) were infected either with a control adenovirus, e.g. an adenovirus expressing only EGFP, or Ad5-RGS4 or Ad5-LscRGS 48 h prior to the assay. As judged by co-expression of EGFP, the efficiency of adenoviral gene transfer (at a MOI of 10) was ≥75% (see Fig. 12a).

For labelling of the myocytes 2.5 µCi/ml [^{3}H]oleic acid was added to the MEM medium 24 h before the assay. Thereafter, the cells were washed once with Hank's balanced salt solution (HBSS, 118 mM NaCl, 5 mM KCl, 1 mM $CaCl_2$, 1 mM $MgCl_2$, 5 mM D-glucose, 15 mM HEPES, pH 7.4) and then allowed to equilibrate for 30 min at 37 °C. The equilibration medium was replaced by fresh HBSS containing 2% ethanol and the indicated stimuli, and incubation was continued for 30 min at 37 °C. Thereaf-

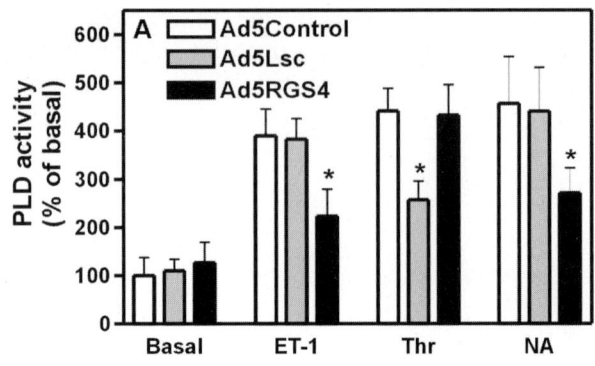
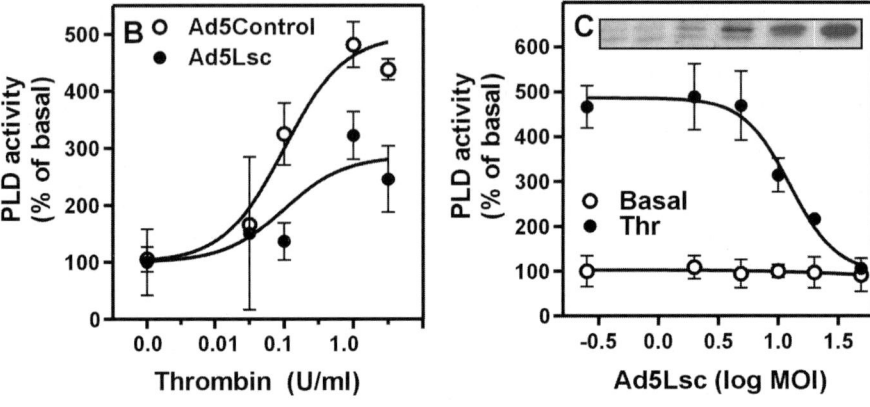

Figure 13a–c
Involvement of distinct G proteins in neonatal rat cardiac myocyte PLD stimulation by endothelin-1, thrombin and noradrenaline. Neonatal rat cardiomyocytes were infected with adenoviruses encoding bacterial galactosidase (Ad5Control, *open bars*) (a,b), Lsc-RGS (Ad5Lsc, *grey bars*) (a–c) or RGS4 (Ad5RGS4, *closed bars*) (a) 48 h prior to the assay if not otherwise indicated at a MOI of 10. The formation of the PLD-specific reaction product [^{3}H]phosphatidylethanol was determined in the absence (Basal) and presence of endothelin-1 (ET-1, 1 µM), thrombin (Thr, if not otherwise indicated 1 U/ml) or noradrenaline (NA, 10 mM in the presence of 1 µM nadolol). Shown are the means ± S.E.M. of n = 6–9 (*$p<0.05$ *vs.* Ad5Control). The over-expression of Lsc-RGS is shown (c, inset)

ter, the incubation medium was replaced by 500 µl ice-cold methanol, cells were scraped off and transferred into a 3 ml tube. The culture dish was washed with an additional 500 µl methanol which were added to the 3 ml tube. Chloroform (1 ml) plus water (0.5 ml) were added and the mixture was vortexed for 30 sec. For phase extraction, the tubes were centrifuged for 10 min at 1180×g. The lower phase was placed in a 1.5 ml Eppendorf tube and the solvent was removed in a vacuum concentrator. The pellet was dissolved in 25 µl chloroform:methanol (1:1). Ten µl were spotted on LK6D silica gel 60 A thin layer chromatography plates (Whatman) and the phospholipids were resolved with a mobile phase consisting of ethyl acetate:isooctane:acetic acid:water (13:2:3:10). A mixture of phosphatidic acid and phosphatidylethanol (50 µg each) was used as standard. The spots containing phosphatidylethanol were scraped off and 10 ml of a scintillation cocktail were added. The formation of the PLD specific product [^{3}H]phosphatidylethanol was quantified in a liquid scintillation counter.

As shown in Fig. 13 endothelin-1, thrombin and noradrenaline (in the presence of the β-adrenoceptor antagonist nadolol) stimulated [^{3}H]phosphatidylethanol formation in the myocytes to a similar extent The over-expression of RGS4 did not alter PLD stimulation by thrombin but blunted the ET_AR- and α_1AR-induced PLD activity by about 50–60% (Fig. 13a). In contrast, thrombin-induced PLD stimulation was significantly blunted, by about 50% in cardiomyocytes over-expressing LscRGS, whereas the stimulation by endothelin-1 and noradrenaline was not affected. The over-expression of LscRGS reduced the maximal extent of thrombin-induced PLD stimulation, without altering the concentration dependency (Fig. 13b). Infection of cardiomyocytes with an increasing MOI of Ad5Lsc resulted in an increased expression of the recombinant protein and a concomitant reduction in thrombin-induced PLD stimulation. At a MOI of 50 the PAR1-induced stimulation of the PLD activity was completely suppressed (Fig. 13c). The data therefore demonstrate that the PAR-1 induced stimulation of cardiac myocytes' PLD is mediated by the $G_{12/13}$-type of heterotrimeric G proteins. In contrast, the ET_AR- and α_1AR-induced PLD stimulation is mediated by the $G_{q/11}$ – phospholipase C – protein kinase C pathway (Fahimi-Vahid et al. 2002; Gosau et al. 2002).

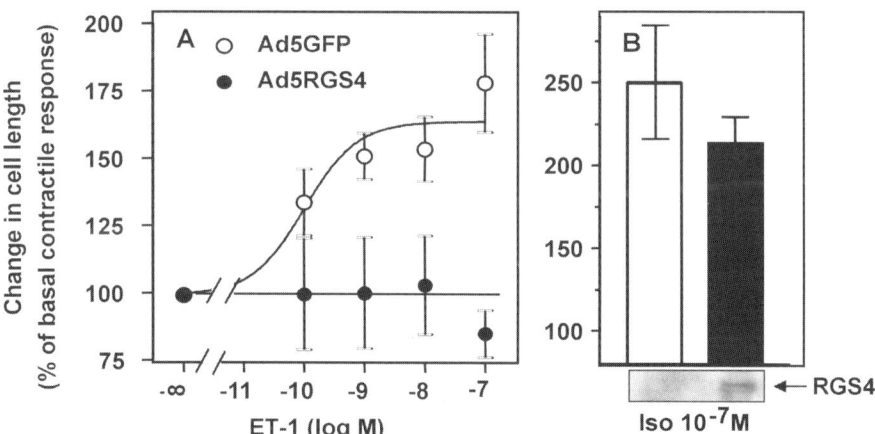

Figure 14a,b
Agonist-induced fractional shortening of adult rabbit ventricular cardiac myocytes. Adult rabbit cardiac myocytes were infected with Ad5GFP or Ad5RGS4 at a MOI of 1 24 h before the assay. Fractional shortening was measured at increasing concentrations of ET-1 (10^{-10}–10^{-7} M) (**a**). At the end of the experiment isoprenaline (0.1 µM) was added (**b**). Basal fractional shortening did not differ: Ad-GFP: 4.1 ± 0.7%, Ad-RGS4: 3.6 ± 0.4%. The over-expression of RGS4 was monitored by immunoblotting

Over-expression of RGS4 Inhibits the $ET_A R$-induced but not b-Adrenoceptor-induced Contractility in Adult Rabbit Cardiac Myocytes

Adult rabbit cardiomyocytes were infected with Ad5-RGS4 or Ad5-EGFP as a control at a MOI of 1 and cultured for 48 h. About 30% of cells showed fluorescence by EGFP (see Fig. 12) and only EGFP positive cells were used. In Ad5-RGS4 infected cells the average over-expression was estimated to reach about 3–6-fold. Myocyte shortening was measured by an edge-detection system (Crescent Electronics) at a stimulation frequency of 0.5 Hz and a sampling rate of 240 Hz. Online and offline analysis was performed with custom-designed Labview software (National Instruments). Cumulative concentration response curves were made with increasing concentrations of endothelin-1 (10^{-10}–10^{-7} M) in both groups. The agonist increased the fractional shortening concentration dependently by about 60–70% in Ad5-EGFP infected cells. No effect was seen in Ad5-RGS4 infected cells (Fig. 14a). In contrast, the β-adrenoceptor agonist isoprenaline (10^{-7} M) given on top of the highest endothelin-1 concentration increased fractional shortening in both groups without significant difference (Fig. 14b). These data demonstrate that the overexpression of RGS4 completely suppresses the $ET_A R$-induced and $G_{q/11}$-mediated increase in myocytes contractility (Mittmann et al. 2002). The G_s-mediated contractile response induced by β-adrenoceptors remains unaffected.

Troubleshooting

Preparation of Neonatal Rat Cardiac Myocytes

1. Sterility of cultures: All materials have to be sterilized and all work has to be performed under aseptic conditions. The extraction of the hearts is most critical. If the cultures become contaminated with fungi, the most likely reason is a contamination of the CBHFF buffer during the chopping up of the hearts.
2. Over-digestion with trypsin: One likely reason for a low number of viable cells from the preparation is an over-digestion with trypsin, which might for example occur after changing the supplier or with a new batch of the enzyme. It is very important to test every new batch of the enzyme before general use. Another possibility for an over-digestion is the use of heated (inactivated) instead of original FCS for trypsin inactivation during the preparation. Additionally, it is a good idea to gradually reduce the volume and exposure time during the repeated digests in the preparation.
3. Mechanical disruption of the tissue: It is very important to perform the triturations with a pipette with a 3 mm wide opening. Regular pipettes have a narrower opening. Thus, the shear forces will probably break the myocytes. It is similarly important to use 40–80 animals for one preparation. With lower animal numbers the number of viable cells obtained from one heart decreases. With higher numbers the efficiency of the procedure decreases. Thus, more animals do not necessarily provide more cells.

4. Non-myocyte contamination: The preparation usually contains less than 5% non-myocytes. The separation relies on the faster adherence of the non-myocytes to the plastic material of the culture dishes. Usually the non-myocytes adhere within 2 h of culture, whereas the myocytes are still floating. Nevertheless, this is a dynamic process and the adherence should be frequently checked during the 60 and 120 min of culture. On the one hand, floating non-myocytes will increase the number of these cells in the final myocyte culture. On the other hand, if the myocytes start to adhere early, they are lost to the planned experiments. It is essential that the myocytes be cultured in the presence of the antimetabolite BrdU. Otherwise the dividing non-myocytes will overgrow the myocytes in the culture and this might cause false results.
5. Plating of the myocytes: The counting of the myocytes is a critical step. If a Neubauer chamber is used, note that the glass plate may crush some myocytes. Thus, too many cells must not be put into the chamber. Otherwise, the number of viable myocytes is underestimated due to mechanical destruction. Cardiac myocytes do not adhere to plastic dishes of all brands. Thus, it is not a good idea to buy dishes from a new supplier without having them tested.

Preparation of Adult Rabbit Myocytes

1. Sterility of cultures: As the rabbit hearts are excised in the open, every material and solution used during the preparation has to be sterile. Otherwise bacterial or fungal contaminations occur frequently.
2. Low number of viable cells: The most sensitive part of this protocol is the enzyme solution. It has to be prepared freshly before use and the pH has to be exactly adjusted. Collagenase, even if bought from the same supplier, differs largely in its activity and every new batch has to be tested. In most cases of a low efficiency of the preparation the collagenase is not working adequately. Another reason for low efficiency is too long a period between extraction of the heart and the start of the perfusion. The perfusion should start within 90–120 s after extraction. If too many cells in hypercontracture appear during the preparation, the Ca^{2+} concentrations have been increased too rapidly. The cells should be allowed to equilibrate at each concentration for at least 5 min.
Additionally, it is a good idea to perform more steps in increasing the Ca^{2+} concentration, e.g. 0.05 mM, 0.0625 mM, 0.078 mM, 0.117 mM, 0.156 mM, 0.235 mM, 0.3125 mM, 0.469 mM, 0.6125 mM.

Amplification and Storage of Recombinant Adenoviruses

1. Unintended viral contamination: During changing of infected cells' medium during the amplification procedure, the virus may contaminate the pipette used and thereby also the stock medium used for feeding. If the same stock medium is used to feed other HEK 293 cells, the virus may contaminate all HEK 293 cells currently in culture. Thus, it is a good idea to prepare an aliquot of the stock medium for feeding infected cells and discard any remnant. If possible, virally infected cells

should be kept in a separate incubator. We also highly recommend the use of an inverse fluorescence microscope to look at virally infected cells. If a regular microscope is used to look at the cells, the covers of the culture dishes have to be removed to focus on the monolayer. The objective of the microscope may get contaminated and spread the virus from dish to dish.
2. Loss of viral titre during storage: Even if the viruses are stored in the recommended high glycerol containing storage buffer at −20 °C, the amount of bioactive virus decreases with time. Therefore repeating the endpoint-dilution assay from time to time to check the virus titre is recommended. Note that freezing and thawing as well as storage at higher temperatures will further reduce the amount of bioactive virus. Therefore the virus stock should be stored in small aliquots adjusted to the volume used in one experiment. If the virus titre falls to less than 50% of its original value, a re-amplification of the virus should be performed.

Infection of Cells and Assay

1. Low number of infected cells: The most common reason is loss of the bioactivity of the virus (see above). Another cause is inhibition of viral infection by high amounts of FCS in the medium used for the infection. A concentration of 2% FCS can be recommended. An alternative procedure that is also tolerated by the cells is addition of the virus in medium without FCS followed by filling up with fresh FCS containing medium after 20 min in the incubator. Viral infection is also dependent on the density of the cells. If more than 3×10^6 neonatal myocytes are plated on a culture dish (∅ 6 cm) the percentage of infected cells will decrease.
2. Consequences of EGFP expression: The expression of EGFP in the infected cells is not independent of the second transgene in the adenovirus. Thus, a lower amount of EGFP expression (for example compared to Ad5-EGFP) does not necessarily indicate a low expression of the protein of interest. The (over)-expression of each protein of interest should therefore be monitored by immunoblotting. Analysis of the time dependence of the transgene expression at different MOIs is recommended to obtain optimal conditions.
3. It has been found that the expression of high amounts of EGFP can impair functions in cardiac myocytes. Therefore, in each experimental setting it must be checked that Ad5-EGFP infected cardiomyocytes do not differ largely in their responses from uninfected cells. In our hands, expression of EGFP under the conditions shown herein did not influence neonatal rat cardiac myocytes' PLD nor single cell fractional shortening in adult rabbit myocytes.
4. "Side effects" of adenoviral gene transfer: To account for side effects of adenoviral infection, the myocytes for the control experiments are usually infected with a recombinant adenovirus encoding only EGFP. Alternatively, a virus leading to the expression of bacterial galactosidase is often used. Nevertheless, the protein of interest itself may cause effects, e.g. induction of apoptosis, which are not readily evident. Such events might however feign an inhibitory effect on the parameter under study. Therefore, appropriate positive controls which are definitely not affected by the (over)-expressed protein are required.

Genetic Analysis of G Protein Function in the Cardiovascular System of the Mouse

Genetic manipulation of the mammalian genome using transgenic or gene targeting techniques provides a powerful tool to characterize the molecular mechanisms underlying cardiovascular function under the conditions of a living organism. The mouse organism has been the principle system where these techniques have been established and refined. Recent advances in the miniaturization of techniques used to study cardiovascular functions in whole animals are now allowing detailed analyses of the effects produced by defined genetic manipulations in the mouse organism (Christensen et al. 1997; Fitzgerald et al. 2003). Several G protein α subunits have been over-expressed in a cardiomyocyte-specific manner, both as wild type or constitutively active forms (Table 7). Also various classical and conditional knockouts of genes encoding murine G protein α subunits have revealed phenotypes in the cardiovascular system (Table 8).

General methods for the generation of transgenic or gene targeted mice have been published in a variety of excellent reviews and books. In the following we would like to give an overview of the different approaches, which have been used to alter gene expression in the cardiovascular system of the mouse and we will give some detailed descriptions of the problems, which may arise when G protein mediated signalling pathways have to be analyzed in mice on a cellular level.

In order to express a transgene constitutively or conditionally in the cardiovascular system various promoters have been used. For cardiomyocyte-specific expression, the α-myosin heavy chain (aMHC) promoter has been used most widely since it results in high level and homogenous expression, both in adult atria and ventricles in a highly cardiac specific manner (Subramaniam et al. 1991). However, other cardiomyocyte-specific promoters, which allow transgene expression before birth have also been successfully used (MLC2a, MLC2v etc.) Several promoters can be used to drive transgene expression in vascular smooth muscle cells. Some promoter fragments of the SM22α-gene have been reported to direct transgene expression to specific parts of the vascular system (Li et al. 1996), and the SMMHC-promoter allows expression in all smooth muscle cells starting from embryonic day 15 (Regan et al. 2000). Specific expression of transgenes in endothelial cells has been achieved using promoter fragments of the *tie1* and *tie2* genes (Korhonen et al. 1995; Schlaeger et al. 1999).

When using plasmid-based transgenes containing short promoter fragments, researchers often observe problems such as integration site dependent effects on the level and specificity of transgene expression. Random integration of foreign DNA can result in position effects that influence the expression of the transgene itself as well as of adjacent endogenous genes. A major improvement in transgenic expression was achieved when large artificial chromosomes containing all the regulatory sequences of a given gene were used for the generation of transgenic vectors. These constructs, which are based on yeast artificial chromosomes (YACs) or P1-derived artificial chromosomes (BACs/PACs) allow position-independent and copy number-dependent transgene expression which guarantees faithful expression of transgenes (Heintz et al. 2001; Giraldo and Montoliu 2001). To better control transgene expression levels, inducible systems have been developed which allow control of the onset, the duration

Table 7
Transgenic expression of wild type or mutant G protein subunits in the cardiovascular system

Transgene	Promoter	Tissue	Phenotype	Reference
$G\gamma_2$(C68S)	αMHC	cardio-myocytes	reduction of $G\beta\gamma$ concentration; parasympathetic heart rate control↓	Gehrmann et al. (2002) Am J Physiol 282: H445–456
$G\alpha_s$ (wt)	αMHC	cardio-myocytes	increased inotropic and chronotropic responses to catecholamines	Gaudin et al. (1995) J Clin Invest 95: 1676–1683, Iwase et al. (1996) Circ Res 78:517–524
$G\alpha_q$ (wt)	αMHC	cardio-myocytes	cardiac hypertrophy, cardiomyopathy	D'Angelo et al. (1997) Proc Natl Acad Sci USA 94: 8121–8126, Adams et al. (1998) Proc Natl Acad Sci USA 95: 10140–10145
$G\alpha_q$ (Q209L) (const. active)	αMHC	cardio-myocytes	cardiac hypertrophy and dilatation	Mende et al. (1998) Proc Natl Acad Sci USA 95: 13893–13898
$G\alpha_q$-peptide (305–359)	αMHC	cardio-myocytes	pressure overload induced ventricular hypertrophy ↓	Akhter et al. (1998) Science 280: 574–577
$G\alpha_q$-peptide (305–359)	SM22α	smooth muscle	phenylephrine-, serotonin-, and angiotensin-induced blood pressure and cardiac hypertrophy ↓	Keys et al. (2002) Hypertension 40: 660–666

MHC myosin heavy chain; *const. active* constitutively active mutant; *wt* wild type form. For details, see text.

and the level of transgene expression. Another advantage of these techniques lies in the possibility of studying an animal before, during and after transient transgene expression, thus allowing comparison of the effect of the expressed transgene with the wild type situation within the same animal. Various systems for inducible and tissue-specific gene expression have been reported. The tetracycline-controlled transacti-

Table 8
Cardiovascular abnormalities in mice lacking α-subunits of heterotrimeric G proteins

Subtype	Expression	Effector	Phenotype	Reference
$G\alpha_{i2}$	wide	AC$\downarrow$;[a] GIRK$\uparrow$[b]	Defective muscarinic regulation of cardiac L-type Ca^{2+} channels; normal basal cardiac function	Nagata et al. (2000) Circ Res 87: 903–909; Chen et al. (2001) Am J Physiol 280: H1989–1995, Jain et al. (2001) Am J Physiol 280: H569–575
$G\alpha_{i3}$	wide	AC$\downarrow$; GIRK$\uparrow$[b]	Defective muscarinic regulation of cardiac L-type Ca^{2+} channels; normal basal cardiac function	Nagata et al. 2000; Jain et al. 2001 (see above)
$G\alpha_o$	neuronal, heart, neuroendocrine	VDCC$\downarrow$;[c] GIRK$\uparrow$	Defective muscarinic regulation of cardiac L-type Ca^{2+} channels	Valenzuela et al. (1997) Proc Natl Acad Sci USA 94: 1727–1732
$G\alpha_q + G\alpha_{11}$	ubiquitous	PLC-β$\uparrow$	myocardial hypoplasia (lethal e11)	Offermanns et al. (1998) EMBO J 17: 4304–4312
$G\alpha_q + G\alpha_{11}$ (cardiomyocyte-restricted)			pressure overload induced hypertrophy $\downarrow$	Wettschureck et al. (2001) Nat Med 7: 1236–1240

[a] AC adenylyl cyclase types I,V,VI; [b] GIRK1-GIRK4 (Kir3.1-Kir3.4), effector is regulated through βγ-subunits; [c] VDCC, voltage dependent calcium channel, P/Q-R-type (Ca$_v$2.1-Ca$_v$2.3), effector is regulated through βγ-subunits; PLC-β, β-isoforms of phospholipase C.

vation (tTA) system is based on the tetracycline-responsive transcriptional regulatory element of *E. coli* (*tetO*) and a mutant bacterial *tet* repressor protein fused to the C-terminal domain of the VP16 protein of the herpes simplex virus (Gossen et al. 1995). Tetracycline-regulated expression of transgenes has been reported in the heart (Yu et al. 1996; Valencik and McDonald 2001), smooth muscle (Ju et al. 2001) and endothelial cells (Sarao and Dumont 1998).

The traditional gene "knock-out" approach results in the loss of gene function in all tissues from early embryonic stages onwards. Since cardiovascular functions are already of great importance before birth, deletion of the genes involved in the devel-

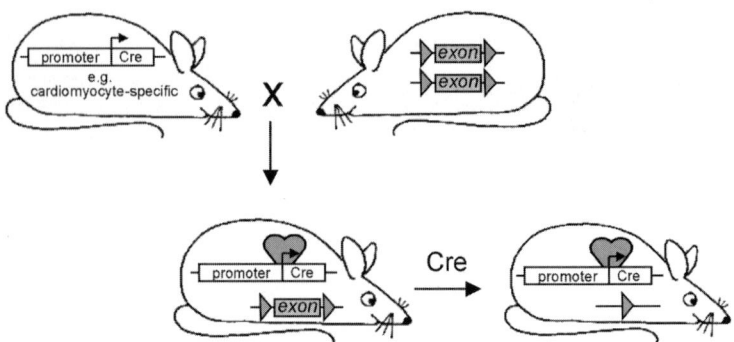

Figure 15
Tissue-specific gene inactivation. Mice carrying the *cre* transgene under the control of a tissue-specific promoter (e.g. cardiomyocyte-specific promoter) are crossed with mice in which an exon of a particular gene is flanked by loxP-sites (red triangles). LoxP-sites were introduced by gene targeting in ES-cells. In mice that carry the *cre* transgene and the "floxed" exon, Cre is expressed in tissues de-fined by the promoter. This will lead to tissue-specific excision of the exon resulting in a deletion of the gene. In tissues that do not express Cre, the gene remains intact

opment or function of the cardiovascular system often results in embryonic lethality (Copp 1995; Conway et al. 2003) preventing the analysis of gene function in adulthood. In addition, lack of a gene product during development or in the adult animal may be offset by the up-regulation of a related gene or may be counterbalanced by more complex compensatory mechanisms. In this case, the phenotype resulting from the deletion of a single gene reflects the result of a complex compensatory reaction of the whole organism and cannot be attributed simply to the missing gene function. To overcome these problems the gene targeting approach has been further developed to restrict gene deletion to specific tissues or to define the onset of gene deletion. The currently favoured techniques rely on the introduction of loxP (locus of crossing over) recognition sites for the recombinase Cre (causes recombination) which recognizes these sites and excises the DNA sequence flanked by two loxP sites leaving one site behind (Le and Sauer 2000). If the targeted gene is flanked by two loxP sites, re-combination and deletion of the gene occurs depending on the site and time of Cre expression. Cre can be transgenically expressed from a specific promoter or after placing its gene downstream of an endogenous promoter (Fig. 15) (Rajewsky et al. 1996).

Tissue-specific gene targeting using Cre/loxP technology has been extended by combining Cre expression with an inducible system which relies on the tet-system or which uses Cre versions whose activity can be regulated by synthetic ligands. In the latter case, Cre recombinase was expressed transgenically under the control of a defined promoter as a fusion protein with a mutated binding domain of the oestrogen or progesterone receptor. The mutation in the binding domain allows only the synthetic compounds tamoxifen or mifepristone to bind with high affinity. In the absence of ligand, the Cre fusion protein is inactive due to binding to the Hsp90 complex. Binding of ligand disinhibits Cre and results in Cre-mediated recombination (Feil et al. 1997; Kellendonk et al. 1999).

Table 9
Mouse lines expressing the recombinase Cre in the cardiovascular system

Promoter driving Cre expression	Expression	Comments	Reference
SM22α (Li et al. (1996) J Cell Biol 132: 849–859)	smooth muscle	constitutive, some preference for vascular SMCs	Holtwick et al. (2002) Proc Natl Acad Sci USA 99:7142-7147
SM22α	smooth muscle	knock-in; inducible (tamoxifen)	Kuhbandner et al. (2000) Genesis 28: 15–22
SMMHC (Madsen et al. (1998) Circ Res 82:908–917)	smooth muscle	transgenic; constitutive	Regan et al. (2000) Circ Res 87: 363–369
MLC2a	cardiomyocytes	knock-in; constitutive, e8.5–10.5	Wettschureck et al. (2001) Nat Med 7:1236–1240
MLC2v	cardiomyocytes	knock-in; constitutive, e8.75	Chen et al. (1998) J Biol Chem 273: 1252–1256
αMHC (Subramaniam et al. (1991) J Biol Chem 266:24613-24620)	cardiomyocytes	transgenic; inducible (RU486)	Minamino et al. (2001) Circ Res 88: 587–592
αMHC (Palermo et al. (1996) Circ Res 78: 504–509)	cardiomyocytes	transgenic; inducible (tamoxifen)	Sohal et al. (2001) Circ Res 89:20–25
αMHC (Subramaniam et al. 1991, see above)	cardiomyocytes	constitutive/postnatal	Agah et al. (1997) J Clin Invest 100: 169–179, Abel et al. (1999) J Clin Invest 104: 1703–1714
Ckmm	muscle cells	transgenic; constitutive; skeletal/heart muscle	Wang et al. (1999) Nat Genet 21: 133–137
Tie-1 (Iljin et al. (1999) FASEB J 13:377–386)	endothelial cells	constitutive, e8	Gustafsson et al. (2001) J Cell Sci 114:671–676

Table 9
Continued

Promoter driving Cre expression	Expression	Comments	Reference
Tie-2	endothelial cells	transgenic; constitutive	Kisanuki et al. (2001) Dev Biol 230: 230–242
Tie-2 (Schläger et al. (1997) Proc Natl Acad Sci USA 94:3058-3063)	endothelial cells	transgenic; inducible (tamoxifen)	Forde et al. (2002) Genesis 33:191–197

A list of published constitutive or inducible Cre mouse lines, which allow the conditional inactivation of genes in the cardiovascular system, is shown in Table 9.

When analyzing genetic mouse models that carry mutations in genes coding for components of the G protein mediated signalling system, a major goal is to relate possible changes in cellular signalling to phenotypical changes of the cardiovascular system. This requires the application of methods for the *in vivo* analysis of cardiovascular functions as well as for the analysis of processes at the cellular or molecular level. Especially when tissue-specific mutants are studied, studies on the cellular level rely on the specificity of the genetic approach as well as on the purity of the cell preparation. A particular problem has been the analysis of cellular functions in adult cardiomyocytes from cardiomyocyte-specific mutants. Only 14% of adult mouse ventricular cells are cardiomyocytes, and 90–95% of these cells are binucleated. This means that 24% of the DNA content of the whole murine ventricle originates from cardiomyocytes (Soonpaa et al., 1996). Thus, methods to isolate and purify adult murine cardiomyocytes are needed to allow the study of cellular processes in a homogenous cell population.

Description of Methods and Practical Approach

Isolation and Purification of Adult Mouse Cardiac Myocytes

Cardiomyocytes from the adult mouse heart are delicate cells and even small alterations in temperature, oxygen levels and nutrient and ion concentrations can affect their viability. Hallmarks of viable cardiomyocytes are their rod-shaped morphology, visible cross-striation and – at least in the first hours after preparation – spontaneous, slow contractions. Several protocols for the isolation of adult mouse cardiomyocytes have been published (Pawloski-Dahm et al. 1998; Kim et al. 1999; Hilal-Dandan et al. 2000) and all are based on the retrograde perfusion of the heart *via* the aorta. Because retrograde perfusion of the aorta leads to closure of the aortic valves, the perfusate is forced into the coronary arteries that branch off from the aorta ascendens immediately above the aortic valves. Distributed *via* coronary arteries, capillaries and veins the perfusate can reach a maximal number of cardiomyocytes, leading to maximal dissociation of cells.

The procedure described here usually results in a quantity of $2–4\times10^6$ cardiomyocytes per heart, with about 70% being rod-shaped, cross-striated and partly contracting cardiomyocytes. The preparations usually contain less than 5% non-cardiomyocytes.

Buffers and Media.
- Perfusion buffer, pH 7.2 at 37 °C (mM)
  NaCl 113, KCl 4.7, KH_2PO_4 0.6, Na_2HPO_4, 0.6, $MgSO_4$ 1.2, $NaHCO_3$ 12, $KHCO_3$ 12, glucose 20, Na^+-HEPES 10, taurine 30, creatine 2, carnitine 2
- Digestion buffer
  Collagenase II (Worthington) 0.08%, trypsin (Invitrogen) 0.1% (w/v), fatty acid free BSA (Sigma) 0.1% (w/v), BDM 10 mM, $CaCl_2$ 0.025 mM in perfusion buffer
- Mincing buffer
  BDM 10 mM in perfusion buffer
- M199 (mM)
  Taurine 30, creatine 2, carnitine 2, heat inactivated FCS 4% (v/v), penicillin 100 U/ml, streptomycin 0.1 mg/ml, in medium 199 (Invitrogen)

Procedure (mod. from Hilal-Dandan et al. 2000).
- Anaesthesia: The mouse is anaesthetized by intraperitoneal injection of ketamine (150 mg/kg) and xylazine (24 mg/kg) in saline. Coagulation is prevented with 100 U heparin i.p.
- Preparation of the heart: After superficial disinfection with 70% ethanol, thoracotomy is performed and the heart is excised with at least 3 mm of aorta ascendens attached to it. The still beating heart is briefly washed in ice-cold Ca^{2+} free perfusion buffer and non-cardiac tissue is removed. The aorta is mounted on a blunted 20 G needle connected to a roller pump and fixed with a thread tied around aorta and needle. During perfusion the heart is suspended in prewarmed perfusion buffer. All perfusion solutions are kept at 37 °C and are bubbled with carbogen (95%O_2; 5%CO_2). Gas bubbles must not enter the tubing. The delay between excision of the heart and the start of perfusion should be kept as short as possible.
- Chemical dissociation of myocardial cells: The heart is first perfused for 4 min with prewarmed, gassed perfusion buffer (3.5–4 ml/min), then for 15 min with prewarmed, gassed digestion buffer at the same speed. After successful perfusion the consistency of the myocardium should be flaccid.
- Mechanical dissociation of cells: The heart is removed from the perfusion apparatus and suspended in perfusion buffer containing 10 mM BDM. Atria are removed and ventricles are minced with scissors or blades. To dissociate cell clumps the suspension is gently pipetted up and down with a pipette tip cut off to give a diameter of about 3 mm. Undissociated clumps are removed by filtration through a 200 µm nylon mesh.

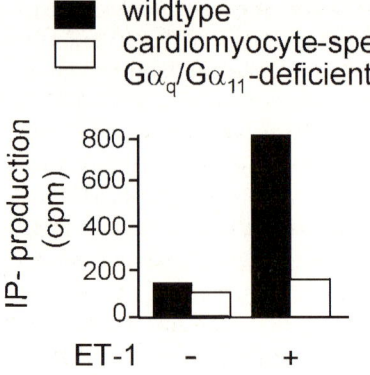

Figure 16
Abrogation of endothelin-1 induced inositol phosphate production in $G\alpha_q/\alpha_{11}$-double deficient mouse cardiomyocytes. Inositol phosphate production in purified, cultured cardiomyocytes after stimulation with 1 µM endothelin-1 (ET-1). In contrast to wild type cardiomyocytes $G\alpha_q/G\alpha_{11}$-deficient cardiomyocytes are unresponsive towards ET-1 stimulation. Basal inositol phosphate production does not differ between the genotypes

- Differential centrifugation to enrich cardiomyocytes: The resulting cell suspension is washed twice in mincing buffer and centrifuged at 50×g for 1 min at room temperature. After the last centrifugation, the pellet is resuspend in 10 ml mincing buffer containing 0.1% fatty acid free BSA
- Recalcification of cardiomyocyte suspension: The calcium concentration is slowly increased to 50, 100, 200, 500, 1000 µM by adding $CaCl_2$ every 4 min from a 1 M stock with gentle shaking.
- Cardiomyocyte culture: The cells are spun down (50×g for 1 min), resuspended in M199, counted and seeded onto laminin-coated dishes (2 µg laminin/cm²) at a density of 3×10^4/cm². Attached cells retain their cardiomyocytic morphology for 12–24 h and then start to detach.

Example

Abrogation of Endothelin-1 Induced Inositol Phosphate Production in $G\alpha_q/G\alpha_{11}$-double Deficient Mouse Cardiomyocytes

Cardiomyocytes from a wild type mouse and an age matched mouse with cardiomyocyte-specific inactivation of the G protein α subunits $G\alpha_q$ and $G\alpha_{11}$ (Wettschureck et al. 2001) were isolated. The yield per heart was 2.7×10^6 for the wild type and 2.4×10^6 cells for the knockout, about 70% of cells showed the typical rod-shaped morphology with cross striation. Cells were seeded at a density of 10^6 cells/5 ml medium on to laminin coated 6 cm dishes (2 plates for each heart) and after 1 h about 70% of cells had adhered. The mouse cardiomyocytes were incubated for 16–20 h with inositol-free medium (Invitrogen) containing 10 µCi/ml *myo*-[³H]inositol. Note that regular medium contains considerable amounts of myo-inositol that would result in poor labelling. Thereafter the *myo*-[³H]inositol containing medium was replaced by inositol-free medium containing 10 mM LiCl to block inositol phosphatase. After 10 min of incubation, one plate of each heart was stimulated with 1 µM endothelin-1 for another 30 min. Thereafter, the medium was replaced by ice cold 10 mM formic acid and water-soluble lipids were extracted during 2 h of shaking at 4 °C. In the meantime ion exchange columns were prepared by loading each column with 0.5 g AG 1–X8 matrix (BioRad) suspended in 3 ml 1 M formic acid. Columns were washed three times with 5 ml H_2O. The formic acid was then extracted three times with ether and once with chloroform to enrich inositol phosphates. The pH of the aqueous extract was adjusted with 25% NH_4OH to pH 7–8 and debris was removed by centrifugation at 12.000 ×g at 4 °C for 2 min. Columns were loaded with the supernatant, washed twice with 10 ml H_2O and inositol phosphates were eluted with 2×2 ml 2 M ammonium formate pH 5.2. After addition of 10 ml scintillation cocktail the production of radioactive inositol phosphates was determined (Fig. 16). In the $G\alpha_q/G\alpha_{11}$-double deficient mouse cardiomyocytes the ET-1 stimulated inositol phosphate production was completely abrogated.

Troubleshooting

Preparation of Adult Mouse Cardiac Myocytes

1. Poor digestion: Air bubbles or precipitations within the tubing of the perfusion system can lead to occlusion of coronary arteries which results in poor digestion. The tip of the blunted needle must not penetrate (or even touch) the aortic valves, for only intact, closed valves will allow proper perfusion of coronary arteries. Different batches of collagenase can have different efficiencies; it might therefore be useful to test several batches. Collagenase B (Roche) or Collagenase II (Worthington) usually work well.
2. Loss of typical morphology: Adult mouse cardiomyocytes easily lose their typical rod-shaped, cross-striated morphology, especially when exposed to high calcium concentrations. Therefore it is crucial to increase calcium slowly during the recalcification step and use gentle shaking. Addition of BDM protects cardiomyocytes from hypercontractions and is therefore essential during enzymatic digestion, cell dissociation and recalcification. Strong shear force during the mechanical dissociation of cardiomyocytes might break cardiomyocytes; this can be prevented by cutting off the tip of the pipette to give a diameter of 3–4 mm.
3. Poor adhesion: In our hands freshly isolated mouse cardiomyocytes adhere well to laminin 10 µg/ml, but only poorly to poly-L-lysine (10 µg/ml), FCS 100%, fibronectin (10 µg/ml) or collagen IV (10 µg/ml).
4. Contamination: To avoid fungal or bacterial contamination the tubing of the perfusion apparatus, instruments and nylon meshes should be rinsed with 70% ethanol and sterile water before and after using. Solutions should be filtered through 0.2 µm sterile filters.

References

Christensen G, Wang Y, Chien KR (1997) Physiological assessment of complex cardiac phenotypes in genetically engineered mice. Am J Physiol 272:H2513–H2524

Conway SJ, Kruzynska-Frejtag A, Kneer PL, Machnicki M, Koushik SV (2003) What cardiovascular defect does my prenatal mouse mutant have, and why? Genesis 35:1–21

Copp AJ (1995) Death before birth: clues from gene knockouts and mutations. Trends Genet 11:87–93

El-Armouche A, Rau T, Zolk O, Ditz D, Pamminger T, Zimmermann WH, Jäckel E, Harding SE, Boknik P, Neumann J, Eschenhagen T (2003) Evidence for protein phosphatase inhibitor-1 playing an amplifier role in β-adrenergic signaling in cardiac myocytes. FASEB J 17:437–439

Fahimi-Vahid M, Gosau N, Michalek C, Han L, Jakobs KH, Schmidt M, Roberts N, Avkiran M, Wieland T (2002) Distinct signaling pathways mediate cardiomyocyte phospholipase D stimulation by endothelin-1 and thrombin. J Mol Cell Cardiol 34:441–453

Feil R, Brocard J, Mascrez B, LeMeur M, Metzger D, Chambon P (1996) Ligand-activated site-specific recombination in mice. Proc Natl Acad Sci USA 93:10887–10890

Fitzgerald SM, Gan L, Wickman A, Bergstrom G (2003) Cardiovascular and renal phenotyping of genetically modified mice: a challenge for traditional physiology. Clin Exp Pharmacol Physiol 30:207–216

Giraldo P, Montoliu L (2001) Size matters: use of YACs, BACs and PACs in transgenic animals. Transgenic Res 10:83–103

Gosau N, Fahimi-Vahid M, Michalek C, Schmidt M, Wieland T (2002) Signalling components involved in the coupling of α_1-adrenoceptors to phospholipase D in neonatal rat cardiac myocytes. Naunyn-Schmiedeberg's Arch Pharmacol 365:468–476

Gossen M, Freundlieb S, Bender G, Muller G, Hillen W, Bujard H (1995) Transcriptional activation by tetracyclines in mammalian cells. Science 268:1766–1769

He TC, Zhou S, Da Costa LT, Yu J, Kinzler KW, Vogelstein B (1998) A simplified system for generating recombinant adenoviruses. Proc Natl Acad Sci USA 95:2509–2514

Heintz N (2001) BAC to the future: the use of bac transgenic mice for neuroscience research. Nat Rev Neurosci 2:861–870

Hilal-Dandan R, Kanter JR, Brunton LL (2000) Characterization of G-protein signaling in ventricular myocytes from the adult mouse heart: differences from the rat. J Mol Cell Cardiol 32:1211–1221

Janssen PM, Schillinger W, Donahue JK, Zeitz O, Emami S, Lehnart SE, Weil J, Eschenhagen T, Hasenfuss G, Prestle J (2002) Intracellular β-blockade: overexpression of $G\alpha_{i2}$ depresses the β-adrenergic response in intact myocardium. Cardiovasc Res 55:300–308

Ju H, Gros R, You X, Tsang S, Husain M, Rabinovitch M (2001) Conditional and targeted overexpression of vascular chymase causes hypertension in transgenic mice. Proc Natl Acad Sci USA 98:7469–7474

Kellendonk C, Tronche F, Casanova E, Anlag K, Opherk C, Schutz G (1999) Inducible site-specific recombination in the brain. J Mol Biol 285:175–182

Kim SJ, Iizuka K, Kelly RA, Geng YJ, Bishop SP, Yang G, Kudej A, McConnell BK, Seidman CE, Seidman JG, Vatner SF (1999) An α-cardiac myosin heavy chain gene mutation impairs contraction and relaxation function of cardiac myocytes. Am J Physiol 276:H1780–H1787

Korhonen J, Lahtinen I, Halmekyto M, Alhonen L, Janne J, Dumont D, Alitalo K (1995) Endothelial-specific gene expression directed by the tie gene promoter *in vivo*. Blood 86:1828–1835

Le Y, Sauer B (2000) Conditional gene knockout using cre recombinase. Methods Mol Biol 136:477–485

Li L, Miano JM, Mercer B, Olson EN (1996) Expression of the SM22α promoter in transgenic mice provides evidence for distinct transcriptional regulatory programs in vascular and visceral smooth muscle cells. J Cell Biol 132:849–859

Mittmann C, Chung CH, Höppner G, Michalek C, Nose M, Schuh A, Eschenhagen T, Weil J, Pieske B, Hirt S, Wieland T (2002) Expression of 10 RGS proteins in human myocardium: functional characterization of an upregulation of RGS4 in heart failure. Cardiovasc Res 55:778–786

Neyroud N, Nuss HB, Leppo MK, Marban E, Donahue JK (2002) Gene delivery to cardiac muscle. Methods Enzymol 346:323–334

Pawloski-Dahm CM, Song G, Kirkpatrick DL, Palermo J, Gulick J, Dorn GW 2nd, Robbins J, Walsh RA (1998) Effects of total replacement of atrial myosin light chain-2 with the ventricular isoform in atrial myocytes of transgenic mice. Circulation 97:1508–1513

Rajewsky K, Gu H, Kuhn R, Betz UA, Muller W, Roes J, Schwenk F (1996) Conditional gene targeting. J Clin Invest 98:600–603

Regan CP, Manabe I, Owens GK (2000) Development of a smooth muscle-targeted cre recombinase mouse reveals novel insights regarding smooth muscle myosin heavy chain promoter regulation. Circ Res 87:363–369

Sarao R, Dumont DJ (1998) Conditional transgene expression in endothelial cells. Transgenic Res 7:421–427

Schlaeger TM, Bartunkova S, Lawitts JA, Teichmann G, Risau W, Deutsch U, Sato TN (1997) Uniform vascular-endothelial-cell-specific gene expression in both embryonic and adult transgenic mice. Proc Natl Acad Sci USA 94:3058–3063

Soonpaa MH, Kim KK, Pajak L, Franklin M, Field LJ (1996) Cardiomyocyte DNA synthesis and binucleation during murine development. Am J Physiol 271:H2183–H2189

Subramaniam A, Jones WK, Gulick J, Wert S, Neumann J, Robbins J (1991) Tissue-specific regulation of the α-myosin heavy chain gene promoter in transgenic mice. J Biol Chem 266:24613–24620

Valencik ML, McDonald JA (2001) Codon optimization markedly improves doxycycline regulated gene expression in the mouse heart. Transgenic Res 10:269–275

Wettschureck N, Rutten H, Zywietz A, Gehring D, Wilkie TM, Chen J, Chien KR, Offermanns S (2001) Absence of pressure overload induced myocardial hypertrophy after conditional inactivation of $G\alpha_q/G\alpha_{11}$ in cardiomyocytes. Nat Med 7:1236–1240

Wiechert S, El-Armouche A, Rau T, Zimmermann WH, Eschenhagen T (2003) 24-h Langendorff-perfused neonatal rat heart to study the impact of adenoviral gene transfer. Am J Physiol 285: H907–914

Yu Z, Redfern CS, Fishman GI (1996) Conditional transgene expression in the heart. Circ Res 79:691–697

Zheng B, Ma YC, Ostrom RS, Lavoie C, Gill GN, Insel PA, Huang XY, Farquhar MG (2001) RGS-PX1, a GAP for $G\alpha_s$ and sorting nexin in vesicular trafficking. Science 294:1939–1942

Recording and Analysing Concentration-Response Curves

Stefan Dhein

Introduction

In many cases it is the goal of a study to evaluate the effect of a physiological mediator or a drug on a given organ, such as the heart or vasculature, under physiological or pathophysiological conditions. This sounds simple, but unfortunately is not. Outlined in the following chapter are the principles of analysing a drug- (or mediator-) effect. The first thing to be proven is that the observed effect truly relates to the drug or mediator (subsequently refered to as drug). The first prerequisite, therefore, is to investigate several concentrations of the drug and to show that the drug's effect is related to the drug's concentration. Increasing concentrations should evoke an increased effect. This is unless there is a second (e.g. toxic) effect that counteracts the desired one at higher concentrations. However, in all cases, a concentration-response curve is needed for the analysis of the effect of a specific drug. To enable analysis, at least five concentration steps should be investigated. A concentration-dependent effect of a drug generally favours the hypothesis that it is related to the drug. However, the next question would be whether this drug effect is specific, i.e. is it related to the drug's action at the receptor or signal transduction system, which it is designed for, or is its effect unspecific (e.g. because of the drug's incorporation into the membrane bilayer)? The first hint of a specific effect can be obtained from analysing the concentration-response curve: the half-maximum concentration EC_{50} should be slightly higher, or at least within the range of the dissociation constant K_D of the drug, at its receptor. A difference, by several orders of magnitude, between EC_{50} and K_D is against the hypothesis that a drug effect is specifically related to a receptor. Further steps in testing the specificity of a drug effect would be to use a competitive antagonist of the drug and perform concentration-response curves in the absence, or presence, of various concentrations of the inhibitor. Assuming a specific drug effect at the receptor system, the competitive antagonist should induce a parallel rightward shift of the concentration-response curve. The magnitude of the shift depends on the affinity of the competitive antagonist, and can be analysed by Schild plot or pA_2-analysis. The method is based on the search for an equally effective concentration of drug A, in the presence of drug B, and analysis of the dose ratio (see below). The pA_2 value should be in the range of the K_D value of drug B in order to prove a specific action of the drug at the believed to be involved receptor.

Another point worth considering is the effect itself. It is often difficult to define an effect exactly, because initial values or basal activity might be present. Very often, the effect is expressed as a percentage of the maximum effect obtainable (with this or with any other drug; although it is necessary to define this exactly). Another possibility is to define the effect as a percentage of the maximum effect possible (regardless of whether this can be achieved with any drug). For example: it might be that a bradycardic effect is investigated in a given model. The maximum effect possible is cardiac arrest, i.e. heart rate = 0, regardless of whether this can be achieved. Thus, the effect is expressed in relation to the maximum effect possible. It is best to define a maximum and minimum effect, and to express all drug effects as a percentage of the difference between maximum and minimum. This is usually performed with vascular preparations: 1) A maximum vasoconstriction is produced with KCl; 2) The preparation is preconstricted with a vasoconstrictor such as noradrenaline, which is then 3) dilated with increasing concentrations of the vasodilatory drug that is being investigated. 4) At the end of the experiment, a maximum dilatation is induced by nifedipine or papaverine (this has to be done at the end of the experiment because it is difficult to wash out the effects of these drugs). The dilator effect of the drug (difference in tone between the noradrenaline-preconstriction and the drug-induced tone), is then expressed as the percentage of the maximal span between KCl and the papaverine-induced tone. Unfortunately, such a procedure is not possible with all preparations and is often impossible to establish *in vivo*. Sometimes (such as with hypertension) the drug effect can be expressed as a percentage 'normalization' (defined as the normal tension) of the current value.

Many preparations or experimental set-ups, show a certain basal activity or initial value. If a drug effect is only related to the initial value, e.g. is expressed as a percentage of the initial value, the results will be hard to compare with, and might vary greatly between, different experiments. It is therefore recommended to define a maximum or minimum effect to which to relate, or to prestretch or preconstrict the preparation, such that the initial values of all preparations are the same.

Description of Methods and Practical Approach

First of all, the classical concentration-response curve is described and analysed. In principle, two types of concentration-response curves can be distinguished: (a) the concentration-response curve of a group or (b) the concentration-response curve of an individual. In the first case, the concentration-response curve (or often dose-response curve) describes the percentage of individuals out of this group who exhibit the desired (or investigated) effect. The underlying mathematics are derived from the Gaussian normal distribution (see Tallarida and Jacob 1979; Tallarida and Murray 1987 for further reading).

Most often in cardiovascular experimental research, concentration-response curves for an individual are actually investigated in a small number of individuals. Therefore, one individual is exposed to increasing concentrations of the drug or mediator that is to be investigated (cummulative concentration-response curve). In some cases it might be necessary to test not more than only one concentration at at time instead of a cumulative dose-response.

The underlying mathematics are closely related to those already known from biochemistry, the Michaelis-Menten kinetics and the Lineweaver-Burk-diagram. To understand the concentration-response curve, one has to assume that everything is related to the interaction of a drug A with a receptor R, yielding the drug-receptor complex [RA], and depending on the drugs affinity constant K_A, according to equation (1):

$$[R] \times [A]/[RA] = K_A \tag{1}$$

$$\text{with } [R_{total}] = [R] + [RA] \tag{2}$$

That means that the fraction of occupied receptors (RA/R_{total}) can be described as:

$$[RA]/[R_{total}] = [RA]/[RA] + [R] \tag{3}$$

Because according to (1)

$$[R]/[RA] = K_A/[A]$$

one can rewrite equation (3) as

$$[RA]/[R_{total}] = 1/\{1 + (K_A/[A])\} \tag{4}$$

This means that the number of occupied receptors depends on the concentration of the agonist. Because the effect of a given concentration of drug A, [A], is related to the effect (E) of this concentration, E_A, and also because E_A should be at its maximum ($=E_{max}$) when all receptors are occupied, equation (4) can be converted to:

$$E_A/E_{max} = [RA]/[R_{total}] = 1/\{1 + (K_A/[A])\} \tag{5}$$

which is equivalent to:

$$E_A = E_{max}/\{1 + (K_A/[A])\} \tag{6}$$

thus relating the effect of a drug to its concentration. Equation (6) is equivalent to the Michaelis-Menten equation known from biochemistry. To obtain the typical sigmoidal concentration-response curve, the effect E is plotted against log ([A]). Now, several values have to be calculated. Firstly, the EC_{50} needs to be determined. This is the concentration of a drug at which its half-maximum effect is observed, or at which 50% of the population exhibit the desired effect. The EC_{50} is related to the potency of the drug. However, it is important to note, that high potency does not mean a great effect, but a high affinity of the drug to its receptor. It is important not to confuse effect with potency. Second, E_{max} needs to be determined by estimating the saturation effect. Moreover, a threshold and saturation concentration, need to be defined.

In some cases, it is not possible to define E_{max} directly from the recorded concentration-response curve. Thus, if the positive inotropic effect of ouabain or other digitalis glycosides is investigated, the positive inotropic effect will be overrun by the toxic arrhythmogenic effect, before reaching saturation. In such cases, one can try to convert the concentration-response curve according to Lineweaver-Burk, in order to obtain a double-reciprocal linear concentration-response-relationship according to the equation:

$$1/[E] = (K_A/E_{max}) \times (1/[A]) + 1/E_{max} \qquad (7)$$

which is of the form $y = a \times x + b$, and can be analysed using simple linear regression. Therefore, the data have to be converted and plotted as $1/E$ against $1/[A]$, and a linear regression can be performed on these data. The y-axis intercept of which E_{max} can be calculated is $1/E_{max}$, whereas the slope is K_A/E_{max}, and the x-axis intercept is $-1/K_A$. Using the E_{max} value, the E_{50} value can be calculated. Following this, $1/E_{50}$ and $1/EC_{50}$ can be read from the curve.

Nowadays, data can usually be fitted to this curve by using non-linear regression algorithms for sigmoidal curves, which are commercially available in computer programs such as GraphPadPrism (GraphPad Inc., San Diego, USA) or SigmaPlot (Jandel Scientific, Erkrath, Germany). However, even when a computer program is used, the steepness of the concentration-response curve (slope), as described by the Hill coefficient, needs to be taken into account. Most computer programs have at least two options (a) Hill slope = 1 or (b) variable slope. This is important, because the slope can be very steep (most often when toxic effects are measured), rather flat, or – and this is the 'normal' case – is ~1. If nothing is known, the slope should be calculated using a 'variable slope' setting in the first analysis. This slope of the concentration-response curve means that in normal curves a doubling of the EC_{50} causes an increase in the effect by 66%, whereas in steep concentration-response curves, this is 75% or even more. The slope is generally evaluated using a Hill plot (which is also derived from biochemistry) by plotting log $(E/(E_{max}-E))$ against log $([A])$, yielding the following linear function:

$$\log(E/(E_{max}-E)) = h \times \log([A]) - \log(K_A) \qquad (8)$$

in which h is the slope of the function. A Hill slope of h = 1 is the 'normal' slope, whereas a Hill slope of ≥1.6 defines a steep concentration-response curve. In biochemistry, this indicates possible cooperation, and is seen when an allosteric modulation is present.

To enable analysis, at least five concentration steps should be investigated. Usually, the steps span several orders of magnitude, and because in most cases the logarithm of the concentration of the drug is plotted, steps are typically 1, 2, 10, 20, 100, 200, 1000, 2000 and so forth, to obtain a plot where intercept points are equal.

A classic method to determine the affinity of a competitive antagonist is the Schild-plot or pA_2-analysis. Here, in the first step, the concentration-response curve for agonist A is recorded. Next, the same concentration-response curve is repeated in the presence of the second antagonist, B, which is being investigated. This is repeated with several concentrations of the antagonist B. For analysis, the concentrations of equal effectiveness are determined, i.e. for a given concentration [A], the concentration of equal effectiveness [A´], in the presence of the antagonist, is sought. The shift of the concentration-response curve for A by B depends on the concentration of B, and its affinity K_B to the receptor.

The dose ratio [A]/[A´] can be described as:

$$[A]/[A´] = 1 + ([B]/K_B) \tag{9}$$

Next, the concentration of B is determined at which the dose-ratio is [A]/[A´] = 2. The equation can be written as:

$$[A]/[A´] = 2 = 1 + ([B]/K_B) \text{ or } [B] = K_B \tag{10}$$

$$pA_2 = -\log([B]) = -\log([K_B]) \tag{11}$$

The higher the value for pA_2, the higher the affinity of B is to its receptor. For graphic analysis, one can plot log (DR–1) against log ([B]), yielding a linear relationship that can be analysed by linear regression. At y = log (DR–1) = 1 the x-value represents pA_2.

The affinity of the antagonist (K_i) to inhibit the agonist-induced effect can be calculated according to the Cheng and Prusoff equation (Cheng and Prusoff 1973):

$$K_i = IC_{50}/([A]/EC_{50}) + 1 \tag{12}$$

which can also be written as:

$$K_i = IC_{50}/([A]/K_D) + 1 \tag{13}$$

IC_{50} is the concentration of antagonist, yielding half-maximal inhibition of the agonist-induced effect; [A] is the concentration of the agonist in the assay; EC_{50} is the concentration of agonist causing 50% of maximal effect.

In many cases, a half-maximum effect is reached before binding to the receptor is half-maximum. This is because an amplifying signal transduction pathway exists between receptor and effector. Therefore, saturation of effect will be achieved before all receptors are occupied, i.e. EC_{50} and BC_{50} (=half maximum binding concentration) will be different. Thus, if for a full agonist $BC_{50} << EC_{50}$, this is the first hint that a receptor reserve (a number of spare receptors) is present.

In some cases, the researcher works with partial agonists that have an intrinsic activity smaller than that of a full agonist. The effect of a partial agonist, however, may depend on the receptor reserve in the assay system. The receptor reserve is defined as the number of receptors that remain unused after the maximun effect is reached. The receptor reserve is usually larger in systems with a multicomponent-signal-transduction system. In systems without an amplifying signal transduction pathway, the receptor reserve is usually small or not present.

When a partial agonist is used, all receptors have to be occupied to obtain the maximum effect. According to the above considerations it can be stated that, if a partial agonist is used in a system with a large receptor reserve, the partial agonist will exhibit an intrinsic activity of 1, whereas in a system with a small receptor reserve, the intrinsic activity of the partial agonist will be considerably smaller than 1.

If the number of receptors used are experimentally so critically reduced (by using an irreversible antagonist) that there is just enough to obtain the maximum effect (100%), the receptor reserve can be determined. The concentration-response curve of the agonist, and the agonist, in the presence of the critical concentration of the irreversible antagonist, can be compared.

Examples

Competitive Antagonism

Firstly, we will consider competitive antagonism. A classic example in cardiovascular research for this type of antagonism is between the β_1-adrenoceptor antagonist betaxolol and the β_1-mediated positive inotropic effect of noradrenaline. Theoretically, we can expect in this case, a rightward shift of the concentration-response curve, which depends on the affinity of the β_1-adrenoceptor antagonist betaxolol to the receptor. To analyse this interaction, a cumulative concentration-response curve is examined on an isolated papillary muscle, and the developing force is recorded.

To characterise the interaction between both drugs, a cumulative concentration-response curve of the agonist is established in the absence or presence of increasing concentrations of the antagonist, that will shift the curve of the agonist to the right (Fig. 1a). Figure 1a shows concentration-response curves of an agonist in the presence of 0, 1, 10 or 100 nM of antagonist; the antagonist shifts the curves to the right in a concentration-dependent manner. Using these concentration-response curves, the dose ratios are determined by calculating the EC_{50} values and defining A´/A, i.e. agonist concentrations of equal effectiveness in absence and presence of the antagonist.

EC_{50} values are now determined yielding, in this example, in values of 10 nM (in absence of the antagonist), 50 nM (in presence of 1 nM antagonist), 300 nM (with 10 nM antagonist) and 2000 nM (with 100 nM antagonist), which means that the dose ratio (DR) is 5, 30 and 200 (and DR−1=4, 29, 199).

Next, the log (DR−1) values are plotted against the negative logarithm of the antagonist's concentrations (Schild-plot) (Fig. 1b). These values should give a straight line, in the case of competetive antagonism, with a slope = 1. It is important that not only a narrow range of the antagonist concentration is investigated, because in some cases (e.g. allosteric modulators) a linear relationship might exist within a narrow range which, with an increasing antagonist concentration, can turn into a saturation curve.

The Schild-plot data can be analysed using linear regression, which yields the X-intercept at (DR−1)=1 (when DR=2), indicating the pA_2 value. In the example the pA_2 value is 2×10^{-10}. A competitive antagonist should give a slope of 1.0 in the Schild-plot. In case of allosteric inhibition the slope of the Schild-plot might differ from 1. However, it is necessary to investigate a dose range that is large enough to evaluate linearity. Allosteric inhibitors might exhibit a linear initial part of the Schild-plot.

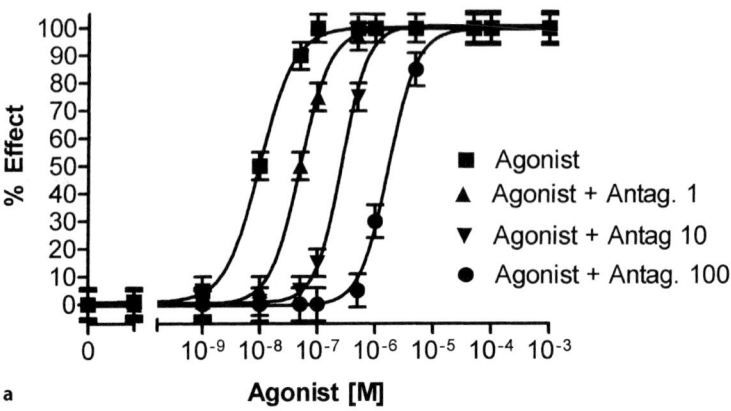

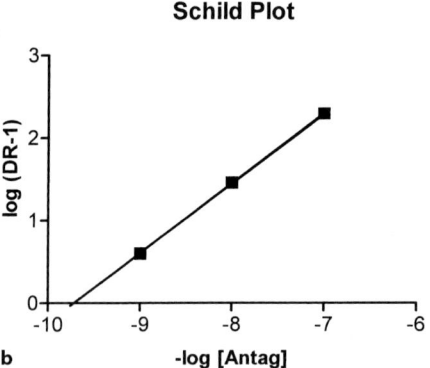

Figure 1a,b
a Typical example for a competitive antagonist. Increasing concentrations of the antagonist cause a parallel rightward shift of the concentration-response curve. b Schild-plot Analysis of the data of panel A, revealing a pA$_2$ value of 9.7 (corresponding to about 2×10^{-10} M) for the antagonist

Non-Competitive Antagonism

Let us now consider a non-competitive antagonism such as phenoxybenzamine and noradrenaline. In the case of a non-competitive antagonism, it is not possible to displace the antagonist by higher concentrations of the agonist, possibly because of covalent binding of the agonist to the receptor or by different binding sites. As a consequence, in the presence of the antagonist, E_{max} is lower than in its absence, even at high agonist concentrations (as shown in Fig. 2). Typically, the EC_{50} is not altered. It is possible to calculate an inhibitor constant according to the methods used in biochemistry.

For this purpose, data should be expressed and plotted as 1/[A] ([A] = agonist concentration) for *x*-values, and 1/E (E=effect) for *y*-values, and plotted as a Lineweaver-Burk diagram both in the presence and absence of inhibitor of various concentrations.

The inhibitor constant K_i can be calculated according to the equation:

$$1/E = [1 + ([I]/K_i)] \times [(K_D/E_{max}) \times (1/[A]) + (1/E_{max})] \tag{14}$$

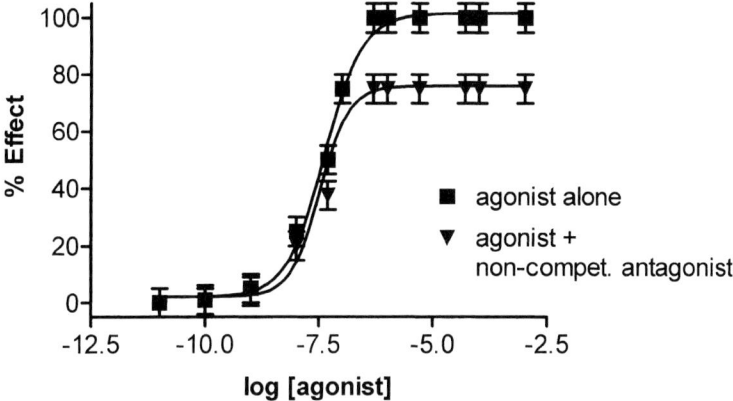

Figure 2
Example of a non-competitive antagonism

With increasing inhibitor concentration [I] the gradient of the linear relationship 1/[A] versus 1/E increases, whereas the X-intercept (in biochemistry=K_M, here =K_D) does not change. The Y-intercept $1/E_{max}$ is typically enhanced, corresponding to a lower E_{max} value.

Functional Antagonism

In many cases the interaction between two compounds is on a functional level, i.e. at two different receptors or signal transduction pathways that are functionally linked. To give an example, one can consider the functional antagonism between adrenaline and acetylcholine with regard to the heart rate. Adrenaline enhances the heart rate via a β_1-adrenoceptor stimulation-dependent increase in adenylylcyclase activity, whereas acetylcholine decreases the heart rate by a M_2-cholinoceptor-dependent inhibition of adenylylcyclase activity, and by inhibition of certain ionic channels, such as the pacemaker current I_f, and by activation of the repolarizing current $I_{K.ACh}$. In these cases, the typical concentration-response curve, in presence of the inhibitor, exhibits a reduced E_{max} and a rightward shift of the curve with increased EC_{50}, as depicted in Fig. 3.

Notice, that depending on the strength of the effect of the full agonist that is under investigation, the functional antagonist might induce a limited rightward shift of an agonist curve with high efficacy, and to a flattening of the concentration-response curve of an agonist with low efficacy.

Type I Synergism

This type of synergism is the opposite of a competitive antagonism. Drug A is a full agonist, and agonistic drug B is given in its presence. For example, if drug B inhibits the inactivation of drug A, this leads to a higher functional concentration of A at the

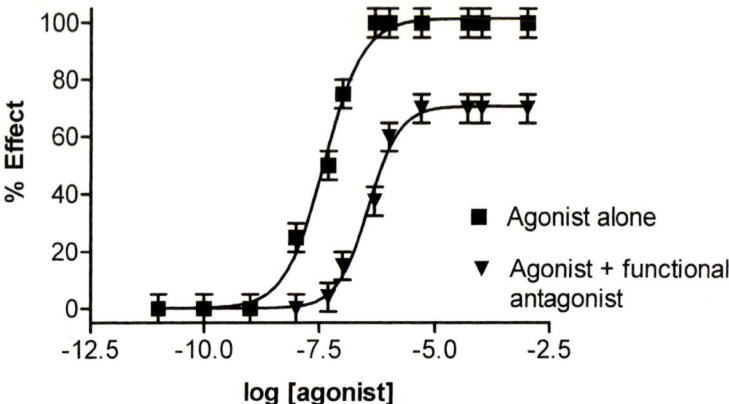

Figure 3
This example shows a typical functional antagonism with a limited rightward shift of the concentration-response curve and concomitant flattening

receptor than in absence of B. As a consequence, the concentration-response curve shifts to the left. A classic example for this type of interaction is between noradrenaline, acting on adrenoceptors, and cocaine or desipramin, which inhibit the uptake of noradrenaline, thereby inhibiting the inactivation of noradrenaline. However, it is necessary to bear in mind that in this case of interaction, the only drug acting at the receptor itself, is drug A.

Type II Synergism

In contrast to type I synergism, type II synergism means that the efficacy of the agonistic drug A is enhanced by the presence of drug B. Typically, this is achieved by drug B acting on the post-receptor signal transduction pathway. The efficacy of isoprenaline, can be enhanced by phosphodiesterase inhibitors, such as 3-isobutyl-1-methylxanthine (IBMX): isoprenaline acts on β-adrenoceptors and enhances intracellular levels of the second messenger cAMP; IBMX inhibits the inactivation phosphodiesterase prolonging the effect of cAMP. This primarily affects the E_{max} of the concentration-response curve of drug A, yielding a higher E_{max}. Because neither the concentration of drug A at the receptor or its affinity are influenced, EC_{50} is typically not altered.

Additive Effects and Complex Interactions

When interactions are investigated it is often necessary to consider basal effects. So might one of the two drugs have an effect and the other drug is tested on top of this (after drug B). For analysis of such effects, it is necessary to plot the total effect of drug A alone, and in combination with drug B, as well as the net effect of drug A in combination with drug B. In such complex interactions, drug B also has a separate effect

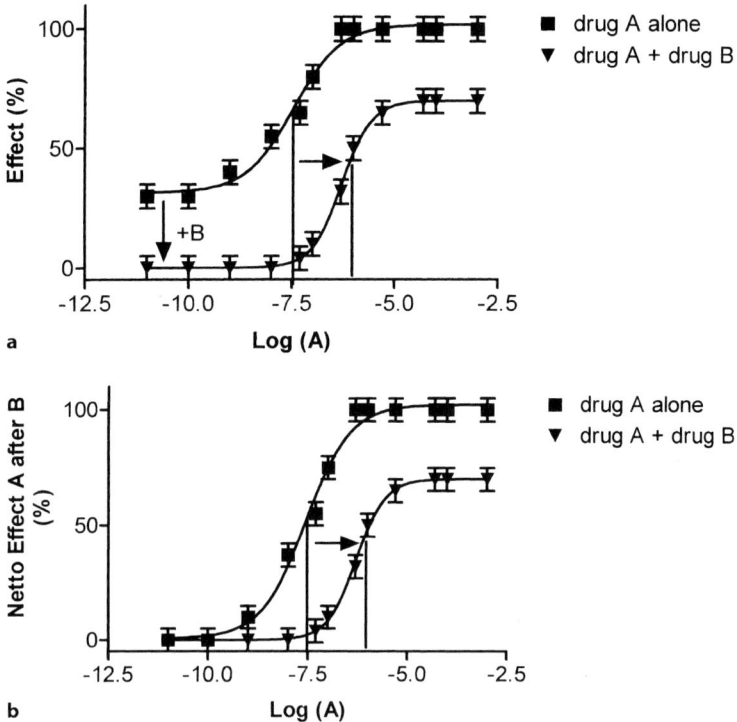

Figure 4
Functional antagonism of two drugs with basal activity of the investigated system. Drug A is given in either the absence or presence of a fixed concentration of drug B that is sufficient to inhibit the basal activity. The second part of the figure shows the net effect of drug A after the addition of drug B

in the absence of drug A. It is therefore necessary to define exactly the maximum effect, if possible, as that which can maximally be achieved in this system with drug A.

Let us consider the following situation (see Fig. 4): in a given system is a basal activity of 30% when drug A is present at low concentrations. This basal activity is completely antagonised by a specific concentration of drug B. When drug A is applied in the presence of drug B, the concentration-response curve of drug A is shifted to the right and flattened. To analyse the interaction in more detail, the net effect of drug A alone is compared with the net effect of drug A after the addition of drug B. In our case, the resulting curve is shifted to the right and the E_{max} is lowered, indicating a type of functional antagonism with similar targets of drug action.

Another type of complex interaction is the independent antagonism. In that case (Fig. 5), we also have a drug A with a basal effect of 30% that is completely antagonised by drug B. When drug A is tested after drug B, the curve is lowered but not shifted to the right. This becomes apparent when the net effect of drug A is analysed following the addition of drug B, yielding an identical curve to the one obtained by adding drug A only. This type of interaction is an independent antagonism and is often observed if two drugs are tested in combinations that have divergent targets of action.

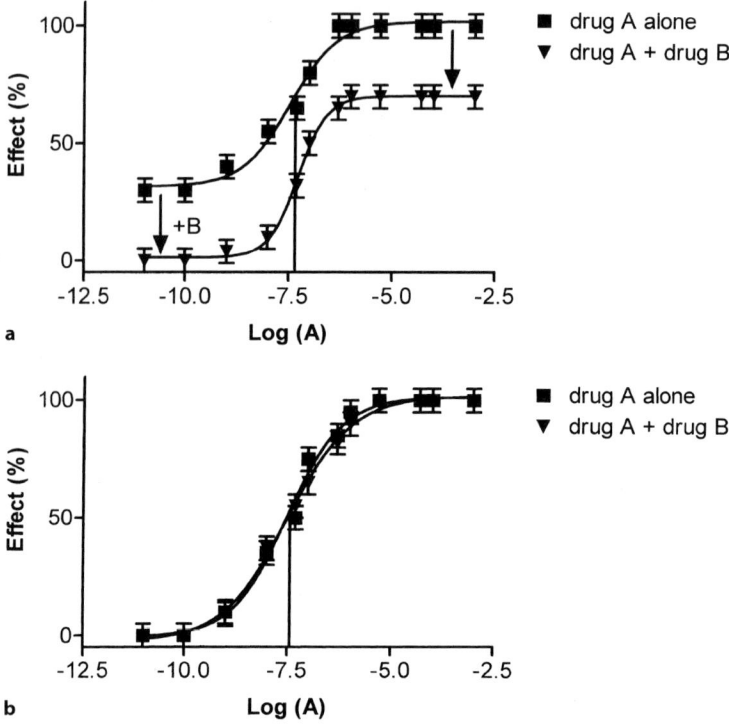

Figure 5
Independent Antagonism of Two Drugs in a System with Basal Activity Similar to that Shown in Fig. 4. Again, drug B is given in a fixed concentration that is sufficient to antagonise the basal activity. However, as seen in the second part of the figure, the net effect of drug A is not altered by the presence of drug B, indicating independent actions

In a similar way, complex synergism might occur (with or without a shift of the EC_{50}) when a second drug is present that exerts its effect in the same direction as drug A. When EC_{50} of the net curve for drug A is changed in presence of drug B (i.e. shifted to the left), we have a functional synergism. An independent synergism is observed when the resulting net curve is identical to the one when drug B is absent.

Thus, regarding independent interactions (synergistic or antagonistic), there is no effect of drug B on the net effect of drug A, hinting at different drug targets and different mechanisms of actions.

In additive effects, the effect of a combination of two drugs might simply be the addition of both effects or at least more or less so (over- or under-additive). If B is equally effective as A, the combined effect of A+B should be 2×A. Meaning that, in the case of a normal concentration-response curve (Hill slope = 1) the effect of A+B should be 2×EC_{50} of A. This is under the assumption that, the effect of 1A is the effect of the EC_{50} of A, and would result in an E_{max} value of 66–67%. In the case of a steep concentration-response curve, E_{max} should be about 75%. Thus, the effect of the combined effect is larger when the concentration-response curve is steeper.

For evaluation purposes, it might be helpful to calculate an additive-concentration-response curve in theory, and compare this with the one being measured. In the case of an independent synergistic interaction, the theoretical curve of the combined effect (in %) can be calculated as:

$$E_{A+B} = E_A + \{E_B \times [(100-E_A)/100]\} \qquad (15)$$

In the case of a normal concentration-response curve (Hill slope = 1), the independent additive synergistic effect is usually larger than the additive effect with similar targets of action (approximately 66–67% of E_{max} at $2\times EC_{50}$ (see above). In the case of a steep concentration-response curve, however, additive and independent effect might be equal or, in the case of a very steep curve, the additive effect might be larger than the independent additive effect.

To construct an additive curve in theory in order to compare it with the registered curve (Fig. 6), the concentration of drug A must first be determined, whose effect is equal to the concentration of drug B. Next, the X-intercept of twice the concentration of A is sought along with the corresponding effect of 2A. In the subsequent step this (the found concentarion of A) is subtracted from the concentration-response curve by shifting it to the right by 1A. The same is carried out for 3A and 4A and so forth, yielding the theoretically-calculated additive curve for a combination of drugs with similar effects. The measured effect can now be classified as additive, over- or under-addi-tive or (see above) as independent. In a similar (but reverse) manner an antagonistic interaction can be classified.

With regard to the interpretation of such effects, great care should be taken and over-interpretation should be avoided. However, in the case of a difference to the simple additive curve, this suggests that the targets of the drug action of drug A and B are not identical. Values of the measured curve that coincide with those of the theo-

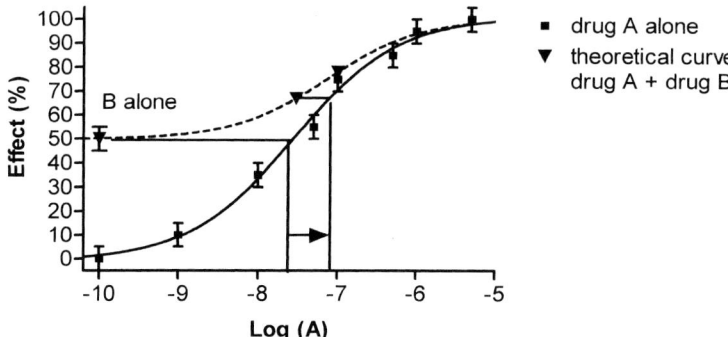

Figure 6
Construction of a theoretically-calculated additive concentration-response curve. First, the concentration of equal effectiveness is determined for drug A. Next, X-intercept of 2A and the corresponding point on the concentration-response curve are determined. From that point, 1A is subtracted and yields the first point of the theoretically-calculated additive curve. The same was done for 2A, 3A, 4A and so forth

retically-calculated additive curve, might indicate similar mechanisms of action for drugs with reversible effects or different mechanisms for drugs with irreversible effects.

An over-additive effect normally contradicts the hypothesis of a similar or identical mechanism of action. Under-additive effects, for example, are observed when a full agonist is tested in the absence and presence of a partial agonist. If the registered effect corresponds to the theoretical independent effect, it might mean that either the effects of both drugs are mediated by different mechanisms and/or that the effects of a combination partner are independent from the effect of the previous dose (as is the case in exponential dose-response curves). However, this does not exclude an effect by a similar or identical mechanism.

Interested readers are referred to the more detailed literature given in the references section.

Troubleshooting

Mathematical analysis of concentration-response curves is now done by a number of computer programs (e.g. GraphPadPrism, SigmaPlot, Origin 6.0 etc.). Generally, the data table has to be generated first, then the data are transformed [concentration to log (concentration)] and thereafter a non-linear fit for sigmoidal curves is performed. If nothing is known about the concentration-response relation, the slope of the non-linear regression curve should be set as variable, otherwise it may be set to 1.0. The software will give the goodness of fit as r^2 which should be higher than 0.85. The Hill slope, also given by the software, is the slope of the concentration-response curve. It is normally about 1.0; in case of toxicity curves, however, it is often steeper (around 1.6 or more). The accuracy of a concentration-response curve can be estimated from the goodness of fit (which should be higher than 0.85), the Hill slope (which should be around 1.0; very flat curves are suspect), EC_{50} and E_{max} as well as the standard deviation of E_{max} and EC_{50}.

A particular problem is incomplete concentration-response curves. They might be due to toxic effects of the investigated drug that do not allow for investigation into the effect of the drug in higher concentrations on the desired parameter. For example, if inotropy is investigated using certain phosphodiesterase inhibitors (such as amrinone or milrinone), these drugs might exert arrhythmogenic effects before reaching a saturation of the concentration-response curve in regard to the inotropic effect. In these cases, it can sometimes be helpful to convert the effect to 1/E and the concentration to 1/C, and to plot 1/E against 1/C according to Lineweaver and Burk. A linear regression yields the Y-intercept as $1/E_{max}$ that can simply be converted to E_{max} (for more details see above).

Occasionally, the measured concentration-response curve does not look like a simple sigmoidal curve but more like a biphasic curve. If this is the case, the first step is to test whether it is truly biphasic or not. Therefore, two fits have to be performed, first the simple sigmoidal fit and second a biphasic fit. In the next step an F-test is performed to find out which fit is best. In the case of a biphasic curve, one has to con-

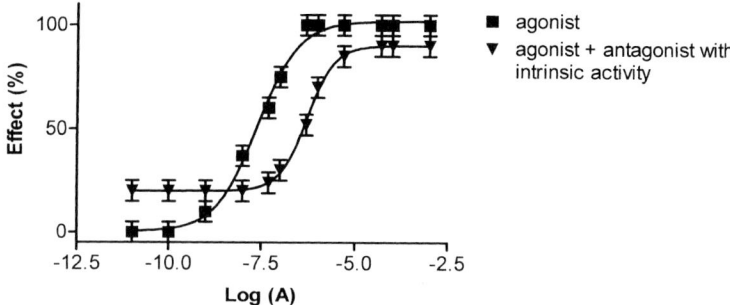

Figure 7
Effect of a partial antagonist with intrinsic activity on the concentration-response curve of a full antagonist. Notice the agonistic effect of the drug in absence or at very low concentrations of the full agonist

sider that the drug might act on two different receptors, or might activate two different mechanisms. If known, one can try to repeat the concentration-response curve in the presence of an inhibitor of one of the receptors. If the inhibited receptor is involved in the biphasic curve, the curve should be converted to a monophasic curve in the presence of the inhibitor.

Some drugs that are used as antagonists might exert intrinsic agonism. This means that the drug binds to the receptor and activates it but does not lead to its full activation. A classic example is the β-adrenoceptor antagonist pindolol. Intrinsic agonism might cause some trouble or confusion when testing it in combination. As outlined above and shown in Fig. 7, the addition of an inhibitor with intrinsic activity causes some agonistic effects that are either detected at very low concentrations or in the absence of a full agonist. At higher concentrations, the antagonist will inhibit the effects of the full agonist because this drug occupies a part of the receptor without activating it fully. This behaviour is similar to a partial antagonism.

When antagonistic effects are investigated, the type of antagonism should be clearly described. With regard to drugs that act at the same receptor: it is possible that an inhibitor competes with the full agonist for the receptor-binding site without activating the receptor, this being a typically competitive antagonist without intrinsic activity. However, it should be kept in mind that this type of drug neither activates nor deactivates the receptor. Thus, in the absence of a full antagonist, this type of antagonist does not exhibit any effect. In the absence of a full agonist, a partial antagonist, a partial agonist or an antagonist with intrinsic activity causes some activation of the receptor but diminishes the effect of a full agonist. Degree of inhibition and shift of the curve depend on the affinity of the full agonist. Besides, another type of antagonist exists: the inverse agonist. An inverse agonist can bind to the receptor and deactivate it. It therefore exerts the opposite action of a full agonist. Thus, in contrast to a competitive antagonist, an inverse agonist will show inhibition of the receptor in absence of a full agonist. A classic example for this type of antagonisms or inverse agonisms comes from the GABA receptor. Benzodiazepines, such as diazepam, act as agonists by binding to the GABA receptor (at a binding site different to the GABA binding site). They activate the receptor and enhance the effect of the endogenous transmitter GABA, thus allowing a chloride current. This action can be completely blocked with the competitive antagonist flumazenil without exerting intrinsic activity. Flumazenil is used in benzodiazepine intoxication and competes with benzodiazepines for their binding site. Bretazenile represents a partial agonist of the GABA receptor. Methyl-6,7-dimethyl-4-ethyl-β-carbolin-3-carboxylic acid (DMCM) acts as an inverse agonist at the GABA receptor, binding to the same binding site as benzodiazepines and reducing the effect of GABA. While the full agonist diazepam leads to sedation and reduces anxiety, the inverse agonist DMCM induces anxiety and agitation.

It might be necessary to characterise a drug as either a receptor-blocker (competitive) or an effector-blocker (non-competitive). In such cases, a dose-ratio test might help. First, a known competitive blocker (A) is tested against a known agonist (C) by measuring the effect of a given concentration of A, compared with the effect of increasing concentrations of C. Subsequently, the unknown blocker B is tested against the agonist C in the same way. Finally, the combined effect of blockers A and B is tested against increasing concentrations of C. If the unknown blocker B is a competitive blocker, the dose ratio follows the equation:

$$DR_{A+B} = DR_A + DR_B - 1 \quad (16)$$

If the unknown drug B is a non-competitive blocker, the dose ratio can be described as:

$$DR_{A+B} = DR_A \times DR_B \quad (17)$$

Sometimes, the duration of drug exposure might influence the effect. Normally, the interaction between drug and receptor is based on weak, reversible binding forces, so that an equilibrium is reached within a short period of time. However, toxic effects are often related to covalent binding or other effects, possibly related to the duration of exposure. In such cases, prolongation of exposure time will yield the true concentration-response curve.

References

Arunlakshana O and Schild HO (1959): Some Quantitative Uses of Drug Anatgonists. Brit J Pharmacol 14: 48-58.
Cheng Y-C and Prusoff WH (1973): Relationship Between the Inhibition Constant (K_i) and the Concentration of Inhibitor Which Causes 50 Percent Inhibition (IC_{50}) of an Enzymatic Reaction. Biochem Pharmacol 22: 3099-3108.
Goldstein A, Aronow L and Kalman SM (1987): Principles of Drug Action: The Basis of Pharmacology. 2nd edition. Wiley, New York, 1974 Kenakin TP: Pharmacologic Analysis of Drug-Receptor Interaction. Raven Press, New York.
Lazarena S and Birdsall NJM (1993): Estimation of Antagonist KB from Inhibition Curves in Functional Experiments: Alternatives to the Cheng-Prusoff Equation. Trends Pharmacol Sci 14: 237-239.
Pöch G and Juan H (1990): Wirkungen von Pharmaka. Thieme Verlag, Stuttgart.
Tallarida RJ and Jacob LS (1979): The Dose Response Relation in Pharmacology. Springer-Verlag, Berlin.
Tallarida RJ and Murray RB (1987): Manual of Pharmacologic Calculations with Computer Programs. Springer-Verlag, New York.
Van den Brink FG (1977): General Theory of Drug-Receptor Interactions. Drug-receptor Interaction Models. Calculation of Drug Parameters. In: Van Rossum JM (Ed): Kinetics of Drug Action. Exp Pharmacol Volume 47, Springer-Verlag, Berlin, pp. 169-254

Measurement of NO and Endothelial Function in Cardiovascular Research

Renate Roesen, Anke Rosenkranz, Dirk Taubert and Reinhard Berkels

Introduction

Furchgott and Zawadzki (1980) demonstrated in their classical experiment that the vascular endothelium liberates NO in response to diverse stimuli, and subsequent activation of soluble guanylate cyclase by NO induces relaxation of the smooth muscle layer (Murad 1994). The significance of NO in blood pressure regulation was recognised early on, since NO is the first and only known dilator associated with an immediate rise in systemic blood pressure when its biosynthesis is blocked. Moreover, NO formation may be induced as a negative-feedback modulator of vasoconstriction: thus the concentration-response curves of vasoconstrictor agonists are shifted to lower concentrations in endothelium-denuded vessels. Over the past two decades, our understanding of the diverse vascular functions of NO has expanded to include the regulation of smooth muscle and endothelial cell growth and apoptosis (Dimmeler et al. 1997). Three isoforms of NO-synthase (NOS) have been identified and characterized (Forstermann et al. 1994). Regulation of the activity and expression of the endothelial isoform, NOS III, appears to be disturbed in nearly all forms of cardiovascular disease. The resultant endothelial dysfunction seems to be a common link in hypertension, atherosclerosis and diabetes mellitus (Cai and Harrison 2000; Vakkilainen et al. 2000; Hink et al. 2001; Cosentino et al. 2002).

Different approaches have been developed to measure NOS expression and activity. Quantification in different cellular compartments is performed either in terms of protein expression using western-blotting techniques, or on an RNA level with RT-PCR (Wassmann et al. 2001; Hecker et al. 1994). Enzyme activity can be determined by measuring the conversion of the NOS substrate L-arginine to L-citrulline (Hirata et al. 1995), or by estimating the formation of NO and/or its stable metabolites nitrite/nitrate (Berkels et al. 2001) in conjunction with the extent of phosphorylation (Hirata et al. 1995; Du et al. 2001). Each of these parameters is of importance and gives different information about the NO signalling cascade.

Endothelial dysfunction is characterized by a diminished NO bioavailability, which is caused in part by an increased production of radical superoxide anions. Endothelial dysfunction is often measured as an impaired relaxation to endothelium-dependent vasodilators such as acetylcholine. However, isolated vessels may also relax in response to an acute application of peroxynitrite. Peroxynitrite is produced during the rapid reaction between NO and superoxide. This also occurs during the decomposition of the so-called NO donor SIN-1, thus vessel tone might not be representative of the true status of endothelial function. It is therefore important to determine the concentration of free NO, however, direct measurement of free NO is difficult given its extremely short half-life (about 5 s), and its accelerated oxidation in the presence of nitrate/nitrite. Moreover, NO undergoes a rapid diffusion-controlled reaction with superoxide anions to form peroxinitrite. Free NO concentrations may, however, be measured electrochemically with Clark-type electrodes (Brovkovych et al. 2001), several different types of which are commercially available. We have experience with different types of NO-electrodes (all from World Precision Instruments, Sarasota), which are characterized by a stable NO signal and a detection limit of 1–5 nmol/l NO in the final solution (Berkels et al. 1996). Although we have not tested them, there are other electrodes available which claim to be more sensitive, from Harvard Apparatus for example.

It is important to bear in mind that a more sensitive electrode is also more likely to be influenced by outside factors, thus background noise will be greater. NO-electrodes are equipped with specialized membranes that allow passage of the NO molecule, but not peroxynitrite or other higher oxidation products of NO (e.g. nitrite or nitrate). NO is then oxidised at the electrode according to its redox potential, the resultant electrical current is proportional to the amount of NO at the membrane surface.

The choice of electrode is dependent on the type of measurement that is to be obtained. Macroelectrodes (2 mm diameter) are recommended for vessels that are open and laid flat, while microelectrodes are more suitable for NO detection in solutions or intact vessels. For this purpose, the L-shaped electrode has been developed, which might be highly useful for concurrent measurement of vessel tone in intact vessels. An alternative possibility is the use of NO spin-trapping agents with concomitant electron spin resonance analysis (Kleschyov and Munzel, 2002), or a specialised Nitric Oxide Analyzer, such as is available from ANTEK Instruments, which measures NO in the gaseous phase.

Description of Methods and Practical Approach

Real-time Measurement of Free NO Concentrations

Endothelial NO formation may be measured under either basal conditions or following specific NOS stimulation by endothelium-dependent vasodilators (including M3-receptor agonists such as acetylcholine or carbachol, NK1-agonists like substance P, or bradykinin), in comparison to measurements obtained when NOS is blocked by nitro-L-arginine (L-NNA) or monomethyl-L-arginine (L-MMA). Receptor distribution for these agonists varies between different vascular beds and species, it is therefore necessary to first verify the presence of these specific receptors in the endothelial preparation under evaluation, and thus identify the optimal tool for stimulating NO formation. Given the variability between tissues obtained even within the same species, it is advisable to examine control and test stimuli within the same vessel.

Calibration of the NO Electrode

The calibration procedure must take into account the NO-gradient that exists at the endothelium, with highest concentrations occurring at the lumen, which fall to zero at distances greater than 1.5 mm. In other words, the final concentration of free NO that is measured by the electrode must correspond with the amplitude of the signal obtained at the endothelium. Such real-time measurement of the acute concentration of free NO released at the precise point at which the electrode tip is placed, differs from measurements of cumulative NO concentrations in solutions. The latter procedure calculates the net NO formation over a period of time by re-conversion of the metabolites nitrite/nitrate in a homogeneous distribution (see below).

Calibration Via Re-Conversion of Nitrite to NO

In this procedure, nitrite (KNO_2) is chemically titrated to generate a standard curve. Nitrite is stoichiometrically converted to NO in the presence of an acidic iodide calibration solution containing (in mmol/l): KI 0.10, K_2SO_4 0.14, H_2SO_4 0.10. The amount of NO generated is calculated according to the equation:

$$2\ KNO_2 + 2\ KI + 2\ H_2SO_4 + 2\ K_2SO_4 \rightarrow 2\ NO + I_2 + 2\ H_2O + 4\ K_2SO_4$$

The electrode is immersed approximately 0.2 cm into 10 ml of calibration solution, followed by the incremental addition of KNO_2 standards, by either (i) delivering increasing amounts of nitrite in increasing volumes to give final NO concentrations in the nanomolar range, or (ii) increasing the concentration by cumulative addition of nitrite in a constant volume. This generates a standard curve for the estimation of final concentration of accumulated NO metabolites in the solution (Berkels et al., 2001). Valid measurements may be obtained if up to 500 µl aliquots are added, although smaller volumes are preferable. No more than a total of 1 ml should be added to the bath to avoid fluctuation in pH and redox capacity of the system. We also found that the calibration curve was not disturbed in the presence of protein (up to 1 mg/ml BSA) or thiol groups (up to 1 mmol/l). Calibration is conducted at room temperature, since higher temperatures are associated with greater background noise and a reduced solubility of NO in aqueous solution. The redox potential of the electrode is too small to reduce nitrate in the solution to nitrite, therefore, nitrate must be enzymatically reduced prior to re-conversion of nitrite to NO. While this may be done using a commercially available nitrate reductor (Nitralyzer™, World Precision Instruments, Sarasota), we found this method was not reproducible.

Calibration with Aqueous NO

An alternative calibration method, which requires specialised facilities due to NO toxicity, employs an aqueous NO standard solution that is prepared under N_2 to exclude contamination by oxygen. First, distilled water is gassed for 60 min. with N_2 (100%) and then saturated with NO gas (1% in N_2) for a further 45 min. Defined volumes (e.g. 4.6 ml) are taken with a gas-tight syringe and added to HEPES solution (100 ml) to yield a final NO concentration of 6.75 mmol/l at 20 °C. Aliquots of this solution are then applied to the electrode to generate a calibration curve in the nanomolar range. Prior to use, all solutions are oxygen-deprived by gassing with 100% N_2.

Experimental Procedure

Isolated Vessels

Vessels are removed from experimental animals (e.g. mice, rats, rabbits) immediately after sacrifice, and carefully cleared of surrounding tissue. Ideally, vessels are continuously perfused *in situ* during preparation, or at least immediately after excision, with Tyrode solution (pH 7.4, room temperature) to prevent stunning from blood clots, to limit contact with hemoglobin and endothelial damage from collapsing vessels. Our normal Tyrode solution contains (in mmol/l): NaCl 136.80, KCl 5.36, $CaCl_2$ 1.80, $MgCl_2$ 1.05, $NaHCO_3$ 23.80, NaH_2PO_4 0.42, D-glucose 5, and saturated with carbogen (5% CO_2 in oxygen). Fat and connective tissue are discarded and freshly prepared tissues are allowed to equilibrate in Tyrode solution continuously bubbled with carbogen at room temperature. For porcine coronary arteries, pig hearts are obtained at the slaughterhouse immediately after death and the coronaries cleared of blood by flushing with ice-cold carbogen-saturated Tyrode solution. Coronary arteries (approx. 8 cm pieces) are excised from hearts on site, transported to the laboratory in Tyrode solution on ice, and treated as above.

It is recommended that the ISO-NO electrode be allowed to pre-equilibrate in the organ bath buffer while tissue sections are prepared for measurement. Vessels are cut into pieces approx. 1 cm in length and opened longitudinally by a single cut. Tissues are transferred to the organ bath and attached at both ends with the luminal site facing upwards. They should lie totally flat and be large enough to allow placement of the macro-electrode in the centre, with cells damaged or disturbed by handling restricted to the borders of the tissue furthest from the electrode. The minimum size of the opened vessel should be at least 4×4 mm, i.e. at least 4 mm in length and with an internal diameter of no less than 1mm. Vessels are incubated with 10 ml HEPES buffered Krebs-Henseleit solution (pH 7.4) containing (in mmol/l): NaCl 140, KCl 5, $CaCl_2$ 2, $MgCl_2$ 1, HEPES 10, glucose 5 and saturated with air (pO_2 150 mmHg). The organ bath system is maintained at 25 °C. The tip of the ISO-NO electrode is then positioned at a constant distance of 1 mm above the endothelial surface, and vessels are again allowed to equilibrate. The incubation solution in the organ bath is renewed after 30 min. Once baseline is established, a reference concentration of an endothelial-dependent vasodilator (e.g. carbachol) is added to the bath. This is then washed out and the signal again allowed to reach baseline.

Cultured Endothelial Cells

We have applied the NO electrode to measure free NO formation in porcine aortic endothelial cells (PAEC) in culture. For these studies, it is essential that the endothelial monolayers are intact and have reached comparable levels of confluency. PAEC cultures were harvested and cultured as previously described (Berkels et al. 1999) and used at passages 1–2. PAEC grown to confluence on glass coverslips are placed into organ baths and free NO in cell monolayers is measured as in vessels (see above).

Estimating NO Formation via Re-Conversion of Nitrite/Nitrate

We found that basal NO formation, in the absence of stimulator agonists, yields NO concentrations that are below the detection level of the electrode. However, basal and stimulated (e.g. by carbachol) NO production may be estimated indirectly by measuring the accumulation of nitrite/nitrate (NO metabolites) over periods of time (Berkels et al. 2001).

The main advantage of this technique is that nitrite/nitrate are stable, thus biological samples may be stored at –80 °C and assayed at a later date. Prior to analysis, nitrate is enzymatically reduced to nitrite (see below), which is then converted stoichiometrically to NO (as detailed above for calibration via re-conversion of nitrite to NO), and quantified. If cumulative NO formation is to be measured in the presence of a NOS inhibitor, it is essential not to use nitro-L-arginine (L-NNA), since decomposition increases the signal.

Following calibration, longitudinally opened vessels are incubated in 500 µl HEPES buffer at 25°C for 30 min. Vessels are removed and a 50 µl mixture of NADPH/FAD (1.5:0.3 mg/ml) is added, followed after 1 min. by 15 µl of nitrate reductase (10 U/ml). Aliquots of the NADPH/FAD solution may be stored frozen, but the activity of NADPH should be tested prior to use. Following a further 30 min incubation at room temperature, aliquots (50–200 µl) of incubation medium are added to the acidic iodide calibration solution for estimation of nitrite content in comparison with a standard curve. Given the variability between preparations, paired control incubations from the same piece of vessel should be conducted in parallel with test substances to allow for valid comparisons. The net rate of NO production over the course of the incubation may be determined from the nitrite concentration using the equation:

$$\text{Rate of NO production} = \text{nitrite concentration (mol/l)} \times \text{volume (l)/incubation time (h)}$$

The amount of nitrite (NO) formed is then corrected for either the wet tissue weight or the luminal surface area of the vessel.

This indirect method may also be applied to measure NO formation in endothelial cells in culture. Defined volumes of the incubation medium (e.g. 500 µl) are treated with FAD/NADPH and nitrate reductase, as described above, then transferred to the acetic iodide solution. The total incubation volume was limited (1.5 ml per 10 cm dish) to maximise the end concentration of nitrite yet adequately cover cell monolayers.

NO formation should be further standardised to cell number, or alternatively be expressed per unit area of cell monolayer, provided that confluency is consistent between experiments.

Practical Considerations

The NO electrode is highly sensitive to outside influences and, as mentioned earlier, increased electrode sensitivity also means increased noise and susceptibility to interference by factors such as the respiratory rate of the experimenter. Laughing in the vicinity of the electrode can induce a signal, just as heavy obstructed breathing can generate artefacts in the recording. Several important factors should therefore be considered to ensure that a meaningful and reproducible signal is obtained. The size of the signal is highly variable between tissues from different species and the agonist used to stimulate NOS. Generally we have found that rabbit aorta yields a better, more sustained NO signal than vessels from rat or pig coronary artery. It is therefore advisable to compare the effects of control and test substances in tissues obtained from the same vessel.

Verification of the NO Signal

The NO-electrode allows for sensitive measurement of free NO, but not its oxidation products, metabolites or other molecules such as CO. However, the simplicity of the system is deceptive. It is therefore essential to verify that increases in the signal are truly attributable to an increase in the formation of free NO. This may involve comparing the signal obtained in both the absence and presence of an NOS inhibitor such as L-MMA, or oxyHb, a NO scavenger that immediately suppresses the NO signal and establishes the absolute baseline of the system. This is problematic if ambient NO is high, for example, in times of peak traffic or smog or as a result of heavy respiration by the experimenter, as the electrode also detects this.

In these conditions, addition of oxyHb will overestimate the contribution of stimulated NO to the detected signal. High ambient nitrites may also complicate the estimation of NO formation via measurement of accumulated nitrite/nitrate, thus it is essential to always conduct a reagent-blank in parallel to correct for nitrite contamination from the air.

Consistent Placement of the Electrode Tip

As mentioned earlier, the concentration of free NO is not homogeneous throughout the organ bath, but is maximal directly at the endothelial surface, with a decreasing NO gradient along the electrode away from the tip. Variation in distance between tissue surface and electrode membrane thus determines the height of the signal obtained. For isolated vessels, the tip of the microelectrode is centred fully within the lumen, so that endothelial surface surrounds the entire electrode at a constant distance from the membrane. This limits variation in the NO concentration detected at the electrode surface and ensures the validity of the calibration. However, the potential effects of contraction and relaxation on the shape and length of the vessel must be taken into account in isometric tension studies. When using macroelectrodes (2 mm diameter) with pieces of vessel opened longitudinally, the electrode tip is placed at a constant distance above the luminal surface. Measurements are integrated across the entire area of the electrode, even the surfaces not in proximity of the endothelium, which leads to an underestimation of the actual NO concentrations that must be taken into account. With microelectrodes, measurement occurs across the entire membrane-encased tip, which must be fully immersed when calibrating in solution.

The addition of test or calibrator solutions to the organ bath must also be standardised in the same way. This involves a fiddly compromise of not placing the pipette in the immediate vicinity of the electrode membrane, yet delivering the aliquot close enough (and with not too much force) to the endothelium to ensure subsequent changes in the NO signal are actually detectable and representative of the stimulatory effects of the agonist.

Detection of Response and Peak Detectable Signal

The maximum height of a transient NO signal is dependent on the response (lag-time) of both the electrode and the detection system. Equipment with a faster response can detect peak transients that are produced rapidly, which would not be distinguishable from background noise, if a detection system with a slower response is used. However, the advantage of the latter system is that noise is dampened and the NO signal is clearer. Such variation in detection response may underlie the differences in peak NO concentrations obtained using commercial electrodes (nanomolar range), as opposed to the faster response electrodes made and used by Malinski and colleagues (micromolar range, Brovkovych et al. 2001), although the lower detection limit is the same for both types of electrode.

The sensitivity of the 2 mm macro-electrodes is dependent on the tolerance or length of the metal sleeve around the membrane as well as the inner carbon fibre to which the membrane is attached. Thus different membranes of the same type may exhibit different sensitivities, making it essential to calibrate the electrode at least every time the membrane is replaced.

When assembling the electrode, gently place the carbon fibre within the sleeve then tighten the nut to attach the sleeve to the main part of the electrode. At this point it is important to hold all components firmly in position and only turn the nut while tightening. Avoid twisting the carbon fibre within the sleeve. While a slight bending of the carbon fibre/membrane stretching increases the sensitivity of the electrode, it also makes the membrane more prone to damage or leaking. It may help to protect the connection-points of the electrode cables (to both plug and electrode), for example, by encasing within a 1000 µl pipette tip and binding with tape for added support.

Organ Bath Conditions

The NO signal is highly sensitive to changes in temperature, and experiments should therefore be conducted out of direct sunlight and preferably removed from windows or sources of variable ventilation. Moreover, temperature differences between the organ bath and the probe should be avoided since even small differences create a signal. The system is maintained at 25 °C, since preliminary studies have shown that increasing the temperature to 37 °C itself produced a signal that made quantitation of stimulated NO formation difficult. A NO-electrode manufactured by Harvard Apparatus is coupled to an intrinsic temperature sensor, which makes it possible to determine if an observed change in the NO signal is caused by a change in temperature. Similarly, volumes added to the organ bath should be standardised and equilibrated to the same temperature as the organ bath, and added with the same speed, force and location each time. Even small volume fluctuations may disturb the baseline, and it is advisable to test the influence of adding a volume of buffer prior to addition of the actual test substance. The diluting effect of larger volumes must also be taken into account.

In addition, electrodes, in particular microelectrodes (70 μm and 30 μm), are sensitive to higher salt concentrations, for example, when 100 mmol/l KCl is applied to depolarise vascular smooth muscle, and often become more susceptible to leaking quickly under these conditions. The same applies to chemical calibration in acidic solutions, thus it is recommended to calibrate in basic solution using the NO donor SNAP in the presence of copper chloride (refer to Instruction Manual, World Precision Instruments, Sarasota).

Ambient Conditions

Variations in ambient conditions may also influence the NO signal. Movement or respiration in the immediate proximity of the electrode can alter heat convection, resulting in a broad deflection of the signal. Similarly, alterations in the NO content of the air within the room or ventilation on different days or at different times during the day, depending on outside traffic or smog, would influence the amount of NO detected by the electrode. It is advisable to test incubation solutions (i.e. HEPES) for possible contamination with nitrite from the atmosphere: if addition induces a positive signal at the NO electrode, solutions should be replaced. Solutions used to dilute test substances should be similarly tested, and the effects of the test substance corrected for the effect of the diluting vehicle.

Examples

Real-Time NO Formation in Rabbit Aorta Stimulated by Carbachol

Carbachol-Induced Free NO Transient in Rabbit Aorta

Sections of rabbit aorta were stimulated with a single addition of carbachol (to final concentration 500 nmol/l) to elicit an immediate rise in free NO at the endothelium that was sustained for over 10 min. (Fig. 1). A prior addition of buffer alone had negligible influence on the NO signal. The initial peak transient was used to determine the maximal NO signal induced by carbachol in the preparation, and subsequently performed concentration-effect curves were expressed relative to this value (% max). We have found that a second addition of the same concentration, following washout, generates a comparable signal that does not differ significantly from the initial response.

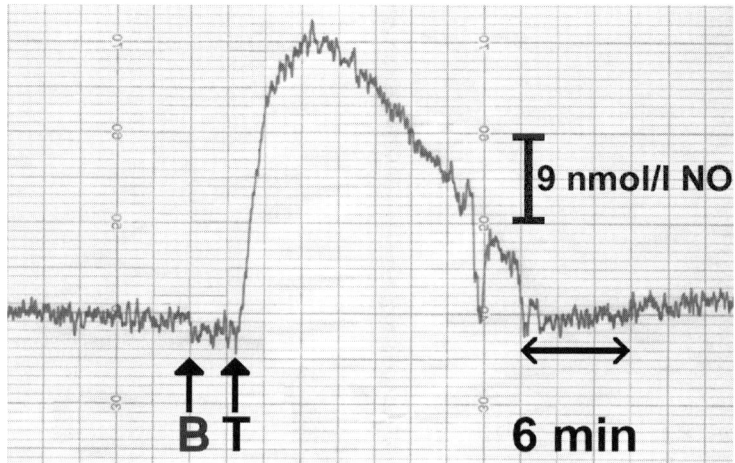

Figure 1
Original trace of real-time NO detection showing a transient rise in free NO induced by carbachol (500 nmol/l) in rabbit aorta. T indicates addition of 50 μl carbachol, B indicates addition of 50 μl buffer alone. This peak was taken as the maximal NO response of the preparation to carbachol. Subsequent concentration-response curves (Figs. 3–4) were expressed relative to this value (% max). Data in Figs. 1–4 was obtained by Isik Kirmizigül, M.D., (unpublished observation, Thesis in preparation, University of Koeln)

Effects of NOS Inhibition on Carbachol-Stimulated NO Formation

Carbachol concentration dependently increased free NO formation in rabbit aorta endothelium (Fig. 2). The concentration-effect curve was completely abolished in the presence of the NOS inhibitor L-NNA (50 μmol/l), confirming endothelial NOS as the source of carbachol-induced free NO formation in this system.

Effects of Superoxide Radicals on Free NO Formation

The effect of extracellular superoxide anions on release of free NO was examined in sections of rabbit aorta. When superoxide radicals were generated with hypoxanthine (0.7 mol/l) plus xanthine oxidase (5 mU/ml), the carbachol-stimulated increase in free NO formation was completely blocked (Fig. 3). This demonstrates that the NO electrode is a useful tool to investigate the interaction between acute NO formation, NO scavenging by reactive oxygen species and endothelial function.

NO Formation in Conditions of Acute Hyperglycaemia

The influence of intracellular oxidative stress was examined by raising the concentration of glucose in the incubation buffer (30 mmol/l). Acute hyperglycaemic conditions significantly attenuated the maximal NO response to carbachol in rabbit aorta (Fig. 4); however, we saw no similar inhibition with the osmolar control mannitol.

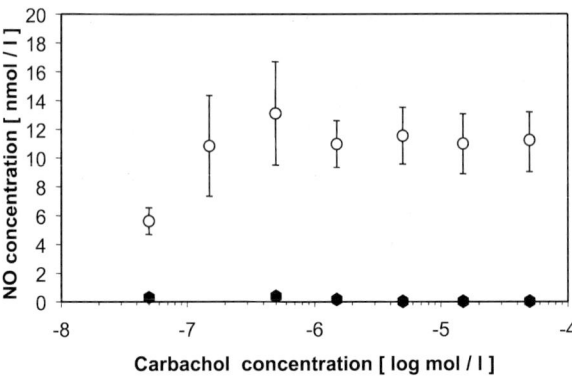

Figure 2
Free NO formation in rabbit aorta stimulated by carbachol alone (○ n=10) and following pre-incubation with 50 µmol/l L-NNA (● n=6). Data represents the local concentration of free NO, and points indicate mean ± SEM

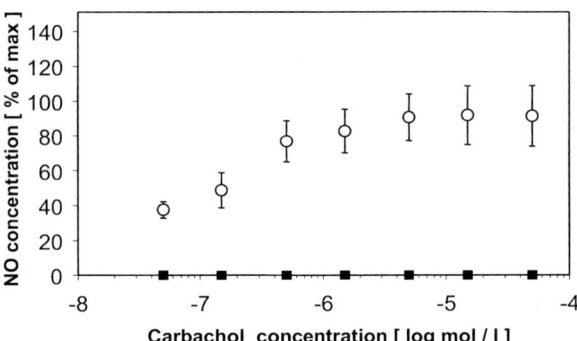

Figure 3
Carbachol-stimulated NO formation in rabbit aorta in the absence (○ n=7) and presence (■ n=4) of 0.7 mol/l hypoxanthine + 5 mU/ml xanthine oxidase. Data is expressed relative to the initial maximal NO peak induced by a single addition of 500 nmol/l carbachol (see Fig. 1) and points represent mean ± SEM

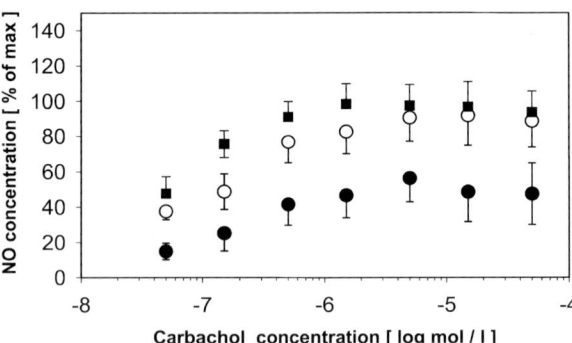

Figure 4
NO formation induced by carbachol following preincubation of rabbit aorta with control (○ n=7), 30 mmol/l glucose (● n=7) or 30 mmol/l glucose ± 5 µmol/l vitamin C (■ n=6). Data is expressed relative to the initial maximal NO peak induced by a single addition of 500 nmol/l carbachol (see Fig. 1) and points represent mean ± SEM

Co-incubation with high glucose plus the antioxidant vitamin C (5 µmol/l) rescued the NO response to carbachol. Thus the NO-electrode may also be used to investigate the influence of simulated pathological conditions and antioxidant substances on NO bioavailabilty and endothelial function.

Free NO Formation in Pig Coronary Artery Stimulated by Substance P

NO Formation Induced by Incremental Increases in Substance P

NO formation in pig coronary artery in response to substance P was measured in real-time using the NO-sensitive electrode (Fig. 5). Note that the peak transients are lower compared to the response observed in rabbit aorta (see Fig. 1) and are reached over a shorter time scale. However the NO-electrode may still be applied to generate reproducible concentration-effect even in a system with a relatively low NO response (Fig. 6).

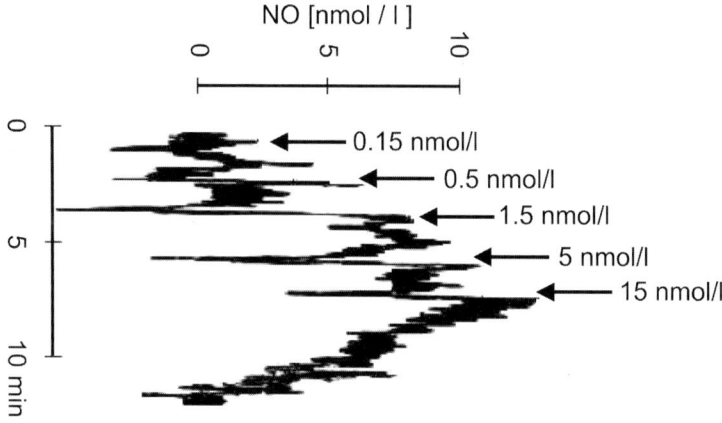

Figure 5
Original trace of real-time NO detection showing time course of NO formation induced by substance P in porcine coronary artery (cumulative addition of substance P indicated by *arrows*)

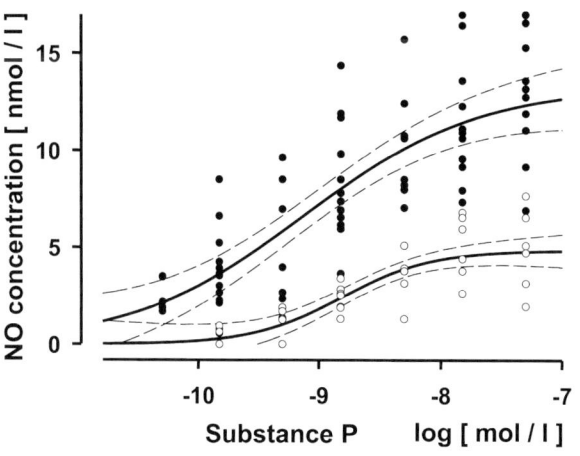

Figure 6
Free NO formation in porcine coronary artery in response to increasing concentrations of substance P (● n=15), and of substance P following pre-incubation with 100 µmol/l L-MMA (○ n=7). Dashed lines indicate 95% confidence limits of fitted curves

Effect of NOS Inhibition on NO Formation in Pig Coronary Artery

Concentration-response curves for substance P were generated in porcine coronary artery (Fig. 6). The effects were examined of NOS inhibition by pre-incubating vessels with L-MMA (100 μmol/l). This was found to depress the maximal NO-responsiveness to substance P. Therefore, the NO-electrode can be used even in less responsive tissues to examine the bioavailability of NO and the role of NOS in endothelial function.

Effect of Shear Stress on NO Formation in Cultured Endothelial Cells

Effects of Shear Stress on Free NO Release from Endothelial Cell Monolayers

As mentioned above, NO formation in unstimulated endothelial cells is below the detection limit of the NO-electrode, therefore, accumulation of the stable metabolites nitrite/nitrate was determined after 30 min incubation as a measure of cumulative NO production.

The influence of endothelial shear stress on NO formation was examined in cultured porcine aortic endothelial cells. PAEC (passage 2) were incubated at 37°C and shear stress applied every 1–2 min by repeatedly (10×) removing 1000 μl of the incubation medium and pipetting it back gently across the cell monolayers. Shear stress induced a marked increase in the free NO signal (Fig. 7) that was only partially prevented by the NOS inhibitor L-MMA (100 μmol/l). These findings highlights that great care must be taken both during incubation and measurement to avoid inadvertent shear forces.

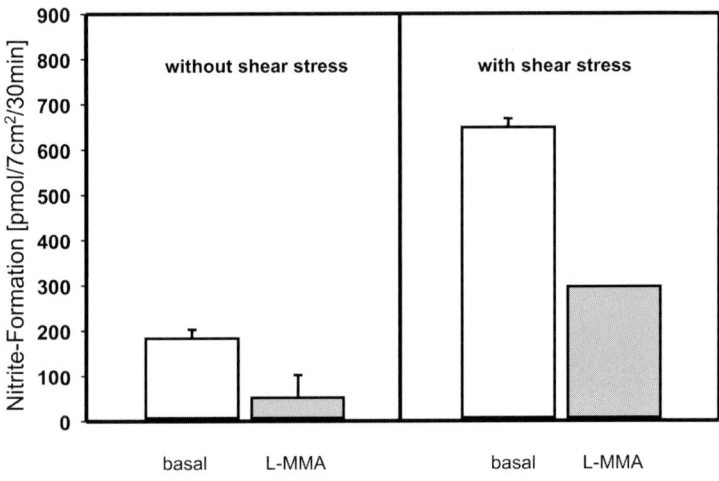

Figure 7
Nitrite accumulation in cultured PAEC (passage 2) under control conditions (left panel) and following shear stress (right panel). Data for basal (open bars) and L-MMA (100 μmol/l)-inhibited nitrite formation (grey bars) represent mean ± SEM from 3 experiments

Troubleshooting

Before mounting the instrumentation equipment, it is essential to determine the most appropriate location. Firstly, the apparatus must be outside the range of possible interference by electric or magnetic fields, and the electrical supply must be shielded. Otherwise, all equipment (incl. incubation buffers!) must share a common grounding. It may also be necessary to place the entire apparatus within a Faraday cage.

No Signal

The electrode should respond to changes in temperature or pH. If not, try to enhance the amplification ("gain"). If there is still no signal, it may be necessary to renew the electrolyte solution in the 2 mm ISO-NO electrode. If using microelectrodes, the tip is likely to be broken. Next, try to obtain a calibration signal (i.e. to NO gas or SNAP), and check the sensitivity of the electrode under calibration conditions. If the electrode is then positioned near an endothelial surface, and there is still no signal (i.e. a straight line, with little noise and no change in response to stimulation), then NO concentrations are likely to be below the detection limit of the electrode, and the incremental increases in NO formation are too small to induce a rise in transient NO concentrations before being oxidised. Thus, try increasing the concentration in larger increments, possibly even adding the highest end concentration of stimulating agent in a single step, to check that the electrode is able to detect NO in this range. Sometimes it may help to add L-arginine (1 mmol/l) to the buffer. When measuring NO via accumulation of nitrite/nitrate, it may help to reduce the incubation volume, or alternatively, increase the size of the aliquot of incubation medium added to the acidic iodate solution.

Baseline Drift or Not Zeroing

A baseline drift may indicate that the ISO-NO electrode is not fully polarised. This may occur when the electrode was detached or if the electrical supply was shut down, for example, by a power-failure. Also, check that there is no continuous change in temperature in the organ bath, as this will also produce a drift in the signal. If there is an extensive drift in the baseline, the membrane is likely to be damaged and needs to be replaced. To determine whether it is indeed necessary to exchange the membrane sleeve, test whether the electrode may be zeroed in a solution of concentrated KCl (100 mmol/l). If zeroing is not possible, then the membrane must be replaced. In this case, however, the electrode will have to be polarized again for at least 12 h before measurements can be resumed.

Noisy Signal

Small air bubbles captured at the membrane while filling the electrode may disturb the signal. Do not tap or shake the electrode to remove the bubbles, but try to "fling" the electrode once in a rapid downward arc. It may also help to tighten the electrode membrane and to check the electrical contacts in the apparatus. The electrolyte solution in the electrode should also be replaced routinely to maintain stable NO measurements.

Signal Not Reproducible

The extreme sensitivity of the electrode makes it essential that the experimental protocol is standardised as much as possible, in particular, the placement of the electrode tip and the addition of substances to the endothelium. Even subtle differences in the force or location of delivery can influence the signal, therefore, shaking or stirring during incubation should be avoided. This applies to both the measurement of real-time NO formation and cumulative production of nitrite/nitrite. In our hands, even gentle shear forces across endothelial cell monolayers resulted in a significant increase in NO signal. Controlled shear stress can be applied as an experimental condition (see examples), however, if it occurs due to inconsistent technique, it can limit the validity and reproducibility of the NO measurement.

References

Berkels R, Bertsch A, Breitenbach T, Klaus W, Rösen R: The Calcium Antagonist Nifedipine Stimulates Endothelial NO Release in Therapeutical Concentrations. Pharm Pharmacol Lett 6: 7578, 1996

Berkels R, Mueller A, Roesen R, Klaus W: Nifedipine and Bay K 8644 Induce an Increase of $[Ca^{2+}]i$ and NO Formation in Endothelial Cells. J Cardiovasc Pharmacol Ther 4(3): 175–181, 1999

Berkels R, Purol-Schnabel S, Roesen R: A New Method to Measure Nitrate/Nitrite with a NO-Sensitive Electrode. J Appl Physiol 90(1): 317–320, 2001

Brovkovych VV, Kalinowski L, Muller-Peddinghaus R, Malinski T: Synergistic Antihypertensive Effects of Nifedipine on Endothelium: Concurrent Release of NO and Scavenging of Superoxide. Hypertension 37(1): 34–39, 2001

Cai H and Harrison DG: Endothelial Dysfunction in Cardiovascular Diseases: the Role of Oxidant Stress. Circ Res 87: 840–844, 2000

Dimmeler S, Rippmann V, Weiland, U, Haendeler J, Zeiher AM: Angiotensin II Induces Apoptosis of Human Endothelial Cells. Protective Effect of Nitric Oxide. Circ Res 81(6): 970–976, 1997

Du XL, Edelstein D, Dimmeler S, Ju Q, Sui C, Brownlee M: Hyperglycemia Inhibits Endothelial Nitric Oxide Synthase Activity by Posttranslational Modification at the Akt Site." J. Clin. Invest. 108: 1341–1348, 2001

Forstermann U, Closs EI, Pollock J, Nakane S, Schwarz M, Gath P, Kleinert H: Nitric Oxide Synthase Isozymes: Characterization, Purification, Molecular Cloning and Functions. Hypertension 23(6 Pt 2): 1121–1131, 1994

Furchgott R and Zawadzki J: The Obligatory Role of Endothelial Cells in the Relaxation of Arterial Smooth Muscle by Acetylcholine. Nature 288: 373–376, 1980

Haller H, Cosentino F, Luscher TF: Endothelial Dysfunction, Hypertension and Atherosclerosis. A Review of the Effects of Lacidipine. Drugs R D 3(5): 311–323, 2002

Hecker M, Mulsch A, Bassenge E, Forstermann U, Busse R: Subcellular Localization and Characterization of Nitric Oxide Synthase(s) in Endothelial Cells: Physiological Implications. Biochem J 299 (Pt 1): 247–252, 1994

Hink U, Li H, Mollnau H, Oelze M, Matheis E, Hartmann M, Skatchkov M, Thaiss F, Stahl RAK, Warnholtz A, Meinertz T, Griendling K, Harrison DG, Forstermann U, Munzel T: Mechanisms Underlying Endothelial Dysfunction in Diabetes Mellitus. Circ Res 88: e14–e22, 2001

Hirata K, Kuroda R, Sakoda T, Katayama M, Inoue N, Suematsu M, Kawashima S, Yokoyama M: Inhibition of Endothelial Nitric Oxide Synthase Activity by Protein Kinase C. Hypertension 25(2): 180–185, 1995

Kleschyov A and Munzel T: Advanced Spin Trapping of Vascular Nitric Oxide Using Colloid Iron Diethyldithiocarbamate. Methods Enzymol 359: 42–51, 2002

Murad F: The Nitric Oxide-Cyclic GMP Signal Transduction System for Intracellular and Intercellular Communication. Recent Prog Horm Res 49: 239–248, 1994

Vakkilainen J, Mäkimattila S, Seppälä-Lindroos A, Vehkavaara S, Lahdenperä S, Groop PH, Taskinen MR, Yki-Järvinen H: Endothelial Dysfunction in Men with Small LDL Particles. Circulation 102: 716–721, 2000

Wassmann S, Laufs U, Baeumer AT, Mueller K, Ahlbory K, Linz W, Itter G, Roesen R, Boehm M, Nickenig G: HMG-CoA Reductase Inhibitors Improve Endothelial Dysfunction in Normocholesterolemic Hypertension via Reduced Production of Reactive Oxygen Species. Hypertension 37(6): 1450–1457, 2001

Biomechanical Stimulation of Vascular Cells In Vitro

Henning Morawietz and Andreas Schubert

Introduction

The cells of the vessel wall *in situ* are constantly exposed to biomechanical forces by the flowing blood. Important mechanical forces are wall shear stress and cyclic mechanical strain resulting in wall stress (Fig. 1). Endothelial cells are preferentially exposed to shear stress, while vascular smooth muscle cells are mainly exposed to mechanical strain in intact vessels (Davies 1995). The shear stress τ at the vessel wall can be derived from Poiseulle's law as:

$$\tau = 4Q \times \eta/\pi \times r^3$$

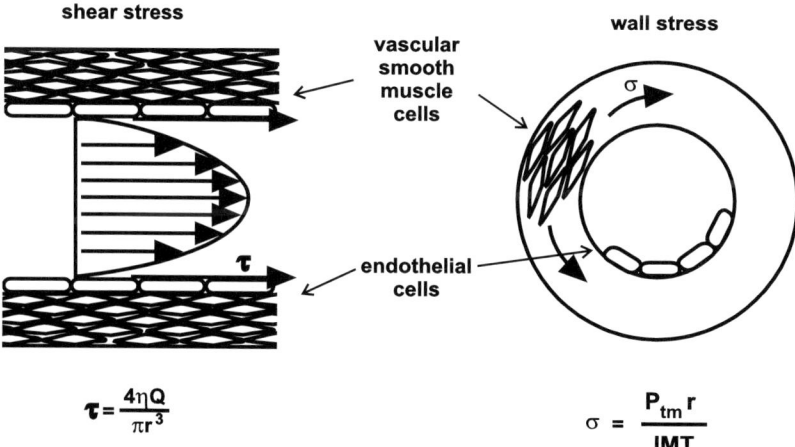

Figure 1
Mechanical Forces in the Vessel Wall. Important mechanical forces are wall shear stress and cyclic mechanical strain resulting in wall stress. Endothelial cells are preferentially exposed to shear stress, while vascular smooth muscle cells are mainly exposed to cyclic mechanical strain in intact vessels. The shear stress τ at the vessel wall can be determined by the formula: $\tau = 4Q \times \eta/\pi \times r^3$, where Q is the fluid flow rate, r the radius, and η the fluid viscosity. The wall stress σ can be calculated as: $\sigma = P_{tm} \times r/IMT$, where P_{tm} is the transmural pressure, r the radius and IMT the intima-media thickness

where Q is the fluid flow rate, r the radius, and η the fluid viscosity. Shear stress causes cell deformation (strain), which increases cytoskeletal tension. In the case of shear stress, the force on a cell acts in one direction, while stretch due to transmural pressure gradients can occur in all directions.

The wall stress σ can be calculated as:

$$\sigma = P_{tm} \times r/IMT$$

where P_{tm} is the transmural pressure, r the radius and IMT the intima-media thickness.

Biomechanical forces can influence structure, growth, and function of vascular cells (Davies et al. 1997; Frangos et al. 2001; Williams 1998). The difference in the magnitude of shear stress has influence on cell shape, molecular adaptation and differentiation of endothelial cells. In response to the degree and direction of shear stress, endothelial cells align their shape and reorganize their cytoskeleton (Franke et al. 1984; Wong et al. 1983).

Several studies show that the type and degree of biomechanical forces acting on the vascular cells play an important role in maintaining vascular integrity and developing vascular diseases. The local hemodynamic forces are considered to be an important stimuli for the localization of atherosclerotic plaques (Davies et al. 2002; Gimbrone et al. 2000). Arterial regions that are exposed to more uniform laminar flow seem to be relatively protected from atherosclerotic lesions (Traub and Berk 1998). However, atherosclerotic lesions develop in the vicinity of arterial branch points and areas of major curvature. These regions are associated with non-laminar flow, flow reversal, and roaming stagnation points (Fig. 2).

The wall shear stress has been determined at different locations in the circulation (Ballermann et al. 1998). Mean shear stress is often ≤ 1 dyn/cm² in large veins. Most authors consider venous levels of shear stress in the range of 1 to 6 dyn/cm². However, in small venules, a shear stress of 20 to 40 dynes/cm² has been described. The mean shear stress in arteries is often described to be in the range of 15 to 30 dyn/cm² (Traub and Berk 1998).

However, studies in human carotid bifurications show that curvature and configuration of the vessel can tremendously affect the shear stress, ranging from 0 dyn/cm² at the outer wall opposite the flow divider to 600 dynes/cm² at the inner wall (Zarins et al. 1983).

In response to mechanical strain, vascular cells can elongate by up to approximately 20% of its initial length in blood vessels (Osol 1995). Augmented mechanical strain has been shown to increase proliferation of vascular smooth muscle cells *in vitro* (Wilson et al. 1993). Therefore, biomechanical strain could be considered as a mitogenic and hypertrophic stimulus in hemodynamic overload and several vascular diseases.

Since the early 1980's, several devices have been developed to apply biomechanical forces on cultured endothelial cells *in vitro* (Dewey et al. 1981). Shear stress is usually applied using cone-and-plate viscometers or parallel flow chambers (Frangos et al. 1985, 1988; Sdougos et al. 1984). Cyclic mechanical strain can be applied by cyclic

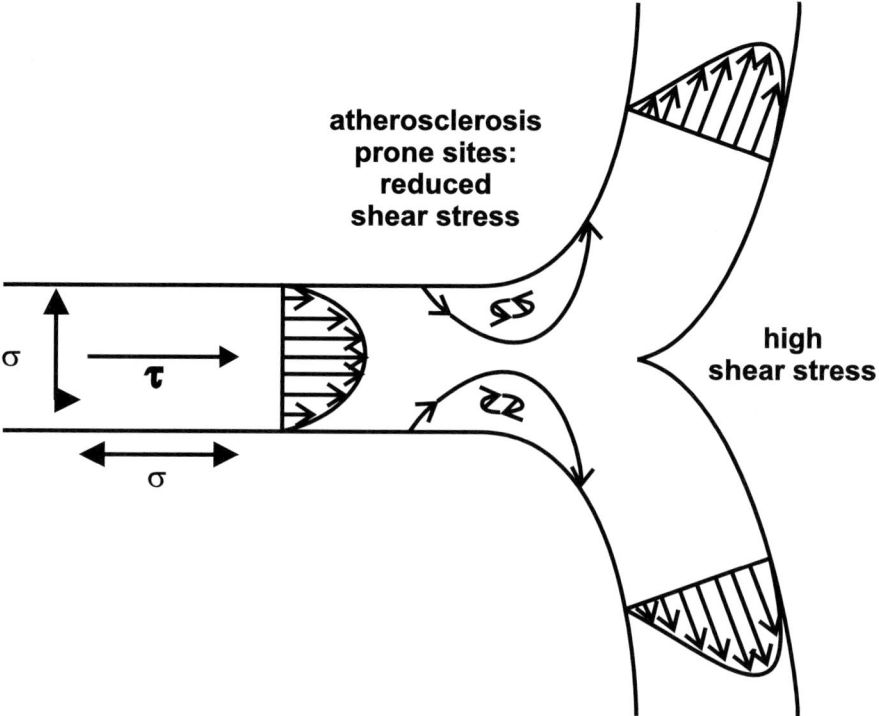

Figure 2
Shear stress and atherosclerosis. The local hemodynamic forces like shear stress τ and strain σ are considered to be involved in the localization of atherosclerotic plaques. Arterial regions that are exposed to more uniform high laminar shear stress seem to be relatively protected from atherosclerotic lesions. However, atherosclerosis prone sites are located in the vicinity of arterial branch points and areas of major curvature. These regions are associated with non-laminar flow, flow reversal, and roaming stagnation points

deformation of cells cultured on distensible elastic membranes (Banes et al. 1985). Biological compression conditions can be simulated using sustained hydrostatic pressure to deform vascular cells cultured *in vitro* (Acevedo et al. 1993).

Our lab started to work on the application of biomechanical forces 9 years ago. We established a cone-and-plate viscometer model to study the impact of laminar shear stress on the endothelin system (Morawietz et al. 2000). Additional projects were focused on the identification of novel genes, downregulated by arterial laminar shear stress (Schubert et al. 2000), and the expression of pro- and antiapoptotic genes in response to shear stress (Bartling et al. 2000). Furthermore, we analyzed in tight cooperation with Harlan Ives' lab at the UCSF, the induction of immediate-early genes in response to cyclic mechanical strain in vascular smooth muscle cells (Morawietz et al. 1999).

Therefore, in this chapter, we would like to focus on the application of shear stress on endothelial cells by a cone-and-plate viscometer, and the application of mechanical strain by cyclic deformation of flexible membranes.

Description of Methods and Practical Approach
Application of Shear Stress on Endothelial Cells

Human Endothelial Cells Culture

Primary cultures of human umbilical vein endothelial cells (HUVEC) are isolated using collagenase IV. In brief, the umbilical veins are washed with 1× HBSS buffer (GIBCO Invitrogen), fixed at the edges and incubated for 12 min at 37 °C with collagenase IV solution (7 mg collagenase IV in 15 ml Dulbecco's PBS, GIBCO Invitrogen). The endothelial cells are eluted with endothelial growth medium, containing medium M199 with 1.25 mg/ml sodium bicarbonate, 100 µg/ml L-glutamine (GIBCO Invitrogen), supplemented with 15 mmol/l HEPES, 100 U/ml penicillin, 100 µg/ml streptomycin, 250 ng/ml fungizone (GIBCO Invitrogen), and 10% calf serum. The endothelial cells are centrifuged at 250×g for 6 min. In order to minimize variations in primary cultures, the isolated HUVEC are pooled every day. The cell number is determined in a cell chamber, and 1.6 to 1.8×10^6 cells are plated in endothelial growth medium with 10% calf serum and 16.7 ng/ml endothelial cell growth supplement (C. C. Pro, Neustadt, Germany) per 60×15 mm tissue culture dish. The dishes are pretreated with 1% (w/v) gelatine for 1 h at 37 °C in an incubator with 5% CO_2, the gelatine solution is removed immediately before the cells are plated. After 90 min, the medium is replaced in order to remove non-adherent cells. Endothelial cells continue to grow under the described conditions and receive fresh medium every second day. Usually, the endothelial cell cultures reach confluence after 4–6 days.

As an alternative, several companies offer commercially available endothelial cells from different human and bovine vessels e.g.:
- Clonetics/BioWhittaker/Cambrex: *http://www.cambrex.com/CatNav.oid.435*
- Cascade Biologics: *http://www.cascadebio.com/index.cfm?fuseaction=home.Content&CID=600*
- PromoCell: *http://www.promocell.com/en/Navigate/product0.php3?target1=50&lang=US*

General Remarks

Cultures of endothelial cells are subjected to laminar shear stress one day after reaching confluence in a cone-and-plate viscometer (Fig. 3). The cone-and-plate viscometer operates in a linear range at any desired rotational speed, to achieve shear stress levels of up to 50 dyn/cm². Increasing levels of shear stress are applied by increasing rotational speed. In order to avoid direct contact of the rotating cone with the edge of the tissue culture dish, a circular area of 91% of the cultured cells is exposed to the indicated amount of laminar shear stress. Laminar shear stress of 1 dyn/cm² (1 dyn/cm² = 0.1 N/m², venous or low shear stress) to 10 dyn/cm² (10 dyn/cm² = 1 N/m²) can be achieved with standard medium. For higher levels of shear stress, e.g. from 15 to 50 dyn/cm² (1.5 to 5 N/m²), the high rotational speed may cause problems such as the medium spilling-over. In this case, 5% dextran (MW 71.400) is added to the cell culture medium to increase the viscosity of the medium 2.95-fold from 0.007 dyn × s/cm² to 0.02065 dyn × s/cm². In these experiments, each cell culture dish should be accompanied by 2 controls from the same HUVEC preparation, incubated under static con-

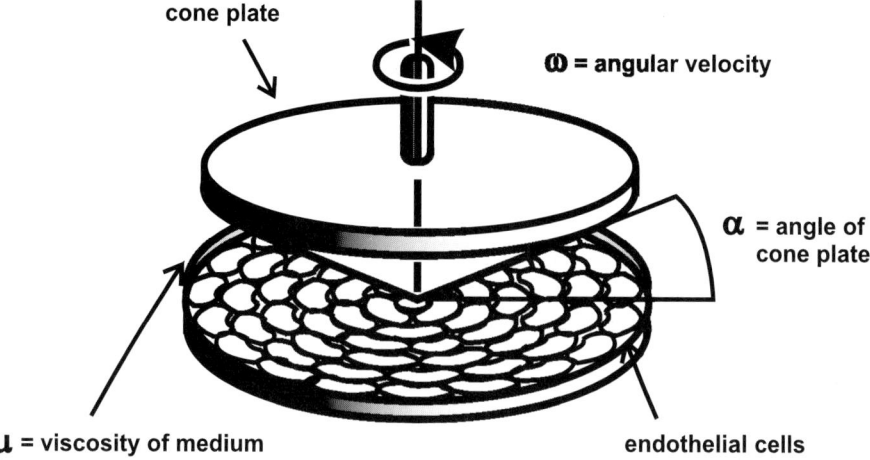

Figure 3
Cone-and-plate viscometer. Cells are subjected to laminar shear stress in a cone-and-plate viscometer. The apparatus consists of a cone with an angle of 0.5° rotating on top of a cell culture dish. The degree of shear stress τ depends on the viscosity of the medium μ, the angular velocity ω, and the angle of the cone α

ditions, with cell culture medium supplemented with or without 5% dextran for the same period of time. Application of laminar shear stress using the cone-and-plate viscometer does not increase the temperature of the cell culture medium (Schubert et al. 2000). In order to balance evaporation of cell culture medium during the 24 h application of shear stress on cells in an open cell culture dish, medium is routinely supplemented at regular intervals with sterile distilled water. The achievement of equal degrees of shear stress at lower rotational speed by using additional dextran, has been shown to give equal results (Malek and Izumo 1992), and does not affect cell viability, detachment or increased release of lactate dehydrogenase (LDH) into the medium as an indicator of cell integrity (e.g. determined by CytoTox 96 Non-Radioactive Cytotoxicity Assay, Promega, Madison, WI). The flow conditions using this approach are laminar, because the parameter R ($r^2\omega\alpha^2/12$) described by Sdougos et al. (1984) is smaller than 4 (e.g. $R_{1dyn/cm}{}^2$: 0.006; $R_{15dyn/cm}{}^2$: 0.03; $R_{30dyn/cm}{}^2$: 0.06; $R_{50dyn/cm}{}^2$: 0.1).

Reagents

- Cell culture medium: standard endothelial growth medium: e.g. medium M199 with 1.25 mg/ml sodium bicarbonate, 100 μg/ml L-glutamine (GIBCO Invitrogen), supplemented with 20% calf serum, 15 mmol/l HEPES, 100 U/ml penicillin, 100 μg/ml streptomycin, 250 ng/ml fungizone (GIBCO Invitrogen), and 16.7 ng/ml endothelial cell growth supplement (C. C. Pro, Neustadt, Germany)
- Medium with dextran: dissolve 5% dextran (MW 71.400, SIGMA) in standard medium in order to increase the viscosity and sterilize by passing through a 0.45 μm pore filter.
- Phosphate-buffered saline (PBS), HBSS

Shear Stress Devices

Commercially available devices: Parallel plate flow chambers or circular flow chambers, e.g. Glycotech, Gaithersburg, MD; Flexcell International Corporation, Hillsborough, NC. For information on the cone-and-plate viscometer shown in Fig. 3, contact Dr. H. Lehnich, Martin Luther University Halle-Wittenberg, Germany, holger.lehnich@medizin.uni-halle.de).

Protocol

1. Confluent cultures of endothelial cells are supplemented with fresh medium and transferred to a CO_2 incubator containing cone-and-plate apparatus. A control dish with endothelial cells from the same preparation is treated in the same way.
2. After 2 h, the lid of one dish is removed and the culture dish transferred into the cone-and-plate apparatus.
3. The cone starts to rotate by adjusting the speed (e.g. 40 rpm).
4. The rotating cone is slowly layered down onto the culture dish and stopped just before the cone touches the cells. This can be monitored on the corresponding scale (e.g. in 10 μm steps).
5. Rotational speed can be adjusted and the shear stress can be applied for the appropriate time. The control dish is incubated under static conditions for the same period of time.
6. During long-term application of shear stress, e.g. 24 h, evaporation of water from the medium has to be replaced. Routinely, slowly add up to 1 ml sterile water twice, to keep the volume of the medium constant.
7. After application of shear stress, the cone is lifted; the culture dish transferred into a sterile flow box and the cells washed twice with PBS. Subsequently, cells can be characterized by standard molecular techniques including RNA or protein preparation, immunofluorescence etc.

Application of Mechanical Strain on Vascular Smooth Muscle Cells

Culture of Vascular Smooth Muscle Cells

Peter Jones established primary cultures of vascular smooth muscle cells from newborn rat aorta (University of Southern California, Los Angeles, CA). From these primary cultures, the cell line R22 D was established, and at passage 15 generously supplied by Dr. Jones (Jones et al. 1979). The cells are maintained in medium with 10% serum (minimum essential medium with 10% fetal bovine serum, 2% tryptose phosphate broth, 50 U/ml penicillin, and 50 U/ml streptomycin) in a humidified atmosphere of 5% CO_2 at 37 °C. Culture medium is changed every other day until cells are confluent. Confluent cells are subcultured with typsin-versene. Cells are used from passages 17–25 for described studies. In most experiments, cells are plated on 6 well (5 cm^2 per well) collagen type I silicone elastomer plates (Flex I, Flexcell International Corporation, Hillsborough, NC) in medium with 10% serum, and cultured until confluent. Three days prior to experimentation, the medium is replaced with serum-free medium (minimum essential medium with 0.5 g/l BSA, 0.5 mg/l apo-Transferrin, 2% tryptose phosphate broth, 50 U/ml penicillin, and 50 U/ml streptomycin). Medium is subsequently replaced with fresh serum-free medium every 24 h, and 3 h prior to the strain experiment. In experiments on different extracellular matrices, confluent cells in conventional plastic flasks are detached with trypsin-versene, and trypsin is then inactivated with serum-containing medium. The cells are then centrifuged for 5 min. at 1.000 rpm, washed once with serum-free medium, and the cells of one 9 cm plastic dish are plated in serum-free medium on one 6-well silicone-elastomere plate coated with collagen type I, pronectin (a fibronectin-like poly RGD matrix) or laminin. Serum-free medium is replaced 24 h later–3 h prior to application of mechanical strain.

As described for endothelial cells, several companies offer commercially available vascular smooth muscle cells from different human and bovine vessels e.g.:
- Clonetics/BioWhittaker/Cambrex: *http://www.cambrex.com/CatNav.oid.486*
- Cascade Biologics: *http://www.cascadebio.com/index.cfm?fuseaction=home.Content&CID=600*
- PromoCell: *http://www.promocell.com/en/Navigate/product0.php3?target1=51&lang=US*

General Remarks

Confluent vascular smooth muscle cells on the silicone elastomer culture plates, are subjected to mechanical deformation with the Flexercell Stress Unit (Flexcell International Corporation, Hillsborough, NC) (Fig. 4). The stress unit is a modification of the unit initially described by Banes and co-workers (Banes et al. 1985; Banes et al. 1990) and consists of a computer controlled vacuum unit and a base plate to hold the cul-

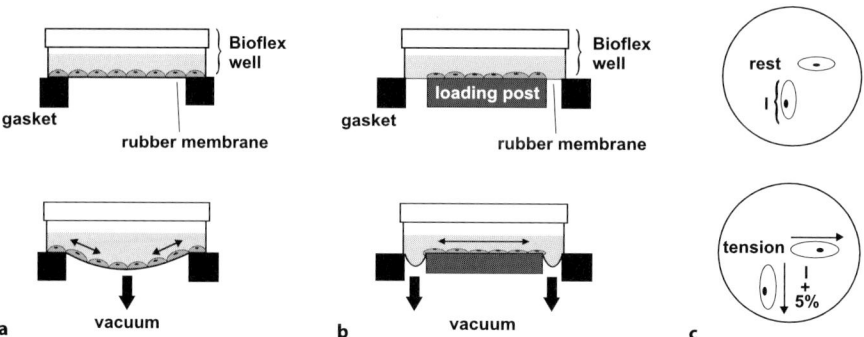

Figure 4a–c
Application of mechanical strain on vascular cells. Endothelial cells are cultured on distensible membranes under static conditions (*top*), or during cyclic application of a vacuum, causing mechanical deformation of membranes and attached cells (*bottom*). The initially described apparatus (**a**), allows the application of mechanical strain of 30% and higher, but has the disadvantage of inhomogeneous cellular deformation (regions of high strain at the periphery and regions of lower strain in the center of the plate). The modified new strain device (**b**) has limitations in respect of the maximally applicable strain, but the advantage of uniform deformation of the cells. Mechanical strain causes cyclic elongation of cells cultured on elastic membranes (**c**)

ture dishes. Vacuum is repetitively applied to the rubber-bottomed dishes via the base plate, which is placed in a humidified incubator with 5% CO_2 at 37 °C. The computer system controls the frequency of deformation and the negative pressure applied to the culture plates. In the initial system, a negative pressure of 20 kPa results in a maximal 25% elongation of cells at the periphery of the dishes (Fig. 4a). The system has been improved (FX-4000T Version or higher) and now allows the application of uniform strain using a loading post (Fig. 4b).

Reagents

- Cell culture medium: standard vascular smooth muscle cell medium with serum: e.g. minimum essential medium with 10% fetal bovine serum, 2% tryptose phosphate broth, 50 U/ml penicillin, and 50 U/ml streptomycin,
- serum-free medium: e.g. minimum essential medium with 0.5 g/l BSA, 0.5 mg/l apo-Transferrin, 2% tryptose phosphate broth, 50 U/ml penicillin, and 50 U/ml streptomycin,
- trypsin-versene or kits for subcultivation of cells available from most commercial cell culture suppliers, Phosphate-buffered saline (PBS),
- Bioflex culture plates (Flexcell International Corporation, Hillsborough, NC).

Strain Devices

Commercially available devices: Flexercell Tension PlusT System, Flexcell International Corporation, Hillsborough, NC. The stress unit is a modification of the unit initially described by Banes (Banes et al. 1985), and consists of a computer controlled vacuum unit and a baseplate to hold the culture dishes. Vacuum is repetitively applied to the rubber-bottomed dishes via the baseplate, which is placed in a humidified incubator with 5% CO_2 at 37 °C. The computer system controls the frequency of deformation and the negative pressure applied to the culture plates (see Fig. 4).

Protocol

1. Confluent vascular smooth muscle cells on Bioflex culture plates (Flexcell International Corporation, Hillsborough, NC) are supplemented with fresh medium without serum, and transferred to a CO_2 incubator containing the baseplate of the Flexercell Tension PlusT System, Flexcell International Corporation, Hillsborough, NC. For application of uniform strain, use the FX-4000T Version (or higher). A control dish with vascular smooth muscle cells from the same preparation or passage is treated in the same way.
2. Follow the Quickstart instructions supplied by the manufacturer. In brief, place four Loading Stations into the four baseplate wells and apply lubricant to the tops of the bottoms. Place four gaskets onto four Bioflex plates and place a Bioflex plate and gasket in each baseplate well.
3. Firstly, turn the FlexLink followed by the computer system on. Double click on the corresponding "FX-4000" icon to start the software.
4. Click on the Users key and register as a user. Afterwards, quit and return to the main window.

5. Using the Regimens, create a regimen by entering values into the appropriate spaces. When completed, save step and then save regimen. Exit the regimen editor.
6. With the assign key, choose the desired baseplate, regimen, and user, then click on the assign icon within the window. Confirm the regimen.
7. If the program is downloaded, you might simulate the regime. If the regimen is correct, click on Stop.
8. Turn on the vacuum system. Click on start to run the regimen. The cells on the plates should begin flexing.
9. Check the water trap to see if water is accumulating. Empty the trap before it is more than half full.
10. You can pause or stop the regime with the corresponding buttons at any time. Usually, the program will stop when the regime is complete.

After application of mechanical strain, the Bioflex culture plates are transferred to a sterile flow box and the cells washed 2× with PBS. Subsequently, cells can be characterized by standard molecular techniques.

Examples

In this paragraph, we will briefly describe studies showing examples of application of shear stress on endothelial cells, and mechanical strain on vascular smooth muscle cells.

Shear Stress

We have performed several studies applying long-term laminar shear stress on human umbilical vein endothelial cells. Application of laminar shear stress, using the cone-and-plate viscometer, does not increase the temperature of the cell culture medium (Schubert et al. 2000).

The achievement of equal degrees of shear stress, at lower rotational speed by using additional dextran, has been shown to give equal results (Malek and Izumo 1992) and did not affect cell viability, detachment or increased release of lactate dehydrogenase (LDH) into the medium as an indicator of cell integrity. In addition, dextran had no effect on control genes like glyceraldehyde 3-phosphate dehydrogenase mRNA expression (Schubert et al. 2000).

After long-term application of laminar shear stress, endothelial cells align in the direction of flow (Fig. 5, center). In contrast, turbulent shear stress does not result in alignment of endothelial cells (Fig. 5, right). On the cellular level, endothelial cells reorganize their microtubular network and their cytoskeleton in the direction of flow (Fig. 6).

The impact of laminar shear stress on the endothelin system was studied in human endothelial cells (Morawietz et al. 2000). In this study, we found a dose-dependent downregulation pre-pro-endothelin-1 mRNA, endothelin-converting enzyme 1 isoform a mRNA expression and of endothelin-1 peptide release into the medium (Fig. 7).

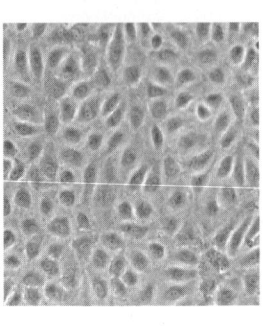 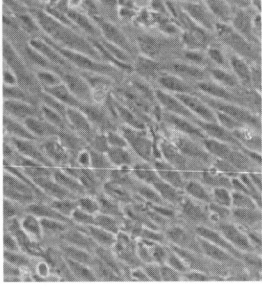 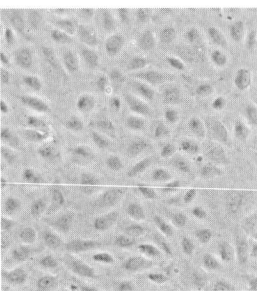

resting cells cells exposed to laminar shear stress cells exposed to turbulent shear stress

Figure 5a–c
Adaptation of endothelial cell shape to the type of shear stress. Human endothelial cells were cultured under standard static conditions (*left*), or subjected to laminar (*middle*), or turbulent (*right*) shear stress of 30 dyn/cm^2 in a cone-and-plate viscometer for 24 h. After application of laminar shear stress cells align in the direction of flow (*middle*). However, turbulent shear stress does not cause alignment of endothelial cells (*right*)

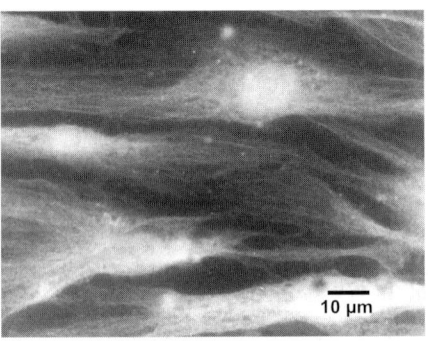

ß-tubulin

Figure 6
Reorganization of endothelial microtubular network in response to shear stress. Human endothelial cells were exposed to laminar shear stress of 30 dyn/cm^2 in a cone-and-plate viscometer for 24 h. The cells were analyzed by immunofluorescence with a human β-tubulin antibody. The cells align in response to shear stress and reorganize their microtubular network in the direction of flow

In another project we cloned a gene differentially downregulated by arterial, compared to venous, laminar shear stress (Schubert et al., 2000). The corresponding gene turned out to be the human homolog of the β-tubulin folding cofactor D. The gene is downregulated by shear stress in a NO-dependent manner.

We analyzed the shear stress-dependent expression of apoptosis-regulating genes in HUVEC (Bartling et al. 2000). In this project, we found that high laminar shear stress (15–30 dyn/cm^2) decreased the susceptibility of HUVEC to undergo apoptosis. This antiapoptotic effect of laminar shear stress could be mediated by decreased expression of the apoptosis-inducing Fas receptor, and increased formation of antiapoptotic soluble Fas isoform FasExo6Del and Bcl-x_L. The upregulation of Bcl-x_L by shear stress is mediated by NO.

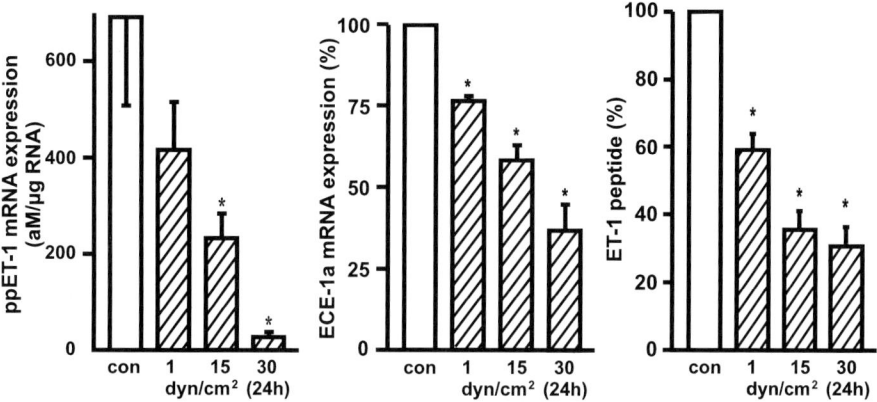

Figure 7
Downregulation of endothelin synthesis and release by long-term laminar shear stress. Human umbilical vein endothelial cells were exposed to laminar shear stress for 24 h. The mRNA expression of pre-pro-endothelin-1 (ppET-1) was quantified by standard-calibrated competitive RT-PCR, of endothelin-converting enzyme isoform 1a by Northern blot analysis and release of endothelin-1 (ET-1) peptide by ELISA. Long-term arterial laminar shear stress results in dose-dependent downregulation ppET-1 mRNA, ECE-1a mRNA and of ET-1 peptide release into the medium (Morawietz et al. 2000)

Furthermore, we analyzed the regulation of genes involved in protein tyrosine sulfation, a widespread post-translational modification. Laminar shear stress causes an isoform shift of the corresponding enzyme tyrosylprotein sulfotransferase (TPST) in HUVEC. Long-term arterial shear stress causes downregulation of isoform TPST1, and upregulation of TPST2 (Goettsch et al. 2002).

Sustained high laminar shear stress is well known to regulate the vascular tone by upregulation of endothelial nitric oxide synthase (Nishida et al. 1992), and downregulation of pre-pro endothelin-1 (Malek and Izumo 1992). Ongoing studies are directed to identify the underlying signal transduction mechanisms, and the transcription factors mediating the differential regulation of genes up- or downregulated by shear stress (Fig. 8).

Mechanical Strain

We analysed, in tight cooperation with Harlan Ives' lab at the UCSF the induction of immediate-early genes in response to cyclic mechanical strain in vascular smooth muscle cells (Morawietz et al. 1999). For application of mechanical strain, the initially used Flexcell apparatus allows the application of mechanical strain of more than 30%. We applied a maximum strain of 25%, which is still in the range described in human circulation (Osol 1995). Even following 24 h of continuous cyclic mechanical strain at maximum level, no increase in lactate dehydrogenase activity (*In vitro* toxicology assay kit, Sigma) was measurable in the supernatant (Morawietz H, Ives HE, unpublished data). Cyclic mechanical strain (1 Hz) increased expression of early growth response gene 1 (Egr-1) and c-jun in vascular smooth muscle cells. Even a single cycle

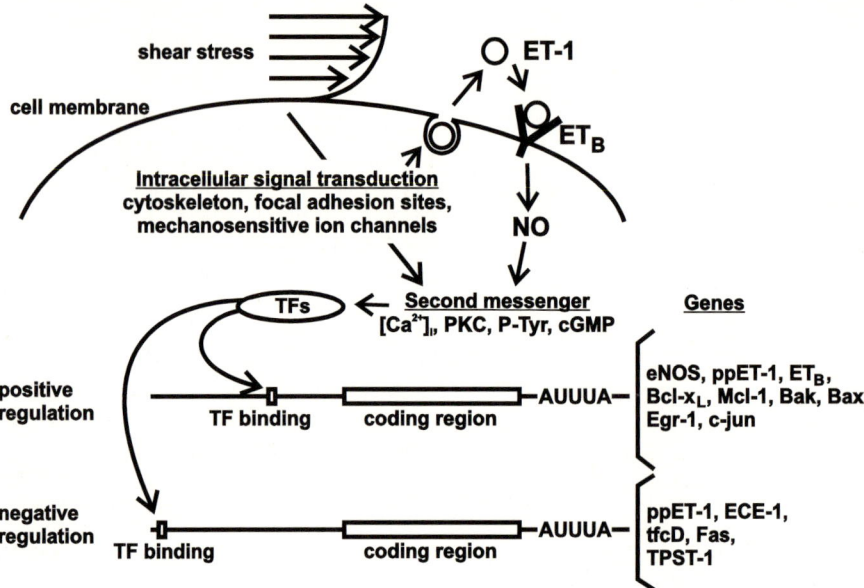

Figure 8
Model of regulation of gene expression by shear stress. Application of shear stress causes intracellular signal transduction in endothelial cells. Cytoskeleton, focal adhesion sites, mechanosensitive ion channels, second messenger and transcription factors (TF) could be involved in the sensing of shear stress and subsequent signal transduction pathways. The mechanosensitive transcription factors can induce or decrease the expression of genes regulated by shear stress. Furthermore, we have indications that an initial release of endothelin-1 (ET-1), binding to its ET_B receptor and NO, could be involved in some changes to the endothelial gene expression pattern in response to shear stress

of mechanical strain lasting only 1 s was sufficient to induce Egr-1 mRNA expression 30 min. later. Strain also induced transiently, transfected Egr-1 promoter-reporter constructs. The extracellular matrix affected the response to mechanical strain. Although not induced on laminin, Egr-1 was induced on collagen I and pronectin. These data suggest that the signal of induction of Egr-1 by mechanical strain might involve specific cell-matrix interactions (Fig. 9).

Other examples of intracellular responses to different dosages of cyclic mechanical strain are increased proliferation (Wilson et al. 1993), or endothelin receptor B-mediated apoptosis of vascular smooth muscle cells (Cattaruzza et al. 2000).

Troubleshooting

Cell Culture

In order to minimize variations of primary cultures, the isolated endothelial cells should be pooled every day and subsequently separated and grown in standard medium under identical conditions. Because the release of growth factor and signalling

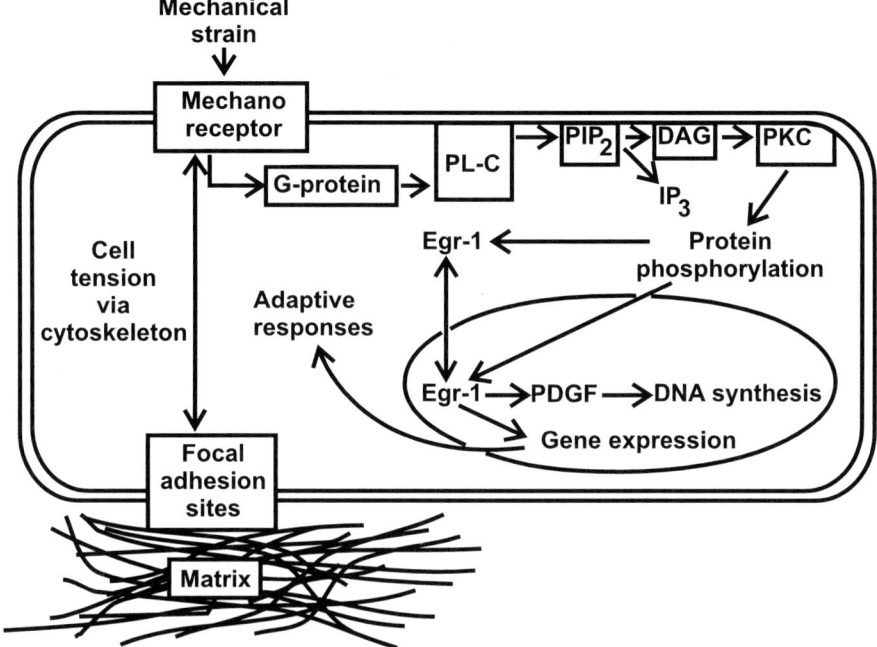

Figure 9
Response of vascular smooth muscle cells to mechanical strain. Exposure of mechanical strain to vascular smooth muscle cells can be sensed by putative mechanoreceptors like stretch-activated cation channels. This process involves an increased cell tension by interactions between the cell surface, focal adhesion sites and extracellular matrix via the cytoskeleton or specific integrins. Further signal transduction pathways might involve second messengers, phosphorylation of target proteins, and activation of transcription factors like early growth response gene-1 (Egr-1). These transcription factors might induce gene expression, e.g. growth factors like platelet-derived growth factor (PDGF) resulting in adaptive responses like proliferation

molecules might vary with cell preparation, growth status and time of incubation, at every time point each experiment is accompanied by an internal control. We recommend standardizing the procedure of adding fresh medium before starting the experiment. Be aware, that even changing the media can induce a variety of genes (e.g. immediate-early genes). The use of dextran to enhance the viscosity of the medium and hence shear stress is feasible, but might cause the problem of changing the osmotic pressure as well. Therefore, some laboratories employ polyvinyl-pyrrolidone instead, which does not pose this problem and at 3% attains a much higher increase in viscosity (typically 10-fold) than dextran.

Application of Shear Stress and Mechanical Strain

Be careful to avoid bubbles when layering the rotating cone onto the culture dish and try to avoid touching the cells. Otherwise, the cells could be scraped off the plate. In order to avoid direct contact of the rotating cone with the edge of the tissue culture dish, a circular area of 91% of the cultured cells is exposed to the indicated amount of laminar shear stress. Therefore, the measured effect of shear stress in the cells harvested for standard biochemical methods might even be slightly underestimated.

In experiments applying turbulent shear stress, due to the geometry of the cone-and-plate viscometer, the parameter R depends on the radius of the cone. Therefore, it should be considered, that a small area in the center of the plate is stimulated with laminar shear stress, while the majority of cells will receive turbulent flow.

Genetic polymorphism in the promoter region might affect the responsiveness of the gene of interest to shear stress in primary cultures of endothelial cells.

During application of mechanical strain, the Bioflex plate and the baseplate should be in tight contact, to ensure the expected deformation by vacuum.

Modifications

The degree of shear stress in the cone-and-plate apparatus $\tau = \mu \times \omega/\alpha$ (τ: shear stress, μ: viscosity of medium, ω: angular velocity, α: angle of cone plate) can be adjusted by varying the rotational speed of the cone. The value n (in rpm) can be calculated in the following way: $n = \tau \times \alpha/2 \times \pi \times \mu$. For example, using a cone of 0.5° ($\alpha = 2 \times \pi \times 0.5°/360° = 0.0087$ rad) and our standard medium ($\mu = 0.007$ dyn $\times$ s/cm^2), the value n in order to achieve a shear stress of 1 dyn/cm^2 (1 dyn/cm^2 = 0.1 N/m^2, low or venous shear stress) is 12 rpm. For the application of higher arterial levels of shear stress ($\geq$15 dyn/cm^2), 5% dextran is added to the cell culture medium to increase the viscosity of our standard medium 2.95-fold, in order to keep the cell culture medium volume constant and to avoid the medium spilling-over, even at a high rotational speed. A 15 dyn/cm^2 level of shear stress (15 dyn/cm^2 = 1.5 N/m^2), using medium with dextran, can be achieved with n = 60 rpm. In this case, the control cells also receive medium with dextran.

The flow conditions using a cone with an angle of 0.5° are laminar, because the parameter R ($r^2 \times \omega \times \alpha^2/12 \times \nu$) (Sdougos et al. 1984) is smaller than 4 in each case. In order to achieve turbulent shear stress, a cone with an angle of 5° can be used. Using this approach, the cone has to rotate with a higher speed, compared to the same degree of laminar shear stress, and the parameter R increases to values higher than 4, resulting in turbulent shear stress (Sdougos et al. 1984).

Alternatively, shear stress can be applied on endothelial cells grown on plain or matrix covered glass cover slips, using parallel plate flow chambers or circular flow chambers, e.g. by Glycotech, Gaithersburg, MD, or by the Flexcell Shear Stress Device or Flexcell Streamer, Flexcell International Corporation, Hillsborough, NC. The Flexcell Shear Stress Device even allows the combination of shear stress and mechanical strain.

Previous versions of the Flexcell device had the disadvantage of inhomogeneous cellular deformation (regions of high strain at the periphery and regions of lower strain in the center of the plate) (see Fig. 4a) (Gilbert et al. 1994). The modified new strain device (e.g. version FX-4000 and higher, Fig. 4b) has limitations in respect of the maximally applicable strain, but the advantage of a uniform deformation of the cells.

Defined pressure can be applied on endothelial or vascular smooth muscle cells using the Flexercell Compression PlusT System, Flexcell International Corporation, Hillsborough, NC.

Suppliers

- Cascade Biologics: *http://www.cascadebio.com*
- Clonetics/BioWhittaker/Cambrex: *http://www.cambrex.com*
- GlycoTech, 7860 Beechcraft Ave., Gaithersburg, MD 20879, phone: +1-800-Glycotk (459-2685), +1-301-738-1080, fax: +1-301-738-1077 *http://www.glycotech.com/apparatus/parallel.html*
- Flexcell International Corporation, 437 Dimmock's Mill Road, Hillsborough, NC 27278, phone: +1-919-732-1591, fax: +1-732-5196, tollfree: (800) 728-3714, e-mail: *flexcell@mindspring.com, www.flexcellint.com/homepage.html*

German distributors:
- Dunn Labortechnik GmbH: *www.dunnlab.de*
- GIBCO Invitrogen Corp.: *www.invitrogen.com*
- Greiner Bio-One GmbH: *www.greinerbioone.com*
- Dr. H. Lehnich, Martin Luther University Halle-Wittenberg, Center of Basic Medical Research, Magdeburger Str. 18, D-06097 Halle, Germany, phone: +49-345-557-1616, fax: +49-345-557-1436, e-mail: *holger.lehnich@medizin.uni-halle.de*)
- PromoCell: *www.promocell.com*

Acknowledgements. This study was supported by the German Research Foundation (Deutsche Forschungsgemeinschaft) (H.M., SFB/TR2 C1: MO 839/S1-1), the German Academic Exchange Service (DAAD) (H.M.), the Oskar Lapp Award of the German Cardiac Society (A.S.), the graduate program of the State Saxony-Anhalt (A.S.), and the German Federal Ministry of Education and Research (BMBF) program NBL3 of the University of Technology Dresden (H.M., Professorship of Vascular Endothelium and Microcirculation). We would like to thank our colleagues at the Institute of Pathophysiology at the Martin Luther University Halle-Wittenberg.

References

Acevedo AD, Bowser SS, Gerritsen ME, Bizios R: Morphological and Proliferative Responses of Endothelial Cells to Hydrostatic Pressure: Role of Fibroblast Growth Factor. J Cell Physiol 157:603–614, 1993

Ballermann BJ, Dardik A, Eng E, Liu A: Shear Stress and the Endothelium. Kidney Int Suppl 67:S100–108, 1998

Banes AJ, Gilbert J, Taylor D, Monbureau O: A New Vacuum-Operated Stress-Providing Instrument That Applies Static or Variable Duration Cyclic Tension or Compression to Cells In Vitro. J Cell Sci 75:35–42, 1985

Banes AJ, Link GW, Jr., Gilbert JW, Tran Son Tay R, Monbureau O: Culturing Cells in a Mechanically Active Environment. Am Biotechnol Lab 8:12–22, 1990

Bartling B, Tostlebe H, Darmer D, Holtz J, Silber RE, Morawietz H: Shear Stress-Dependent Expression of Apoptosis-Regulating Genes in Endothelial Cells. Biochem Biophys Res Commun 278:740–746, 2000

Cattaruzza M, Dimigen C, Ehrenreich H, Hecker M: Stretch-Induced Endothelin B Receptor-Mediated Apoptosis in Vascular Smooth Muscle Cells. FASEB J 14:991–998, 2000

Davies PF: Flow-Mediated Endothelial Mechanotransduction. Physiol Rev 75:519–560, 1995

Davies PF, Barbee KA, Volin MV, Robotewskyj A, Chen J, Joseph L, Griem ml, Wernick MN, Jacobs E, Polacek DC, et al.: Spatial Relationships in Early Signalling Events of Flow-Mediated Endothelial Mechanotransduction. Annu Rev Physiol 59:527–549, 1997

Davies PF, Polacek DC, Shi C, Helmke BP: The Convergence of Haemodynamics, Genomics, and Endothelial Structure in Studies of the Focal Origin of Atherosclerosis. Biorheology 39:299–306, 2002

Dewey CF, Jr., Bussolari SR, Gimbrone MA, Jr., Davies PF: The Dynamic Response of Vascular Endothelial Cells to Fluid Shear Stress. J Biomech Eng 103:177–185, 1981

Frangos JA, Eskin SG, McIntire LV, Ives CL: Flow Effects on Prostacyclin Production by Cultured Human Endothelial Cells. Science 227:1477–1479, 1985

Frangos JA, McIntyre LV, Eskin SG: Shear Stress Induced Stimulation of Mammalian Cell Metabolism. Biotechnol Bioeng 32:1053–1060, 1988

Frangos SG, Knox R, Yano Y, Chen E, Di Luozzo G, Chen AH, Sumpio BE: The Integrin-Mediated Cyclic Strain-Induced Signalling Pathway in Vascular Endothelial Cells. Endothelium 8:1–10, 2001

Franke RP, Grafe M, Schnittler H, Seiffge D, Mittermayer C, Drenckhahn D: Induction of Human Vascular Endothelial Stress Fibres by Fluid Shear Stress. Nature 307:648–649, 1984

Gilbert JA, Weinhold PS, Banes AJ, Link GW, Jones GL: Strain Profiles for Circular Cell Culture Plates Containing Flexible Surfaces Employed to Mechanically Deform Cells In Vitro. J Biomech 27:1169–1177, 1994

Gimbrone MA, Jr., Topper JN, Nagel T, Anderson KR, Garcia-Cardena G: Endothelial Dysfunction, Hemodynamic Forces, and Atherogenesis. Ann N Y Acad Sci 902:230–239, 2000

Goettsch S, Goettsch W, Morawietz H, Bayer P: Shear Stress Mediates Tyrosylprotein Sulfotransferase Isoform Shift in Human Endothelial Cells. Biochem Biophys Res Commun 294:541–546, 2002

Jones PA, Scott-Burden T, Gevers W: Glycoprotein, Elastin, and Collagen Secretion by Rat Smooth Muscle Cells. Proc Natl Acad Sci U S A 76:353–357, 1979

Malek A, Izumo S: Physiological Fluid Shear Stress Causes Downregulation of Endothelin-1 mRNA in Bovine Aortic Endothelium. Am J Physiol 263:C389–396, 1992

Morawietz H, Ma YH, Vives F, Wilson E, Sukhatme VP, Holtz J, Ives HE: Rapid Induction and Translocation of Egr-1 in Response to Mechanical Strain in Vascular Smooth Muscle Cells. Circ Res 84:678–687, 1999

Morawietz H, Talanow R, Szibor M, Rueckschloss U, Schubert A, Bartling B, Darmer D, Holtz J: Regulation of the Endothelin System by Shear Stress in Human Endothelial Cells. J Physiol (Lond) 525:761–770, 2000

Nishida K, Harrison DG, Navas JP, Fisher AA, Dockery SP, Uematsu M, Nerem RM, Alexander RW, Murphy TJ: Molecular Cloning and Characterization of the Constitutive Bovine Aortic Endothelial Cell Nitric Oxide Synthase. J Clin Invest 90:2092–2096, 1992

Osol G: Mechanotransduction by Vascular Smooth Muscle. J Vasc Res 32:275–292, 1995

Schubert A, Cattaruzza M, Hecker M, Darmer D, Holtz J, Morawietz H: Shear Stress-Dependent Regulation of the Human b-Tubulin Folding Cofactor D Gene. Circ Res 87:1188–1194, 2000

Sdougos HP, Bussolari SR, Dewey CFJ: Secondary Flow and Turbulence in a Cone-Plate Device. J Fluid Mech 138:379–404, 1984

Traub O, Berk BC: Laminar Shear Stress: Mechanisms by Which Endothelial Cells Transduce an Atheroprotective Force. Arterioscler Thromb Vasc Biol 18:677–685, 1998

Williams B: Mechanical Influences on Vascular Smooth Muscle Cell Function. J Hypertens 16:1921–1929, 1998

Wilson E, Mai Q, Sudhir K, Weiss RH, Ives HE: Mechanical Strain Induces Growth of Vascular Smooth Muscle Cells via Autocrine Action of PDGF. J Cell Biol 123:741–747, 1993

Wong AJ, Pollard TD, Herman IM: Actin Filament Stress Fibres in Vascular Endothelial Cells In Vivo. Science 219:867–869, 1983

Zarins CK, Giddens DP, Bharadvaj BK, Sottiurai VS, Mabon RF, Glagov S: Carotid bifurcation atherosclerosis. Quantitative Correlation of Plaque Localization with Flow Velocity Profiles and Wall Shear Stress. Circ Res 53:502–514, 1983

Measurement of Function and Regulation of Adrenergic Receptors

Marc Brede, Melanie Philipp and Lutz Hein

Introduction

Transgenic and gene-targeted mouse models have significantly advanced our understanding of the physiology and pharmacology of the adrenergic system. The adrenergic system comprises the following molecular components: 1) the enzymes involved in the biosynthesis of the endogenous catecholamines, 2) the receptors which mediate the biological effects of adrenaline and noradrenaline, 3) the transporter proteins which are required for presynaptic and extraneuronal transport of neurotransmitters, and 4) the enzymes involved in the metabolism of catecholamines (see Fig. 1).

Adrenaline and noradrenaline (and also dopamine) belong to the endogenous catecholamines. The biosynthesis of these catecholamines starts with the precursor amino acid tyrosine. In further sequential steps, tyrosine is first converted to L-DOPA by the rate-limiting enzyme in this pathway, tyrosine hydroxylase, followed by generation of dopamine by the aromatic L-amino acid decarboxylase (dopa decarboxylase). Dopamine itself is transported into synaptic vesicles by a vesicular monoamine transporter (VMAT). Inside these vesicles, dopamine β-hydroxylase converts dopamine to noradrenaline, which is stored as the major neurotransmitter of the sympathetic system. Only in the chromaffin cells of the adrenal medulla (and a few nuclei of the central nervous system) is noradrenaline further enzymatically transformed to adrenaline. Upon depolarization of sympathetic nerves or chromaffin cells, noradrenaline and adrenaline are released into the synaptic cleft or into the blood stream, respectively. Most of the released noradrenaline is recycled back from the synaptic cleft into the synaptic vesicles, where it is available for release again by noradrenaline-(NAT) and vesicular monoamine-(VMAT)transporters. A small fraction of the recycled catecholamines is destined for degradation by the enzymes monoamine oxidase (MAO) and catechol-O-methyltransferase (COMT).

As noradrenaline and adrenaline do not readily penetrate cellular membranes, their biological actions are sensed and transferred into the cells by plasma membrane receptors, which belong to the superfamily of G protein-coupled receptors (GPCR). Based on pharmacological properties, these receptors were initially subdivided into α_1-, α_2-, and β-adrenergic receptors. Later, more pharmacological ligands and, most importantly, molecular cloning led to the identification of 9 adrenergic receptor subtypes altogether: α_{1A}, α_{1B}, α_{1D}, α_{2A}, α_{2B}, α_{2C}, β_1, β_2, β_3 (Bylund et al. 1998). These receptors have been identified and cloned from species including human, rat, mouse, rabbit and many others.

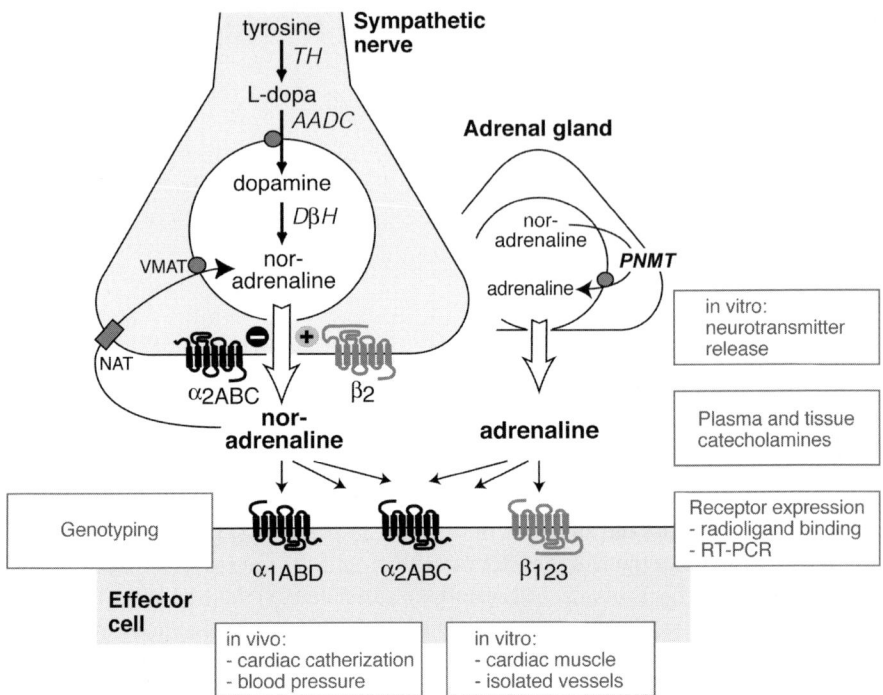

Figure 1
The adrenergic system and methods for studying adrenergic receptor function and regulation. Upon activation of sympathetic nerves or adrenal chromaffin cells, noradrenaline and adrenaline are secreted and can activate adrenergic receptors on surrounding cells (sympathetic nerves) or enter the blood circulation (adrenaline released from the adrenal gland). Release of noradrenaline from nerve terminals is controlled by presynaptic inhibitory α_2- and activating β_2-adrenergic receptors. Actions of noradrenaline are terminated by uptake into nerve terminals and synaptic vesicles by active transporters (NAT, VMAT) and by uptake into neighboring cells (not shown). In this review, several methods are described (see boxes) to investigate the function of the adrenergic system in transgenic and gene-targeted mouse models. Abbreviations: *AADC* aromatic L-amino acid decarboxylase; *DβH* dopamine β-hydroxylase; *NAT* nordadrenaline transporter; *PNMT* phenylethanolamine-N-methyltransferase; *TH*, tyrosine hydroxylase; *VMAT* vesicular monoamine transporter

Due to lack of sufficiently subtype-selective ligands, the precise physiological function of the adrenergic receptors has not been fully explored until recently. The development of molecular genetic methods has greatly advanced the field by cell type-specific overexpression ("transgenic mice") or targeted deletion ("knockout mice") of individual adrenergic receptor subtypes (for recent reviews, see Rohrer et al. 2000; Philipp et al. 2002; Engelhardt and Hein 2003). In addition, several transgenic mouse models were generated to study the function of the biosynthetic enzymes, transporters and metabolic enzymes of the adrenergic system (for review, see Carson and Robertson 2002).

During the course of the investigation of transgenic mouse models, an array of methods has been developed or adapted for application in mice. In this chapter, an overview of the methods, which are required to study the adrenergic system in genetically modified mouse models (see Fig. 1) will be provided. Primarily, methods and strategies which have been useful to identify the physiological functions of α_2-adrenergic receptor subtypes will be described. Wherever possible, experimental details or references will be given for the study of α_1- and β-receptor subtypes. The methods, described will cover a complete phenotyping array, starting with genotyping of mice, followed by *in vivo* cardiac catheterization and blood pressure measurements, *in vitro* organ bath methods and biochemical and receptor expression assays. Wherever methods are discussed in greater detail in another chapter of this book, cross-references will be provided.

Description of Methods and Practical Approach

Genotyping and Isolation of Genomic DNA

Although it may be best to perform cardiovascular experiments in transgenic mice with an investigator who is blinded with respect to the genotype of the animals, genotyping is an essential tool for mating of the mice and identifying a group of animals which are suitable for a particular experiment. Usually, the genotype of transgenic or knockout mice can easily be determined by PCR analysis of genomic DNA isolated from small tissue biopsies (Fig. 2a). For this purpose, a small biopsy may be taken from the animals tail (1–2 mm) or from the ear at the age of 3 weeks.

Biopsies are incubated in 200 µl Chelex-100 buffer in Eppendorf tubes (see below) with the addition of 5 µl proteinase K (concentration 20 mg/ml) for 3–12 h at 55 °C in a rotating shaker. Chelex-100 (Biorad, Munich) is a chelating resin with a high affinity for polyvalent metal ions and is used in forensic studies to obtain DNA from small tissue or blood samples (Walsh et al. 1991). Best results are achieved after overnight incubation of the tissue biopsies. After proteinase K digestion of the samples, the tubes are briefly vortexed and centrifuged for 30 s at 13000 rpm in a tabletop centrifuge followed by heating to 100 °C for 8 min to melt the Chelex. After heating, the samples are centrifuged again at 13000 rpm for 3 min. The supernatant can be directly used for PCR analysis. Usually 1 µl of the supernatant will give a clear PCR result, but sometimes a 1:10 dilution of the supernatant before PCR analysis may help to achieve more robust PCR amplification.

Wild type and transgenic or knockout alleles may be distinguished by using allele-specific primers (see Fig. 2a). Several primer sets for genotyping of mice lacking or overexpressing adrenergic receptors have been described (Engelhardt et al. 1999; Kaumann et al. 2001; Brede et al. 2002) or are available from the authors of this chapter upon request.

Chelex buffer

- 0.1 M NaCl
- 0.5% Na-lauroylsarcosine
- 5% Chelex-100
- in water

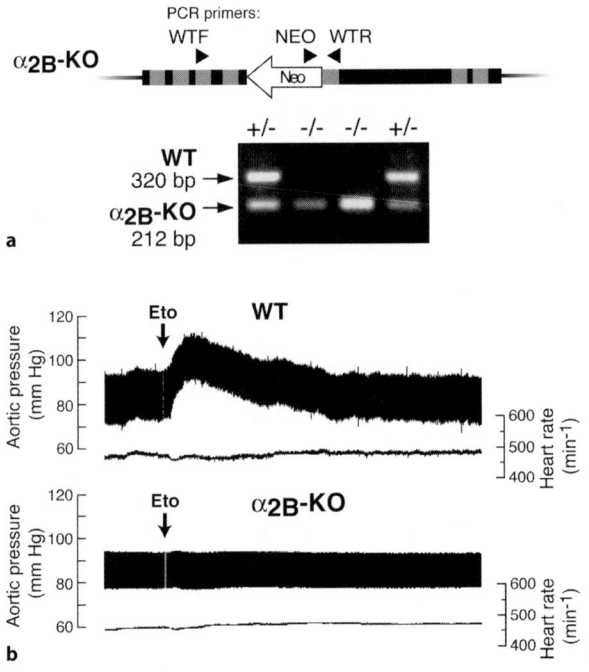

Figure 2
Etomidate can activate α_{2B}-adrenergic receptors.
a Genotyping of α_{2B}-receptor knockout mice. The upper scheme shows the coding sequence of the mouse α_{2B}-adrenergic receptor gene (black, gray boxes represent transmembrane domains of the α_{2B}-receptor), which was disrupted by insertion of a neomycin resistance cassette (Neo). For genotyping of mice, the wild-type allele (WT) can be amplified from genomic DNA with the primers WTF and WTR, resulting in a 320 bp DNA fragment, which is visualized in the agarose gel. The knockout allele is amplified using the primer pair NEO – WTR, yielding a 212 bp long DNA product. b) Aortic pressure (upper traces) and heart rate (lower traces) were determined under anesthesia in wild type or α_{2B}-KO mice. Etomidate elicits a transient hypertensive response in WT but not in α_{2B}-KO mice. Data adapted from Paris et al. (2003)

In vivo Cardiovascular Function

Left Ventricular Catheterization

In order to examine *in vivo* cardiovascular function in transgenic mice, several methods may be used. Non-invasive methods use echocardiography or rapid magnetic resonance imaging (e.g. Wiesmann et al. 2001). Invasive methods use fluid-filled or catheter-tip pressure transducers or implantable Doppler flow probes. Here, we will describe direct left ventricular catheterization of mice using a small catheter-tip pressure-volume transducer, e.g. manufactured by Millar Instruments (Houston, USA). These catheters are available in different sizes, with the 1.4 F and 1.8 F sizes being best for application in mice. The 1.4 F catheter has a tip diameter of 0.47 mm and may be used for left ventricular catheterization in mice with a body weight of at least 18–20 g (Fig. 3a). The 1.8 F catheter is mechanically more robust, but may only be used for larger mice >25–30 g body weight. Both catheters are available for pressure measurements or for combined pressure-volume determination.

For routine cardiac catheterization, mice have to be anesthetized for approximately 30 min (maximal duration 60 min). Several anesthetics may be used for this purpose, however one has to be aware that all anesthetic agents may be cardiodepressive. Despite the fact that ketamine-xylazine is a widely used combination for anesthe-

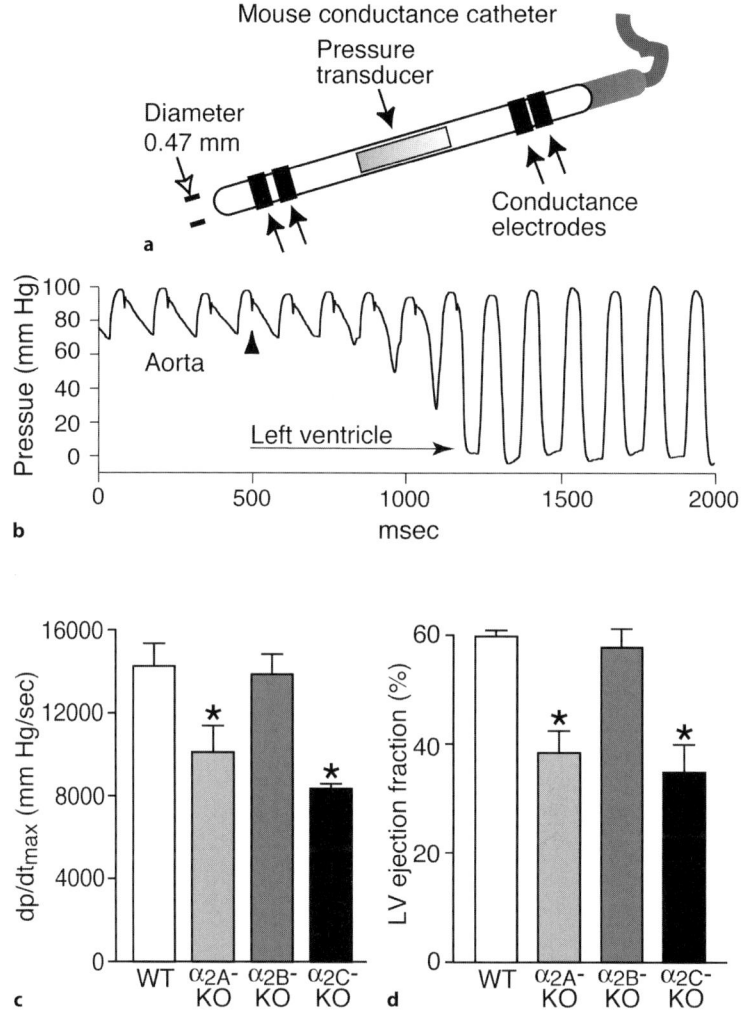

Figure 3a–d
Left ventricular catheterization of α_2-adrenergic receptor knockout mice. a A 1.4F conductance catheter can be inserted into the carotid artery of an anesthetized mouse. b) Original pressure recording showing typical aortic and left ventricular pressure curves in the mouse. c, d) After experimental left ventricular pressure overload, mice lacking α_{2A}- or α_{2C}-adrenergic receptors have lower left ventricular contractility (dp/dt_{max}) and ejection fraction. Data in c, d are adapted from Brede et al. (2002)

sia, it should not be used to investigate the adrenergic system *in vivo* as xylazine is an agonist of α_2-adrenergic receptors and thus lowers central sympathetic tone and decreases presynaptic noradrenaline release. Of all available methods, Avertin (tribromoethanol) by i.p. injection or isoflurane inhalation gave the best and most reproducible results when studying adrenergic receptors *in vivo*. Both methods of anesthesia result in heart rates around 450 min^{-1} and left ventricular contractility (dp/dt_{max})

values of 8000–10000 mm Hg/s in normal adult wild-type mice (Brede et al. 2002). Avertin should be prepared in stock solutions which are stored at –20 °C in small aliquots (Hogan et al. 1986). Long-term storage at room temperature may cause formation of toxic tribromoethanol derivatives, which may cause severe, lethal peritonitis in mice 5–7 days after i.p. injection (Nicol et al. 1965). However, this side effect of old Avertin solutions can be completely avoided if one uses fresh solutions, which may be used for a few days if they are stored at 4 °C overnight. Alternatively, isoflurane (3.0 vol% for induction, 1.5–2.0 vol% for maintenance of anesthesia) may be applied *via* a nose cone. For both methods of anesthesia, mice may breath spontaneously.

Avertin solution

- 2 g 2,2,2-tribromoethanol
- 2.5 ml tertiary amylalcohol
- warm in water bath
- dilute to 80 ml with distilled water
- stir until tribromoethanol is dissolved
- store in aliquots at –20 °C until use
- inject 13–15 µl/g body weight

After induction of anesthesia, mice are placed on a heating plate to prevent lowering of body temperature during anesthesia. A small midline incision (1.5–2 cm) is made through the skin along the trachea. Using small forceps, pretracheal muscles are moved to the side and the right carotid artery, which can be found in the immediate vicinity of the trachea, is exposed. Next, two 7.0 silk sutures are placed around the common carotid artery, leaving approximately 1 cm space between the sutures. The distal suture, which is just below the bifurcation of the common carotid artery, may be tied immediately and the ends of the suture fixed with adhesive tape to the heating plate. Closure of the distal carotid suture will guarantee that no retrograde blood flow through the cerebral circulation will occur when the artery is cut open for insertion of the catheter. The proximal suture is left open, and the thread is pulled with a small clamp towards the feet of the animal. Between the stretched sutures, the carotid artery may be cut open with a small pair of scissors of the type used in ophthalmological surgical procedures. Through this incision, which should not extend over more than 50% of the artery's circumference, the catheter is inserted into the lumen of the carotid artery and advanced into the aorta. In larger mice (which have a wider lumen of the carotid artery), the proximal suture should be tied when the catheter is pushed through the vessel in order to avoid bleeding from the site of arterial incision. At this stage, the catheter should be connected to the recording system to monitor the pressure curve. Normally, the catheter should now reside in the proximal carotid artery or aorta, which should result in the appearance of the typical arterial pressure curve with systolic and diastolic pressures of 90–120 mm Hg and 70–80 mmHg, respectively (see Figs. 2b, 3a). The next step will be to advance the catheter further in the direction of the left ventricle. Frequently, one may sense a small resistance during the advance of the catheter which indicates that the catheter tip has reached the aortic valve. At this point, the catheter may be carefully pushed forward and backward until the resistance disappears and the tip slides into the lumen of the left ventricle. Correct positioning of the catheter inside the left ventricle may be controlled by observing the pressure curve on the monitor (see Fig. 3a). Inside the left ventricle, the diastolic pressure should drop to values of 0–5 mm Hg. At this stage, one allows the pressure curve, heart rate and contractility to stabilize for a few minutes to obtain baseline values (see Fig. 3b).

In order to assess function of cardiac (or other) adrenergic receptors during left ventricular catheterization, an intravenous line for application of agonists or antagonists may be conveniently placed into the left jugular vein. The vein is prepared on the left side of the mouse in order to avoid disturbances to the pressure catheter on the right side. As described above for the carotid artery, the left jugular vein is prepared, two sutures are placed around the vein, and a small PE-10 polyethylene tube is advanced through a very small incision into the vein. Through this PE-10 tubing, one may apply bolus injections or continuous infusions of drugs to activate or inhibit adrenergic receptors. Direct intravenous drug application has several advantages over i.p. injection. Most importantly, i.v. injection allows very precise control of the timing and the dose which is applied. As a routinely used drug to activate cardiac β-adrenergic receptors and thus assess maximal positive inotropic stimulation, dobutamine may be i.v. infused in increasing concentrations as follows. First, a stock solution of 2 mg/ml dobutamine is prepared in water, followed by 1:100 dilution in physiological saline. This dobutamine solution (0.02 mg/ml) is then infused by a microinfusion pump at rates between 7.5 µl/min and 375 µl/min to achieve dobutamine infusion rates of 5–200 µg/kg/min. The infusion pump may be started at the lowest rate (7.5 µl/min) and the infusion rate constantly increased in 1 min intervals until the maximal rate is achieved. In this situation, one has to be careful not to overload the circulatory system of the mouse with volume. Thus, for smaller mice (<25 g body weight) the concentration of dobutamine should be increased to avoid volume overload. In a similar way, β-adenergic receptor antagonists may be applied to determine basal cardiac contractility in the absence of noradrenaline or adrenaline stimulating left ventricular β-receptors (Engelhardt et al. 2001). At the end of the experiment, the mice may be killed by an overdose of anesthesia and blood and tissues may be prepared for biochemical analysis.

From these measurements, several parameters of cardiac function may be derived, including heart rate, diastolic and systolic pressures and maximal rates of left ventricular contraction and relaxation (dp/dt_{max} and dp/dt_{min}). These parameters may all be helpful in investigating the function of cardiac adrenergic receptors. However, cardiac contractility may only be assessed from these parameters with great caution. In particular the dp/dt_{max} value may be very much dependent on the heart rate, with higher heart rates resulting "automatically" in higher dp/dt_{max} values. For *in vivo* determination of left ventricular contractility, a pressure-volume catheter (Millar Instruments, Houston, USA) may be helpful. This catheter combines a pressure transducer with two pairs of electrodes which determine the conductance of the surrounding medium (see Fig. 3a). As the conductances of blood and solid tissue differ, this approach may be used to derive left ventricular volume parameters. However, great care must be used to convert conductance values to absolute volume parameters. Details of this procedure are described in the instructions of the manufacturer of the pressure-volume catheter and in several original papers published by Kass and coauthors (see e.g. Georgakopoulos et al. 1998). In order to derive parameters of cardiac contractility which are (largely) independent of the heart rate, a set of pressure-volume loops has to be obtained with different levels of cardiac preload. However, changing cardiac preload acutely in anesthetized mice requires additional surgical procedures, i.e. opening of the abdominal cavity to transiently occlude the vena cava between liver and diaphragm. As one may rupture the diaphragm and thus open the thorax during this procedure, the mice should be ventilated for conductance catheterization. Several groups have tried to use pharmacological agents to lower preload, but all agents used also lowered afterload by interfering with arterial vasoconstriction. Examples of rate-independent measures of left ventricular contractility are ejection fraction and preload-recruitable stroke work (Georgakopoulos et al. 1998).

Invasive Blood Pressure Measurement in Conscious Mice

A similar technique for vascular access as described above may be used to investigate blood pressure regulation in conscious, unrestrained mice (Desai et al. 1997; Link et al. 1996). For this purpose, a saline-filled PE-10 catheter is inserted into the right carotid artery of an anesthetized mouse. The PE-10 catheter (total length 10 cm) is then firmly fixed by several sutures to the carotid artery and to the surrounding muscles. The intraluminal tip of the catheter should ideally be positioned in the very proximal part of the common carotid artery in close vicinity to the aorta. The remaining part of the catheter is then tunnelled to the back of the mouse, where the closed end of the catheter is kept in a small subcutaneous pouch. The skin wounds are then closed by sutures and the mouse allowed to recover from surgery for at least 24 h. After recovery, the PE-10 catheter may be removed from the subcutaneous pouch and can be connected to a pressure transducer and infusion pump for intravascular application of drugs. In order to avoid rupture or tearing of the PE-10 tubing, the catheter can be pushed through PE-50 tubing before connection to the pressure transducer. With this setup, blood pressure and heart rate can be measured directly and adrenergic agonists and antagonists may be applied without disturbing the mice. At the end of each experiment, the PE-10 catheter may be briefly rinsed with heparin to avoid clotting of blood at the catheter tip and the catheter can be stored again in the subcutaneous pouch until the next day. This procedure may be repeated for a number of days (Desai et al. 1997), but on average 1–3 catheter days are the maximum which may be achieved in a large group of mice.

In vitro Organ Bath Methods

In vitro Cardiac Preparations

In vitro organ bath studies are essential to determine the function of adrenergic receptors, as these are important regulators of cardiac contractility and rhythm. Thus, isolated, intact cardiac preparations (e.g. Langendorff hearts, isolated working hearts), cardiac tissue specimens (left and right atria, papillary muscle, ventricular strips) and isolated cardiac myocytes may be used to determine functional parameters of adrenergic regulation. For details on these methods, the reader is referred to the relevant chapters of this book.

In vitro Investigation of Adrenergic Signaling in Isolated Mouse Blood Vessels

Adrenergic receptors are ubiquitously expressed in all parts and cell types of the vascular system. To complement *in vivo* hemodynamic studies, *in vitro* methods for investigation of vascular smooth muscle cell contraction or endothelial function are essential. A large variety of arterial and venous blood vessels prepared from adult mice may be investigated with a small vessel myograph, including conducting arteries (aorta, carotid artery, femoral artery), distributing arteries (renal, mesenteric, coronary, cerebral arteries) and veins (pulmonary vein, vena cava, portal vein) (for details, see Chruscinski et al. 2001).

For studies on isolated blood vessels, adult mice (3–6 months old) are sacrificed by cervical dislocation and various vessels are dissected from the animal. The vessels are placed in a physiological salt solution consisting of 118 mM NaCl, 4.7 mM KCl, 2.5 mM $CaCl_2$, 1.18 mM $MgSO_4$, 1.18 mM KH_2PO_4, 25 mM $NaHCO_3$, 0.03 mM EDTA and 10 mM glucose. Vessels are stored at 4 °C before being placed in the myograph organ-bath. The vessels are dissected from the surrounding tissue and cut into 2 mm long pieces. A single tungsten wire (40 μm diameter) is passed through the lumen of each vessel segment with care taken not to damage the endothelium. This single wire is then attached to one of the supports on a computer-controlled, automated small vessel myograph (Myo500A, J.P. Trading, Aarhus, Denmark). A second tungsten wire is passed through the lumen of the vessel and attached to the second support. One of the supports is attached to a drive motor and micrometer, allowing for control of movement and measurement of distances between the two wires. The second support is connected to a force transducer to measure the wall tension developed by the contracting/relaxing vessel. During the time that the vessel is being mounted, physiological salt solution is present in the myograph bath, maintained at 37 °C and bubbled by $5\%O_2/95\%CO_2$. A computer-assisted normalization protocol is then performed to determine the optimal pre-tension and vessel diameter as described previously (Mulvany and Halpern 1976). Briefly, to determine the length-tension relationship for each vessel, the computer adjusts the support connected to the micrometer. Based on this relationship, it is possible to estimate the diameter (L_{100}) that the vessel would have if it experienced a transmural pressure of 100 mmHg. For arterial vessels, the diameter of the vessel was set to $0.9 \times L_{100}$ for optimal pretension. Because venous and pulmonary pressures are much lower than the pressure of the systemic circulation, venous vessels are normalized to a transmural pressure of 30 mmHg.

After the standardized normalization procedure, vessels are challenged with a high potassium-solution consisting of 42.7 mM NaCl, 80 mM KCl, 2.5 mM $CaCl_2$, 1.18 mM $MgSO_4$, 1.18 mM KH_2PO_4, 25 mM $NaHCO_3$, 0.03 mM EDTA and 10 mM glucose to determine whether the vessel is viable. Only vessels that demonstrate a contraction in response to the high potassium solution can be used for further studies. Afterwards the solution is replaced again by the low-potassium solution and the vessel is equilibrated for 30 min. After the equilibration period, vessels are precontracted by adding 10 µM phenylephrine or 3 µM prostaglandin $F_{2\alpha}$. Various vessels show different sensitivity to the precontracting substances described above (Chruscinski et al. 2001). To determine the vasoconstrictive effect of a receptor ligand, increasing concentrations are added to the organ-bath without precontraction of the vessel to create concentration-response curves for the substance. Various substances can be tested after each other in a single set-up.

At the end of the experiment, vessels can be fixed in the organ-bath with 4% paraformaldehyde for standard histological and morphometric analyses (see e.g. Brede et al. 2001).

Neurotransmitter Release from Isolated Tissues

Release of noradrenaline from sympathetic nerves and of adrenaline from the adrenal gland is an important determinant of cardiovascular function. Thus, methods have been developed which allow the determination of release of noradrenaline from tissues which are innervated by sympathetic nerves, including the heart and blood vessels. In addition, we will discuss methods to measure catecholamine levels in blood, urine and tissues of transgenic mice.

Release of noradrenaline can be determined *in vitro* from any tissue which contains sympathetic nerves (most peripheral tissues and organs) or adrenergic neurons (most parts of the central nervous system). For this purpose, small pieces of tissue are incubated in physiological buffer containing radioactive, i.e. [^{3}H]-labelled, noradrenaline. The presynaptic transporters will take up the radioactive transmitter into the synaptic vesicles (see Fig. 1). Pieces of mouse atria, ductus deferens or spleen or 0.3 mm thick brain slices (2 mm diameter pieces of cortex, hippocampus etc.) are incubated for 30–60 min in superfusion buffer (see below) containing 0.2 µM [^{3}H]noradrenaline (2 µl of radioactive stock solution/ml buffer) at 37 °C. During the incubation, the solution is gassed with 5% CO_2/95% O_2 *via* small polyethylene tubing. To remove extracellular radioactive noradrenaline, the tissue pieces are rinsed 5 times in superfusion buffer and transferred to the superfusion chambers. The chambers are perfused with buffer at a constant flow of 0.6–1.5 ml/min. After 30 min, the tissues are electrically stimulated but the radioactivity from this first stimulation period is discarded.

After 60 min of superfusion in the chamber, tissues may be electrically stimulated with different rectangular pulses every 20 min and adrenergic agonists or antagonists can be added to the superfusion media to inhibit (α_2-agonists) or increase (β_2-agonists) electrically evoked release of [^{3}H]noradrenaline (see Fig. 4). Peripheral tissues, including atria, are electrically stimulated with 18 pulses (1 ms pulse width, 47 V/cm) at 3 Hz. Single pulses are not sufficient to release enough radioactivity from the sympathetic nerves into the superfusion medium, thus one has to use multiple stimuli which are applied rapidly in order to avoid inhibition of relase by the endogenous noradrenaline (so called "pseudo one pulse" stimulation). Tissue pieces of the brain contain enough transmitter to measure [^{3}H]noradrenaline release after sti-mulation with single rectangluar pulses. In order to prevent reuptake of released transmitter into the presynaptic nerve, 1 µM desipramine should be added to the superfusion

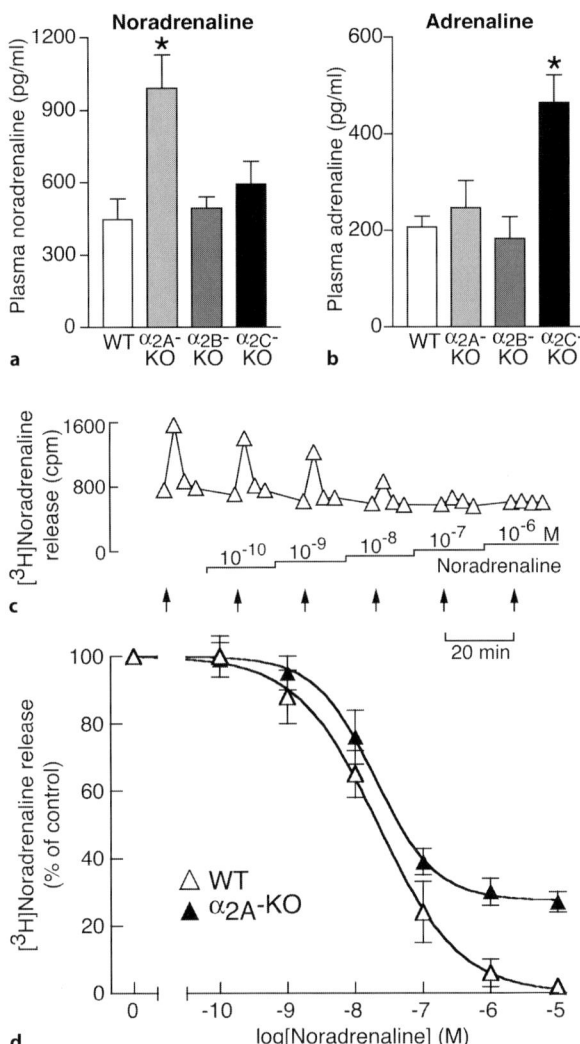

Figure 4a–d
Plasma catecholamines and noradrenaline release from isolated tissues of a_2-knockout mice. **a, b** Mice with targeted deletion of the α_{2A}- or α_{2C}-receptor have elevated plasma levels of noradrenaline and adrenaline, respectively. **c, d** Determination of noradrenaline release from sympathetic nerves in isolated mouse atria. Tissues were incubated with [^{3}H]noradrenaline and electrically stimulated (*arrows*). Release of radioactive transmitter (**c**) can be completely abolished by addition of noradrenaline (*via* presynaptic α_2-adrenergic receptors). **d** The inhibitory effect of noradrenaline is blunted in atria from mice lacking α_{2A}-receptors as compared with wild-type atria. Data are adapted from Hein et al. (1999) and Brede et al. (2003)

media to block presynaptic noradrenaline transporters. Superfusion media are collected in 1–2 min intervals and radioactivity is determined after addition of scintillation fluid in a β-counter. At the end of the stimulation period, tissues are dissolved in 0.1 M NaOH, 2% SDS and radioactivity still contained in the tissue is determined.

Electrically stimulated release at each period of stimulation is then calculated as % of tissue radioactivity released. Basal values (in the absence of drugs) are normalized to 100% and effects of adrenergic agonists and antagonists normalized to this basal value (Fig. 4d). Usually, 4–8 superfusion chambers are sufficient to derive high quality concentration-response curves for most agonists.

Superfusion medium:
118 mM NaCl	1.3 mM $CaCl_2$ (brain, 2.5 mM for atria)
4.8 mM KCl	1.2 mM $MgSO_4$
25 mM $NaHCO_3$	11 mM D-Glucose
1.2 mM KH_2CO_3	0.57 mM ascorbic acid
0.03 mM Na-EDTA	1 µM ascorbic acid

Determination of Plasma and Tissue Catecholamines

Plasma Catecholamines

Catecholamines can be determined from tissues, plasma or urine samples of transgenic mice. Noradrenaline in the blood plasma results from spillover into the blood of transmitter which has been released from peripheral sympathetic nerves. In order to determine resting catecholamine concentrations in the blood, it would be ideal to obtain blood samples for analysis from conscious mice, which are resting and are not aroused. However, even routine handling of the mice results in a stress response which is accompanied by large increases in plasma noradrenaline and adrenaline. Thus, the only possible method for determination of basal plasma catecholamine levels is to obtain blood from anesthetized mice. For this purpose, mice are anesthetized and placed on a warming plate and 200 µl blood is drawn through a small skin incision from the carotid artery at a defined time after induction of anesthesia. Blood is collected in heparinized 1.5 ml Eppendorf vials and centrifuged for 5 min at 14000 rpm in a table top centrifuge. The supernatant plasma is frozen in liquid nitrogen and stored at –80 °C until further analysis.

Catecholamines are determined by HPLC combined with electrochemical detection as described (Hein et al. 1999; Brede et al. 2002, 2003). For this method, the following solutions are combined:
- 100 µl mouse plasma
- 500 µl 1% EDTA, 1.25% Na_2SO_3
- 900 µl water
- 100 µl dihydroxybenzylamine (from 10 ng/ml standard solution)
- 300 µl 2 M Tris-HCl (pH 8.2)
- 20 mg aluminum oxide (Al_2O_3)

The mixture is incubated for 5 min on a rotating wheel followed by centrifugation at 1000 rpm at 4 °C for 1 min. The aluminum oxide pellet is washed twice with distilled water and bound catecholamines are eluated with 0.1 M $HClO_4$. The eluate is directly used for HPLC-electrochemical detection of noradrenaline, adrenaline, dopamine, L-DOPA and DOPAC as described (Halbrugge et al. 1988).

Urine Catecholamines

Total body catecholamine excretion can be determined by collecting mouse urine in metabolic cages for periods of 24 h (mouse metabolic cage, Tecniplast, Italia). 3 to 4 adult mice of the same genotype are grouped in one metabolic cage and urine from these mice is collected in 1 ml 0.4 M perchloric acid, which is covered by 0.5 ml mineral oil to avoid evaporation of the sample. After 24 h, the urine volume is measured followed by centrifugation of the urine samples (5 min at 14000 rpm). Catecholamines are extracted as described above for plasma samples.

Tissue Catecholamines

For determination of tissue catecholamines, small tissue specimens (50–100 mg) are frozen in liquid nitrogen. Specimens are wrapped in tinfoil and crushed with a pestle and mortar. The weight of the fine-ground tissue is determined and 500 μl 0.4 M perchloric acid is added, followed by homogenization of the tissue with an Ultraturrax at maximal speed. 30 μl of a solution containing standardized concentrations of catecholamines and metabolites is added and the mixture is incubated overnight at 4 °C. Next morning, the samples are centrifuged for 10 min at 14000 rpm and the supernatant is used for catecholamine extraction and detection as described above.

Adrenergic Receptor Expression Analysis

Radioligand Binding

Determination of α_2-adrenergic receptors by radioligand binding should always be performed with freshly prepared tissue membranes. Storage of membranes of murine origin leads usually to protein degradation and therefore to misleading results. However, dissected tissue can be stored at –80 °C after shock freezing in liquid nitrogen. Fresh or frozen tissue is disrupted in a hypotonic lysis buffer with an Ultraturrax (Janke & Kunkel). Nuclei and larger cell debris are removed by centrifugation at 1500×g at 4 °C. An additional 30 min centrifugation step at 45 000×g pellets cell membranes and vesicles, which are resuspended in binding buffer and thoroughly homogenized with a Dounce homogeniser. The protein concentration in the suspension should now be determined. The amount of membrane suspension for the radioligand binding study will be chosen depending on the expected density of adrenergic receptors. In most cases 100 μg of membrane protein are a good starting point. For exact measurements a saturation curve should be generated including measurements for at least 5 concentrations of radioligand, e.g. the α_2-receptor antagonist [^{3}H]RX821002 at 0.3 nM, 0.6 nM, 1 nM, 2 nM, 4 nM. Additionally, the nonspecific binding has to be measured in order to calculate the specific binding. For this purpose a non-radioactive ligand is used, which has the same or higher affinity for the receptor as the radioligand. In the case of α_2-adrenergic receptors 1 μM atipamezole or phentolamine work perfectly.

	total binding	nonspecific binding
membrane suspension	50 μl	50 μl
radioligand	50 μl	50 μl
non-radioactive ligand		50 μl
binding buffer	100 μl	50 μl

After incubation for 1 h at room temperature, the suspension is vacuum-filtered over GF/B filters, which had been prewetted with 25 mM glycylglycine pH 7.5, and washed 3 times with 5 ml ice-cold glycylglycine. The filters are then transferred into scintillation vials and covered with at least 4 ml of scintillation liquid. It is necessary to wait for equilibration before measuring the samples in a β-counter.

Hypotonic lysis buffer:
- 2 mM EDTA
- 5 mM Tris-HCl
- pH 7.4

Binding buffer:
- 4 mM EDTA
- 4 mM EGTA
- 32 mM Hepes
- 80 mM NaCl
- pH 7.6

Determination of mRNA Expression by RT-PCR

Whenever radioligand-binding analysis is not possible due to extremely small tissue samples or low expression of adrenergic receptors, RT-PCR allows one to determine whether a particular cardiovascular tissue or cell-type expresses mRNA for the adrenergic receptor(s) of interest. If PCR of the same reverse transcription reaction (RT) is performed for a housekeeping gene (i. e. β-actin, GAPDH) semi-quantitative results can also be obtained. The preparation of the RNA can be done using a silica-based extraction method or the common, rather time-consuming method by Chomczynski and Sacchi (1987). Most important for the whole experiment is absolutely clean working practice to avoid contamination with RNases and thereby to prevent degradation of the RNA. Thus all solutions have to be made with DEPC-treated water and the glass has to be baked. As all the α_2-adrenergic receptors are encoded by intronless genes, it is not possible to design primers that span introns and allow simple distinction between PCR products derived from cDNA (i.e. corresponding to RNA) or from genomic DNA. Therefore, a digest of the RNA samples with DNase I is recommended for 30–60 min at 37 °C. To check the integrity of RNA, denaturing agarose gel electrophoresis may be used. 500 ng RNA is mixed with RNA loading buffer and denatured for 5 min at 65 °C. Immediately after denaturation, the samples have to be cooled on ice before loading onto a 1.2% agarose gel containing 1.8 vol% formaldehyde and 0.5 µg/ml ethidium bromide. The electrophoresis is performed at 70 V in RNA-running buffer. If the RNA is still intact, two bands appear at the positions of 1.9 and 4.7 kb indicating murine 18s and 28s rRNA. The reverse transcription is performed with up to 1 µg of RNA, but best results will be obtained with a minimum of 300 ng RNA. Depending on the gene of interest, an oligo-dTTP primer consisting of 15 to 18 dTTPs, oligo-hexamers or a gene-specific primer will be used for reverse transcription.

To give an example for expression analysis of α_{2A}- and α_{2B}-receptors, we used 20 μl of RT-mix (see below), which was incubated for 15 min at 42 °C, then boiled for 5 min and placed on ice immediately afterwards. The PCR was performed with 2 μl of reverse transcription mix. Because of the intronless structure of α_2-receptors a control reaction without adding reverse transcriptase should be done to see whether the amplified fragment by PCR is due to expression of the RNA or caused by residual genomic DNA in the sample.

However, for the detection of α_{2C}-receptors a slightly modified protocol was used. The RT-mix containing an α_{2C}-specific primer was incubated for 10 min at 70 °C and chilled afterwards. After adding 200 U of reverse transcriptase, the RNA was transcribed for 1 h at 42 °C. Then again a final denaturation step (10 min at 95 °C) and fast chilling on ice were performed.

10 × RNA-gel buffer:
- 10 mM EDTA
- 50 mM Na-acetate
- 200 mM MOPS
- pH 7.0

RNA-running buffer:
- 1× RNA-gel buffer with 0.75% formaldehyde

RNA-loading buffer:
- 16 μl saturated bromophenolblue solution
- 80 μl 0.5 M EDTA pH 8
- 100 μl DEPC-water
- 720 μl 37% formaldehyde
- 2 ml glycerol 100%
- 3084 μl formamide
- 4 ml 10× RNA-gel buffer

RT-mix for $\alpha_{2A/B}$-receptor:
- 2.5 μM oligo-dTTP
- 1 mM dNTP
- 5 mM DTT
- 1× Superscript buffer
- 2–4 U RNasin RNase inhibitor
- 20 U Superscript reverse transcriptase

RT-Mix:
- 2.5 μM RT-primer for α_{2C}
- 500 μM dNTP
- 5 mM DTT
- 1× Superscript buffer
- 2–4 U RNasin RNase inhibitor

Examples

Etomidate Activates α_2-Adenergic Receptors

The intravenous anesthetic etomidate exhibits structural similarities to specific α_2-adrenergic agonists. In order to test whether etomidate may also interact *in vivo* with α_2-adrenergic receptors, we investigated the hemodynamic profile of etomidate in wild type and α_2-receptor knockout mice (Paris et al. 2003). Figure 2 shows an example of the genotyping procedure to distinguish between wild type and α_{2B}-KO mice. For generation of the α_{2B}-receptor knockout mice (Link et al. 1996), a neomycin resistance cassette was integrated into the coding sequence of the murine α_{2B}-receptor gene (see Fig. 2a). Using primers which are specific for the wild type receptor's sequence or the neomycin cassette, one can amplify DNA fragments from genomic DNA which differ in size between wild type and α_{2B}-KO mice. Heterozygous knockout mice display DNA bands for both wild type and knockout alleles.

In order to determine the effects of etomidate on resting blood pressure, mice were anesthetized with Avertin and a microtip catheter was inserted into the aorta as described above. Intravenous injection of etomidate resulted in a transient rise in arterial blood pressure in wild type mice (see Fig. 2b, WT traces). Etomidate did not affect blood pressure in α_{2B}-KO mice (see Fig. 2b, lower traces). These findings were further supported by additional experiments with recombinant α_{2B}-receptors expressed in HEK293 cells. Taken together, these results demonstrate that etomidate acts as an agonist at α_2-adrenoceptors, which is apparent *in vivo* primarily as an α_{2B}-receptor-mediated increase in blood pressure (Paris et al., 2003). This effect of etomidate may contribute to the cardiovascular stability of patients after induction of anesthesia with etomidate.

Deletion of α_2-Adrenergic Receptors Results in Heart Failure

Elevated plasma norepinephrine levels are associated with increased mortality in patients and in animal models with chronic heart failure. In order to test which α_2-adrenoceptor subtype(s) operate as presynaptic inhibitory receptors (see Fig. 1) to control noradrenaline release in heart failure, we have investigated the response of gene-targeted mice lacking α_2-adrenoceptor subtypes to chronic left ventricular pressure overload. Experimental heart failure was induced in mice by transverse aortic constriction. Three months after aortic banding, survival was dramatically reduced in α_{2A}-KO and α_{2C}-KO mice as compared with wild type and α_{2B}-deficient animals (Brede et al. 2002). Using direct left ventricular catheterization in anesthetized mice (see Fig. 3) as described in the Methods section of this chapter, decreased survival of knockout mice after aortic constriction was associated with reduced left ventricular contractility (see Fig. 3c) and lower left ventricular ejection fraction (see Fig. 3d).

The primary cause for the enhanced heart failure phenotype in α_2-deficient mice was the absence of these receptors in the sympathetic neurons. As described in the introduction, α_2-receptors operate as feedback inhibitors of noradrenaline release from sympathetic nerves (α_{2A}) or adrenal chromaffin cells (α_{2C}, Fig. 1). In anesthetized mice, plasma noradrenaline and adrenaline levels were selectively elevated in mice lacking α_{2A}- or α_{2C}-receptors, respectively (see Fig. 4a, b; Brede et al. 2003). In isolated tissues, e.g. cardiac atria, the defect in presynaptic feedback regulation can be directly determined by radioactive neurotransmitter assays (see Fig. 4c,d). In atria from wild type mice, exogenous noradrenaline can completely inhibit electrically induced release of [^{3}H]noradrenaline (see Fig. 4c). However, in α_{2A}-KO atria the inhibitory effect of noradrenaline is significantly smaller (see Fig. 4d; Hein et al. 1999). Thus, α_2-receptors are essential for feedback control of noradrenaline and adrenaline release. Genetic defects in these inhibitory regulators leads to enhanced circulating catecholamine levels which predispose the mice for the development of severe heart failure.

Vascular Remodeling in Angiotensin AT2 Receptor-Deficient Mice

Angiotensin II activates two distinct G protein-coupled receptors, termed AT_1 and AT_2 receptors. Most of the known cardiovascular effects of angiotensin II are mediated by the AT_1 receptor subtype. In order to determine the cardiovascular functions of AT_2-receptors, we investigated mice lacking these receptors (Hein et al. 1995; Brede et al. 2001). *In vivo* pressure responses to angiotensin II or the α_1-adrenergic receptor agonist phenylephrine were greatly enhanced in AT_2-KO mice. Deletion of the angiotensin AT_2 receptor did not lead to a compensatory increase in the activity of the circulating renin-angiotensin system, and arterial blood pressure was identical between wild type control mice (WT) and AT_2-KO mice (Brede et al. 2001). Cardiac contractility as assessed by left ventricular catheterization did not differ between AT_2-KO and WT mice. However, isolated femoral arteries from AT_2-KO showed enhanced vasoconstriction to noradrenaline and K$^+$ depolarization when compared to WT arteries (Fig. 5a,b). Morphometric analysis of large and small femoral arteries revealed a significant hypertrophy of media smooth muscle cells (Fig. 5c,d). Phospho-P70S6 kinase levels were significantly increased in aortae from AT_2-KO mice as compared with WT mice. These results indicate that vascular AT_2-receptors inhibit the activity of and hence, hypertrophic signalling by the P70S6 kinase *in vivo* and thus are important regulators of vascular structure and function.

Troubleshooting

Many details should be carefully observed when analyzing phenotypes in transgenic mice. As the adrenergic system is not only an essential regulator of the cardiovascular system but also controls the response to stress and increased metabolic needs of the body, alterations in several physiological systems may significantly affect adrenergic signaling in the cardiovascular system. The release of noradrenaline and adrenaline from sympathetic nerves and from the adrenal gland is easily affected by surrounding noise, frequent cage changes, novel animal caretakers, and prolonged handling of the animals. Thus, catecholamine levels in the plasma and excretion in the urine should only be investigated in groups of mice which have been adapted to a controlled and quiet environment for a few days.

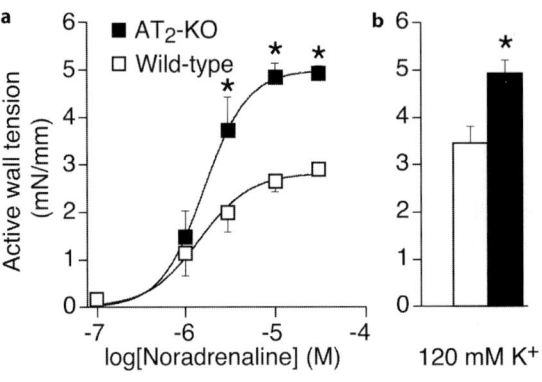

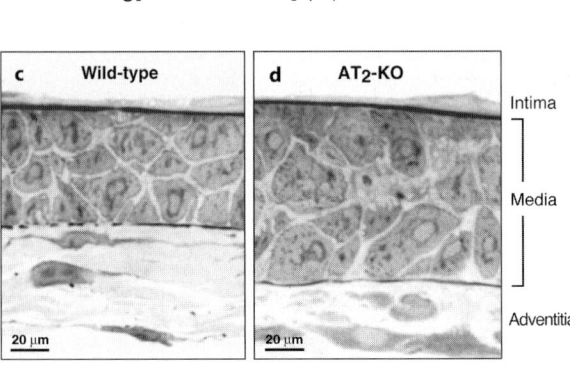

Figure 5a–d
Enhanced adrenergic vasoconstriction in angiotensin AT_2-receptor knockout mice. **a** Isolated femoral artery segments from mice lacking AT_2-receptors show enhanced vasoconstriction in response to noradrenaline (displayed as active wall tension) as compared with vessel segments from wild type littermates. **b** Depolarization of vascular smooth muscle cells with 120 mM K$^+$ also causes stronger vasoconstriction in AT_2-KO than in WT vessels. **c,d** After pressure-controlled fixation femoral arteries *in situ*, vascular myocyte hypertrophy becomes apparent in AT_2-KO vessels as compared with WT femoral arteries (Brede et al. 2001)

As increased circulating catecholamine levels may effectively alter postsynaptic receptor signaling and cause desensitization, receptor phosphorylation and downregulation, the development of a chronic phenotype, e.g. cardiac hypertrophy and heart failure, may be indirectly influenced by the surroundings. Attention should be paid to the gender of the animals; frequently male mice have higher levels of catecholamine release than female mice. Thus, heart failure and hypertensive phenotypes may develop more easily in male mice than in groups of female mice. Aggression between male animals housed in a single cage should be observed and prevented by separating animals early before aggressive behavior results in long-term stress. In particular, male mice of the FVB/N strain of mice, which is frequently used for pronuclear injection to generate transgenic mice, may suddenly exhibit aggressive behavior (which is sometimes mostly apparent during the activity period of the mice at night).

Furthermore, the genetic background of transgenic and knockout mice used for experimental cardiovascular studies may be very important. Frequently gene-targeted mice are maintained for some time on a mixed genetic background containing genes from the embryonic stem cells (129Sv mouse strain) and of the C57BL6 strain. It may be advisable to cross the deleted ("knockout") allele onto a C57BL6 background for 8–10 generations to obtain "congenic mice" which only differ in one gene. Sometimes, the genetic background may decide between life and death, i.e. the deleted gene or transgene may be lethal on one genetic background but may yield surviving mice on a different or on a mixed background (Philipp et al. 2002). If no optimal control mice are available which perfectly match with the genetic background of transgenic or knockout mice, a compromise might be to cross heterozygous mice to yield wild type and knockout littermates, which will then be used for one set of experiments. In conclusion, achieving homogeneity in experimental design, environmental conditions and genetic mouse strain backgrounds will be one of the important goals when investigating the adrenergic system in genetically engineered mouse models.

The authors' work was supported by grants from the Deutsche Forschungsgemeinschaft (SFB355, SFB487, Bonn, Germany).

References

Altman JD, Trendelenburg AU, MacMillan L, Bernstein D, Limbird L, Starke K, Kobilka BK, Hein L. (1999) Abnormal sympathetic α_2-autoreceptor function in α_{2A}-adrenergic receptor knockout mice. Mol. Pharmacol. 56, 154–161

Brede M, Hadamek L, Meinel L, Wiesmann F, Peters J, Engelhardt S, Simm A, Lohse MJ, Hein L (2001) Vascular hypertrophy and increased P70S6 kinase in mice lacking the angiotensin II AT_2 receptor. Circulation 104, 2602–2607

Brede M, Wiesmann F, Jahns R, Hadamek K, Arnolt C, Neubauer S, Lohse MJ, Hein L (2002) Feedback inhibition of catecholamine release by two different α_2-adrenoceptor subtypes prevents progression of heart failure. Circulation 106, 2491–2496

Brede M, Nagy G, Philipp M, Sørensen J, Lohse MJ, Hein L (2003). Differential control of adrenal and sympathetic catecholamine release by α_2-adrenergic receptor subtypes. Mol. Endocrinol. 17, 1640–1646

Bylund DB, Bond RA, Clarke DE, Eikenburg DC, Hieble JP, Langer SZ, Lefkowitz RJ, Minneman KP, Molinoff PB, Ruffolo RR, Strosberg AD, Trendelenburg UG (1998) Adrenoceptors. In: The IUPHAR compendium of receptor characterization and classification, IUPHAR Media. London, pp 58–74

Carson RP, Robertson D (2002) Genetic manipulation of noradrenergic neurons. J Pharmacol Exp Ther 301: 410–417

Chomczynski P, Sacchi N (1987) Single-step method of RNA isolation by acid guanidinium thiocyanate-phenol-chloroform extraction. Anal Biochem 162. 156–159

Chruscinski A, Brede ME, Meinel L, Lohse MJ, Kobilka BK, Hein L (2001) Differential distribution of β-adrenergic receptor subtypes in blood vessels of knockout mice lacking β_1- or β_2-adrenergic receptors. Mol Pharmacol 60: 955–962

Desai KH, Sato R, Schauble E, Barsh GS, Kobilka BK, Bernstein D (1997) Cardiovascular indexes in the mouse at rest and with exercise: new tools to study models of cardiac disease. Am J Physiol. 272, H1053–H1061

Engelhardt S, Hein L, Wiesmann F, Lohse MJ (1999) Progressive hypertrophy and heart failure in β_1-adrenergic receptor transgenic mice. Proc Natl Acad Sci USA 96: 7059–7064

Engelhardt S, Boknik P, Keller U, Neumann J, Lohse MJ, Hein L (2001a) Early impairment of calcium handling and altered expression of junction in hearts of mice overexpressing the β_1-adrenergic receptor. Faseb J. 15: 2718–2720

Georgakopoulos D, Mitzner WA, Chen CH, Byrne BJ, Millar HD, Hare JM, Kass DA (1998) *In vivo* murine left ventricular pressure-volume relations by miniaturized conductance micromanometry. Am J Physiol 274, H1416–H1422

Halbrugge T, Gerhardt T, Ludwig J, Heidbreder E, Graefe KH (1988) Assay of catecholamines and dihydroxyphenylethyleneglycol in human plasma and its application in orthostasis and mental stress. Life Sci. 43, 19–26

Hein L, Barsh GS, Pratt RE, Dzau VJ, Kobilka BK (1995) Behavioural and cardiovascular effect of disrupting the angiotensin II type-2 receptor gene in mice. Nature 377, 744–747

Hogan B, Costantini F, Lacy E (1986) Manipulating the mouse embryo. A laboratory manual. Cold Spring Harbor Laboratory, 1986

Kaumann AJ, Engelhardt S, Hein L, Molenaar P, Lohse M (2001) Abolition of (-)-CGP 12177-evoked cardiostimulation in double β_1/β_2-adrenoceptor knockout mice. Obligatory role of β_1-adrenoceptors for putative β_4-adrenoceptor pharmacology. Naunyn Schmiedeberg's Arch Pharmacol 363: 87–93

Link RE, Desai K, Hein L, Stevens ME, Chruscinski A, Bernstein D, Barsh GS, Kobilka BK (1996) Cardiovascular regulation in mice lacking a_2-adrenergic receptor subtypes b and c. Science 273, 803–805

Mulvany MJ, Halpern W (1976) Mechanical properties of vascular smooth muscle cells *in situ*. Nature 260, 617–619

Nicol T, Vernon-Roberts B, Quantock DC (1965) Protective effect of oestrogens against the toxic decomposition products of tribromoethanol. Nature 208, 1098–1099

Paris A, Philipp M, Steinfath M, Tonner P, Lohse MJ, Scholz J, Hein L (2003) Activation of α_{2B}-adrenoceptors mediates cardiovascular effects of etomidate. Anesthesiology 99: 889–895

Philipp M, Brede M, Hein L (2002) Physiological significance of α_2-adrenergic receptor subtype diversity: one receptor is not enough. Am J Physiol 283: R287–R295

Rohrer DK (2000) Targeted disruption of adrenergic receptor genes. Methods Mol Biol 126: 259–277

Walsh PS; Metzger DA, Higuchi R (1991) Chelex-100 as a medium for simple extraction of DNA for PCR-based typing from forensic material. BioTechniques 10: 506–513

Wiesmann F, Ruff J, Engelhardt S, Hein L, Dienesch C, Leupold A, Illinger R, Frydrychowicz A, Hiller KH, Rommel E, Haase A, Lohse MJ, Neubauer S (2001) Dobutamine stress magnetic resonance microimaging in mice: Acute changes of cardiac geometry and function in normal and failing murine hearts. Circ. Res. 88, 563–569

Measurement of Function and Regulation of Muscarinic Acetylcholine Receptors

Björn Kaiser and Chris J. van Koppen

Introduction

The G protein-coupled receptors (GPCRs) including the muscarinic acetylcholine receptors (mAChRs) constitute a family of seven transmembrane spanning proteins. These proteins respond to an array of sensory and chemical stimuli, e.g. light, hormones, and neurotransmitters. The receptors transmit extracellular stimuli into the cell interior via stimulation of heterotrimeric guanine nucleotide binding proteins (G proteins). GPCR activation represents a co-ordinated balance of molecular mechanisms governing receptor signalling, desensitization, and resensitization (Ferguson, 2001). Five distinct mAChR subtypes (M_1–M_5) have been identified in different mammalian tissues with different expression patterns and each receptor subtype being the product of one of the five different genes (Bonner, 1989). In general, the M_1, M_3 and M_5 mAChR subtypes couple preferentially via $G_{q/11}$ proteins to phospholipase C (PLC) with subsequent formation of inositol 1,4,5-trisphosphate and diacylglycerol, whereas M_2 and M_4 mAChRs couple preferentially via pertussis toxin-sensitive G_i proteins leading to inhibition of adenylyl cyclase. The mAChRs are differentially distributed in the nervous system and peripheral organs like the heart, exocrine glands and smooth muscle tissues (Caulfield 1993). In the mammalian heart of various species, including human, the predominant mAChR subtype is of the M_2 subtype. Stimulation of the M_2 mAChR mediates negative chronotropic and inotropic effects of acetylcholine. Besides M_2 mAChRs, M_1 and M_3 mAChRs exist in the heart. For example, the M_1 mAChR has been detected by using RT-PCR detection of the corresponding mRNA and by protein detection with specific antibodies in the guinea-pig and rat heart (Sharma et al. 1997). In the human heart, there is some evidence from functional, biochemical and molecular biological studies that another mAChR subtype, one different from the M_2 subtype, exists, at least in the right atrium; the functional importance of this receptor still remains to be elucidated (for reviews, see Dhein et al. 2001; Brodde and Michel 1999). Multiple mechanisms regulate the signalling pathways of the five members of G protein-coupled mAChRs. Strong or persistent activation of mAChRs can induce receptor internalization and down-regulation, which proceed in a highly regulated manner depending on receptor subtype and cell type (see for a review, van Koppen and Kaiser, 2003). We have developed a model of clathrin-mediated internalization of mAChRs in the experimental cell system of HEK-293 cells (van Koppen and Kaiser 2003). Following agonist binding to M_1 (or M_3 and M_4) mAChRs, the receptor is phosphorylated by receptor kinases (e.g. G protein-coupled receptor kinases and casein kinase 1α; Krupnick and Benovic 1998; Tobin et al. 1997), followed by binding of β-arrestin to the phosphorylated receptor. β-Arrestin recruits and activates the cytosolic tyrosine kinase c-Src. In addition, β-arrestin interacts with clathrin and the clathrin adapter complex AP-2, leading to immobilization of the receptor-β-arrestin-c-Src complex in the clathrin-coated pit. Activated c-Src phosphorylates dynamin, which leads to activation of dynamin, and activated dynamin molecules polymerize as a collar around the neck of the endocytic pit containing the receptor and catalyze the fission of the vesicle from the plasma membrane. After release of dynamin, clathrin and β-arrestin, the receptors are thought to recycle back to the plasma membrane. Internalization of the M_2 mAChR appears to be regulated distinct from the M_1, M_3 and M_4 mAChR subtypes in HEK-293 and other cells. It also requires functionally active dynamin but it proceeds in an apparent β-arrestin-, c-Src-, and clathrin-independent manner. In addition, the M_2 mAChR does not recycle back to the plasma membrane but is down-regulated (van Koppen and Kaiser 2003). In many cells, persistent activation of mAChRs over hours induces a loss of total number of cellular receptors. This process, also termed receptor down-regulation, can only be overcome by *de novo* receptor synthesis. In this chapter, we describe various methods of analyzing the function and regulation of mAChRs in intact cells and membrane homogenates.

Description of Methods and Practical Approach

Radioligand Binding Assays to Measure mAChRs on the Cell Surface of Intact Cells and in Cell Membrane Homogenates

Introduction

In this subchapter, we describe two different radioligand binding assays. One binding assay to measure the number of mAChRs on the cell surface of intact cells and a second binding assay to determine the total number of mAChRs in crude membrane homogenates of the cells. The number of cell surface mAChRs is measured by the binding of the high affinity quaternary muscarinic receptor antagonist [^{3}H]N-methylscopolamine ([^{3}H]NMS) (K_d-value of ~300 pM), whereas total mAChR number (i.e., intracellular and plasma membrane-located) is determined with the membrane-permeable high affinity muscarinic receptor antagonist [^{3}H]Quinuclidinyl benzilate ([^{3}H]QNB (K_d-value of ~50 pM).

[³H]NMS Binding Assay to Intact Cells

Measuring of cell surface mAChRs is accomplished by the binding of the positively charged muscarinic receptor antagonist [^{3}H]NMS to intact cells. Because [^{3}H]NMS cannot cross the plasma membrane at 4 °C, it can only bind to mAChRs on the cell surface of cells. For this reason, [^{3}H]NMS is useful in determining the internalization

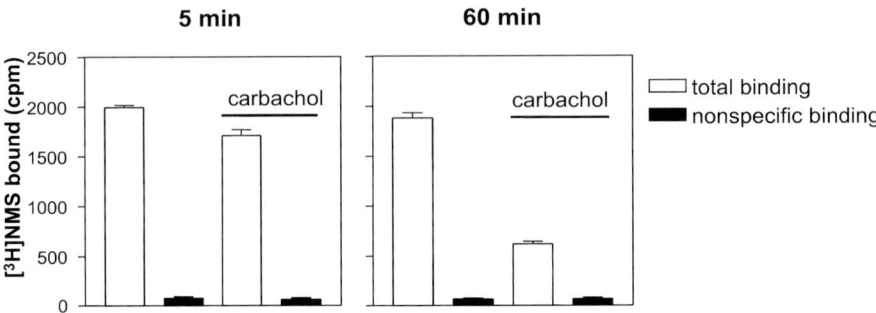

Figure 1
Total and nonspecific binding of [³H]NMS to intact HEK-293 cells expressing M₂ mAChRs. Effect of agonist treatment. Intact HEK-293 cells expressing M₂ mAChRs were incubated for 5 and 60 min in the absence and presence of 10 µM carbachol. Thereafter, cells were washed to remove agonist. Total and nonspecific binding of [³H]NMS to the cell surface was determined by incubation of the cells with 2 nM [³H]NMS in the absence and presence of 30 µM atropine for 4 h at 4 °C, respectively

of receptors following agonist treatment of the cells. For this, cells expressing the mAChRs are subcultured on 24 well plates. The wells should be coated with 0.1 mg/ml poly-L-lysine (molecular weight >300,000; Sigma) before plating out the cells because the cells are easily washed away. On the day of the binding experiment, the culture medium is removed and the cells are washed once with Hank's balanced salt solution (HBSS) (118 mM NaCl, 5 mM KCl, 1 mM CaCl$_2$, 1 mM MgCl$_2$, 15 mM HEPES, 5 mM glucose, pH 7.4) at 37 °C. After incubation of the cells in 500 µl HBSS with or without carbachol (1 µM – 10 mM) for 0–60 min at 37 °C, medium is rapidly removed by suction. Then, cells are rinsed three times with 500 µl ice-cold HBSS. Thereafter, cells are incubated in 500 µl HBSS containing a receptor-saturating concentration of 2 nM [³H]NMS (specific radioactivity of ~80 Ci/mmol) at 4 °C. Atropine (final concentration

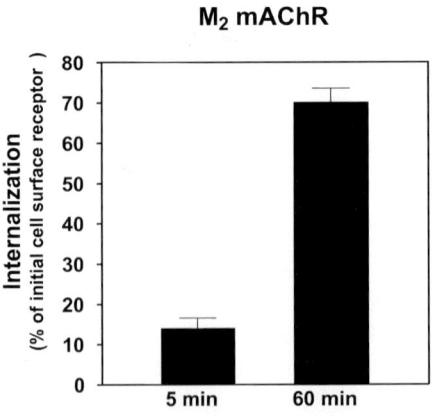

Figure 2
Internalization of M₂mAChRs in HEK-293 cells. HEK-293 cells expressing M₂ mAChRs were incubated with or with-out 10 µM carbachol for 5 or 60 min at 37 °C. Thereafter, cells were washed to remove agonist and incubated for 4 h at 4 °C in the presence of 2 nM [³H]NMS binding in the absence or presence of 30 µM atropine. Internalization is expressed as (1-quotient of cell surface receptors of car-bachol-treated and untreated cells) × 100%

10-50 µM) is included in parallel incubations to measure non-specific binding of [³H]NMS. It is important that incubation with [³H]NMS and subsequent washing are carried out at 4 °C because internalized receptors may return to the cell surface at incubation temperatures higher than 10 °C. After 4 h, cells are washed twice with 500 µl of ice-cold HBSS to wash away non-specifically bound [³H]NMS. The cells are then solubilized in 1% Triton X-100 and scraped off the plates. The cell lysates are transferred into scintillation vials, which receive 3.5 ml scintillation fluid (Packard Emulsifier-Scintillator Plus). After vortexing for 10 s, radioactivity is measured by tritium counting in a liquid scintillation counter. Total [³H]NMS binding is determined in quadruplicate whereas non-specific binding of [³H]NMS is measured in duplicate (Fig. 1).

Care should be taken that depletion of radioligand by binding to specific and non-specific binding sites is less than 15% of total radioligand added. Internalization of mAChRs is expressed as (1- quotient of cell surface receptors of carbachol-treated and untreated cells) × 100% (Fig. 2).

[³H]QNB Binding Assay to Cell Membranes

The total number of mAChRs is determined by the lipophilic membrane-permeable muscarinic receptor antagonist [³H]QNB (specific radioactivity of ~45 Ci/mmol) to crude cell homogenates. Following culturing on 6 well plates, cells are carefully washed with 5 ml ice-cold HBSS. Then, cells from 6 wells are scraped from the plates with ice-cold 6 × 1 ml HBSS and homogenized together in a ground glass homogenizer by hand with 10 – 20 strokes. Thereafter, the crude cell homogenates are placed on ice for subsequent [³H]QNB binding assay but the cell membranes may also be stored as pellet at –80 °C after centrifugation at 10,000 g at 4 °C. If loss of mAChRs by agonist-induced receptor down-regulation is to be investigated, the cells on the 6 well plates can be pre-treated with or without carbachol (1 µM – 10 mM) for 0–12 h at 37 °C in HBSS followed by three washes with ice-cold HBSS to remove agonist. Then, 800 µl of crude cell homogenate is added to a 3.5 ml polypropylene tube and mixed with 100 µl [³H]QNB (approximate receptor-saturating final concentration of 600 pM) in HBSS, 100 µl HBSS with or without atropine (final concentration 10-50 µM) and incubated while shaking in a water bath at 37 °C. After 60–90 min, the binding reaction is terminated by vacuum filtration of the incubation mixture through Whatman GF/C glass-fiber filters and washing of the filters twice with ice-cold 6 ml HBSS. Filters are transferred into scintillation vials containing 3.5 ml fluid scintillation solution.

Radioactivity in the filter is determined after vortexing of the vials for 10 seconds. Total and non-specific binding of [³H]QNB is determined in quadruplicate and duplicate, respectively. Again, care should be taken that radioligand depletion by binding to specific and non-specific binding sites is less than 15% of total radioligand added. Protein content of the membrane homogenates can be determined according to method of Bradford (1976). The total mAChR number is to be expressed as fmol receptor/mg protein.

Muscarinic Acetylcholine Receptor-Stimulated [^{35}S]GTPγS Binding to G Proteins

Introduction

The next step in mAChR signaling is the activation of heterotrimeric guanine nucleotide-binding proteins (G proteins). Agonist binding to the mAChR activates various heterotrimeric G proteins, which results in the exchange of guanosine 5'-diphosphate (GDP) for guanosine 5'-triphosphate (GTP) bound to α subunit (Neer, 1995). The M_1, M_3 and M_5 mAChRs couple preferentially to the G_q family of G proteins whereas the M_2 and M_4 mAChRs preferentially couple to the G_i family of G proteins (Caulfield 1993). To study G protein activation by mAChRs in a quantitative manner, the radiolabeled GTP analogue guanosine 5'-O-(γ-[^{35}S]thio)triphosphate ([^{35}S]GTPγS, specific radioactivity of ~1250 Ci/mmol) is taken. This GTP analogue is strongly resistant to hydrolysis and has a high affinity for all types of G protein α subunits. Here, we describe the isolation of HEK-293 cell membranes and the measurement of M_2 mAChR-induced specific binding of [^{35}S]GTPgS to these membranes. For more background details on [^{35}S]GTPγS binding, the reader is referred to Wieland and Jakobs 1994.

Isolation of HEK-293 Cell Membranes

Three confluent 145 mm tissue culture dishes with HEK-293 cells (80–100% confluency) are necessary to isolate sufficient membranes. The plates are rinsed 3–4 times with 10 ml ice-cold HBSS and the cells are collected in a total volume of 18 ml ice-cold HBSS and centrifuged in a Sorvall SS-34 centrifuge for 10 min at 2,000 g (4,500 rpm) at 4 °C. The pellets are resuspended in 5 ml buffer A (140 mM NaCl, 10 mM triethanolamine hydrochloride (TEA), pH 7.4). After centrifugation for 10 min at 2,000 g, the pellets are resuspended in 20 ml buffer B (250 mM sucrose, 10 mM Tris-HCl 1.5 mM $MgCl_2$, 1 mM ATP, 3 mM benzamidine, 100 µM phenylmethylsulfonyl fluoride, 1 µM leupeptin, pH 7.5). The cells are cracked in nitrogen atmosphere under high pressure (20 bar) for 30 min at 4 °C. Next, ice-cold 500 µl 50 mM EGTA (final concentration 1.25 mM) is added to the cell suspension and the tubes are centrifuged for 15 min at 1,000 g (3,200 rpm) at 4 °C in a Sorvall SS-34 centrifuge. Then, the supernatant is filtered over two layers of cheese cloth and centrifuged for 15 min at 10,000 g (13,000 rpm) at 4 °C. The pellets are resuspended in 2 ml buffer C (20 mM Tris-HCl, 1 mM EDTA, 1 mM ATP, 3 mM benzamidine, 100 µM phenylmethylsulfonyl fluoride, 1 µM leupeptin, 1 mM dithiothreitol, pH 7.5). The membrane suspension is centrifuged again for 15 min at 10,000 g at 4 °C, taken up in 1 ml buffer C, recentrifuged for 15 min at 10,000 g at 4 °C and then resuspended in 350 µl buffer C. Aliquots of 50 ml of the membrane fraction are then quick-frozen at -70 °C.

Measurement of M_2 mAChR-induced [^{35}S]GTPγS Binding to Heterotrimeric G Proteins in Membranes from HEK-293 Cells

The following filtration assay for the measurement of [^{35}S]GTPγS binding to membranes from HEK-293 cells has been described previously (Wieland and Jakobs 1994). HEK-293 cell membranes (see above) are resuspended in freshly made buffer D to a final volume of 200 µl (final membrane protein concentration 0.5–1.0 µg/µl) and held on ice. Buffer D contains 50 mM TEA, 150 mM NaCl, 5 mM $MgCl_2$, 1 mM EDTA, 1 mM dithiothreitol at pH 7.4. The reaction mixture for measuring [^{35}S]GTPγS binding contains buffer D, 1 µM GDP (Roche), 0.4 nM [^{35}S]GTPγS (about 1×10^6 cpm), with or without 1 mM carbachol and 10 µl of the diluted membranes in a total volume of 100 µl. The incubation in 3 ml reaction tubes is started by addition of membrane suspension to the pre-warmed reaction mixture and is carried out in quadruplicate for 15–20 min at 30 °C. Non-specific binding is measured in the presence of 10 µM unlabeled GTPγS (Roche) in the reaction mixture. The reaction is terminated by rapid filtration through Whatman GF/C glass-fiber filters, after which the filters are rapidly washed with 2×12 ml ice-cold 50 mM Tris, 5 mM $MgCl_2$, pH 7.4. The filters are put into 8 ml scintillation vials after which 3.5 ml scintillation fluid is added. After shaking for 30 min at room temperature, radioactivity is measured in a liquid scintillation counter. The results are expressed as fmol specific [^{35}S]GTPγS binding per mg protein or, optionally, per fmol M_2 mAChRs. This assay is suitable to determine desensitization of M_2 mAChR-mediated activation of the heterotrimeric G proteins. For this, intact cells on the plates are first pretreated with or without 1 µM–1 mM carbachol for 1–15 min in HBSS. Thereafter, the cells are rinsed 4 times with 10 ml ice-cold HBSS and the membranes are collected as described above.

Determination of M_2 mAChR-Mediated Inhibition of cAMP Accumulation in Intact Cells

Introduction

Accumulation of intracellular cAMP in response to M_2 or M_4 mAChR stimulation can be used as a convenient means to determine the functional responsiveness of these mAChR subtypes. The procedure described here represents a relatively simple method for the determination of intracellular cAMP levels following stimulation of mAChRs.

Determination of mAChR-Mediated Inhibition of cAMP Accumulation

Cells are cultured to near confluency on 60 mm poly-L-lysine-coated tissue culture dishes and culture media. Before starting the assay, cells are washed three times with HBSS at 37 °C. Then, 2 ml of HBSS containing 5 mM theophyllin is added and the plates are placed in a 37 °C incubator for 20 min. Then, forskolin (dissolved in 50% ethanol) is added to the plates (final concentration of 50 µM). Forskolin stimulates adenylyl cyclase directly. Receptor agonists (e.g. carbachol) are added to the cells simultaneously with forskolin in the same solution and the cells are incubated for 5–15 min at 37 °C. Then, plates are rinsed twice with ice-cold HBSS, followed by addition of ice-cold 2 ml 5% (w/v) trichloroacetic acid. The cell lysates are scraped off the plates and transferred into test tubes on ice. A recovery standard consisting of 0.7 nCi [2,8-^{3}H]cAMP (specific radioactivity of ~30 Ci/mmol) is added and the tubes are centrifuged at 2,700 g for 15–30 min at room temperature. One ml cation-exchange columns (AG 50W-X4, 200-400 mesh, Bio-Rad) are shortly regenerated before use by two column volume washes with 1 M HCl, twice with 0.5 M NaOH and six times with distilled water. The columns can be regenerated 3–4 times. The supernatant of the cell lysates is then poured over the cation-exchange columns to partially purify cellular cAMP from the extract. The pellet is saved for protein determination. Columns are subsequently washed with 3–3.5 ml of water and cAMP is eluted with further addition of 3–4 ml of water. The efficiency of cAMP recovery from the column can be determined by mixing 1 ml of column eluate with scintillation fluid and comparing the radioactivity in the eluate with radioactivity from the [^{3}H]cAMP recovery standard. The protein pellet is hydrolyzed with 1 M NaOH at 60–70 °C and the protein amount can be measured by a modification of the Lowry protein assay method (Peterson 1977). cAMP is quantitated from column eluants by the competitive protein-binding assay of Gilman et al. (1970). For this, in a final assay volume of 200 μl, 10–160 μl of eluant is added. The volume of the eluant is dependent on the cell type, length of time that the cells were incubated with forskolin and the agonist used and should be able of competing away 75% of [^{3}H]cAMP added to the assay. In addition to column eluant, 30 μl of an assay mix containing 3.3 mg/ml bovine serum albumin (BSA), 0.3 M sodium acetate, pH 4, and 1 pmol [^{3}H]cAMP is added and the reaction is initiated by addition of approximately 3 μg of the regulatory subunit of protein kinase A (Sigma). The regulatory subunit of protein kinase A should be able to bind approximately 30% of the [^{3}H]cAMP in the assay mix in the absence of competing cAMP. In parallel, a standard curve is made by substituting column eluant with varying amounts of unlabeled cAMP of known concentration (0.5–30 pmol) in the assay tubes. The amount of accumulated cAMP in the cells can be determined by using this standard curve. The assay tubes are incubated on ice for 2–4 h and the reaction is terminated by addition of 1 ml of ice-cold 20 mM KH_2PO_4, pH 6.0. The assay volume is then filtered over 0.45 μm nitrocellulose followed by 3 washes of 3 ml of ice-cold 20 mM KH_2PO_4, pH 6.0 each. Filters are subsequently dissolved in Packard Emulsifier Scintillator Plus scintillation fluid and counted in a scintillation counter. Triplicate plates are performed for each treatment and each plate is assayed in triplicate in the binding assay.

Determination of mAChR-Induced Stimulation of Phospholipase C

Introduction

Activation of phospholipase C (PLC) leads to breakdown of phosphatidylinositol 4,5-bisphosphate in the plasma membrane into the two second messengers: inositol 1,4,5-trisphosphate (IP_3) and diacylglycerol (DAG). IP_3 can subsequently be dephosphorylated into inositol. A convenient assay to measure mAChR-induced PLC stimulation is to measure the production of total inositol phosphates (IP_x) in the presence of 10 mM LiCl. The inclusion of 10 mM LiCl prevents dephosphorylation of [^{3}H]inositol phosphates by inhibiting inositol phosphatases and allows accumulation of inositol 1-phosphate (IP_1), inositol 1,4-bisphosphate (IP_2), and inositol 1,4,5-trisphosphate (IP_3) over the period of the carbachol treatment. Total inositol phosphates

(= IP_3, IP_2 and IP_1) can then be determined by using anion-exchange chromatography. The PLC assay is particularly suitable for the measurent of function and regulation of the M_1, M_3 and M_5 mAChR subtypes, which strongly increase PLC activity via pertussis-insensitive G proteins of the G_q family (Caulfield 1993). M_2 and M_4 mAChR subtypes stimulate PLC activity to a much smaller extent.

Phospholipase C Assay in Intact Cells

Measurement of mAChR-induced PLC stimulation is based on the formation of cellular [^{3}H]inositol phosphates from [^{3}H]phosphatidylinositol 4,5-bisphosphate in intact cells prelabelled with *myo*-[^{3}H]inositol. A nearly confluent (70–80%) monolayer of cells on poly-L-lysine-coated 35 mm culture dishes are labelled overnight by incubation of the cells with 0.5–1 µCi/ml radiolabeled *myo*-[^{3}H]inositol (specific radioactivity of ~24 Ci/mmol) in DME/F12 medium with serum for 16 h at 37 °C in 5% CO_2. It is wise to take aliquots of 20 µl immediately after addition of *myo*-[^{3}H]inositol for measurement of total radioactivity added to the plates and at the end of the labelling procedure to determine the cellular uptake of *myo*-[^{3}H]inositol. If receptor-induced PLC activation is weak, one can use custom-made inositol-free DME medium (available from Invitrogen/BRL) or label the cells for 48 h instead of 16 h. After labeling, the medium is removed and [^{3}H]inositol-labeled cells are equilibrated with 1 ml HBSS (37 °C) supplemented with 10 mM LiCl for 15 min at 37 °C. Then, carbachol (1 nM–10 mM) is added to the medium for 0–60 min in HBSS with 10 mM LiCl. The reaction is stopped by removal of the buffer and addition of 1 ml ice-cold methanol to the plates. The cells are rapidly scraped from the dishes and transferred immediately into 3.5 ml reaction tubes on ice. Protein content of the cells is determined by the method of Bradford (Bradford 1976) using separate non-radioactive culture dishes. All experiments are run in triplicate. If desensitization of mAChR-stimulated PLC is to be determined, cells are first pretreated with or without 1 µM–10 mM carbachol for 0–60 min in HBSS without 10 mM LiCl. The plates are then rinsed 3–4 times with 2 ml warm (37 C) HBSS without 10 mM LiCl to remove mAChR agonist. Next, the cells are preincubated for 5–10 min in HBSS containing 10 mM LiCl to block inositol phosphatases after which the agonist is added to the plates.

Isolation of [^{3}H]inositol Phosphates from the Cell Extract

The quantification of PLC-mediated *myo*-[^{3}H]inositol phosphates formation is accomplished by anion exchange chromatography. For this, 2 ml from a 1:1 aqueous solution of Bio-Rad AG 1-X8 200-400 mesh, formate form is applied to a series of columns. Before loading the samples, the columns are equilibrated (or regenerated) with 6 ml 2 M ammonium formate + 0.1 M formic acid and rinsed twice with 6 ml distilled water. The columns can be regenerated in 6 times. Dried columns are best stored at 4 °C following regeneration with 2 M ammonium formate + 0.1 M formic acid to prevent growth of mould. [^{3}H]inositol phosphates are isolated from the cell extracts by separating the aqueous phase of the cell extract by chloroform-methanol extraction. For this, the methanol extracts of the cells (1 ml) are mixed with 1 ml ice-cold chloroform and 0.5 ml ice-cold distilled water. The mixture is vigorously vortexed and centrifuged for 10 min at 2,400 rpm (Heraeus Megafuge 1.0 R) at 4 °C. The complete (1 ml) upper, aqueous phase of the cell extract is applied to the columns. After loading the columns and washing off free myo-[^{3}H]inositol and [^{3}H]glycerophosphoinositol with 6 ml dH$_2$O and 5 ml 50 mM ammonium formate, the collection vials are changed. Then, the [^{3}H]IP$_3$, [^{3}H]IP$_2$ and [^{3}H]IP$_1$ fractions are eluted together from the column by adding 6 ml 1 M ammonium formate + 0.1 M formic acid. From these eluates, 1 ml aliquots are counted by liquid scintillation spectrometry after addition of 3.5 ml liquid scintillation fluid. Inositol phosphate formation is normalized for protein content and given as radioactivity (counts per minute) per mg protein. Sometimes, it may be necessary to measure the formation of IP$_3$ instead of total inositol phosphates. In such cases, the cells should be activated in the absence of LiCl and to isolate IP$_3$ separately from IP$_2$ + IP$_1$, the following procedure should be followed. After elution with 6 ml H$_2$O and 5 ml of 50 mM ammonium formate, collection vials are changed. Then, 10 ml of 0.4 M ammonium formate + 0.1 M formic acid solution are added to the column to elute IP$_1$ and IP$_2$. Then, after changing collection vials again, 6 ml 1 M ammonium formate + 0.1 M formic acid solution are added and IP$_3$ is eluted from the column. Again, 1 ml aliquots from the eluate are taken for radioactivity counting.

mAChR-Induced Activation of Phospholipase D in HEK-293 cells

Introduction

Stimulation of phospholipase D (PLD) is a signal transduction pathway which is involved in diverse cellular functions (Singer et al. 1997). PLD preferentially hydrolyzes the main plasma membrane-embedded phospholipid phosphatidylcholine into phosphatidic acid (PA) and choline. PLD can also catalyze a transphosphatidylation reaction in which H$_2$O can be substituted for by a primary alcohol, in most cases ethanol, leading to the generation of metabolically stable phosphatidylalcohols. Like other phosphatidylalcohols, phosphatidylethanol (PtdEtOH) can serve as an unambiguous marker of PLD activation. The M$_1$ and M$_3$ mAChRs couple much more efficiently to PLD than the M$_2$ and M$_4$ mAChRs. Interestingly, mAChR-mediated PLD activation desensitizes completely within 1–5 min. It is believed that this rapid desensitization of mAChR-mediated PLD activation is due to rapid inactivation by an as yet undefined mechanism (van Koppen and Kaiser 2003).

Phospholipase D Assay in Intact Cells

For the measurement of mAChR-induced stimulation of PLD activity, cells on 35 mm poly-L-lysine-coated plates are labelled by adding [^{3}H]oleic acid (specific radioactivity of ~24 Ci/mmol, 2 µCi/ml) to the culture medium. After 24 hours, culture medium is removed and the cells are equilibrated for 10 min at 37 °C in HBSS. Then, cells are incubated with HBSS containing 400 mM ethanol at 37 °C with or without different concentrations of carbachol to measure [^{3}H]PtdEtOH formation. The reaction is stopped after removal of the medium and addition of 1 ml ice-cold methanol to the dishes. Cells are scraped off from the culture dishes and transferred into 6.5 ml reaction tubes on ice. The cell lysates are mixed thoroughly with 0.5 ml of ice-cold water and 1 ml of ice-cold chloroform followed by centrifugation for 10 min at 3,400 rpm (4 °C). The lower organic phase containing [^{3}H]PtdEtOH is pipetted into a 3.5 ml reaction tube and dried by vacuum centrifugation at room temperature. The phospholipids are redissolved in 25 µl chloroform/methanol (1:1; by volume) and spotted in 10 µl aliquots on pre-coated Silica Gel 60C plates (Merck) pre-loaded with the non-radioactive lipid standards PA (Sigma) and PtdEtOH (Avanti). As mobile phase, we use the organic mixture of ethylacetate/isooctane/acetic acid/water (13:2:3:10 by volume; take upper phase after mixing). The phospholipids are detected by iodine (Merck) staining and identified by the lipid standards. The pencil marked radioactive lipids on the plates are sprayed with water, scraped from the Silica Gel plates and mixed with 3.5 ml liquid scintillation fluid for radioactivity counting. Measurement of PLD activity in the absence of ethanol is used to determine background radioactivity. Radioactivity in these samples should be lower than the radioactivity determined in samples of plates incubated in the presence of ethanol without carbachol. Protein amount is measured by the method of Bradford (Bradford, 1976) in separate culture dishes which contain no radioactivity. The formation of [^{3}H]phosphatidylethanol is expressed as percentage of total labelled phospholipids spotted on the plate.

Immunocytochemical Localization of M_2 mAChRs in HEK-293 Cells

Introduction

The following immunocytochemical method has been developed to visualize the internalization of myc-tagged M_2 mAChRs in HEK-293 cells using a commercially available anti-myc antibody. In our hands, fixation and permeabilization of the cells with methanol preserves the antigenicity of the proteins and cell morphology much better than formaldehyde. It is obvious that in cellular systems in which internalization of the endogenously expressed mAChRs is to be studied, antibodies against the native mAChRs have to be used .

Immunocytochemical Staining

HEK-293 cells stably expressing myc-tagged M_1 or M_2 mAChRs are grown on poly-L-lysine-coated 18×18 mm glass coverslips for 24 h in culture medium. The culture medium is aspirated and the cells are treated with or without carbachol (1 µM to 10 mM) in 500 µl HBSS at 37 °C for 0–60 min. Cells are washed twice with phosphate-buffered saline (PBS) (148 mM NaCl, 3.5 mM Na_2HPO_4, 3 mM KCl, 1.5 mM KH_2PO_4, pH 7.4), fixed and permeabilized with 500 µl ice-cold methanol for 5 min at 4 °C. Then, cells are washed three times with PBS for 5 min each at room temperature and incubated in Tris-buffered saline (TBS; 10 mM Tris-HCl, 150 mM NaCl, pH 7.4) containing 0.5% fatty acid-free BSA to saturate non-specific binding sites at room temperature. After 45 min, cells are incubated for 1–2 hours at room temperature with the anti-c-myc 9E10 monoclonal mouse antibody (5 µg/ml; Roche) diluted in TBS containing 0.5% BSA, followed by washing of the cells three times with TBS plus 0.5% BSA for 5 min at room temperature. Subsequently, cells are incubated either with a fluorescein isothiocyanate-labeled (FITC) secondary anti-mouse sheep antibody or a tetramethyl rhodamine isothiocyanate-labeled (TRITC) secondary anti-mouse sheep antibody for 1 h at room temperature in the dark. After three washes with TBS plus 0.5% BSA for 5 min each and once in TBS for 5 min, the coverslips are mounted on glass slides using Mowiol 4-88 solution (2.4 g Mowiol 4-88 (Calbiochem), 6 g glycerol, 6 ml distilled water, 12 ml 0.2 M Tris-HCl, pH 8.0). Immunofluorescence is detected using a Zeiss Axiophot fluorescence microscope equipped with standards filter for the above mentioned secondary antibodies. Background staining of the cells should be determined by immunofluorescence of methanol-fixed non-transfected cells or by immunofluorescence of methanol-fixed transfected cells incubated with only secondary antibody. This background staining should be marginal compared with the positive controls.

Examples

Total and Non-Specific Binding of [^{3}H]NMS to Intact HEK-293 Cells Expressing M_2 mAChRs

As we have described above, mAChRs on the cell surface can be determined by measuring the binding of [^{3}H]NMS to intact cells. Figure 1 shows the internalization of M_2 mAChRs after 5 and 60 min of incubation with 10 µM carbachol. It is obvious that the level of nonspecific binding of [^{3}H]NMS should remain constant and independent of the time of incubation and carbachol treatment. In addition, total binding of [^{3}H]NMS to cells incubated without carbachol treatment should also remain constant. Figure 2 displays the extent of internalization of M_2 mAChR as percentage of initial cell surface receptor number. A 5 min incubation with 10 µM carbachol reduces cell surface receptor number by 14±3 %, with 70±4% of the initial number of receptors are internalized after 60 min of incubation with 10 µM carbachol.

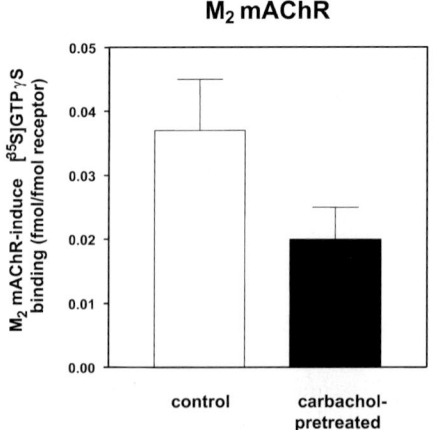

Figure 3
Carbachol-induced desensitization of M_2 mAChR-induced specific [^{35}S]GTPγS binding in membranes of HEK-293 cells. HEK-293 cells expressing M_2 mAChRs were incubated with or without 1 mM carbachol for 1 min at 37 °C. Then, cells were washed to remove agonist and partially purified membranes were made. M_2 mAChRs-induced specific [^{35}S]GTPγS binding was determined by incubating membranes of control and carbachol-treated cells with or without 1 mM carbachol for 15 min at 30 °C

M_2 mAChR-Induced [^{35}S]GTPγS Binding to Heterotrimeric G Proteins

Above, we have described a [^{35}S]GTPγS binding assay to determine M_2 mAChR-induced activation of heterotrimeric G proteins in isolated membranes from HEK-293 cells. As shown in Fig. 3, pre-treatment of HEK-293 cells with 1 mM carbachol for 1 min at 37 °C leads to a ~50% loss in M_2 mAChR-induced [^{35}S]GTPγS binding in isolated membranes upon a second receptor challenge with 1 mM carbachol for 15 min at 30 °C. This assay is therefore helpful in analyzing the initial steps in mAChR signal transduction with regard to the mechanism of G protein activation as well as regulation of mAChRs.

Immunocytochemical Localization of M_2 mAChR in HEK-293 Cells

We have used immunocytochemistry to determine the internalization of M_2 mAChRs in HEK-293 cells. For this, M_2 mAChR were tagged with a c-myc epitope at the extracellular amino terminus after the N-terminal methionine. As shown in Fig. 4, M_2 mAChRs in untreated HEK-293 cells can be found predominantly at the cell surface.

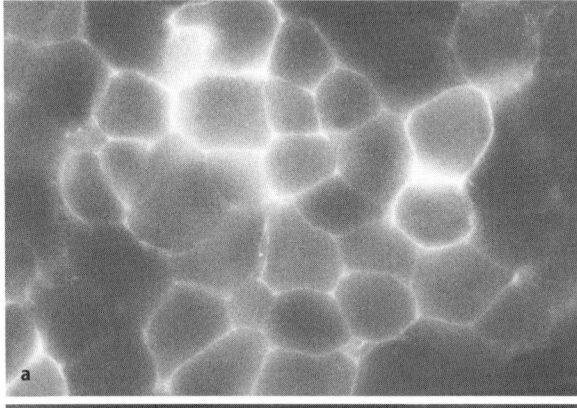

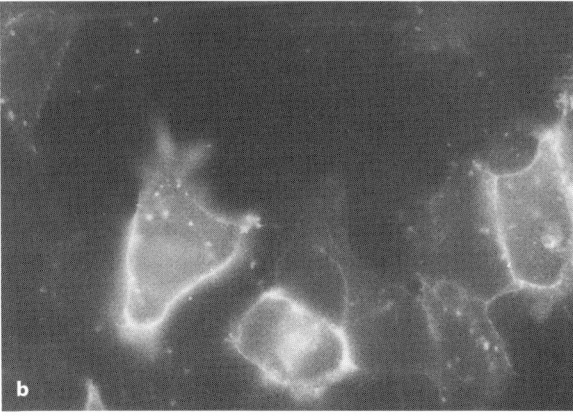

Figure 4a,b
Visualization of M_2 mAChR internalization in HEK-293 cells by immunofluorescence microscopy. HEK-293 cells stably expressing *myc*-tagged M_2 mAChRs were incubated in the absence (a) and presence (b) of 1 mM carbachol for 60 min at 37 °C. Then, cells were fixed and permeabilized with methanol and incubated with mouse anti-*myc* antibody followed by incubation with anti-mouse fluorescein isothiocyanate-labeled sheep secondary antibody and immunofluorescence was detected using a Zeiss Axiophot fluorescent microscope

After 60 min of incubation with 1 mM carbachol, M_2 mAChRs are subsequently found in the cell interior indicating that they have been translocated from the plasma membrane into the cytoplasm.

Troubleshooting

Radioligand Binding Assays

In principal, the length of incubation with the radioligand should be sufficiently long to attain steady-state equilibrium between radioligand association to and dissociation from the receptor. [^{3}H]QNB is the most widely used muscarinic receptor radioligand and incubation with [^{3}H]QNB is usually carried out at 37 °C for 60–90 min. However, as the binding of this slowly dissociating radioligand [^{3}H]QNB theoretically requires incubation periods of extreme length, the commonly used incubation period for [^{3}H]QNB represents a compromise between obtaining steady-state equilibrium and preventing mAChR degradation. In the case of [^{3}H]NMS, this is not an issue because [^{3}H]NMS dissociates much more rapidly at 37 °C. However, as [^{3}H]NMS binding assays are performed with intact cells, it is important that incubation with [^{3}H]NMS and washing of the cells are carried out at temperatures below 10 °C. At these temperatures, receptor transport does not take place.

M_2 mAChR-Stimulated Binding of [^{35}S]GTPγS to Heterotrimeric G Proteins

It is evident that the membrane isolation procedure should be rapid and carried out at 4 °C while storage of the membrane aliquots should be immediately at -70 °C. It is important to note that receptor-induced [^{35}S]GTPγS binding to G_i proteins is much more readily to detect than [^{35}S]GTPγS binding to $G_{q/11}$ proteins. For more details on optimizing the [^{35}S]GTPγS assay procedure, the reader is referred to Wieland and Jakobs (1994).

mAChR-Mediated Inhibition of cAMP Accumulation in Intact Cells

In general, inhibition of cAMP accumulation by M_2 and M_4 mAChRs is carried out in the presence of forskolin, which stimulates adenylyl cyclase directly, and a phosphodiesterase inhibitor, i.e., theophyllin. Under these conditions, the effects measured are based on the regulation of adenylyl cyclase activity by G_i proteins alone. While M_2 and M_4 mAChRs will usually alter cAMP levels by inhibition of adenylyl cyclase activity, in some cells M_1 and M_3 mAChRs may increase intracellular cAMP levels by stimulation of calmodulin-dependent adenylyl cyclases or via activation of G_s proteins. In other cell types, M_1 and M_3 mAChRs may, in the absence of phosphodiesterase inhibitors, also decrease intracellular cAMP levels due to stimulation of calmodulin-dependent phosphodiesterases. Thus, experiments on changes in cAMP accumulation in intact cells must be well planned and interpreted with careful attention to the assay conditions used.

mAChR-Mediated PLC-Activation

Basal and receptor-stimulated levels of phospholipase C can be critically dependent on cell density depending on the cell lines. So, careful attention to plating densities, growth and media conditions is necessary. In general, cellular uptake of myo-[^{3}H]inositol should be above 25%. In case of insufficient uptake, incorporation of myo-[^{3}H]inositol in the cells can be increased by using inositol-free medium or extending the labelling time.

Immunocytochemical Localization of mAChRs

The most obvious problems during immunocytochemical localization of mAChRs are the absence of specific immunofluorescence and the occurence of high non-specific labelling of the cells. It is possible that the primary antibody cannot recognize the native antigen. This may occur when the antibody has been raised against a denatured form of the antigen. When the immunofluorescence signal is weak, it also possible that the glass slides have not been stored in the dark prior to microscopy. On the other hand, bright spots of fluorescence can result from inadequate washing of the slides after immunolabelling with the antibodies or by the presence of unconjugated fluorochrome deposits. These spots may be avoided by centrifugation of the antibody stock solutions for 5 min at 13,000 g. When the labelling appears specific but the background staining is still high, it may be helpful to reduce antibody concentration and check whether the primary or secondary antibody bind with sufficient selectivity to the antigen.

References

Bonner TI, Buckley NJ, Young AC, Brann MR (1987) Identification of a family of muscarinic acetylcholine receptor genes. Science 237: 527–532
Bradford MM (1976) A rapid and sensitive method for the quantitation of microgram quantities of protein utilizing the principle of protein-dye binding. Anal Biochem 72: 248–254
Brodde OE, Michel M (1999) Adrenergic and muscarinic receptors in the human heart. Pharmacol Rev 51: 651–690
Caulfield MP (1993) Muscarinic receptors-characterization, coupling and function. Pharmacol Ther 58: 319–379
Dhein S, van Koppen CJ, Brodde OE (2001) Muscarinic receptors in the mammalian heart. Pharmacol Res 44: 161–182
Ferguson SSG (2001) Evolving concepts in G protein-coupled receptor endocytosis: The role in receptor desensitization and signaling. Pharmacol Rev 53: 1–24
Gilman AG (1970) A protein binding assay for adenosine 3':5'-cyclic monophosphate. Proc Natl Acad Sci USA 67: 305–312
Krupnick JG, Benovic JL (1998) The role of receptor kinases and arrestins in G protein-coupled receptor regulation. Annu Rev Pharmacol Toxicol 38: 289–319
Neer EJ (1995) Heterotrimeric G proteins: Organizers of transmembrane signals. Cell 80: 249–257
Peterson GL (1977) A simplification of the protein assay method of Lowry *et al.* which is more generally applicable. Anal Biochem 83: 346–356

Sharma VK, Colecraft HM, Rubin LE, Sheu SS (1997) Does mammalian heart contain only the M2 muscarinic receptor subtype? Life Sci 60: 1023–1029

Singer WD, Brown HA, Sternweis PC (1997) Regulation of eukaryotic phosphatidylinositol-specific phospholipase C and phospholipase D. Annu Rev Biochem 66: 475–509

Tobin AB, Totty NF, Sterlin AE, Nahorski SR (1997) Stimulus-dependent phosphorylation of G-protein-coupled receptors by casein kinase 1a. J Biol Chem 272: 20844–20849

van Koppen CJ, Kaiser B (2003) Regulation of muscarinic acetylcholine receptor signaling. Pharmacol Ther 98: 197–220

Wieland T, Jakobs KH (1994) Measurement of receptor-stimulated guanosine 5'-O-(γ-thio)triphosphate binding by G proteins. Meth Enzymol 237: 3–13

Cytometry in Cardiovascular Research

Attila Tárnok

Introduction

Almost 150 years after Rudolf Virchow's first publication on Cellularpathologie in 1859 (Virchow, 1859), cytological analyses still plays a fundamental role in clinical routine and decision-making. Besides conventional histology and cytology, cytometric assays are established standard procedures for numerous applications. Cytometry is a technological and analytical approach to quantitatively and rapidly analysing individual cells in heterogeneous populations, in order to stoichiometrically determine their constituents, which have been labelled with fluorescent dyes. The general principle of cytometric analysis is that, for a high number of individual cells within a (mixed) cell population, such as blood leukocytes, the total fluorescence intensity (integral fluorescence) is measured. The value of the integral fluorescence, is proportional to the brightness of a cell at a given fluorescence colour, and is therefore a direct measure of the number of fluorescent dye molecules per cell. These systems are multiplexed, as the cells can be labelled simultaneously with many different fluorescent dyes targeting different cell constituents. Cytometric systems are high throughput instruments that allow the collection of data of thousands of individual cells within seconds.

Cytometric analysis of biological samples are realised in two types of instruments:
- Flow Cytometers (FCM) and
- Slide Based Cytometers (SBC).

For analysis by both systems, samples that have been labelled with fluorescence dyes are excited by laser light or a mercury arc lamp. The generated fluorescence light is then detected by photomultipliers (PMTs), which convert the light signals into electronic signals. The amplitude of these electronic signals corresponds to the brightness of the objects. The difference between FCM and SBC is that, whereas FCM measures cells in suspension, SBC cells are fixed or adhere to a solid light-transmitting surface (glass or plastic). Therefore, FCM is most suitable for the measurement of blood and other bodily fluids, and SBC is more suited to tissue cultures and sections. Furthermore, whereas in FCM the cells are lost after analysis, in SBC they remain on the slide and may be subdued to additional preparatory steps or reanalysis. SBC is also best suited for hypocellular or precious specimens.

Cytometry instruments are intended to detect many different fluorescence colours. The only restrictions in the dyes used, is whether they are excited by the laser lines available, and the fluorescence signals are detectable by the optical filters of the respective instrument. With lasers, the most common excitation lines are blue excitation at 488 nm (with an Argon (Ar) ion laser) and red excitation around 630 nm (with a diode or a Helium Neon (HeNe) laser). This restricts the use of fluorescence labels to those excitable in the blue or red. The most common label for staining of proteins such as antibodies, are the 488 nm excitable dyes: fluorescein-isothiocyanate (FITC), phycoerythrin (PE, RPE), peridinin chlorophyll protein (PerCP™ trademark of BD Biosciences), and tandem dyes that rely on fluorescence resonance energy transfer (PE, TexasRed, PE-Cy5, PE-Cy5.5, PE-Cy7 etc.). With red excitation, the dyes allophycocyanine (APC) and the fluorescence resonance energy transfer dyes APC-Cy5.5 and APC-Cy7 may be used. In addition, there are a great variety of dyes for DNA, RNA, and protein labelling, as well as for cell function (for an overview see Haugland 2002). The fluorescence colours that are detected by the PMTs are defined by the optical filters (usually dichroic and bandpass filters) that are placed in the optical path.

One important characteristic of cytometry is the way the data are stored. This is done in a standardised form, so called "list mode" data, that is in agreement with the flow cytometry standard format FCS (Shapiro 2003). In brief, in list-mode format, values of every measured event (i.e. every cell) are stored separately in a list and can later be retrieved for each individual event with all values measured. By using this approach, values may be displayed in any possible data combination, which in multi-colour experiments allows the detection of cells with unique combinations of antigen expression. In FCS format, in addition to the primary data, also key information about the measurement such as the exact instrument setting, date and time of the analysis, number of events and comments are archived, and may be retrieved at a later time.

Two typical ways to display list-mode data are the dot-plot display (as an example see Fig. 1a), and the histogram display (Fig. 1b). In a dot-plot, the values of two different parameters of an event are shown in a two dimensional display. Each dot on this graph displays the values for one cell or particle. In the histogram display, the cell values are displayed versus their frequency (cell count). In both displays, regions can be drawn in the graph and the statistics for the events inside this region (i.e. cell count, frequency, integral fluorescence value) can be displayed. In addition, the events within this region can be separately displayed in another histogram or dot-plot. This process is termed "gating", and allows scrutiny of the data for populations within higher than two-dimensional hierarchies.

Figure 1 ▶
Typical calibration of fluorescence intensity scaling of cytometry instruments with spherotech rainbow™ microbeads. a Dot-plot displaying forward versus sideward light scatter. The particles gated in R1 are used for subsequent analysis. b Intensity distribution histogram of beads with six (FCM) or eight (LSC) intensity populations. The left two histograms display intensity distribution in the FITC channel, the right in the PE channel. The numbers in each histogram correspond to the molecule numbers per bead population as provided by the manufacturer. c Calibration curves for FITC (*left*) and PE (*right*). Molecule numbers versus Integral fluorescence measured by LSC (open symbols, left vertical scale) or FCM (FACSCalibur BD Biosciences, closed symbol, right vertical scales)

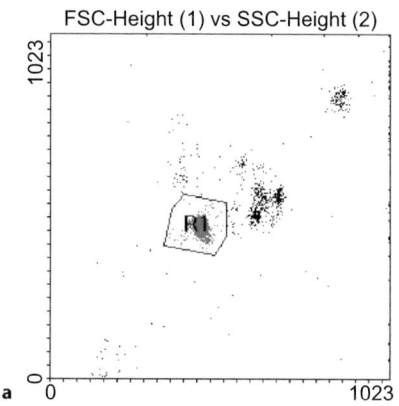

Calibration of the Cytometry with fluorescent beads

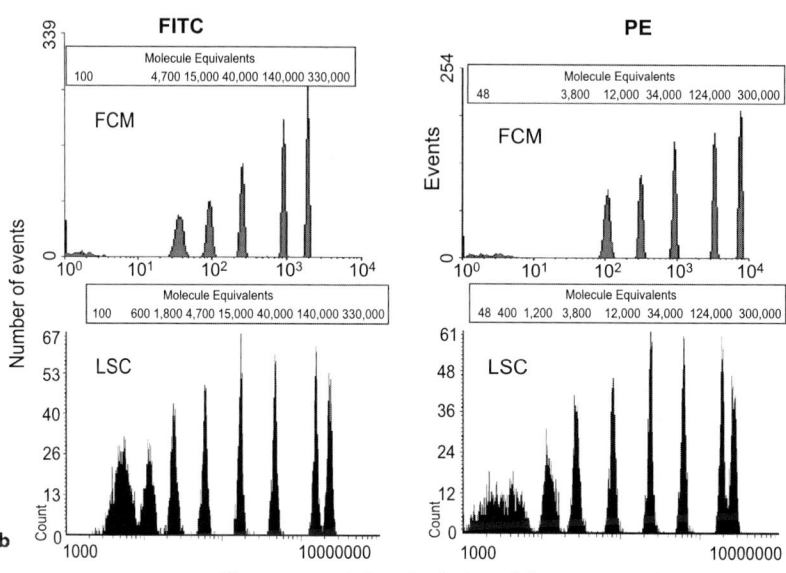

Flurescence intensity (integral fluorescence)

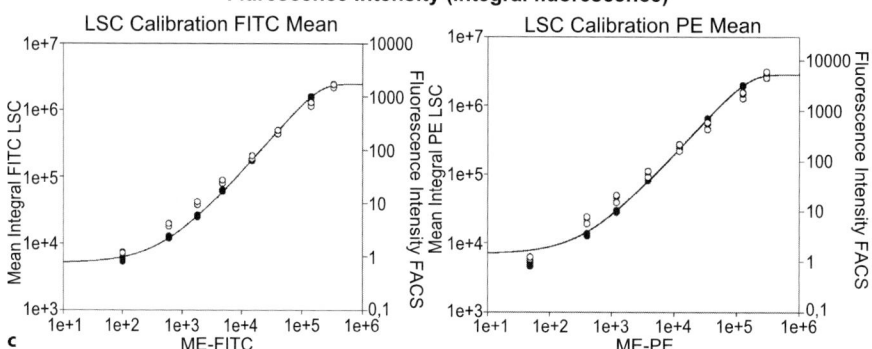

Flow Cytometry

Since the introduction of commercially available flow cytometers in the 1960's for clinical diagnosis (ICP-11 by Phywe GmbH; Dittrich and Göhde 1969), this technology became the most commonly applied multiparametric fluorescence analyses of cells in suspension (Dittrich and Göhde 1970). Flow cytometry (FCM) allows the detection of minor cell sub-populations at high speed, and their discrimination based on two morphological parameters (forward and sideward or orthogonal light scatter, FSC and SSC, respectively) and a multitude of expression patterns. Rapid throughput and standardisation, makes FCM a versatile routine clinical diagnostic tool. Common fields of application for FCM are DNA-ploidy, cell cycle analysis of tumours, and immunophenotyping of leukaemia, immune deficiency and graft vs. host disease, among others. The ability to monitor the cells' morphology by FCM, however, is limited to FSC and SSC, but morphological information is of particular interest in pathology. In the 70's, this handicap led to the implementation of the electrostatic cell sorter into FCM (Crissman et al., 1975), and the development of mechanical cell sorters. Cell sorting allows the purification of cells of interest, but is technically demanding, expensive and in most settings, not applicable for routine clinical purposes. Therefore, the demand for technologies soon arose that would combine the advantages of both rapid multiparametric analysis and cell morphology (Kachel et al. 1997; Kamentsky and Kamentsky 1991). Today, several high quality instruments are commercial available, which are able to routinely analyse four to nine colours at a time.

Slide Based Cytometry

Although the concept of SBC dates back into the mid 80's, the Laser Scanning Cytometer (LSC) was the first instrument to come up years later. The LSC was introduced in the early 1990's (Kamentsky and Kamentsky 1991), and became commercially available in 1996. It is a microscope-based instrument, which fills the gap between high throughput multiparametric cytometry and morphological analysis and documentation. Instrumentation and software of the LSC is explained elsewhere (Kamentsky and Kamentsky 1991; Tarnok and Gerstner 2002). In brief, the instrumentation is built around a routine epi-fluorescence microscope, which is equipped with a motorised stage that holds the microscope slide. The specimen is immobilised on a conventional glass slide and analysed by excitation with either one or two single laser beams. The actual set-up of the LSC allows excitation with blue (488 nm, argon laser) or red (630 nm, helium neon laser) light. The instrument can be upgraded with a violet (405 nm) diode laser that measures co-linearly with the HeNe laser, and can be very useful for measuring DNA staining with dyes such as 4',6-diamidion-2-phenylindole (DAPI) and HOECHST (bisbenzimid).

The area on the glass slide to be measured is scanned stepwise. The fluorescent light emitted is guided to an optical bench equipped with four PMTs. With this equipment, four fluorescent colours can be distinguished with a single excitation. Above all, data recently presented show that, with appropriate minor modifications in the filter settings, the instrument is able to detect and quantify up to six different fluorochromes simultaneously (Gerstner et al. 2002). Moreover, the excitation light scattered by the specimen, is detected by a photodiode below the slide producing a signal called "forward scatter", a parameter related to the cells' morphology. After each step of the scan, a digital image is created for each PMT (i.e. for each fluorescence). Analysis can be performed with the proprietary software (WinCyte™), according to the operator's settings.

A unique feature of the LSC, is its function to review each cell of a measurement, due to the x-y recording of the position of each measured event. With this feature, each cell can be visualised in a light or microscopic manner, and even its fluorescence can be recorded any time during, and even after the end of the measurement. With the aid of this function, it is possible to verify the measured data, particularly:
- If objects are single cells, doublets, debris or artefacts
- Document the cells morphology or fluorescence

By cytometry in general, irrespective if by FCM or SBC, any cellular parameter can be analysed by itself or in combination with other parameters, as long as these cell properties can be tagged in some way to fluorescent dyes. Among the most important applications of cytometry, are the determinations of:
- Cell surface or intracellular antigen expression
- Cell physiology (intracellular free Ca2+, intracellular pH, oxidative burst etc.)
- Apoptosis (annexin V assay, mitochondrial membrane potential, DNA fragmentation a.o.)
- Intracellular cytokine expression
- Molecular biology (DNA content, fluorescence *in situ* hybridisation, etc.)

It is beyond the scope of this chapter to detail all the different applications of Cytometry in Cardiology. For a comprehensive overview of methods and applications, the reader is referred to the appropriate textbooks (Robinson et al., 2003). For more detailed information on Cytometry technologies refer to standard works on cytometry (e.g. Shapiro 2003).

In cardiology cytometry, FCM particularly has been used in various fields of clinical research. Among others, leukocyte activation was determined during cardiosurgical trauma. The following chapter focuses on the quantitative analysis of leukocyte activation marker expression by FCM.

Determination of Leukocyte Activation Marker Expression by FCM

The measurement of the expression level of adhesion molecules and activation markers on circulating leukocytes has been used in the recent years in various aspects of cardiology, for example, the analysis of leukocyte activation during cardiovascular surgery (Hambsch et al. 2002), and early detection of sepsis. It has also been used in different aspects of predictive medicine (Valet and Tarnok 2003), such as, pre-operative assessment of patients at risk of post-operative capillary leak syndrome (Tarnok et al. 2001), detection of patients with unstable coronary artery disease (Mazzone et al. 1993), and risk assessments of patients with early in-stent restenosis (Rahimi et al. 2003). This chapter will focus on the approach of quantitating cell surface expression of adhesion molecules on leukocytes, e.g. in patients with coronary artery disease, for predictive medicine. In principle, this assay is applicable for all assays, where antigen expression determination is a key issue.

Despite the progress in coronary stent implantation, clinical success is still limited by restenosis (Fishman et al. 1994). In-stent restenosis is mainly caused by neointimal proliferation, as an inflammatory reaction to the mechanical wall injury (Bittl 1996). However, it is still unknown why stenting leads to reactions of differing extent among patients. Taking specific risk factors into consideration may have the potential of reducing the restenosis rate, by choosing an individualised treatment. Besides lesion-related risk factors, such as lesion length, vessel diameter and length of the stent, three patient-related prognostic factors for restenosis after stenting were identified: systemic inflammatory status, diabetes mellitus and deletion polymorphism of the ACE gene (Buffon et al. 1999).

Clinical studies have shown a subsequent activation of adhesion molecules on leukocytes in patients with restenosis after intervention (Kamijikkoku et al. 1998). Adhesion molecules, i.e. interacting selectins, integrins and their ligands, facilitate the recruitment of circulating leukocytes, leading to their transient rolling along the endothelium, diapedesis and subsequent transmigration to sites of inflammation (Springer 1994). L-Selectin, is constitutively expressed on leukocytes and often shed after activation. This leads to up-regulation of the β_2-integrin complex, (CD11/CD18) (Lefer 1997), which is required for a stronger attachment to the endothelium and subsequent transmigration. Ligands of integrins are the intercellular adhesion molecules, i.e. ICAM-1 (Springer 1994). The activation of adhesion molecules after coronary intervention, confirms the induction of a systemic inflammatory response by coronary angioplasty and subsequent stent implantation (Azar et al. 1997).

The role of adhesion molecules, however, and their pre-procedural levels in the multifactorial process of restenosis is not yet well known. Our group demonstrated the predictive potential of pre-operative adhesion molecule expression on monocytes and granulocytes in risk assessment for postoperative inflammatory reactions (Tarnok et al. 2001).

In the present example, it will be demonstrated how pre-procedural adhesion molecule expression on leukocytes and their expression levels directly correlate with restenosis, and subsequently can be assessed to identify patients with an increased risk of restenosis. This example is based on recently published material investigating L-selectin (CD62L), LFA-1 (CD11a/CD18), Mac-1 (CD11b/CD18), ICAM-1 (CD54) and MHC II (HLA-DR) expression on leukocytes, in patients before angiography and in healthy volunteers as control (Rahimi et al. 2003).

Cytometric analysis is an ideal technological platform for the novel clinical concept of predictive medicine. Predictive medicine aims at the detection of changes in patient's disease state, prior to the manifestation of deterioration or improvement of the current status. Such instances may concern multi organ failure in sepsis or non-infectious posttraumatic shock in intensive care, or the pre-therapeutic identification of high-risk patients in surgical therapy (overview in Valet and Tárnok 2003). Individualised disease course predictions for currently envisaged standard therapies would definitively allow, in many instances, early curative interaction by specific therapeutic measures, prior to the occurrence of irreversible tissue destruction with its inherent potential to incapacitate the patient, in many instances, on a longer run. Predictive medicine is based on the analysis of the CYTOME of an individual patient. Cytome/Cytomics, is the multimolecular cytometric analysis of the cellular heterogeneity of cytomes (cellular systems/organs/body) accessing a maximum of information on the apparent molecular cell phenotype in disease. The term Cytomics carries a disciplinary aspect. It was coined by molecular botanists in analogy to Genomics and Proteomics, describing the analyses of the genome, the Proteome and the Cytome (http://www.genomicglossaries.com/content/omes.asp). Although the term is method independent, Cytometry technologies provide typical CYTOMICS platforms (Valet 2002).

Endothelial Progenitor Cell Quantitation by SBC

This method deals with one of the typical applications of SBC, focusing on one of its major advantages in cytometric sample analysis, the multiplexed analysis of adherent cells in culture (Lenz et al. 2003). For more on clinical applications of SBC see Tarnok and Gerstner (2002).

The dogma that vasculogenesis (i.e. proliferation of entirely new vessels into tissues) is limited to embryogenesis, was shattered by the evidence of endothelial progenitor cells (EPCs) in the peripheral blood of adults by Asahara et al. (1997) and Lin et al. (2000). Studies with human patients, showed a higher incidence of putative precursor cells of EPCs (mononuclear cells that were CD34$^+$ and expressed endothelial markers) in the peripheral blood of infarct patients, compared to a group of healthy control patients (Takahashi et al., 1999). In culture, these putative progenitors formed clusters, and cells were positive for endothelial cell lineage markers such as CD31 (PECAM), vascular endothelial cadherin, and kinase insert domain receptors. Myocardial and lower extremity-ischemia-induced angiogenic growth factors, and a resulting appearance of EPCs, was shown by Kalka et al. (2000) in animal experiments. In another study molecular- and cytobiologic assays indicated that several growth factors stimulated the mobilisation of the EPCs from the bone marrow (Takahashi et al. 1999). However, the amount of mobilised EPCs and their migration to the site of an ischemia, as a reaction to an ischemic insult, seems not to be adequate for a curative neovascularisation. Also, when ex vivo expanded EPCs were injected locally into an area of insufficient blood supply, this led to a dramatic improvement of the local blood support.

Concurrently, it was shown in athymic mice with hind limb ischemia who received ex vivo expanded human EPCs, that the capillary density in the ischemic area was higher and the rate of limb loss was significantly reduced, against a control group of animals without human EPCs (Kalka et al. 2000). The authors proposed the use of EPCs for therapeutic neovascularisation (Kalka et al. 2000; Strauer et al. 2002). The first experiments that have been performed in humans recently (Strauer et al. 2002), clearly showed the potency of this novel therapeutic approach in treating and curing sites of infarct and improper blood supply. These very promising results, may in future lead to standardised therapy of infarct patients, by ex vivo expanding their own EPCs isolated from their peripheral blood mononuclear leukocyte fraction, and reinjection directly into the sites of a seizure.

Although the clinical and experimental developments are very promising, there is a need for standardisation of the analytical part of the therapeutic protocols. In infarct patients, as well as in patients with diabetes mellitus, the number of ex vivo expandable EPCs varies highly by a factor of 10 or even more (Tepper et al. 2002; Shintani et al. 2001). Therefore, under standardised culture conditions, the number of reinjected EPCs may vary by an order of magnitude, depending on the patients EPC yield. In order to have a sufficiently reliable way to quantify the number of EPCs that will be reinjected, quantitative cytometric methods are necessary. The assays used so far to quantify the number of expanded EPCs are clearly insufficient. In the short-term (i.e. 4–7 d) cultures that are used for reimplantation into the patient, the residual cell population consists of a mixture of different cells types (not only EPCs but also surviving leukocytes and possibly other cells). In order to unequivocally characterise EPCs in culture, it is unavoidable to use simultaneously different markers for EPCs (e.g. DiI LDL, and VEGF-receptor) and for residual leukocytes (e.g. by CD45 the pan-leukocyte antigen). Manual analysis of specimens labelled by three different colours is not only tedious but also inaccurate.

Above all, all publications so far estimated ("quantified") the number of EPCs in the culture chambers by manually counting the number of cells in about four "arbitrary" regions. Quantification of cells in this way is highly unreliable, and certainly not useful therapy monitoring. The arbitrary positioning of the counting areas is inaccurate because the cells in culture are discontinuously distributed over the dish (Tepper et al. 2002). Therefore, it is important to count all cells of interest in a culture dish for standardised quality control.

One method in quantifying EPCs is by FCM as the golden standard for immunophenotyping of peripheral blood leukocytes. This is due to the high throughput, multiparametric analysis, possibility to detect rare events and weak signals, and the availability of standardised preparation and analysis protocols worldwide. Thus, it fits for the determination of the very rare putative precursor cells. In contrast, it is not possible to measure immobilised cells with FCM without removing them from the culture dishes by rigorous mechanical and enzymatic treatment. This obstacle may be overcome by applying SBC as an analytical tool for the quantitation of the attached cells in culture (Lenz et al. 2003). This technology was chosen to estimate the cultured EPCs in the culture dishes (Lenz et al. 2003).

For this study, the special features of the LSC allow the measurement of cultured cells on the slide and verification of the results. This novel slide based approach, for the standardised quantitation of EPCs may be suited for routine clinical use in future.

Description of Methods and Practical Approach
Standardisation and Calibration

Calibration

For the quantitative and reproducible analysis of antigen expression levels (i.e. molecule numbers per cell), it is crucial that instrument performance and sample preparation are highly standardised. In particular, if expression levels are monitored over time, if absolute expression levels are measured for comparison between patients or, if experiments are performed at different institutions or using different instruments, it is pivotal to ensure that a measured fluorescence intensity always equals a comparable number of fluorescent molecules. On the one hand, the position of a cell on the scale reflecting its brightness is not absolute but depends on the instrument setting, in particular on the PMT voltage and optical filters. Therefore, a cell may be positioned on any value of fluorescence intensity by changing the instrument set-up. On the other hand, even if the instrument settings are identical, measurements of identical samples may differ substantially between instruments. These differences are due to product dependent variations in the performance of the instruments (e.g. sensitivity of the PMTs, type of optical filters) or loss of instrument sensitivity with time e.g. due to dirtying of the optical path, among others. It is therefore evident, that for instrument independent analysis, daily instrument calibration is necessary.

In principle, there are two ways for instrument standardisation: internal or external calibration. For internal standardisation standard calibration particles (microbeads) are stained with the antibodies of interest i.e. a cell. These beads contain a defined number of anti-mouse immuno-globuline antibodies on their surface, and are stained like the cells with fluorescence labelled mouse anti-human antibodies. Under saturating conditions, the brightness of the stained beads can be directly translated into molecule numbers per cell (Bikoue et al. 2002). An even better internal standard are the antigens on the cells to be analysed. As reference antigens, those with known and relatively stable surface numbers are suited. These are, for example, lineage markers such as CD45, CD3 and CD4 among others (Bikoue et al. 2002). Antigens indicating cell activation are inappropriate. Following staining with the appropriate anti-CD antigen at saturating concentrations, the measured brightness per cell at any given colour can be directly translated into molecule numbers, and even be used to construct calibration curves.

Although not as accurate as the internal calibration, external calibration is a simple and reproducible way to standardise instrument set-up. Here, standard microbeads that are stable and labelled with fluorescent dyes are used. These types of beads are commercially available from several providers. Best suited, are beads that consist of several bead populations of different brightness. One type of beads, Rainbow™ beads from Spherotech (Libertyville, IL, USA), is available in sets of eight or six different levels of brightness. For analysis, the particles are diluted 1/10 in phosphate buffered saline (PBS Sigma-Aldrich Chemie GmbH, Deisenhofen, Germany), and data of about 10,000 events are collected at the identical instrument setting as that for the cells.

For further analysis, the data are displayed as a dot-plot of FSC versus SSC. These events are displayed as histograms of each fluorescence (e.g. see Fig. 1b), by placing a gate around the major population (see Fig. 1a). The events that fall outside the gate are mostly bead aggregates, and non-bead events such as crystals. The fluorescence intensity values may be used to calculate a calibration curve to translate fluorescence intensity values into fluorescence molecule equivalents per cell (see Fig. 1c). This calculation is done by four parametric logistic or four parametric sigmoidal regression, using commercial software packages (SPSS, Canyon Lake, TX), or the calculation program provided by the bead manufacturer.

Once the cytometry instrument has been calibrated, during subsequent analysis of the samples of interest, PMT settings must not be changed. Otherwise, the calibration curve is not applicable for the determination of antigen numbers.

Titration of Antibodies and Dyes

New monoclonal antibodies should be titrated to determine the saturation concentrations. In order to determine the saturation concentrations of antibodies, a given number of cells are stained with varying antibody concentrations and the respective fluorescence intensities are recorded. By increasing the concentration, the fluorescence intensity of labelled cells should increase up to a maximal level and plateau. This is the saturation concentration. It is also important to take non-specific binding into account, as this will increase with increasing antibody concentration. Non-specific binding can either be checked within the test sample on cells that should not be stained (e.g. when testing a T-cell marker B-cells may be used as control cells), or alternatively, so called control antibodies (see below) may be used, or the binding of the specific antibody is blocked by pre-staining with excessive amounts of unlabelled antibody of the identical specificity. The specific fluorescence intensity is the difference of the brightness of antibody labelled cells subtracted by the respective back ground. The antibody concentrations used in the experiments should be slightly above saturating concentrations in order to take variations in cell numbers into account.

Negative Control

For every cytometry measurement, it is crucial to also measure the brightness of the cells that are not specific to the respective antibody. This may be done, by simply measuring unlabelled cells that were otherwise treated as the stained cells. A better choice is to use control antibodies. Control antibodies for anti-human antibodies, are pre-absorbed against the antigens of humans, and should therefore only bind non-specifically. Fluorescence intensities of cells stained with these control antibodies reflect background staining. Control antibodies should be selected so that they are from the same species and have the identical immunoglobuline subclass (if possible) as the respective specific antibodies.

The position on the scale of the cells stained with control antibodies serves as the threshold for the discrimination of labelled and unlabelled cells. The specific brightness (fluorescence intensity or Integral fluorescence), is calculated as the difference of the brightness of cells labelled with specific and control antibody.

FCM Analysis of Leukocyte Activation Markers

Sampling and Blood Preparation

Peripheral blood from the antecubital vein is sampled just prior to angiography, between 7 and 8 a.m. with a 21-gauge needle, from randomly recruited patients e.g. with stable angina and healthy volunteers. Standardised sampling time is important in order to minimise the effect of circadianic variations of antigen expression on the circulating leukocytes. EDTA anti-coagulated whole blood is immediately processed. Four tubes are filled with 40 µl blood each and incubated with monoclonal antibodies (mab) in the dark for 15 min at 20 °C. Red blood cells are lysed by 1 ml lysing solution (BD Biosciences, San Jose, CA). Cells are mixed and incubated in the dark for another 10 min at 20 °C. After centrifugation at $1,400 \times g$ for 15 min, cells are washed using 1.5 ml PBS (Sigma-Aldrich Chemie GmbH), subsequently centrifuged at 1,400 G for 10 min. and resuspended for fixation in 0.5 ml of 0.5% paraformaldehyde (Sigma) in PBS, freshly filtered through a 0.22 µm pore filter and stored in the dark at 4 °C. Measurements should be performed within 2–3 h after sampling.

Monoclonal Antibodies (mab)

Isotype anti-murine (mu) mab anti-mu-IgG_1 [FITC], anti-mu-IgG_{2a} [PE], anti-mu-IgG_1 [PerCP] and anti-mu-IgG_1 [APC] serve as control. For staining, commercially available fluorescence-dye labelled anti-human-mab may be used:
  anti-CD18 [FITC] clone MHM23 (Dako, Golstrup, Denmark), anti-CD11a [PE] clone HI111 (Pharmingen, San Diego, CA), anti-CD3 [APC] clone S4.1 (Caltag, Hamburg, Germany), anti-CD11b [PE] clone D12 (BD Biosciences), anti-CD16/anti-CD56 [TRC] clone 3G8 and NKI-nbl-1 (Caltag), anti-CD62L [PE] clone Dreg-56 (Pharmingen), anti-CD54 [FITC] clone 84H10 (Immunotech, Marseille, France), anti-HLA-DR [PerCP] clone L243 (BD Biosciences), CD3 [APC] clone S4.1 (Caltag). Antibodies from other providers may also be used, but need testing prior to application.

Measurement by FCM

Analysis in the presented example was performed by a FACScalibur™ (BD Biosciences) flow cytometer. Routine daily procedure of these instruments includes performance testing and calibration using standard reference Spherobeads (Spherotech Inc.) as outlined above. New monoclonal antibodies should be titrated to determine the saturating concentrations.
  Cell analysis is usually triggered on forward light scatter (FSC). Both FSC and SSC are measured on a linear scale. The threshold level is set so that all leukocytes, including small lymphocytes, are included, but erythrocytes and platelets are excluded from the analysis. Care should be taken that the threshold value is positioned neither too tight to the cell population with the lowest FSC values, (lymphocytes) nor too far to the left. In the first case, cells of interest will be lost from the measurement because all events below the threshold will not be recorded. In the latter case, data of too many events of non-leukocyte origin (crystals, cell debris, red blood cells, platelet aggre-

gates) will be collected. All fluorescence is measured on a logarithmic scale. Typically, in total, data of about 50,000 events are collected. It is recommended that staining and measurement of each sample is duplicated.

Analysis and Data Display of FCM Measurements

Analysis of FCM data is performed by the instrument's proprietary analysis software (e.g. CellQuest™, BD Biosciences). Alternatively, other commercial analysis software or shareware can be used. Nowadays, FCM data are highly standardised and belong to either the FCS2.0 or FCS 3.0 standard. Therefore, FCM data analysis software is generally able to analyse data obtained on any newer FCM instrument.

To analyse the data obtained from whole blood measurements, the initial procedure is to identify and gate for the major leukocyte subsets as shown in Fig. 2a. Lympho-, mono- and granulocytes are distinguished by FSC versus SSC (i.e. particle size versus granularity; Fig. 2a). These gates are used to exclude doublets and debris from smaller cells that were accidentally included into the first gate, i.e. are above the threshold. Lymphocytes can be sub-classified by the lineage markers CD3/CD16+ CD56 (T- and NK-cells) determination (not shown). Expression of adhesion molecules (CD11a, CD11b, CD18, CD54, CD62L and HLA-DR) is measured on each subpopulation as the difference between the specific assays, and the mean intensity of control antibody-stained assay, and calculated using calibration beads as standard. Data can be expressed as mean fluorescence intensity (MFI). Alternatively, the molecule numbers per cell population can be calculated using the calibration curve that has been generated with e.g. the standard beads.

These data may then be further subdued to sophisticated statistical analysis. Typically within, and between, group comparisons with parametric or non-parametric statistics are performed (among others Kruskal-Wallis test, Mann-Whitney test (SPSS, Version 8.0, Canyon Lake, TX)). Of particular interest for predictive medicine (Valet and Tarnok 2003), are statistics for group discrimination with data-mining capabilities, such as multivariate discriminant analysis (SPSS) or CLASSIF 1 (Valet 2002).

LSC Analysis of EPCs

Blood Sampling

Peripheral blood is obtained from e.g. healthy young adult volunteers. A volume of 12 ml venous blood is taken in EDTA-containing syringes. The cells are prepared for short-term cultures, which are then analysed by the LSC.

Short-Term Cell Culture and Staining

According to the method of Vasa and colleagues (2001), mononuclear cells are isolated from the obtained EDTA supplemented blood samples by density gradient centrifugation of peripheral blood over a Ficoll-Hypaque density gradient (Gibco BRL., Gaithersburg, MD, USA). After isolation, 2×10^6 cells are plated on gelatine coated

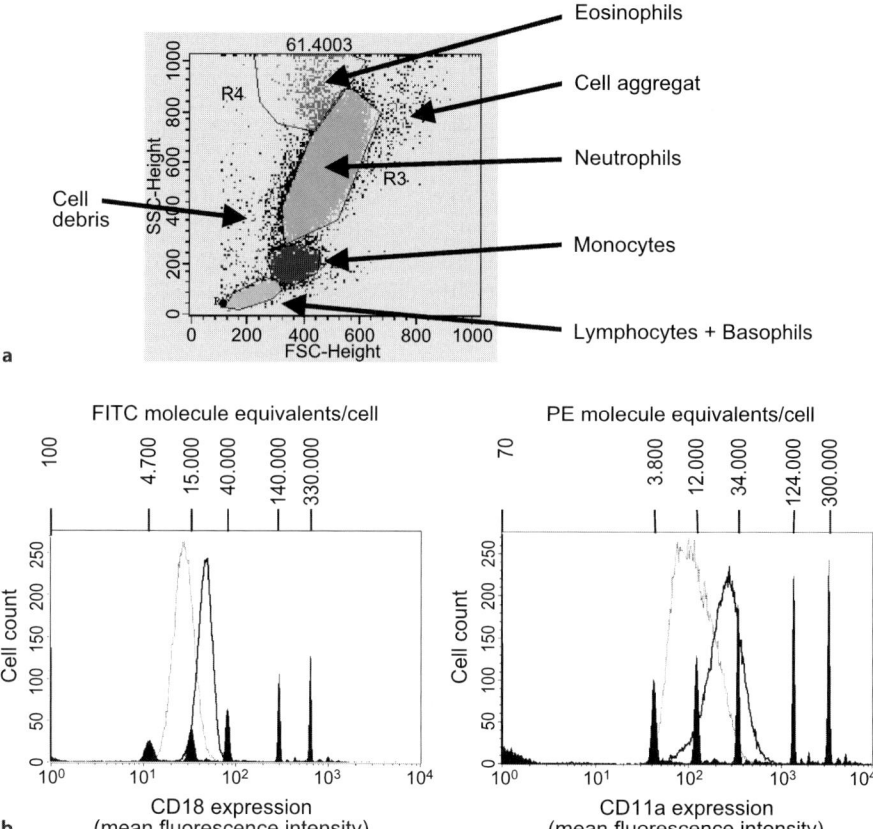

Figure 2a,b
Flow cytometric analysis of peripheral blood leukocytes for the determination of adhesion molecule expression (LFA-1: CD11a/CD18). In the *top* figure (a) cell morphology (FSC versus SSC) is displayed for all leukocytes. In this display four different clusters can be distinguished as indicated by the gates. These clusters can be assigned to different leukocyte sub-populations. In the *bottom* two histograms (b) the fluorescence intensity of neutrophils as gated in the top figure is displayed for a patient with relatively low (*hatched lines*) and high antigen expression (*through lines*). The overlaid black bars display the position of the calibration particles. The bottom image shows that the difference in the mean antigen number is about 20,000 for CD18 and 30,000 for CD11a

4-well chamber slides (NUNC, Wiesbaden, Germany) in medium (medium 199, containing 20% calf serum, Gibco) and growth factor supplement (CCpro, Neustadt, Germany) and antibiotics (Pen/Strept, Gibco). After four days in culture on the slide non-adherent cells are removed by rinsing with culture medium. For EPC staining the residual adherent cells are incubated for 1 h at 37 °C with 2.4 mg/ml DiI-LDL (1,1 dioctadecyl-3,3,3,3-tetramethylindocarbocyanine-labeled acetylated low density lipoprotein, Molecular Probes, Eugene, OR, USA), diluted 1/300 in culture medium. The staining is performed in three of the four chambers. One is left DiI-free as a negative control. Fixation with paraformaldehyde (2% in PBS) for 10 min is followed by incubation with UEA-1 (FITC-labelled Ulex europaeus agglutinin I, Sigma, Deisenhofen, Germany) for 1 h. Optimal UEA-1 concentrations are tested by titration. Again, only three chambers are stained (the two DiI labeled and the one unlabeled as a negative control for DiI), one chamber is left lectin-free as a negative control for FITC. After a final rinsing with cell culture medium, the plastic chambers of the chamber slide are removed, and the samples are covered with a fluorescent mounting medium (DAKO) and covered with a coverslip. The specimens should be analysed on the Laser Scanning Cytometer (LSC, Compucyte Corp.) within the next 24 h. The measurement is affected by the length of storage, but in our hands the results were virtually identical, even after up to two weeks of storage in the dark at 4 °C.

EPC Sample Analysis

The microscope slide with the specimen is placed onto the motorised stage of the microscope. Data acquisition is performed using the proprietary software of the LSC, WinCyte™ (Compucyte Corp.) Using the software, four rectangular scan regions are created per slide (Fig. 3). Each of these scan areas covers one of the four chambers of the chamber slide. Positioning of the areas is checked microscopically. The scan areas have to cover a slightly greater area than that of the bottom of a chamber. This is necessary in order to ensure that all cells of the respective chamber are measured. For excitation, the 488 nm line of the Ar-Laser is used. Triggering signals for cell detection are both the FITC fluorescence (green, measured in the detector FL1) of the lectin, and the orange fluorescence of the DiI (measured in Fl2). Both signals are combined into a so-called Add parameter. An Add parameter combines the signals from different detectors that are excited by one laser (in our case Ar). The maximum number of Add signals with Ar is five (four types of fluorescence and light scatter). Parameters from two different lasers cannot be added. This add parameter is then regarded as a novel parameter and can be used for triggering. The minimum area per cell is set to 10 μm^2 in order to exclude cell debris and other smaller artefacts from the analysis. The data

Figure 3 ▶
Analysis and gating strategy of EPCs on chamber slides. All analysed cells are displayed in an X-Y-dot-plot (*top left*). In this display, the data are seen as a virtual slide showing events in the four stripes corresponding to the four chambers on the chamber slide. Cells in the left and second left stripe were stained with lectin-FITC or DiI-LDL alone, and served as single colour controls. The second two stripes were stained with both dyes and served as specimens for EPC enumeration. The data from each stripe were then displayed as a dot plot of DiI-LDL Integral fluorescence versus FITC-lectin Integral fluorescence (*bottom dot-plots*). The control samples were used to construct a quadrant that contained less than 1% double positive cells for both control samples. The cells in this quadrant were determined with the doubled stained samples. As an example, patient 1 is a patient with low EPCs, whilst patient 2 has a relatively high number of EPCs.
An alternative gating strategy is that data are first displayed as a dot-plot of cell area versus Forward Scatter Max pixel (not shown). In this display, a gate can be created including cells with intermediate Max Pixel values and an area of around 150 μm^2. Dots with lower Max Pixel value are cell debris. (By courtesy of Dr. V. Adams, Dept. of Cardiology, Herzzentrum Leipzig GmbH, University of Leipzig, Germany)

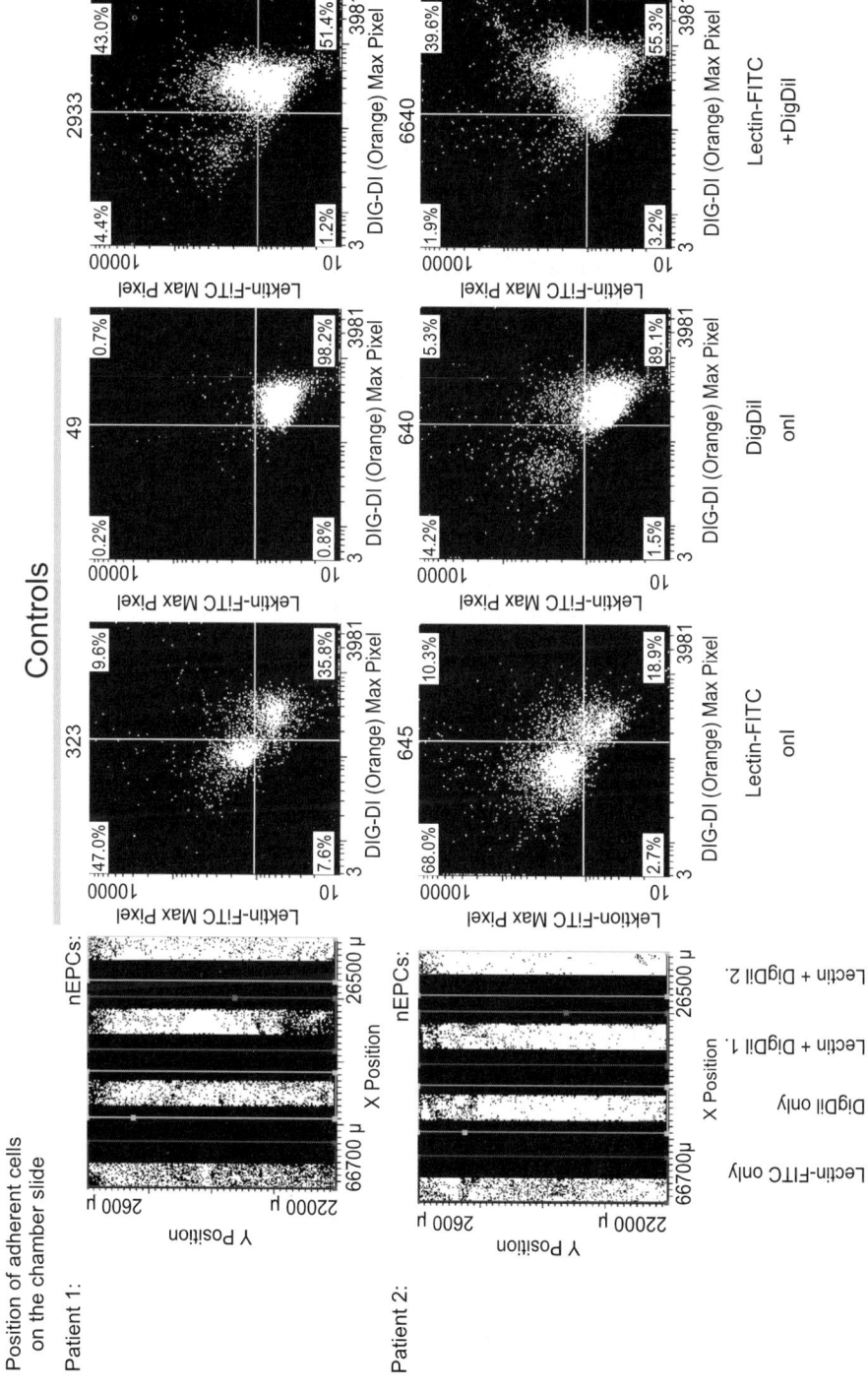

acquisition is started, and the scan data images that are produced by the PMTs for FITC, DiI and the Add parameter are checked for proper recognition by the software in the scan data image display (not shown). If not all cells are recognised, or too many cells are merged into one object, the threshold value has to be modified accordingly. It is also important to adjust the PMTs so that stained cells are in scale but are not over-modulated. This is best checked by, displaying the fluorescence max pixel for each colour of interest in a histogram, and regulating the PMT voltage. Fluorescence max pixel is the brightest pixel intensity value in a measured object. Checks should be made at the beginning of the analysis, that the fluorescence max pixel values do not exceed the upper limit of the scale in any of the fluorescence channels.

For proper triggering by an Add parameter, it is important that the light signal coming from the cell is free, and therefore negative background is identical for all primary parameters. If, as an example, the setting for the FITC signal is selected so that the background is much brighter than that of the DiI signal then the Add parameter will show mostly the FITC but not the DiI image. In this case, triggering will basically be identical if the FITC data or the Add parameter is used. When the instrument setup has been optimised, the four regions of the chamber slide are measured and the resulting data file is saved as an FCS 3.0 format document.

EPC Data Analysis

LSC, like other cytometry instruments, also generates list-mode data in FCS data-file format. However, due to the more complex data that are generated by the image analysis as compared to FCM, these data are best analysed with the instrument's proprietary software. For data analysis, the primary data are gated on a two-parameter display of cell area versus scatter max pixel. A region is then created around the intact cells (not shown). These cells are recognised as a separate cluster of dots in the display with an area around 50 μm^2 and moderate Max Pixel values. Cell debris and artefacts generally have low size and Max Pixel. The correct positioning of the analysis gate is checked, by replacing the slide with which the respective analysis was performed and relocating the cells in the analysis gate. For further analysis, only cells in this region are taken into account.

In order to quantitate the number of DiI and FITC double positive cells, which are regarded as EPCs in a dot-plot display, DiI integral fluorescence is displayed versus the FITC integral fluorescence. Quadrant statistics are set up using the single dye stained control samples (see Fig. 3). The quadrants are positioned with the control samples, so that less than one percent of the cells appear double positive. As a result, the absolute number of double positive cells in this quadrant is determined for both double stained areas of a slide.

In additional experiments, more antibodies stained with different fluorochromes such as APC, a red light excitable and emitting dye, may be added. As an example, the pan leukocyte antigen CD45 may be used in order to simultaneously visualise leukocytes in the sample. The data acquisition is performed as shown for the two colour experiments, with the exception that both the Ar- and the HeNe-lasers are used for the measurement (example not shown). As shown elsewhere (Gerstner et al. 2002) up to six colours at least can be detected simultaneously with the LSC, up to four additional antigens can be detected in a single run with i.e. the combination FITC and DiI staining. Note, that if the instrument is run in the dual laser mode, the time needed for data accquisition doubles.

Examples
Calibration

A typical calibration of a FCM and SBC instrument is shown in Fig. 1b. In these examples, two different types of beads were used (both types were Rainbow™ beads from Spherotech Inc.). One set of beads, used in the FCM instrument (top row) consists of six bead populations of different brightness. The other set of beads used in the LSC, consists of populations of eight different intensities (middle row). Both sets of beads are also suitable to calibrate in the red (PerCP, PE-Cy5) emission channels. For calibration of the APC channel, for which the red excitation (HeNe or photodiode) is used, separate sets of calibration particles are available.

With both instruments best resolution at 488 nm excitation is achieved in the green (FITC) or the orange (PE) emission range. As can be seen in Fig. 1b and c, the LSC is also able to discriminate very dim fluorescence with less that 500 fluorescence molecules on a single event from the background. This means that the dyes PE or FITC are best suited to cytometrically detect antigens of low frequency. It is recommended, that the instrument set-up is adjusted with the beads, so that the brightness of positively stained cells will fall into the central part of the logarithmic scale (2nd and 3rd log). In this region the PMT linearity, sensitivity and resolution are optimal. Resolution and linearity are decreased in the first and last decade of the logarithmic scale.

Using the calibration beads the measured fluorescence intensities can be assigned to the number of fluorescence molecules per bead population, as provided by the manufacturer. With these data calibration lines can be constructed, and subsequently used to calculate molecule numbers per cell from fluorescence intensities (Fig. 1, bottom row). The calibration curve can either be calculated with the aid of a program provided by the manufacturer, or manually by fitting the data to a four parametric sigmoidal regression line (SPSS).

FCM Analysis of the Antigen Expression

Figure 2 shows a typical antigen expression pattern on neutrophils of patients with different adhesion molecule expression. Histograms are overlaid, with the respective calibration particle data. The data show that significant differences exist among the investigated groups in expression of LFA-1 (CD11a/CD18) and Mac-1 (CD11b/CD18) on monocytes and neutrophils (Rahimi et al. 2003). The restenosis group shows a higher expression of CD11a on monocytes and neutrophils, compared to the no restenosis and control groups prior to stent implantation. Similar results are found for CD11b on monocytes. These results suggest that preliminary activation status of CD11a and CD11b may play a role in the subsequent development of restenosis.

In the displayed example (Fig. 2) LFA-1 (CD11a/CD18) expressions are shown on neutrophils as gated, played in the dot-plot. As can be seen, substantial differences in the expression level exists between the two individuals displayed. Importantly, peripheral blood from both patients was drawn, stained and analysed on the same day, with an identically calibrated instrument. This indicates that expression levels may differ by nearly an order of magnitude or even more. In this example, the calculated antigen numbers were about 30,000 molecules of CD11a and 20,000 CD18 different between patients. As detailed elsewhere, these differences between groups of patients having chronic restenosis and no restenosis, can be exploited for early prediction of risk (Rahimi et al. 2003).

LSC Analysis of EPCs

The analysis of adherent EPCs, following short-term culture by the LSC, is of substantial support in EPC enumeration. On the one hand, the cells have been preselected by the density gradient centrifugation and growth, in a medium supporting EPC growth. Therefore, many more cells in the culture are positive for EPC markers, and quantitation is therefore reliably performable with a lower number of analysed cells, than by FCM of the precursors not cultivated (not shown). The cells do not usually grow homogeneously on the slide, but often regions of higher and lower cell density are observed (compare the cell densities in the two double stained chambers in Fig. 3). Therefore, the total culture well is analysed. The LSC provides the opportunity for cell visualisation whereby the cells can also be judged by their appropriate morphology. Multiplexed assays can also be performed to exclude a leukocyte origin of cells. In culture, single staining is insufficient for unequivocal recognition of EPCs. As exemplified in Fig. 3, many cells are single positive either for LDL or lectin, but only a subset of them expresses both characteristics. The same results are found with other endothelial markers such as KDR or PECAM, among others (not shown).

By labelling with the pan-leukocyte marker CD45 cell cultures can be tested to test if in fact the cultures also contain leukocytes. This antigen can be stained in addition to the DiI and FITC labels in a three-colour approach using the red excitable and far red emitting fluorochrome APC as a label for the anti CD45 antibody. The sample is than analysed in the dual-laser mode. Typically, the majority of these cells are either double negative for DiI-LDL and FITC-lectin, or single positive for one dye, but hardly ever double positive. Importantly, the morphology of the CD45 labelled cells is smaller and round, in contrast to that of typical EPCs, which are large and irregular in shape. These experiments should be used to test if by using DiI-LDL in combination with FITC-lectin the double positive population is contaminated by leukocytes.

LSC, and other quantitative SBC assays, have so far not been used to quantitate EPCs in culture. EPC quantitation is superior over their scoring by flow cytometry for two reasons. On the one hand, more EPCs are present following the short-term culture so that statistical evaluations are more reliable, but their removal for FCM analysis leads to cell loss and obstruction. On the other hand, due to the difficulties in unequivocally characterising these cells by antigen expression alone in circulation, the additional information on their morphology is crucial. LSC is a reliable way to quantitate cells, compared to manual scoring of "arbitrary" fields on the slide.

Troubleshooting

For specific troubleshooting with the various instruments that were available on the market, the reader is referred to the respective manuals or should contact the manufacturer. In the following, some of the most common problems that may arise when doing cytometric analysis with FCM, or SBC, will be shown. For a comprehensive overview of the specific assays, see Robinson et al. (2003) or ask the technical service. Troubleshooting with respect to cell culture, staining and related topics are beyond the scope of this chapter. In cases of technical problems, the reader is kindly asked to refer to appropriate protocols and textbooks.

FCM

- Beads are not measurable or only at very low count rates:
    - Increase bead concentration or increase count rate on the instrument setting.
    - Check threshold value. Calibration beads are often lower in diameter than leukocytes for better discrimination. Decrease the FSC threshold value for the beads if necessary.
    - Sample line of the instrument may be clogged. Perform cleaning procedure as recommended by the manufacturer.
    - Count rate is too high
- Decreased count rate setting of the instrument:
    - Increase dilution of cells or beads.
    - Check if the sheath fluid tank is filled with sheath fluid and is sealed airtight.
- No signals are detectable:
    - Check that sample line is not clogged and seals are airtight.
    - Check sample in the microscope.
    - Check if the FCM instrument and the computer are properly connected. Turn down both instruments
- Populations (clusters) of signals move over the screen:
    - Movement of signals is most often due to unstable sheath or sample pressure. This can be due to dirt, air bubbles or obstructed sample lines or sheath tank.
    - Check that sample line is not clogged and seals are airtight. Remove air bubbles from the tubing.
    - Check if the sheath fluid tank is filled with sheath fluid and is sealed airtight. Change sheath tank if necessary.
    - Check that the correct type of sample tube is being used and whether it seals airtight.

- No staining detectable:
    - Check your sample with the fluorescence microscope. It is recommended to always have a fluorescence microscope near the flow cytometry, so that sample staining and cell morphology can be counterchecked.
    - Check if protocol for the PMT settings has been loaded and if the PMTs are on. Check laser power.
    - Note that fluorescent dyes are light sensitive and fluorescence emission intensity may go down due to photobleaching. Therefore, protect the dyes and the stained samples carefully from light.
- Negative (i.e. unstained) cells are below baseline:
    - Care should be taken, that cells stained with control antibodies or unlabelled cells are still in scale. Otherwise, it is not possible to calculate specific binding above background, or to position analytical gates properly.
    - Increase PMT voltage until cells get in scale. Otherwise check compensation.
- Wrong compensation:
    - Fluorescence dyes are not only visible in one, but usually in several detectors; a phenomenon termed "fluorescence spill-over". This is due to the relatively broad emission spectrum of most of the dyes. Particularly problematic are the fluorescence resonance energy transfer dyes like PE-Cy5, PE-Cy7, APC-Cy7 (Gerstner et al. 2002). These dyes emit deep red (Cy5 or Cy7), due to the fact that the donor dye PE or APC, is directly excited by the laser and transfers its energy via resonance energy transfer to the acceptor dye. These dyes are very useful, because they allow the combination of more colours. However, they tend to emit not only in the respective acceptor, but also sometimes substantially in the donor colour.
    - In order to take this spill over into account fluorescence compensation is performed, by subtracting a certain percentage of the dye producing a spill over (e.g. FITC into PE), from the fluorescence of the dye of interest (e.g. PE), by using the instrument software. It is possible for mistakes to be made here, by either over- or under-compensation. In overcompensation, too much is subtracted from the fluorescence of the dye of interest, and negative cells will be out of scale. With under-compensation, the opposite is the case (details see Shapiro 2003; Robinson et al. 2002).
    - Compensation should be adjusted separately for each single colour labelled cell. It is noteworthy, that this adjustment should be performed with any new set of antibodies or if the antibody provider is changed. Different providers have slightly different formula for the fluorochromes and therefore the products may vary with respect to their emission spectra. Different dyes measured in the same channel could need different compensation values.

LSC

- Light scatter signals are not visible:
  Light scatter of EPC is generally lower than that of adhering leukocytes, because they flatten on the surface of the culture dish, which leads to a reduced contrast. This obstacle may be overcome in part fine adjusting the condenser and the obscuration bar below the microscope stage above the photo-diode (details see product manual).
- Light scatter signals are too high:
  If the background in the scan data image of the light scatter is too high, inappropriate data are collected. Optimise light scatter that reaches the light scatter detector by focussing the condenser and adjusting the obscuration bar (details see manual).
- In scan data image of light scatter cells appear dark against light background or are distorted:
  In particular, if light scatter is used as a triggering signal or for further analysis, cells must appear as bright particles above a dark background and should be morphologically intact in shape. Optimise obscuration bar settings.
- Count rate is too low:
  - Check threshold and minimal area settings on the scan data image and modify the values until optimal results are obtained. This step always needs to be done before starting the measurements.
  - The count rate in the LSC instrument also depends on the cells density on the microscope slide and the magnification of the objective used. At a given magnification the same number of fields of vision are always analysed. The count rate, can therefore only be increased, by seeding more cells.
- No specific staining detectable:
  - Check staining with the fluorescence microscope of the instrument.
  - Check if fluorescence detection is done in the correct channel with the appropriate optical filters. Increase PMT voltage if necessary.
  - pH indicators in culture media such as phenol-red, are fluorescent and excitable by UV and blue light. Their emission is in the range of FITC and PE and may therefore completely overlay FITC or DiI fluorescence. Wash cells thoroughly in PBS before staining. Better: use phenol-red free culture medium.
- DiI is not visible in double stained specimens:
  - This is most often due to an excess of FITC-lectin in the sample. Reduce FITC lectin concentration and check with samples.

Acknowledgement. The author thanks Dr. Dominik Lenz and Dr. Jozsef Bocsi, both Dept. of Paediatric Cardiology, Cardiac Centre, university of Leipzig, Germany, for critical reading of the manuscript and helpful comments, and the Interdisciplinary Centre for Clinical Research, IZKF, Leipzig, for support.

References

Asahara T, Murohara T, Sullivan A: Isolation of Putative Progenitor Endothelial Cells for Angiogenesis. Science. 275: 964–967, 1997

Azar RR, McKay RG, Kierman FJ, Seecharran B, Feng YJ, Fram DB, Wu AH, Waters DD: Coronary Angioplasty Induces a Systemic Inflammatory Response. Am J Cardiol 80:1476–1478, 1997

Bikoue A, Janossy G, Barnett D: Stabilised Cellular Immuno-Fluorescence Assay: CD45 Expression as a Calibration Standard for Human Leukocytes. J Immunol Methods 266:19–32, 2002

Bittl JA: Advances in Coronary Angioplasty. N Engl J Med 335:1290–1302, 1996

Buffon A, Liuzzo G, Biasucci LM, Pasqualetti P, Ramazzotti V, Rebuzzi AG, Crea F, Maseri A: Preprocedural Serum Levels of C- Reactive Protein Predict Early Complications and Late Restenosis After Coronary Angioplasty. J Am Coll Cardiol 34:1512–1521, 1999

Crissman HA, Mullaney PF, Steinkamp JA: Methods and Applications of Flow Systems for Analysis and Sorting of Mammalian Cells. Methods Cell Biol 9:179–246, 1975

Dittrich W, Göhde W: Impulszytophotometrie bei Einzelzellen in Suspension. Z Naturforsch B 24:221–228, 1969

Dittrich W, Göhde W: Phase Progression in Two Dose Response of Ehrlich Ascites Tumour Cells. Atomkernenergie 15-36:174–176, 1970

Fischman DL, Leon ml, Baim DS, Schatz R, Ricci D, Renn I, Detre K, Veltri L, Almond D, Teirstein P, Fish R, Colombo A, Brinker J, Moses J, Shaknovich A: A Randomized Comparison of Coronary-Stent Placement and Balloon Angioplasty in the Treatment of Coronary Artery Disease. N Engl J Med 331:496–501, 1994

Gerstner A.O.H., Lenz D, Laffers W, Hoffmann RA, Steinbrecher M, Bootz F, Tárnok A: Near-Infrared Dyes for Six-Color Immunophenotyping by Laser Scanning Cytometry. Cytometry 48:115–123, 2002

Hambsch J, Osmancik P, Bocsi J, Schneider P, Tarnok A: Neutrophil Adhesion Molecule Expression and Serum Concentration of Soluble Adhesion Molecules During and After Pediatric Cardiovascular Surgery With or Without Cardiopulmonary Bypass. Anesthesiology 96:1078–85, 2002

Haugland RP: Handbook of Fluorescent Probes and Research Products. 9th Edition. Molecular Probes Inc., Eugene OR, 2002

Kachel V, Benker G, Lichtnau K, Valet G, Glossner E: Fast Imaging in Flow: A Means of Combining Flow-Cytometry and Image Analysis. J Histochem Cytochem 27:335–341, 1997

Kalka C, Masuda H, Takahashi T, Kalka-Moll WM, Silver M, Kearney M, Li T, Isner JM, Asahara T: Transplantation of Ex Vivo Expanded Endothelial Progenitor Cells for Therapeutic Neovascularization. Proc Natl Acad Sci USA 97:3422–3427, 2000

Kamentsky LA, Burger DE, Gershman RJ, Kamentsky LD, Luther E: Slide-Based Laser Scanning Cytometry., Acta Cytologica 41:123–143, 1997

Kamentsky LA, Kamentsky LD: Microscope-Based Multiparameter Laser Scanning Cytometer Yielding Data Comparable to Flow Cytometry Data. Cytometry 12:381–387, 1991

Kamijikkoku S, Murohara T, Tayama S, Matsuyama K, Honda T, Ando M, Hayasaki K: Acute Myocardial Infarction and Increased Soluble Intercellular Adhesion Molecule-1: A Marker of Vascular Inflammation and a Risk of Early Restenosis? Am Heart J 136:231–236, 1998

Lefer AM: Selectins: Vital Vasculotropic Vectors Involved in Vascular Remodelling. Circulation 96:3258–3260, 1997

Lenz D, Lenk K, Adams V, Boldt J, Hambrecht R, Tárnok A: Detection of Endothelial Progenitor Cells by Flow and Laser Scanning Cytometry. In: Nicolau DV, Enderlein J, Leif RC, Farkas DL (eds) Manipulation and Analysis of Biomolecules, Cells, and Tissues. Proceedings of SPIE 4962:384–394, 2003

Lin Y, Weisdorf DJ, Solovey A: Origins of Circulating Endothelial Cells and Endothelial Outgrowth from Blood. J Clin Invest 105:71–77, 2000

Rahimi K, Maerz HK, Zotz RJ, Tarnok A. Pre-Procedural Expression of Mac-1 and LFA-1 on Leukocytes for Prediction of Late Restenosis and Their Possible Correlation with Advanced Coronary Artery Disease. Cytometry 53B:63–69 2003

Robinson JP, Darzynkiewicz Z, Hyun W, Orfao A, Rabinovitch P (Eds.). Current Protocols in Cytometry. John Wiley and Sons, Inc. New York, 2003

Shapiro HM : Practical Flow Cytometry. John Wiley and Sons Ltd. New York, 2003

Shintani S, Murohara T, Ikeda H, Ueno T, Honma T, Katoh A, Sasaki K, Shimada T, Oik, Y, Imaizumi T : Mobilization of Endothelial Progenitor Cells in Patients with Myocardial Infarction. Circulation 23:2776–2779, 2001

Springer T: Traffic Signals for Lymphocyte Re-Circulation and Emigration: The Multistep Paradigma. Cell 76:301–314, 1994

Strauer BE, Brehm M, Zeus T, Kostering M, Hernandez A, Sorg RV, Kogler G, Wernet P: Repair of Infarcted Myocardium by Autologous Intracoronary Mononuclear Bone Marrow Cell Transplantation in Humans. Circulation 106:1913–1918, 2002

Takahashi T, Kalka C, Masuda H, Chen D, Silver M, Kearney M, Magner M, Isner J, Asahara T: Ischemia- and Cytokine-Induced Mobilization of Bone Marrow-Derived Endothelial Progenitor Cells for Neovascularization. Nature Medicine 5:434–439, 1999

Tárnok A, Bocsi J, Pipek M, Osmancik P, Valet G, Schneider P, Hambsch J: Preoperative Prediction of Postoperative Edema and Effusion in Pediatric Cardiac Surgery by Altered Antigen Expression Patterns on Granulocytes and Monocytes. Cytometry 46:247–253, 2001

Tárnok A, Gerstner AO: Clinical Applications of Laser Scanning Cytometry. Cytometry 50:133–143, 2002
Tepper OM, Galiano RD, Capla JM, Kalka C, Gagne PJ, Jacobowitz GR, Levine JP, Gurtner GC: Human Endothelial Progenitor Cells from Type II Diabetics Exhibit Impaired Proliferation, Adhesion, and Incorporation into Vascular Structures. Circulation 106:2781–2786, 2002
Valet G: Predictive Medicine by Cytomics: Potential and Challenges. J Biol Regul Homeost Agents 16:164–167, 2002
Valet GK, Tárnok A. Cytomics in Predictive Medicine. Cytometry 53B: 1–3, 2003
Van Lente F: Markers of Inflammation as Predictors in Cardiovascular Disease. Clin Chim Acta 293:31–52, 2000
Vasa M., Fichtlscherer S, Adler K, Aicher A, Martin H, Zeiher AM, Dimmeler S: Increase in Circulating Endothelial Progenitor Cells by Statin Therapy in Patients with Coronary Heart Disease. Circulation 103:21–26, 2001
Virchow R: Cellularpathologie. Berlin: August Hirschwald, 1859

Molecular Biology in Cardiovascular Research

7 Molecular Biology Techniques
— 889

7 Molecular Biology Techniques

7.1 Real-Time PCR Analysis of Cardiac Samples — 891
Dalton A. Foster and Steven M. Taffet

7.2 Use of cDNA Arrays to Explore Gene Expression in Genetically Manipulated Mice and Cell Lines — 907
Dumitru A. Iacobas, Sandra Iacobas and David C. Spray

7.3 Using Antibody Arrays to Detect Protein-Protein Interactions — 916
Heather S. Duffy, Ionela Iacobas, David C. Spray and Anthony W. Ashton

7.4 Surface Plasmon Resonance as a Method to Study the Kinetics and Amplitude of Protein-Protein Binding — 936
Brian D. Lang, Mario Delmar and Wanda Coombs

7.5 How to Solve a Protein Structure by Nuclear Magnetic Resonance – The Connexin43 Carboxyl Terminal Domain — 948
Paul L. Sorgen

7.6 Managing a Transgenic Mouse Colony: A Guide for the Novice — 959
Robert H. Quinn and Karen L. Vikstrom

Real-Time PCR Analysis of Cardiac Samples
Dalton A. Foster and Steven M. Taffet

Introduction

A proper understanding of the workings of the heart requires an appreciation of the engines that make cardiac excitation and contraction possible. These ion channels, pumps and exchangers are all central to this process, and are in turn regulated by many other proteins which assist them in governing membrane current flow. Further regulation is provided by the autonomic nervous system, which exerts a profound effect on cardiac function as a whole by controlling the activity of proteins that affect both heart rate and contractility. Pathologies often arise as a result of aberrant or inappropriate protein expression and the subsequent destruction of equilibrium. As such, the profiling of protein expressions in both diseased and normal states can yield important clues as to how diseases evolve. Moreover, it can allow researchers to identify proteins critical to the development of certain pathologies, and target them for pharmacological intervention. A first step in this process can be the careful study and comparison of the RNA expression profiles of diseased and normal hearts. Comparing RNA levels is often used, as the expression of a given protein often follows closely the expression of its RNA.

The methods available for analyzing mRNA expression levels are diverse. The factors used when deciding upon the best approach are equally varied and depend in part upon the type of data the researcher is seeking. The type of sample material available, the quantity of the material, and technical proficiency of the lab must all be taken into consideration. Northern blotting, *in situ* hybridization, RNase protection assays, cDNA arrays and RT-PCR are all tried and true techniques when comparative data are sought. For the researcher requiring data that is more exacting, quantitative PCR is the method of choice. There have been three basic incarnations of "quantitative" PCR to date: Semi-quantitative PCR, competitive quantitative PCR and Real-Time PCR (Bustin 2000; 2002; Ong and Irvine 2002; Overbergh et al. 2003). What is the advantage of performing quantitative PCR vs. normal PCR in acquiring quantitative data? To answer this question one must first appreciate the limitations inherent in classical polymerase chain reactions.

During the initial phase of a PCR reaction, the concentration of reagents i.e. the primers, and dNTP's is in great excess. Conversely, the concentration of template and amplicons is relatively low. This small amount of product helps to drive the reaction forward, eventually leading to the accumulation of amplicons at an exponential rate.

At a certain point, the rate of product formation plateaus and becomes minimal. Exactly when this happens for a given primer template combination is extremely variable, but we do know that it occurs when the accumulated product effectively becomes a feedback inhibitor of the very reaction that produces it. More specifically, product begins to preferentially re-anneal with itself as opposed to primer, thereby causing the production of new amplicons to slow. This is typically the phase many PCR reactions are in when they are halted and the samples removed for analysis. Yet, because the reaction is no longer exponential, it is the least likely point at which to obtain credible quantitative data. This is because analysis of samples during the exponential phase, results in quantitative data that is extremely reproducible, and provides the researchers with several orders of magnitude of dynamic range over which to analyze the data. Only in the exponential phase can the amount of gene expression be made readily available to the researcher, and as a result the overall relevance of a given gene in the expression profile for a specific pathology be assessed. The three basic types of quantitative PCR address this challenge of acquiring data from the exponential phase by using different approaches.

Semi-quantitative RT-PCR is the least sophisticated of the three techniques mentioned. In semi-quantitative PCR, a researcher monitors product accumulation during the exponential phase, by interrupting the amplification at a cycle that was predetermined, as a result of an optimization process that is sometimes laborious. More specifically, the exponential phase for a given reaction is determined, by halting PCR reactions at the end of each cycle and assessing the amount of product formed. While useful, semi-quantitative RT-PCR is limited by a relatively small dynamic range,

Quantitative-competitive PCR obtains quantitative data by a different means. It involves the simultaneous amplification of both the target and a competitor (internal standard) in the same tube. This internal standard is usually DNA, which can be amplified with primers specific for the target sequence, but can be distinguished from the target by size or internal sequence. The amount of target template is, therefore, quantified by the titration of an unknown amount of target template against a dilution series of known amounts of the competitor sequence. Quantitative-competitive PCR is limited by the inherent difficulty in designing a functional competitor, as well as the labor involved in optimizing the technique. Additionally, there are no guarantees that absolute quantification will be achievable using the internal standard, because differences in the amplification efficiencies between the control and target DNA can go undetected.

The post-amplification steps required to detect PCR products, further complicate acquiring quantitative data from either semi-quantitative or quantitative-competitive PCR. Ethidium bromide staining of agarose gels, the use of fluorescence labeling, radioactive labeling, southern blotting etc. all require numerous steps which are both laborious and time consuming. Many of the techniques also pose hazards to both the researcher and the environment, whether from toxic molecules or radiochemicals. Additionally, these techniques require imaging the result and quantifying the image. This is a significant source of error in obtaining a quantification of the result.

Quantitative Real-Time PCR manages to overcome all of the troubles associated with the pursuit of quantitative data. Real-Time PCR allows for the procurement of quantitative data during the critical exponential phase of amplification reaction, with-

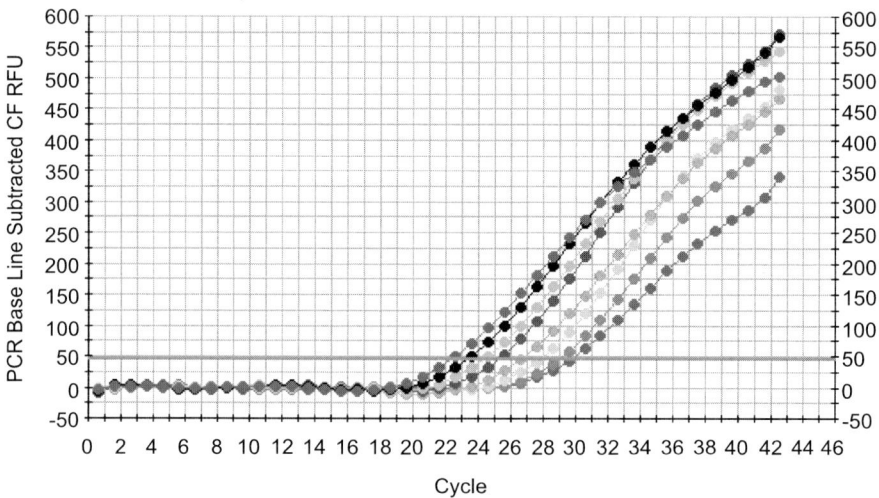

Figure 1
Example of a Real-Time PCR Result: A sample result was extracted from the iCycler software tutorial. Multiple dilutions of primers were used to create a set of values. The Ct (threshold cycle) increases with greater dilution. *For coloured version see appendix*

out requiring the optimization steps required of semi- and competitive-quantitative PCR, or the post-amplification steps required for both methods in order to visualize the PCR products. Real-Time PCR is, therefore, the method of choice because it provides for speed, a reduced risk of contamination and the acquisition of quantitative data.

Just what is Real-Time PCR? Real-Time PCR is based on the detection and quantification of signal generated by a fluorescent reporter, the intensity of which is designed to increase in direct proportion to the amount of PCR product yielded during amplification. The amount of fluorescence produced at each cycle or the delta Rn is derived from the equation Rn+ (fluorescence emission of PCR product at each cycle) – Rn– (the fluorescence emission of the baseline). The delta Rn collected at each cycle is then used to construct amplification plots. The fluorescence emissions data are plotted versus cycle number.

During the early phase of the reaction, the delta Rn values do not exceed threshold, which is arbitrarily set at ten times the standard deviation of the baseline set from cycles 3–15. The resulting curve (Fig. 1), allows for the determination of what is know as the threshold cycle (C_T) or the cycle number at which the amount of fluorescence generated by PCR products becomes detectable above background. By using both a threshold cycle and a standard curve, quantitative information can be generated. The relative levels of fluorescence produced can be accessed while the reaction progresses in real-time. Most important, are the levels recorded during the exponential phase, which is then correlated with the initial amount of template in the reaction tubes.

Description of Methods and Practical Approach
Chemistries

The fluorescence-based methods developed to detect the accumulation of PCR products can be either nonspecific or sequence specific. Nonspecific detection methods make use of fluorescent dsDNA intercalating dyes such as SYBR® green and ethidium bromide. Additionally, they are the simplest and most cost effective methods available. Ethidium bromide helped demonstrate the feasibility of monitoring reactions as they progress in real time. Higuchi et al (Higuchi et al. 1993), using ethidium bromide and a CCD camera, introduced the world to the concept of real time quantitative PCR. Due to ethidium bromide's hazardous nature, a less non-toxic alternative SYBR green is in use by most laboratories today. SYBR® green has an additional benefit of fluorescing only when incorporated into double stranded DNA (Fig. 2). The greatest advantage of a non-specific detection system is its flexibility. SYBR green can be used with any primer pair to amplify any target. Therefore it is a very cost effective and safe way to generate quantitative data. This flexibility, however, is a double-edged sword. SYBR green lacks sequence specificity, and it will detect non-specific PCR products and primer-dimers as well as the legitimate amplicons. This can result in the overestimation of the target DNA concentration. A combination of techniques can be used to circumvent this drawback. Firstly, melt curve analysis should be performed, enabling the differentiation of fluorescence originating from target DNA and that produced by primer-dimers or spurious PCR products. Additionally, careful design of primers and reaction optimization are fundamental to the proper function of any PCR reaction, and can also reduce non-specific fluorescence. Lastly, a Hot-Start protocol should be employed to minimize the amplification of illegitimate PCR products.

Specific detection methods rely on the principle of Fluorescence Resonance Energy Transfer or FRET, which is based on the transfer of energy from a donor molecule to an acceptor molecule. The degree of energy transfer is directly proportional to the distance between the moieties. In the case of two fluorophores with overlapping excitation and emission spectra, excitation of the donor molecule will result in a corresponding increase in fluorescence from the acceptor molecule, if the two molecules are in close enough proximity. When this principle is applied for sequence specific

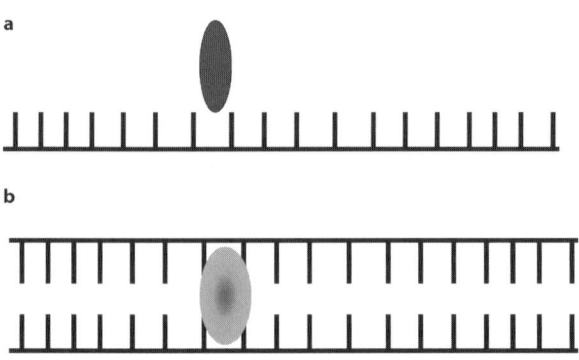

Figure 2a,b
Illustration of the SYBR green reaction: **a** SYBR green does not fluoresce when free or associated with single stranded DNA. **b** SYBER green fluorescens when bound to double-stranded DNA. *For coloured version see appendix*

detection in Real-Time assays, donor and acceptor molecules are placed at either side of a probe complimentary to the target sequence. The technique has been further modified by the replacement of the fluorogenic acceptor with a non-fluorogenic acceptor molecule or quencher. Therefore, when the donor and acceptor molecules are in close proximity, no fluorescence will be detected. However, when the distance between the two is increased, the reporter dye will fluoresce unimpeded. Fluorescent reporter dyes commonly used include FAM (6-carboxyfluorescein), TET (tetrachloro-6-carboxyfluorescein), Joe (2,7-dimethoxy-4,5-dichloro-6-carboxyfluorescein), HEX (hexachloro-6-carboxyfluorescein) and VIC. DABCYL and TAMRA are both popular quenchers, and have been used widely and effectively in Real-Time PCR applications. These quenchers, however, suffer from well-known individual weaknesses, such as the poor excitation and emissions overlap of DABCYL with the fluorescent dyes, or the auto fluorescence of TAMRA. New and improved quenchers called "Black Hole Quenchers" have been developed and are being marketed. Black Hole quenchers unlike DABCYL can quench over the entire range of the visible spectrum and unlike TAMRA do not autofluoresce.

Two specific detection methods, "Molecular Beacons" and "Scorpion primers", achieve separation between reporter and quencher dyes by hybridization with target DNA during the annealing phase of the amplification cycle. TaqMan assays, on the other hand, achieve separation through the enzymatic cleavage of the probes during the extension phase of the PCR reaction. Regardless of the method or technique used, FRET allows for the real-time monitoring and quantification of PCR product accumulation in a sequence specific manner.

TaqMan probes are based on 5' nuclease assay technology. TaqMan probes are comprised of a target sequence specific probe labeled at the 5' end, with a fluorescent reporter dye and at the 3' end with a quencher. Little, or no fluorescence, is emitted by the TaqMan probe, in either the hybridized or unhybridized states, due to the closeness of the reporter and quencher moieties. Hybridization of probe to target sequence during PCR renders the probe accessible to the 5'-3' exonuclease activity of Taq polymerase. The degradation of the probe results in the separation of the fluorophore from the quencher, allowing it to fluoresce freely (Fig. 3). Therefore, as more PCR product is generated, more probe are degraded, and the level of fluorescence increases proportionally.

Molecular Beacons (Marras et al. 1999; Tyagi et al. 1998; Tyagi and Kramer 1996) like TaqMan probes, possess a reporter dye at the 5' end and a quencher at the other. Unlike TaqMan probes, Molecular Beacons adopt a stem-loop configuration to bring the reporter and quencher in close proximity, which facilitates FRET. Fluorescence of the reporter dye is achieved when the probe anneals with its target sequence and is in an extended configuration. The increased distance between reporter and quencher prevents FRET from occurring, allowing the accumulation of PCR product to be monitored as an increase in fluorescent emissions from the hybridized probe. Molecular Beacons have a higher specificity than TaqMan probes, which is partly due to the stem loop structure they adopt in the unhybridized state (Fig. 4). They are, therefore, especially useful for SNP analysis, as they can distinguish between targets differing by a single nucleotide and have been employed extensively in the area of mutation detection.

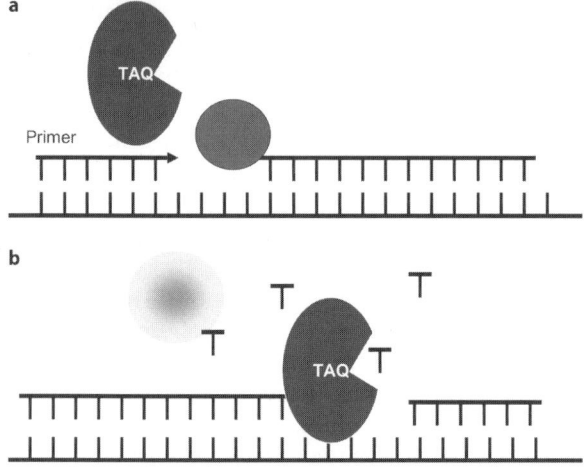

Figure 3a,b
Example of a TaqMan Reaction: **a** Taqman probes allow energy transfer from the fluorescent emitter and the quencher when intact. **b** Taq polymerase has exonuclease activity that digests the probe allowing the emitter to freely fluorescence. *For coloured version see appendix*

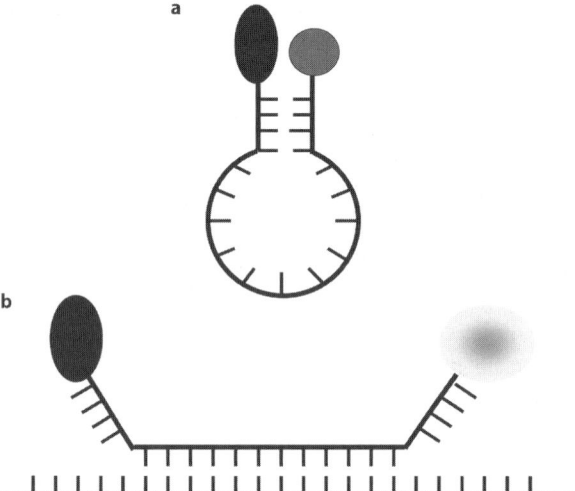

Figure 4a,b
Example of a Molecular Beacon: **a** The native structure of free Molecular Beacon probes brings the emitter and quencher close together inhibiting fluorescence. **b** When product is available, the probe binds to the target, forcing the emitter to separate from the quencher allowing the emitter to freely fluorescence. *For coloured version see appendix*

Scorpion primers (Taveau et al. 2002; Thelwell et al. 2000) represent the next step in the evolution of sequence detection methods. They improve sequence specificity and increase the speed and efficiency of Real-Time PCR assays. Scorpion primers are comprised essentially of a Molecular Beacon with a sequence specific primer attached at the 3' end of the stem-loop configuration. The primers contain a modification called a PCR stopper (typically hexethylene glycol) at their 5' end, which unites the beacon and primer, and prevents the PCR reaction from copying the step loop portion of the Scorpion primer. The molecular beacon portion of the Scorpion primer is designed to bind complimentarily with the extension products of the primer to which it is attached. During the annealing phase of the PCR cycle, the probe sequence curls back to hybridize the target sequence in the amplicon (Fig. 5). This results in the se-

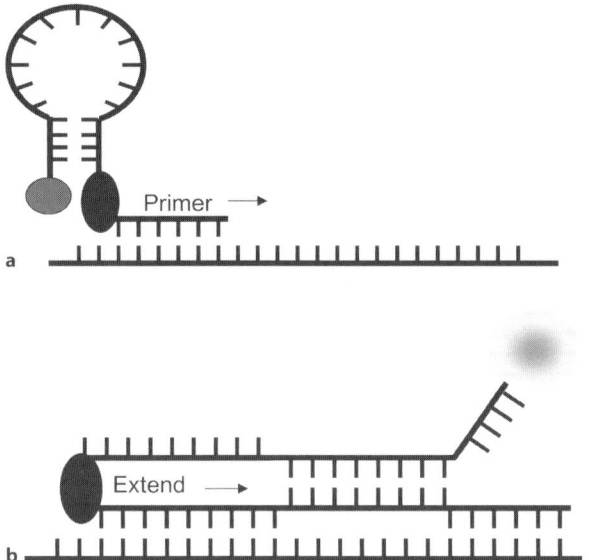

Figure 5a,b
Scorpion Primers. Scorpion primers are able to act as a combination of a PCR primer and Molecular Beacon. **a** The native structure of the scorpion probe brings the emitter and quencher close together inhibiting fluorescence, whilst the other end of the molecule can act as a PCR primer. **b** After extension of a PCR product, the probe binds to the target forcing the emitter to separate from the quencher, allowing the emitter to freely fluoresce. The target is the product of extension of the primer end of the molecule making the detection intramolecular. *For coloured version see appendix*

paration of the fluorescent dye and quencher at either end of the stem loop configuration, preventing FRET, and allowing for increases in fluorescence in a sequence specific manner.

The uni-molecular configuration of Scorpion primers imbues them with a kinetic advantage over TaqMan and Molecular Beacons because probe-target interaction becomes an intra-molecular event. Therefore, unlike TaqMan and Molecular Beacon assays, fluorescent signal generation is no longer dependent upon the chance meeting of a probe, normally present in low concentrations, with its target. This allows for the use of more rapid cycling conditions, and more importantly, the production of greater signal strengths, as more probe is able to anneal with its corresponding target per given cycle. Scorpion primers possess an additional advantage over TaqMan assays, which they share with Molecular Beacons; PCR reactions using Scorpion primers are performed at the optimal temperature for polymerase activity, whereas TaqMan assays are performed at lower temperatures, which allows for the 5' nuclease activity of the enzyme to function. Scorpion primers have been further tailored to overcome some quenching of reporter dye fluorescence that may occur even in the open configuration. Duplex Scorpion primers achieve greater signal strength by placing dye and quencher on separate complimentary oligonucleotides. The primer, PCR stopper, and probe comprise one half of the duplex Scorpion probe. The other half consists of an oligonucleotide complimentary to the probe sequence with a quencher linked to its 3' end. As with regular Scorpion primers, duplex Scorpion primers retain the kinetic advantages of intra-molecular binding of probe to its target following denaturation and polymerization. During the PCR cycle annealing phase, interaction between probe and primer extension products is favored kinetically over probe-quencher oligonucleotide binding. As a result, greater distances between fluorophore and quencher at the time of signal detection are achieved, thus yielding significantly greater signal intensity with lower background fluorescence levels when compared to the normal Scorpion primer format. Additionally, duplex Scorpion primers are much easier to design and synthesize, as each oligonucleotide requires only one dye be attached, and neither requires the engineering of a stem-loop structure duplex. This significantly reduces the labor required to design these probes, and the effort required to produce them.

Hybridization probes are one of the more complicated applications designed for Real-Time PCR. For this system a total of four oligonucleotides are required: two primers and two probes. Each probe is labeled with either a donor or acceptor dye, and both probes are designed to hybridize to the target in a head to tail manner. This brings the donor and acceptors in close proximity allowing FRET to occur. Unlike Molecular Beacons, TaqMan assays or Scorpion primers, hybridization probes do not utilize a quencher, therefore, the signal produced from the acceptor dye is what is used to track the amount of DNA produced during the PCR reaction.

Peptide nucleic acid (PNA) oligomers have also been used as probes for real-time PCR assays. They are similar in structure to DNA in that they possess a repeating N-(2-aminoethyl)-glycine backbone which mimics the phosphate backbone of DNA. They make excellent highly specific probes because they are non-charged, and therefore require no salt in order to stabilize the duplexes that can form with either RNA or DNA. The melting temperature of PNA/ DNA or PNA/RNA duplexes is, therefore, much higher than those formed by DNA/DNA interactions. This allows duplex formation to occur at low salt conditions while preserving high specificity. The higher melting temperature of PNA's, permits design to be shorter if need be, as a 15-mer PNA probe will possess a similar melting point as a DNA 25-mer. However, specificity will be diminished as probe length decreases, and this must be kept in mind when designing PNA probes.

Instrumentation

Presently there exists a wide variety of instrumentation designed for Real-Time PCR from which to choose. They all overcome the inherent deficiencies in conventional-reverse transcription-PCR, and are capable of monitoring increases in fluorescence during a reaction in real-time. They all attempt to reduce the cost associated with real-time by minimizing the amount of reagent and template needed. The machines will vary primarily in terms of cost, the light source used to stimulate the fluorophores, the amount of samples which can be processed during a typical run, multiplexing capabilities, and the overall friendliness of the user interface.

The ABI 7700 from Applied Biosystems is one of the better known Real-Time PCR machines, primarily because it was the first to become commercially available. Applied Biosystems has followed up the ABI 7700 with the Gene Amp 5700 and the 7900HT, which differs from the ABI 7700, in that up to 384 samples can be processed at a time. Although old in comparison to many other machines, the ABI 7700 remains a viable choice for many researchers. It can be used for 5' nuclease assays (TaqMan), Molecular Beacon assays, as well as non-specific sequence detection methods (SYBR green). The ABI 7700 and the ABI 7900HT are limited perhaps only by the light sources which they use to excite fluorescent dyes. Both instruments rely on a single excitation laser as a light source, which exposes the two weaknesses of the ABI 7700 and the ABI 7900HT. With a limited excitation range of 488-514, there are fewer dyes available from which the researcher can choose. Additionally, the laser light source, while intense, provides less uniform excitation of fluorophores over a given range. This limitation becomes important when multiplexing or amplifying more than one target in the same tube, and monitoring both reactions via fluorescent emissions from probes labeled with different fluorophores. Therefore, when using the ABI 7700 or ABI 7900HT for multiplexing, it is critical that fluorophores with a dissimilar absorbance and emission spectra be chosen. In the Gene Amp 5700, the excitation laser is replaced with a halogen lamp, which provides uniform excitation over a much broader spectrum of wavelengths. The 5700 does retain the flexibility of the 7700 in terms of the sequence detection chemistries which can be used, but it falls short in that it can only detect one single wavelength, and is therefore incapable of multiplexing.

The LightCycler from Roche Molecular Biochemical's has a very unique approach to Real-Time PCR both in terms of light source, sample containers and thermocycling. It is a very compact machine and utilizes borosilicate capillary tubes to accommodate samples. A blue-light emitting diode is used as a light source, and the resulting emissions are interpreted by three silicon photodiodes that can filter out various wavelengths, which allows the researcher to perform multiplexing reaction with the LightCycler. For thermocycling, air is used as the heating medium, which along with the high surface area to volume ratio of the borosilicate tubes, means that a PCR run of 30–40 cycles can be performed in 20–30 min compared to 2 h. Apart from the obvious advantage of speed, the LightCycler is relatively inexpensive when compared with other machines. Its disadvantages include the required use of capillary tubes as opposed to regular PCR tubes. Additionally, its speed is somewhat negated by the small sample format, in that only 32 reactions can be performed at a given time. This deficiency limits the scope of studies in which a large number of samples must be compared during a single run.

The Biorad iCycler, like the LightCycler, is also a very compact real-time PCR machine. It is a modular machine in that the thermocycler module is not permanently attached to the optics component. They can be and are sold separately. The iCycler uses a halogen tungsten lamp and can amplify up to 96 samples at once. The sample capacity of the iCycler can be extended up to 384 samples for those requiring additional throughput.

The Rotor-Gene from Corbett Research, like the LightCycler, represents a radical departure from other Real-Time PCR machines in terms of design. The Rotor-Gene employs LED light sources, four in number, to excite the fluorescent dyes. Subsequent emissions are monitored via six filters and photomultipliers. The most unique element of the Rotor-Gene is that the real-time reactions are carried out in PCR tubes placed in a 36 or 72 well rotor that spins at 500 rpm during the run. The centrifugal motion is said to reduce temperature equilibration times, and sample-to-sample nonuniformity, thereby improving consistency and reliability.

The Smart Cycler is a recent entry into the Real-Time PCR machine marketplace. It is manufactured by Cephid, and can use TaqMan, Molecular Beacons, Scorpion primers, hybridization probes as well SYBR® green I. It is uniquely flexible, in that each of its 16 sample wells can be operated independently. This means that up to 16 separate reactions, requiring different thermocycling parameters or optical settings, can be performed simultaneously. The major disadvantage of the Smart Cycler system is the limited sample size format, which may be inadequate for quantitative studies.

The Stratagene MX4000 is also a relatively new option available to researchers in the market for a Real-Time PCR machine. The MX4000 uses a quartz-tungsten halogen lamp and can be used with all of the sequence detection chemistries detailed earlier in this discussion. Its 96 well block can accommodate samples in many formats i.e. tubes or plates. The MX4000 is sold with an integrated personal computer which functions and stores data separately from the Real-Time PCR machine itself, thereby providing protection from possible loss of data if the PCR machine is damaged or disabled.

Example

To determine the utility of Real-Time PCR, we designed a Molecular Beacon probe and primers for use in the Biorad I-cycler. A specific probe for the Kir 2.1 potassium channel was designed and dually labeled with the reporter dye FAM at the 5' end, and the Black Hole Quencher at the 3' end (International DNA Technologies, IDT). For quantification, a standard curve was constructed with Kir 2.1 amplicons that was generated by the primers designed to be used in combination with the probe. A commercially available TET-labeled Cylcophilin probe and primer set (Amersham) was chosen as the internal control for correcting variations in RNA input, and inefficiencies in reverse transcription.

RNA Extraction

There are many choices of systems for isolation of RNA from mammalian tissue. Our own experience has been with TRI Reagent (Molecular Research Center, Inc). This is one of a group of reagents that are composed of a mono-phase mixture of phenol and guanidine thiocyanate (Chadderton et al. 1997; Mannhalter et al. 2000). TRI Reagent is sometimes marketed as TRIzol, an alternative formulation is sold as RNAzol or RNA-Bee by Iso-Tex Diagnostics, Inc. Although we have no experience with this product it should be similar to TRI reagent in its effectiveness. Both reagents utilize phenol and guanidine thiocyanate to inhibit RNAse and denature proteins. Chloroform or an alternative reagent, bromo-chloro-propane (BCP) is then added to separate the pha-ses. RNA is isolated from the upper (aqueous) phase by alcohol precipitation. RNA is quantified spectrophotometrically.

Specific protocol for the isolation of RNA from heart tissue:
1. Dissect and weigh 300 mg of heart tissue
2. Add 3 ml of TRI Reagent (Molecular Research Center, Inc.)
3. Homogenize for 10 s, put on ice for 2 min, repeat 2× more

4. Store the homogenate at room temperature for 5 min
5. Add 0.3 ml of BCP, shake vigorously for 15 s
6. Store sample at room temperature for 10 min
7. Centrifuge at 12,000 g for 15 min
8. Transfer upper aqueous phase to new tube
9. Add equal volume of isopropanol, mix and store at room temperature for 10 min
10. Centrifuge at 12,000 g for 8 min at 4 °C
11. Remove the supernatant and wash RNA pellet by adding 3 ml of 75% ethanol and centrifuge at 7,500 g for 5 min at 4 °C
12. Remove the ethanol and air-dried pellet for 5 min
13. Dissolve RNA in DEPC-water

cDNA Synthesis

There are numerous reverse transcription systems to choose from. These systems vary in their primers, enzyme, as well as other reagents. Further variability is the one-tube/two-tube reaction issue. One-tube systems, in which the reverse transcription reaction and amplification takes place in a single tube, are clearly more convenient, however, that convenience is gained at the expense of flexibility and some sensitivity. Reagent mixes that work for both the reverse transcription step and the PCR step, are generally a compromise not optimized for either step. In this example we have chosen to run two separate reactions. The choice of the reverse transcription system is crucial to the Real-Time quantitation of specific mRNA, as the cDNA product must accurately reflect the input mRNA. Choosing a system with the sensitivity to amplify a rare mRNA, and also has the dynamic range to show differences in content, is therefore critical

The mechanism of priming is one of the most important considerations in setting up the cDNA synthesis. Oligo dT anneals to the poly A tail of mRNA to prime the reverse transcription of mRNA. This would result in some full-length transcripts and preferentially transcribe from mRNA. One obvious problem with this mechanism is that it would miss the transcripts that do not have poly A tails. There is also a tendency for incomplete reverse transcription, which results in fragments that have a higher proportion of the three prime end of transcripts and lower representations of the five prime ends. Random oligonucleotides will, by their nature, produce smaller fragments of cDNA and there may be an over-representation of the five prime ends. It may then be useful to use a mixture of oligo dT and random oligonucleotides to produce templates for real time PCR. While some of the transcripts will be incomplete, the products analyzed by PCR are relatively small (less than 200 bp) and will be well represented.

While every molecular supply company has a brand of reverse transcriptase, there are only two types of reverse transcriptase used in most assays. These are MMLV (Moloney murine leukemia virus) and AMV (avian myeloblastosis virus). Both enzymes contain RNAse H in the native form, but MMLV reverse transcriptase has much less of this RNAse. Mutated forms of MMLV are available as recombinant molecules that have reduced or absent RNAse H activity. MMLV represents the more commonly utilized reverse transcriptase. The presence of RNAse H, reduces the amount of full-length product produced. However, the effect of RNAse H on the final sensitivity of reverse transcription and PCR analysis of transcripts is unclear. There are clearly manufacturers that claim it is harmful, and others that can show that it increases the sensitivity of the reaction. We have chosen to use the iScript reverse transcription system for our reactions, which is an RNAse H+, MMLV derived enzyme. As kit contents may vary, a detailed procedure for the reverse transcription step will not be presented.

In the current example, we utilized 2 µg of RNA from either the right or left ventricle, and reverse-transcribed, using the iScript cDNA synthesis kit (Biorad). A positive control containing RNA provided with the kit, and a negative control containing no reverse transcriptase, were cycled along with the test samples. The success of the reverse transcription reaction was assessed by PCR using the Kir 2.1 specific primers, and primers provided with the reverse transcription kit for the positive control.

Primer and Probe Design

Primer and probe design are complicated processes that require multiple parameters to be considered. The size of the product and the optimal design of both probes and primers are just starting points. The most important parameter concerning primer and probe design is the Tm gap that should exist between primer melting and probe melting. The Tm value of the primers should be between them 58–60°, whilst that of the probe should be 7–10° above that of the primers. The optimal GC contents and the ideal lengths of the primers and probes, the most favorable length of the amplicons, and the spacing that should exist between the end of the primers and the probe on the sequence to be amplified, can complicate the design process. Several commercially available software suites are available, but online sites are also available and free to use. Two such sites, which we have used, are available from Stratagene and International DNA Technologies:
- *http://labtools.stratagene.com/*
- *http://biotools.idtdna.com/gateway/*

Both programs are easy and simple to use. One simply has to cut and paste the template sequence and designate the sites one wishes the probe and primers to anneal to. The Stratagene suite enables the researcher to also design probes and primers for use in multiplexing reactions. The IDT suite does not provide this convenience, but it does allow the researcher to directly blast the chosen probe primer set to ensure their specificity for the sequence of interest, independent of the software utilized. Fortunately both software suites have their default parameters set to the ideal values for the concerns listed above, which greatly simplifies the design process even for a novice.

The Kir 2.1 primer and probe pair was designed using free web-based software provided by Stratagene. To ensure their specificity, we performed a blast search against the relevant databases. We chose to label the Kir 2.1 probe with FAM at the 5' end, and the Darkhole quencher BHQ-1 at the 3' end. Our choice of fluorophore was for practical reasons. Firstly, the Biorad I-cycler we were using had the appropriate filters to monitor FAM and TET wavelengths. Secondly, since we anticipated multiplexing with a TET labeled cyclophilin internal control, we wanted to choose a fluorophore for the Kir 2.1 probe that would have no significant spectral overlap with TET.

Amplification

There are many enzymes available for the amplification step. These are mostly based on Taq (Thermus aquaticus) polymerase, however, others are based on mutated forms of Taq, vent polymerase (Thermococcus litoralis) and Pfu (Pyrococcus furiosus) polymerase. Taq has the highest processivity, but vent and Pfu have better fidelity, due to the presence of 3' to 5' proof reading activity. Some mutants of Taq have higher fidelity. One way to improve specificity in PCR is to utilize a hot start procedure. Most reactions are assembled at room temperature where primers may bind to DNA sequences with little specificity. As the reaction is heated to denaturation temperature, the polymerase becomes active, extending these mismatched products. Taq polymerase may be as much as 70% active at 50 °C. Mismatches can be eliminated, by preventing polymerase activation at lower temperatures (Chou et al. 1992). Many early implementations of this technique were cumbersome with wax pellets surrounding the enzyme, or the necessity of adding the polymerase after denaturation, when the reaction was already in the cycler. New implementations of hot start utilize inhibitors that are denatured at higher temperatures. Monoclonal antibodies that inactivate the enzyme are the most common mechanism (Kellogg et al. 1994). These antibodies inactivate at temperatures above 70 °C, allowing the enzyme to activate. Other implementations involve chemical inhibitors that no longer inhibit at higher temperature. However, hot start enzymes are preferable in any real time application.

In our example, PCR reactions were run using the Brilliant Core Quantitative PCR reagent (Stratagene). This cloned Taq polymerase is chemically inactivated at lower temperatures. This polymerase, as many others, comes as a "master mix", with all reagents except template, primer and probe. These mixes reduce the variability in the assay. It is useful to prepare a more complete mix with your specific probe and primers, helping to further reduce pipetting error and tube-to-tube variability.

Optimization of Probes and Primers

The molecular beacon concentration was optimized by using a standard primer concentration of 200 µM per primer and varying the final concentration of beacon from 200–500 nM.

The optimal concentration of primers for use with the molecular beacon are determined by finding the lowest concentration of forward and reverse primers which yield the lowest Ct values and adequate fluorescence. The primer concentrations are determined by holding the beacon concentration, and concentrations of either the forward or reverse constant at 200 µM, while varying the other from 200–600 nM. After finding the lowest concentration for one of the primers, the optimal concentration for the other is found varying its concentration against the low concentration found for the first.

Multiplexing

If a researcher decides to multiplex, or amplify more than one target DNA in the same tube, the task of optimizing the Real-Time PCR reaction becomes more complex. The goal is to balance the efficiencies of the competing reactions and prevent one from completely inhibiting the other(s). For our purposes, we multiplexed the Kir 2.1 reaction and the internal control cyclophilin reaction, to minimize variability from amplifying the target and normalizing reaction in separate tubes. The Kir 2.1 and cyclophilin reactions were optimized separately, before running both reactions in the same tube. In our hands, the cylcophilin cDNA present in the right ventricle and left ventricle samples was significantly greater than that for the Kir 2.1 channel. So much so, that the cyclophilin reaction reached its exponential phase well ahead of the Kir 2.1 reaction, and thus completely inhibited the amplification of Kir 2.1. To solve this problem we created a serial dilution of the optimized cylcophilin primer concentration. We then added a master mix containing sample cDNA to the primer solution, the optimized Kir 2.1 primers and probe, as well as the optimized concentration of cyclophilin probe. By monitoring the amplification of both targets on the FAM and TET channels, we were able to determine a dilution of cyclophilin primers that could efficiently amplify its target, without preventing the concurrent amplification of Kir 2.1.

PCR Cycling Parameters

For control and experimental reactions the cycling parameters used were:
- 10 min denaturation at 95 °C
- 30 s at 95 °C
- 1 min at 55 °C X 40
- 30 s at 72 °C

Data Analysis

Relative quantification may in the end rely on the choice of a standard by which to compare the result. A variety of housekeeping genes have been used to standardize RNA analysis and there is no clear-cut advantage to any one of the standard RNA. rRNA can be used, but may not be the best choice. The amount of rRNA is higher than any expressed gene, and amounts of rRNA may vary from the amount of mRNA. There are further complications due to the lack of rRNA in purified mRNA preparations and the lack of priming by oligo-dT. The other common choices are also not perfect. These include β-actin, GAPDH, cyclophilin, β-2 microglobulin, HPRT1, and a long list of others. All of these do vary in concentration from tissue to tissue, and may also vary due to treatment protocol. Perhaps the best approach is to measure several housekeeping genes and average their content (Vandesompele et al. 2002).

The results from the reactions in our lab are normalized against cyclophilin, and quantified using a standard curve generated from Kir 2.1 DNA. The software that accompanies many Real-Time PCR machines has the capacity to quantify target DNA relative to the standard curve automatically. Additionally, some software suites allow for automatic exportation of the Ct values into Excel for further statistical analysis. Details of the analysis software will vary by cycler and version.

Troubleshooting

Preventing Contamination

PCR in general and reverse transcription, and PCR in particular, are highly sensitive to contaminated DNA in the reaction. The two primary sources of DNA contamination are genomic DNA, which co-precipitated with the RNA, and products of other PCR reactions you may have run. To prevent the corruption of experiments, every precaution must be taken to minimize genomic DNA contamination and cross contamination between experiments. The problem of genomic is a particular one. A strategy is to design primers that span exon-exon junctions. The result is that genomic DNA will not be an effective template for the reaction. This not always practical and other mechanisms are required. Contamination of Genomic DNA can be minimized, by treating RNA samples with RNase-free DNase. This will remove the contamination, but requires total elimination of the DNase before the reverse transcription. Even trace amounts may reduce the sensitivity of the reaction.

Contamination of reactions with the products of previous ones has always been a problem with PCR. It becomes a greater problem when less abundant products are being assessed. In some ways, this problem is eliminated in Real-Time PCR, as the reaction can be tested without opening the reaction tube. However, good technique requires care in separate PCR preparation. The use of separate areas, reagents and pipettes for template preparation and amplification setup are important. Even more important, is to isolate any product from the setup reagents. The use of aerosol resistant pipette tips provides further protection, so that the product does not contain dTTP, the AmpErase system uses dUTP in the PCR reaction. UNG (Uracil-N-glycosylase) is then used, following the reverse transcription, which produces cDNA with dTTP. UNG recognizes and catalyses the destruction of DNA strands containing deoxyuridine, but not the DNA containing thymidine, preventing carryover. Thus, any DNA produced in previous amplifications can be destroyed, while the template produced for this reaction will remain intact. UNG is inactive at the temperature of a PCR reaction (greater than 50 °C).

One way to assess the level of DNA contamination in the RNA samples, is to perform a PCR reaction using total RNA that has not been reverse transcribed as a template. It is important to note that the critical parameter is not the absence of an amplification product, but that the level of product amplified from contamination is significantly less than the reverse transcribed signal. This may be achieved with careful preparation of samples and isolation of PCR products from starting reagents.

General Considerations

As with any new technique, there are critical parameters one should be aware of to ensure success. Specificity is of paramount concern, as the amplifying of incorrect product completely nullifies PCR's utility. Since Real-Time PCR is effectively PCR with a fluorogenic probe added, all factors that could affect "non real-time amplifications" are in play. Magnesium chloride concentration and buffer composition are both factors that must be considered. Particular consideration must be made with primer composition, specificity of primer action, probe structure and melting point. Many of these parameters are controlled by the mix preparation purchased. The amounts of primers and probes as well as cycling parameters are also critical and may vary when multiplexing. In the end, the most important factors are the skill, care and consistency of the individual setting up the reactions.

References

Bustin, S.A., (2000) Absolute Quantification of mRNA Using Real-Time Reverse Transcription Polymerase Chain Reaction Assays. J. Mol. Endocrinol. 25, 169–193

Bustin, S.A., (2002) Quantification of mRNA Using Real-Time Reverse Transcription PCR (RT-PCR): Trends and Problems. J. Mol. Endocrinol. 29, 23–39

Chadderton, T., Wilson, C., Bewick, M., Gluck, S., (1997) Evaluation of Three Rapid RNA Extraction Reagents: Relevance for Use in RT-PCR's and Measurement of Low Level Gene Expression in Clinical Samples. Cell Mol. Biol. (Noisy - le-grand) 43, 1227–1234

Chou, Q., Russell, M., Birch, D.E., Raymond, J., Bloch, W., (1992) Prevention of Pre-PCR Mis-Priming and Primer Dimerization Improves Low-Copy-Number Amplifications. Nucleic Acids Res. 20, 1717–1723

Higuchi, R., Fockler, C., Dollinger, G., Watson, R., (1993) Kinetic PCR Analysis: Real-Time Monitoring of DNA Amplification Reactions. Biotechnology (N. Y) 11, 1026v1030

Kellogg, D.E., Rybalkin, I., Chen, S., Mukhamedova, N., Vlasik, T., Siebert, P.D., Chenchik, A., (1994) TaqStart Antibody: "Hot Start" PCR Facilitated by a Neutralizing Monoclonal Antibody Directed Against Taq DNA Polymerase. Biotechniques 16, 1134–1137

Mannhalter, C., Koizar, D., Mitterbauer, G., (2000) Evaluation of RNA Isolation Methods and Reference Genes for RT-PCR Analyses of Rare Target RNA. Clin. Chem. Lab Med. 38, 171–177

Marras, S.A., Kramer, F.R., Tyagi, S., (1999) Multiplex Detection of Single-Nucleotide Variations Using Molecular Beacons. Genet. Anal. 14, 151–156

Ong, Y.L., Irvine, A., (2002) Quantitative Real-Time PCR: A Critique of Method and Practical Considerations. Hematology. 7, 59–67

Overbergh, L., Giulietti, A., Valckx, D., Decallonne ,R., Bouillon, R., Mathieu, C., (2003) The Use of Real-Time Reverse Transcriptase PCR for the Quantification of Cytokine Gene Expression. J. Biomol. Tech. 14, 33–43

Taveau, M., Stockholm, D., Spencer, M., Richard, I., (2002) Quantification of Splice Variants Using Molecular Beacon or Scorpion Primers. Anal. Biochem. 305, 227–235

Thelwell, N., Millington, S., Solinas, A., Booth, J., Brown, T., (2000) Mode of Action and Application of Scorpion Primers to Mutation Detection. Nucleic Acids Res. 28, 3752–3761

Tyagi, S., Bratu, D.P., Kramer, F.R., (1998) Multicolor Molecular Beacons for Allele Discrimination. Nat. Biotechnol. 16, 49–53

Tyagi, S., Kramer, F.R., (1996) Molecular Beacons: Probes That Fluoresce Upon Hybridization. Nat. Biotechnol. 14, 303–308

Vandesompele, J., De Preter, K., Pattyn, F., Poppe, B., Van Roy, N., De Paepe, A., Speleman, F., (2002) Accurate Normalization of Real-Time Quantitative RT-PCR Data by Geometric Averaging of Multiple Internal Control Genes. Genome Biol. 3, 34

Use of cDNA Arrays to Explore Gene Expression in Genetically Manipulated Mice and Cell Lines

Dumitru A. Iacobas, Sandra Iacobas and David C. Spray

Introduction

Mutations and altered expression of specific genes have been shown to be responsible for a number of cardiovascular disorders, including chronic hypertension, coronary heart disease, stroke, and rheumatic heart disease as well as arrhythmias, congenital defects and diseases of the vessel wall. For many of these disorders, changes in gene expression leads to deleterious alterations of protein concentrations that may be compensated by therapeutic treatment. Identification of such changes in disease states may thus help indicate treatment strategies to prevent the disease or diminish its severity. An important tool for determining the impact of altered expression of selected genes is the genetically manipulated animal model, in which one or more genes are knocked out or knocked in. A relatively recent interest of our group has been to evaluate alterations in gene expression in various tissues of mice, in which the coding region of particular gap junction proteins (connexins) is disrupted by homologous recombination and in cultures of connexin-deficient cell lines transiently or stably transfected with connexins.

This chapter presents a summary of the cDNA microarray technology that we have used to explore alterations in gene expression patterns in connexin null mice and in transfected cells. In addition, we summarize analytical tools that we have developed to mine the data obtained in microarray experiments.

Overview of the cDNA Microarray Technique

The cDNA microarray technique (for general reference see Rampal 2001; Schena 2000) typically uses two-color labeling (generally red (r) vs. green (g) fluorescent Cy5 and Cy3 dyes) to provide ratios of thousands of individual gene expression levels in two sources of RNA (see Fig. 1a). The detection elements (i.e. the cDNA microarray chips) are produced by robotically printing tens of thousands of selected cDNA clones obtained from libraries containing millions of expressed sequence tags (ESTs) on chemically treated 1"×3" glass slides. For example, the mouse cDNA microarrays produced by the Microarray Facility of the Albert Einstein College of Medicine (*http://microarray1k.aecom.yu.edu*), contain 27,400 cDNA selected mouse ESTs and 192 bacterial controls, in 4×12 (48) blocks, each block containing 598 spots

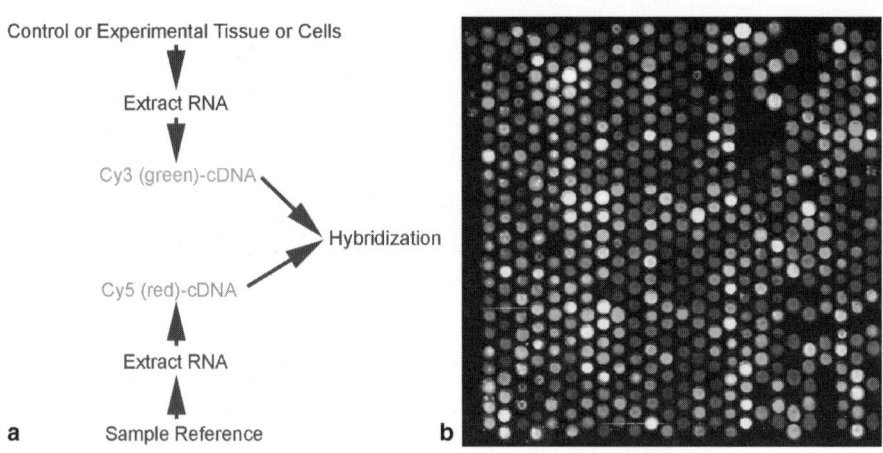

Figure 1a,b
The simplified scheme of the cDNA microarray method, and part of the 8-bit pseudo-color image of a hybridized 27.4k cDNA microarray chip, produced by the Albert Einstein College of Medicine Microarray Facility. **a** The green-labeled heart extract of the connexin deficient mouse was co-hybridized with the red-labeled mouse reference. **b** Yellow spots indicate that mRNA abundance is similar in the two samples, while red/green spots indicate that a labeled source contains more mRNA. *For coloured version see appendix*

110 µm in diameter and printed by the same pen. A dual laser scanner quantifies the red and green fluorescence in each individual spot and the two 16-bit images are merged into a pseudocolor 8-bit composite image that should appear yellow when mRNA abundance is similar in the two samples and be biased towards red or green if one labeled source contains more mRNA than the other (see Fig. 1b).

Description of Methods and Practical Approach

Methodological Details Regarding cDNA Microarrays

RNA Extraction, Reverse Transcription and Hybridization with the Microarray

Total RNA is extracted in Trizol (Gibco, following the method of Auffray and Rougeon 1980) from each of the tissues/cell cultures to be compared. When the RNA extraction cannot be performed immediately after the tissue isolation, the specimen can be preserved at 4°C up to 1 month in a special medium such as RNA-later™ (Ambion Cat#7020), or at –80 °C for longer periods. 60 µg total RNA is precipitated to eliminate the ethanol, then re-suspended in 17 µl DEPC-H_2O, 2 µl oligo dT is added and the resulting 19 ml solution is incubated for 5 min at 65 °C to anneal the RNA. In order to obtain labeled cDNA, 21 µl fluorescent mix (4 µl 0.1 M DTT + 4 µl 10× low dT dNTP + 4 µl Cy3 (green-emission) or Cy5 (red-emission) dUTP + 5× first strand buffer) and 2 µl Superscript-RT (Gibco) are added. After 1 h incubation at 42 °C, 2 µl Superscript-

RT is added again followed by a second incubation at 42 °C for another hour and heating at 94 °C for 3 min. Fluorescent cDNA probes are cleaned from the RNA and concentrated. 1 µl blocking solution and 40 ml hybridization buffer are added, denatured at 94 °C for 2 min and incubated at 50 °C for approximately 1 h. Hybridization takes place overnight, at 50 °C, against an amino-silane coated microarray spotted with 27,400 selected mouse cDNA sequences. The chip is then washed at room temperature, using solutions containing 0.1% SDS (sodium lauryl sulfate) and 1% SSC (3 M NaCl + 0.3 M sodium citrate) to remove the non-hybridized fluorescent cDNAs.

Scanning, Data Acquisition and Normalization

The hybridized microarray is scanned with a dual laser system that converts the red and green fluorescent emissions of each pixel separately from the array surface into 16 bit signals. The size of the pixel depends on the scanner resolution, generally 5 or 10 µm. In addition to the specific hybridization with the spots, the slide coat may also adsorb labeled cDNAs non-specifically. Therefore, the user must subtract the background signal (B) from the foreground signal (F). This operation depends on the assumption that B within the spots is the same as in the pixels surrounding the spots; however, fluorescent intensity is not uniform across the pixels either within or outside the spots. The best way to overcome this problem is to subtract the median of B from the median of F. In order to avoid false hits, spots with excessive local imperfections (customarily flagged by the acquisition program, such as GenePix™ Pro 4.1, www.axon.com), those where the median of F is not statistically significantly ($p < 0.001$) greater than the median of B, and those where the signal is saturated, are eliminated from subsequent analysis.

The intensity of the recorded signals depends on the acceleration voltages in the two photo multiplier tubes of the scanner. By modifying these settings, the color of the spot in the 8-bit composite image can be changed. Therefore, it is necessary to normalize the data so that comparison with biological significance can be made. In order to decide whether the observed expression regulation is statistically significant (i.e. it exceeds the normal biological variability and the potential technical noise), one has to replicate the experiment several times in order to evaluate both the expression variability within the compared types of specimens, and the maximum signal error for each spot due to technical differences across the chips. We have developed an iterative procedure by which the background subtracted raw data are calibrated, alternating intra-chip and inter-chip normalization, until the average correction becomes less than the pre-established threshold (5%). The intra-chip normalization balances the readings of the two channels within-print tip groups (pen-domains) for each chip, while the inter-chip normalization balances the readings of the same channel ("red" or "green") for all chips. Both normalizations are carried out in three successive steps to: i) balance the total net fluorescence of valid spots (global normalization), ii) correct the intensity-dependent bias (usually referred to as "lowess normalization") and iii) establish a standard distribution (mean 0 and standard deviation 1) for the log ratios (scale normalization). In cases where multiple spots on the array represent the same gene, the fluorescence value used is the weighted average of the calibrated inten-

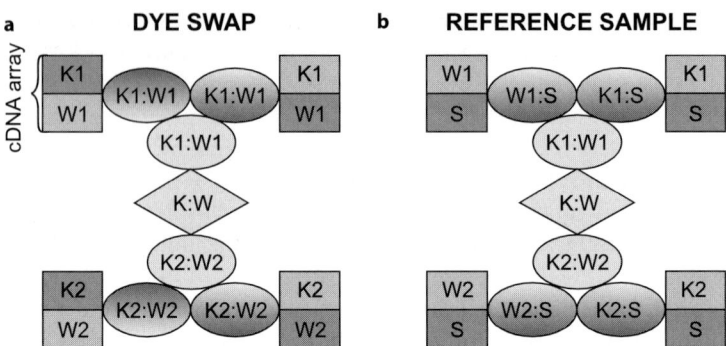

Figure 2a,b
Experimental designs. Each rectangle of two squares represents a single cDNA array, as indicated in the upper left corner of the figure. Symbols within squares indicate hybridized extracts: S = reference, W = wildtype heart, K = Cx43 null heart, with colors indicating whether the dye label was red (Cy5) or green (Cy3). Ovals indicate: K:W = expression ratio in K compared to W, K:S = expression ratio in K compared to S, W:S = expression ratio in W compared to S, with color indicating the type of ratio: red-to-red, green-to-green, green-to-red, red-to-green, or the geometric average of the red and green ratios (*yellow*). *For coloured version see appendix*

sities of the corresponding spots; thus, the contribution of each of the spots increases with the number of identities, between the spotted sequence and the probed gene, and decreases with the length of the query.

Experimental Design

The traditional ratiometric cDNA microarray method of determining gene expression uses different dyes to label control and experimental RNA. However, this introduces additional variables, as the dyes differ in their incorporation of the RNA samples, their hybridization efficiency with the microarray and their fluorescence yields (Butte 2002; Iacobas et al. 2002a). In order to correct the inherent bias towards one or other probe, two strategies (and their variants) are currently in general use (Churchill 2002; Holloway et al. 2002; Kerr and Churchill 2001). Dye-swapping, in which the same RNA samples are labeled with each of the fluorescent tags and then their ratios are averaged (Fig. 2a), and Reference Sample, in which control and experimental samples are all labeled with the same tag (Fig. 2b) and then co-hybridized on separate arrays with an identical reference RNA sample (labeled "S" in Fig. 2b). We have used each of these strategies and summarized their advantages and disadvantages (Iacobas et al. 2002b).

Co-hybridization of control samples to a constant reference allows calculation of what we consider to be a critical parameter of gene expression control, the correlation between the expression of one gene and of all others, under normal conditions. In our view, this possibility of correlation analysis makes the reference method the strategy of choice between these alternatives. However, a potential problem with this strategy is that it depends on the Reference RNA being constant (requiring preparation of sufficient amounts for all experiments at one time), whereas, at least some degradation might be expected to occur over time, even when the reference is optimally maintained at −80 °C.

Quantification and Identification of Genes With Regulated Expression

Detection of Significant Expression Alterations

Quantification of spots that are regulated in experimental specimens as compared to controls, requires measurement of both the average fluorescence of each spot in control and in experimental groups, and calculation of the variance within each group to determine whether changes are statistically significant. Our analysis of background-corrected signals calculates the mean and variance for each spot on all control and experimental specimens (see Fig. 3a), and averages the regulations detected by different spots probing the same gene. In order to generate statistically meaningful data sets, we generally compare samples from four distinct control and four experimental tissues or cell cultures. Significantly altered genes are considered to be those rejected by the two-tailed t-test for equality of means with an assigned p-value (examples in Iacobas et al. 2003).

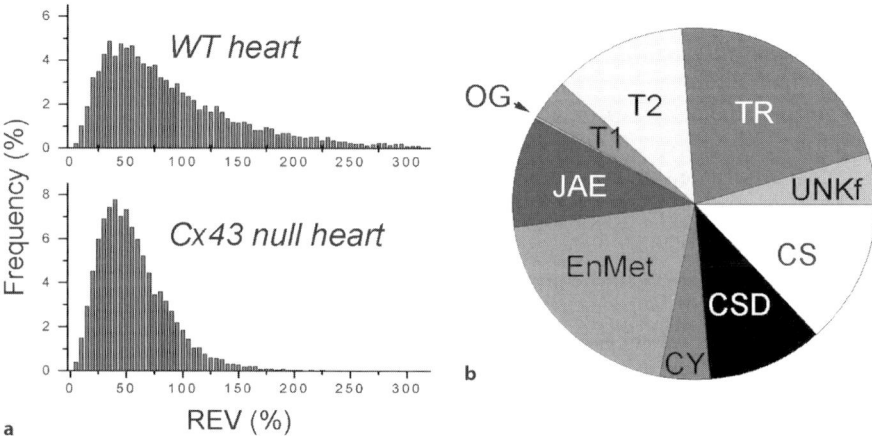

Figure 3
Detection of statistically altered gene expression. **a** Histograms showing the range and relative frequency of variation in gene expression for all spots on the arrays for wildtype (WT) and Cx43 null hearts. These distributions are quite different (p-val <10^{-30}); for WT hearts the mean Relative Estimated Variability (REV) was 90.5 ± 62.6 (SD) with skewness 1.3 and kurtosis 1.7, while mean REV for Cx43 null heart was 57.9 ± 34.4, with skewness 2.0 and kurtosis 8.8. **b** Distribution of functions of significantly regulated genes in Cx43 null compared to wildtype hearts. Note that the functions of altered genes include transcriptional (TR), Junction-Adhesion-Extracellular Matrix (JAE), Energy and Metabolism (EnMet), as well as signaling, transport and cytoskeleton. Abbreviations for all functional classes are given in text. *For coloured version see appendix*

It should be noted that the Reference Sample strategy provides measurement of variance for each spot in the multiple arrays hybridized with cDNA from both control and treated samples. This not only allows determination of whether apparent differences are statistically significant, but it also allows comparison of the degree of stability of expression of each gene in the control and experimental groups. This stability varies markedly: some genes show variability as low as a few percent of the average expression level among four specimens, while others vary several-fold (Iacobas et al. 2003; see also Fig. 3a). We have defined the Relative Estimated (transcription) Variability (REV) that evaluates the statistically significant limit of expression variability within a homogeneous batch of specimens and accounts for the stringency of the transcription control, with low REV values indicating high control (Iacobas et al. 2003).

Identification of Genes Corresponding to Spotted Sequences

A complication of the cDNA array technique is that, while many sequences chosen for spotting correspond to genes with known encoded proteins, others correspond to expressed sequences that remain without known protein product. Gene annotation of the arrays is thus a dynamic process, requiring continuous updating through websites such as: *http://genome-www5.stanford.edu/cgi-bin/source//sourceBatchSearch*. This website provides information about Clone ID, GenBank Accession, dbEST cloneID, UniGene ClusterID, UniGene gene name, UniGene gene symbol, Gene aliases, Locus Link ID, Representative mRNA Acc, Representative Protein Accession, Chromosome location, Cytoband, Gene ontology, Enzymatic function and Sub cellular locations for human, mouse and rat genes. The continuous annotation updating, and the existence of millions of sequences that can be spotted, gives rise to another complication, which is that most genes represented on the microarray are probed by multiple spots, with different bit-scores derived from the raw alignment of the spotted sequence to the analyzed gene. Although this redundancy provides assurance that genes are truly regulated, the multiple values of spots for the same gene requires averaging; as noted above, we use a weighted average considering the degree of homology.

Classification of Functions of Regulated Genes

Because a large number of genes are generally regulated in genetically modified mice or following transfection, it is useful to categorize the functions of the proteins encoded by the regulated genes, in order to begin to determine functional changes. One simple classification scheme that we found useful is based on cell biological functions (Alberts et al. 1994): Junction-Adhesion-Extra cellular Matrix (JAE: antigens, globulins, integrins, claudins, cadherins, connexins, desmosomal components, laminin, proteoglycans, etc), Cytoskeletal (CY: intermediary filaments, microtubules, centrioles, actin, and their associated proteins), Transport into the cell (T1: channels, transporters, and ionotropic receptors), Transport within the cell (T2: proteins of vesicles, cellular motors, endosomes, lysosomes, nuclear transport, protein folding, etc), Cell Signaling (CS: G-protein coupled receptors, protein kinases, SH2 and SH3 domain proteins, calcium binding proteins, etc), Cell Cycle-Shape-Differentiation (CSD:

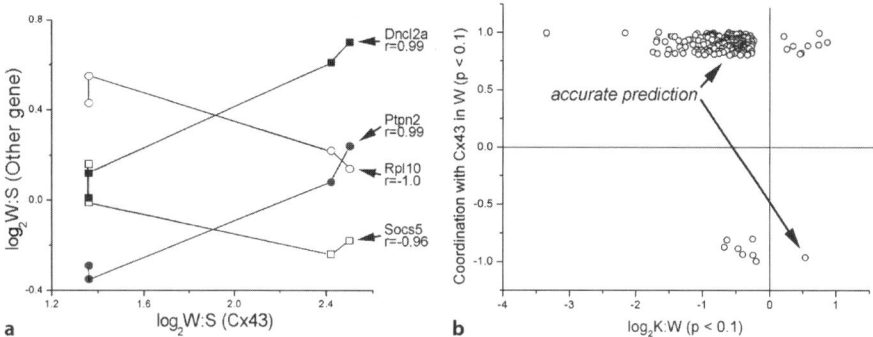

Figure 4a,b
Coordination of the expression of other genes with that of Cx43. **a** Binary logarithm of expression ratios for Cx43 were plotted against that of every other gene, for the four separate arrays, using wildtype hearts. Examples are shown of synergistic expressions (Dncl2a = dynein cytoplasmic light chain 2A and Ptpn2 = protein tyrosine phosphatase, non-receptor type 2) and antagonistic expressions (Rpl10 = ribosomal protein 10 and Socs5 = suppressor of cytokine signaling 5). Note the high correlation coefficients (r values). **b** The coordination analysis of other genes with Cx43 in wildtype hearts plotted as a function of the $\log_2$ ratio of gene expression in Cx43 null heart (K) compared to wildtype (W) heart. Note the accurate prediction of the up- or down- type of regulation for 92.5% of the significantly regulated genes in the Cx43 null heart that were also significantly coordinated (synergistically or antagonistically) with Cx43 expression in the wildtype heart. This finding provides evidence of normal linkage of expression of these genes with Cx43

growth factors, apoptosis-related genes, cytokines, etc.), Transcription (TR: DNA binding proteins, DNA repair, RNA, transcription factors, oncogenes, etc), Energy and Metabolism (EnMet: oxidants, peroxisomes, respiratory chain, glycolysis and glycogenesis, enzymes, etc), Organelle Genetics (OG: mitochondrial genes), and genes encoding proteins for which function is presently unknown (UNKf).

One advantage of such a scheme is the small number of categories, readily allowing subdivision to reflect greater similarities (e.g., Cell Signaling genes that encode protein kinases or phosphatases). Alternatively, genes may be grouped according to signaling pathways, where both target proteins and those that function to alter its function are clustered within a category (see, for example, Iacobas et al. 2003, for apoptosis-related genes and Iacobas et al. 2004, for cell motility). Such a scheme may be of particular utility when attempting to define correlation of related gene expression patterns, as indicated below.

Transcription Coordination and Identification of Functional Pathways

The hybridization of control/experimental samples against a standard reference (see Fig. 2b) allows direct comparison of the expression values for pairs of genes in each array within a series. Calculation of the Pearson correlation coefficient (Iacobas 1977) across the series of arrays used for every type of specimen can be used to determine whether two genes are synergistically ($r > 0.9$), antagonistically ($r < -0.9$) or independently ($-0.05 < r < 0.05$) expressed (see examples of synergistically and antagonistically expressed genes with Cx43 in Fig. 4a).

Application of These Methods to Determine Gene Expression Changes in Hearts of Connexin43 Null Mice

Connexin43 (Cx43) is the most widespread gap junction protein found in mammals, occurring in almost every tissue (Chen et al. 1995); it is a primary component of intercellular gap junction channels in cardiac tissue, where it is the most abundant gap junction protein in ventricular myocytes (see Spray et al. 2001). Recent evidence suggesting a genetic linkage to hypoplastic left heart syndrome (Dasgupta et al. 2001), and post-infarction ventricular arrhythmias are considered to be largely gap junction diseases (Severs 2001; Kano and Saffitz 2001). Cx43 null mice die at birth due to a developmental cardiac abnormality, where hyperplasia blocks blood flow exiting from the right ventricular outflow tract to the lungs (Reaume et al. 1995).

In order to determine the extent to which Cx43 deletion affected other cardiac genes, we used the AECOM 27,400 mouse cDNA arrays to compare hearts from four neonatal Cx43 null mice and four wild type littermates. For these studies, we used the Reference Sample Method (see Figs. 1 and 2b), with Cy3 (green) incorporated into control and test RNA, and Reference labeled with Cy5 (red).

The significant decrease of the mean value of the Relative Estimated Variability (REV) in hearts of Cx43 null mice as compared to the wild type mice (see Fig. 3a), indicates more stringent transcriptional control in the mutant, presumably as a compensatory effect to the alterations induced by the Cx43 disruption. This observation is consistent with decreased mean REV values in other organs of genetically manipulated animals (brains of Cx43 -/-, Cx43 +/- and Cx32 -/- mice, and livers of Cx32 -/- mice) as well as in the brain, heart and kidney of mice subjected to various stresses such as chronic and cyclic hypoxia or mechanical stress (Iacobas et al., unpublished results).

When array data was further processed, we found that 586 out of 5613 adequately quantified distinct genes with known protein products were significantly ($p < 0.05$) regulated in Cx43 null hearts of newborn mice. 93% of the affected genes were down regulated. When affected genes were categorized according to function (see Fig. 3b), the greatest percentages were transcription factors (22%) and energy-metabolism (20%). However, genes encoding proteins with all types of cellular functions were affected, indicating that altered expression of this gap junction gene leads to widespread changes in expression of other genes.

These results suggest that phenotypic changes arising from gene deletion may not only reflect absence of the functional protein that this gene encodes, but will also extend to altered expression of other proteins whose gene expression is linked to that of the deleted gene.

We have also explored whether genes regulated in the connexin43 null tissue exhibited expression variation in normal tissue that was coordinated with the expression of Cx43. We found that 92.5% of the coordinately (synergistically and antagonistically) expressed genes with Cx43 in the heart of WT mice accurately predicted the regulation type in the heart of Cx43 null mice (see Fig. 4b).

This finding suggests that the altered expression detected for many genes in the Cx43 null heart may reflect the coordinated expression of these genes with Cx43 in the normal heart.

Conclusions

Genetically manipulated mice are useful tools to mimic genetic disorders in humans, and thus in understanding the complexity and intricacy of the processes triggered by disruption of single genes. Important phenotypic changes have been attributed to the absence of intercellular gap junction channels in tissues where they are normally expressed. Findings from our studies of Cx43 null mice indicate that gap junction genes regulate other genes controlling multiple cellular functional pathways.

Acknowledgements. Supported in part by National Institutes of Health grants NS42807, NS41282, and MH65495.

References

Alberts B, Bray D, Lewis J, Raff M, Roberts K, Watson JD. (1994). Molecular Biology of the Cell, 3rd ed., New York and London: Garland Publishing
Auffray C, Rougeon F. (1980) Purification of Mouse Immunoglobulin Heavy-Chain Messenger RNAs From Total Myeloma Tumor RNA. Eur. J. Biochem. 107:303–314
Butte A, (2002). The Use and Analysis of Microarray Data. Nat Rev Drug Discov. 1(12): 951–60. Review
Chen ZQ, Lefebvre D, Bai XH, Reaume A, Rossant J, Lye SJ. (1995). Identification of Two Regulatory Elements Within the Promoter Region of the Mouse Connexin 43 Gene, J Biol Chem. 24;270(8):3863–3868
Churchill GA. (2002). Fundamentals of Experimental Design for cDNA Microarrays, Nat Genet. 32 Suppl:490–5. Review
Dasgupta C, Martinez AM, Zuppan CW, Shah MM, Bailey LL, Fletcher WH. (2001). Identification of Connexin43 (alpha1) Gap Junction Gene Mutations in Patients With Hypoplastic Left Heart Syndrome by Denaturing Gradient Gel Electrophoresis (DGGE), Mutat Res. 479(1–2):173–86
Holloway AJ, van Laar RK, Tothill RW, Bowtell DD. (2202). Options Available—from Start to Finish—for Obtaining Data From DNA Microarrays II, Nat Genet. 32 Suppl:481–489. Review
Iacobas DA. (1997). Medical Biostatistics. 3rd Engl. Ed. Bucharest, Bucura Mond.
Iacobas DA. (2000). Exploring the Gene Eexpression. In DA. Iacobas: "Ideas and Methods in the Physics of Living", pp.273-305, 4th Engl Ed, Constanta: Tilia Press Int.
Iacobas DA, Urban M, Massimi A, Spray DC. (2002a). Improved Procedures to Mine Data Obtained from Spotted Cdna Arrays, J Biomol Tech. 13(1), 5–19
Iacobas DA, Urban M, Massimi A, Iacobas S, Spray DC. (2002b). Hits and Misses from Gene Expression Ratio Measurements in cDNA Microarray Studies.) J Biomol Tech. 13(3), 143–157
Iacobas DA, Scemes E, Spray DC (2004). Gene Expression in Connexin43 Null Astrocytes Extended Beyond the Gap Junction, Neurochem. Intl., in press
Iacobas DA, Urban M, Iacobas S, Scemes E, Spray DC. (2003). Array Analysis of Gene Expression in Connexin43 Null Astrocytes, Physiol Genomics. 15: 177–190
Kanno S, Saffitz JE (2001) .The Role of Myocardial Gap Junctions in Electrical Conduction and Arrhythmogenesis, Cardiovasc Pathol. 10(4):169–77
Kerr M.K., Churchill G.A. (2001). Statistical Design and the Analysis of Gene expression Microarrays, Genetical Research, 77:123–128
Rampal J.B. (Editor) (2001). DNA Arrays. Methods and Protocols. (2001). Methods in Molecular Biology, Volume 170. Humana Press, Totowa, New Jersey
Reaume A.G., de Sousa P.A., Kulkarni S., Langille B.L., Zhu D., Davies T.C., Juneja S.C., Kidder G.M., Rossant J. (1995). Cardiac Malformation in Neonatal Mice Lacking Connexin43, Science, 267:1831–1834
Schena M. (editor). (2000). Microarray Biochip Technology, Eaton Publishing, Natick, MA.
Severs NJ. (2001) Gap Junction Remodeling and Cardiac Arrhythmogenesis: Cause or Coincidence? J Cell Mol Med. 5(4):355–66
Spray, D.C., Suadicani , S., Srinivas, M. Gutstein, D.E., and Fishman, G.I. (2001). Gap Junctions in the Cardiovascular System. Handbook of Physiology: Section 2: The Cardiovascular System. Vol. 1: The Heart: Gap Junctions in the Cardiovascular System. Oxford University Press New York, pp.169–212

Using Antibody Arrays to Detect Protein-Protein Interactions

Heather S. Duffy, Ionela Iacobas, David C. Spray and Anthony W. Ashton

Introduction

The antibody array technique is a step in the direction of high-throughput screens, similar to the cDNA or oligonucleotide arrays that have been developed for gene profiling. Antibody arrays allow for rapid screening of multiple potential interactions, confirmation of which is relatively simple, given the state of technology now available for co-immunoprecipitation, confocal immunolocalization and mass spectrometry. In this Chapter we review this powerful method, using as an example the study of protein-protein interactions involving connexin, the protein subunit that forms gap junction channels.

Gap junction channels have traditionally been thought to function solely as conduits for transport of ions and small molecules between adjacent cells. Consequently, much of the previous work in this field has focused on properties of the channel itself or on factors controlling expression or function of gap junction channel proteins (connexins). However, protein-protein interactions are being increasingly appreciated as playing major roles in regulating functions of other membrane proteins (Sheng et al. 2001).

Recent evidence suggests that protein-protein interactions are a novel mechanism for gap junction regulation as well. The binding of multiple protein partners indicates that there is a large complex of proteins associated with gap junctions; composition of these complexes (or Nexus) may change under physiological and pathological conditions and may vary depending on the tissue and intracellular compartments in which they are found (see Duffy et al. 2001 for review).

Most connexin-interacting proteins identified to date have been discovered through immuno-co-localization and verified through co-immunoprecipitation, although higher throughput methods such as yeast two-hybrid screens, and mass spectometric analysis of proteins pulled down with connexin antibodies or tagged connexin constructs, are presently being used by several laboratories.

An alternative method by which to look for multiple binding partners for a given protein is the Antibody Array. This technology utilizes multiple antibodies, directed against a wide variety of proteins, spotted onto nitrocellulose membranes. Antibody-spotted membranes are incubated with lysates from cultured cells or whole tissues to allow for binding of the proteins to the antibodies. Probing with an HRP-tagged an-

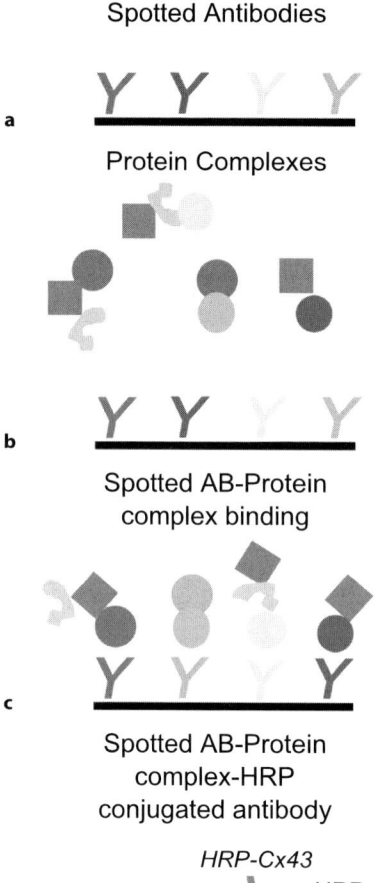

Figure 1a–d
Cartoon depicting the antibody array method: Antibodies are spotted onto PVDF membrane (**a**), incubated with cell or tissue lysates (**b**). Antibodies capture their epitopes, bringing entire protein complexes with them (**c**). These complexes are then detected with HRP conjugated antibodies directed at a protein of interest (**d**), in this case an antibody directed against Connexin43 (HRP-Cx43)

tibody to a protein of interest, such as Connexin43, allows detection of this protein within the complex bound to the antibody array (Fig. 1). In essence, these arrays can allow hundreds of individual co-immunoprecipitation studies to be done simultaneously. The antibody array is a simpler technique than western blot, and gives more information than immunoprecipitation regarding a single potential binding partner.

Description of Methods and Practical Approach

Making an Antibody Array

Antibody arrays are commercially available (e.g. Hypromatrix; Worchester, MA) that give excellent, highly reproducible results; alternatively, arrays with selected antibodies may be generated using the protocol described below. Advantages of pre-made arrays include simplicity of use, high variety of signal transduction pathways probed, and high reproducibility due to homogeneous spotting of the antibodies on the membranes. Disadvantages of commercial arrays include, limitations of examination to proteins that may not make any biological sense or be of little interest, the considerable cost involved in purchasing multiple arrays to reproduce the data, and lack of information regarding properties of the proprietary antibodies spotted on the arrays. Therefore, it is advantageous to produce arrays within individual laboratories or core facilities to supplement the commercial arrays. Arrays can be produced relatively simply using an array spotter such as the Bio-Rad "Bio-Dot" apparatus (Bio-Rad, Hercules, CA). This apparatus consists of a 96 well plate, where each well is open-ended, for spotting antibodies onto membranes. To use, cut PVDF membrane (Millipore, Bedford, MA) to fit array base, and hydrate membrane with methanol followed by rinsing 3 times, for 10 min each time, in PBS at pH 7.4. Sandwich the membrane between the lower base of the Bio-Dot apparatus and the upper 96 well plate. Add 100 µl of antibody diluted in PBS to each well. Each well should contain either a different antibody or a replicate of an antibody used elsewhere in the array (for determining consistency). Rock the entire array apparatus for 5 min at room temp. on a rotating shaker, then evacuate solution through the membrane, through the attached vacuum manifold. Follow this with 3 rinses PBS at pH 7.4 (400 µl each), remove PVDF membrane and air-dry overnight.

Tissue or Cell Preparation

Tissues or cell culture samples can be prepared by lysis in 500 µl of 1% NP-40 lysis buffer [50 mM Tris-HCl pH 7.4, 1% NP-40 or Triton-X 100, 0.25 mM Na-deoxycholate, 150 mM NaCl, 2 mM EGTA, 0.1 mM Na_3VO_4, 10 mM NaF, 1 mM PMSF and 1 tablet of "Complete" protease inhibitor cocktail (Roche Laboratories, Palo Alto, CA)] and sonicated for 10 s. After sonication, incubate lysates 30 min on ice and then spin at 4 °C for 10 min at 12,000 rpm. Remove supernatant and determine protein levels using a standard protein assay (e.g. BioRad Protein Assay system BioRad, Hercules, CA). Rehydrate dried antibody arrays by 10 s rinse in methanol followed by rinsing in PBS at pH 7.5 3 times for 10 min. Incubate arrays in TBST (150mM NaCl, 25mM Tris-HCl, 0.05% Tween20, pH 7.5) for 5 min at room temperature and block with 5% skimmed milk in TBST for 1 h at room temperature Following block, incubate with protein samples (250 µg/ml) in 5% skimmed milk/TBST for 1 h at room temperature. Following three 10 min washes in TBST, incubate the array with antibody directed against a protein of interest, conjugated to HRP (Pierce EZ Link Kit, Pierce Bio.) in TBST with

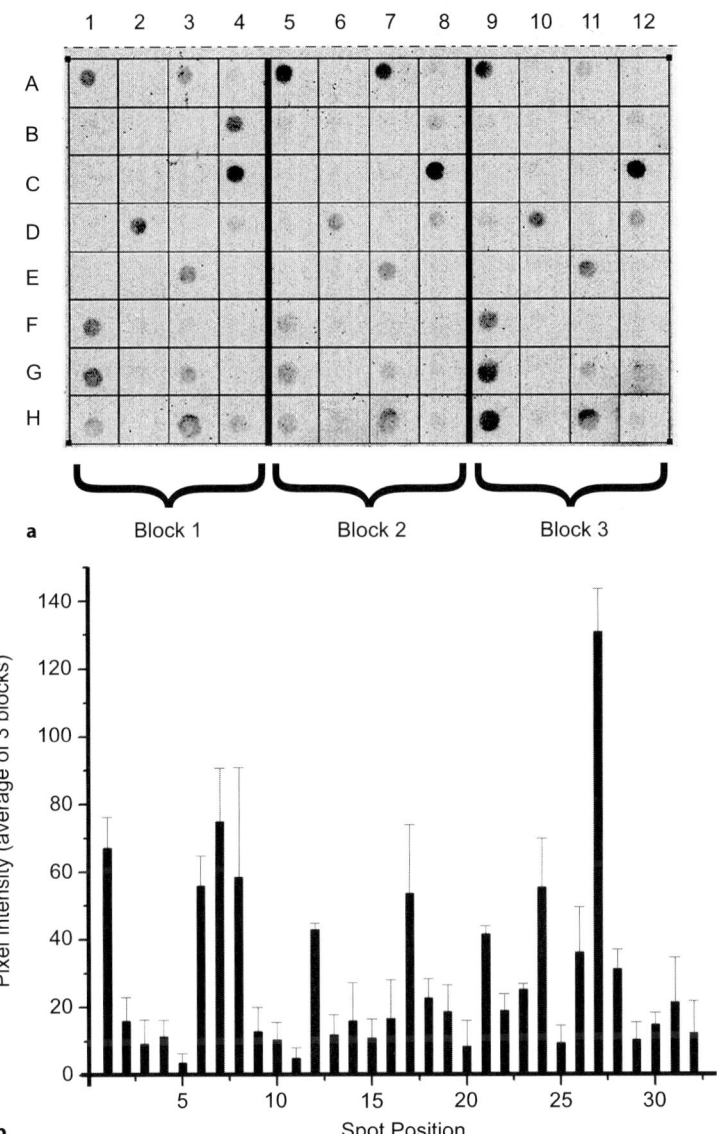

Figure 2a,b
Homemade antibody array of lysates obtained from whole heart tissue probed with HRP-conjugated anti-Cx43 (polyclonal, Zymed, S. San Francisco, CA). Thirty-two individual antibodies were spotted alphabetically in the first four columns of the array. This pattern was repeated for rows 5–8 and 9–12 to determine reproducibility of binding. a Note that with few exceptions, the spots are of similar size and the signals are similar between corresponding spots in blocks of the array. b The array data was analyzed with densitometry and the intensity of each spot averaged. Average signal from each of the 32 antibodies used is shown

5% skimmed milk for 1 h. Following 3×10 min TBST, expose arrays to ECL HRP detection kit (Amersham) and expose on X-ray film. An example of results obtained with such a homemade array is shown in Fig. 2. Here, we spotted 32 different antibodies onto the first four columns of the array, and repeated this pattern of antibodies again in columns 5–8 and 9–12, to determine the reproducibility of the technique. Lysate was obtained from heart tissue and Cx43 binding was probed using HRP-conjugated Cx43 polyclonal antibody (Zymed, S. San Francisco, CA).

Densitometry

Quantitative analysis of antibody array data sets is highly desirable, as determination of which spots are positive can be confounded by high background levels, giving a poor signal to noise ratio. We have used scanning densitometry (Personal Densitometer SI; Molecular Dynamics) to determine the spots with signal intensities that are above background. The resolution was set at 12 bits with a pixel size of 100 µm, and we calibrated the scanner using blank, pre-exposed film. The densitometer provides raw optical density (intensity) of each spot as well as determining spot perimeter, number of pixels, width, intensity and background. For data analysis we used Image QuaNT 5.2 for Windows software. Analysis of scanned films included digital subtraction of the local background around each individual spot, thus controlling for alterations in background levels over different areas of the array (Fig. 2). Comparison of spots within an array (Intra-array normalization) and comparison of spots between two arrays (Inter-array normalization) are considered separately below.

Intra-Array Normalization

Although the global background is eliminated from data by calibration of the scanner, local variations between different areas may occur. Thus, we boxed each spot into identically sized rectangular cells (400 boxes for Hypromatrix array, 96 boxes for home-made array) and considered each cell as a separate field. Using ImageQuaNT we computed the local median of the intensities of the pixels at each cell's border, giving an estimation of local background. We chose the median, instead of the arithmetic average, to avoid extreme values that might artificially affect the background value. The background of each cell is subtracted from the intensity of the array spot allowing for direct comparison between spots. An example of densitometry data can be seen in Fig. 2b. Here the average intensity of the signal from each antibody spot is plotted as a histogram. Note that many of the antibodies give reproducible results. When using the larger, commercial arrays (Fig. 3), it can be seen that whilst there are many spots above background, there are relatively few spots of high intensity (Fig. 3a). If an arbitrary cut-off value of 20 pixel units is used (Fig. 3a), only the highest intensity spots (16 out of 400 or 4.0%) are detected (Fig. 3a), thus narrowing the list of potential binding partners to a manageable level. Candidate protein-protein interactions are then verified through complementary techniques such as co-immunoprecipitation, and subcellular localization of these interactions is determined with immunostaining.

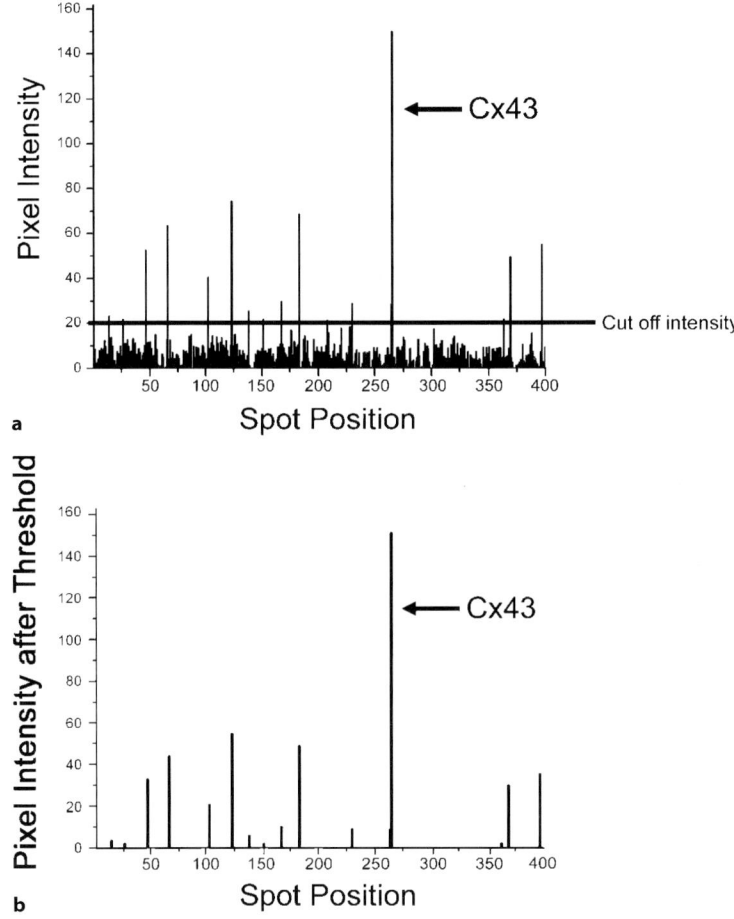

Figure 3a,b
Histograms of positive hits on the antibody array: **a** All points histogram of the data from a Hypromatrix array incubated with lysates from whole heart. Densitometric analysis shows multiple potential positive hits, with Cx43 being the highest intensity hit. To determine the hits with the highest probability of specific interaction with Cx43, an arbitrary cut off of 20 intensity units is imposed. **b** The hits above 20 intensity units show 16 hits, including Cx43 itself, indicating possible interaction of Cx43 with 15 other proteins

Inter-Array Normalization

Antibody arrays can be used to compare protein-protein interactions under a variety of cellular conditions by direct comparison of two arrays. To control for variation between arrays, normalization is required. Except for local differences that intra-array normalization corrects, overall variation could be due to membrane variations or experimental variables (see troubleshooting section below). For the arrays to be com-

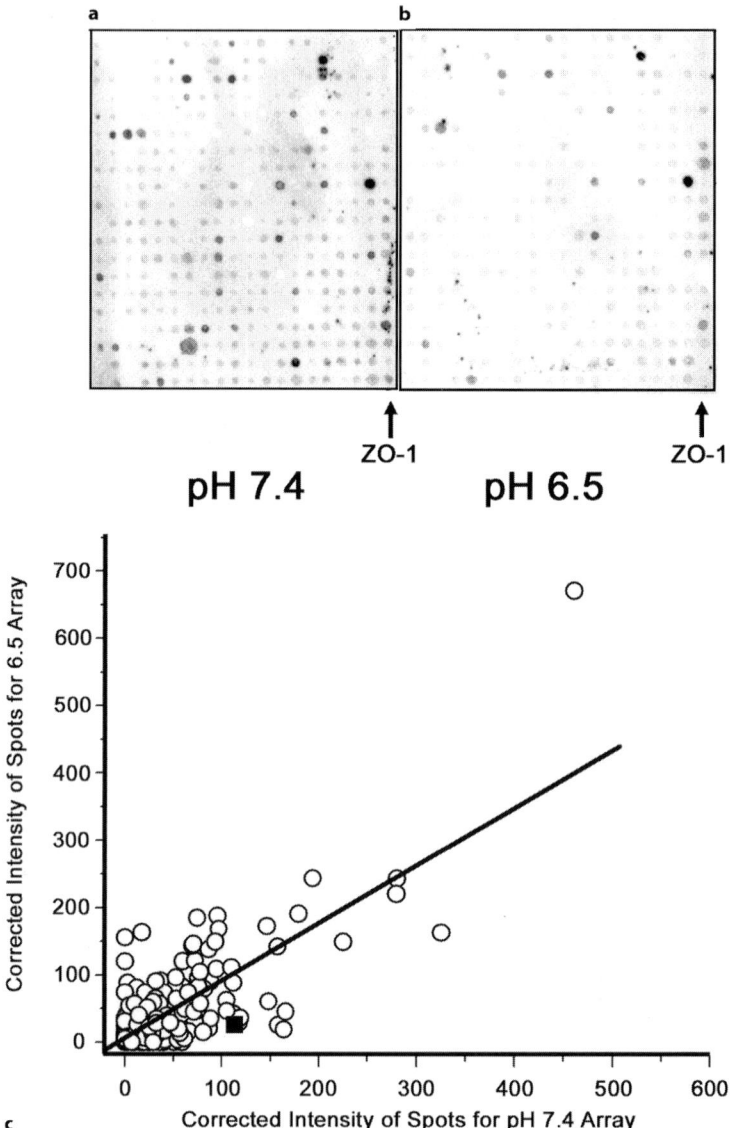

Figure 4a–c
Comparison of antibody arrays from astrocytes maintained at intracellular pH 7.4 or 6.5 for 30 min. Cultured astrocytes, which utilize Cx43 as their main gap junction protein, were subjected to 30 min of low intracellular pH, antibody arrays were performed to examine changes in binding partners for Cx43 under conditions of acidification. At pH 7.4 (**a**) multiple binding partners were found to be potential interacting partners with Cx43, including a known binding partner ZO-1 (*arrow*). However, the number of binding partners for Cx43 following 30 min. of intracellular pH was greatly decreased (**b**). Alterations in the binding partners included a loss of interaction with ZO-1, an event we have shown to occur under conditions of intracellular acidification (Duffy et al. 2004). **c** The potential binding partners for Cx43 in cells maintained at pH 7.4 are plotted against the potential binding partners in cells maintained at pH 6.5. The data point corresponding to ZO-1 is noted by the black filled square. It can be seen that the position of the ZO-1 data point is below the correlation line, indicating a decrease in the interaction of ZO-1 with Cx43 in cells maintained at low intracellular pH

parable, they need the same number of spots and spot sizes. To compare intensities of the same spot on two separate arrays A_1 (i) and A_2 (j), we begin by introducing a global coefficient, C:

$$C = \frac{\sum_{i=1}^{n}(I_i - B_i)}{\sum_{j=1}^{n}(I_j - B_j)}$$

I_i-B_i represents the intensity of the spot i (on array A_1) after subtraction of the local background under and surrounding spot I, and I_j-B_j represents the intensity of the spot j (on array A_2) after subtraction of the local background under and surrounding spot j, where n is the total number of spots on an array. Comparison of $I_i - B_i$ with $(I_j - B_j) \times C$ provides corrected intensities of two identical spots on two separate arrays. Statistical analysis of average intensities after such correction can be used to determine if a given sample has more or less binding to a given spot. One application of the inter-array normalization is shown in Fig. 4, where binding partners for Cx43 are compared at normal and reduced intracellular pH (Fig. 4A pH 7.4, Fig. 4B pH 6.5). Graphic representation comparing intensities of two identical spots in separate arrays (Fig. 4C) shows that alteration of intracellular pH changes the binding partners of Cx43.

Technical Considerations in Antibody Arrays

Issues in Array Design: Choice of Support Matrix

The solid support used greatly determines the quality of array analysis, as it influences efficiency of antibody attachment, degree of nonspecific binding and accessibility of antibodies to widely differing antigens. With these parameters to consider, the solid support used for the development of protein and antibody arrays must meet three key requirements. First, the support used must combine optimal binding under quasi-physiological conditions with high binding capacity; second, it must be suitable for high-throughput screening and easy to manufacture; and third, it must provide a non-denaturing environment which preserves protein structure. One of the key uses of antibody arrays is the study of interacting protein partners; however, many proteins unfold upon immobilization, which causes a loss of any activity/binding that is dependent on 3-dimensional structure. Thus, while it is difficult to define general immobilization strategies that do not discriminate between proteins, the structural similarity of antibodies greatly reduces variability, making antibody arrays easier to design.

For membrane-style antibody arrays, PVDF is the support of choice, as it best fulfils the above three conditions. The protein binding capacity of PVDF is among the highest of all membrane-style supports. Also, the high capacity protein binding of PVDF is achieved without the need to enhance the support with additional surface chemical modifications to immobilize and stabilize the antibodies. While other membrane supports (such as nylon and nitrocellulose) may have binding capacities equivalent to PVDF, our experience indicates that the signal-to-noise ratio of PVDF is superior to these other membranes. Other membranes we have tried (such as nitrocellulose), result in background signal so strong that arrays are un-interpretable. PVDF filter membranes also have superior mechanical strength compared to nitrocellulose, and provide a non-denaturing environment for immobilization of antibodies. PVDF binds and immobilizes proteins by passive adsorption to the membrane, and our results indicate that protein function is well preserved, and antigenicity retained, even when arrays are made up to 4 weeks in advance. In addition, strength of protein bonding to PVDF results in highly stable arrays that allow multiple re-probing reactions, increasing throughput and decreasing the cost of making the arrays.

Antibody Spot Size

Ekins (1998) predicted that smaller spot sizes increase the fractional occupancy of immobilized antibody, and therefore equilibrium is reached more rapidly. We have used two different spot sizes, 1.5 mm diameter on the Hypromatrix array and 3 mm diameter on our own arrays (a 4× difference in spot density). We have found similar relative binding to these different sized spots. These data are consistent with the findings that spot diameters between 200 and 1500 µm had similar antibody occupancy and association rates with a soluble antigen, whereas signal intensity decreased when spot size fell below 200 mm (Sapsford et al. 2001). Our studies and those of Sapsford et al. were performed using flow or agitation, which minimizes diffusion time in determining association kinetics between antibody and antigen. Thus, as long as antibody arrays are probed under non-static conditions, spot size is not critical in array design.

One advantage of using larger spot sizes is the ease of creating a uniform distribu-tion of antibody across the spot area and a decrease in percentage of malformed spots. Using a dot-blot apparatus to form arrays incurs problems inherent to the device itself. Drying of the membrane and trapping of air bubbles in wells during array preparation can both result in non-homogeneous distribution of the antibody over the spot area (halos), where antibody gets trapped in the well periphery leaving the center devoid of binding capacity. Whilst a disadvantage of larger spots is the requirement of greater amounts of antibody, the larger well format allows easier manipulation of sample volumes, minimizing non-homogeneities such as those considered above.

Variation in Signal Strength

Using the methodology outlined here, we have observed remarkably uniform signal intensities of different spots containing the same antigen within an array (see Fig. 2). When present, such variability may reflect non-uniform immobilization chemistry across the surface of the arrays or errors made with the pipette.

Choice of Antibodies as Components on the Array

The minimum antibody concentration required to produce consistent results was previously determined to be 8×10^{-11} g of antibody in a 100 mm diameter spot (Kuzenow et al. 2003). Extrapolating this concentration to the average spot used to create our arrays (3 mm), the minimum concentration should be 72 ng of antibody per spot. We obtained reliable results using 250 ng of antibody per spot, although signal intensity is reduced compared to arrays using 500 ng or 1 μg antibody. More importantly, using less antibody limits the ability to re-probe the membranes, thereby increasing the cost and time spent making arrays. We find that arrays made with 250 ng of antibody can only be probed once, while those made with 500 ng or 1ug of antibody per spot can be stripped and re-probed up to 8×. Conversely, using too much antibody can result in steric hindrance of antibody binding by antibodies adjacently immobilized on the same surface. When we examined saturation curves with different concentrations of capture antibody, no decrease in signal intensity was observed up to 1 mg per spot. No further increases in binding resulted from use of more than 800 ng of antibody per spot. In the final analysis 500 ng per spot is a good compromise between usefulness and frugality, and we suggest using this concentration.

In addition to deciding upon the concentration of antibody to use, a number of factors must be considered when choosing antibodies to be used for array synthesis:

- While many antibodies work well in Western blot analysis, many peptide antibodies require denaturation of the protein to be active, as the native conformation of the protein may mask the antigenic site for the antibody. Thus, antibodies against full-length epitopes, or those confirmed to work in immunoprecipitation/ELISA, are preferred for use in antibody arrays. Antibodies recommended for immunohistochemistry and immunofluorescent analysis may work in the array format, as both assays require recognition of proteins in their native conformation, however, empirical validation is still recommended.

- Antibodies should be checked for specificity and cross-reactivity to determine their suitability for use in an antibody array format. To avoid a high rate of false-positive results inherent in the design of other protein-protein interaction screens (such as yeast two hybrid), antibodies used to make arrays should be highly specific when used in immunoprecipitation assays.

- Monoclonal versus Polyclonal antibodies. The fact that polyclonal antibodies recognize multiple different epitopes within a single target in polyclonal sera, is both a strength (polyclonals can be used in all experimental formats and will recognize a target protein, even if one binding site is covered by a protein partner), and a weakness (numerous interactions may lower overall signal). Similarly, unique reactivity of monoclonal antibodies provides great specificity in a capture antibody unless the binding site is obscured by complex interrelationships of proteins within the complex. Whilst a balance can be hard to strike, using a monoclonal antibody as the capture antibody, and a polyclonal as the detecting antibody, gives optimal results. With this format the monoclonal antibody is less likely to obscure the antigen for the detecting antibody.

- One very important consideration is that the antigen-antibody interaction should not alter the structure of protein-protein complexes. One such case was initially reported in the binding of connexin43 to the junctional protein ZO-1. In this case, the Cx43 antibody did not co-immunoprecipitate ZO-1, as it precluded the binding interaction, despite this interaction being confirmed by blotting for Cx43 after ZO-1 immunoprecipitation (Giepmans and Moolenaar 1998). To avoid this, it is best to choose capture antibodies whose epitope is distinct from the major sites of protein-protein interaction (such as an extracellular domain of a membrane protein).

- Issues in execution of array experiments: Spotting antibodies to membranes: Spotting buffer composition can influence protein binding capacity of a surface, stability of proteins and quality of the spots produced. We find that PBS is best for spotting antibodies. Surprisingly, the pH of the spotting buffer seems to have little effect on antibody stability or preservation of antigenicity, as PBS at pH 7.0, 7.4 and 8.0 all produced equally viable arrays in our hands. This result is similar to those of others who found the stability of spotted antibodies was independent of the pH of the spotting buffer over a pH range of 5.5–8.0 (Kusnezow et al. 2003).

HRP Conjugation of Antibodies

Chemical modification and attachment of bulky reporter moieties (such as HRP) to the detecting antibodies used in array experiments can have a number of serious consequences, especially if binding sites cannot be guaranteed to be protected from these changes. The use of amine- and thiol-reactive reagents to label antibodies can result in chemical modification of binding sites or steric hindrance of binding sites by the reporter group. One alternative is to attach an enzyme group to the carbodydrate chains in the Fc portion of the molecule, preferably through sidechain oxidization. Another is to use gentle conjugation chemistries to protect reactivity of the antibody being conjugated. We have found that EZ-link activated peroxidase reagent (Pierce Biotechnology Inc.) offers gentle conjugation chemistries that produce a stable, covalent conjugate. In addition, a great degree of control can be exerted over the level of HRP incorporated onto the antibody through varying the molar ratios, buffer composition and pH. We use the high pH coupling protocol, which generates Ig-HRP, and conjugates with greater specific activity.

Irrespective of the coupling chemistry used, the behavior of all detecting antibodies should be unchanged post-conjugation. To determine this, an aliquot of the antibody obtained prior to conjugation should be compared in Western blot analysis to activity of the conjugated antibody. The chosen antibody should be highly specific for the protein of interest, preferably with high affinity. Such antibodies should yield a strong signal against the protein of interest in western blots, and the conjugated antibody should give the same mono-specific banding pattern as the unconjugated antibody, indicating that specificity and signal strength have been maintained.

Finally, in conditions where no mono-specific antibody against the protein of interest exists, the protein can be expressed as a fusion with one of the many commercially available protein tags (6× His, Flag, Myc or GST). Antibodies against these tags are normally very specific, have high avidity for the target, and can be purchased pre-conjugated to HRP. The disadvantage of this strategy, is that the tag may become hidden within the interior of a protein complex, and be unavailable for binding by the antibody. In addition, the presence of a tag may alter the interactions of the protein of interest (Giepmans and Moolenaar 1998).

Protein Extraction

Consideration should be given to optimize extraction of the protein of interest from tissue without disrupting the complex interactions of proteins in their native state. For this function the choice of detergent, or indeed whether or not to use a detergent, is crucial. Non-membrane bound proteins do not necessarily require a detergent to liberate them from cells. Therefore, their interactions can be examined in lysates without detergent. However, extraction of most proteins from cells and tissues, especially membrane bound and cytoskeletal proteins, requires use of detergents. Some proteins, such as Bax detergents like NP-40 and TX-100, induce conformational changes that enable formation of protein-protein interactions where none previously existed (Hsu and Youle 1998). Use of other detergents, such as SDS, CHAPS, Brij35 and deoxycholate, is clearly contraindicated for studies of protein-protein interaction, as they are recommended for separation of protein complexes. An additional parameter to consider is solubility of the target protein in the detergent of choice. Multiple proteins are insoluble in some detergents, most notably Triton X-100. Since the choice of detergent should optimize protein recovery, these detergents are not recommended for these proteins. We find that NP-40 is a reliable choice that provides mild conditions under which most proteins are solubilized in their native conformation with their interactions intact.

Hybridization of Protein Complexes/Cell Lysates to Arrays

For array studies, sensitivity and selectivity of the assay are largely determined by the amount of signal generated, which in turn is controlled by the amount of lysate added, stringency of hybridization, and concentration of the detecting antibody.

Amount of Lysate Used in the Hybridization

After extraction of protein complexes from tissues or cells, the concentration of lysate to use for hybridization must be determined. Because ninety percent of the mass of the proteome is contributed by approximately 10% of the proteins (Kusnezow et al. 2003), concentration of lysate used should be sufficient to detect interactions with proteins of low abundance. Studies using simple protein solutions as ligands have placed the lower detection limit of antibody arrays at approximately 10 nM (Leuking et al. 1999) with reliable, reproducible signal detected over a concentration range of 1–1000 µg/ml (Kukar et al. 2002). However, systems to detect interactions in complex lysates, such as the ones used here, require greater sensitivity. We have observed low backgrounds and good signal strength in our system, within a range of lysates concentration of 250–1000 µg of protein per ml of hybridization solution, with most of our studies performed at 250 µg/ml. We have not extended the lower limit of our system any further, as this is a protein concentration that can be readily achieved from most cells and tissues, and offers a robust signal for subsequent analysis.

Stringency and Blocking

Stringency of the hybridization can be altered to determine the affinity of any set of interactions. A strategy we have used in the above protocol, to maximize the number of binding partners detected, is to reduce the amount of milk in the hybridization step to 1% (w/v) as opposed to 5% used in the blocking step. The amount of milk used in hybridization buffers can interfere with binding, such that raising it to 2.5 or 5% will increase stringency of the hybridization, thereby revealing only the strongest interactions.

While increasing the concentration of skimmed milk as a blocking agent increases stringency of hybridization, it may also influence the strength of antibody-antigen interactions. For antibody arrays, a common technique to alter stringency is to wash the membrane with increasing salt concentrations (Ge 2000). Low salt washes (with 100–150 mM KCl) maximize detection of possible interacting proteins, whilst high salt washes (500 mM KCl) limit detection and reveal only highly specific, high affinity interactions.

No additional benefit is gained by using salt concentrations above 500 mM. Our protocol uses 150 mM NaCl, which is quite gentle and facilitates detection of all potential interactions. Because antibody-antigen interactions are hardly affected by salt concentration, membranes can be washed in 500 mM NaCl or KCl after detection and re-probed to determine the higher affinity interactions.

During hybridization, detergents can be used to reduce interactions of hydrophobic proteins with the array support, especially for hydrophobic supports like PVDF. Only Tween-20 should be used for washing steps, as SDS, NP-40 and Triton X-100 may remove protein membranes. However, we recommend that high salt washes be used to control stringency, and that controlling hybridization through use of detergents be used only as a last resort.

Antibody Concentrations and Detecting the Protein of Interest

The final consideration is the amount of detecting antibody to use. Recommended concentrations vary from 1.5–10 µg/ml and 50–100 µg/ml for high affinity and weak affinity antibodies respectively. We found a robust signal with no background when using 0.5 µg/ml to 1 µg/ml antibody conjugated using the high pH protocol that creates a more highly labeled Ig molecule. The compromise in raising antibody concentration is the potential to increase background binding, which reduces the relative signal strength.

In some cases, where the antibody is not particularly avid, a lower concentration of antibody can be used in combination with secondary amplification. In this protocol, the detection antibody is conjugated to biotin instead of HRP and strepavadin-HRP used to amplify the signal. This step extends the procedure for only an extra 60 min (30 min with avadin-HRP and 3×10 min washes). One complication is that cells contain endogenous biotin-binding proteins, especially in the nuclear compartment; thus, the use of biotinylated antibodies may result in more false positives than using antibodies directly conjugated to HRP.

Detecting the Interacting Proteins

The studies in the literature indicate that most proteins are parts of larger complexes of multiple protein-protein interactions, either direct or indirect. Thus, the expected result of any antibody array experiment should be that a number of spots give signals of varying intensity with little or no background. However, experiments do not always give the expected results. The following are a list of problems, their potential causes and ways of resolving them to improve array results

Troubleshooting

A number of potential problems may occur during preparation of array membranes due to problems with the blotting apparatus. Some potential problems and their causes are listed below:

Leakage from Individual Wells or Cross-Well Contamination

1. Improper assembly of the apparatus. Check that all connections are sufficiently tight and that the apparatus and membrane are sufficiently well opposed.
2. Improper rehydration of the membrane. Always re-hydrate the membrane prior to application of samples. Drying of membranes, especially highly hydrophobic membranes such as PVDF, occurs rapidly and is easily prevented.

No or Uneven Filtration

Presence of aggregates or debris: Molecular polymers, aggregates or debris can plug the pores in the membrane. This is especially prevalent when using membranes with pore size <0.45 µm. Antibodies should always be centrifuged before sampling to decrease the amount of aggregated antibody spotted to the membrane.

Bubbles are obstructing filtration. To fix this problem triturate liquid in the wells up and down to displace bubbles.

Halos and Incomplete Spots

1. Membrane is not properly rehydrated before applying samples: Always re-hydrate membrane with PBS prior to applying any sample.
2. Excessive concentrations of sample are loaded or sample was loaded in an insufficiently large volume: When too much sample is present, wicking into the membrane around the well occurs. A fluid depth of 0.25 cm (200–300 µl in most commercial dot-blot apparatus) will ensure even distribution of the sample across the well and decreased occurrence of halos and incomplete spots.

Poor Detection Sensitivity or No Reactivity

1. Conjugation of detecting antibody is not satisfactory:
   The array technique uses a directly conjugated antibody for detection. Thus, less than optimal conjugation ratios yield an antibody with weak signal and poor sensitivity. Before using any conjugated primary antibody in antibody array assays, it should be tested in regular Western blot assay. The conjugated antibody should work well in western blotting and sensitivity should be comparable to that of un-

conjugated antibodies. To determine extent of HRP incorporation, compare enzyme activity of the conjugated antibody to that of a known standard (such as a commercially available pre-conjugated antibody).

2. Enzyme conjugate or the substrate in inactivated:
   During storage the conjugation of HRP to the detecting antibody can become unstable, separating the HRP and antibody or inactivating the HRP enzyme. Testing for enzyme activity using a known substrate is important. If enzyme activity is robust, check that the HRP is still bound to the antibody by substrate cleavage after immobilization of the antibody on protein A beads. Washing the beads will remove any unbound HRP and enzyme activity will be lost if the two are no longer conjugated. As long as Tween 20 is used, detergents in reactions and washes should not inhibit HRP activity. Lastly, avoid using sodium azide to store HRP conjugated antibodies. Azide is a potent inhibitor of HRP and should be removed from antibody preparations prior to conjugation.

3. Primary Antibody is not sensitive enough or epitope is hidden:
   Low levels of amplification due to use of directly conjugated antibodies that requires high affinity antibodies be used to generate detectable signals. If low affinity of the antibody is a problem, either switch to an antibody with higher affinity or increase antigen concentration by increasing amounts of protein extract utilized. Alternatively, the antigen on your protein may be denatured or obscured by another protein. To circumvent this make sure you use gentle lysis buffers that maintain native protein conformation or try switching to another antibody that detects a different region of the protein.

4. The protein of interest and its interacting proteins are not extracted or complexes are dissociated during extraction:
   Vary the extraction conditions. Some proteins are more soluble in some detergents than others. In addition, some complexes are more labile than others. Western blot should be performed to optimize the conditions for the extraction of the protein of interest. If the extraction conditions are optimized and low sensitivity persists, try decreasing incubation time and shortening duration of incubations, especially wash steps, to enhance the number of complexes retained.

5. Poor binding to or immobilization of antibodies on the membrane:
   This can result from a number of factors. SDS, NP-40 and Triton X-100 will remove protein from the membrane. If these detergents are required, reduce the concentration of detergent and duration of any washes. Tween 20 is preferable, as it will not denature protein complexes and is compatible with HRP-based detection strategies.

   Another source of problems may be loss of binding capacity by the membrane. PVDF has a shelf life, like any other support matrix, which can expire with a rapid loss of binding capacity and avidity. The loss of binding capacity reduces the amount of antibody immobilized to the membrane and subsequent loss during wash steps and incubations. The result will be very small spot sizes on the final exposure quite often accompanied by a dramatic increase in background staining. If this occurs, dispose of the remaining membrane and remake the array using new PVDF.

6. Sample load was insufficient:
   Since 90% of the mass of any proteome is contributed by approximately 10% of the proteins, the amount of lysate used in the analysis should be chosen that is sufficient to detect interactions with proteins of low abundance. A negative or weak signal may reflect the fact that the protein complexes were at too low a concentration to be detected. Increase the concentration of antigen applied, antibody concentration and reaction times for lysate hybridization.

High Background After Incubation with Labeled Probes

Non-specific background signal is one of the most serious problems encountered in protein array technologies, compared to their nucleic acid counterparts. Some sources of background and their possible solutions are listed below:
1. Blocking is not complete:
   Block the array with increased concentrations of blocking reagent or for longer times, such as overnight at 4 °C. It is important to note, however, that increasing concentrations of either BSA or non-fat dry milk can reduce signal intensities obtained in the subsequent analyses. TopBlock (Sigma-Aldrich Pty. Ltd.), a mixture of small proteins ($³3$ kDa), is reportedly better at reducing background signal while preserving signal intensity in situations where antibodies or lysates require higher levels of blocking (Kusnezow et al. 2003). In this study, the background produced by using 3% TopBlock was found to be about four times lower than results obtained with 3% BSA or 4% skimmed milk powder.
2. Cell lysate or detecting antibody is too concentrated:
   Dilute the antibodies and lysate concentrations separately in order to optimize the signal-to-noise ratio. In addition, increase the number and/or duration of the washes.
3. Antibodies contain reactivities against components in blocking reagents:
   This is especially true for antibodies against phospho-tyrosine residues or in cases where the blocking reagent is not pure protein. In addition, match the blocker with the detection system, i.e., hemoglobin reacts with horseradish peroxidase, BSA may contain IgG contaminants. Either pre-incubate antibodies with blocking reagents or perform wash steps in the presence of blocking reagent. Alternatively, changing the blocking reagent may work best.
4. Excess free HRP in conjugated antibody solution:
   Mix conjugated antibody with glycerol (1:1) for 10 min at room temp. prior to dilution of antibody in blocking solution, to minimize sticking of non-conjugated HRP to the membrane.
5. Excessive reaction time in the substrate:
   Remove the blot from the substrate reaction when the signal-to-noise level is acceptable. Last, always include a surfactant in wash solutions to decrease the low affinity charge and hydrophobic interactions that can add to non-specific binding. We have always used Tween-20 in the antibody and blocking buffers and find it is very compatible with the array format.

Removal of the Probe from the Array for Re-Probing

One advantage of creating membrane-based antibody arrays is that they can be stripped and re-probed, which increases throughput and decreases the costs of the arrays production. However, the stripping protocol used should be gentle enough to leave the antibody on the array surface in a viable, active conformation. While a number of methods may meet these criteria, we have found that two protocols work particularly well. The first protocol is to incubate in a buffer containing 50 mM Tris (pH 6.8) containing 2% SDS and 0.7% 2-mercaptoethanol for 10 min at room temperature. Alternatively, incubation in 1 M $(NH_4)_2SO_4$ and 1 M urea at room temperature for 15 min (Ge 2000) works equally well. Stripped arrays need to be re-equilibrated with PBS-Tween 20 before being incubated with another probe.

Interpretation of Array Results

It is generally appreciated that most biological events are mediated by "protein machines" that are comprised of anywhere from several up to 100 different polypeptides (Alberts 1998). With this in mind, the expected result of any array experiment is that a number of spots on the array give a signal of varying intensity, indicating the cognate ligands in a complex with the protein of interest. However, the array technology can generate false positives and negatives like any other mass analysis assay.

False Positives

Some proteins have complex interrelationships with other proteins; however, if the array seems to have generated too many positive spots (i.e. a pattern of interactions seem too complex for the protein of interest), then an array probing the lysate from a null cell or tissue should be performed as a control. This control examines signal generation in the absence of the target protein and controls for non-specific activities of the detection antibody, such as reactivities against the capture antibodies used to make the array. If the antibody is found to be reactive against a negative control, either change or affinity-purify it.

False Negatives

While Antibody arrays are better than many assays for analysis of protein interactions, they may still generate false positives, thus failing to identify potential interactions. One reason is that the majority of antibodies on any array will have to compete with native factors present in lysates that bind to target proteins. Depending on the relative affinity of the immobilized antibody and the native competitor, this competition will result in only a fraction of the target protein binding to the array. In addition, some proteins may not bind at all if the antibody-binding site is occluded in the interior of a stable complex and inaccessible to the capture antibody. To determine the extent of protein-protein interactions being missed on an array, it is important for the array to contain a number of controls including:

1. An antibody against the target protein. This serves as a positive control for the capture and detection antibodies and provides assurance that the system is working.
2. Antibodies against one or more proteins already known to be in a complex with the protein of interest. For connexin43 the obvious choice was ZO1, as the two proteins had been previously reported to interact (Geipmans and Moolenaar 1998; Toyofuku et al. 1998: Duffy et al. 2004). In the absence of such information, the positive control in point #1 will have to suffice.

Interpretation of Data

Multiple spots are expected to give positive signals (see Fig. 4a), indicating that several proteins interact with the protein of interest. Once the specificity of the array results is demonstrated, the data needs to be organized in such a way that biological functions can by hypothesized for such protein-protein interactions. One such strategy is to group proteins that are positive hits on the array into families of proteins known to participate within individual signaling pathways. Many proteins in cells exist as preformed complexes required for coordinated regulation of signaling, such as NFκB and IκB and cyclin E/Cdk2 and their cognate inhibitors, p21 and p27. Therefore, an interaction of the protein of interest with cyclin E should also detect an interaction with Cdk2 and also p21 or p27. In this way, predictions of biological function can be made from more than just one interaction. The greater the number of hits in a single pathway, the greater the chance that the protein being detected will impact the function of that particular signaling cascade.

Of course, all potential interacting proteins need to be confirmed by immunoprecipitation analysis. Further, interactions may be direct or indirect, e.g., through a third protein. Therefore the nature of the interaction must also be determined using direct interaction screens with recombinant proteins, such as pull-down assays or *in vitro* assays such as Surface Plasmon Resonance (Duffy et al. 2001).

Cautionary Note on Interpreting Relative Affinity by Intensity

It is tempting to draw conclusions on the strength of the interaction between the protein of interest and its cognate binding partner based on intensity of the spot identified on an array. However, this is not possible for several reasons. The target protein will often be a part of a multi-protein complex. In such circumstances, multiple copies of the captured protein may interact with the target protein, resulting in adjacent antibodies being occupied by a single complex. The reverse is also true, where multiple copies of the target protein may interact with the captured protein producing very high signal for rare complexes. Thus, for all but binary interactions, uncertainty of the stoichiometry, results in a breakdown between the relationship between signal intensity and affinity/degree of complex formation.

Another reason that intensity and affinity do not correlate is that in a multi-protein complex, antigenic sites for the capture and detection antibodies may be obscured. In this case, inaccessibility of the antigen to antibody in one complex may limit the signal generated. Conversely, in a complex where affinity of the interaction is lower, a more open conformation may result in a higher degree of antibody binding, thereby resulting in increase signal generation.

Furthermore, the amount of the protein of interest captured by another protein is dependent not only on the strength of binding but also on the amount of protein present. If expression of one binding partner is greater than another, then the law of mass action dictates that the protein of interest will complex more often to the more highly expressed protein. Greater numbers of complexes will obviously result in a stronger signal on the array, resulting in an analysis skewed toward a non-representative estimate of interaction strength.

Lastly, the more concentrated a ligand for the capture antibody, the more quickly the binding reaches equilibrium (Sapsford et al. 2001). Therefore, a less highly expressed protein (or one where fewer antigenic sites are exposed) displays a linear relationship between antigen binding and time, long after the more highly expressed proteins have reached saturation for their antibodies. The result is that less numerous complexes will take longer to equilibrate and reach maximum signal strength. Thus, even the highest affinity interactions may result in weak signal, if the complexes are rare and insufficient time is given for the binding to the capture antibody to reach equilibrium.

For these reasons, comparison of binding affinity based on spot intensity between two different complexes on the same array is not appropriate. What is more acceptable is a comparison of the binding intensity of the same complex between two different arrays. Having said this, different pathological conditions can produce changes in protein structure and function (such as phosphorylation, glycosylation and fatty acylation) that result in altered protein conformations that may change the antigenicity of the complex and signal strength, without significant changes in affinity of one protein for another. While still a more reliable comparison, even this analysis must be undertaken with a degree of caution.

Conclusion

As a high-throughput screen, antibody arrays can give a wealth of information regarding the protein-protein interactions of connexins, or any other protein of interest. When used with more traditional biochemical methods such as co-immunoprecipitation and fluorescence immunolocalization, antibody arrays can give information on novel binding partners, and interactions of proteins within previously unknown cellular pathways. The quality of the data and the care in which the data are interpreted can greatly decrease the amount of false positives or negatives in the data set, leading to new information on protein function within cells and tissues. Understanding the function and regulation of these interactions can open the doors to a deeper understanding of protein function and may aid in novel drug designs that target protein function.

Acknowledgements. This research was funded in part by grants from National Institutes of Health to HSD (Training Grant NS07098), DCS (MH65495, NS41282), and AWA (0020186T, 0335416T).

References

Alberts, B. (1998). The Cell as a Collection of Protein Machines: Preparing the Next Generation of Molecular Biologists. Cell 92(3): 291–4

Duffy, H.S., Ashton, A. W., O'Donnell, P, Coombs, W., Taffet, S. M., Delmar, M. and Spray, D.C. (2004) Regulation of Connexin43 Protein Complexes by Intracellular Acidification. Circ Res 94: 215–222

Duffy, H.S., Delmar, M., Coombs, M., Taffet, S.M., Hertzberg, E.L. and Spray, D.C. (2001). Functional Demonstration of Connexin-Protein Binding Using Surface Plasmon Resonance. Cell Commun Adhes. 8(4–6): 225–9

Ekins, R. P. (1998). Ligand Assays: From Electrophoresis to Miniaturized Microarrays. Clin Chem 44(9): 2015–30

Ge, H. (2000). UPA, A Universal Protein Array System for Quantitative Detection of Protein-Protein, Protein-DNA, Protein-RNA and Protein-Ligand Interactions. Nucleic Acids Res 28(2): e3

Giepmans, B. N. and Moolenaar, W. H. (1998). The Gap Junction Protein Connexin43 Interacts with the Second PDZ Domain of the Zona Occludens-1 protein. Curr Biol 8(16): 931–4

Hsu, Y. T. and Youle, R. J. (1998). Bax in Murine Thymus is a Soluble Monomeric Protein that Displays Differential Detergent-Induced Conformations. J Biol Chem 273(17): 10777–83

Kukar, T., Eckenrode, S., Gu, Y., Lian, W., Megginson, M., She, J. X. and Wu, D. (2002). Protein Microarrays to Detect Protein-Protein Interactions Using Red and Green Fluorescent Proteins. Anal Biochem 306(1): 50–4

Kusnezow, W., Jacob, A., Walijew, A., Diehl, F. and Hoheisel, J. D. (2003). Antibody Microarrays: An Evaluation of Production Parameters. Proteomics 3(3): 254–64

Lueking, A., Horn, M., Eickhoff, H., Bussow, K., Lehrach, H. and Walter, G. (1999). Protein Microarrays for Gene Expression and Antibody Screening. Anal Biochem 270: 103–111

Sapsford, K. E., Liron, Z., Shubin, Y. S. and Ligler, F. S. (2001). Kinetics of Antigen Binding to Arrays of Antibodies in Different Sized Spots. Anal Chem 73(22): 5518–24

Sheng M. 2001. Molecular Organization of the Postsynaptic Specialization. Proc Natl Acad Sci U S A. 2001 Jun 19;98(13): 7058–61

Toyofuku T Yabuki M, Otsu K, Kuzuya T, Hori M, Tada M (1998). Direct Association of the Gap Junction Protein Connexin-43 with ZO-1 in Cardiac Myocytes. J Biol Chem 273(21): 12725–31

Surface Plasmon Resonance as a Method to Study the Kinetics and Amplitude of Protein-Protein Binding

Brian D. Lang, Mario Delmar and Wanda Coombs

Introduction

The topic of protein-protein interactions has become a major research area in recent years. The reductionist approach of identifying individual genes and proteins is now being matched by the analysis of the interactions that individual players undergo. One could intuitively argue that molecules in a cell are absent of function if they cannot associate and interact with others. The product of a gene is a character in a play, not the play itself. It is in the way the players interact that a function is achieved. Here, we review the basic theory and some of the practical aspects in the application of a technique called "surface plasmon resonance" (SPR) to study intermolecular interactions *in vitro*.

Theory

Surface Plasmon Resonance

Surface plasmon resonance (SPR) is a spectroscopic method to determine binding amplitude and kinetics in real time. The ligand of interest (commonly a purified, recombinant protein) is covalently bound to a matrix, which is fixed over a thin film of gold. An incident beam of light is focused on the metal film, and the reflected light is collected by a sensor. Various angles of incidence of light are scanned. There is a particular angle of incidence at which the photons in the light resonate with the electrons in the gold. The device detects the angle of incidence suited for resonance as a decrease in the amplitude of the reflected light. The angle of incidence at which resonance occurs is highly sensitive to changes in the molecular content occurring in the immediate vicinity of the matrix. Thus, binding of a ligate (added to the flow chamber) to the matrix-bound ligand is sensed immediately as a shift in the angle of incidence required for resonance. As a result, a plot of angle of incidence (in arc seconds), as a function of time, directly represents the amplitude and kinetics of ligate-ligand binding in real time.

Mirror Resonance Spectroscopy

An alternative method is called mirror resonance spectroscopy. This technique takes advantage of the change in direction suffered by a light wave when moving between two media of different refractive indices. For waves traveling from high to low refractive index materials, there is a particular incident angle at which the wave is completely reflected (total internal reflection). If a region of high refractive index material is bound on both sides ("cladded") by low index material, the light will be constrained within the high index material through successive total internal reflections. This "guiding" will occur only at a discrete angle "θ", which is in turn extremely sensitive to the physical parameters of the system. The principle of this biosensor is that protein binding at or near the surface of the cladding material changes the value of θ. Under this principle, a ligand is immobilized to the surface of a cuvette. A potential binding partner is added. If the two molecules do bind, it is reported as a change in the value of θ (in arc-sec). As in the case of surface plasmon resonance, this method allows for real time measurement of protein-protein interactions and a direct measurement of binding kinetics.

Comparison between Surface Plasmon Resonance and Mirror Resonance Spetroscopy

SPR-based instruments and resonant mirror-based instruments both allow detection of biomolecular interactions in real-time. In practice, the main difference between these two commercially available platforms ("Biacore" for SPR; "Iasys" for MRS) is how the samples are delivered to the detection surface. In the SPR-based instrument, the sample is injected in a continuous flow, using computer-controlled microfluidics. In contrast, the mirror resonance platform utilizes a cuvette-based system. Cuvettes are open to the air, and therefore introduce evaporation as a potential problem. Evaporation may lead to fluctuating analyte and buffer concentrations. Additionally, it may be difficult to control precisely the temperature at the sensor surface, leading to unstable baseline data, as the refractive index of water is highly sensitive to changes in temperature. Since the flow cells in the SPR-based instrument are closed, evaporation is not a concern and the temperature is kept stable.

Additionally, in a cuvette system the analyte is introduced in a single fixed volume injection, possibly causing depletion of analyte during the course of a binding analysis. Since Biacore is a continuous flow instrument, analyte is refreshed during an injection, preventing analyte depletion. The open cuvette system has the advantage that analyte can stay in contact with the sensor surface for an unlimited period of time. This allows binding events to reach equilibrium even if they are extremely slow. Since Biacore injections are done in a continual flow, the length of an injection is limited by the flow rate and volume of the injection tubing. To allow extended injection times on a Biacore instrument, several labs have attempted modifications of the injection system (Abrantes et al. 2001; Schuck et al. 1998). In this chapter, we focus our attention on the use of the Surface Plasmon Resonance-based instrument. Many of the concepts expressed here can be transported to the use of mirror resonance-based technology.

Description of Methods and Practical Approach

Ligand Immobilization

In any Biacore experiment, one interactant (the ligand) must be immobilized on the surface of a sensor chip. There are many methods for ligand immobilization, the choice of which depends on the nature of the biomolecule, the presence of any tags, and the specific application. Approaches for immobilization can be classified into three main categories: direct coupling, high affinity capture, and hydrophobic adsorption.

Direct Coupling

In a direct coupling approach, the ligand molecule is linked covalently via carboxyl groups on the sensor chip surface (Fig. 1). Amine coupling, discussed elsewhere in this chapter, is commonly used for protein immobilization, as most proteins contain several surface-exposed amine groups. Amine coupling is optimized, by taking advantage of the overall negative charge of the dextran surface, in a technique called preconcentration (Fig. 2). When a protein is prepared in a buffer with a pH below the isoelectric point (pI) of the protein, electrostatic attraction will drive the ligand into the matrix and enhance the efficiency of the coupling by increasing the local concentration. However, for acidic proteins (pI<3.5), this technique will not be effective, as carboxyl motifs on the dextran will be protonated in very low pH buffers. Moreover, many proteins will be adversely affected if exposed to acidic buffers for extended periods.

While amine coupling is relatively simple to perform, a possible disadvantage is the generation of a heterogeneous surface. Since there may be many accessible amine residues, the molecules can be oriented randomly. In some cases, amine containing residues may be critical for activity of a binding site, and this coupling chemistry may lead to altered activity. One alternative to amine coupling is thiol-disulphide exchange (Johnsson et al. 1995). This coupling can be performed in two orientations, ligand thiol or surface thiol. In ligand thiol, an active disulphide is first created on the sensor chip by derivatizing carboxyl groups with NHS/EDC followed by PDEA (2-(2-pyridinylthio)ethanamine hydrochloride). This active disulphide will exchange spontaneously with intrinsic thiol groups on the ligand molecule. Disulphides that remain active are then blocked with a cysteine solution.

A ligand thiol approach can be used for molecules that lack intrinsic thiol groups. In this case, an active disulphide is created on the ligand molecule by incubating the molecule with PDEA and EDC. Thiol groups are created on the sensor chip surface by injection of EDC/NHS, followed by cystamine and DTT (dithiothreitol). The PDEA-modified ligand is injected over the thiol-containing surface, and excess thiols are deactivated by injecting PDEA. Since ligands are attached by a disulfide bond, the linkage will be sensitive to reducing conditions; therefore, buffer additives such as DTT must be used at low concentrations.

Surface Plasmon Resonance

ALDEHYDE CHEMISTRY

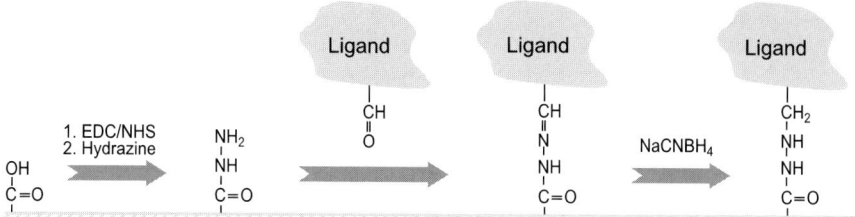

AMINE COUPLING CHEMISTRY

LIGAND THIOL CHEMISTRY

SURFACE THIOL CHEMISTRY

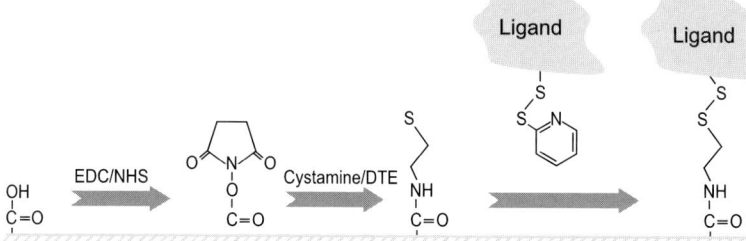

Figure 1
An illustration of common chemistries used to directly couple biological molecules to a sensor chip surface

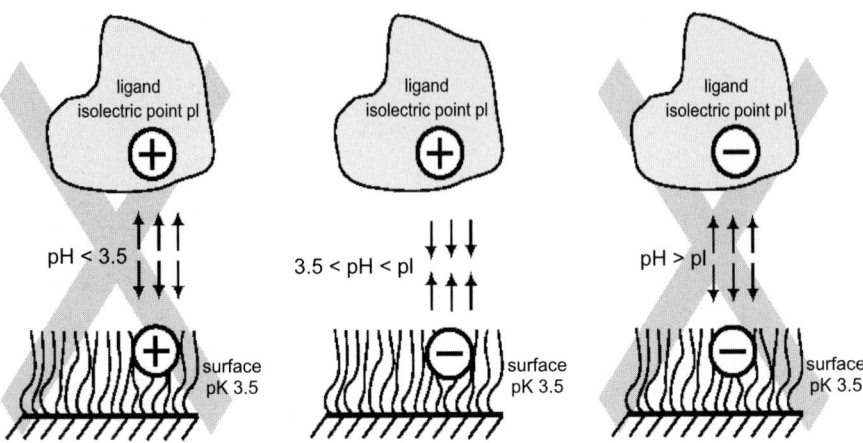

Figure 2
Preconcentration: The solvent is buffered at a pH below the isolelectric point (pI) of the ligand, to drive the ligand into the matrix

An advantage of thiol coupling is that most protein molecules contain less thiols than amine groups; therefore, a more homogeneous surface can be generated as compared to amine coupling. Thiol coupling can also be useful for ligand molecules with very low pIs (<3.5). As thiol coupling is more efficient than amine coupling, preconcentration is not always necessary.

A third type of direct coupling uses aldehyde chemistry (Johnsson et al. 1995). This procedure is convenient for carbohydrates, glycoproteins or glycolipids. For aldehyde coupling, the dextran surface is first activated with NHS/EDC, followed by hydrazine to create an active hydrazide on the surface. Due to the toxic nature of hydrazine, the less toxic carbohydrazide can be substituted. Ligands containing aldehyde groups will react with the activated surface. If a carbohydrate ligand does not contain native aldehydes the groups can be formed by oxidizing cis-diol groups with periodate.

High-affinity Capture

For high-affinity capture, covalent binding of the ligand molecule is not required. Rather, the ligand is bound via a second molecule that has been coupled directly to the surface (Fig. 3). There are many examples of capture systems; one of the most common is antibody-antigen interaction, such as rabbit anti-mouse IgG, used to capture mouse monoclonal antibodies.

There are two sensor chips available from Biacore designed for specific capture systems. The first, Sensor Chip NTA, utilizes the metal chelator nitrilotriacetic acid to capture proteins containing 6X histidine tags (Nieba et al. 1997). When using the NTA surface, Ni^{+2} cations must be injected prior to capturing the ligand. At the end of the

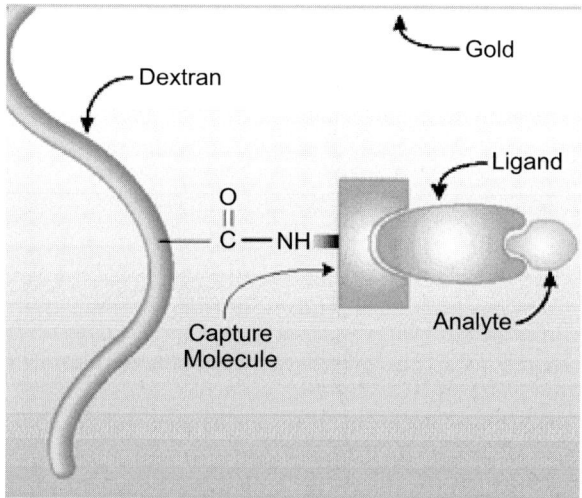

Figure 3
Schematic illustrating the basic configuration of a high affinity capture immobilization

cycle, ethylenediaminetetraacetate (EDTA) is injected to regenerate the surface. The second, Sensor Chip SA, contains pre-immobilized streptavidin for capturing ligands modified with biotin (Johnsson et al. 1995).

There are several advantages for using high-affinity capture as compared to direct coupling. First, if a ligand molecule is sensitive to covalent modification (e.g. the binding site contains free amine groups), direct coupling may significantly affect binding activity. Capture approaches require no covalent modification of the ligand, and therefore should not affect activity. Second, direct coupling has the potential to generate a heterogeneous surface, while high-affinity capture will orient the ligand molecules homogeneously. Third, a fresh ligand surface is created with every cycle; therefore, the ligand is not required to stay active on the surface through long assays, with multiple regeneration injections. However, this is not the case for the biotin-SA system. Once a biotin-containing ligand is immobilized, it is not possible to remove the ligand without damaging the SA surface. Finally, since many capture systems utilize well-characterized interactions, regeneration conditions for the surface may already be known.

Hydrophobic Adsorption

Biacore produces two sensor chips for working with hydrophobic molecules. Sensor Chip HPA possesses a flat, hydrophobic thiol-alkane surface for the preparation of lipid monolayers. Once a lipid monolayer is created, ligands such as peripheral membrane proteins can be immobilized via their interaction with the lipid environment. Alternatively, the lipid monolayer can be created with micelles that already contain the ligand of interest. The surface of Sensor Chip L1 contains carboxymethylated dextran, as well as long-chain lipophilic tails. The tails are able to insert themselves into the hydrophobic layer of liposomes, which allows the liposomes to be captured intact, or "opened up" to form a lipid bilayer (Rich and Myszka 2000).

Example

This example describes the surface preparation procedure for amine coupling of a purified ligand to the Biacore sensor chip CM-5. These are general purpose chips coated with carboxymethylated dextran to which proteins (and other biomolecules) can be covalently bound. The dextran matrix also provides a hydrophilic environment suitable for protein interaction.

The present protocol was modified from "Biacore Basics," edited by Biacore, Inc.
1. Equilibrate sensor chip and all buffers and reagents to room temp. Sterile filter (through 0.22 µm filter) and degas all buffers for 20 min.
2. Dock CM-5 sensor chip.
3. Prime equipment using filtered and degassed HBS-EP buffer pH 7.4 (commercially available through Biacore). Do this three times.
4. Run sensorgram (plot of response in RU (response units) vs. time, showing progress of interaction). Sensorgram is displayed on the computer during course of analysis.
5. Set flow rate at 5 µl/min. over flow cells 1 and 2. Flow cell 2 (FC-2) will be the experimental cell and flow cell 1 (FC-1) will be the reference or blank cell.
6. Dilute ligand of interest in appropriate buffer (buffer selected after pH scouting experiment).
7. Mix NHS (N-Hydroxysuccinimide) and EDC (1-Ethyl 3-3-dimethylaminopropyl carbodiimide) 1:1 just before use. (Reagents from Amine Coupling Kit- Biacore #BR-1000-50)
8. Inject 35 µl of NHS/EDC mixture for a total of 7 min contact time, to activate surface, to give reactive succinimide esters.
9. Change flow path to FC-2 only. This will bypass FC-1 to avoid coupling ligand to reference cell.
10. Choose MANUAL INJECT to control the desired amount of ligand bound to matrix. Enter a volume of 50 µl. Load sample loop with ligand. In this step, ligand is passed over the activation surface and the esters react with amine groups to link the ligand covalently to the dextran.
11. To monitor level of immobilization, place a report point just prior to ligand injection and designate that point as baseline. Place another report point after an injection of 1-3 µl of ligand. Stop and start injection until the desired amount of RUs is achieved. Do not inject more than the volume loaded. Monitor this by watching "accumulated volume" amount. The desired amount of ligand bound is application specific.
12. Change flow path to FC-1 and FC-2.

13. Inject 35 µl of Ethanolamine Hydrochloride-NaOH pH 8.5 for a total of 7 min contact time. This step deactivates remaining esters.
14. Insert report points to indicate final immobilization level in RUs.
15. Save immobilization sensorgram.

This chip can now be used to screen binding partners to the ligand of interest. The chip can be also be undocked and stored in the refrigerator, in a 50 ml conical tube with a small amount of water, for later use. Depending on the properties of the particular immobilized molecule, the surface will be stable for several weeks or more stored this way.

Troubleshooting

No Binding Response

When setting up a new system in Biacore, one of the first problems that may be encountered is a lack of binding activity upon injection of analyte. One possibility is that the ligand molecule is negatively affected by the immobilization procedure (e.g. amine coupling). In this case, it may be necessary to try a different coupling chemistry, or a capture system if available. Another possible solution is to reverse the system, and immobilize the analyte molecule.

Low or negative responses can also be a result of the nature of interactants being used. Referring back to the equation for calculating R_{max}, the response of an injected analyte is directly proportional to the molecular weight of the analyte divided by the molecular weight of the ligand. Therefore, if an analyte molecule is many times smaller than the ligand molecule, very low responses can be expected. By using the equation for R_{max}, it is possible to determine a sufficient amount of ligand in order to immobilize and get a measurable analyte binding response. Alternatively, in such a situation, it may be better to immobilize the smaller of the two molecules, if possible.

Finally, the affinity of the interactants will also determine the level of binding response. An injection of analyte at a concentration equal to the equilibrium dissociation constant, K_D, will give a response at equilibrium equal to one-half of R_{max} (Fig. 4). Therefore, injections at concentrations much lower than K_D will give accordingly low responses. It is recommended, when testing a new surface, to use very high analyte concentrations (10-fold above the expected K_D). If the K_D is not known, injections of progressively increasing concentrations of analyte (beginning with ~250 nM) may be necessary before a signal is detected.

It should also be mentioned that the quality of the reagents should be confirmed prior to analysis by Biacore. If direct coupling is used, ligand preparations must be >95% pure. Immobilization of impurities will decrease the observed activity of the surface. Also, it is beneficial to have an estimate of the active concentration of each component, as some preparations may contain a high percentage of inactive molecules.

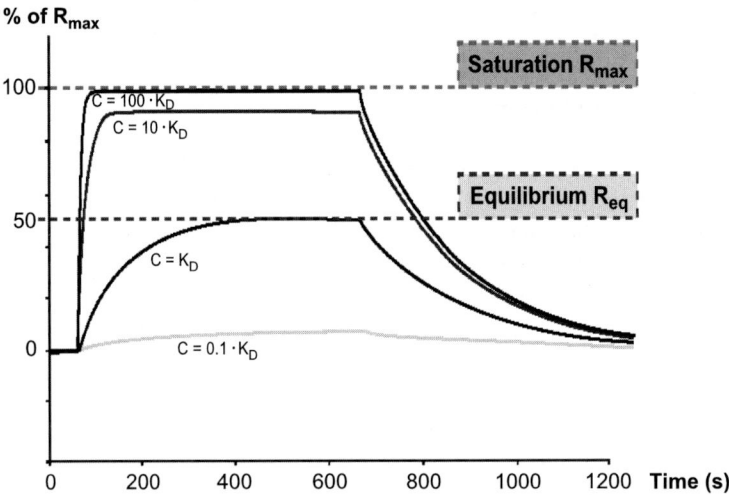

Figure 4
Responses at equilibrium (R_{eq}) for an interaction are proportional to the equilibrium dissociation constant (K_D) for the interactants. In these sensorgrams, response is normalized to percentage of saturation (R_{max})

Non-specific Binding

In any Biacore experiment, it is highly recommended to include a reference surface as a negative control. At least, this is to correct for bulk refractive index changes caused by differences between the analyte and running buffer composition. The reference surface is also necessary for diagnosing non-specific binding. If the analyte has an affinity for the dextran surface, this will be apparent from examining the sensorgrams generated from the reference surface. Ideally, reference sensorgrams will only reflect bulk refractive changes, and possess a rectangular shape. If the shape of the curve during injection appears to be increasing, or the response does not return to baseline at the end of the injection, non-specific binding is likely occurring.

Once diagnosed, there are several methods of reducing non-specific binding. If the binding is due to the overall negative charge of the surface, increasing the salt concentration of analyte and running buffers may be beneficial. Another solution is to use a different sensor chip. For example, Sensor Chip CM4 has fewer carboxymethyl groups than Sensor Chip CM5, and therefore has a less overall negative charge.

Non-specific binding may also be due to attraction to the dextran. In this case, surface binding may be reduced by including soluble dextran in analyte and running buffers; a concentration of 1 mg/mL of soluble dextran is usually sufficient. Again, use of sensor chips other than Sensor Chip CM5 may also be helpful. The length of dextran on Sensor Chip CM3 is one-third the length of Sensor Chip CM5 and Sensor Chip C1 contains no dextran at all. Finally, other modifications of buffers should be tested. Common modifications include the addition of detergents such as surfactant P20, and the use of salts other than NaCl.

Regeneration

Once specific binding activity has been demonstrated, it may be necessary to determine conditions for removing bound analyte (regeneration) of the surface. Proper optimization of a regeneration protocol is critical for carrying out a high-quality Biacore experiment. An ideal regeneration protocol will remove all bound analyte, while leaving the immobilized ligand intact and active. If the inherent dissociation rate constant of an interaction is relatively fast (>0.01 s-1), analyte will dissociate rapidly, and regeneration is not necessary. However, for very stable interactions, a regeneration buffer is essential.

When scouting regeneration buffers, the analyte must be injected between each regeneration buffer tested, regardless of how much analyte is removed. This is to test if the regeneration buffer has affected the activity of the surface. Another important point is to always begin by testing the mildest regeneration conditions. Common regeneration buffers include acidic or basic solutions (e.g. glycine pH 3.0, 10 mM HCl, 20 mM NaOH), high salt (2.5 M NaCl), or solvents such as ethylene glycol. In some cases, combinations of buffers that disrupt multiple types of interactions, such as ionic and hydrophobic, may be much more effective than two separate injections.

Difficulty in Fitting Kinetic Data to a 1:1 Model

In a kinetic analysis, proper experimental design is essential in order to achieve quality curve fitting and determination of kinetic rate constants. If the quality seems poor when evaluating the overall quality of a fit, there are several possible causes.

The first possible cause is mass transport limitation. In the flow cells of a Biacore instrument, the analyte must diffuse to the dextran surface before ligand binding can take place. In an ideal experimental system, this diffusion is not limiting, and therefore the rate of interaction can be measured accurately. However, under certain conditions, diffusion does become limiting and sensorgrams will no longer fit a simple 1:1 Langmuir model (Karlsson et al. 1994). The preferred method of avoiding mass transport limitation is to immobilize very low levels of ligand. Ideally, the maximum response of analyte binding at saturation should not exceed 150 RU. Due to the high sensitivity of Biacore instruments, maximum responses of less than 30 RU are routine. On high-density surfaces (> 150 RU for R_{max}), the large number of binding sites available may lead to depletion of analyte near the surface of the sensor chip. Therefore, association rate constants will appear artificially smaller. Similarly, during dissociation, analyte molecules will have a greater probability of re-binding to another ligand molecule, leading to the observation of slower dissociation rate constants.

Additionally, it is recommended to run kinetic analyses at relatively fast flow rates (>30 μL/min). Increased flow rates decrease the distance analyte molecules must diffuse, and therefore mass transport occurs more rapidly (Karlsson et al. 1994). A simple test to detect mass transport in an experiment involves injecting an identical analyte concentration for the same amount of time, at three different flow rates, 15, 30 and 75 μL/min (Fig. 5). If mass transport is not limiting, these three sensorgrams should overlay. If the three curves appear different (the initial binding rate increases, maxi-

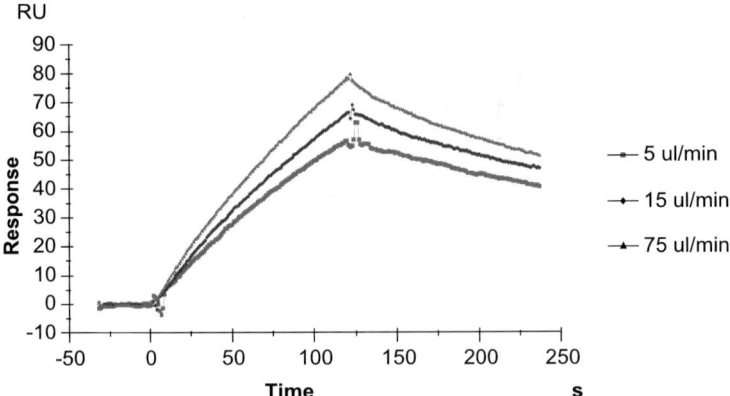

Figure 5
Overlay of sensorgrams illustrating a flow-rate test for detection of mass-transport limitation in a binding interaction

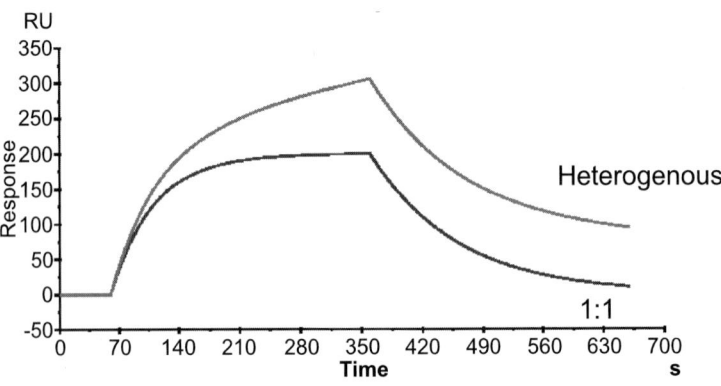

Figure 6
Representative sensorgrams showing the difference between a 1:1 binding interaction and an interaction displaying heterogeneity

mum binding level increases, or dissociation rate increases), there is most likely mass transport limitation. In cases where ligand density is already at very low levels, it may be necessary to use a binding model that incorporates mass transfer limitation. This model is included in the BiaEvaluation software package 4.

Another cause of poor agreement between experimental data and calculation fit is heterogeneity in either the ligand or analyte. Heterogeneity can usually be detected in sensorgrams by a biphasic association and/or dissociation. If there is heteroge-neity in the ligand, this may be observed by injecting high analyte concentrations (10-100-fold above the expected K_D). In these cases, curves will appear to reach equilibrium; however, there will be a slow rise in the sensorgram, rather than a flat, horizontal line (Fig. 6). During dissociation, a rapid dissociation phase may be followed by a slower phase, with a signal that appears to run parallel to the baseline. As mentioned above, heterogeneity may be introduced by direct immobilization. Therefore, an alternative immobilization strategy may be necessary. Another source of heterogeneity is impurities in the ligand or analyte preparations. Additional purification steps may be necessary to remove potentially interfering molecules.

However, heterogeneity may be an inherent property of the interactants. The BiaEvaluation software contains binding models for heterogeneous ligand, bivalent analyte, and conformational change (Karlsson and Falt 1997). These models should be used where appropriate. However, if these properties are not known beforehand, achieving a better fit by using these models is not sufficient cause to justify their use. Properties such as bivalency, or conformational change, must be confirmed using alternative methodologies.

References

Abrantes M, Magone, MT, Boyd, LF, Schuck, P (2001) Adaptation of a Surface Plasmon Resonance Biosensor with Microfluidics for Use with Small Sample Volumes and Long Contact Times. Analytical Chemistry 73(13): 2828-35

Johnsson B, Lofas, S, Lindquist,G, Edstrom, A, Muller Hillgre, R-M, Hansson, A (1995) Comparison of Methods for Immobilization to Carboxymethyl Dextran Sensor Surfaces by Analysis of the Specific activity of monoclonal antibodies. Journal of Molecular Recognition 8:125-131

Karlsson, R, Falt, A (1997) Experimental Design for Kinetic Analysis of Protein-Protein Interactions with Surface Plasmon Resonance Biosensors. Journal of Immunological Methods 200:121-133

Karlsson, R, Roos, H, Fagerstam, L, Persson, B (1994) Kinetic and Concentration Analysis using BIA Technology. Methods 6:99-110

Nieba, L, Nieba-Axmann, SE, Persson, A, Hamalainen, M, Edebratt, F, Hansson, A, Lidholm, J, Magnusson, K, Karlsson, AF, Pluckthun, A (1997) BIACORE Analysis of Histidine-Tagged Proteins Using a Chelating NTA Sensor Chip. Analytical Biochemistry 252:217-228

Rich, RL, Myszka, DG (2000) Advances in Surface Plasmon Resonance Biosensor Analysis. Current Opinion in Biotechnology 11:54-61

Schuck, P, Millar, DB, Kortt AA (1998) Determination of Binding Constants by Equilibrium Titration with Circulating Sample in a Surface Plasmon Resonance Biosensor. Analytical Biochemistry 265(1): 79-91

How to Solve a Protein Structure by Nuclear Magnetic Resonance – The Connexin43 Carboxyl Terminal Domain

Paul L. Sorgen

Introduction

Nuclear magnetic resonance, or NMR, as it is usually called, has become a power tool in biology for solving protein structures at atomic resolution. Since the first NMR derived three-dimensional (3D) solution structure of a small protein was determined in 1985, over 2,000 structures have been deposited in the Protein Data Base. The 2002 Nobel Prize in chemistry was given to Kurt Wuthrich for his work on "Three dimensional Structure of Biomolecules". New advancements for structural determination by NMR (i.e. higher field magnets and cryoprobe technology) have increased the molecular weight threshold close to 100 kDa. Liquid-state NMR has other far-reaching applications in chemical and biological research. Some of these applications include the constitution and conformation of organic molecules, 3D structure of nucleic acids, conformational dynamics and mobility of biomacromolecules in solution, chemical and conformational exchange, enzyme mechanism and chemical reactions, mapping protein-protein interactions, folding studies, and rational drug design. While many laboratories can utilize these applications, I believe a major hurdle for most scientists is the "black box" between a purified protein on an SDS-PAGE gel and the answer to their particular scientific question, i.e. the NMR. What I hope to accomplish in this chapter, is explain how spectroscopists go about solving a protein structure by NMR methods. This overview will incorporate a sampling of theory, sample preparation, data collection, processing, analysis, structure generation, and deposition into the appropriate data banks, thus defining what is inside the "black box." The solution structure of the carboxyl terminal domain from the cardiac gap junction protein Connexin43 (Cx43CT) will be used as the test sample. Cx43CT examples are embedded in the descriptions of methods to better illustrate what is to be expected from each step during structure determination by NMR.

What I would like to do before getting started, is define a few NMR terms that will be discussed in this chapter:

- $B0$: The static magnetic field. The magnetic flux density is expressed in tesla (T), or often, as an equivalent ^{1}H resonance frequency (for example, 600 MHz for a 14.1 T magnet).
- Chemical shift: This is the interaction of the nuclear spins with the electronic field surrounding it. Different chemical groups in the molecule have characteristic chemical shifts and making the resonance assignment to these chemical groups

will be used for structural determination. The chemical shift parameter is denoted δ and quoted in ppm (parts per million).
- Larmor frequency: The magnetic moment of each nucleus precesses around B0 at a unique frequency.
- Magnetic moment: The nucleus has a positive charge and is spinning. This generates a small magnetic field. The nucleus therefore possesses a magnetic moment, μ, which is proportional to its spin, I.
- Nuclear spin: Designated by I, its values are positive integers (ex. 0, 1, 2…) and half-integers (ex. 1/2, 3/2, 5/2…). NMR can only observe nuclei with I>0. If an element has a spin-1/2 nuclide, this is generally the one preferred for NMR analysis, because it will tend to give narrower resonances. Nuclei with I>1/2 has a quadruple moment, which usually results in broader peaks.
- Probe: The sample tube sits within an inductor coil, which transmits radio frequency pulses and receives resonance signals. In a fixed-frequency probe, the resistance and capacitance, are set so that the circuit is only in resonance at a particular frequency, corresponding to the Larmor frequency of the nuclide to be detected. In a tunable or broadband probe, both are adjustable to make the circuit respond to a desired frequency (within a specified range). In this way, a wide variety of nuclides can be observed with a single probe.
- Signal-to-noise ratio (S/N): Ratio of the height of a line or signal (usually the largest) to the noise. Signal increases as n (the number of repetitions) but noise only increases by $\sqrt{n}$ so S/N increases by $\sqrt{n}$.
- Spin-spin coupling: This is the interaction of one nuclear spin with the other through chemical bonds. Coupling patterns are crucial to identify spin systems in a molecule and for the determination of its chemical structure
- T1: Spin-lattice relaxation time-constant. Relates to the time taken for excited spins, in the presence of $B0$, to loose energy to their surroundings and return to their equilibrium state.
- T2: Spin-spin relaxation time-constant. Relates to the time for a conserved exchange of energy between spins.

Theory

Though I want to dive into the exciting part of NMR, structural determination, I must take a quick step back to explain some theory. The physical mechanism of NMR involves atomic Nuclei in a Magnetic field who's Resonance occurs at a well-defined energy. The magnetic resonance phenomenon occurs as a result of the quantum mechanism property of spin. The spinning can be visualized as a rotating charge that generates a small magnetic field. Many atoms (such as ^{12}C) have paired spins against each other, such that the nucleus of the atom has no overall spin. However, some atoms (^1H, ^{13}C, ^{15}N, and ^{31}P) posses an overall spin of ½ that has two possible orientations, a low-energy α-state and a high-energy β-state. In the absence of an external magnetic field, these orientations have equal energy. After inserting the sample into the static magnetic field ($B0$), the spins in the ensemble of molecules in the NMR tube are either in the α- or β-state (Fig. 1). At thermal equilibrium, the population of the

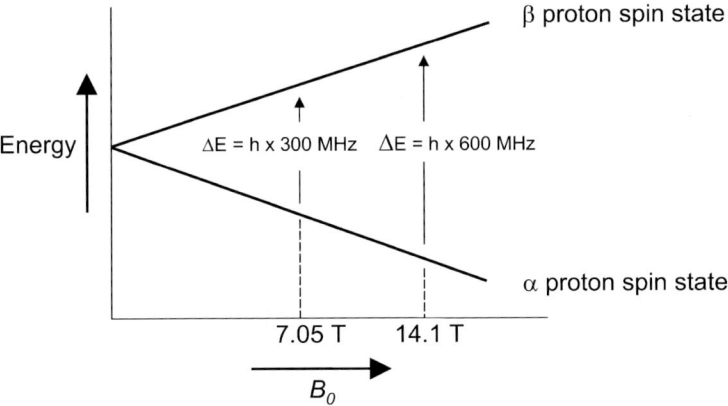

Figure 1
Graphical relationship between field B0 and frequency v. The energy difference (ΔE) between the spin states is proportional to the strength of B0. B0 is the strength of the external homogeneous magnetic field. The actual population ratio is given by the Boltzmann equation that relates the population ratio to ΔE and the absolute temperature. h is Planck's constant

α- and β-states, according to the Boltzmann distribution, are almost equal (10^{-5} difference) since the energies involved are fairly small. Thus the lower energy level will contain slightly more nuclei than the higher level. This is the reason why NMR is often called an 'insensitive' technique.

Electromagnetic radiation is used to excite these nuclei into the higher energy level. The frequency of radiation needed is determined by the difference in energy between levels (Larmor frequency). The higher energy state nuclei return to the lower state by two different relaxation processes: Spin-lattice (longitudinal) relaxation (T1) or Spin-Spin (transverse) relaxation (T2). Spin lattice relaxation is caused by components of the sample having equal frequency and phase to the Larmor frequency of the nuclei of interest, thus causing the higher energy state to lose energy and return to the lower state. Spin-spin relaxation is caused by an exchange of energy states caused by neighboring nuclei, however, the net energy populations do not change, but the average lifetime of a nucleus in the exited state will decrease.

Of great importance to what was described above, is the time between excitation and full relaxation in which the NMR signal is detected and data recorded. If an external radio frequency in a direction perpendicular to the magnetic field (right hand thumb rule applies), for example the X-axis, will tilt the nuclear spins, also called bulk magnetization from, Z-axis to the direction of Y-axis (Fig. 2), we can place our detector along this axis and detect the NMR signal. The combined precession of many spins generates a small but detectable excess oscillating magnetic field in the X-Y plane perpendicular to the external magnetic field. These oscillations induce an alternating voltage (the NMR signal) in a detection coil. Signal is fed into a preamp that provides an initial stage of amplification to the NMR signal. Signal is mixed with the transmitter frequency to produce an audio signal and sent through an audio filter that restricts the frequency bandwidth of the instrument (reduce noise). Filtered audio signal is sent to an analog-to-digital converter so the computer can handle the digitized signal. Processing of this signal will be described later.

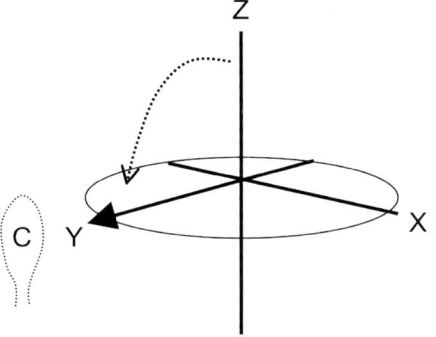

Figure 2
A 90° pulse rotates the equilibrium magnetization down to the Y-axis. Radio frequency coils (C) create the field that rotates the net magnetization in a pulse sequence. They also detect the transverse magnetization as it precesses in the XY plane

Description of Methods and Practical Approach

Sample Preparation

One would be surprised, but for an NMR spectroscopist, a major hurdle to solving a protein structure is having your protein of interest, under the right conditions, to be placed in the magnet. Proteins >10 kDa in size must be isotopically labeled with ^{15}N, ^{15}N^{13}C, and/or ^{15}N^{13}C^{2}D. For protein labeling, minimal media such as M63 or M22 are used so the only nitrogen, carbon, and deuterium sources come from ^{15}N-ammonium chloride/sulfate, ^{13}C-glucose, and D$_2$O, respectively. Growth times usually increase with minimal media. The other problem is that protein yields can decrease as compared to enriched medias such as Luria Broth. For example, the Cx43CT yielded 4 in Luria Broth and 3 in M63 media. From experience, when cells are grown in 100% D$_2$O, they need to be acclimated into the D$_2$O media by overnight growths in 20%, then 40%, 60%, and 80% D$_2$O (the most problematic jump is from 80–100%).

Fortunately, the price of labeled material has decreased to an average of $30/gram for ^{15}N, $125/gram for ^{13}C, and $175/L for D$_2$O (Cambridge Isotopes Laboratory or Spectra Stable Isotopes). A typical one-liter of minimal media contains 1 gm of ^{15}N and 2 gm of ^{13}C. The difference in price between ^{15}N and ^{13}C is the reason why sample preparation and initial NMR experiments are performed with ^{15}N only. The optimal NMR solution conditions are >90% purity at 1–2 mM and sample stability for greater than 1 week. NMR glass tubes (ex. Wilmad 512) would require 550 µL of solution, but specialized glass tubes (Shigemi tubes) whose magnetic susceptibility is adjusted to that of water (in order to maintain good resolution) can decrease the required volume to 280 µL. If possible, the pH and salt should be as low as possible. A lower pH will reduce the proton exchange from the amide proton. Many of the NMR experiments use this proton during detection and rapid exchange will decrease the signal intensity. The problem with salt (>500 mM) is that more power is needed in the coils during pulsing of the sample that will introduce unwanted heat. Heat will change the location of resonance peaks as well as cause sample degradation. Another condition that will need optimization is temperature (typical ranges from 7–42 °C). Changing the temperature may affect the exchange rates between three-frequency ranges; slow, intermediate, and fast. Finally, added to the H$_2$O solution is 5–10% deuterium, used as a lock from magnetic drift, 1 mM sodium azide to curtail bacterial growth, and

3-(Trimethylsilyl)- Propionic acid-D4 (TSP) as an internal reference. The optimal solution condition for the Cx43CT was 1.5 mM in PBS (pH 5.8) buffer at 7 °C. Sample half-life was two months.

Data Collection and Processing

The two main vendors to supply spectrometers in the United States are Varian, Inc. and Bruker. Magnets consist of solenoid of super conducting wire (the main coil NbSn-NbTi) in a Dewar containing liquid helium, so that the wire is below its Tc and remains super conducting. The coil is charged with current (~100 amps) to generate the desired field and the energy stored in the coil is >1 MJ (can boil 7 lbs of water). The current will flow as long as the temperature is kept below a critical level, which is achieved by immersion in a bath of liquid helium, at temperature of 4.2 K (−270 °C). Surrounding the liquid helium is a bath of liquid nitrogen to decrease the evaporation rate. The nitrogen needs to be refilled every two weeks and the helium every two months.

My experience with data collection on both magnets does not lend me to favor one over the other. Each has a unique philosophy towards how the data is collected (and cost), but in the end, a 600 MHz magnet is a 600 MHz magnet. The upper field strength magnets are now at 900 MHz, with the average institution having a 600 MHz instrument. As mentioned earlier, a major advancement with spectrometers is cryoprobe technology. Cryoprobes cool the detection circuitry to very low temperatures while maintaining the sample itself at ambient temperatures. Current cryoprobes provide a factor of 3× improvement in signal-to-noise ratio, which means about a factor of ten reduction in data collection time. Data to solve the Cx43CT structure was collected on a Bruker DRX-600 MHz magnet.

Once the sample is placed in the magnet, the first order of business is to tune the probe and shim the magnet. The shims are small electromagnets that can be adjusted to cancel out errors (gradients) in the static magnetic field. Shimming is the process of adjusting these fields to produce a magnetic field that is uniform over the whole of the sample. After downloading the pulse sequence(s) to run the NMR experiment(s), certain parameters will need to be optimized (i.e. pulse lengths, pulse powers, sweep width, scans, gain, carrier position, and number of increments). When the experiment(s) are ready to start, either type go (Varian) or zg (Bruker). The average cost per hour for NMR time is 10 $. One-dimensional (1D) ^{1}H and two-dimensional (2D) ^{1}H^{15}N-Heteronuclear Single Quantum Coherence (HSQC) experiments are the initial spectra collected to check for protein concentration, folding, and overall feasibility for determining a protein structure. An NMR ^{1}H^{15}N-HSQC spectrum of a protein provides a fingerprint for each amino acid except proline (Fig. 3).

The total time for data acquisition for a protein structure determination is about 4 weeks. The chemical shift assignments can be obtained from as little as one week to several months (and for membrane proteins, years). A standard experimental procedure section will look as follows: Backbone sequential assignments will be obtained using the following 3D experiments: HNCACB (Wittekind and Mueller 1993), CBCA(CO)NH (Grzesiek and Bax 1993), HNCA (Kay et al. 1992), HNCO (Muhan-

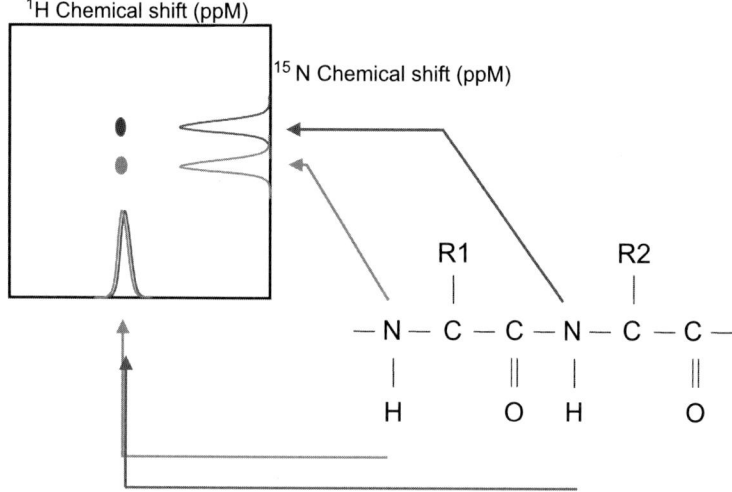

Figure 3
$^1H^{15}N$-Heteronuclear Single-Quantum Correlation (HSQC). Represented are two peaks (ovals) in a $^1H^{15}N$-HSQC spectrum and where their resonances are coming from in the amino acid sequence

diram and Kay 1994), HNCACO (Engelke and Ruterjans 1995), HNHA (Vuister and Bax 1993), and HCACO (Power et al. 1991). Side chain chemical shifts will be obtained from a 3D HCCH-TOCSY (Kay et al. 1993) and ^{15}N-TOCSY-HSQC (Zhang et al. 1994). Distance constraints will be derived from NOEs observed in ^{15}N-NOESY-HSQC and ^{13}C-NOESY-HSQC (Zhang et al. 1994) spectra. Constraints for backbone torsion angles will be derived from the HNHA spectrum (Vuister and Bax 1993).

Both Varian and Bruker have programming to process NMR data, but a more commonly used program, NMRPipe, can convert data from both companies to more powerful analysis programs (Delaglio et al. 1995). NMRPipe system is a Unix pipeline-based software environment tailored for processing multidimensional data. In a nutshell, streams of NMR data flow through a pipeline of processing programs engineered to maintain and exploit accurate records of data size, detection mode, calibration information, and processing parameters in all dimensions. Examples of processing functions are FT, Fourier Transformation; LP, Linear Prediction; SP, Sine to Power Window; and POLY, Polynomial Baseline Correction. A graphical interface program, NMRDraw, provides facilities for inspecting raw and processed data via 1D and 2D slices or projections from all dimensions.

Correctly processed data will allow us to move to the more time consuming step, assigning all the chemical shifts and interatomic distances observed by the nuclear Overhauser effect (NOE). The NOE allows the transfer of magnetization from one spin to another through space, and scales with distance r between the two spins [NOE $\sim 1/r^6$ (r=distance); interproton distances ≤ 5 Å will be detected]. Therefore, the NOE is related to the 3D structure of a molecule. NMRView is one of the programs used for visualization and analysis of the NMR datasets (Johnson 1994). The program allows multiple spectra to be analyzed together along with automated peak picking and identification. It took approximately 5 months to assign the backbone resonances for Cx43CT (132 amino acids). Observed for Cx43CT were: 401 intra-residue (i), 471 sequential (i-i+1), 304 medium (i-i+2,3,4), and 1 long-range distance restraints ($\geq i$-i+5) for a total of 1,177. NMRView will output files in the proper format for structural generation programs. Additional constraints used for structural determination were coupling constants, hydrogen bonding, chemical shifts, residual dipolar coupling, and T1/T2 ratios.

Structure Generation

As we close in on a final solution structure, a quick review of protein structure is in order:
- Primary structure – the sequence of amino acids in the chain. It always starts from N terminal (NH2) to C terminal (CO group);
- Secondary structure – the way the amino acid chains are arranged locally (examples like α-helix, β-sheet, and β-turn); and
- Tertiary structure – tells how all the elements of the secondary structure come together in solution (how the whole protein folds (or not) in solution).

The ultimate goal is to find all conformations consistent with restraints and standard covalent geometries (bond lengths, bond angles, and van der Waals radii). While we would dream of only one conformation meeting all these criteria, in reality we find a group of almost equally good solutions. The reason for multiple solution conformations are that proteins in solution are dynamic (i.e. not just in one fixed structure), have more than one major conformation in solution, or there might not be enough restraints to uniquely define the conformations. Generation of the initial structures (based on the restraints mentioned above) can be performed by distance geometry (Havel et al. 1983a,b) (ex. DG II, XPLOR), variable target function algorithms (Braun and Go 1985) (ex. DIANA/DYANA), or torsion angle dynamics (Stein et al. 1997) (ex. Crystallography & NMR Systems or CNS).

Model structures for Cx43CT were calculated by simulated annealing, using torsion angle dynamics as implemented in the program CNS (accomplished in 3 months for the Cx43CT structure). CNS was developed for macromolecular structure determination by X-ray crystallography or solution NMR spectroscopy (Bunger et al. 1998). CNS meets the demands of solving larger and larger macromolecular structures. NOE cross-peaks from ^{15}N-NOESY-HSQC and ^{13}C-NOESY-HSQC experiments are classified as strong, medium, and weak and converted into distance restraints of 1.8–2.5 Å, 1.8–3.5 Å, and 1.8–5.5 Å, respectively. When CNS generates structures, the program tries to accommodate (i.e. find the lowest energy) each restraint (i.e. NOE connectivity's assigned) placed in the restraint files. The time to generate 100 Cx43CT structures was 5 hours. Each structure is accompanied with a text file describing the deviations and violations for the various experimental and chemical restraints. This information will be used to return to the initial NMR experiments to find any missassignments.

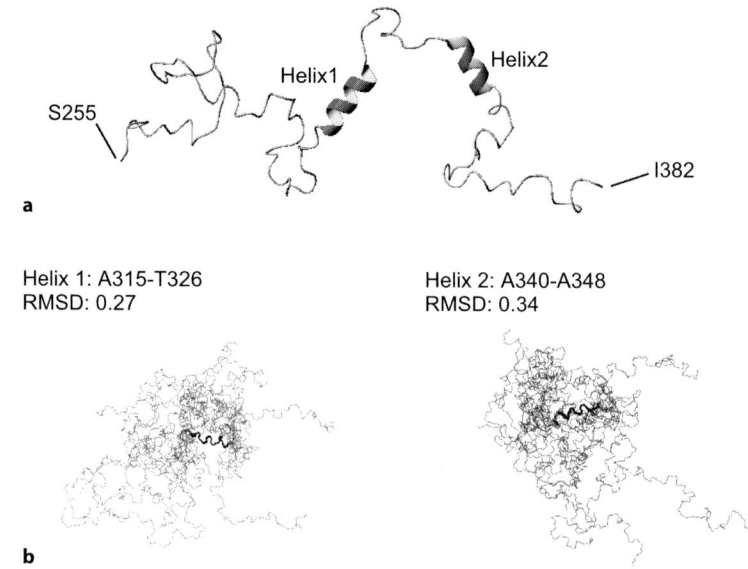

Figure 4
Solution structure of the Cx43CT in PBS buffer (pH 5.8) at 7°C. A: Lowest energy structure with amino acids comprising the α-helix colored red. B: Backbone traces of the 10 Cx43CT NMR conformers that best represent the structure are aligned by superimposing the backbone atoms (bold) of residues A315-T326 and D340-A348.

The macromolecular structures generated by CNS can be displayed and analyzed using the program MOLMOL (Konradi et al. 1996). A few of the advantages that MOLMOL provides are different visualization possibilities (ex. interatomic distances and hydrogen bonds), different conformations of a molecule can be superimposed and quantitative comparisons made by root mean square deviations, and the generation of high-quality pictures. Another useful feature from MOLMOL is that all the distance restraints less than 5 Å can be generated for a particular structure from CNS. This list should be identical to the list inputted into CNS, however, this is not always the case and the explanations can always be found back in the original NMR spectra. The differences can occur from assignment mistakes, mistaken NOE assignments, over-lap, overly narrow distance range constraints, or multiple conformations in solution. Finally, the resulting structures that fitted the constraints best, and had the lowest calculated energy, were further refined by molecular mechanics (energy minimization). In total, the RMSD between backbone atoms and all non-hydrogen atoms in the different structures are typically 0.3–0.8 Å and 0.8–1.5 Å, respectively.

The overall structure of the Cx43CT was mainly random coil, however, two regions of helical structure are present. These helical regions were superimposed on the basis of backbone coordinates from 315A-326T and 340D-3348A. The total RMSD for these alignments were 0.27 Å and 0.34 Å, respectively (Fig. 4).

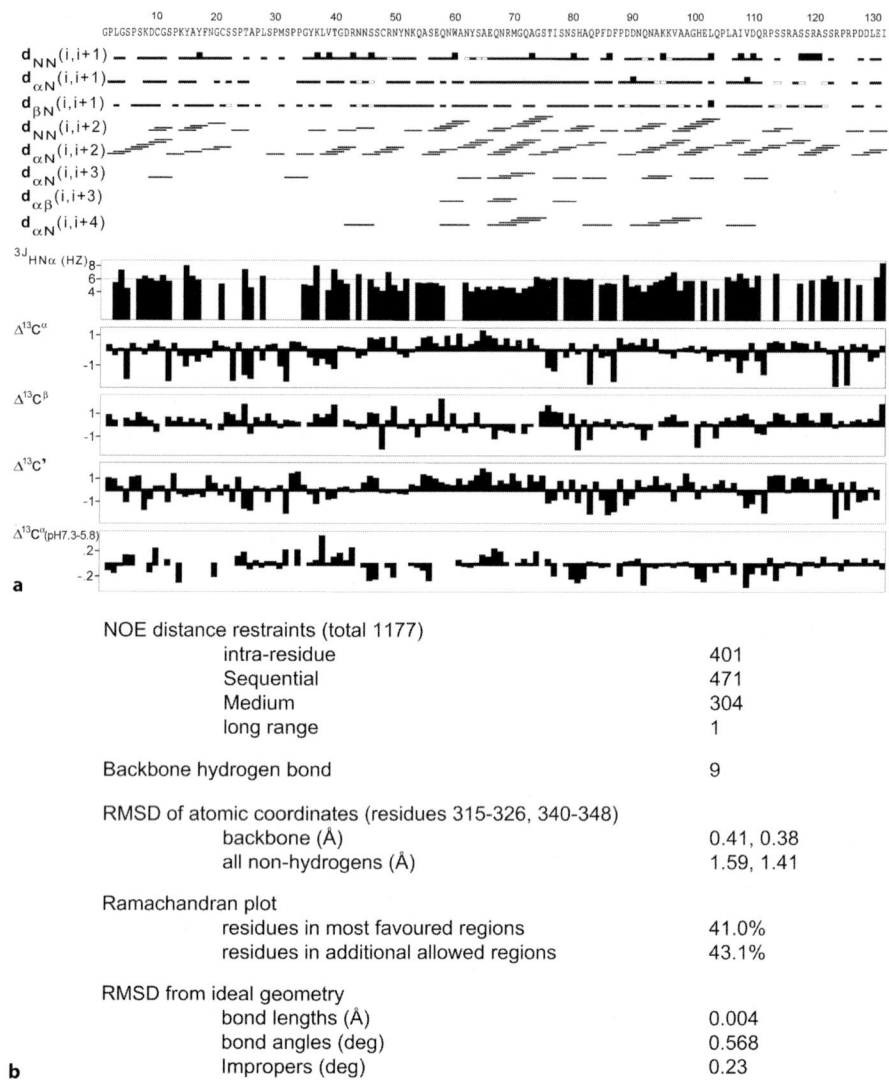

Figure 5
NMR data reported from structure determination. a Backbone NOEs, ^{3}JHN coupling constants, and secondary shifts of ^{13}C', ^{13}C$^\alpha$, ^{13}C$^\beta$ for the low pH form of Cx43CT. b Structural statistics of the 10 lowest energy Cx43CT structures

Check and Deposit

The experiments have been performed, assignments made, and structures generated, so how do you know your structure is correct? Independent structural evaluation programs check the number, average, maximum, and patterns of violations from refinement programs before the structures can be deposited into the Protein Data Bank.

Two such checking programs, AQUA/PROCHECK_NMR (Laskowski et al. 1996) and Whatif (Vriend 1990), report on values of structural quality, bond length and angles, backbone dihedral angles in favorable regions of Ramachandran plot, torsion angles, and favorable van der Waals packing. The ideal conditions (acceptable upper limit) are to have no violations of constraints, maximum NOE violations of < 0.5 Å and torsion angle violations < 5°.

The International Union of Pure and Applied Chemistry (IUPAC) published recommendations for the presentation of NMR structures of proteins and nucleic acids (Markley et al. 1998). Parameters that should be reported are the experiments, data acquisition, processing, referencing, assignments (method, extent), and a secondary structure figure, summary of constraints (Fig. 5a), method of calculation and refinement, and structural statistics (Fig. 5b). The NMR data (chemical shifts, etc.) for Cx43CT were deposited at the BioMagResBank (5431) and coordinates at the Protein Data Bank (1R5S).

Troubleshooting

Many excellent books have been written to provide a comprehensive treatment of the principles, practice, and problems associated with biomolecular NMR spectroscopy (Cavanagh et al. 1996; Freeman 1998; Levitt 2001; Evans 1995). Additionally, the Internet has NMR web pages (i.e. NMR Information Server; *http://www.spincore.com/nmrinfo/*) to connect users for the purpose of discussing common problems. While this troubleshooting is related to the NMR, I would like to mention briefly sample preparation. This is less an issue of troubleshooting and more about optimization. Finding conditions to 1) increase protein yields in minimal media will dramatically cut costs, 2) increase of the final protein concentration will cut down the data collection time, 3) decrease in salt will allow for lower power pulses (less introduction of heat which can cause sample degradation), and 4) optimization of temperature and pH will improve the signal to noise ratio, allowing for easier data analysis (e. g. see Duffy et al. 2002; Krueger-Koplin et al. 2003; Sorgen et al. 2002a,b).

Concluding Remarks

Hopefully I have provided a brief, but thorough look at the process of structural determination by solution NMR. I have presented the methods and computer programs that I used to solve the structure of Cx43CT, but there are many alternative programs to reach the same conclusions which I did not have time to discuss. A major time investment for solving NMR structures (other than the theory) is learning the vast amount of computer programs.

I always tell new spectroscopists that solving your first structure would take half the time if you were to do it all over again. Once these tools have been mastered, as I mentioned in the introduction, the information that NMR can provide (not just solving structures) can be invaluable.

References

Braun, W., Go, N. (1985) Calculation of protein conformations by proton-proton dustance constraints. A new efficient algorithm. J Mol Biol 186, 611–626

Brunger, A. T., Adams, P. D., Clore, G. M. et al. (1998) Crystallography & NMR system: A new software suite for macromolecular structure determination. Acta Crystallogr D Biol Crystallogr 54 (Pt 5), 905–921

Cavanagh, J., Fairbrother, W. J., Palmer III, A. G., and Skelton, N. J. (1996) Protein NMR Spectroscopy, Academic Press, San Diego

Delaglio, F., Grzesiek, S., Vuister, G. W., Zhu, G., Pfeifer, J., and Bax, A. (1995) NMR-Pipe: a multidimensional spectral processing system based on UNIX pipes. J Biomol NMR 6, 277–293

Duffy, H. S., Sorgen, P. L., Girvin, M. E., O'Donnell, P., Coombs, W., Taffet, S. M., Delmar, M., and Spray, D. C. (2002) pH-dependent intramolecular binding and structure involving Cx43 cytoplasmic domains. J Biol Chem 277, 36706–36714

Engelke, J., and Ruterjans, H. (1995) Sequential protein backbone assignments using an improved 3D-HN(CA)CO pulse scheme. J. Magn. Reson. Ser. B 109, 318–322

Freeman, R. (1998) Spin Choreography. Oxford University Press, New York

Grzesiek, S., and Bax, A. (1993) Amino acid type determination in the sequential assignment procedure of uniform 13C/15N-enriched proteins. J. Biomol. NMR 3, 185–204

Havel, T. F., Kuntz, I. D., and Crippen, G. M. (1983a) The combinatorial distance geometry method for the calculation of molecular conformation. II. Sample problems and computational statistics. J Theor Biol 104, 359–381

Johnson, B. A. a. B., R. A. (1994) NMR-View: A Computer program for the visualization and analysis of NMR data. J. Biomol. NMR 4, 603–614

Kay, L. E., Ikura, M., Tschudin, R., and Bax, A. (1992) Three-Dimensional Triple-Resonance Spectroscopy of Isotopically Enriched Proteins. J. Magn. Reson. 89, 496–514

Kay, L. E., Xu, G. Y., Singer, A. U., Muhandiram, R., and Forman-Kay, J. D. (1993) A Gradient-Enhanced HCCH-TOCSY Experiment for Recording Side-Chair and 13C Correlations in H_2O Samples of Proteins. J. Magn. Reson.Ser. B 101, 333–337

Koradi, R., Billeter, M., and Wuthrich, K. (1996) MOLMOL: a program for display and analysis of macromolecular structures. J Mol Graph 14, 51–55, 29–32

Krueger-Koplin, R. D., Sorgen, P. L., Krueger-Koplin, S. T. et al. (2003) An evaluation of detergents for NMR structural studies of membrane proteins. J. Biomol. NMR.

Laskowski, R. A., Rullmannn, J. A., MacArthur, M. W., Kaptein, R., and Thornton, J. M. (1996) AQW and PROCHECK-NMR: programs for checking the quality of protein structures solved by NMR. J Biomol NMR 8, 477–486

Levitt, M. (2001) Spin Dynamics, John Wiley & Sons, LTD, Chichester

Evans, J. (1995) Biomolecular NMR Spectroscopy, Oxford University Press, New York Markley, J. L., Bax, A., Arata, Y., Hilbers, C. W., Kaptein, R., Sykes, B. D., Wright, P. E., and Wuthrich, K. (1998) J Mol Biol 280, 933–952

Muhandiram, R., and Kay, L. E. (1994) Gradient-enhanced triple-resonance NMR experiments with improved sensitivity. J. Magn. Reson. Ser. B 109, 203–2216

Power, R., Gronenborn, A. M., Clore, G. M., and Bax, A. (1991) Secondary structure of the ribonuclease H domain of the human immunodeficiency virus reverse transcriptase in solution using three-dimensional double and triple resonance heteronuclear magnetic resonance spectroscopy. J. Magn. Reson. 94, 209–213

Sorgen, P. L., Cahill, S. M., Krueger-Koplin, R. D., Krueger-Koplin, S. T., Schenck, C. C., and Girvin, M. E. (2002a) Structure of the Rhodobacter sphaeroides light-harvesting 1 beta subunit in detergent micelles. Biochemistry 41, 31–41

Sorgen, P. L., Duffy, H. S., Cahill, S. M., Coombs, W., Spray, D. C., Delmar, M., and Girvin, M. E. (2002b) Sequence-specific resonance assignment of the carboxyl terminal domain of Connexin43. J Biomol NMR 23, 245–246

Stein, E. G., Rice, L. M., and Brunger, A. T. (1997) Torsion-angle molecular dynamics as a new efficient tool for NMR structure calculation. J Magn Reson 124, 154–164

Vriend, G. (1990) WHAT IF: a molecular modeling and drug design program. J. Mol. Graph. 8, 52–56

Vuister, G. W., and Bax, A. (1993) Quantitative J Correlation: A New Approach for Measuring Homonuclear Three-Bond J(HNHa) Coupling Constants in 15N-Enriched Proteins. J. Magn. Reson. 96, 432–440

Wittekind, M., and Mueller, L. (1993) J. Magn. Reson. Ser. B 101, 201–205ang, O., Kay, L. E., Olivier, J. P., and Forman-Kay, J. D. (1994) HNCACB, a high-sensitivity 3D NMR experiment to correlate amide-proton and nitrogen resonances with the alpha- and Beta-carbon resonances in proteins. J Biomol NMR 4, 845–858

Managing a Transgenic Mouse Colony: A Guide for the Novice

Robert H. Quinn and Karen L. Vikstrom

Introduction

Although the mouse has long been an important model organism for experimental biology, mouse models have played only a minor role in basic cardiovascular research for most of the 21st century. However, since the late 1980s the use of mouse models in cardiovascular research has expanded tremendously mainly due to the development of murine transgenic technology. Although genetic models in larger animals, such as rabbits, have significant physiological and anatomical advantages over the mouse in cardiovascular research, the greater difficulty in genetically modifying them, and the significantly greater expense in maintaining their breeding colonies, has slowed their use as genetic models. Moreover, many transgenic mice suitable for cardiovascular research are already available through commercial sources or through collaborative arrangement. Consequently, it is often possible for an investigator to obtain a suitable transgenic mouse model for his/her research program without creating it from scratch. In addition, programs are currently underway to identify mutant mice resulting from chemical mutagenesis (Brown and Hardisty 2003). The mutagenesis programs are likely to significantly increase the number of murine models with cardiovascular phenotypes that are available. Thus, for the foreseeable future, it is likely that the use of mutant mice in cardiovascular research will continue to increase and that additional researchers will begin to use murine models for at least a proportion of their research endeavors. This chapter is intended as a guide for individuals who have no practical experience in mouse animal husbandry and are contemplating obtaining established transgenic mouse models for their research programs.

The majority of transgenic mice currently available to the cardiovascular research community were created using technology developed during the 1980s that stemmed from two important findings 1) when foreign DNA is microinjected into the pronucleus of a fertilized mouse egg, it is capable of stably incorporating into the mouse genome (Gordon et al. 1980; Brinster et al. 1981) and 2) after targeted modification of the genome in pluripotent embryonic stem cells (ES cells), the modified ES cells can be introduced into blastocysts and subsequently contribute to the germ line. These findings provided the basis for the two most common types of transgenic animals used today: those with gain-of-function mutations and those with gene targeted mutations. Gain-of-function transgenics, often referred to as "overexpressors", were the first to gain widespread use and are still frequently used. To produce this type of

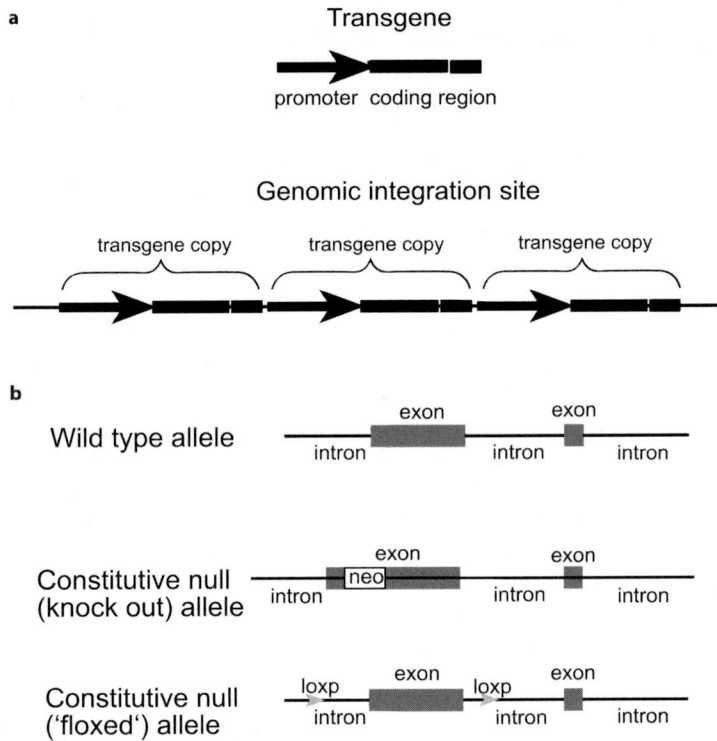

Figure 1a,b
Gain-of-function transgenics and targeted mutations. **a** Gain-of-function transgenics result from the stable incorporation of a transgene, a 'mini-gene' containing regulatory sequence (promoter) sufficient to direct expression of the 'mini-gene' *in vivo*. By using promoters that restrict transgene expression to specific cell types, transgene expression can be directed to specific cell populations. A well-characterized example is the murine α myosin heavy chain promoter (Gulick et al. 1991), which drives robust transgene expression in the cardiac myocyte. **b** Gene targeted mutations use homologous recombination in ES cells to modify a locus within the mouse genome. The most common type of targeted mutation creates a constitutive null allele by inserting exogenous DNA into an exon so that it results in premature transcriptional or translational termination. Animals with two copies of this type of mutation never make the wild type gene product and constitute a constitutive null or a knockout animal. In contrast, conditional null alleles are silent unless a viral recombinase is provided to excise the sequence between the recombinase recognition sites (loxp sites in this example). The ability to use gain-of-function transgenics to drive expression of recombinase allows the loss of the gene product to be targeted to a specific cell type or during different developmental stages

transgenic, a mini-gene consisting of transcriptional regulatory sequences (the promoter) and protein coding sequences, constitutes the transgene (Fig. 1a). This transgene is introduced into the mouse genome by physical injection of the transgene DNA into the pronucleus of a fertilized mouse egg. Some of the mice that develop from the injected eggs will have integrated the transgene DNA into their genome, typically as a concatamer (Fig. 1a), and will transmit this DNA to subsequent generations of mice.

In transgenic mice with gene-targeted mutations, mutations are directed to a specific gene using homologous recombination in ES cells. The incorporation of the mutant ES cells into mouse blastocysts will lead to animals that transmit the targeted mutation to subsequent generations, as long as their germline contains cells derived from the ES cells. Depending on the nature of the recombination events, targeted mutations can take a number of forms. The most common example is the creation of a constitutive null allele (Fig. 1b). The null allele is produced through the introduction of exogenous sequence (for example, sequence coding for antibiotic resistance [neo], GFP, or β-galactosidase) into a crucial exon, such that the introduced sequence causes premature transcriptional or translational termination. An animal with two copies of the null allele is commonly referred to as a knockout mouse. A conditional null allele results when the target sequences for a viral recombinase are introduced so that they flank a crucial exon. In the example illustrated in Fig. 1b, the loxP sites recognized by the Cre recombinase are found flanking an exon producing a floxed allele. In the absence of the Cre recombinase, this targeted mutation is silent and should not interfere with the production of a wild type gene product. However, if the Cre recombinase is supplied in trans, the genomic sequence between the loxP sites will be excised, resulting in a null allele. The most common way to supply the Cre recombinase, is by crossing mice with the floxed allele with gain-of-function transgenics that express the Cre recombinase in a specific cell population. If the Cre recombinase is expressed only in specific cell types (for example, cardiac myocytes or vascular smooth muscle cells) the exon will only be excised in those cell types. While these are the most commonly encountered forms of targeted mutations, homologous recombination can be used to produce other types of mutations such as subtle change in the endogenous locus, point mutations (a.k.a. knock in) or the production of chimeric genes. A number of excellent articles and manuals are available that provide much greater detail on these methods (Lewandowski 2001; Pinkert 2002).

Description of Methods and Practical Approach

Obtaining Mice from Non-Commercial Sources

Although many institutions have developed their own programs and facilities for creating transgenic mice, the vast majority of investigators use animals developed at other research institutions or from commercial sources. The distinct advantages of this type of use, are that the animals are often fairly well characterized phenotypically (such that the husbandry requirements are already known) and there is an easily replenished source of animals, therefore, the receiving institution does not (necessarily) need to be concerned with maintaining the line. The disadvantages are that the receiving institution now has to deal with health concerns and/or importation regulations when receiving animals from noncommercial sources, and the investigator may encounter significant expense and delays when obtaining cryopreserved animals from commercial sources.

Importation

Since rats and mice bred for research are not covered under the Animal Welfare Act (USDA, 2002), there are no specific requirements that apply to importation of these animals into the US. According to the United States Department of Agriculture Animal and Plant Health Inspection Service (APHIS), USDA importation permits **are not required** for live laboratory mammals if: (1) a health certificate signed by a licensed veterinarian stating that the animals are clinically healthy accompanies live mammals and (2) there is a statement from the shipper/producer indicating that the animals have not been exposed to or inoculated with any livestock or poultry disease agents exotic to the United States; and have not originated from a facility where work with exotic disease agents affecting livestock or poultry is conducted. Therefore, essentially the only requirement to bring transgenic mice into the United States is that they are legally exported from the country of origin. The export requirements of other countries vary widely, so these will not be specifically addressed here. Commercial rodent suppliers dealing in worldwide markets can be a valuable resource regarding these regulations and some even offer brokerage services to arrange shipments from other countries. The only exception to the above is, when the animals constitute a biological hazard requiring containment above Animal Biosafety Level 1, as defined by the Centers for Disease Control (CDC). In this instance, numerous importation regulations may apply from the Public Health Service, Department of Transportation, U.S. Postal Service, Occupational Health and Safety Administration, and others. The specific regulations that may apply can be found in the CDC Biosafety Guidelines, Appendix C (USDHHS, 1999).

Quarantine

Receiving animals from other institutions always constitutes a risk to the resident animals at the receiving institution. Even if the receiving institution does not have stringent standards and maintains colonies with some baseline level of disease, the introduction of new animals may bring agents to which the resident animals have not previously been exposed. This can lead to devastating outbreaks throughout entire facilities. Therefore, it is good practice, to subject all animals obtained from non-commercial sources to a quarantine period for a minimum of 4–6 weeks. The goal of a good quarantine program is to ensure that animals leaving quarantine are healthy and do not constitute a vector for disease prior to introduction into established colonies. This 4–6 week period addresses this goal in a number of ways. First, it provides adequate time to observe the animals for indications of clinical disease and to determine any special husbandry requirements for ensured health. Second, if the animals are harboring a contagious virus, this will probably be adequate time for the viral infection to run its course and for the quarantined animals to develop protective immunity, thus no longer presenting a hazard to other animals. Thirdly, it allows time for the development of an antibody response to any sub-clinical infections that may then be detected by serological testing. However, it is imperative to use standard, known immunocompetent mice as contact and/or dirty-bedding sentinels to test, since the immune response (and possibly course of infection) is unknown in most transgenic animals (Rehg 2001). Otto and Tolwani (2002) provide a comprehensive blueprint for a good quarantine program that permits continuous receipt of animals from various sources in a limited quarantine space. The most important aspect of a good quarantine program is physical separation between quarantine and colony animals. It is best to limit human traffic into a quarantine area to only those individuals required to care for the animals. When developing a quarantine program, careful attention should be directed toward traffic patterns of both humans and equipment, particularly ensuring that nothing travels from the quarantine area into any colony areas (or at least not without being thoroughly disinfected first). Animals in quarantine should not be used experimentally until after the quarantine period has expired. Although this delay can be frustrating to the investigators, it is an important safeguard to the health of established breeding colonies at the institution. This delay also allows the animals an adjustment period to recover from the stress of shipping and to adjust to other changes in their environment (such as husbandry differences between institutions).

Maintaining a Mouse Colony

Housing Considerations

The care of transgenic mouse colonies is an ever-moving target. The multitude of genetic modifications and potential phenotypic results are innumerable. From a practical standpoint, this translates into a spectrum of husbandry requirements ranging from standard, "conventional" housing to a sterile "isolator"-type environment for severely immunosuppressed strains. There is a common misconception that "transgenic animals" must be maintained under "barrier conditions." This misconception arose during the early days of genetic manipulation and it has been perpetuated ever since. To understand why this misconception continues, one must merely look at the circumstances under which it was developed.

When transgenic animals were first being created more than 20 years ago, it was common that the colonies from which these animals were developed fell under the definition of "conventional." Twenty years ago "conventional" housing often meant that there was no formal health-monitoring program or any effort to exclude or eliminate common rodent pathogens. Therefore, when a single founder animal was identified (and it's status immediately changed from "standard laboratory mouse" to "irreplaceable genetic model of human disease"), there was often an immediate need to "protect" this animal from the resident infectious agents. This was most often accomplished by secluding the animal in a "barrier", using techniques that had been developed for gnotobiotic ("germ-restricted") animal housing. Once these animals were "clean" inside a barrier, it was considered safer and easier to maintain them in the barrier rather than risk exposing them to the "conventional" conditions with their unknown immune status. The standards of laboratory animal husbandry have improved significantly in the last 20 years. Conventional colonies have given way to specific-pathogen-free (SPF) colonies, which exclude a wide host of infectious organisms. In addition, standard housing techniques have changed to include filter-topped isolator caging, improved sanitation requirements, limited personnel access, and improved food and water sources. These improvements have resulted in "standard" housing environments that are acceptable for a great many genetically altered strains. Although there are transgenic strains with immunosuppressive phenotypes that require strict barrier housing, it should not be assumed that all transgenic animals need this type of environment to survive.

The specific husbandry requirements of any transgenic strain should be determined during the period of phenotypic characterization. Since the phenotype of any newly created transgenic animal is essentially unknown, it is always advisable to create these animals in very "clean" background stock and under the strictest barrier conditions. It is imperative to protect these founder animals from infectious agents until the colony is well established. At that point, barring any phenotypic alterations indicative of severe immunosuppression, some animals may be removed from the barrier and placed in standard housing for a trial period, to determine if they have any increased susceptibility to nonpathogenic organisms within this type of housing environment. If the mouse model of interest is not immunosuppressed, there are advantages to maintaining the colony in a conventional housing facility. Cost is the most obvious advantage. In most facilities, "barrier" housing costs up to twice (or more) the rate of standard housing. Since a large number of cages may be necessary to maintain a breeding colony, the cost differential can be significant. The second advantage is access. It is often difficult to conduct experiments within a barrier facility due to space constraints for equipment, special apparel requirements, and inability to remove and return animals from the barrier. Finally, removing animals to be used for experimentation from the barrier facility actually provides protection for the barrier itself. Moving experimental procedures outside of the barrier decreases traffic into the barrier, thus the integrity of the barrier will be much stronger (Gordon 2002). Although other means of protecting valuable genetic strains should be employed (such as embryo cryopreservation), it is common to maintain a small breeding contingent within a barrier-housing unit to serve as replacements in the event of a catastrophic loss within the main colony. However, if these mouse strains are also being maintained at other institutions, this may be unnecessary.

Breeding Strategies

The nature of the mutation, as well as the mouse's phenotype, will determine whether mutant animals are bred to each other or crossed with a wild type mouse. Gain-of-function transgenics are often used as heterozygous animals. If that is the case, crossing the mutant animal with a wild type mouse of the appropriate strain (see section on congenic animals below) should produce approximately equal numbers of wild type and heterozygous-transgenics. For most knockout models, animals with two targeted alleles are needed for experiments. If the presence of two null alleles does not produce a lethal phenotype, or an animal with significant fertility problems, it may be possible to maintain the line by crossing homozygous animals. Otherwise the line will need to be perpetuated by breeding heterozygous mice. In this case, assuming that the homozygous knockouts do not exhibit reduced viability, approximately 25% of the offspring will have the desired genotype. If production of the animal of interest results from crosses between mouse-lines with distinct mutations (such as producing animals with a conditional null allele and a cre-transgene) the percentage of pups with the correct genotype is even lower. It must be emphasized that producing significant numbers of animals with the correct genotype is not a trivial endeavor. For instance, take the example of producing knockout animals through heterozygous crosses. If the average size of a litter were 6 (litter size will vary) producing 6 knockout animals from heterozygous crosses would require 4 litters (~24 pups). Of course, if gender-matched animals are required, the number of pups required will double. If the experimental population needs to be age-matched, additional breeding animals may be needed to ensure the required number of productive mating during the target period. In any case, knowledge of the breeding characteristics of the transgenic line, as well as the desired number of animals to be produced, will determine the number of breeding stock required.

Once the breeding stock is available, the colony can be expanded to provide animals for experimentation as well as replacement breeding stock. Setting up monogamous breeding pairs in which one male and one female animal are continuously housed together is the simplest approach. In many cases this will result in the birth of a new litter every three weeks, due to mating during the post-partum estrus cycle. Since the presence of an older litter in a cage diverts maternal resources away from the new litter, and the excess number of animals may result in the rapid accumulation of unacceptable levels of urine and feces, it is advisable to wean the first litter before the birth of the second litter. Most pregnant dams do not appear obviously pregnant until the third week of gestation. If the dam appears pregnant when the current pups are ~2½ weeks of age it is likely that she will drop a litter within a day or two of weaning the current pups. If the genetic model exhibits reduced reproductive performance, decreased neonatal viability, or the colony needs to be expanded rapidly, you may need to increase the number of potential litters through harem mating (one male housed with 2–3 females) or by rotating a stud male through several cages of females. If harem mating is pursued, the investigator must take care to ensure that sufficient females are removed from the cage once pregnant to prevent overcrowding due to multiple litters. If the male mouse is overly aggressive, it also is advisable to remove him prior to the birth of the litter. Once removed, the male should not be returned to the cage until the litter is weaned, due to the risk to the pups.

Weaning and Screening

Most mouse pups can be weaned when they are 18–20 days old, although weaning should be delayed if the pups are unusually small or exhibit reduced vigor. Unless the mutant mouse strain is maintained by crossing homozygous animals, the genotype of each mouse must be determined empirically. In virtually all cases, this is accomplished through analysis of genomic DNA isolated from each animal. The most common source for the genomic DNA is a small piece of tail that is removed at the time of weaning (animal welfare issues involved in tail "biopsies" and alternative tissue sources are discussed later in this chapter). As animals are genotyped, they must also be permanently marked for later identification (also see below). Although the use of PCR-based methods has dramatically shortened the time needed for genotyping, it is still a time consuming and costly process.

Efficient genotyping requires some skill in genomic DNA isolation and molecular analysis. The techniques involved are not difficult, but if DNA based methodology is new to the investigator, it is advisable to find a laboratory that routinely uses DNA-based methods for assistance. The first step in the process is isolating the genomic DNA from the tissue sample. For the purpose of this discussion we will assume that tail biopsies are being used. Methods to extract genomic DNA from tail biopsies have evolved significantly since the mid 1980s. Prior to the development of PCR, routine genotyping of transgenic mice required micrograms of genomic DNA suitable for use in Southern blot analysis. A typical protocol involved proteinase K digestion of the tissue sample, multiple phenol extractions and alcohol precipitation followed by collection of the DNA precipitate by spooling or centrifugation (Hogan et al. 1986). Although there are situations in which screening by Southern blot analysis is still appropriate (such as verifying transgene integrity in new lines or determining transgene copy number), PCR-based methods have become the norm for routine genotyping. The advantages of using PCR-based screening are faster turnaround (<1 day vs. >3 days), greater sensitivity and lower expense. PCR –based genotyping also requires only small amounts of DNA (20–100 ng), so a smaller piece of tissue can be used to prepare the DNA sample. This is much preferable from an animal welfare perspective. Phenol extractions should not be necessary to prepare tail DNA of sufficient quality for PCR analysis and phenol-free methods have been published in laboratory manuals (Spector et al. 1998) and are available on the Jackson Laboratory website (*http://www.jax.org/imr/supp_proto.html*). Another option is to use commercially available kits. A number of companies sell kits for purifying genomic DNA from cells and tissues. Although the kit approach is more costly than purifying DNA from scratch, using a kit may be more accessible for individuals without prior experience of purifying DNA. One of the most crucial steps in purifying the DNA sample is the tissue lysis. Due to the high collagen content of the rodent tail, lysing tail samples is much more difficult than lysing lymphocytes or less collagen-rich tissues. Consequently, when choosing a kit, make certain that it has been optimized for isolation of DNA from tail samples.

The goal of genotyping is to unambiguously distinguish the possible genotypes in the litter being screened. If the screening protocol is robust, it should work consistently and very few samples should require repeat screening. Genotyping a heterozygous gain-of-function transgenic is straightforward since the PCR is used to distinguish the presence or absence of the transgene. PCR primers (Fig. 2a; P1 and P2) that amplify a transgene-specific DNA fragment will amplify the appropriately sized band from the transgenic animals' DNA, but not from the nontransgenic littermates. However, using only transgene-specific PCR primers in the screening protocol has a significant drawback. The absence of the transgene-specific band usually indicates a non-transgenic animal, however, it may also be the result of poor DNA quality, low DNA concentration or investigator error. If non-transgenic littermates are used as the experimental control population, a false negative could result in a transgenic animal being placed in the control group and lead to significant experimental error. To control for false negatives, a second primer pair that should amplify a band in every sample can be included in the reaction. In this case, a PCR product should be present in every sample (Fig. 2b) and the genotype of the animal is determined by the size of the amplified products.

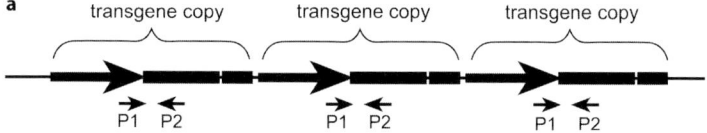

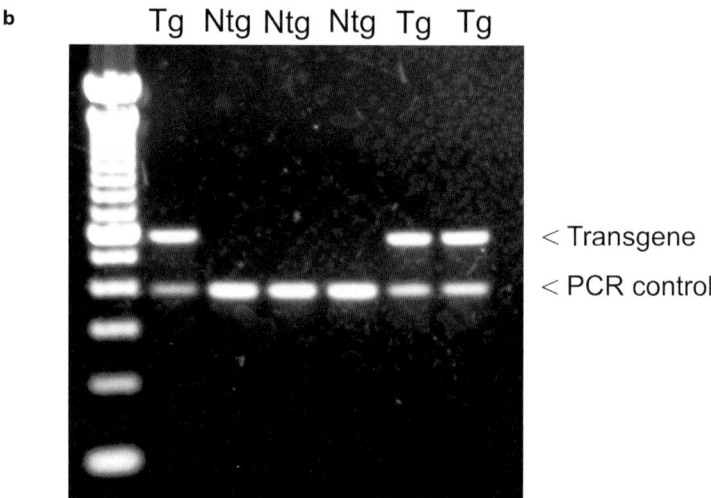

Figure 2a,b
Screening gain-of-function transgenics by PCR. **a** Genotyping a gain-of-function transgenic by PCR is a matter of determining the presence or absence of the transgene. PCR primers (P1 and P2) that are specific to the transgene will amplify an appropriately sized DNA fragment in the transgenic animals but not in the non-transgenic littermates. **b** False negatives are a significant risk in PCR based screening. Although the absence of the transgene-specific band usually indicates a non-transgenic animal, it may be the result of poor DNA quality, low DNA concentration or investigator error. To control for false negatives, a second primer pair that should amplify a band in every sample can be included in the reaction. This internal control greatly reduces the risk of false negatives. In the example shown here, the screening protocol results in two PCR products in the transgenic animals (Tg), a transgene specific band and a band for the internal control. Only the control PCR product is present in the non-transgenic littermates (Ntg). If no amplification product is detected the genotyping is inconclusive

Screening gene-targeted mutations by PCR is slightly more complicated. In this case, the screening protocol must not only distinguish the presence or absence of the targeted allele, it must also determine if the animal is heterozygous or homozygous for the mutation. For a constitutive 'knockout' allele, one approach is to use 3 primers for the PCR: 2 primers that anneal to genomic sequences flanking the antibiotic selection cassette (Fig. 3a, P1 and P2) and one primer that anneals to sequence located within the antibiotic selection cassette (Fig. 3a, P3). If the mouse is wild type, only a P1-P2 product will be amplified. If the mouse is heterozygous both P1-P2 and P1-P3 pro-

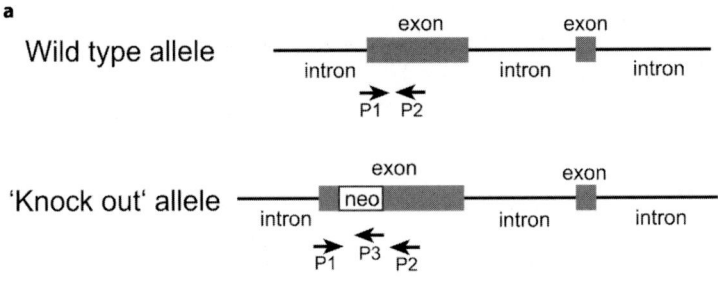

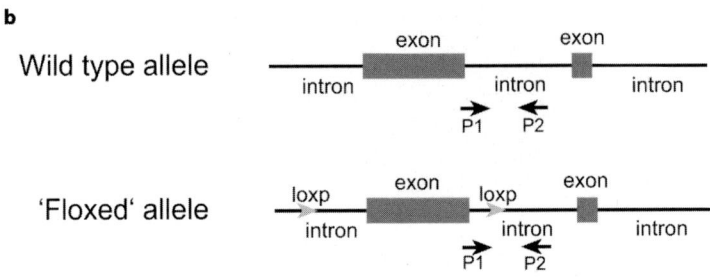

Figure 3a,b
Screening gene targeted mutations by PCR. **a** When screening a constitutive null allele by PCR the protocol must distinguish between 0, 1 or 2 copies of the targeted allele. One approach uses 3 primers for the PCR: 2 primers that anneal to genomic sequences flanking the antibiotic selection cassette (P1 and P2) and one primer that anneals to sequence located within the antibiotic selection cassette (P3). If the mouse is wild type (0 copies of the targeted allele), only a P1-P2 product will be amplified. If the mouse is heterozygous both P1-P2 and P1-P3 products will be amplified. In a homozygous knockout, the P1-P3 product will be amplified and any P1-P2 product that is amplified will be much larger than the wild type P1-P2 amplicon, due to the amplification of sequence from the selection cassette. **b** The presence of the 32 bp loxP site in a conditional null allele, provides a means to distinguish the wild type and mutant alleles since PCR primers flanking one of the loxP sites will amplify PCR products of slightly different sizes from the wild type and mutant alleles

ducts will be amplified. In a homozygous knockout, the P1-P3 product will be amplified. Although the P1 and P2 sequences are present in the homozygous knockout, the intervening selection cassette will result in a larger amplification product than seen with the wild type mouse and this larger product may not amplify efficiently. If the mice are being screened for the presence of a floxed (conditional null) allele, PCR primers that flank one of the loxP sites will amplify PCR products of slightly different sizes from the wild type and mutant alleles (Fig. 3b).

Colony records

As mentioned above, as animals are genotyped, they should be permanently identified for pedigree records and/or selection into experimental groups. Information about each mouse (date of birth, identification code, genotype, dam, and sire) should be re-

Colony logs

Mouse #	DOB	Sex	Sire	Dam	Genotype	Cage #	ID code	Notes

Breeding logs

Male Female		Date set up:		Retire by:			
Litter #	DOB	# Born	Date weaned	Number each sex		Remarks	
				Males	Females		
1							
2							
3							
4							
5							
6							

Figure 4
Keeping careful records is an important aspect of maintaining a transgenic mouse colony. In addition to the animal's date of birth, gender and genotype, important information to note include parentage, the identification markings for that animal (ear punch code, tattoo, etc.) and the eventual use of the animal. In the case of breeding pairs, careful records help to evaluate the reproductivity of breeding animals and facilitate the timely replacement of the stock

corded in a colony log. For an example of a colony log sheet, see Fig. 4. Most Institutional Animal Care and Use Committees (IACUC) require a yearly account of the number of animals used. Noting the date of euthanasia in the colony log, and indicating if the animal was excess stock or used in an experiment, can simplify the yearly accounting. Maintaining accurate records of the breeding stock is also important (Fig. 4). Most inbred mouse strains are sexually mature by 8 weeks of age and healthy female mice usually reproduce well until 8–10 months of age. Although females may remain reproductively active after 8–10 months of age, the production of viable litters is greatly reduced. The reproductive performance of male mice also drops with increased age. Moreover, animals with significant cardiovascular dysfunction may show decreased reproductive performance at an earlier age than wild type animals. It behooves the investigator to keep track of the age of the breeding stock as well as the number of litters produced by both the male and female. Unless a substantial population of young animals is always on hand, replacement-breeding stock should be identified before the current breeders stop producing litters. To do otherwise puts the breeding colony at risk and may force the investigator to obtain replacement animals from outside the colony (and become subject to all the inherent delays).

Congenic Versus Noncongenic Strains

Inbred mice, such as C57BL/6 or DBA, are genetically homogenous animals resulting from numerous generations of inbreeding. Due to the resulting accumulation of genetic polymorphisms, the characteristics of inbred strains, including such characteristics as heart rate, heart size or body size, may vary. An example of the impact of these strain differences can be seen in their response to exercise (Lerman et al. 2002). Most transgenic animals have a mixed strain background when they are produced. For gain-of-function transgenics, the oocytes used for microinjection are often isolated from animals that are a cross between two inbred strains. Gene targeted animals are typically produced using ES cells derived from the 129-mouse strain, which are then introduced into C57BL/6 derived blastocysts. As mentioned above, in each case the genetic variability in the resulting transgenic line has the potential to impact on the phenotype of that line. One way to account for these differences experimentally is to use the wild type littermates for experimental control groups since these animals should have essentially the same genetic makeup as the mutant animals. However, the most rigorous approach is to minimize the genetic variability within the transgenic line. To remove the genetic heterogeneity in the transgenic requires many generations of backcrossing to a specific strain of inbred mice (most often the C57BL/6 strain). For example, 10–14 generations of backcrossing a transgenic line to the C57BL/6 strain would result in the transgenic line becoming congenic with C57BL/6. In other words, the transgenic line would have essentially no genetic difference from the backcross strain except for the transgene locus. Traditionally, making a transgenic line congenic requires several years of effort. However, the use of marker-assisted selection strategies can significantly shorten that time frame (Markel 1997).

Examples

The number of transgenic models available to the cardiovascular researcher is expanding rapidly. Consequently, any print list of transgenic mouse models pertinent to the cardiovascular research community is seriously outdated by the time it is published. However, both the Jackson Research Laboratory and the NIH maintain online, searchable databases of genetic resources that are periodically updated. These databases are a good place to look for the most up-to-date listing of transgenic mouse models. Information about these resources is provided in Table 1.

Table 1
Major portals to Internet resources for transgenic animals with cardiovascular phenotypes

Organization	Description	Site
The Jackson Laboratory	The Jackson Laboratory website contains information about various inbred strains, mouse genome informatics, and a searchable database of transgenic mice (tbase). There is much more extremely useful information on this site than is readily apparent from the site map. Luckily, the search function works well.	http://www.jax.org/ http://tbase.jax.org/
NIH	The NHLBI maintains a searchable database of genetic models related to heart, lung, blood or sleep disorders. In addition, both the trans-NIH mouse initiative and NHLBI-sponsored Program for Genomic Initiatives maintain an extensive list of links of interest including links to additional databases of mutant mice.	http://www.nhlbi.nih.gov/resources/medres/transgen.htm http://www.nih.gov/science/models/mouse/ http://www.nhlbi.nih.gov/resources/pga/index.htm

Troubleshooting

Special Husbandry Considerations

Aside from concerns over the immuno-competency of a newly developed strain, there are often other phenotypic changes that may impact upon the animal's husbandry needs (Monastersky and Geistfeld 2002). Although an investigator may be altering a very specific genetic sequence, with expected results extrapolated from the known function of the gene, the actual and total phenotypic alterations that will occur are always unknown (Morton and Hau 2003). This exemplifies why it is so important to characterize the phenotype of these animals as quickly as possible.

Food

Genetic alterations often lead to (or are associated with) decreased lactation, smaller pup weights, smaller weaning weights, weaker pups, and/or animals with tooth abnormalities. These changes may need to be addressed with delayed weaning, providing softened food, providing food on the cage floor, or special diets.

Water

Some animals may require longer watering tubes (if the animals are small) or even water dishes if they have ambulatory difficulties.

Bedding

Smaller pups or those with metabolic disturbances may need increased bedding to provide extra warmth, especially when housed in cages with accessory ventilation. Some animals may show neurological abnormalities leading to ingestion of bedding and alternative methods of housing may need to be employed.

Grouping

Transgenic mice are often created on a C57BL/6 genetic background. This strain has a tendency to be aggressive (especially between males) and genetic manipulation may actually exacerbate this behavior. Smaller groups, separation of aggressors, and/or even individual housing may be required. Females of this strain are also notoriously poor mothers, often neglecting or cannibalizing their pups, especially on first litters, thereby necessitating 'cross-fostering' onto other dams (Monastersky and Geistfeld 2002).

Institutional Animal Care and Use Committee (IACUC) Issues Concerning Genetically Modified Animals

The use of genetically modified animals often involves issues that are of particular concern to IACUCs. These include common procedures used in transgenic colonies (that may or may not be used in other colonies) such as tissue collection for genotyping and individual animal identification methods. Breeding colonies complicate the consideration of animal numbers used in research. Transgenic disease models raise issues of health and welfare. All of these issues must be defined and approved by the IACUC when working with these models.

Tissue Collection for Genotyping

Genotyping is most commonly performed using DNA derived from a "tail biopsy" in mice. Traditionally, this involved restraining the animal and quickly removing between 0.2 and 1 cm of tail with a sharp scalpel or scissors. Although animals often exhibit only brief indications of pain and/or distress, performing this procedure on un-anesthetized animals has increasingly come under the scrutiny of IACUCs (Flecknell and Silverman 2000). Currently there are no federal regulations or guidelines that require the use of anesthesia for tail biopsy. By definition then, this regulation defaults to the guidelines established by the IACUC for each institution. The most common position of IACUCs, is to assume that this procedure is painful and require anesthesia +/– analgesia, unless there is adequate scientific justification for withholding it. Another common IACUC requirement is that this procedure only be performed in neonatal animals (usually up to 30 days of age) since ossification of the tail is incomplete until this time (Pinkert 2003). Another common source of tissue for genotyping is ear pinna that is removed during ear notching for identification (Chen and Evans 1990). This usually does not provide adequate tissue for southern blot analysis, but is often sufficient for PCR based analysis. IACUCs tend to favor the use of this tissue, since its collection appears to be less traumatic than tail snips and provides the dual purpose of genotyping and animal identification. Newer, less invasive methods of sample collection for genotyping are being developed all the time (Pinkert 2003). Samples such as saliva, feces, oral swabs, vaginal swabs, rectal swabs, fur clippings, and blood have all been reported. Since IACUCs are mandated to ensure that alternatives are considered, it is not uncommon for an IACUC to require that an investigator provide scientific justification for why these less invasive procedures cannot be used prior to approving tail biopsy. The most distinct disadvantage of these alternatives is that they usually require a very sensitive method of detection since the sample quantity or concentration is so low.

Individual Animal Identification

General research using standard rodent models is often approached from a group basis whereby there is no need to identify individual animals. Often the identification of these groups occurs at cage level, not by individual animal. This is often not the case with transgenic animals, especially if there is a breeding colony involved. Once animals are genotyped, it is usually imperative that each animal be permanently identified for pedigree records and/or selection into experimental groups. All permanent methods of identification in rodents are invasive to some degree. Much like sample collection for genotyping, most IACUCs prefer (or require) that the least invasive methods be considered and justifiably rejected prior to approval of more invasive methods. Traditionally, the removal of sections of digits from the front feet in neonatal animals, according to a numbering code (toe clipping), was the method of choice. The most recent versions of the Guide for the Care and Use of Laboratory Animals ("Guide") (NRC, 1996) and the Public Health Service Policy (OLAW, 2000) mandate that this procedure only be performed after determining that other means of identification "are not feasible". Ear notching is another traditional means of identification that is still largely in favor today. This involves using a special "ear punch" to remove a small circle from the center and/or notch from the edge of the ear pinnae (with or without anesthesia), again according to a standardized code. This method provides the added benefit of a tissue sample for genotyping (see above). Adjunct to this, a number of manufacturers make numbered ear tags for use in small rodents, although inflammatory reactions and loss of tags can be a problem. Less invasive methods of permanent identification in mice are being developed all the time. Methods such as digital tattooing, tail tattooing, and subcutaneous microchip implantation are becoming more popular and preferred by IACUCs. The major disadvantage is that each of these methods requires specialized equipment for marking and/or reading the identification method.

Animal Number Justification

Breeding colonies of transgenic rodents present challenging accounting issues for the investigator and the IACUC. The "Guide" specifies that IACUCs must consider "Justification of the species and number of animals requested." Most IACUCs interpret this to mean justification for the approximate number of animals to be used in experimental protocols. For knockout mice, it is often only the homozygote animals that are of interest, yet, due to fertility problems in homozygotes, the line may need to be perpetuated by breeding heterozygotes. Following Mendelian genetics, this means that up to 75% of the animals created may not be useful experimentally, although wild-type littermates are usually used as controls. Most IACUCs do not require strict accounting of these extraneous animals, only the animals that are actually used in experimental protocols. Irregardless, the creation of these animals within the institution still falls under the purview of the IACUC, and therefore most committees require at least an explanation of the breeding scheme, estimate of the total animals to be created, method of genotyping, and method of disposal of the extraneous animals. Genotyping is currently a "gray zone", in that some committees consider this as "experimental use" and therefore require accounting of all animals, while some committees do not. In addition, some committees consider even the creation of transgenic animals with subnormal phenotypes as "use" and require strict accounting.

Significant Disease Models

As the use of transgenic mice in research has expanded, IACUCs have had to deal with an ever-increasing need to define appropriate endpoints and interventions to address pain and distress issues in animals that spontaneously develop serious health conditions (Morton and Hau 2003). Although IACUCs have always had to deal with these issues for induced models of disease, these situations were somewhat simpler since induction and course of the disease was usually well known and controlled. In transgenic animals, there is often an insidious onset with a gradual increase in severity. This may result in the IACUC having to develop some type of health scoring system (usually specific for the model), which defines the precise point at which intervention must occur. Another complexity for the IACUC from this standpoint is in the generation of new transgenic models. Since the phenotypic effects are unknown until the model is characterized, the IACUC may have to deal with continuously evolving welfare issues as these lines are produced. Unfortunately, like many other aspects of research, transgenic models do not easily conform to regulatory oversight and standard procedures.

References

Brinster RL, Chen HY, Trumbauer M, Senear AW, Warren R, Palmiter RD (1981) Somatic Expression of Herpes Thymidine Kinase in Mice Following Injection of a Fusion Gene into Eggs. Cell 27:223-231

Brown SD, Hardisty RE (2003) Mutagenesis Strategies for Identifying Novel Loci Associated with Disease Phenotypes. Seminars in Cell & Develop. Biol. 14:19-24, 2003

Spector DL, Goldman RD, Leinwand LA (eds). (1998). Cells: A Laboratory Manual. Cold Spring Harbor Laboratory Press, Cold Spring Harbor NY

Chen SZ, Evans GA (1990), A Simple Screening Method for Transgenic Mice Using the Polymerase Chain Reaction. Biotechniques 8: 32-33

Flecknell P, Silverman, J (2000), Pain and Distress. In: The IACUC Handbook. Silverman J Suckow MA Murthy S (eds) CRC Press, Boca Raton, FL, Pp. 221-249

Gordon JW, Ruddle FH (1981), Integration and Stable Germ Line Transmission of Genes Injected into Mouse Pronuclei. Science 214:1244-1246

Gordon JW (2002), Barrier Facilities for Transgenic Rodents in Academic Centers – A Two-Edged Sword. Comp. Med. 52(5): 397–402

Gulick J, Subramaniam A, Neumann J, Robbins J (1991), Isolation and Characterization of the Mouse Cardiac Myosin Heavy Chain Genes. J.Biol.Chem. 266:9180–9185, 1991

Hogan B, Costantini F, Lacy E (1986), Manipulating the Mouse Embryo. A laboratory Manual. Cold Spring Harbor Laboratory Press, Cold Spring Harbor NY

Lerman I, Harrison BC, Freeman K, Hewett TE, Allen DL, Robbins L, Leinwand LA (2002), Genetic Variability in Forced and Voluntary Endurance Exercise Performance in Seven Inbred Mouse Strains. J.Appl.Physiol. 92:2245–2255, 2002

Lewandoski M (2001), Conditional Control of Gene Expression in the Mouse. Nature Reviews Genetics 2:743–755

Markel P, Shu P, Ebeling C, Carlson GA, Nagle DL, Smutko JS, Moore KJ (1997) Theoretical and Empirical Issues for Marker-Assisted Breeding of Congenic Mouse Strains. Nat.Genet. 17:280–284

Monastersky GM, Geistfeld JG (2002), Transgenic and Knockout Mice. In: Laboratory Animal Medicine, 2nd Ed., Fox JG Anderson C Loew FM Quimby FW (eds) Academic Press, San Diego, Pp. 1135–1141

Morton DB, Hau J. (2003) Welfare Assessment and Humane Endpoints. In: Handbook of Laboratory Animal Science, 2nd Ed.,. Hau J, Van Hoosier JL, Jr., eds. CRC Press, Boca Raton, FL, Pp. 478–486

National Research Council (NRC) (1996) Guide for the Care and Use of Laboratory Animals. National Academy Press, Washington, D.C

Office of Laboratory Animal Welfare [OLAW]. (2000) Public Health Service Policy on Humane Care and Use of Laboratory Animals. National Institutes of Health, Bethesda, MD

Otto G, Tolwani RJ (2002) Use of Microisolator Caging in a Risk-Based Mouse Import and Quarantine Program: A Retrospective Study. Contemp. Top. Lab. Anim. Sci. 41: 20–27

Pinkert CA. (2003) Overview: Transgenic Animal Technology: Alternatives in Genotyping and Phenotyping. Comp. Med. 53: 126–139

Pinkert CA (ed), Transgenic Animal Technology. A Laboratory Handbook. 2nd ed. (2002). Academic Press, San Diego, CA

Rehg JE, Blackman MA, Toth LA. (2001), Persistent Transmission of Mouse Hepatitis Virus by Transgenic Mice. Comp. Med. 51: 369–374

Silver LM. (1995) The Mouse Genome. In: Mouse Genetics: Concepts and Applications. Oxford University Press, Oxford, UK

United States Department of Agriculture (USDA) (2002) United States Code Title 7, Chapter 54: Animal Welfare Act and Animal Welfare Regulations. U.S. Government Printing Office, Washington, D.C

United States Department of Health and Human Services (USDHHS) (1999) Appendix C: Transportation and Transfer of Biological Agents. In: Biosafety in Microbiological and Biomedical Laboratories, 4th Ed., U.S. Government Printing Office, Washington, D.C., pp. 214–218

Appendix

Colour Plates
— 979

Index
— 997

Colour Plates

Chapter 1.3

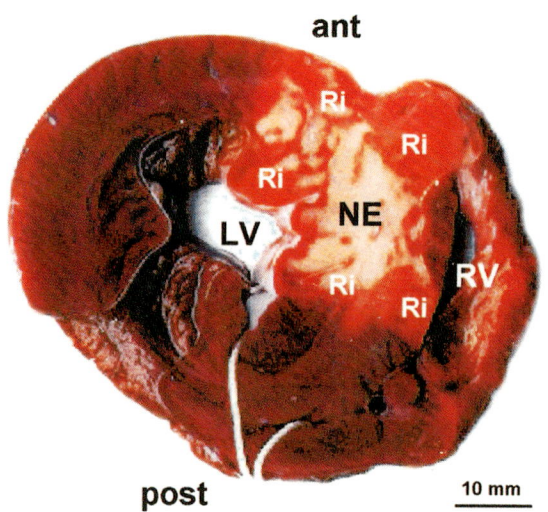

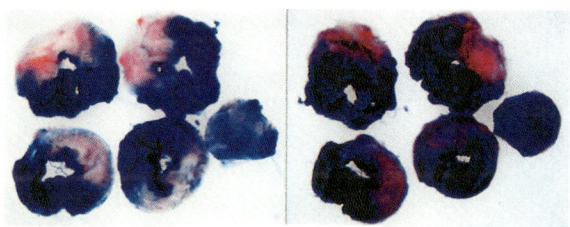

Figure 3

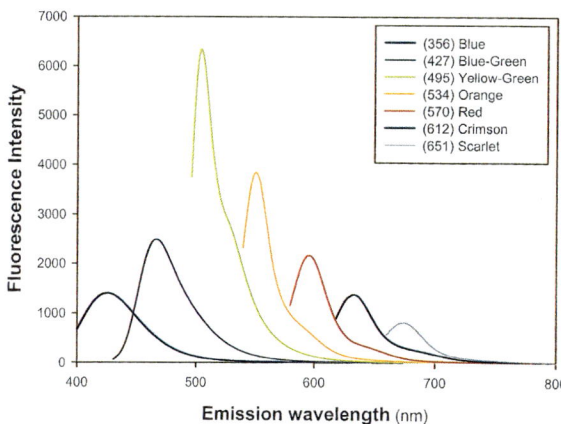

Figure 4

Chapter 1.4

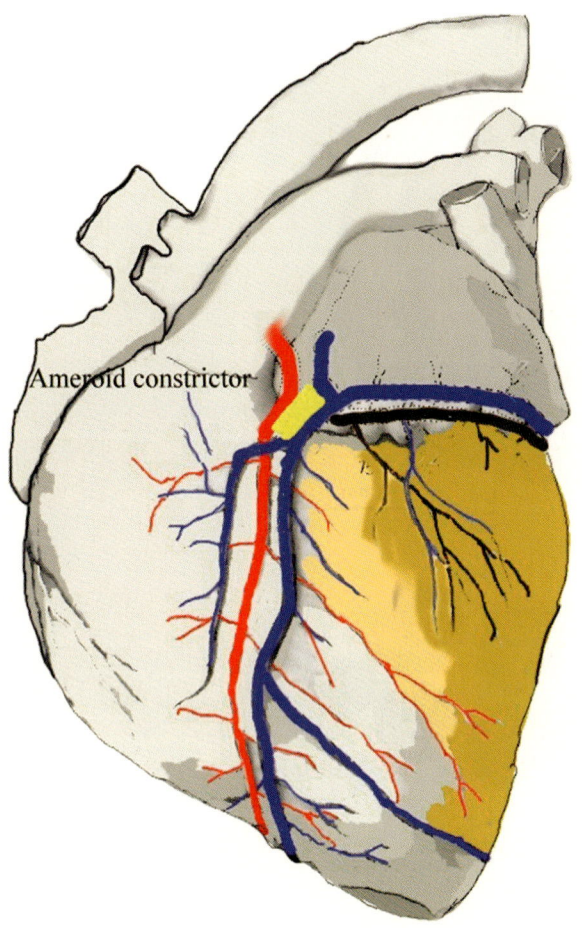

Figure 1

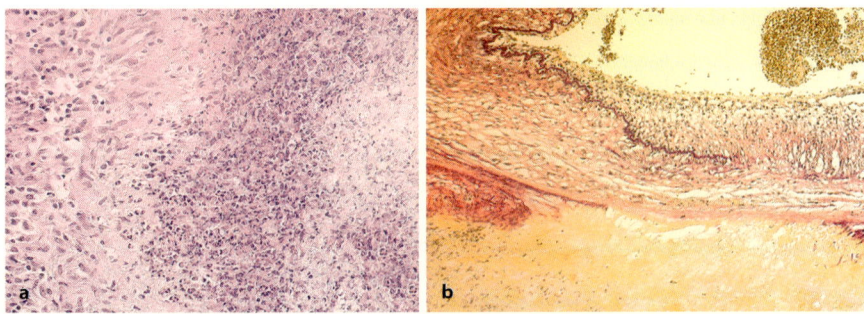

Figure 3

Chapter 1.8

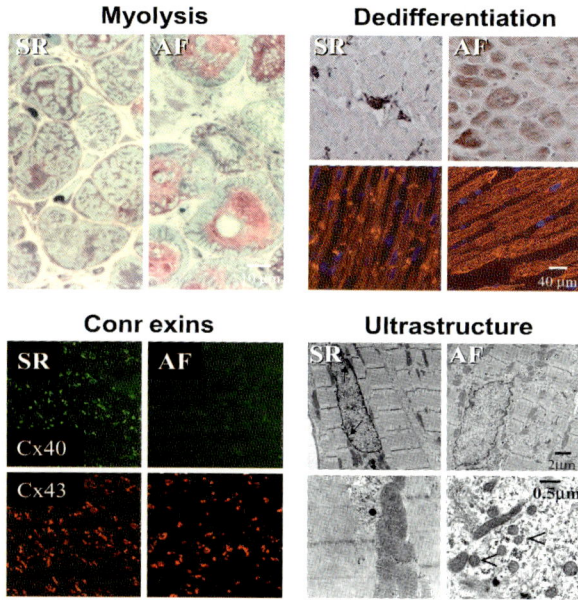

Figure 5

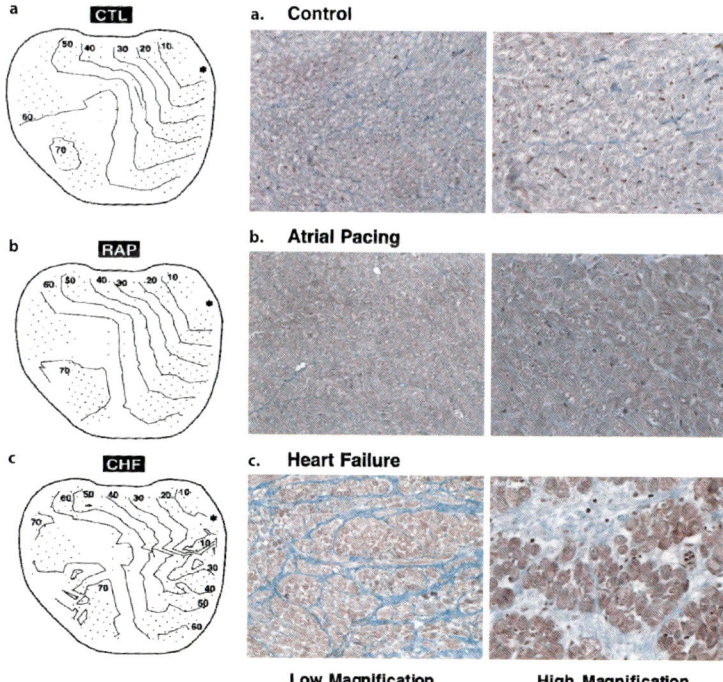

Figure 7

Chapter 2.2

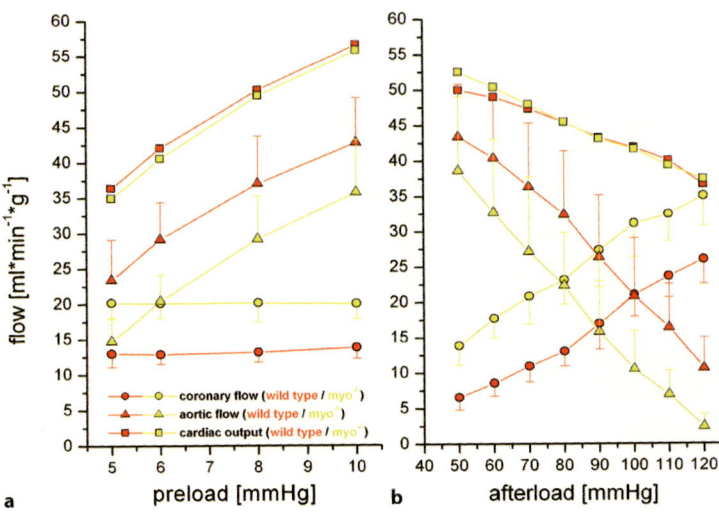

Figure 3

Chapter 3.1

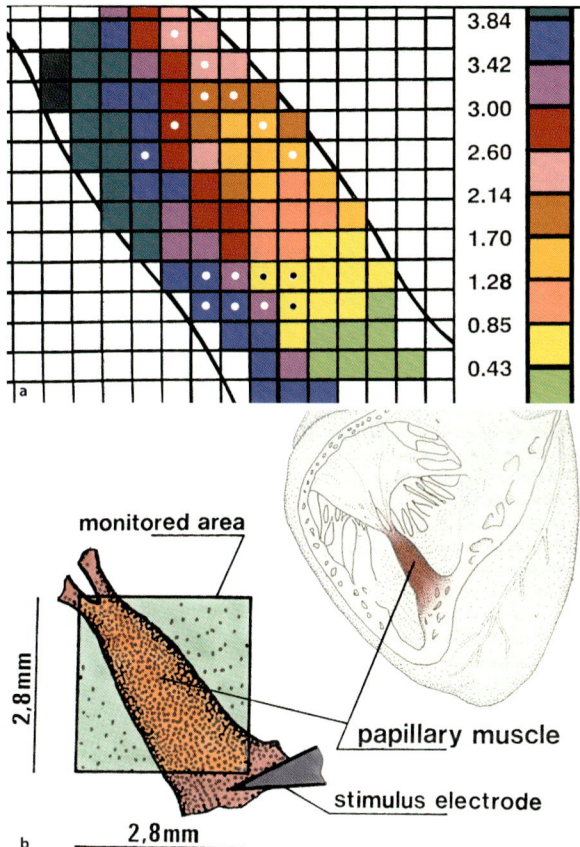

Figure 7

Chapter 3.2

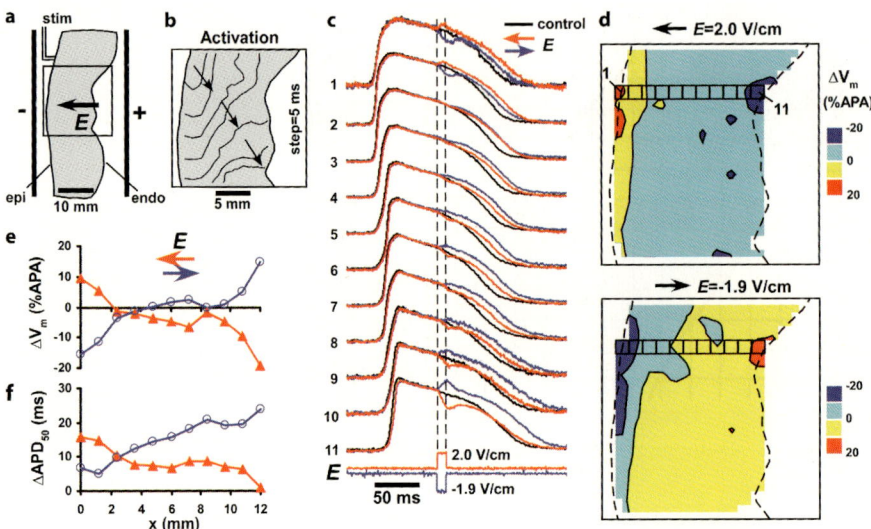

Figure 5

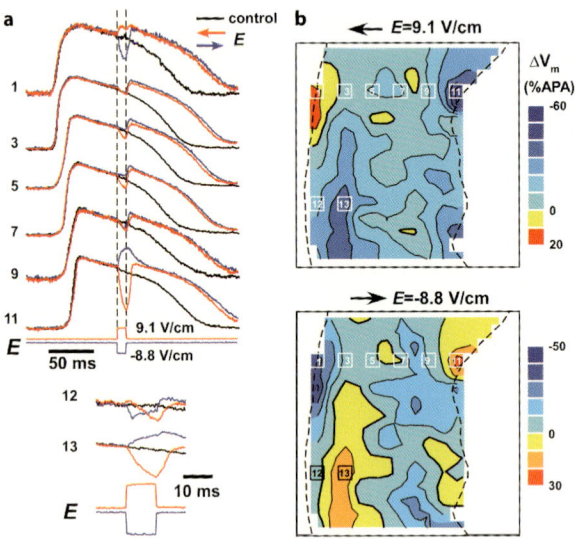

Figure 6

Chapter 3.7

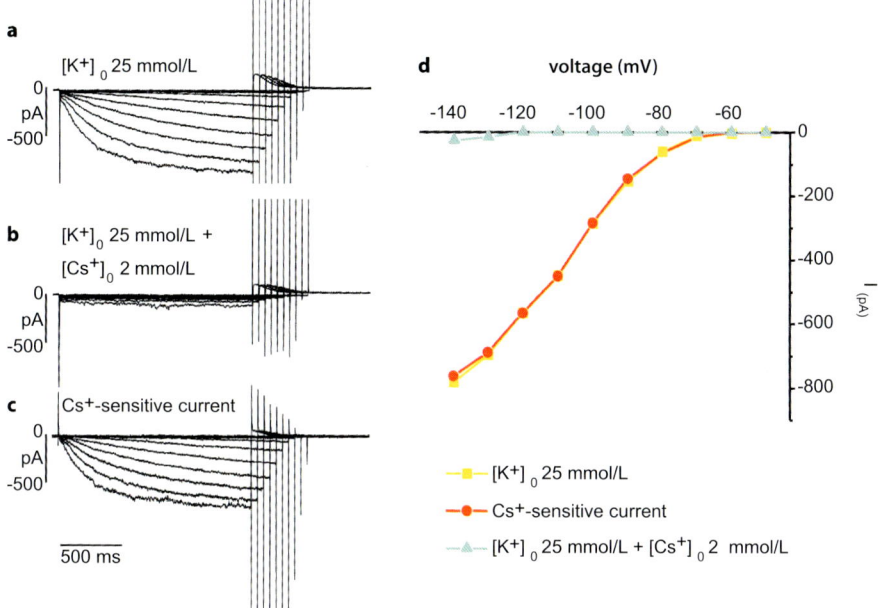

Figure 9

Chapter 3.10

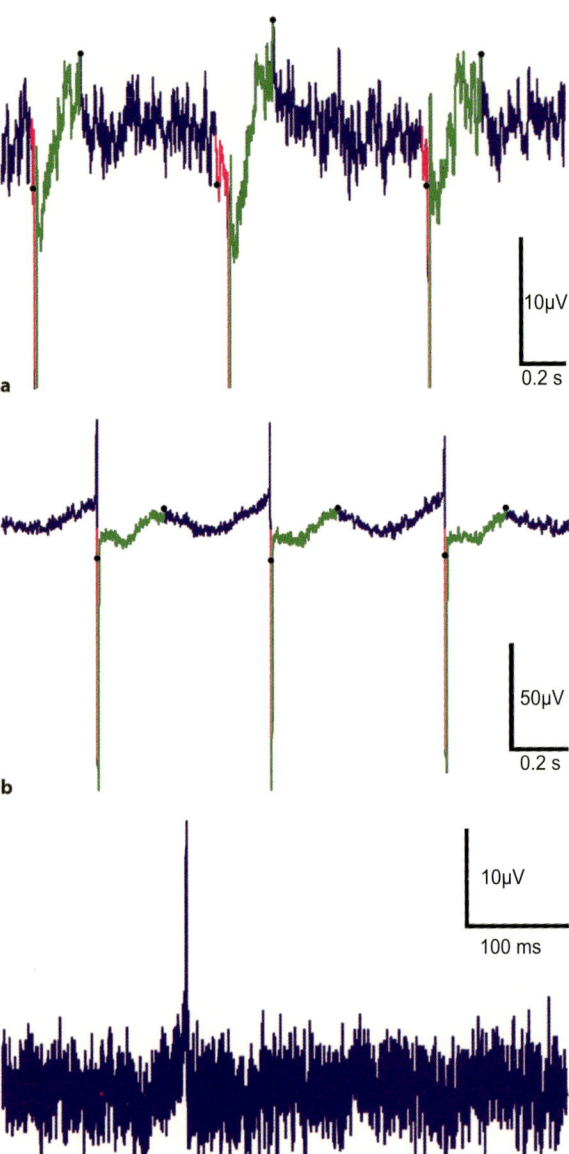

Figure 3

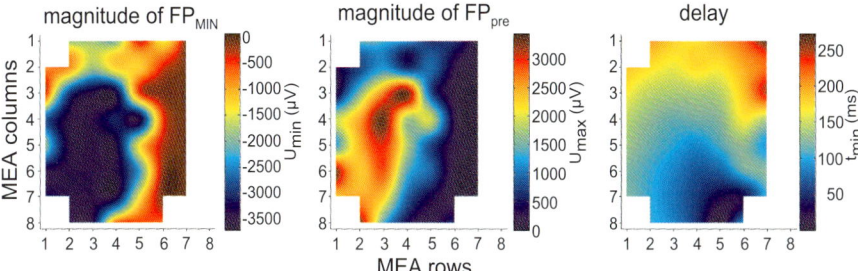

Figure 4

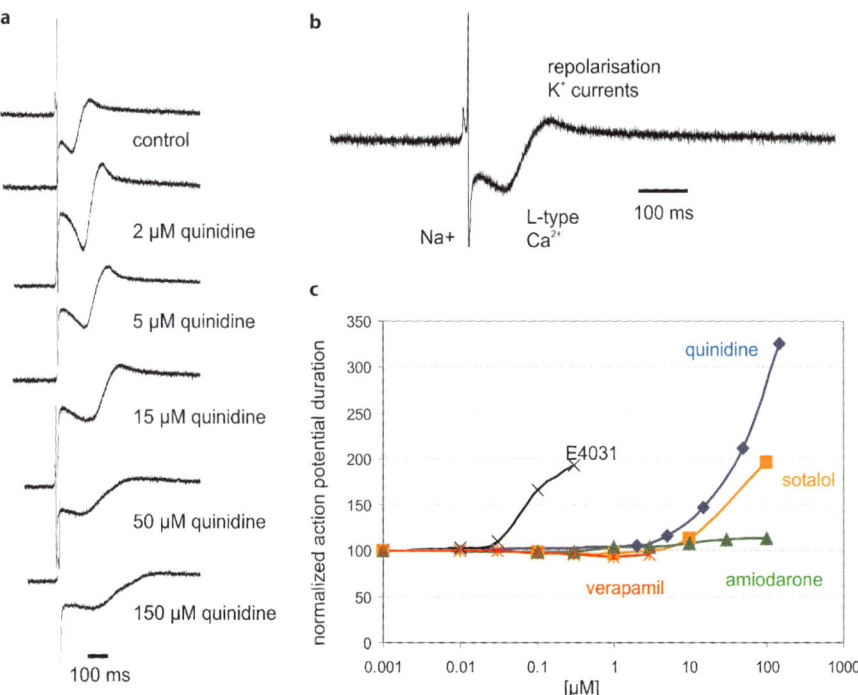

Figure 6

Chapter 4.5

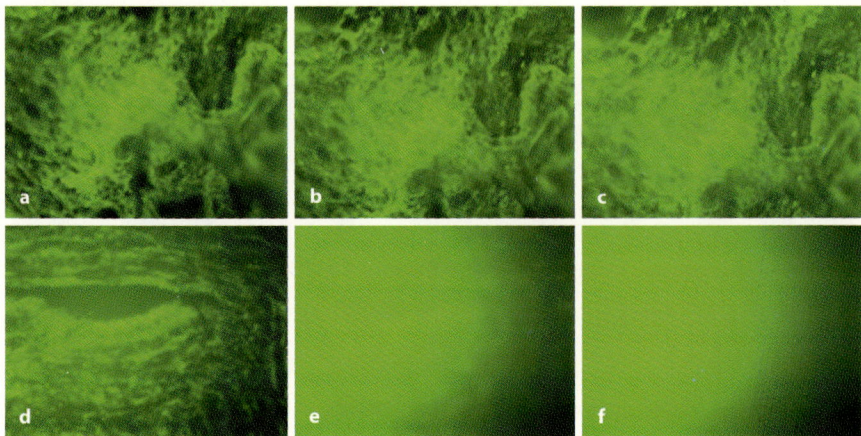

Figure 3

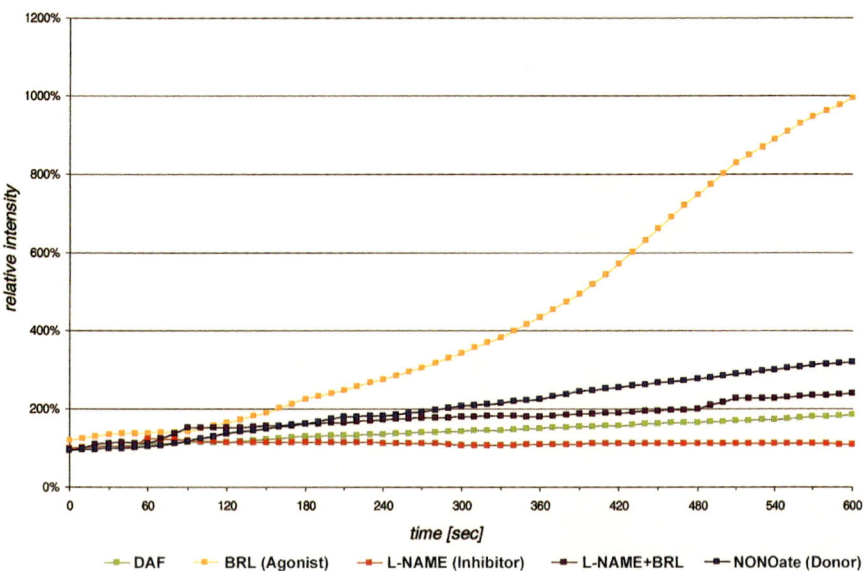

Figure 4

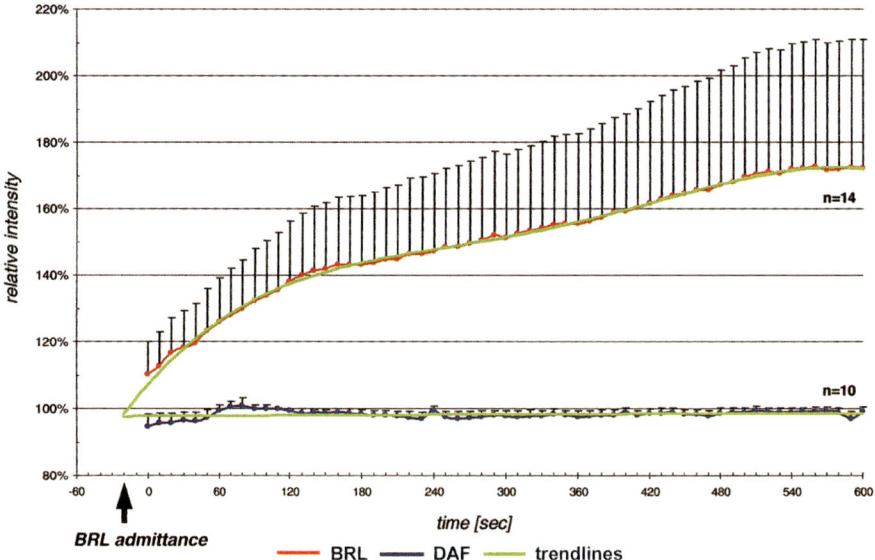

Figure 5

Chapter 5.2

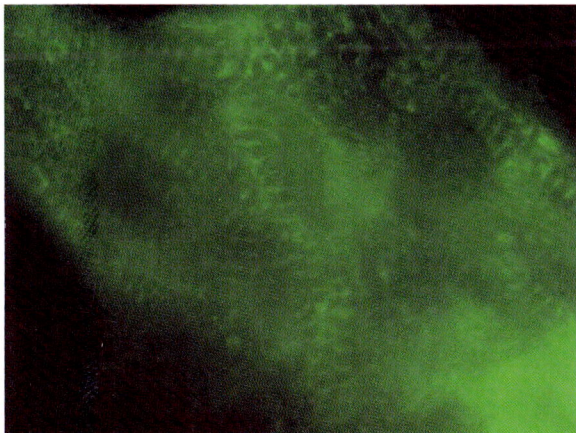

Figure 1

Chapter 5.5

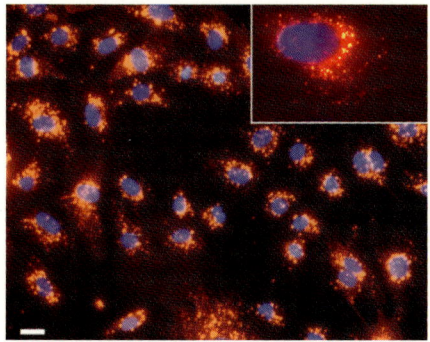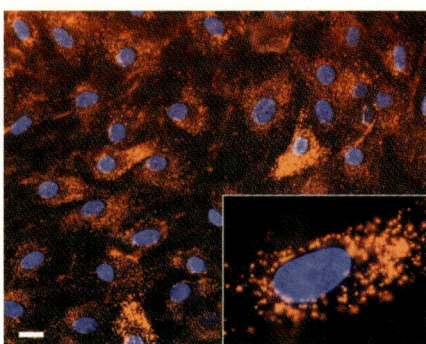

Figure 3

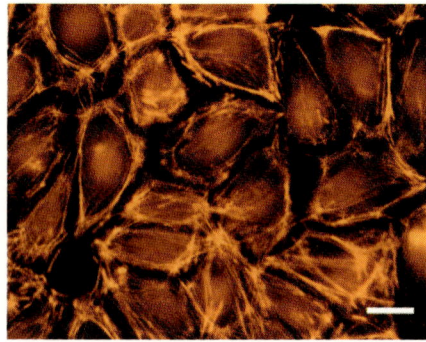

Figure 4

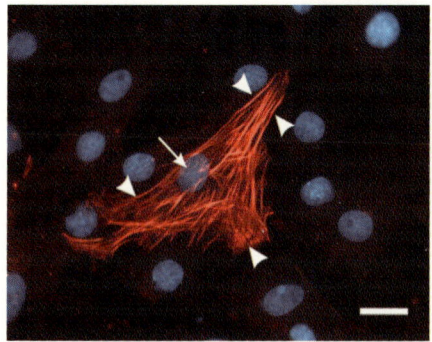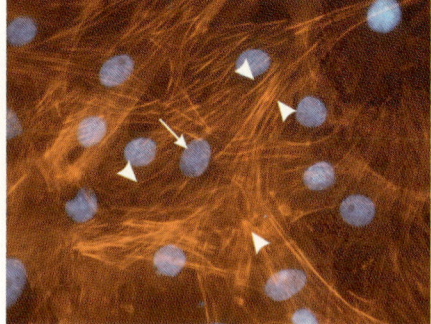

Figure 5

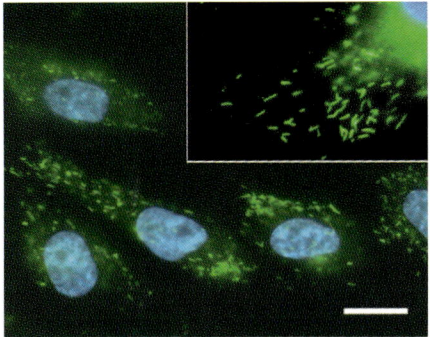

Figure 6

Chapter 5.6

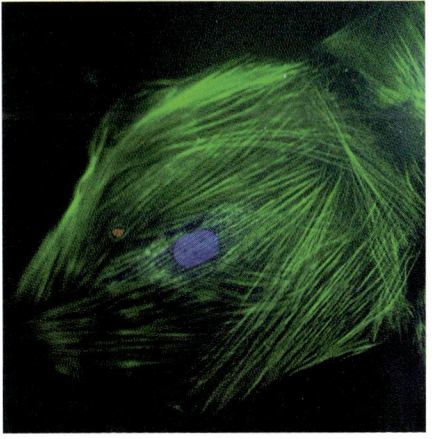
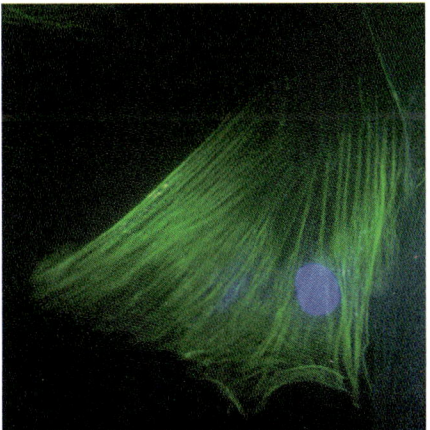

Figure 2

Chapter 7.1

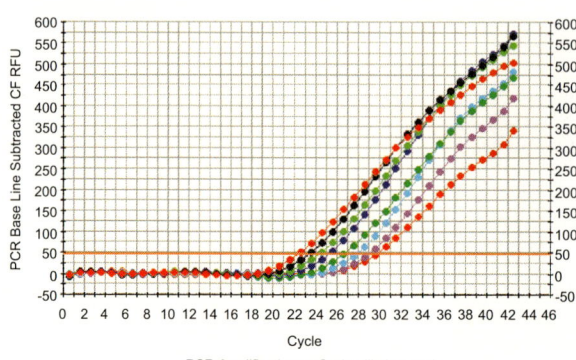

Figure 1

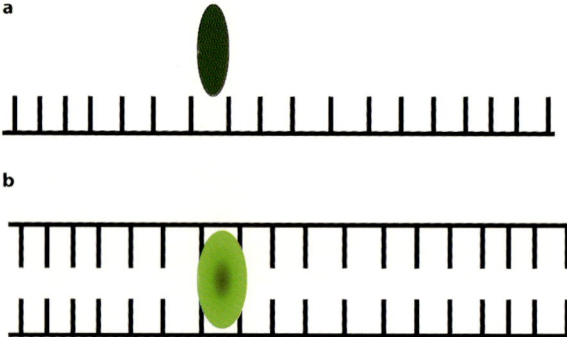

Figure 2

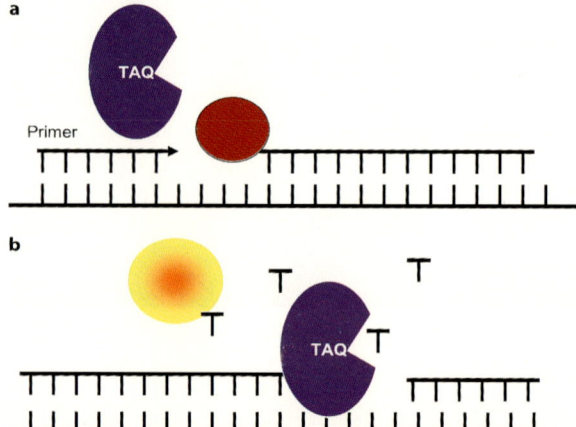

Figure 3

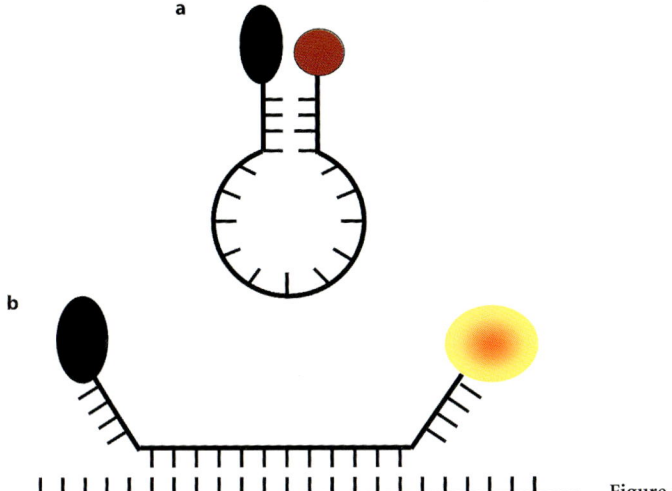

Figure 4

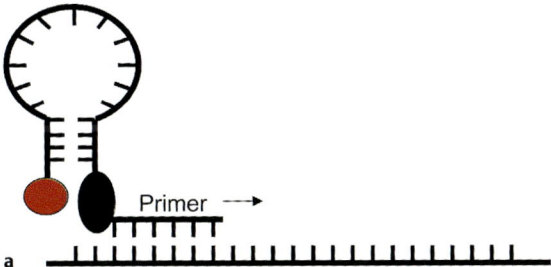

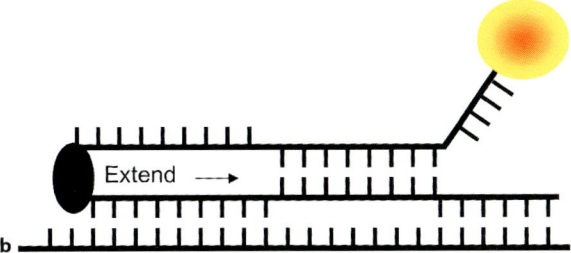

Figure 5

Chapter 7.2

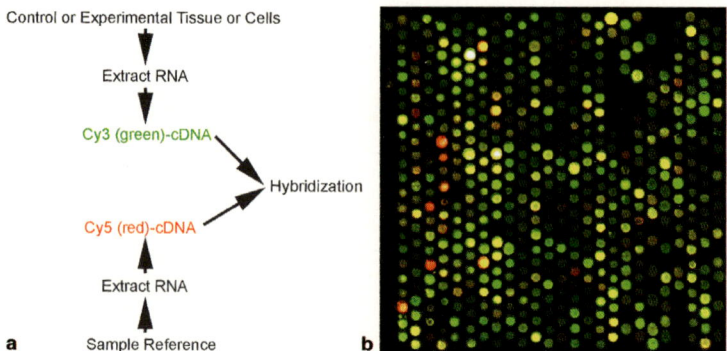

Figure 1

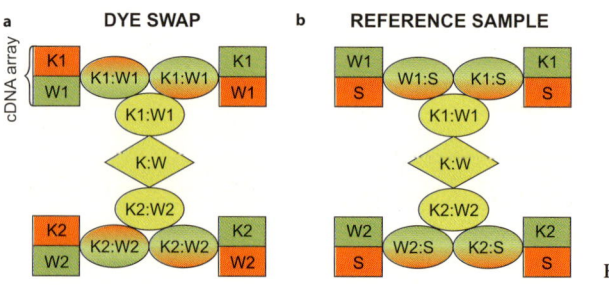

Figure 2

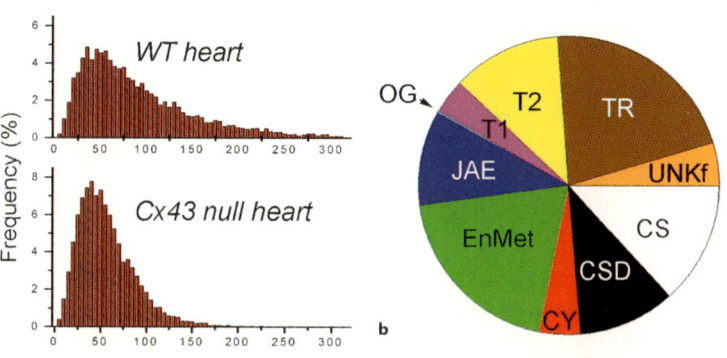

Figure 3

Index

Index

A

absolute value optimum (AVO) 282
acepromazine 12
acetone 460
– fixation 622
acetylcholine 138, 144, 208
acid fuchsin 490
acrylamide 697
actin 635
– polymerization 234
action potential 191, 397
– amplitude (APA) 248
– clamp 318
– propagation 266
– recording 194
activated clotting time (ACT) 36
activation 358, 362
– kinetics 329
– pattern 258, 259
– propagation 265
– recovery interval (ARI) 258, 266
– sequence 259
– time point 258, 265, 268
– vector 259
acute
– hyperglycaemia 807
– myocardial ischemia 118
additive-concentration-response 795
adenovirus 771
adhesion molecule 868
adrenal chromaffin cells 844
adrenaline 829, 835
adrenergic receptor 833
α_1-adrenoceptor 732
α_2-adrenoceptor 732
β-adrenoceptor 732
– β_3-adrenoceptor 550
– blockade 121
adult stem cells 597
afterload 174
aged hearts 268
alanine 342
albumin 571
aldehyde 458
– aldehyde-based fixatives 459
alizarin red 486
alkaline 488
– phosphatase (AP) 465, 466
– – reaction 708
allosteric modulation 787, 789

alpha-sarcomeric actin 515
Amanita phalloides 623
American Type Culture Collection (ATCC) 579
ameroid constrictor 58, 61, 90
– placement 63
Amido black staining 711
amine coupling 938
3-amino-9-ethylcarbazole (AEC) 467
amino acid 327
4-aminopyridine 367, 387
amphotericin 320
amplicon 894
amplifier 277, 318
anaesthesia 758
– general anaesthesia 5
– inhalation anaesthesia 5, 9, 13, 18, 21
– – dogs 16
– – sheep 12
– intravenous anaesthesia 5, 20
– – pigs 8
– – rabbits 17
– mechanical ventilation 48
– neuroleptanaesthesia 6
– of dogs 15
– of rabbits 16
– of rats 20
– of sheep 12
– short anaesthesia 5
analog-to-digital converter 243, 950
angiogenetic factor 59
angiogenic growth factor 58
angiogenin 60
angiopoetin 60
angiostatin 60
angiotensin II 845
animal
– experiment 105
– model 111
anisotropic ratio 266
anisotropy 256, 257, 260, 267, 398
anomalous mole fraction effect (AMFE) 328
anthracycline 100
anti-aliasing analog filter 247
anti-arrhythmic drug 111, 194, 423
anti-sense strand 508
antibiotics 10, 261, 575
antibody array 916, 923

antibody-antigen interaction 928
antidepressant 749
antigen expression 871
antihistaminic drugs 261
antimycotics 575
antioxidant substance 808
aortic
– cannulation 168, 184
– flow 179
– valve
– – insufficiency 171
– – stenosis 78
AP-analysis 295
AP-recording 293
apoptotic cell death 564
aqueous NO 801
Araldite 530, 532, 544
– embedding 497
argon ion laser 219
β-arrestin 849
arrhythmia 45, 171, 197, 256, 258, 439
– drug-induced 261
– induction 423
– management 129
arterial
– cannulation 30, 31
– hypertension 72
arterio-venous fistula 95
artery damage during implantation 70
ascorbic acid 571
K-aspartate 387
asymmetrical signals 413
atherosclerosis 630
atherosclerotic lesion 814
atipamezol 17
ATP-sensitive potassium channel activation 124
atrial
– dilatation 142
– fibrillation 129
– – heart failure 141
– flow 179
– myocytes
– – structural remodeling 135
– tachyarrhythmia 136
atrioventricular conduction time 163
atropine 851
autologous endothelial progenitor cell 61
autonomic neural regulation 111

auxotonic setup 190
Avertin solution 834
avian myeloblastosis virus 901
avidin 467
– avidin-biotin-peroxidase complex (ABC) 466
azaperone 6, 8, 9, 49
azathioprine 657

B

Ba^{2+} current 340
Bachman's bundle 139
background staining 463, 464, 710
banding 77
BAPTA 123
baroreceptor reflex sensitivity 117, 136
basic cycle length (BCL) 263
Bay K 8644 340
beat rate variability 444
beat-to-beat variability 259
beating cell 587
benzodiazepines 74
benzodiazocine 339
benzothiazepine 335, 337, 343
benzoylpyrrole 339
Bessel filter 244
bevellers 306, 312
bicaval cannulation 31
bicinchoninic acid (BCA) assay 692
binning 246
biophysical properties 328
biopsy 410
biotin 465, 500, 505, 941
– biotin-streptavidin (BSA) 466
– biotin-streptavidin-HRP system 706
bis-acrylamide 696
Biuret-reaction 693
Bjerrum buffer 701
Blalock-Taussig shunt 77
blocking agents 707
blocking solution 706
blood cardioplegia 79
blot stripping 711
blotting
– membrane 700
– time 703, 704

Bolt buffer 703
Boltzmann
– distribution 408, 950
– function 300, 302, 349
bone marrow derived stem cells 593, 607
border zone 259
bovine serum albumine (BSA) 649
Boyle Marriott bottle 166
Bradford assay 692, 694
bradycardia 6
bradykinin 538, 540
breakthrough-points (BTP) 259
bridge amplifier 278, 279
bromo-chloro-propane (BCP) 900
bromodeoxyuridine (BrDU) 67
bronchial hypersecretion 6
bronchospasm 6
Brugada syndrome 423
buffer 472, 507, 689
buprenorphine 16
2,3-butanedione monoxime 234, 764

C

Ca^{2+}
– channel 324
– currents 301
cacodylate buffer 527
calcium
– calcium-dependent in-activation 330
– calcium-tolerant cell 561
– channel antagonist 123
– ions 330
– permeation 328
caldesmon 635
calibration 879
calmodulin 330
calponin 636
cAMP 316
– accumulation 860
cannulated vessel segment 198, 202, 208
cannulation
– arterial 31
– bicaval 31
– two-stage 31
capacitive feedback technique 290

carbachol 120, 651, 803, 858
carbon dioxide 614
CARD 467
cardiac
– arrhythmia 251
– Arrhythmia Suppression Trial 226
– excitation pattern 444
– failure 72
– function 173
– glycosides
– – analysis by HPLC 677
– output 174
– rhythmogenesis 382
– tissue 272
– – engineering 640
– troponins 43
Cardiac Myocyte Populated Matrix (CMPM) 641
cardioactive drugs 443
cardiomyoblast 569
cardiomyocytes 579
– isolation 411
cardiomyoplasty 579
cardiopulmonary bypass 9
cardiotomy reservoir 26
CARTO 427
catecholamine 840, 846
– analysis by HPLC 674
catheter-based manometer 44
caveolae 304
CBFHH 644
cDNA 909
– microarray 907
cell
– aggregate 439
– cell-attached configuration 291, 292
– cell-membrane resistance 292
– culture 433, 436, 874
– – coating 435
– – sample 918
– lysis 686, 688
– pairs 411
cellulose nitrate coating 436
centrifugal pumps 29
channel
– conductance 410
– phosphorylation 334
– selectivity 358
charge-coupled device
– array 220
charge-coupled device (CCD)
– camera 245

Chelex buffer 831
Cheng-Prusoff equation 738, 788
chloralose 48, 758
chloroform 768
7-β-OH cholesterol 575
chondroitin 489
chromanol 372
chromatography 663
chronic ischemia 58
chymotrypsin 570
ciclosporine A 657
circular casting mould 646
circumflex coronary artery 90
class III antiarrhythmics 261
closed extracorporeal perfusion system 34
CMRL 1415ATM 570
cocaine 122, 757
collagenase 410, 569
– buffer 560
– solution 411, 572, 612
collateral 67
– blood vessels 62
– development 69
– growth 61
colloid osmotic pressure 258
competition binding experiment 736, 742
competitive antagonism 784, 789
competitive antagonist affinity 787
complete obstruction 63
complex
– interaction 792
– synergism 794
compliance chamber 179
computer-assisted planimetry 43
concentration-response curve 784, 785
conductance 399
conduction 265
– velocity 196
cone-and-plate viscometer 814, 816
congestive heart failure 83
connexin 397
Connexin43 914, 918, 933, 948
connexon 397
continuous buffer 701
controller setup 282
Coomassie blue staining solution 694, 699, 705

coordinated expression 914
coronary
– angiography 67
– circulation 89, 173
– – resistance 156
– flow 173, 258
– occlusion 42
– perfusion 41
– thrombosis 42
coupling 399
cre
– recombinase 961
– transgene 965
creatine kinase (CK) 43
critical micelle concentration (CMC) 689
cross-circulation 26
crosslinking aldehyde fixatives 502
crude membrane 752
cryoconversation medium 583
cryofixation 525
cryopreservation 637
cryoprobe 952
cryoprotection 461, 473
cryosection staining 636
cultured cell 568, 802
current
– characteristics 297
– clamp 280
– – recording 278
– density 703, 704
– reversal potential 389
– voltage relation 298, 303, 358, 360, 375
cuvette system 937
cyclic
– GMP 120
– nucleotide-binding domain (CNBD) 382
– nucleotides 385
cyclophilin 904
cytochalasin D 234
cytometry 863
CYTOMICS 869
cytoplasm 294, 315, 487
cytoplasmatic protein 686, 688
cytoplasmic access resistance 414
cytosol 218
cytosolic
– protein 686
– resistance 406

D

DABCYL 895
DAF 547
DAF-FM fluorescence 551
Dahl salt sensitive rat (DSS) 85
data acquisition 185, 318
– hardware 242
de-staining solution 705
defibrillation 126
– procedure 116
– shock 250
densitometry 550, 920
density gradient centrifugation 691
depolarisation 223, 273
– voltage 390
dermatan sulphate 489
desipramine 751
desmethoxyverapamil 342
detergents 688, 689
– ionic 689
– non-ionic 689
– zwitterionic 689
dexpanthenol 20
dextran 171, 817, 823, 825, 938
di-4-ANEPPS 234, 236, 251
diabetic cardiomyopathy 496
diameter measurement 205
3,3'-diamino-benzidine (DAB) 467
diazophenylthioether (DPT) membrane 700
dichroic mirror (DM) 240
diethylether 6
differential attachment 575
– technique 569
differential centrifugation 686, 690
diffusion 191
digestion 569, 781
digoxigenin 500, 505
1,4-dihydropyridine 335
dihydropyridine 337, 338, 342, 350
Dil-Ac-LDL-uptake 622
diltiazem 335, 337, 343
dimethyl sulphoxide 219, 235
dimethylarsinic acid 527
direct coupling 938
discontinuous
– buffer 702
– single electrode voltage clamp amplifier 399

dislocation of electrodes 270
dispersion 256, 259, 266
dissociation constant KD 784
DMSO 588, 596
DNA 966
dobutamine 835
dopamine 829
Doppler flow transducer 113
dose ratio (DR) 789
double cell voltage clamp method 399
Dounce homogeniser 687
doxorubicin 102
Dulbecco's wash solution 573
Dunn carbonate buffer 701
dynamic cardiomyoplasty 105
dynamin 849

E

E-modulus (elasticity modulus) 190
E4031 444
EC50 786, 789, 791
echocardiography 74
Edman degradation 717
EDTA 352
effective refractory period (ERP) 418
EGFP expression 772
elastase 570
electric resistance 281
electrical
– defibrillation 427
– noise 254, 268
– pacing 565
– properties 275
– stimulation 280
electroblotting 686, 699
electrocardiogram 160
electrochromism 218
electrode 163
– resistance 403
– shielding 288
electrolyte solution 344
electromagnetic flow probe 161
electrometer amplifier 278
electron microscopy 543
electronmicroscopical method 70
electrophoresis 715
– buffer 697

electrophysiological
– measurement 45, 192
– recording 310, 320
electrophysiology 191, 265
electrospray-ionisation (ESI) 717
ELISA 715
elution efficacy 701
Emax 786, 791
embedding 461
embryo extract 570
embryoid bodies (EBs) 578
embryonal carcinoma cell 593
embryonic
– chick heart 570
– stem 477
– stem cell 592
end-diastolic LVP (EDP), 258
end-diastolic pressure (EDP) 163
endostatin 508
endothelial
– cell 571, 610
– progenitor cell (EPC) 593, 869
endothelin 823
endothelium 837
endotoxin 620
endpoint dilution assay 765
Engineered Heart Tissue (EHT) 640
enhanced
– chemiluminescene (ECL) detection 710
– green fluorescent protein (EGFP) 764
eNOS 462, 471, 538
envelop-of-tails test 372
enzymatic disaggregation 633
enzyme-based cytochemistry 467
eosin 488
– Y staining solution 698
epicardial
– electrocardiogram (ECG) 163
– mapping 268
– multielectrode mapping 256
– potential mapping 258
Epon 530, 532
ethanol 219, 460
ethidium bromide staining 892
2-ethoxyethylacetate 47
ethyl ether 157
ethylene glycol 945
ethylenediaminetetraacetate (EDTA) 941
etomidate 844
euthanasia 614

Evans Blue 44
excitation-contraction coupling 303
exercise plus ischemia test 115
experimental chamber 308, 309
external fast perfusion 313
extracellular
– matrix 68, 824
– potassium concentration 394
– potentials 233
– solution 401
extracorporeal
– circuit 26
– circulation (ECC) 7, 75
extravidin 467

F

F-actin staining 623
Faraday's cage 308, 312
Fas receptor 822
fast perfusion system 314
feeder cell culture medium 583
Feng medium 410, 411
fentanyl 6, 7, 10, 17, 115, 157
FGF family, 60
fibrillation pacemaker 131
fibroblast 571, 640
fibronectin coating 436
filament 306
Fischer 344 rats 656
FISH 515
– technique 514
FITC-labelled dextran 205
fixation 527
fixative 472
flecainide 194, 227
flow
– chamber 814
– cytometers (FCM) 863
– meter 188
– of injury current 266
– probe 46
fluid viscosity 814
flumazenil 17
fluorescence 873
– dye 468
– labelling 500
fluorescent signal 517
fluorochromes 467
fluorophores 899
fluosol-43 171

foetal calf serum (FCS) 562, 569, 570, 644
foetal rat serum 570
formaldehyde 459
– binding 460
formalin 462, 506
forskolin 854
FP shape analyses 440
Frank-Starling mechanism 168, 268
free NO concentration
– real-time measurement 800
functional antagonism 210, 791, 793

G

G protein 759, 780, 852
– coupled receptors (GPCRs) 759, 848
– heterotrimeric 859
GABA transporter 749
gain-of-function transgenics 970
galanin 512
gap junction 397, 914, 918
– channel 398
– conductance 405
gap junctional
– coupling 265
– uncoupling 267
garden hose phenomenon 170
gating currents 326
gel electrophoresis 686, 696
gelatine 571, 582
gene
– expression 907
– transfer 60, 648
– – adenovirus mediated 656
gene-targeted
– mouse model 829
– mutation 961
general anaesthesia 5
genetic polymorphism 826
genomic DNA 831
genotyping 972
Giga-ohm seal 345
Glanzstreifen 398
glibenclamide 124
glucocorticoid 571
glucose 199
K-glutamate 387
glutamine 337
glutaraldehyde 459

glutardialdehyde 528
glycogen 498
glycylglycine 842
gold-silver staining 466
Goldmann-Hodgkin-Katz equation 391
Goldner staining 490, 492, 496
goretex foil 11
gramicidin 320
graphite electrodes 703, 705
green fluorescence protein (GFP) 461, 648
grounding 257, 438
GTPase-activating proteins (GAPs) 761
guanosine 5'-triphosphate (GTP) 852
guanylyl cyclase 517
guinea pig 157, 191, 299, 316, 412
– myocytes 373
– ventricular cardiomyocytes 296

H

haematopoietic stem cells 593, 605
Hagen-Poiseuille's law 31, 156
half-maximum concentration EC50 784
haloperidol 263, 370
halothane 6, 48, 55, 157, 408
Hamamatsu array 243, 244
Ham's F10 570
Hank's salt solution 597, 850
Harbor Extracellular Matrix (ECM) 643
hardshell reservoir 30
HCN1/2 channels 383
He-Ne laser 219
heart
– explantation 184
– failure 141
– rate (HR) 66, 163, 173, 258
HEK-293 cell 859
hematoxylin-eosin (HE) staining 485, 487
hemodynamic 68
– measurement 74
heparan 489
heparin 157
hepatocytes 607

HEPES 199, 346, 539
heptanol 407, 410
HERG 371
– channel 444
heterogeneity 946
hexethylene glycol 896
hibernation 136
High Efficiency Particulate Air filter (HEPA-filte 611
high voltage amplifier 285
high-affinity capture 940
high-performance liquid chromatography (HPLC) 661
high-pressure liquid chromatography 663
Hill
– coefficient 787
– slope 787
His bundle
– ablation 143
– electrogram 163
histological examination 170
histology 863
HIV1-alpha 60
HMR 1556 372
homogeneity 259
homogenisation 687, 688, 731
– buffer 688, 690
homozygotes 974
hormonally defined media 571
horse serum 569, 570, 655
horseradish peroxidase (HRP) 44, 467, 505, 709, 710
HPLC
– analytical 671
– electrochemical detection 668
– instrument 664
– mobile phase 665, 681
– phase systems 670
– sample preparation 672
– troubleshooting 681
human
– embryonic kidney (HEK 293) 765
– umbilical cord 620
– umbilical vein endothelial cells (HUVEC) 816
hybridisation 927
– probe 898
– solution 504
hydraulic occluder 90, 126
hydrophobic
– adsorption 941
– interaction 464
– protein 928

hydrostatic pressure 158
hydroxyl 459
hydroxymethyl 459
– starch 171
hyperpolarisation 223
– activated inward current 381
– potential 387
hypertension 140
hypertrophy 78
hypotension 16
hypothermia 56
hypromatrix array 924

I

IACUC 973
IC_{50} 788
ICAM 610
ice crystals 461
ICI 118,552 122
immunoassay 715
immunocytochemical staining 857
immunodetection 706
immunoelectron
– labelling 535
– microscopy 525
immunofluorescence signal 861
immunogold
– silver staining 465, 468
– staining 537
immunohistochemical method 70
immunohistochemistry 457
immunostaining 920
in situ hybridisation 500
inactivation 362
incomplete concentration-response curve 796
independent
– additive effect 795
– antagonism 794
infarct size 258
infarction 58
infinity corrected optics 242
inflammatory response 868
inhalation anaesthesia 5, 9, 13, 16, 24
– rabbits 18
– rats 21
inhibitor constant Ki 790
inhomogeneity 256
inositol phosphate 781, 856

inositol-free medium 780
inotropic effect 190
input resistance 406
instantaneous conductance 408
integral membrane protein 688, 689
integrating headstage 290
inter-electrode distance 265
intercalated disk 397
internal perfusion 315
interstitial fibrosis 136
intra-array normalization 920
intracellular solution 402
intracoronary thrombosis 41
intramyocardial transplantation 61
intravenous anaesthesia 5, 8
– rabbits 17
– rats 20
intraventricular pressure 162
intrinsic
– activity 789
– agonism 797
inverse
– agonist 797
– microscopy 549
inward rectification 357, 369, 370, 376
iodine solution 112
iodophenol system 707
ion channel 601
ion-exchange purification system 567
ion-pair chromatography 671, 683
ionic current 296
ionophore 319
irbesartan 141
ischemia 257, 258, 428
– border zone 266
– center zone 266
– reperfusion 256
– – arrhythmia 257, 261, 263
ischemic
– area 256, 265
– centre 259
isochrone 224, 260, 269
– plot 267
isoflurane 6, 9, 48, 55
isolated 190
– cardiac myocytes 308
– heart 173
– trabecular strips 756
– vessel 802

isolation of pairs of cardiomyocytes 410
isometric 192
– contraction 439
– force recording 192
– transducer 160
isoprenaline 331, 650, 653, 770
isoproterenol 331, 350
isotonic
– force
– – recording 193
– – transducer 160
– setup 190
isovolumetric measurement of force 162
isradipine 339
ivabradine 392

K

ketamine 6, 12, 17, 49, 74, 649, 758, 832
Ki-67 antigen 67
kinase 471
knockout mice 186, 612, 830, 961
Krebs-Henseleit solution 164, 527, 754
krypton laser 219
Kyhse-Andersen buffer 702

L

L-arginine 546
L-glutamine 581
L-type calcium channel 329, 330, 339, 387
lactate dehydrogenase (LDH) 43
– activity 823
Laemmli sample buffer 698
laminin adhesion 314
Langendorff 155, 174
– heart 421, 761
– – constant flow 155
– – preparation 157, 159
– – setup 157
– perfusion system 558
– technique 257, 261, 412
Larmor frequency 950

laser emission 219
latissimus dorsi muscle 112
Laurière buffer 702
law of mass action 725
lead citrate staining 534
leak currents 377
left anterior descending artery
– ligation of 88
left anterior descending
  coronary artery 88
left circumflex artery (LCX) 63
left ventricular
– catheterization 832
– dysfunction 89
– hypertrophy (LVH) 72
– pressure (LVP) 163, 258
– volume parameter 835
lethal
– air embolism 55
– arrhythmia 117
leukemia inhibitory factor (LIF) 580
leukocytes 863
lidocaine 11, 194
ligand immobilization 938
Lin-c-kitPOS 600
linear
– gradient polyacrylamide gel 698
– optimum (LO) method 282
Lineweaver-Burk diagram 786, 790
lipophilic path 338
liposomes 942
liquid
– helium 952
– nitrogen 553, 588
LocaLisa system 427
long-term drug effects 439
long-term monitoring 433
longitudinal
– propagation 266
– velocity 267
Lowry assay 692, 693, 854
LR White resin 532
Ludwig, Carl 190
luminol system 707
lusitropic effect 190
lymphocytes 874
lysis
– buffer 688, 691
– – high-salt 691
– – no-salt 691
– – single detergent 691
– – triple detergent 691

M

M199 570
mAChR 849, 851
MALDI 716
manipulators 316
MAP signal
– computer-aided analysis 425
– fidelity 427
MAPC 598
mapping 221, 224
– system 257
marginal branches 90
mass spectrometry (MS) 716
Masson staining 490
Matsudaira buffer 702, 703
maximum contraction velocity
  (dP/dt_{max}) 163
maximum relaxation velocity
  (dP/dt_{min}) 163
Mayer's haemalum 488
[^{3}H]-mazindol 751
MEA 434
– preparing for cell culture 434
– recording setup 437
measurement of free NO 800
mechanical
– force 190
– noise 253
– ventilation 37
medetomidine 6, 15, 17, 157
megakaryocytes 625
membrane
– capacitance 283, 304, 388
– channel 303
– depolarisation 324, 329
– membrane-bound protein 688
– potential 272, 363
– potential signal 285
– protein 686, 688
– resistance 404, 415
mercury (Hg) lamp 239
mercury/xenon arc lamp 219
merocyanine 218
mesenchymal stem cells (MSC) 593, 604
metaiodobenzylguanidine (MIBG) 750
metal ion affinity chromatography (IMAC) 715
metamizol 10, 16
methanol 460
– fixation 622
methoxyverapamil 342

methylene blue 485, 489
– solution 533
– staining 497
mibefradil 301
mice
– clinical and blood parameters 24
– genetically altered 173
Michaelis-Menten kinetics 786
microelectrode 191, 194, 215, 274
– array 432
– capacitance 276, 307
– fabrication 305
– glass 305
– resistance 275
microforges 307
micromanipulator 309
microscopic mapping 249
microscopy 308
microsphere 46, 47, 56
– colored 67
– measurement 52
microvascular coronary EC from rat 616
mid-sternal thoracotomy 40
midazolam 6, 7, 17, 49, 53
mini-pig 7
minimized perfusion system 32
MinK-related peptide 1 383
mirror resonance spectroscopy 937
mispriming 523
mitochondria 541
mitotic cycle 569
mitral
– insufficiency 96
– regurgitation 90
modulus hugging 283
Moloney murine leukemia virus 901
monoclonal antibodies 872
monophasic action potential (MAP) 45, 163, 417
MOPS 199
morphine sulfate 112
motion artifacts 439
mouse
– blastocyst 961
– ES cells 606
multi-protein complex 933
multiplexing 904
multiplicity of infection (MOI) 648
murine fibroblast 583

muscarinic receptor 732
mutagenesis 959
myocardial
- blood flow (MBF) 53
- function 68
- infarct 89
- - size 51
- infarction 72, 125, 141, 142, 496
- injury
- - markers 56
- - plasma markers 43
- ischemia 37, 39, 58
- laser revascularisation 59
- necrosis 61
- perfusion 68
- protection 31
- reperfusion 37
myogenic autoregulation 170
myoglobin 43, 186
myopathy
- stress-induced 69
myosin light chain 2 600

N

N_2O 6
Na
- current 299
- pyruvate 164
$NaHCO_3$ 200
naloxon 17
Nd:YVO4 laser 240
neoangiogenesis 60
neodymium YAG laser 219
neonatal rat cardiomyocytes 568, 762
- cultivation 569
neovascularisation 61, 869
Nernst equation 316
neuroleptanaesthesia 6
neuroleptanalgetics 17
neuroleptic drugs 261
neuronal rhythmogenesis 382
nifedipine 131, 337, 338
nimodipine 338
[³H]-nisoxetine 751
nitrate 801
nitrendipine 335
nitric oxide (NO) 546
nitrite 801
- re-conversion 801
nitro blue tetrazolium 258

nitrocellulose 700
- membrane 918
NMR 948
NO
- electrode 800
- - calibration 801
- metabolite 801
non-cardiomyocytes 571, 575
non-competitive antagonism 790
non-crosslinking fixatives 460
non-specific binding 706, 729
noradrenaline 201, 207, 748, 829, 835
- [³H]-noradrenaline uptake 750
- transporter 748
norepinephrine 844
Northern blot 522
NOS inhibition 807
nuclear
- magnetic resonance 948
- Overhauser effect (NOE) 953
numerical correction for series resistance 405
nylon membrane 700
nystatin 319

O

occlusivity adjustment 29
oedema 170, 270
offset potential 276
Ohm's Law 283, 307
oligomerization 523
oligonucleotide 503
onset of block 359
open extracorporeal perfusion system 33
open-chest
- preparation 40
- surgery 37
operational amplifier OPA121 243
optical
- action potential 237
- filter 240
- magnification 221
- mapping 233, 236
- signal 248
organ perfusion 627
oscillation 950
oscilloscope 254

osmium tetroxide solution 528
osmolarity 438
outward rectifiers 357
over-additive effect 796
over-staining 481
oxonol 218
oxygenation 165, 182

P

P wave 130
p-formaldehyde 170
P19 EC cells 593, 596, 606
pA_2 789
- analysis 784
pacemaker 439, 450
- cell 384
pAdEasy-1 764
paraffin 461, 468, 506
paraformaldehyde 473, 475, 507, 527, 528, 621
partial
- agonist 788, 796
- antagonism 797
passive constraints 104
patch clamp 288, 405
- amplifier 289
- electrode 291
pathway of excitation propagation 442
PCR
- cycling parameter 904
- primer 966
PE-10 catheter 836
peak conductance 299
peak-current amplitude 327
penicillin 581
- penicillin/streptomycin solution 573
pentobarbital 6
pentobarbitone 49
peptide nucleic acid (PNA) oligomer 898
perforated patch 319
perfused heart 173
perfusion 41
- pressure 160, 178
- system 311
- - closed extracorporeal 34
- - minimized 32, 35
perfusion-contraction-matching 41
pericardiotomy 54

pericardium 39
peripheral
– blood 869
– membrane protein 688
peristaltic pump 312
peroxidase 464, 465, 466
– anti-peroxidase (PAP) 466
peroxynitrite 546
Petri dishes 571
pharmacology 256
phenol-chloroform extraction 508
phenylalkylamine (PAA) 335, 342
– anti-peroxidase (PAP) 337
phenylephrine 838
phosphatase 471
phosphate
– anion 209
– buffered saline (PBS) 572
phosphoamino acid analysis 715
phosphoinositide 3-kinase pathway 334
phospholamban 653
phospholipase
– C (PLC) 854
– D (PLD) 856
phosphopeptide mapping 715
phosphorylated amino acid 713
phosphorylation 470
– specific antibody 714
phosphoserine 714
phosphotyrosine antibody 714
photobleaching 248
photodetector 241, 242
photodiode array 242, 246
photodiodes 245
photomultipliers (PMTs) 863
phototoxicity 240
physical exercise 59
physiological saline solution 199
picric acid 490
Picro-Sirius red staining 493
pie shaped constrictor 63
piezo stepper 317
piezoelectric crystals 133
pig 6, 7, 58, 411
– clinical and blood parameters 11
– coronary artery 809
piglet 7
pipette 401
– solution 402
piritramide 53
plasma catecholamine 840
platinum 705

Pluronic F-127 236
pneumothorax 75, 81
Poiseulle's law 813
polarisation 268
– macroscopic 253
poly-L-lysine 565, 850
polyethylenimine 435
polymerase chain reaction (PCR) 503
polymorphic tachycardia 229
polysaccharide antigens 458
Ponceau S 706
pore region 325
positive endexpiratory pressure (PEEP) 650
post-embedding 529
post-perfusion digestion 560
postoperative
– analgesia 19
– treatment 10, 18, 22
potassium 389, 392
– channel 355
– currents 303
– solution 202, 837
Potter-Elvejhem homogeniser 687
Powell medium 560
pre-embedding immunostaining 531
pre-pro endothelin-1 823
preabsorption of the antiserum 474
predictive medicine 868
prednisolone 657
preload 174
premedication 8, 9, 18, 21, 63
pressure
– constant Langendorff heart 155
– overload 77
primary cell culture 574
primer 902
– oligomerization 506
pro-arrhythmic activity 256
probe design 902
Proliferating Nuclear Antigen (PCNA) 67
proline 329
pronase 570
propagating wave 256
propagation 397
– velocity 442
propofol 15
proportional-integral (P-I) controller 281

propranolol HCl 121
propylene oxide 530
prostaglandin 838
protease 569
protein
– A 707
– A-kinase anchoring protein 335
– analysis by HPLC 679
– concentration 691
– extraction 926
– kinase 712, 713
– pellet 854
– phosphatase 713
– phosphorylation 712
– protein-protein interaction 918
– synthesis 564
proteinase inhibitor 687
proteolysis 687
pseudo-one pulse stimulation 838
PtdEtOH 857
puller 305, 306
pulmonary
– congestion 81
– edema 81
– valve stenosis 73
Purkinje fibres 384
PVDF blotting membrane 700
PXI chassis 245
pyridinium 218
pyruvate 199

Q

QRS complex 258, 270
QT interval 443, 444
QTc 263
quarantine 962
quartz-glass pipette 315
quinidine 266, 444

R

R-R-interval 130
rabbit 157, 257, 411
– aorta 806
– clinical and blood parameters 19

radioligand binding 841
rapid
- outward rectifier I_{Kr} 369
- ventricular pacing 97
rat 157, 191
- phaeochromocytoma 748
re-probing 932
Real-Time PCR 891
receptor
- expression assay 831
- reserve 788
- theory 725
recombinase Cre 776
recording membrane capacitance 304
recovery
- from block 359
- from inactivation 359, 365
reentrant arrhythmia 265, 266
refractory period 194
relative mobility 696
relative molecular mass 696
Rentrop score 67
reperfusion 39
- injury 50
repolarization 227, 248
- pattern 265
- repolarization-related arrhythmia mechanism 417
- time point 258, 270
resin 468
resting membrane potential 191
retrograde perfusion 174
retroorbital punction 20, 22
reversal potential 365
RH-237 234, 236
rhodamine 218
right coronary artery (RCA) 141
ring vessel segment 198, 200, 207
RNA 521, 842, 891
- extraction 900
- loading buffer 843
- running buffer 843
rodent heart 627
roller pumps 28
Rosenthal plot 735, 741
RT-PCR 522, 891
- semi-quantitative 892
rubidium 389
ruminant 13
rundown 415

S

safety pharmacology 256
saline solution 219
sample preparation 714
- for HPLC 672
sampling rate 445
sarcoplasmic reticulum calcium 124
saturation binding experiment 732, 740
Scatchard plot 735
scatter factor 60
Schäfer-Nielsen buffer 701
Schild plot 784, 787, 789
Scorpion primers 897
SDS-PAGE 719
sedation 614
selenium 571
semi-dry
- apparatus 703
- blot 700, 705
semithin 532
sense strand 508
separating gel 696, 697
separation of different ionic currents 296
series resistance 399, 413
serum-free medium 571, 819
SEVC
- amplifier 293, 304
- system 287
sevoflurane 48
shear stress 810, 813, 821
sheep 411
- clinical and blood parameters 14
short anaesthesia 5
shunt model 76
signal-to-noise ratio 237, 253, 450, 923
silicon photodiodes 899
silver impregnation 493
simulated ischemia 196
single cell
- electrophysiology 601
- recording 221
- RT-PCR 320
single detergent lysis buffer 691
single electrode clamp 286
sink current 421
sino-atrial node (SAN) cell 384
Sirius red 490

slide based cytometers (SBC) 863
SM22a gene 773
smooth muscle
- α-smooth muscle actin 624
- myosin heavy chain (SM-MHC) 635
sodium 391
- channel-blocking drugs 266
- propionate 197
softshell reservoir 30
solid-phase extraction 673
sonomicrometry 45, 51
- array 90
sotalol 444
source current 421
SP cells 599
spatio-temporal pattern 439, 444
specific binding 729
spontaneously hypertensive rats (SHR) 84
spotting buffer 926
ST
- deviation 260
- elevation 256, 258, 259, 263, 270
- segment 171
stacking gel 696, 697
staining procedures 485
stainless steel electrodes 705
steady state
- activation 300, 362
- conductance 408
- inactivation 364
stem cell
- research 514
- therapy 61
stenosis 41
sterile pericarditis 139
sternotomy 80
stimulus
- electrode 226
- generator 318
- isolator 280
streptavidin-biotin system 467
streptomycin 581
stress avoidance 69
stripping buffer 711
stroke 72
styryl 218
sub-xiphoid transdiaphragmal approach 74
subcellular
- fraction 690
- molecular distribution 477

substance P 809
subtotal ischemia 41
sucrose 687
sudden cardiac death 72, 111
superoxide anion 807
surface plasmon resonance (SPR) 936
Svoboda buffer 702
swine model 59
switch clamp amplifiers 400
Sylgard 347
symmetrical optimum (SO) 282
synergism 791, 792
synthetic oligonucleotide probes 503
Syrian cardiomyopathic hamster 85

T

T-tubule 304, 313
T-wave 258, 270, 423
tachycardia-remodeled cardiomyocytes 132
tail current 362, 369
– amplitude 300
TAMRA 895
tandem mass spectrometry (MS/MS) 717
tank blot 700, 704
tannic acid 528
TaqMan assay 895
target
– protein 932
– validation 652
tedisamil 367
telemetric transfer of ECG 66
telemetry unit 65
temperature control 310
teratocarcinoma 593
tertiapin 378
test battery approach 463
tetracycline 775
tetrazolium 43, 50
tetrodotoxin 296, 300, 387
TEVC
– A/B system 285
– system 288
TGF
– α 60
– β 60
thalamus 384
thermoregulation 10

thiol coupling 940
thiopental 6, 7, 9
thiopentone sodium 49
thoracic aorta 632
thoracotomy 40
threonine 714
thrombosis 42
tissue
– catecholamines 841
– dissociation 615
– embedding 473
– preservation 458
– sectioning 473
TNF-α 60
toe clipping 973
toluidine blue 485, 489
torsade de pointes 261
– arrhythmia 257, 428
Towbin buffer 700, 701, 703
tracer technique 747
transcription factors 603
transducer 188
transfer buffer 700
transferrin 571
transgene DNA 960
transgenic mice 562, 830, 972
– colony 963
– in heart failure 85
– model 829
transient
– outward current 357, 359
– staining 706
transjunctional current 409
transmembrane domain 749
transverse
– propagation 267
– velocity 267
trapanal 12
treadmill ergometer 66
triazole-fluorescein 547
tribromoethanol 834
trichrome staining 487, 489
Tris 728, 752
– buffered saline 649
troponin 51, 56
troubleshooting
– HPLC 681
trypsin 570, 645, 819
trypsinization 638
Tungsten-halogen lamp 219, 239, 254
TV-densitometry 469, 475
two-dimensional (2D)-HPLC 716
two-electrode voltage clamp 284

two-stage cannulation 31
tympania 13
Tyrode solution 164, 191, 294, 314, 527, 548
tyrosine phosphorylation 714
tyrosylprotein sulfotransferase (TPST) 823

U

UL-FS49 392
ultra rapid
– delayed rectifier 357
– outward rectifier I_{Kur} 375
ultramicrotome 533
ultrasonic crystal 163
ultrathin sectioning 533
Ultraturrax 687, 690
uncomfortable wrapping 69
uncoupling 197, 259, 265
under-additive effect 796
underfeeding 69
unpurified bone marrow 604
uracil-N-glycosylase 905
uranyl acetate 528
– solution 534
– staining 534
urine catecholamines 840
use-dependency 367

V

van Gieson
– solution 490, 491
– staining 496
vascular smooth muscle cell 815
– culture 818
– dysfunction 630
VC systems tuning 283
VCAM 610
vector 259
VEGF family 60
vein damage during implantation 70
Velcro-covered glass tubes 643
velocity 259
venous
– cannulae 30
– reservoir 30

ventricular
- afterload 173
- extrasystole 266
- fibrillation 11, 111, 120, 230, 421
- force 160
- function 173, 174
- remodelling 88, 89
- tachyarrhythmia 111, 115
verapamil 335, 337, 444
- analysis by HPLC 662
vessel
- isolation 200
- mounting 200
viability test 209
vibration isolation table 317
vignetting 242
Viokase 570
viral contamination 771
virtual electrodes 252
virus dilution 765
vitamin C 808
voltage
- clamp 272, 280, 311, 399
- - pattern 298
- voltage-dependent inactivation 402, 406
- voltage-gated calcium channels 324
- voltage-sensitive dye 234
volume overload 96
Von Kossa's silver staining 495
von Willebrand factor (vWF) 625

W

Weible-Pallade bodies 625
Weigert's iron-hematoxylin 491
Western blot 481, 686, 699, 704, 705, 715, 925
- analyses 464
- recycling 711
whole-cell
- configuration 292
- mode 292
Wollenberger clamp 551, 553
working heart 173
wound infection 69

X

xanthine oxidase 807
xenogenic protein 656
Xenon (Xe) lamp 239
Xenopus oocytes 285, 371, 383
- expression systems 281
xylazine 6, 12, 15, 17, 157, 649, 832

Y

yeast artificial chromosome 773

Z

ZO-1 925

Printing: Krips bv, Meppel
Binding: Litges & Dopf, Heppenheim